Sexually Transmitted Infections and Sexually Transmitted Diseases

Gerd Gross • Stephen K. Tyring
(Editors)

Sexually Transmitted Infections and Sexually Transmitted Diseases

Springer

Editors
Prof. Dr. Gerd Gross
Department of Dermatology
and Venereology
University of Rostock
Strempelstraße 13
18057 Rostock
Germany
gerd.gross@med.uni-rostock.de

Stephen K. Tyring, MD, PhD
Clinical Professor
Center for Clinical Studies
Department of Dermatology
University of Texas, Health Science Center
6655 Travis Street, Suite 100
Houston TX 77030-1317
USA
styring@ccstexas.com

ISBN 978-3-642-14662-6 ISBN 978-3-642-14663-3 (eBook)

DOI 10.1007/978-3-642-14663-3

Springer Heidelberg Dordrecht London New York

Library of Congress Control Number: 2011921948

Cover design: eStudioCalamar, Figueres/Berlin

Printed on acid-free paper

Springer is part of Springer Science+Business Media (www.springer.com)

Foreword

"Medicine, to produce health, has to examine disease, and music, to create harmony, must investigate discord." Plutarch (AD 46–120), Translation by John Dryden (1631–1700).

Strictly speaking a foreword or preface are introductory remarks, especially by another than the author of the book. Dear reader, please excuse this once, the foreword from a contributor to this work. This field of medicine which examines pathology, clinical studies, sociology, diagnosis, prevention and treatment of an aspect of one of the results of humanity, the erotic or sexual life, has been much studied. But its passage ensues. Thus in the nature of endeavours of mankind, the study of sexually transmitted infections and sexually transmitted diseases will need to continue. This work the result of five years labour by two editors from two continents has resulted in sixty-three chapters, the products of many more minds cooperating and writing about the essentials of studies, research and clinical observation of the subject to instruct the reader who wishes to learn more about sexually transmitted infections and sexually transmitted diseases.

By the time one is asked to write a foreword, realisation dawns of the rapid passage of professional life. It seems not long ago but in fact it was almost fifty years when as a medical student at Charing Cross Hospital, London, who realised he did not know how to make a Gram stain, a prerequisite in the bacteriology final exams in those days, he ventured into the department for venereal diseases where not only did he learn how to pass his practical, but learned about those the same age as himself who were treated with devotion, respect and the best contemporary knowledge of the subject. This time the summer of 1964 made me want to study sexually transmitted diseases for my career. Little did I know then what a wonderful journey it would be for the rest of my life. Dear reader, especially for those at the start of their professional journeys, I hope aspects of this book will also make you think you would like to help others by devoting some of your energy and intellect to adding to the corpus of knowledge about sexually transmitted infections.

Since then so much has been added to sexually transmitted infections. Syphilis had been studied for five hundred years. We thought it would become a rare disease. We realise now we were mistaken and it weaves into all the other sexually transmitted infections. Antibiotic resistance in gonorrhoea has increased as would be expected but applied research into effective chemotherapy has lagged. Knowledge of Chlamydia trachomatis at that time only known to a few is now an everyday matter, but it affects the fertility of so many young people. The diagnosis of microbial infection has been enormously furthered by techniques of applied DNA hybridisation. We had no cure and little understanding of the effects of genital herpes. There is still so much to be done in that field. We were beginning to understand the complexity of human genital papilloma virus infection. We were at the start of its relationship in some aspects to cervical and ano-genital neoplasia. The vaccine was many years away. In the 1970s, the sexual aspects of hepatitis B and then later the other hepatitises were established. A visit to San Francisco in 1975 was enough to show me how public health medicine took as a matter of serious concern, enteric diseases transmitted through sexual contact in men who had sex with men.

Then AIDS came to the Western World. For those of us in the field at the time we saw for the first time in the post-antibiotic era our fellow humans terribly suffering from a disease which at the start we did not know the cause. We saw ambulant patients, in my country mostly previously healthy men and later women and infants, visibly failing in health in front of us before dying. For all of us deep into our specialty, we saw dying patients, friends, loved ones, colleagues, for AIDS spared very few infected with the human immunodeficiency virus (HIV) in its early years. No specialty can work in isolation. The epidemic of HIV brought in extra magnificent and welcome minds and manpower into sexually transmitted infections. It introduced much needed governmental, international aid and private finance for prevention, and applied research. It rapidly brought the might of the pharmaceutical industry to manufacture within a comparatively short time highly active anti-retroviral therapy. Yet in that field so much more still needs to be done. I have travelled much to continents outside the West to see what devastating effects HIV/AIDS has on developing countries not only in the loss to human life but to the structure of countries and their social and economic well-being. So much still needs to be done.

Our knowledge of prevention of sexually transmitted infections is still in its infancy. There is far more to be done in the field of the development of immunisation to prevent sexually transmitted infections. In nineteenth century Europe there was a concept of immunisation for syphilis. This has not yet been achieved.

A glory of this work has been German–American cooperation in medical science. This follows a long and hallowed tradition in Europe and America. In the nineteenth century post-graduate students flocked to Vienna and Berlin to learn from the great men of medicine in those times. One such was the great William Osler, though born in Canada and making his career as a professor at Johns Hopkins and Oxford. In Vienna they would learn dermatology still a basic specialty of sexually transmitted infections from masters such as Hebra, Sigmund, Neumann and Kaposi. In Berlin the pupil would learn from the giants of general medicine and pathology such as Traube, Frerichs, Johannes Muller and Rudolph Virchow. It was not only in medicine that this cooperation flourished. Bismarck was much influenced by various friendships with American intellectuals of his day. Even the catastrophe of 1933 meant that American medical science would be enriched by refugees from Germany and Austria. However we must not forget this work is truly international from some of the best minds in the subject from around the world.

The editors Gerd Gross and Stephen Tyring are to be congratulated in seeing their concept reaching fulfilment. It is not an easy task to shepherd the contributors of a post-graduate medical comprehensive multi-authorship book towards finalisation of their copy in not too long a time. It is a happy achievement for all authors in such a book to have written their allotted chapters to the best of their ability. One so much hopes this book will encourage and assist towards knowledge of sexually transmitted infections and sexually transmitted diseases.

Michael Waugh, FRCP, FRCPI, FAChSHM
Emeritus Consultant Physician Genitourinary
Medicine Leeds General Infirmary,
United Kingdom.

Preface

Sexually transmitted diseases (STDs), previously known as venereal diseases, have been a topic of major concern for centuries as they are considered very important risk factors for morbidity and mortality both in poor and in industrialised countries.

Great steps have been made during the last two centuries to combat STDs. The introduction of penicillin was a major breakthrough in the treatment of syphilis. In the late twentieth century HIV was documented as the cause of AIDS, and the association between genotypes of HPV and genitoanal cancer was documented. These events paved the way to the production of many classes of antiretroviral drugs and to the development of prophylactic HPV vaccines.

We now have a far better understanding of numerous sexually transmitted infections. Recent developments in diagnostic techniques not only have permitted more accurate diagnosis but also have widely improved our understanding of the natural history of STDs. It is only through such understanding that the feasibility of specific therapies and preventive methods can be determined, but much remains to be learned regarding STDs.

When planning this text an important consideration was to identify the audience to whom it is directed. It should be of value to the widest audience of physicians and scientists interested in sexually transmitted infections and STDs. However it is not intended only for clinicians and laboratory scientists. It is not a compendium of diseases and information about how they should be treated. Rather it attempts a synthesis of these areas, discussing the clinical, diagnostic, epidemiologic, pharmacologic, molecular biologic and immunologic interrelationships of pathogenic agents, antibiotics, antifungals, antivirals and disease.

The book is intended for those who will most need it in the coming years: the medical student and resident who are interested in infectious diseases, the clinician who diagnoses and treats STDs and the microbiologist who will advance new developments in the field.

We hope that the text will be of interest to readers who are concerned in any way with patients suffering from STDs and associated public health problems, e.g. physicians, nurses, counsellors, students, laboratory personnel, public health workers and politicians. It is also intended for the research scientist who hopefully will be encouraged to do further work in the field of STDs and sexually transmitted infections.

In order to reach such a wide and diverse audience, all aspects of sexually transmitted infections and STDs are covered in this text. We are grateful to the contributors from all parts of the world with their different backgrounds and recognised expertise compiling this manifold book.

There are many instances of overlap in the book, but this is not considered to be undesirable. In many instances it is done for completeness and emphasis. The reader will notice that the individual chapters vary somewhat in terms of length, organization and style. These variations arise from the differing natures of the topics being discussed. We have decided to maintain these differences, since the state of the art varies widely from one area to another.

This book not only covers diagnosis and treatment, but also emphasizes prevention. Education is the cornerstone of prevention and is the goal of this book. Recently the first vaccines to prevent STDs, i.e. for hepatitis B and HPVs, have been added to the list of preventative interventions ranging from condoms to abstinence. It is anticipated that vaccines to prevent other STDs will be added to this list in the future. Education regarding both prevention and treatment should result in better control of STDs. We hope that the book will contribute to increased awareness and knowledge of sexually transmitted infections and STDs emphasizing their important role in human medicine.

April 2011

Prof. Dr. Gerd Gross
Director Department of Dermatology and
Venereology, Medical School,
University of Rostock, Germany, 1996-today.
President, German STD-Society 1998-2010
Vice President, Paul-Ehrlich-Society 2008-2010
Honorary Member or fellow of corresponding
societies of dermato-venereology in Poland,
Hungary and Chile and of the Baltic
Association of Dermatovenereology (BADV)

Stephen K. Tyring, MD, Phd
Clinical Professor of Dermatology,
Microbiology/Molecular Genetics and
Internal Medicine University of Texas Health Science
Center Houston, Texas USA

Acknowledgements

We would like to thank all the authors for their contributions and input to our book. The production of this volume is due to the generous support of Springer Publishers which is gratefully appreciated. A special thanks to Martina Himberger, Gurunathan Karthikeyan and the editorial staff of Springer Publishers for their encouragement and continuous cooperation in assisting the publication of this book.

We very much appreciate the support of the German STD Society, the Paul Ehrlich Society and the International Union Against Sexually Transmitted Infections (IUSTI). We extend special thanks to Sissy Gudat (Rostock, Germany) for her efficient secretarial organization. Dr. Tyring wishes to thank his wife, Patricia Lee, MD, for her support during the production of this book.

The Editors

Contents

Part XII Psychosocial Issues

Part XIII Economical and Political Issues

Part I

Basic Elements

History of Sexually Transmitted Infections

1

Michael Waugh

Core Messages

- A basic knowledge of the history of sexually transmitted infections (STIs) is important not only for professionals but also for the general public.
- This knowledge enables the reader to understand the development of STIs, which have had such an enormous impact on the behaviour and health of the human race. This history has been studied and written about by medical and general historians for 500 years.
- STIs have been described since the beginning of recorded history in Europe and Asia, in handwritten manuscripts until the invention of the printing press by Gutenberg in 1454. The history of STIs for the next 500 years followed the growth of medical and scientific discoveries and thus knowledge. STIs were affected by many human activities: travel, trade, war, colonial expansion, migration, industrialization, increasing public education, prostitution, the emancipation of women, slaves, and men who have sex with men.
- This chapter describes the history of STIs from the ancient times of gonorrhoea, into the era of syphilis and all the other sexually transmitted diseases, and now HIV/AIDS.

1.1 Definition

In this chapter, a sexually transmitted infection (STI) is defined as an infection passed from one person to another as a result of a sexual act. This definition includes sequelae passed from an infected mother to a child (congenital infection).

1.2 Aims

This chapter aims to give a concise history of STIs from ancient to modern times. It comprises the following historical eras:

1. The ancient times prior to the outbreak of syphilis in sixteenth-century Europe.
2. The development of the concept of venereal diseases (VD) until nineteenth century.
3. The development of a scientific basis for sexually transmitted diseases (STDs) from the nineteenth century.
4. The impact on society before and after the discovery of AIDS.
5. Scientific achievements since the advent of chemotherapy.

1.3 Sexually Transmitted Infections in Ancient Times

There are records of STIs – most notably urethral discharge that was probably gonorrhoea – from the earliest times [1]. For example, STIs have been

M. Waugh
Emeritus Consultant Genitourinary Physician, General Infirmary, Consultant Genito-urinary Medicine,
Nuffield Hospital, 151, Roker Lane, LS28 9ND Leeds, UK
e-mail: mike@mawpud.fsnet.co.uk

G. Gross and S.K. Tyring (eds.), *Sexually Transmitted Infections and Sexually Transmitted Diseases*,
DOI: 10.1007/978-3-642-14663-3_1, © Springer-Verlag Berlin Heidelberg 2011

described in the Ebers papyrus [2]; the Old Testament in Leviticus 15:2–33 ("The running issue," "Clothing needing washing as did the man himself," "All infected persons had to keep themselves apart from others for 7 days," "and if any man's seed of copulation go out from him then he shall wash all his flesh in water…the women also with whom man shall lie with seed of copulation…", "And the women if she have an issue she too…and she shall be put apart for 7 days") [1]. The Greek and Roman authorities described STIs, including Hippocrates, Celsus, Galen (who gave us the word *gonorrhoea*, meaning a flow of semen), Arateus of Cappadocia (who distinguished vaginal gonorrhoea from simple discharge), and Soranus (who described the condition) [1]. The Golden Age of Islam (900–1100 AD) [3] is exemplified by Abu Ali al Hussein ibn Sina Avicenna (980–1037), who was less remarkable as a physician than as a philosopher and physicist. His gigantic Canon of Medicine (al-Qānūn fī'ṭ-Ṭibb), which dealt with the whole of systemic medicine, recommended irrigations for urethral discharge. Later, Maimonides of Cordoba (1135–1204), who spent most of his active life in Cairo, in "Aphorisms" described gonorrhoea as fluid escaping without erection or feeling of pleasure, doughy, and the result of disease including amorousness and excesses [4].

During the Middle Ages in Europe, advances in the knowledge of gonorrhoea were made. Roger of Salerno (1180) and William of Salicet (1210–77) wrote on the causality and natural history of gonorrhoea; John of Gaddesden (1280–1361) recognised urethritis, epididymitis and vaginitis [1]. The contagiousness of gonorrhoea was generally recognised, as shown by rules for preventing infected prostitutes from plying their trade in Southwark, London in 1162 [1], Avignon in 1347 [1, 5], and Hamburg, Strasbourg, Cologne and Ulm in the eleventh to fifteenth centuries [6].

Other STIs, including scabies and pediculosis pubis, have also been recognised since ancient times [4], although the concept of different causes for skin diseases has only developed in the last 300 years [7]. Genital human papilloma virus infection (HPV; i.e., genital warts) have been recognised for 2000 years [4, 8]. Anal warts resulting from anal intercourse were exemplified by Juvenal in his satires. Much later, they were described by the English surgeon Richard Wiseman in 1676 [9] and the French physician Jean Astruc in 1736 [10].

1.4 The Development of the Concept of Venereal Diseases Prior to the Nineteenth Century

The Renaissance showed that any change in medical knowledge is as much influenced by outside social, geopolitical and economic forces as it is from within medicine [11]. So it was with venereal diseases (VD). Syphilis is among the most interesting of diseases from a historical standpoint, not only because of arguments about its origin, but because of its influence on morality and measures towards public health [4, 8, 10, 12]. Its origin has been controversial. The pre-Columbian view is that syphilis was endemic in Europe before the invasion of Italy by Charles VIII in 1494, and with the disbandment of mercenaries it spread sexually all over Europe [4, 8, 13].

The Columbian (Americanist) view is that syphilis was acquired by the sailors of Christopher Columbus and spread after 1493 through Europe [10]. Both these views have their advocates, who usually claim skeletal remains from America or Europe (now aided by genotyping) to further their arguments. Another idea is that of Hudson (1946) [14], who emphasized the evolutionary relationships of yaws, pinta, endemic syphilis, and sporadic syphilis. He regarded them as variants of the same disease that originated in sub-Saharan Africa.

There is a great amount of literature not only on syphilis's effect in Italy [11, 13, 15], but also on its progress, discoveries and consequences throughout Europe [4, 8, 16] after 1494. By the end of the fifteenth century, most of its immediate consequences, including congenital syphilis [17, 18], had been described.

However, some controversies surrounded syphilis for many years. The Diet of Worms (7th August 1495) was the first printed document to mention this new severe disease: "There have been severe diseases and plagues of the people, to wit 'bösen Blattern' which have never occurred before nor been heard of within the memory of man" [15]. In the Latin translation, this new type of disease [12], "bösen Blattern," is called *Malum Francicum* – a French name that is still used today in many countries of Asia (farengi) [19]. The French called it the Neapolitan disease [12]. By some, syphilis was considered to be a pox due to the wrath of God [4, 8, 12] and a punishment for immorality. Even astrological explanations were given for it [12, 13].

However, the venereal origins of syphilis were quickly realised and bluntly stated by Andrew Boord in 1547: "It may come when one pocky person doth synne in lechery the one with another. All the kyndes of the pockes be infectiouse" [4]. The term *venereal disease* (lues venerea) was used by Jacques de Bethencourt of Rouen in 1527 [4, 8, 10, 12]. In 1530, Girolamo Fracastoro of Verona [20] wrote "Syphilus sive morbus gallicus"; a swineherd or shepherd was thought smitten with the disease when he refused to make sacrifices to Apollo [4]. Guaiacum, a wood recently imported from South America, was popularised as a treatment because of its sudorific properties by Fracastoro [12]. Also used was mercury in ointment, pill and fumigation forms. It had been used in scabies grossa in Italy for hundreds of years after being inherited from Arabic medicine, so it continued to be used for the new disease syphilis [13].

Cautery of the primary sore was also utilised as treatment, as shown on contemporary watercolours [11]. It has erroneously been taught that Gabrielle Fallopius (1523–1562) [11, 16] recommended the condom as a preventive measure. In fact, Fallopius recommended that his students at Padua prevent contagion by making a wash using active ingredients of guaicum, mercury, copper and gentian root; this wash was to be applied in a bag at the bottom of one's culottes after coitus [16]. He described the typical indurated primary sore and also noticed syphilis was more frequent in men with long prepuces [11, 12, 16], as well as being rare in Jews (who were of course circumcised). It was actually Daniel Turner (1717) who advocated the use of the "condum" (Latin for "condere to protect") to prevent from VD [21].

Jean Fernel (1506–1588) rejected the Galenic concept that genital lesions were secondary to humoral disorders arising in the liver. He taught that morbus Gallicus was caused by a virus usually acquired through intercourse. He stated that midwives may contract it through the hand and the wet nurse through her nipple. He also noted that oral and anal moist lesions were contagious and that the virus could not pass through intact skin. He taught about a long incubation period, prolonged latency, and exacerbations. He also referred to lues venerea- venereal plague (De lues venereae curatione perfectissimo, 1556) [4, 8, 10, 16]. The confusion between the causation of syphilis and gonorrhoea seems to have been compounded by Paracelsus (1493–1531), who called morbus gallicus "French gonorrhoea." He divided it into states–simple and virulent, which developed constitutional symptoms [12, 17]. This was the start of two viewpoints on the diseases: monists [10, 22] believed that gonorrhoea and syphilis were part of the same disease, whereas dualists [23, 24] thought they were separate.

Lancisi (1654–1720) posthumously correlated dilatation of the heart with syphilis "aneurysma gallicum" in 1728 [25]. In the same year, Boerhaave (1668–1738) in Leiden implicated syphilis as a cause of cardiovascular disease as well as considering it to be part of generalised neurological decay [4]. In 1736, Jean Astruc (1684–1776), in "De morbis veneriis libri sex," summarized all there was to know about VD to that time. He believed in its American origin, but shared the belief of the monists [10]. He provided clinical descriptions of several conditions, including genital herpes, condylomata acuminata, phimosis, and balanoposthitis.

Van Swieten (1700–1772), a pupil of Boerhaave called to Vienna after 1749, popularised more liberal treatment of syphilitics, as well as the introduction of graduated dosage with mercury to prevent side effects such as oversalivation (ptyalism), the shakes (tremors), and renal disease [4].

John Hunter (1728–1793) wrote "A Treatise on the Venereal Disease" in 1786, but it was not one of his best works. His error was to adhere to the monist doctrine. In an experiment in 1767, he tried to prove that gonorrhoea and syphilis had a single cause. Gonococcal pus was inoculated onto the prepuce and glans penis. Unfortunately, the inoculum was chosen from a patient suffering from syphilis as well as gonorrhoea. As the inoculum was not put in the urethra, no gonorrhoea, only syphilis, resulted. This caused the faulty deduction that the result depended on the nature of the surface of the inoculum–gonorrhoea for moist surfaces and ulceration for a cutaneous surface [4, 8, 22]. In Edinburgh, Benjamin Bell (1749–1806)–following the teachings of Morgagni (1682–1771) in 1793 (Treatise on gonorrhoea virulenta and lues venerea)–refuted Hunter's ideas after inoculation experiments on students [23]. The French venereologist Philippe Ricord (1800–1889) in 1838 [24] used 2,500 inoculation experiments performed between 1831–1837 to show conclusively that gonorrhoea and syphilis were different diseases (Traité Pratique des Maladies Vénériennes). Although ethical standards in those days were different, when others in France tried similar experimentation on patients, cases were taken before the courts.

After the French Revolution, postreform medical teaching had an immense impact globally [26]. Ricord [8, 12] exemplified this teaching. He was born in Baltimore and obtained a teaching position in Paris from 1831. Ricord was an excellent and witty teacher; he was considerate women with VD and was a proponent of the vaginal speculum. He was also the classifier of syphilis in primary, secondary and tertiary stages, although he still did not recognise the separate entity of chancroid–which was left to his pupil Leon Bassereau (1810–1887) [27]–or that secondary syphilis was contagious. His pupils, such as Paul Diday and Alfred Fournier (1832–1914), were worthy successors to his school and its teaching traditions.

There were some other smaller advances in knowledge in those times. In 1814, Thomas Bateman's fourth edition of "A Practical Synopsis of Cutaneous Disease" described Herpes praeputalis [7], with an excellent clinical description but stating that a practical mistake with serious consequences for the patient would be made if syphilis was wrongly diagnosed for then mercury would be prescribed. In 1818, Benjamin Brodie (1783–1862) wrote a textbook on diseases of the joints [28] and described the syndrome. This was later described by Launois in 1899 [8] and by Hans Reiter (1881–1969) in 1916 [29], with the main triad being urethritis, arthritis and conjunctivitis. In 1835, Wallace (1791–1837) in Dublin introduced potassium iodide into the treatment of syphilis following contemporary interest in the chemistry of the halogens [30].

1.5 The Development of a Scientific Basis for Sexually Transmitted Disease from the Nineteenth Century

The Industrial Revolution brought with it movement of populations into cities, which also contributed to increasing STD rates. The Industrial Revolution also was the lever for advances in engineering and the natural sciences, which would have effects throughout medicine. Nations that considered themselves to be civilised also enabled public health medicine, as well as provided medical education to middle-class citizens to increase manpower for providing these services. The fields of epidemiology and microscopy; the reorganisation of medical education in great centres such as Paris [26], Vienna [31], London [4] and New York; and later advances in microbiology, serology, immunology [31] and organic chemistry led to recognition of causal agents for syphilis, chancroid, gonorrhoea, lymphogranuloma venereum, and advances in the microbiology of STDs–and ultimately cures for them.

1.5.1 Epidemiology

The concept of the nation-state and the regulation by the state of various aspects of a citizen's life meant that the relationship of VD took on a new importance in this era [4]. Parent-Duchatelet (1790–1836) [32] was a pioneer in epidemiology. Posthumously in 1837, he tabulated where prostitutes lived in Paris, where they came from, and their former trades. He also noted that syphilis, gonorrhoea, scabies and uterine cancers were more frequent in them than in other women. This was the start of many epidemiological and sociological studies on the relationships of society, women, prostitution, and VD throughout the nineteenth centuries and to present times. Such studies were highlighted by Flexner (1914) [33] and the British Royal Commission on Venereal Diseases (1916) [34]. Colonial policies on sex and its influence on STDs and society thus needed to be formulated [19].

Chancroid. It was left to Bassereau (1852) [27] to publish his clinically based observations that the sore of chancroid was a separate entity from syphilis and that it did not lead to spread in the body as did syphilis with constitutional symptoms. Augusto Ducrey (1860–1940) [35], working in the department of Paul Gerson Unna (1850–1924) in Hamburg, discovered the organism of chancroid in the pus from its lesions in 1889.

Congenital syphilis. By 1854, Diday [12, 36] had described all that was known on congenital syphilis to that time. From 1857–1863, Jonathan Hutchinson (1828–1913) in London described his triad of interstitial keratitis and labyrinthine disease, which were all later codified by the successor to Ricord in Paris, Alfred Fournier, in "La syphilis heriditaire tardive" in 1886 [4, 12, 36].

Neurosyphilis. Fournier (1875) [4, 37] proposed that syphilis was the cause of general paralysis (GPI), tabes dorsalis, tabo-paresis, and primary optic atrophy. But it was not until 1913 that Hideyo Noguchi (1876–1928) and Moore [38], who were working at the Rockefeller Institute in New York, were able to demonstrate spirochaetes in the brains of a series of paretics.

Gonorrhoea. Microbiology made amazing progress in the latter part of the nineteenth century, led by Louis Pasteur (1822–1895) and Robert Koch (1843–1910). Using Koch's techniques, Albert Neisser [39] (1855–1916), at the age of 23 in 1879 with a Zeiss Microscope and an Abbe condenser, was able to demonstrate the micrococci of gonorrhoea from cases of purulent urethritis and ophthalmia neonatorum, but reserved his judgement until culture and inoculation experiments had been performed. In 1882, he stated: "Gonococci are absolutely constant in every case of gonorrhoea... and they are not found in any other disease...furthermore, gonococci are the only organisms found in gonorrhoeal pus" [8]. Carl Crédé (1819–92), in 1883 in Leipzig, published his procedure where instillation of 2% silver nitrate prevented ophthalmia neonatorum [40]. Succeeding workers elaborated on diagnostics of gonorrhoea, as summated by Vienna's Ernest Finger (1856–1939) in "Die Blennorrhoe der Sexualorgane und ihre Complicationen" in 1888 [5].

1.5.2 Syphilis: Causation, Serology and the Magic Bullet

Between 1875–1877, Edwin Klebs (1834–1914) in Prague had observed spirochaetes in human syphilitic material and may have transmitted the disease to monkeys [4]. Experimental syphilis was reinvigorated by Elie Metchnikoff (1845–1916) and Pierre E. Roux (1853–1933), who showed that syphilis could be transmitted to chimpanzees [41]. On March 3, 1905, at the Charite in Berlin, dermatologist Erich Hoffman (1868–1959) and protozoologist Fritz Schaudinn (1871–1906) demonstrated spirochaetes (later called *Treponema pallidum*) from preparations of patients with early syphilis with fresh and Giemsa-stained preparations [42]. In the same year, Aldo Castellani (1877–1971) [43], working in Ceylon, described the spirochaete (now *T. pertenue*) in yaws. By 1906, Karl Landsteiner (1868–1943) and Viktor Mucha (1877–1933) were able to demonstrate *T. pallidum* by dark field methods [44].

The earlier work of Jules Bordet (1870–1961) and Octave Gengou (1875–1961) [45] defined the complement fixation test (CFT) in 1901, in which an infection could be diagnosed by finding its antibody in the serum. August von Wassermann (1866–1925) was able to show in 1906 the value of the CFT in the diagnosis of syphilis [46], which was later evaluated by Landsteiner and Rudolf Muller in 1907 [47]. The introduction of the first test for a specific antibody to exclude false-positive results did not come until 1949 with the introduction of the treponemal immobilization test by Robert Nelson and Manfred Mayer [48].

Until the advent of the arsenicals, mercury was still the main treatment for syphilis [12]. In 1895, Adolph Jarisch (1850–1902) [8] from Innsbruck described a phenomenon that was well recognised in patients with secondary syphilis with mercury inunctions, in which the first few hours there was an exacerbation of symptoms. This was later recorded in more detail by Karl Herxheimer (1861–1944) [49].

Paul Ehrlich (1854–1915) had for many years been working on synthetic agents to control trypanosomal infections. In 1909, it was found that 606-arsphenamine (Salvarsan) was effective when given intravenously for syphilis in animals. By 1910, it was found to be effective in the cure of syphilis in humans and was thus the magic bullet – "Therapia sterilis magna" [50].

Malarial therapy was introduced in 1917 for the treatment of GPI by Julius Wagner von Jauregg (1857–1940) an Austrian neuropsychiatrist [51] who had noticed patients improved after being given a controllable source for a fever. It was used later with penicillin until the 1950s. Although not as active as arsenicals, bismuth was found to effective for syphilis by R. Sazerac and Constantin Levaditi (1874–1953) in 1921 [52], and it was used until the 1960s.

1.5.3 Chlamydial Trachomatis Oculogenital Infection

In the 1900s, Neisser had worked on experimental syphilis in orangutans in Java [8]. While there, some members of his team – Ludwig Halberstaedter (1876–1949) and Stanislaus von Prowazek (1875–1915) [53] – also researched conjunctival scrapings from patients with trachoma by inoculating them into orangutan and reporting inclusion bodies (1907). This work was continued by Lindner [54], who reported inclusions in urethral specimens from 3 of 10 men with nongonococcal urethritis.

With the advent of penicillin, it was noticed that some men with urethral discharge did not respond to penicillin. This resulted in the 1950 work of Arthur Herbert Harkness (1889–1970), who recognised nongonococcal urethritis as a separate entity [55]. From 1959, when it was first isolated from genital material *Chlamydia trachomatis* and later recovered from the eyes of a baby with inclusion conjunctivitis and the mother's cervix by Jones and his team at the Institute of Ophthalmology in London [56], the organism has been increasingly recognised and is the most frequent bacterial STD in industrialised countries.

Donovanosis. This tropical STD was described by Kenneth Macleod (1844–1922) of The Indian Medical Service in 1881[57]. Its causality was identified in 1905 by Charles Donovan (1863–1951) [58] from Madras, who identified intracellular bodies from stained biopsies of the granulating lesions. In 1945, members of Goodpasture's team [59] at Vanderbilt University in Tennessee were able to propagate them in eggs. Thus the organism has been named *Calymmatobacterium granulomatis*.

1.5.4 Impact on Society Before and After the Discovery of AIDS

Few diseases have had such an impact on society as STIs. After all, these infections have an enormous impact on those who contract them – both physically and psychologically. If not treated, STIs may cause serious ill health and even death – especially viral STIs, which can develop from HIV to AIDS, from human genital papilloma virus to anogenital cancers, from herpes genitalis to morbidity and recurrences, and from hepatitis B or C to morbidity and mortality through long-term disease of the liver. It has been a short time in human history from from the advent of antibiotics, which to the general public seemingly allowed for instant cure of bacterial STDs, to the discovery of HIV – not withstanding infertility caused by pelvic inflammatory disease or epididymo-orchitis as a result of gonococcal or chlamydial infections. This chapter has already alluded to STIs and their impact on conventional morality. However, if a study is made of great literature in the last 400 years, the argument for chastity for the individual does not seem to make any impact for very long: from Voltaire in *Dictionnaire Philosophique*,"Venereal diseases are like the fine arts – it is pointless to ask who invented them,". to Alexander Pope in *Satires of Dr Donne*, "Time that at last matures a clap to pox-Whose gentle progress makes a calf an ox," and to Henrik Ibsen in *Ghosts*, who had little effect in modern times, "I never asked you for life. And what sort of life have you given me?" Rather the reaction is usually more like James Boswell in the *London Journal*, "When I got home, though, there came Sorrow. Too plain was Signor Gonorrhoea."

The financial strain put on a nation may be more impactful, considering the cost of STI morbidity to a large section of its young workforce. The final report of the British Royal Commission on Venereal Disease in 1916 demonstrated the high mortality from syphilis, with mortality statistics showing 10% of London working-class males infected; 25% of infantile blindness was found to be due to ophthalmia neonatorum [34]. More recently, Thailand realized in the 1990s that if HIV disease was allowed to spread, apart from mortality, too many of the young productive workforce would be ill, thus causing a drain on the nation's finances apart from it damaging the tourist trade (World Bank, 1997) [60].

AIDS was first recognised in 1981 [61] in men who had sex with men (MSM) in New York and California; thus, it unfortunately was called "the gay plague." However, very soon it was realised that it was also transmitted through infected blood and by birth processes as well as sexually. The greatest numbers of cases have been reported in heterosexuals in sub-Saharan Africa and South Asia, the former being one of the most under-resourced parts of the world [60]. Paradoxically, AIDS has challenged societal attitudes to the morality of sexual behaviour, especially same-sex relationships, the rights of women, the needs of Africa, and international affairs between industrialised donor countries and much poorer countries. It has also acted as catalyst to increase medical and industrial research in basic sciences, pharmaceuticals, health and community education, and very many ethical and social problems that were involved with an epidemic that now is globally pandemic [60].

These pragmatic realities are a profound argument for expert epidemiology of STIs, continued public education to prevent them, the continued use of the condom in all casual sexual encounters, and further research into development of preventive vaccines for STIs – in addition to the presently available hepatitis A, hepatitis B, and HPV vaccines.

1.5.5 Scientific Achievements since the Advent of Chemotherapy

Ehrlich [50] had been a pioneer in treating infectious diseases with synthetic compounds. However, with the exception of treponemata, it was thought that bacteria were not susceptible to chemotherapy. Research on penicillin and sulphonamides was to change this. In 1935, Gerhard Domagk (1895–1964) [62], who was working with IG Farbenindustrie, reported that Prontosil (one of the azo dyes he had tested) was curative against haemolytic streptococcal infections in animals. It was soon shown that the activity of Prontosil was due to the liberation of sulphanilamide, which can be easily manufactured. In 1937, studies on its use in gonorrhoea appeared in Germany, Great Britain, and the United States [63]. By the start of World War II, it was the main treatment of gonorrhoea in all opposing military forces. However, by 1944 resistant strains of *N. gonorrhoea* had occurred in up to 75% of cases [8]. Sulphonamides combined with streptomycin were used in the treatment of nongonococcal urethritis in some cases until the 1970s, or in combination with trimethoprim in the treatment of chancroid, donovanosis, and lymphogranuloma venereum in some instances.

The story of the discovery and development of penicillin is one of the great romances of medicine, with the 1945 Nobel Prize awarded to Alexander Fleming (1881–1955), Howard Florey (1898–1968) and Ernst Chain (1906–1979). The use of penicillin in the treatment of syphilis was first reported by John F. Mahoney (1889–1957) and his team in 1943: "Four patients with primary lesions were treated with 25,000 units of the drug intramuscularly at 4-hour intervals night and day for 8 days. The chancres all became darkfield negative within 16 hours" [64]. Penicillin was also found to be effective in gonorrhoea, although by 1958 it was evident that resistance was developing. In the following years, this became a major problem [8]. Although the resistance of gonorrhoea to most antimicrobials sooner or later was reported, the resistance of *T. pallidum* to penicillin has not yet occurred.

The course of untreated syphilis had been studied in detail in Oslo, Norway by Caesar Boeck (1845–1913), followed up by his successor Bruusgaard, and reported in 1955 by Gjestland [65]. In all, 30% of patients developed complications of one sort or another [8].

In 1932, the US Public Health Service had studied the course of untreated syphilis on black people in Tuskegee, Alabama. This study continued for 30 years. Patients with early syphilis were treated with arsenicals, but the remainder of patients with a history suggestive of syphilis and positive serological tests were left untreated. This study was conducted long after penicillin had been shown to be effective and informed consent was never obtained from the patients [66]. Medical ethics, like most human development, does not remain static. Therefore, any long-term medical research should be monitored for changing attitudes to contemporary ethics.

Tetracyclines have been the mainstay therapy of nongonococcal urethritis (NGU) caused by *C. trachomatis* or *U. urealyticum* since their development and introduction after 1948 [67]. An underrecognised development, which ended years of suffering of women with chronic vaginal discharge caused by trichomoniasis and also paved the way to therapy of anaerobes, was the effectivity of metronidazole [68].

It is always difficult to decide when to finish a history. In this case, this chapter ends before the advent of modern treatment for candidiasis, herpes genitalis, genital HPV infection, and HIV/AIDS, as well as the introduction of effective vaccines for some STIs. However, these topics will be discussed elsewhere in this book.

Take-Home Pearls

- Knowledge about the development of any subject is important, so that one can learn not only about the subject's general impact but also its achievements and failures.
- These achievements and failures may enable the reader to formulate ideas for research that may have impact on scientific progress in sexually transmitted infections (STIs).
- Knowledge of the history of STIs is necessary for historical purposes and future research. Sometimes it is controversial; sometimes contemporary medical ethics are challenged. But without these challenges, knowledge of the past will not help mankind in the future.

References

1. Morton, R.S.: Gonorrhoea. WB Saunders, London, Philadelphia, Toronto (1977)
2. Joachim, H.: Papyros Ebers. Das älteste Buch über Heilkunde, aus dem Ägyptischen zum erstenmal vollstandig ubersetzt von. Joachim. G. Reimer, Berlin (1890)
3. Arnold, T., Guillaume, A.: The Legacy of Islam, 1st edn. Oxford University Press, London (1931)
4. Waugh, M.A.: History of clinical developments in sexually transmitted diseases. In: Holmes, K.K., Mardh, P.A., Sparling, P.J., Wiesner, P.F. (eds.) Sexually Transmitted Diseases, 2nd edn, pp. 3–16. Mc Graw Hill, New York (1984)
5. Finger, E.A.F.: Die Blenorrhoea der Sexualorgane und ihre Complicationen. F. Deuticke, Leipzig (1888)
6. Sanger, W.W.: The History of Prostitution. The Medical Publishing Co, New York (1919)
7. Bateman, T.: A Practical Synopsis of Cutaneous Diseases, 4th edn. Longman, Hurst, Rees, Orme, Brown, London (1814)
8. Oriel, J.D.: The Scars of Venus A History of Venereology. Springer-Verlag, London, Berlin, Heidelberg, New York (1994)
9. Wiseman, R.: Several Chirurgical Treatises. R. Royston, London (1676)
10. Astruc, J.: De morbis venereis libri sex. G. Cavalier, Paris (1736)
11. Arrizabalaga, J., Henderson, J., French, R.: The Great Pox. Yale University Press, New Haven, London (1997)
12. Jeanselme, E.: Histoire de la syphilis. G. Doin, Paris (1931)
13. Sudhoff, K., Singer, C.: The Earliest Printed Literature on Syphilis. R. Lier, Florence (1925)
14. Hudson, E.H.: Treponematosis. Oxford University Press, New York (1946)
15. Sudhoff, K.: Graphische und Typographische Erstlinge der Syphilis Literatur aus den Jahren 1495 und 1496. Carl Kuhn, Munich (1912)
16. Quetel, C.: History of Syphilis. Polity Press, Cambridge (1990)
17. Paracelsus: von der französischen Krankheit drey. Bücher. H Gulfferich, Frankfurt am Main (1553).
18. Torrella, C.: Tractatus cum consiliis contra pudendagram seu morbum gallicum. Pietro della Turre, Rome (1497)
19. Lewis, M., Bamber, S., Waugh, M.: Sex, Disease and Society A Comparative History of Sexually Transmitted Diseases and HIV/AIDS in Asia and the Pacific. Greenwood Press, Westport, London (1997)
20. Fracastoro, G.: Syphilus sive morbus gallicus. S. Nicolini da Sabbio, Verona (1530)
21. Turner, D.: Syphilis A Practical Dissertation on the Venereal Disease. Walthoe, Wilkin, Bonwicke, Ward, London (1728)
22. Hunter, J.: A Treatise on the Venereal Disease. W. Bulmer and Co, London (1786)
23. Bell, B.: Treatise on Gonorrhoea Virulenta and Lues Venerea. J Watson & G Mudie, Edinburgh (1793)
24. Ricord, P.: Traité pratique des maladies vénériennes ou récherches critiques et experimentales sur inoculation appliqué a l'etude de ces maladies, pp. 5–198. Rouvier et le Bouvrier, Paris (1838)
25. Lancisi GM (1728) De motu cordis et aneurysmatibus. Naples
26. Ackerknecht, E.H.: Medicine at the Paris Hospital 1794–1848. Johns Hopkins Press, Baltimore (1967)
27. Bassereau, L.: Traité des affections de la peau symptomatiques de la syphilis, p. 197. J-B Bailliere, Paris (1852)
28. Brodie, B.C.: Pathological and Surgical Observations on Diseases of the Joints, pp. 51–63. Longman, London (1818)
29. Reiter, H.: Über eine bisher unerkannte Spirochateninfektion (Spirochaetosis arthritica). Dtsch. Med. Wochenschr. **42**, 1535–1536 (1916)
30. Wallace, W.: Treatment of the venereal disease by the hydriodate of potash, or iodide of potassium. Lancet **2**, 5–11 (1835)
31. Lesky, E.: The Vienna Medical School of the 19th Century. Johns Hopkins University Press, Baltimore, London (1976)
32. Parent-Duchatelet, A.J.B.: De la Prostitution de la ville de Paris. JB Bailliere, Paris (1836)
33. Flexner, A.: Prostitution in Europe. The Century Co., New York (1914)
34. Royal Commission on Venereal Diseases: Final Report of the Commissioners. His Majesty's Stationery Office, London (1916)
35. Ducrey, A.: Experimentelle Untersuchungen über den Asteckungsstoff des weichen Schankers und über die Bubonen. Mschr. Prakt. Derm. **9**, 387 (1889)
36. Fournier, A.: La syphilis hereditaire tardive. G. Masson, Paris (1886)
37. Fournier, A.: De l' ataxie locomotrice d'origine syphilitique. Ann. Dermatol. Syphiligraph **1**, 7 (1875)
38. Noguchi, H., Moore, J.W.: A demonstration of *Treponema pallidum* in the brain in cases of general paralysis. J. Exp. Med. **17**, 232–238 (1913)
39. Neisser, A.: Über eine der Gonorrhoe eigentümliche Micrococcusform. Centralb. Med. Wochenschr. **17**, 497–500 (1879)
40. Crédé, C.S.F.: Die Vehütung der Augenentzündung der Neugeborenen. Arch. Gynaek. **21**, 179–195 (1883)
41. Metchnikoff, E., Roux, P.: Etudes experimentales sur la syphilis. Ann. Inst. Pasteur **17**, 808–821 (1903). 1904. 18: 1–6
42. Schaudinn, F., Hoffmann, E.: Vorlaufiger Bericht uber das Vorkommen von Spirochaeten in syphilitischen Krankheitsprodukten und bei Papillomen. Arb. K. Gesundhamt **22**, 527–534 (1905)
43. Castellani, A.: On the presence of spirochaetes in 2 cases of ulcerated parengi (yaws). Br. Med. J. **1**, 1280 (1905)
44. Landsteiner, K., Mucha, V.: Technik der Spirochaetenuntersuchung. Wien. Klin. Wochenschr. **19**, 1349 (1906)
45. Bordet, J.J.B.V., Gengou, O.: Sur l' existence de substances sensibilisatrices dans la plupart des serums antimicrobiens. Ann. Inst. Pasteur **15**, 289–302 (1901)
46. Wassermann, A., Neisser, A., Bruck, C.: Eine serodiagnostiche Reaktion bei Syphilis. Dtsch Med. Wochenschr. **32**, 745–746 (1906)
47. Landsteiner, K., Muller, R.: Zur Technik der Spirochaenuntersuchung. Wien. Klin. Wochenschr. **20**, 1565 (1907)
48. Nelson, R.A., Mayer, M.N.: Immobilisation of *Treponema pallidum* in vitro by antibody produced in syphilitic infection. J. Exp. Med. **89**, 369–393 (1949)
49. Herxheimer, K., Krause: Über eine bei syphilitschen vorkommende Quecksilberreaktion. Dtsch. Med. Wochenschr. **28**, 895–897 (1902)

50. Ehrlich, P., Hatta, S.: Die experimentelle Chemotherapie der Spirillosen. Julius Springer, Berlin (1910)
51. Wagner von Jauregg, J.W.: Die Behandlung der progresssiven Paralyse und Tabes. Wien. Med. Wochenschr. **71**(1106), 1210 (1921)
52. Sazerac, R., Levaditi, C.: Traitement de la syphilis par le bismuth. C. R. Acad. Sci. Paris **173**, 338–339 (1921)
53. Halberstaedter, L., von Prowazek, D.: Über Zelleinschlüsse parasitärer Natur beim Trachom. Arb K Gesundh Amt **26**, 44–47 (1907)
54. Lindner, K.: Zur Ätiologie der gonokokkenfreien Urethritis. Wien. Klin. Wochenschr. **23**, 283–284 (1910)
55. Harkness, A.H.: Non-Gonococcal Urethritis. Livingstone, Edinburgh (1950)
56. Jones, B.R., Collier, L.H., Smith, C.H.: Isolation of virus from inclusion blennorrhoea. Lancet **1**, 902–905 (1959)
57. MacLeod, K.: Precis of operations performed in the wards of the First Surgeon, Medical College Hospital, during the year 1881. Indian Med. Gaz. **17**, 113–123 (1882)
58. Donovan, C.: Medical cases from Madras General Hospital: ulcerating granuloma of the pudenda. Indian Med. Gaz. **40**, 414 (1905)
59. Anderson, K., de Monbreun, W.A., Goodpasture, E.W.: An etiologic consideration of Donovania granulomatis cultivated from granuloma inguinale (3 cases) in embryonic yolk. J. Exp. Med. **81**, 25–39 (1945)
60. World Bank: Confronting AIDS Public Priorities in a Global Epidemic. Oxford University Press, New York (1997)
61. Centers for Disease Control: Pneumocystis pneumonia – Los Angeles. Morb. Mortal Weekly Rep. **30**, 250–252 (1981)
62. Domagk, G.: Ein Beitrag zur chemotherapie der bakterielle Infekionen. Dtsch. Med. Wochenschr. **61**, 250 (1935)
63. Kampmeier, R.H.: Introduction of sulphonamide therapy for gonorrhoea. Sex. Transm. Dis. **10**, 81–84 (1983)
64. Mahoney, J.F., Arnold, R.C., Harris, A.: Penicillin treatment of early syphilis – a preliminary report. Am J Publ Health **33**, 1387–1391 (1943)
65. Gjestland, T.: The Oslo study of untreated syphilis: an epidemiological investigation of the natural course of syphilitic infection based on a restudy of the Boeck- Bruusgard material. Acta Derm – Vener **35**(Suppl 34), 1–368 (1955)
66. Rockwell, D.H.: The Tuskegee study of untreated syphilis. Arch. Intern. Med. **114**, 792–797 (1964)
67. Willcox, R.R., Findlay, G.M.: Urethritis, gonococcal and nonspecific, treated by aureomycin. Brit. Med. J. **2**, 257 (1949)
68. Durel, P., Roiron, V., Siboulet, A., Borel, J.Q.: Systemic treatment of human trichomoniasis with a derivative of nitroimidazole. Brit. J. Vener. Dis. **36**, 21–26 (1960)

Epidemiology of Sexually Transmitted Infections

2

Aron Gewirtzman, Laura Bobrick, Kelly Conner, and Stephen K. Tyring

Core Messages

- Sexually transmitted infections (STIs) are commonplace worldwide and may be caused by bacteria, fungi, protozoa, parasites, or viruses.
- Epidemiology involves the study of incidence and prevalence of disease in large populations as well as detection of the source and cause of epidemics of infectious disease.
- Acute diseases tend to have high incidence and low prevalence; chronic diseases may have high prevalence even if incidence is low.
- Developing nations have the largest proportion of STIs, while most industrialized countries have low or falling rates of infection.
- Prevention is the best tool to decrease morbidity and mortality of STIs.

2.1 Introduction

Sexually transmitted infections (STIs) are extraordinarily commonplace, with an estimated 340 million new cases of "curable" infections occurring each year (see Table 2.1) worldwide in men and women aged 15–49 years [1]. These infections include those caused by bacterial, mycological, and protozoal agents that have been treated by appropriate antibiotics and chemotherapeutic agents for more than 40 years (namely syphilis, gonorrhea, chlamydia, and trichomoniasis). In spite of adequate available therapy, such STIs have continued to be a public health problem in both industrialized and developing countries. In addition to the "curable" STIs, there are also millions of viral STIs that occur annually (including human immunodeficiency virus [HIV], herpesviruses, human papilloma viruses, and hepatitis B viruses) that cannot be eradicated through currently available medication.

The largest proportion of STIs occur in developing nations, led by South and Southeast Asia, followed by sub-Saharan Africa, Latin America, and the Caribbean [2]. An equilibrium has been reached in most industrialized countries with low (and often still falling) rates of infection. In contrast, the equilibrium reached in many developing countries has been with highly endemic levels of disease [3].

STIs are not only a cause of acute morbidity in adults, but may result in complications including male and female infertility, ectopic pregnancy, cervical cancer, premature mortality, congenital syphilis and fetal wastage, low birth weight, and prematurity and ophthalmia neonatorum [3].

Care for the sequelae of STIs accounts for a large proportion of tertiary healthcare costs in terms of screening and treatment of cervical cancer, management of liver disease, investigation for infertility

A. Gewirtzman and L. Bobrick
Center for Clinical Studies, Houston, TX, USA

K. Conner
University of Texas Health Science Center, Houston, TX, USA

S.K. Tyring (✉)
Department of Dermatology, University of Texas Health Science Center, 6655 Travis Street, Suite 100, Houston, TX 77030, USA
e-mail: styring@ccstexas.com

G. Gross and S.K. Tyring (eds.), *Sexually Transmitted Infections and Sexually Transmitted Diseases*,
DOI: 10.1007/978-3-642-14663-3_2,

Table 2.1 Worldwide incidence of common "curable" sexually transmitted infections

Infection	Worldwide Incidence/ Prevalence
Trichomonas	170–190 million incident cases
Chlamydia	Over 90 million incident cases
Gonorrhea	Over 62 million incident cases
Syphilis	12 million incident cases
Chanchroid	6–7 million incident cases

causes, care for perinatal morbidity, childhood blindness, pulmonary disease in children, and chronic pelvic pain in women [1]. The costs increase further when the cofactor effect of other STIs on HIV transmission is taken into consideration [1, 2]. The economic burden of STIs is huge, especially for developing countries where they account for 17% of economic losses caused by ill health [4].

Many STIs are asymptomatic and therefore can be difficult to recognize and control. Thus, the worldwide incidence of new cases of STIs may be even higher than the estimated 340 million mentioned above. For example, it is estimated that actual reported cases of STIs represent only 50–80% of reportable STIs in the United States, reflecting limited screening and low disease reporting [5].

Several risk factors exist that make certain populations more prone to STIs than others (see Table 2.2). While these risk factors are not shared by all STIs, there are many commonalities. Young age, for example, is a risk factor common to many STIs. Adolescents and young adults (15–24 years old) make up only 25% of the sexually active population, but represent almost 50% of all new acquired STIs [5]. This may be confounded by the fact that this age group is more prone to engage in high-risk sexual activity (another risk factor) than the older population. Other groups known to participate in high-risk sexual activity (such as sex with multiple partners and unprotected sex) include prostitutes, intravenous (IV) drug users, and prison inmates. Not surprisingly, these groups are also known to be at higher risk for STIs than the general population. Additional risk factors for several STIs include lack of male circumcision, low socioeconomic status, and poor hygiene.

Epidemiology is the branch of medicine dealing with the incidence and prevalence of disease in large

Table 2.2 Major risk factors of sexually transmitted infections

Infection	Young Age	High-Risk Sexual Behavior	Low Socioeconomic Status	Poor Hygiene	Other Specific Risk Factors
Trichomonas		X	X	X	Increased age
Chlamydia	X	X			Female gender
Gonorrhea	X	X	X		
Syphilis	X	X			MSM population
Chancroid	X	X		X	Lack of male circumcision
Donovanosis	X	X	X		
Herpes simplex		X	X		
Human papillomavirus		X	X		Bimodal age distribution, lack of male circumcision
HIV/AIDS		X	X		MSM population (in the United States), perinatal infection, IV drug use
Hepatitis B		X			Lack of childhood vaccination, vertical transmission, IV drug use
Molluscum contagiosum	X	X			
Scabies/pubic lice		X	X	X	

populations and with the detection of the source and cause of epidemics of infectious disease. The terms incidence and prevalence are often confused even in scientific literature. Technically, incidence refers to the number of new cases of a disease in a population over a period of time (usually a year). Prevalence, on the other hand, refers to the total number of cases of a disease in a given population at a specific time. Acute diseases or those with high mortality rates tend to have a high incidence and low prevalence, since those who acquire the disease either get better or expire; either way they are unlikely to be infected with the disease at any particular point in time. Chronic diseases may have high prevalence even if incidence is low, as those with the disease never get rid of it and are added to the number of incident cases each year. The remainder of this chapter will focus specifically on several of the most common STIs, for which the epidemiology is best described in previous literature.

2.2 Epidemiological Trends of Common Sexually Transmitted Infections

2.2.1 *Trichomonas Vaginalis*

2.2.1.1 Burden of Disease

Trichomonas vaginalis, a pathogenic protozoan, is the most common nonviral cause of STI worldwide. It is frequently asymptomatic in men, or may cause a short-lived course of nongonococcal urethritis, but it is significant because the parasite is easily transmitted to women during the short period of infection. Women infected with *T. vaginalis* may also be asymptomatic (up to 30% of cases), but the majority experience vaginitis. Additionally, *T. vaginalis* infection may be responsible for significant reproductive health sequelae including pelvic inflammatory disease and adverse outcomes of pregnancy (such as preterm labor and low birth weight) [6, 7]. Perhaps most importantly, *T. vaginalis* infection has been implicated as one of the most important cofactors in amplifying HIV transmission, particularly in the African American population of the United States [8].

2.2.1.2 Incidence and Prevalence

The World Health Organization (WHO) estimates an incidence of 170–190 million new cases of *T. vaginalis* infection worldwide each year. However, these estimates may be low, since they are based on wet mounts that are not as sensitive as new polymerase chain reaction (PCR) technology [9]. Extensive data are available regarding the prevalence of *T. vaginalis* infection but can be difficult to interpret due to variation in diagnostic technique, study settings, populations studied, and whether symptoms were present or absent in participants. Overall, prevalence rates have ranged from 5% to 10% in women in the general population to as high as 50–60% in high-risk populations such as prison inmates and commercial sex workers [10]. Prevalence in males similarly has a high degree of variation depending on the population studied, ranging between 0% in low-risk asymptomatic men to 58% among adolescent males at high risk for sexually transmitted diseases (STDs).

An estimated 7.4 million new cases of *T. vaginalis* infection are reported in the United States each year. Prevalence ranges between 2.2% for young women (≤20 years) compared with 6.1% in women ≥25 years. Male prevalence was lower for both age categories, with a reported 0.8% among men≤ 20 and 2.8% in males ≥25 years [6]. In Northern Australia, a study of indigenous women found a similar increase in prevalence with age, although the overall prevalence (25%) was higher than that seen in US studies [6, 11].

Amongst pregnant women in Latin America and the Caribbean, trichomoniasis prevalence rates ranged from 2.1% in Brazil to 27.5% in Chile [12, 13]. In Africa, pregnant females had prevalence rates ranging from 9.9% in the Central African Republic to as high as 41.4% in South Africa [14, 15].

2.2.1.3 Risk Factors

Unlike chlamydia and gonorrhea, young age is not a risk factor for trichomoniasis. Prevalence of *T. vaginalis* infection appears to increase with age for both males and females, possibly due to its frequent asymptomatic nature of the infection and therefore persistence of untreated infections [6].

Studies in developed nations have found high prevalence of trichomoniasis in prison inmates, IV drug users, and sex workers [6]. A common trend in these three risk groups is that they are more likely to engage in high-risk sexual behavior than the general population. Unprotected sex with multiple partners increases the chance of *T. vaginalis* infection, as with any STD. In a study by Tyndall et al. of IV drug users with high HIV prevalence, 57% of female participants reported more than 100 lifetime partners. Condoms were generally not used with regular partners, used about half of the time with casual partners, and used about 80% of the time with paying partners [16].

There is no doubt that protected sex with a condom helps prevent *T. vaginalis* infection as well as other STIs (see Chap. 55). Sex workers in countries such as Australia, where there is a decriminalized regulated system, have a much lower incidence of trichomoniasis than do street sex workers [17, 18]. This is likely because street sex workers are less likely to use protection than those who work in a regulated brothel.

Other risk factors that have been described include subjects with poor personal hygiene and low socioeconomic status [10].

2.2.2 *Chlamydia*

2.2.2.1 Burden of Disease

Chlamydia trachomatis is responsible for more cases of STD than any other bacterial pathogen, and is therefore an enormous worldwide public health problem. Since asymptomatic infection is common, it can easily be passed unknowingly between sexual partners. In addition to sexual transmission, the organism can be transmitted by droplets, hands, contaminated clothing, flies, and by passage through an infected birth canal.

In females, chlamydia primarily presents as a cervical infection following exposure to an infected partner. Initial infection may either be asymptomatic or cause a self-limited acute inflammatory response. However, repeated or untreated infection may cause chronic inflammation, irreversible tissue damage, and scarring (i.e., pelvic inflammatory disease) that may lead to infertility or increased risk of ectopic pregnancy. There is a four- to sixfold increased risk of pelvic inflammatory disease and a two- to fourfold increased risk of ectopic pregnancy associated with recurrent infections [19].

In men, chlamydia is the commonest cause of nongonococcal urethritis. Almost 50% of men with chlamydia experience urethritis associated with pain and penile discharge, but those with asymptomatic infection may serve as carriers of the disease. Men rarely suffer long-term health problems as a result of chlamydia infection.

Contamination of the hands with genital discharge may lead to a conjunctival infection following contact with the eyes. Babies born to mothers with infection of their genital tract frequently present with chlamydial eye infection within a week of birth (chlamydia "ophthalmia neonatorum"), and may subsequently develop pneumonia.

Worldwide, the most important disease caused by *C. trachomatis* is trachoma that affects the inner upper eyelid and cornea and is one of the commonest infectious causes of blindness (an estimated seven to nine million people are blind as a result of trachoma). The disease is particularly prevalent and severe in rural populations living in poor and arid areas of the world where people have limited access to water and personal hygiene is difficult. In the United States, Native Americans are most commonly infected.

Another disease caused by *C. trachomatis* is lymphogranuloma venereum (LGV), a condition characterized by painful lymphadenopathy. LGV is caused by the L1, L2, and L3 serovars of *C. trachomatis* and begins as a painless ulcer that is usually self-limited. The secondary stage of LGV is the painful lymphadenopathy, most commonly of the inguinal or femoral lymph nodes; these nodes may coalesce to form buboes that can rupture in as many as one third of patients. The tertiary stage of LGV is caused by fibrosis that can result in lymphatic obstruction, edema, abscesses, and strictures.

2.2.2.2 Incidence and Prevalence

The WHO estimates that over 90 million new cases of chlamydia are diagnosed each year [20]. Various studies have estimated that there are four to five million new cases of chlamydial infection each year in the United States alone. Prevalence varies greatly depending on the type of population studied, as several factors (to be discussed in detail below) greatly increase the risk for chlamydia. For example, in the US adolescent female population, prevalence varies from 5% among suburban adolescent females to as high as 25–30% among urban adolescents, resulting in an overall prevalence of 12% in the adolescent population as a whole in the United States [20–22]. Worldwide prevalence rates are similar to that of the United States, ranging between 5% and 15% for most of Europe, Australia, Africa, and Japan [23–26]. In certain countries in which intensive chlamydia control programs have been instituted, significant reduction in prevalence has been observed. For example, the number of cases of chlamydia was reduced by over 50% over a 7-year period in Sweden with similar declines seen in the US Pacific Northwest and Wisconsin following the institution of control programs [27, 28].

2.2.2.3 Risk Factors

Young age is the strongest predictor of chlamydia. The highest rates have been consistently found among young sexually active women, particularly adolescents [29]. In a large surveillance study performed in Germany, the highest prevalence of chlamydia was found among 15–19-year-old females, with prevalence significantly decreased after 25 years of age [20].

Prevalence among females appears to be up to three or four times greater than that of males. This may be due to anatomical factors, as the cervix of adolescent females is not sufficiently developed and is therefore particularly susceptible to STIs [20, 30]. This would also partially explain the particularly high rate of chlamydia in adolescents. However, the reported gender disparity is likely at least partially due to the greater frequency that females access health care through routine Pap smear screening, family planning services, and other services related to reproductive health care.

In the United States, non-white race and Hispanic ethnicity have been associated with higher prevalence than in other groups. In the United States, the Center for Disease Control (CDC) data show that rates among African Americans are several-fold higher than other racial and ethnic groups [31]. Some of these data may be skewed due to confounding by socioeconomic status. As previously mentioned, urban adolescent females in the United States have a significantly higher prevalence of chlamydia infection when compared to their suburban counterparts. Worldwide, the greatest number of chlamydia infection cases was detected among individuals of the black Caribbean race [20].

As with most STIs, several sexual behavior risk factors exist. For chlamydia, these include frequency of intercourse, multiple partners, a new partner in the past 2 months, a partner with an STD diagnosis, young age at first intercourse, and failure to use barrier contraception [31–33]. Hormonal contraception use may be associated with a higher risk of chlamydia [34], perhaps due to a lesser likelihood of using barrier contraception in conjunction with hormonal contraception. The significantly greater prevalence of chlamydia among female prostitutes in Central Africa compared to that of male and female students in Africa (38.3% versus 3–7%, respectively) exemplifies the degree of risk that sexual behavior can have on the epidemiology of this disease [23, 25, 35]. Chlamydia and other inflammatory STDs are also associated with increased susceptibility to and transmission of HIV infection [36].

2.2.3 Gonorrhea

2.2.3.1 Burden of Disease

Neisseria gonorrhoeae is a gram-negative diplococcus responsible for infection through contact with the penis, vagina, mouth, or anus regardless of ejaculation. Although gonorrhea can also spread from mother to baby during delivery it is commonly transmitted through sexual contact. The bacterium develops and multiplies in the cervix, uterus, and fallopian tubes of women, within the urethra of both males and females, and secondarily in the mouth, throat, eyes, and anus.

In females, gonorrhea is frequently asymptomatic, often misdiagnosed as bladder or vaginal infections [37]. Alternatively, infection may result in painful or burning urination, increased vaginal discharge, or vaginal bleeding. Further complications include pelvic inflammatory disease and increased risks of infertility, ectopic pregnancy, postpartum endometriosis, cystitis, and mucopurulent cervicitis.

Males experience epididymitis, urethritis, and white, yellow, or green penile discharge. Symptoms typically appear 2–5 days after infection, but the infection may lie dormant for up to 30 days. Similar to chlamydia, the effects of gonorrheal infection in males are commonly short term; however, infection is 1.5 times greater than in females [38].

Gonorrhea is more likely to transmit from asymptomatic carriers than people with evident infection. Approximately 1% of gonococcal occurrences begin as anorectal and pharyngeal infections in women who have sex with men as well as men who have sex with men (MSM). Disseminated gonococcal infections (DGIs) develop into a skin rash and asymmetrical septic polyarthritis.

Pregnant females with active infection may transmit the disease to the baby during delivery as it passes through the birth canal. This transmission may cause potentially fatal blood, joint, or conjunctival infections (gonococcal ophthalmia neonatorum), which result in rapid blindness [39]. Pneumonia may also occur and symptoms appear 5–12 days after birth. The transmission of HIV also increases in people with gonorrhea infection.

2.2.3.2 Incidence and Prevalence

Over 62 million people are infected worldwide annually with 700,000 incidences in the United States [40]. Gonorrhea is prevalent in both developed and developing nations and is frequently concomitant with chlamydia infection. In 1999 the greatest incidence of infection occurred in South Asia followed by sub-Saharan Africa and Latin America and the Caribbean. Per 1,000 people the rate of new infection was highest in sub-Saharan Africa, where pregnant women were infected with gonorrhea at rates ranging from 0.02% in Gabon to 3.1% in the Central African Republic and 7.8% in South Africa [41].

Throughout the 1990s the highest prevalence rates (3% or greater) in the Western Pacific were in Cambodia and Papua New Guinea [42]. Vietnam, China, and the Philippines reported rates of 1% or less [43]. A significant increase in gonorrhea incidence occurred in eastern Europe between 1995 and 1999 with highest rates in Estonia, Russia, and Belarus [44]. Western Europe reported a significant decline from 1980 to 1991 with the rate below 20 infections/100,000 people. Between 1981 and 1995 Canada experienced a tenfold reduction from 226 infections/100,000 persons to 19 infections/100,000 [45].

The US CDC estimates that only 50% of gonorrheal infections are actually reported since the disease often illustrates few or no symptoms. The CDC reported 358,366 cases of gonorrhea in the United States in 2006 with the rate of infection at 120.9/100,000 persons. Significant control programs throughout the 1970s resulted in a national decline from 1975 to 1997; however, 2006 marked the second consecutive year of increased incidence [37, 46].

In the United States infections are highest in young adults and African Americans; however, the rate of cases per 100,000 population declined by 7.7% in African Americans between 2002 and 2006 (from 713.7 to 658.4, respectively) [47]. Between 2005 and 2006 all racial and ethnic groups except Asian/Pacific Islanders saw slight increases in gonorrhea infections. American Indian/Alaska Natives experienced the greatest increase of 22.9%, followed by 17.7% among Caucasians, and 11.8% among Hispanics. A decrease of 1.4% was observed among Asian/Pacific Islanders [48, 49].

2.2.3.3 Risk Factors

Those with the highest rate of gonococcal infection tend to be of young age (<24), live in high-density urban communities, have multiple sex partners, and engage in unprotected sexual intercourse. Women contract gonorrhea 50% of the time they engage in sexual relations with an infected male although men only contract infections 20% of the time they have sexual relations with infected females [49].

In 2006, approximately 69% of total reported cases of gonorrhea in the United States occurred among African Americans with a rate 18 times greater than that among Caucasians. African American men and women aged 15–19 had increased incidences for the second consecutive year from 2005 to 2006. African American males were infected 25 times more than Caucasian males while African American females were infected 14 times more frequently than Caucasian females. Among all racial, ethnic, and age categories, African Americans aged 15–19 and 20–24 years experienced the highest rates of gonorrhea in 2006. The infection rate per 100,000 African Americans was 658.4, compared to 36.5, 77.4, and 138.3 for Caucasians, Hispanics, and American Indian/Alaska Natives, respectively [37, 39, 50]. These racial disparities are likely confounded by socioeconomic and cultural factors.

Social behavior significantly affects gonorrhea rates as multiple sexual partners and unprotected sexual activity contribute to higher rates of infection. Latex condoms and other barrier methods reduce the risk of spreading the infection through vaginal intercourse or mouth-to-penis, oral–anal, and mouth-to-vulva contact. Ocular infection of gonorrhea occurs if discharge containing the disease meets the eye during sex or with direct hand-to-eye contact. Persons previously treated with gonorrhea can be reinfected if exposed again and sexual partners can continue to pass the disease back and forth if neither seeks adequate treatment. Although gonorrhea is commonly treated with fluoroquinolone antibiotics throughout the world, the CDC reports an increase of resistant *N. gonorrhoeae* and therefore recommends only administering cephalosporin antibiotics in the United States [51].

2.2.4 Syphilis

2.2.4.1 Burden of Disease

Syphilis is an STI caused by the spirochete *Treponema pallidum*. The infection has been frequently referred to as the "great imitator" due to the great variety of clinical presentations that arise in infected patients that may mimic or resemble a variety of other infectious and autoimmune etiologies. The infection is transmitted by sexual contact or through vertical transmission from an infected mother to her baby.

Syphilis passes through a series of frequently overlapping stages – primary, secondary, latency, and tertiary. Primary syphilis is characterized by a single, painless chancre that begins about 21 days after exposure as a macule that becomes a papule, which then ulcerates. The chancre frequently is overlooked by infected patients because it is temporary and painless. Secondary syphilis presents with an array of dermatological lesions and eruptions that can occur 4–10 weeks after exposure. Other symptoms include fever, meningismus, myalgias, weight loss, anorexia, hair loss, arthralgias, mucous patches, and condylomata lata. It is the secondary stage that gives syphilis the nickname the "great imitator" because of its wide array of presentations. In the latent stage of syphilis the *Treponema* spirochete is seemingly clinically silent and is detected only by serological testing. The tertiary stage involves other organ systems and may lead to devastating cardiovascular and neurological complications [52].

If left untreated during pregnancy, syphilis may contribute to stillbirth, preterm labor, and intrauterine growth restriction. Congenital syphilis, while rare in developed countries, may cause hepatosplenomegaly and failure to thrive in the newborn. A child infected with congenital syphilis may manifest a range of neurological disorders later in life [53].

Fortunately *T. pallidum* is sensitive to penicillin and its devastating consequences are largely avoidable if the diagnosis is made promptly. Despite the availability of effective treatment and the potential for prevention, syphilis remains a major scourge of the modern world.

2.2.4.2 Incidence and Prevalence

The WHO estimated that in 1999 there were approximately 12 million new cases of syphilis [2]. Of these new cases of syphilis, over two-thirds occurred in sub-Saharan Africa and Southeast Asia. Recent outbreaks have been described in several countries across the world. For example, in the United States rates of syphilis have increased from 2.9/100,000 in 2005 to 3.3/100,000 in 2006.

WHO estimates of syphilis incidence in 1999 (in millions)

Region	Males	Females	New cases in 1999
Australia/ New Zealand	0.004	0.004	0.008
North America	0.054	0.053	0.107
Eastern Europe and Central Asia	0.053	0.052	0.105
Western Europe	0.069	0.066	0.136
North Africa and Middle East	0.167	0.197	0.364
Latin America and Caribbean	1.294	1.634	2.928
Sub-Saharan Africa	1.683	2.144	3.828
Southeast Asia	1.851	2.187	4.038
Total	5.29	6.47	11.76

There was a steady decline in the incidence of syphilis in both Europe and the United States during the second half of the last century, leading to suggestions that endemic syphilis might even be eradicated in these countries. The past few years, however, have seen an upsurge in syphilis in Europe and North America. The reasons underlying this reversal are complex but include migration of people from high-prevalence countries, population mixing, and changes in risk behavior including the use of the Internet to meet partners, use of recreational drugs, and a reduction in safe sex practices in gay men [54].

The prevalence of syphilis varies widely depending on the type of population being studied and associated risk factors. The National Health and Nutrition Examination Surveys showed that the prevalence of syphilis seroreactivity was low (0.71%) in the general US population of 18–49-year-olds while epidemiological studies in parts of Africa reveal prevalence rates in pregnant women of 4–15% [53, 55].

2.2.4.3 Risk Factors

In the United States the most frequent age group to be infected with syphilis is the 25–29 range. Men (5.7/100,000) are infected more frequently than women (1.0/100,000) in the United States and this has been linked to the rising prevalence of MSM-associated syphilis. In fact, the CDC estimates that 64% of new cases in the United States are linked to MSM. Epidemiological studies in other countries, however, have shown women to be at greater risk of becoming infected [54].

Syphilis in pregnant women can have devastating consequences. In Africa, the prevalence rate in pregnant women has been estimated to be as high as 15%. In pregnancy, untreated early syphilis will result in a stillbirth rate of 25% and will be responsible for 14% of neonatal deaths. This results in a perinatal mortality rate of about 40%.

2.2.5 *Chancroid*

2.2.5.1 Burden of Disease

Chancroid is the soft chancre caused by *Haemophilus ducreyi* and is endemic in many developing and resource-poor countries. It presents as an acute ulcerative disease, usually of the genitals, and is often associated with inguinal adenitis or buboes [56]. It is differentiated from syphilis by the soft, irregular borders of the ulcerations that are painful [57]. Most infections are clinically apparent (few asymptomatic carriers). Chancroid is easily spread; it is estimated that the probability of transmitting chancroid from an infected to an uninfected person during a single sexual exposure is between 35% and 70% [56, 58]. From a public health perspective, the most important consequence of *H. ducreyi* is not the ulcerative disease itself, but the strong association between chancroid and HIV infection.

2.2.5.2 Prevalence and Incidence

Worldwide estimates range between six and seven million new cases of chancroid each year [57, 58]. However, due to the lack of availability of diagnostic tests, these numbers are often based on the prevalence of syphilis and are therefore not entirely accurate. When determined by multiplex PCR (the most accurate diagnostic test, although not commercially available), the prevalence of chancroid in cases of genital ulcerative disease ranged between 23% and 56% in endemic areas of Asia, Africa, and the Caribbean. This compares to 0.9% of the ulcers from an STD clinic in the Netherlands and similarly low prevalence in other European countries [58]. In a test of genital ulcer etiology in ten US cities, chancroid was found to be the cause of 12% of ulcers in Chicago and 20% in Memphis, whereas no cases were found in any of the other eight cities [59].

2.2.5.3 Risk Factors

The major risk factors for chancroid transmission are unprotected sex, lack of male circumcision, and poor hygiene. While use of antibiotics has certainly been a boon to the decline of chancroid in developed nations, it is not solely responsible for the 80-fold decrease seen in the US population between 1947 and 1997 [57]. Social factors including shifting patterns of prostitution, more frequent condom use, and better hygiene have decreased the potential reservoir of *H. ducreyi* and thus prevented its spread.

There is no nonhuman reservoir for *H. ducreyi* and therefore the organism is not sustainable outside the most active human sexual networks [57]. This is due to the relatively short duration of infectivity (about 5 weeks on average), which requires frequent contacts to spread within a population. It is estimated that the sexual partner change rate required to maintain *H. ducreyi* in a population is 15–20/ year when using an average duration of infection of 5 weeks and a transmission rate of 70% [57, 58]. Therefore, sex trade workers are often responsible for the continued presence of chancroid in the population. This is exemplified by the decreased prevalence of chancroid in Thailand. Through the 100% condom campaign, a multifactorial intervention that included promotion of condom use for commercial sex acts (as well as treatment services and other modalities), the annual prevalence of chancroid fell from over 30,000 cases to fewer than 2,000 cases [58, 60].

Circumcision has been found to decrease the spread of multiple STDs, including chancroid, syphilis, and HIV. A recent systematic review found circumcision to be protective against chancroid in six out of seven studies [61]. There is a plausible reason for the protective effect of circumcision from a biological standpoint. Pathogens can replicate within the warm, moist area under the foreskin, allowing for an increased load of the pathogenic organism. Additionally, uncircumcised men may be at increased risk as the result of entry of pathogens through the inner surface of the foreskin and frenulum, or through micro-abrasions occurring during intercourse [61].

Lack of hygiene is another potential risk factor in the spread of chancroid. During World War I, simple washing with soap and water within a few hours of sexual exposure was effective in reducing risk of chancroid [57, 62]. Troops exposed to prostitutes were encouraged to attend post-coital centers where local prophylaxis was applied, including soap and water (which is effective even in the presence of skin abrasions). Omission of soap and water was identified as the cause of failed prophylaxis for chancroid amongst the American Expeditionary Forces in Paris during the World War I [62]. The ideal hygienic regimen involves both pre-exposure application of soap and water (including beneath the foreskin in uncircumcised males) as well as post-exposure washing.

2.2.6 Donovanosis (Granuloma Inguinale)

2.2.6.1 Burden of Disease

Donovanosis (Granuloma inguinale, GI) is caused by the gram-negative bacillus *Klebsiella granulomatis*. The primary mode of transmission is through sexual contact, although a fecal route and vertical transmission by passing through an infected birth canal have also been described. The disease is characterized by chronic genital ulceration that usually affects the genital region (90% of cases) or inguinal region (10%). There are four classic presentations of donovanosis: (a) ulcerogranulomatous (the most common type) resulting in beefy red, non-tender ulcers that bleed readily to the touch; (b) hypertrophic or verrucous ulcers that may resemble warts; (c) necrotic deep ulcers that cause tissue destruction; and (d) cicatricial lesions that are dry and sclerotic [63].

2.2.6.2 Incidence and Prevalence

Prior to the antibiotic era, donovanosis was prevalent worldwide, but nowadays significant numbers are found in only a few developing countries, with the main foci being Papua New Guinea, KwaZulu-Natal, Transvaal, Zimbabwe, parts of India and Brazil, and among the Aboriginal population of Australia [63–65].

Papua New Guinea was previously among the worst-affected regions; in 1980 donovanosis accounted for 46% of genital ulcers in women and was the second most common cause of genital ulcer disease after herpes in 1989–1990 [63, 64]. However, a 2000 WHO report found that donovanosis has become rare in Papua New Guinea, with only infrequent cases reported [66].

In Durban (KwaZulu-Natal), case reports of donovanosis increased from 212 in 1988 to 3,153 in 1997, accounting for 11–16% of cases of genital ulcers [63, 64]. A similar percentage (14%) of genital ulcer cases due to donovanosis has been seen in South India. However, in Brazil (0.3%) and Jamaica (4.1%), donovanosis is responsible for a much small percentage of cases seen at STI clinics [63].

2.2.6.3 Risk Factors

Like many STIs, the most frequent age range of patients who acquire donovanosis is 20–40 years, most likely due to sexual practices. Unprotected sex and multiple sexual partners are both risk factors for donovanosis. There appears to be a racial predilection in several countries, but this is thought to be due mostly to socioeconomic status rather than a true racial susceptibility. For example, the incidence is higher in blacks than in whites in the United States, higher in natives than in Europeans in New Guinea, and higher in the Aboriginal population than in whites in Australia.

2.2.7 Herpes Simplex

2.2.7.1 Burden of Disease

Genital herpes is one of the most common ulcerating diseases of the genital mucosa. It results from infection with herpes simplex virus (HSV), more commonly HSV-2 but also HSV-1. The virus is transmitted through skin-to-skin contact, especially through sexual contact with new partners. The initial presentation is accompanied by genital ulcers, tender local inguinal lymphadenopathy, dysuria, fever, and malaise. Alternatively, the infection may be mild or asymptomatic. Patients with genital HSV infection can suffer considerable morbidity with frequent painful recurrences that may be associated with significant psychosocial distress [67].

Ulcerating genital diseases such as those resulting from HSV-2 infection have also been linked to a higher risk of HIV infection due to mucosal breakdown [68]. Vertical transmission from an infected mother to her baby at delivery can result in meningitis, disseminated infection, or death of the infant. Studies consistently show that less than a quarter of infected people know that they have genital herpes. Therefore, most people are infected when they have sexual contact with asymptomatic, unsuspecting carriers who are shedding the virus [69].

2.2.2.2 Incidence and Prevalence

The prevalence of HSV-2 seropositivity varies widely with generally higher rates in developing countries. The National Health and Nutrition Examination Survey (NHANES) III, which was conducted between 1988 and 1994, collected serological data on over 40,000 individuals in the United States. HSV-2 antibody was assessed with an immunodot assay specific for glycoprotein gG-2 of HSV-2 [70]. This survey showed a 30% increase in prevalence over the previous survey, the NHANES II, which spanned 1976–1980. The overall prevalence of HSV-2 among study participants was 21.9%, which corresponds to over 45 million people in the general US population.

Prevalence in other countries can vary from 2% to 74% according to the country, age, gender, and urban versus rural areas. In sub-Saharan Africa, for example, 30–80% of women and 10–50% of men were found to be seropositive for HSV-2. Central and South America had rates from 20% to 40%. Developed countries typically had lower rates of HSV-2 seropositivity. France, for example, had a rate of 17.2% while the United Kingdom had even lower rates of around 3.3% in males and 5.1% in females [71]. The yearly incidence in the United States has been estimated to be 4.6/1,000 to 8.4/1,000 [72].

2.2.7.3 Risk Factors

In the United States, overall prevalence is higher in women (25.6%) compared with men (17.8%) and in blacks (45.9%) compared to non-Hispanic whites (17.6%). Seroprevalence increases rapidly in younger age groups and then stabilizes around age 30. Additional contributing variables include increased number of lifetime partners, early age of sexual debut, poverty, cocaine abuse, and less education. Other populations with a higher prevalence include those attending an STD clinic, those testing positive for HIV, and sex workers [73].

2.2.8 Human Papillomavirus

2.2.8.1 Burden of Disease

At present, human papillomavirus (HPV) infections are the most commonly diagnosed STD worldwide.

HPVs are species-specific and are only known to infect humans. The viruses are spread by person-to-person direct contact and infect epithelial tissues of skin and mucous membranes. Viral transmission may occur even in the absence of visible lesions and many patients may be unaware that they are infected.

Manifestations of infection occur as cutaneous disease such as common, plantar, and flat warts. Sexual contact may result in condylomata acuminata, or genital warts, which are painless, fleshy lesions that have a predilection for warm, moist surfaces. Other presentations of the viral infection may also occur such as respiratory papillomatosis and focal epithelial hyperplasia of the oral cavity. The infection may be obvious clinically or completely asymptomatic [74].

HPV is recognized as a causal agent in the pathogenesis of cervical cancer, the second most common malignancy in women and representing 9.8% of all female cancers [75]. It has also proven to be the cause of other anogenital cancers. Colonization with certain subtypes of HPV is associated with high-grade squamous intraepithelial lesions (HSIL). These lesions are associated with an increased risk of invasive cervical cancer.

It is estimated that around 290 million women are infected with HPV [74, 76]. Guidelines recommend commencement of screening at 21 years of age or within 3 years of onset of sexual activity, whichever comes first. Despite no currently available cure for HPV infection, colonization may be reversed by normal immune processes.

2.2.8.2 Incidence and Prevalence

Multiple world surveys and population studies reveal a greater than tenfold variation in the worldwide prevalence of HPV. A meta-analysis conducted by de Sanjosé et al. estimated a worldwide HPV prevalence in women with normal cervical cytology to be approximately 10%. Africa had the highest estimated prevalence (31.6%) while Southeast Asia (6.2%) and southern Europe (6.8%) had the lowest estimated HPV prevalence [76].

HPV prevalence adapted by Sanjosé et al. meta-analysis

Location	HPV prevalence
Global	10.4%
Africa	*22.1%*
Eastern	31.6 %
Northern	21.5%
Southern	15.5%
Western	17%
Americas	*13%*
Central	20.4%
South	12.3%
North	11.3%
Europe	*8.1%*
Eastern	29.1%
Northern	7.9%
Southern	6.8%
Western	8.4%
Asia	*8%*
Eastern	13.6%
Japan/Taiwan	7.0%
Southeast	6.2%
South-central	7.5%

2.2.8.3 Risk Factors

There is a clear age-specific pattern of HPV prevalence for all the major world regions. Prevalence is highest in women younger than 34 and then decreases in the 35–44 age group. An increase in prevalence also occurs in older women, aged 45–54 [76]. This rise in prevalence occurring in the post-menopausal age group has an unclear etiology. It is postulated that changes in hormonal and immunological status facilitate the detection of previously unidentified latent infections. However, studies have indicated that an additional number of sexual partners in middle age or changes in sexual habits may also play a role in the upward trend of HPV prevalence in this age group [77].

A survey conducted in the United States, the NHANES, found a 26.8% overall prevalence of HPV infection in self-collected vaginal samples from women 14–59 years old [78]. Race and socioeconomic status seem to be risk factors for HPV acquisition. One US study found that 39% of black women, compared with 24% of Mexican American and 24% of white women, were positive for any HPV. In that same study, women who were identified to be living in poverty were twice as likely to be infected with HPV as women of higher socioeconomic status. Marriage appears to be a protective factor. Women who were married had noticeably lower rates of HPV infection than unmarried women. Higher rates were identified in women who were widows, divorcees, separated, or living with a partner [79].

The prevalence of HPV infections is believed to be lower in men than in women, but one study of 18–70-year-old men attending an STD clinic found a 28.2% prevalence of HPV infection [80]. Circumcision may be an independent protective factor in men. One study revealed a prevalence of penile HPV colonization of 20% in uncircumcised men while the prevalence in circumcised men was 5.5% [81].

The distribution of various HPV types has also been studied. Certain subtypes of HPV are known to be of higher risk for inducing malignant transformation such as types 16 and 18. HPV subtype 16 is the most frequently isolated type in the world. It is present in 12.3%, 18.4%, 21.4%, and 25.5% of HPV-positive women from Africa, Asia, South America, and Europe, respectively [82].

2.2.9 HIV/AIDS

2.2.9.1 Burden of Disease

HIV is a Group VI retrovirus with four stages that evolves into acquired immunodeficiency syndrome (AIDS). HIV begins as a primary infection, becomes clinically asymptomatic, and then symptomatic before advancing to AIDS. HIV attacks the immune system by destroying critical CD4 cells and AIDS significantly increases the risk of life-threatening opportunistic infections [42, 83]. HIV infection is a pandemic in humans that has claimed more than 25 million people worldwide since first recognized in December 1981 according to the WHO and the Joint United Nations Program on HIV/AIDS (UNAIDS) [44, 84]. AIDS is a collection of symptoms and infections that progressively destroy the immune system and create susceptibility for opportunistic infections and malignancies. HIV evolves to AIDS after 10–15 years of infection in 90% of cases [85].

HIV/AIDS affects both genders and all racial/ethnic groups similarly in terms of virology but infects genders, races/ethnicities, and inhabitants of industrialized versus developing nations at disproportionate rates. HIV destroys T cells, macrophages, and dendritic cells by viral killing of infected cells, increasing rates of apoptosis in infected cells or through CD8 cytotoxic lymphocytes, all of which eventually result in loss of cell-mediated immunity [47].

HIV is transmitted through sexual contact with an infected person, sharing needles/syringes with an infected person, or through HIV-infected blood given through transfusions, though this medium is less common as donated blood is frequently screened for HIV antibodies. Babies born to HIV-infected women may acquire the disease before or during birth or through breastfeeding [86]. In significantly fewer instances healthcare workers acquire HIV from needle sticks containing HIV-infected blood.

The opportunistic infections in HIV/AIDS-infected people include bacterial, protozoal, fungal, and viral diseases in addition to HIV-associated malignancies as defined in the various stages by the WHO. Persistent generalized lymphadenopathy occurs in Stage I, and weight loss, respiratory tract infections (sinusitis, tonsillitis, otitis media, pharyngitis), herpes zoster, oral ulcerations, and pruritic eruptions are evident in Stage II. Severe weight loss (over 10% of body weight), chronic diarrhea, persistent fever, oral candidiasis, tuberculosis, and oral hairy leukoplakia occur in Stage III along with more severe conditions. Pneumonia, empyema, meningitis, acute necrotizing stomatitis, and bacteremia are also characteristic in this stage. The progression from HIV to AIDS is associated with chronic herpes simplex infection, Kaposi sarcoma, central nervous system toxoplasmosis, disseminated mycosis, recurrent septicemia, and nephropathy [83]. In women, HIV/AIDS produces recurrent vaginal yeast infections, severe pelvic inflammatory disease, and cervical cancer [83, 87]. The fungal infection *Pneumocystis jiroveci* that causes pneumonia is the most prevalent opportunistic infection in persons with AIDS and the leading cause of death [87].

2.2.9.2 Incidence and Prevalence

As of November 2007, 33.2 million people worldwide were infected with HIV/AIDS and the virus claimed approximately 2.4–3.3 million lives in 2005 alone. HIV/AIDS infections have increased from 8 million in 1991 to the current total [2]. Sub-Saharan Africa experiences one third of all HIV/AIDS-related deaths with 21.6–27.4 million persons infected. The WHO noted that 2.9 million people became HIV/AIDS-infected in 2007 of which 2.5 million were adults and 0.42 million children. Over 2.1 million people succumbed to AIDS including 1.7 million adults and 0.33 million children [15, 87, 88]. Women account for 50% of all HIV infections and persons under 25 years total half of all new HIV infections [14].

Statistics vary based on region, gender, age, race/ethnicity, and social behaviors (including sexual preferences). South/Southeast Asia is second to sub-Saharan Africa with four million HIV/AIDS-infected people and 270,000 deaths in 2007. Latin America and eastern Europe/Central Asia both host 1.6 million infected with 58,000 and 55,000 deaths, respectively. Western and Central Europe and East Asia both have between 750,000 and 800,000 persons infected although East Asia's deaths were significantly greater at 32,000 compared to 12,000 in European nations [42, 89]. Over 1.3 million HIV/AIDS-infected people lived in North America as of 2007 with a reported 21,000 deaths [90]. HIV/AIDS is the leading cause of death in African American women aged 25–34 years [91].

2.2.9.3 Risk Factors

Age is a significant factor in HIV/AIDS incidences worldwide with persons aged 25–34 comprising the largest proportion of newly diagnosed cases in the United States [92]. Persons aged 50 or older total 15% of new diagnoses but comprise 35% of all AIDS-related deaths [93]. Young adults transmit the virus at greater rates than average due to sexual risk behavior and insufficient testing or diagnosis. Prevalence in the United States is greatest among MSM followed by 80% of people engaging in high-risk heterosexual contact [94]. Almost 75% of HIV/AIDS diagnoses in 2006 were of adolescent and adult males; however, 9,708 women were infected in the United States [21].

African Americans are disproportionally infected, accounting for 55% of all HIV infections among persons aged 13–24 [95]. The infection rate for black women (45.5/100,000) is 23 times greater than of white women (2/100,000) and 4 times greater than Hispanic women (11.2/100,000) [39]. Factors attributed to higher rates suggest that overall greater amount of poverty, STDs, and social stigma create more illnesses (49% of all HIV/AIDS cases in the United States) and shorter survival rates among African Americans [96].

Hispanics and Latinos comprised 18% of new HIV/AIDS diagnoses in 2006 and 17% of total people living with HIV/AIDS infection [97]. Lack of access to adequate health care and antiviral therapies contributes to their increase in transmission and conversion. Sexual contact between males, injection drug use, and high-risk heterosexual contact are the three most common methods of transmission for Hispanic and Latino males.

MSM, regardless of their sexual identity, have comprised 500,000 AIDS infections with over 300,000 deaths since the beginning of the epidemic [98]. Two-thirds of all men living with HIV contracted the infection from sex with men although only 5–7% report sexual relations with other males [99]. Research is unclear as to whether statistics are higher in this population due to increased testing or an actual increase in HIV infections since 53% of new HIV/AIDS cases are MSM-related.

Pregnant women with HIV/AIDS infection risk transmission to their child during pregnancy, birth, or afterwards through breastfeeding. An estimated 142 children under 13 years of age were diagnosed with HIV/AIDS from perinatal infections in 2006 [100]. Over 6,051 perinatally infected people were living with HIV/AIDS at the end of 2005 [86]. Early detection and treatment are critical and highly effective in preventing transmission of HIV/AIDS from infected mothers to their children [101].

Social behavior factors are the single greatest indicator of variations in HIV/AIDS infections. MSM, high-risk heterosexual intercourse, injection drug usage, and sexual intercourse with multiple partners without protection are all significant risk factors for transmission. The use of latex condoms, mutual monogamy with an uninfected partner, clean needle/syringe usage without sharing, and frequent testing can minimize transmission rates [102].

2.2.10 Hepatitis B

2.2.10.1 Burden of Disease

Hepatitis B virus (HBV) is one of the most serious and common causes of viral hepatitis. HBV infections can lead to the development of acute fulminate hepatitis, chronic hepatic insufficiency, cirrhosis, hepatocellular carcinoma, and death due to liver failure. It is estimated that chronic HBV infection is associated with 60–80% of the world's hepatocellular carcinomas, the fifth most common cancer that is responsible for 300–500,000 deaths/year [103, 104].

The WHO estimates that approximately 2 billion people have been infected with HBV worldwide and more than 350 million are chronic HBV carriers. It is the tenth leading cause of death worldwide and results in 500,000–700,000 deaths annually [105, 106]. The virus is very resilient, resists breakdown outside of the human body, and is transmitted through infected body fluids such as blood, saliva, and semen. HBV may be transmitted through sexual contact, contact with bodily fluids such as through contaminated injections and transfusions, or through perinatal transmission [107].

2.2.10.2 Incidence and Prevalence

The prevalence of HBV infection varies widely in different areas of the world. The highest prevalence of HBV infection is found in areas of sub-Saharan Africa, Southeast Asia, eastern Mediterranean countries, the interior of the Amazon basin, and certain parts of the Caribbean. In these areas it is estimated that greater than 8% of the population is seropositive for HBsAg and up to 20% of the population may be chronically infected. A moderate prevalence of 2–8% is found in many areas of Asia, eastern and southern Europe, Russia, and Central and South America. A lower prevalence of less than 2% HBsAg seropositivity is found in developed areas of North America, western Europe, Australia, and New Zealand [106, 108].

Incidence rates vary widely but frequently are correlated with the local prevalence rates. The CDC reports that there were an estimated 46,000 new infections in the United States in 2006 [109]. HBV vaccination of children has reduced incidence to a large extent among younger age groups. However, higher incidence rates continue among adults, particularly males aged 25–44 years, reflecting the need to vaccinate adults at risk for HBV infection [110].

2.2.10.3 Risk Factors

In areas with high prevalence rates, the majority of infections occur from mother to child vertical transmission and horizontal transmission such as from child-to-child contact in household settings. Since the introduction of childhood HBV vaccination programs in most developed countries, areas with lower prevalence rates have exhibited more cases due to sexual contact and contaminated needles rather than prenatal or childhood transmission [105, 107]. The pattern of transmission is directly correlated with geographical prevalence because prenatal or early childhood acquired HBV infection has a greater risk of chronicity than infection acquired later in life due to drug abuse or sexual contact. The most common risk factors are sexual exposure (sexual contact with a person known to have hepatitis B, multiple sex partners, and MSM) and injection drug use.

2.2.11 Molluscum Contagiosum

2.2.11.1 Burden of Disease

Molluscum contagiosum is caused by the poxvirus Molluscipox (MCV) which was previously a disease primarily in children but has now evolved into an STI in adults. MCV has four types (MCV-1 to MCV-4) with MCV-1 the most prevalent and MCV-2 sexually transmitted in adults [111, 112]. The infection affects the skin and mucous membranes, producing a benign self-limited papular eruption of multiple umbilicated cutaneous tumors present on the thighs, buttocks, groin, lower abdomen, and occasionally external genital or anal region. It is transmitted by skin-to-skin contact of lesions in addition to sexual contact, although MCV may also pass through water (swimming pools and baths) occupied by infected persons or touching towels/clothing in contact with lesions [112]. Persons already infected risk autoinoculation if they touch lesions and then touch unaffected body parts. The incubation period averages 2–3 months and may last 1 week to 6 months. Untreated lesions generally remain between 2 weeks to 4 years although the average is 2 years [113, 114].

2.2.11.2 Incidence and Prevalence

Molluscum infections are not limited to any geographical region but are more common in warm, humid climates with high-density populations. Since 1966 there is a reported increase of cases in the United States; however, incidences are not routinely monitored since infections typically resolve without treatment [115].

AIDS-infected or other immune-compromised people are subject to frequent, extensive outbreaks. Approximately 10–20% of symptomatic HIV/AIDS-infected people experience progressive molluscum symptoms although the exact incidence remains unknown. The range is higher (25–35%) in HIV-infected persons with a CD4 count less than 200 cells/mm^3 [116, 117].

2.2.11.3 Risk Factors

Age is a significant factor for MCV infection as transmission between children is common due to frequent contact in communal areas (school, daycare centers, parks, pools, etc.) and lack of proper hygiene. Any person is susceptible to molluscum contagiosum regardless of sexual activity [118]. The CDC recommends that infected persons refrain from contact sports, swimming, shaving areas with active lesions, sharing personal items including hair brushes and soap, and abstain from sexual contact [119, 120].

The highest incidence of molluscum contagiosum infection is in HIV-infected patients and characterized by larger size, greater number, more rapid growth, and atypical locations. The lesions are uncharacteristic from the usual dome-shaped molluscum evident in healthy children. Central umbilication is unapparent as patients with advanced HIV disease experience giant, tumor-like, nodular lesions exceeding 1 cm in diameter, often causing significant deformation and even necrosis [121, 122]. Disseminated molluscum develops as several hundred lesions in a pattern resembling disseminated cryptococcal disease [123]. The unusual manifestation of molluscum in persons with immune suppression is only cosmetic and proves no systemic effect.

People engaging in sexual activity risk infection with skin-to-skin contact; therefore latex condoms and other moisture barriers used for vaginal, oral, and anal sex greatly reduce transmission. MCV does not require mucous membrane contact in order for the virus to spread and moisture barriers do not protect contact from all potentially infected areas including the scrotum [124]. Abstinence from sexual activity and mutual monogamy with one uninfected partner are significant preventable measures. Typically as with other skin-to-skin STIs (scabies and pubic lice) molluscum contagiosum incidences are greater in people who engage in unprotected sex with one or multiple partners [125].

2.2.12 Scabies/Pubic Lice

2.2.12.1 Burden of Disease

Scabies, the microscopic mite *Sarcoptes scabiei*, is prevalent worldwide affecting all ages and racial/ethnic groups. Common areas of infection are webs of fingers/toes, pubic/groin area, axillae, umbilicus, breasts, palms of hands, and soles of feet [126]. Fewer than ten mites typically infest unless a person has crusted (Norwegian) scabies, which is highly infectious and generates thousands of mites; however, these incidences are reported in the elderly, HIV-infected, and other immune-compromised people [127, 128]. Female parasites burrow under the skin, lay eggs within a few hours following infestation, and continue to lay two to three eggs daily. Scabies eggs hatch and become adults after 10 days, when the cycle restarts; however, symptoms do not appear until 4–6 weeks following new infection. Persons previously exposed experience symptoms 1–4 days after infection and both new and recurrent infections are active until successfully treated. Mites only survive between 48 and 72 h unattached from humans, but adult females live up to 1 month [128]. Sexual transmission is through close physical contact and more likely when partners share a bed or spend the night together rather than through sexual activity [129]. Crowded conditions are ideal for rapid infection including hospitals, institutions, childcare facilities, and nursing homes where skin-to-skin contact is frequent. Scabies spreads within households due to prolonged contact with infested objects including linens, furniture, and clothing [130].

Pubic lice, also known as crabs, is the parasite *Phthirus pubis*, which infests the human genital area and undergoes a life cycle in three stages [131]. They are spread through sexual contact although they can rarely infest through linens or clothing, similar to scabies. Pubic lice attach to pubic hair but can transmit to other coarse body hair on legs, axillae, mustache, beard, eyelashes, or eyebrows [132]. Lice eggs or nits are not visible to the naked eye, but are whitish in color and attach firmly to the hair shaft, taking 6–10 days to hatch and laying 30–90 eggs during their lifetime. Nymphs are baby lice that survive off blood and reproduce approximately 2–3 weeks after hatching. Adult lice resemble ocean crabs with six legs and are tan to grayish white in color. Female lice are larger than males but all fully grown lice are as large as 4.5 mm long; however, 1.25–2 mm is common. Lice only survive 1–2 days upon detaching from humans or losing access to a blood supply [131]. Although body lice may transmit typhus, relapsing, or trench fevers, which have high mortality rates especially in colder climates or in overcrowding, pubic lice infection results only in severe itching. Upon injecting saliva into the host during feeding, pubic lice may also cause pruritus resulting in severe scratching [133].

2.2.12.2 Incidence and Prevalence

Once considered a "disease of the poor" in industrialized nations, scabies affects 300 million people worldwide in all socioeconomic classes and in all climates [134]. Poverty, sanitation, poor water supply, and densely populated regions attribute to scabies epidemics. Personal hygiene and adequate clean water supply are critical to prevent and control the spread of scabies [135]. Numerical data are scarce because scabies is frequently unreported and predominately treated using home remedies.

Due to mandatory reporting of scabies in Slovenia since 1969, a study observing epidemic trends for 30 years until 1999 proved major peaks of infection during World War II and post-war years (1941–1946), 1972, and 1982 until stabilizing [136]. There were 432 cases/100,000 in 1972 and 220 cases/100,000 in 1982 until the steady decline toward approximately 50 cases/year as reported in 1993 and thereafter [137]. The demographics with greatest incidence are alcoholics, drug addicts, homeless persons, refugees, small children in day care centers, disabled persons, and the elderly in nursing homes [136, 138].

Other statistics are available as a result of military documentation of soldiers' health conditions and various studies indicate higher incidences associated with communal living quarters including shared personal items/toiletries as well as close physical contact during missions [139]. An observation of 2,481 soldiers in Skopje, Yugoslavia, during 1969–1971 reported 15% overall infection within the initial month of service, 42.2% after 2 months, and 72.5% of soldiers infected with scabies after 6 months [140]. From 1968 to 1981 the Army Health Branch Epidemiology Department of the Israeli Defense Force documented occurrences based on routine screenings (in addition to mandatory reporting) and observed two epidemics from 1973 to 1985 and 1972 to 1987 with increases of 17.7- and 3.9-fold, respectively. Sharp declines were noted in studies between 1981 and 1999 and 1984 and 1999 with morbidity decreasing 113.6- and 13.6-fold, respectively. The Israeli–Lebanese War of 1982 is partially attributed as the cause of the first epidemic [140, 141].

Pubic lice affect millions worldwide and the American National Institute for Allergy and Infectious Diseases (NIAID) estimates three million new cases annually in the United States. More than 1% of the population acquires pubic lice infection although the figure could be much higher if reporting were mandatory [135, 142]. Over 10–12 million Americans are infested with lice each year with head and pubic as the most reported forms. Case reports observe pubic lice in sexually active persons between ages 14 and 40 [143]. A study published in 2006 indicated a decreasing trend in pubic lice attributed to the increase of hair depilatory in many Western nations. The lack of habitat for lice to attach and survive in lowered rates of transmission to women and subsequently incidences in males decreased too [144].

2.2.12.3 Risk Factors

The general population of any geographical region is at risk for scabies and pubic lice although increased awareness of personal hygiene and specific social behavior may reduce the risk of exposure [126]. Early detection of both STIs is critical in order to receive effective treatment and halt potential transmission.

The CDC advises persons with scabies infection to notify all sexual partners and household members, discontinue intimate or sexual contact until the condition resolves, and quarantine/disinfect all infested articles including clothing, linens, and furniture [143]. All standard guidelines for safe sex and STD/STI prevention apply; however, mutual monogamy will not alter the risk of contracting or spreading scabies, but can result in recurrent infection. Condoms also prove ineffective as sexual intercourse or ejaculation is irrelevant to scabies transmission [131, 145]. Pubic lice prevention follows similar guidelines to that of scabies in order to reduce transmission or recurrent infection. Abstaining from sexual contact entirely or abstaining until the infestation is treated or resolved is the only effective method of prevention.

2.3 Summary

STIs are widespread throughout the world. These infections range from minor nuisances (e.g., pubic lice or molluscum) to life-threatening or deadly diseases (e.g., HIV). Many infections, such as those caused by bacteria for which antibiotics are known and effective, are curable while viral diseases such as HSV, HPV, and HIV have no current cure. Prevention is the best tool to decrease the morbidity and mortality of STIs. Understanding the epidemiology of each infection, particularly modifiable risk factors, is imperative in order to aid prevention and eradication efforts. The epidemiology of STIs will continue to change in our era of easy travel and economic globalization and therefore needs to be updated constantly in order to keep up with disease trends worldwide.

Take-Home Pearls

- Several infectious caused by bacterial, mycological, and protozoal agents can be treated successfully, whereas viral STIs cannot be eradicated with currently available medications.
- Many STIs are asymptomatic and can be difficult to recognize and control.
- Risk factors such as age, socioeconomic status, and high-risk sexual behavior make certain populations more prone to STIs than others.
- Adolescents and young adults are responsible for almost 50% of all newly acquired STIs.
- Groups known to participate in high-risk sexual activity are at higher risk for STI.
- *Trichomonas vaginalis*, a protozoa, is the most common non-viral cause of STI worldwide.
- *Chlamydia trachomatis* is the most common bacterial cause of STI.
- Gonorrhea is frequently concomitant with Chlamydia infection.
- Over two-thirds of worldwide syphilis infections occur in sub-Saharan Africa and Southeast Asia, although there has been an upsurge in cases in the United States and Europe over the past few years.
- HPV infections are the most commonly diagnosed STIs worldwide. In addition to cutaneous manifestations such as warts and condyloma, HPV is recognized as a causal agent in the pathogenesis of cervical cancer.
- Most HSV infections are spread through sexual contact with asymptomatic, unsuspecting carriers who shed the virus.
- Ulcerating genital disease such as HSV-2 is a risk factor for HIV infection due to mucosal breakdown.
- Condom use, mutual monogamy with an uninfected partner, and clean needle/syringe use can minimize transmission rates of HIV/AIDS.

References

1. Global Strategy for the Prevention and Control of Sexually Transmitted Infections: 2006-2015: Breaking the chain of transmission. WHO Press, Geneva (2007)
2. Global Prevalence and Incidence of Curable STIs: World Health Organization (WHO/CDS/CDR/EDC/2001.10), Geneva (2001)
3. WHO/UNAIDS: Sexually transmitted diseases: policies and principles for prevention and care [cited]. www.who.int/hiv/pub/sti/en/prev_care_en.pdf
4. Mayaud, P., Mabey, D.: Approaches to the control of sexually transmitted infections in developing countries: old

problems and modern challenges. Sex. Transm. Infect. **80**(3), 174–182 (June 2004)
5. Da Ros, C.T., Schmitt Cda, S.: Global epidemiology of sexually transmitted diseases. Asian J. Androl. **10**(1), 110–114 (Jan 2008)
6. Johnston, V.J., Mabey, D.C.: Global epidemiology and control of Trichomonas vaginalis. Curr. Opin. Infect. Dis. **21**(1), 56–64 (2008 Feb)
7. Cotch, M.F., Pastorek 2nd, J.G., Nugent, R.P., Hillier, S.L., Gibbs, R.S., Martin, D.H., et al.: Trichomonas vaginalis associated with low birth weight and preterm delivery. The Vaginal Infections and Prematurity Study Group. Sex. Transm. Dis. **24**(6), 353–360 (1997 Jul)
8. Sorvillo, F., Smith, L., Kerndt, P., Ash, L.: Trichomonas vaginalis, HIV, and African-Americans. Emerg. Infect. Dis. **7**(6), 927–932 (Nov–Dec 2001)
9. Van der Pol, B.: Trichomonas vaginalis infection: the most prevalent nonviral sexually transmitted infection receives the least public health attention. Clin. Infect. Dis. **44**(1), 23–25 (2007 Jan 1)
10. Krieger, J.N., Alderete, J.F.: Trichomonas vaginalis and trichomoniasis. In: Holmes, K.K., Sparling, P.F., Mardh, P., Lemon, S.M., Stamm, W.E., Plot, P., et al. (eds.) Sexually Transmitted Diseases, 3rd edn, pp. 587–604. McGraw-Hill, New York (1999)
11. Bowden, F.J., Paterson, B.A., Mein, J., Savage, J., Fairley, C.K., Garland, S.M., et al.: Estimating the prevalence of Trichomonas vaginalis, Chlamydia trachomatis, Neisseria gonorrhoeae, and human papillomavirus infection in indigenous women in northern Australia. Sex. Transm. Infect. **75**(6), 431–434 (1999 Dec)
12. Simoes, J.A., Giraldo, P.C., Ribbeiro Filho, A.D., et al.: Prevalencia e fatores de risco associados as infeccoes cervico-vaginais durante a gestacao. Rev. Bras. Ginecol. Obstet. **18**(6), 459–467 (1996)
13. Franjola, R., Anazco, R., Puente, R., Moraleda, L., Herrmann, F., Palma, M.: Trichomonas vaginalis infection in pregnant women and newborn infants. Rev. Méd. Chile **117**(2), 142–145 (1989 Feb)
14. Blankhart, D., Muller, O., Gresenguet, G., Weis, P.: Sexually transmitted infections in young pregnant women in Bangui, Central African Republic. Int. J. STD AIDS **10**(9), 609–614 (1999 Sep)
15. Sturm, A.W., Wilkinson, D., Ndovela, N., Bowen, S., Connolly, C.: Pregnant women as a reservoir of undetected sexually transmitted diseases in rural South Africa: implications for disease control. Am. J. Publ. Health **88**(8), 1243–1245 (1998 Aug)
16. Tyndall, M.W., Patrick, D., Spittal, P., Li, K., O'Shaughnessy, M.V., Schechter, M.T.: Risky sexual behaviours among injection drugs users with high HIV prevalence: implications for STD control. Sex. Transm. Infect. **78**(suppl 1), i170–i175 (April 2002)
17. Morton, A.N., Wakefield, T., Tabrizi, S.N., Garland, S.M., Fairley, C.K.: An outreach programme for sexually transmitted infection screening in street sex workers using self-administered samples. Int. J. STD AIDS **10**(11), 741–743 (Nov 1999)
18. Lee, D.M., Binger, A., Hocking, J., Fairley, C.K.: The incidence of sexually transmitted infections among frequently screened sex workers in a decriminalised and regulated system in Melbourne. Sex. Transm. Infect. **81**(5), 434–436 (Oct 2005)
19. Shafer, M.A., Pantell, R.H., Schachter, J.: Is the routine pelvic examination needed with the advent of urine-based screening for sexually transmitted diseases? Arch. Pediatr. Adolesc. Med. **153**(2), 119–125 (1999 Feb)
20. Kucinskiene, V., Sutaite, I., Valiukeviciene, S., Milasauskiene, Z., Domeika, M.: Prevalence and risk factors of genital Chlamydia trachomatis infection. Medicina (Kaunas) **42**(11), 885–894 (2006)
21. Bunnell, R.E., Dahlberg, L., Rolfs, R., Ransom, R., Gershman, K., Farshy, C., et al.: High prevalence and incidence of sexually transmitted diseases in urban adolescent females despite moderate risk behaviors. J. Infect. Dis. **180**(5), 1624–1631 (1999 Nov)
22. Burstein, G.R., Gaydos, C.A., Diener-West, M., Howell, M.R., Zenilman, J.M., Quinn, T.C.: Incident Chlamydia trachomatis infections among inner-city adolescent females. JAMA **280**(6), 521–526 (1998 Aug 12)
23. Buve, A., Weiss, H.A., Laga, M., Van Dyck, E., Musonda, R., Zekeng, L., et al.: The epidemiology of gonorrhoea, chlamydial infection and syphilis in four African cities. AIDS **15**(suppl 4), S79–S88 (2001 Aug)
24. Imai, H., Shinohara, H., Nakao, H., Tsukino, H., Hamasuna, R., Katoh, T.: Prevalence and risk factors of asymptomatic chlamydial infection among students in Japan. Int. J. STD AIDS **15**(6), 408–414 (2004 Jun)
25. Ngandjio, A., Clerc, M., Fonkoua, M.C., Thonnon, J., Njock, F., Pouillot, R., et al.: Screening of volunteer students in Yaounde (Cameroon, Central Africa) for *Chlamydia trachomatis* infection and genotyping of isolated *C. trachomatis* strains. J. Clin. Microbiol. **41**(9), 4404–4407 (Sept 2003)
26. Williams, H., Tabrizi, S.N., Lee, W., Kovacs, G.T., Garland, S.: Adolescence and other risk factors for Chlamydia trachomatis genitourinary infection in women in Melbourne, Australia. Sex. Transm. Infect. **79**(1), 31–34 (2003 Feb)
27. Stamm, W.E.: Chlamydia trachomatis infections of the adult. In: Holmes, K.K., Sparling, P.F., Mardh, P., Lemon, S.M., Stamm, W.E., Plot, P., et al. (eds.) Sexually Transmitted Diseases, 3rd edn, pp. 407–422. McGraw-Hill, New York (1999)
28. Mardh, P.A.: Is Europe ready for STD screening? Genitourin. Med. **73**(2), 96–98 (April 1997)
29. Wilson, J.S., Honey, E., Templeton, A., Paavonen, J., Mardh, P.A., Stray-Pedersen, B.: A systematic review of the prevalence of Chlamydia trachomatis among European women. Hum. Reprod. Update **8**(4), 385–394 (July–Aug 2002)
30. Sedlecki, K., Markovic, M., Rajic, G.: Risk factors for Chlamydia infections of the genital organs in adolescent females. Srp. Arh. Celok. Lek. **129**(7–8), 169–174 (July–Aug 2001)
31. Cates Jr., W., Wasserheit, J.N.: Genital chlamydial infections: epidemiology and reproductive sequelae. Am. J. Obstet. Gynecol. **164**(6 Pt 2), 1771–1781 (June 1991)
32. Burstein, G.R., Zenilman, J.M., Gaydos, C.A., Diener-West, M., Howell, M.R., Brathwaite, W., et al.: Predictors of repeat Chlamydia trachomatis infections diagnosed by DNA amplification testing among inner city females. Sex. Transm. Infect. **77**(1), 26–32 (Feb 2001)
33. Hillis, S.D., Nakashima, A., Marchbanks, P.A., Addiss, D.G., Davis, J.P.: Risk factors for recurrent Chlamydia

trachomatis infections in women. Am. J. Obstet. Gynecol. **170**(3), 801–806 (Mar 1994)
34. Louv, W.C., Austin, H., Perlman, J., Alexander, W.J.: Oral contraceptive use and the risk of chlamydial and gonococcal infections. Am. J. Obstet. Gynecol. **160**(2), 396–402 (1989 Feb)
35. Kaptue, L., Zekeng, L., Djoumessi, S., Monny-Lobe, M., Nichols, D., Debuysscher, R.: HIV and chlamydia infections among prostitutes in Yaounde, Cameroon. Genitourin. Med. **67**(2), 143–145 (1991 Apr)
36. Eron Jr., J.J., Gilliam, B., Fiscus, S., Dyer, J., Cohen, M.S.: HIV-1 shedding and chlamydial urethritis. JAMA **275**(1), 36 (1996 Jan 3)
37. Fox, K.K., Whittington, W.L., Levine, W.C., Moran, J.S., Zaidi, A.A., Nakashima, A.K.: Gonorrhea in the United States, 1981-1996. Demographic and geographic trends. Sex. Transm. Dis. **25**(7), 386–393 (Aug 1998)
38. Hook, E.W., HH, H.: Gonococcal infections in the adult. In: Holmes, K.K., Sparling, P.F., Mardh, P., Lemon, S.M., Stamm, W.E., Plot, P., et al. (eds.) Sexually Transmitted Diseases, 3rd edn, pp. 451–466. McGraw-Hill, New York (1999)
39. CDC: Sexually Transmitted Disease Surveillance, 2006 [cited; 192]. http://www.cdc.gov/std/stats/pdf/Surv2006.pdf(Nov 2007)
40. DeSchryver, A., Meheus, A.: Epidemiology of sexually transmitted diseases: the global picture. WHO Bull. OMS **68**, 639–653 (1990)
41. Costello Daly, C., Wangel, A.M., Hoffman, I.F., Canner, J.K., Lule, G.S., Lema, V.M., et al.: Validation of the WHO diagnostic algorithm and development of an alternative scoring system for the management of women presenting with vaginal discharge in Malawi. Sex. Transm. Infect. **74**(suppl 1), S50–S58 (June 1998)
42. WHO: STI/HIV status and trends of STI, HIV and AIDS at the end of the millennium [cited] http://www.who.int/hiv/strategic/en/wpr_millenium.pdf (1999)
43. Handsfield, H.H., Sparling, P.F.: Neisseria gonorrhoeae. In: Mandell, G.L., Bennett, J.E., Dolin, R. (eds.) Principles and Practice of Infectious Diseases, 6th edn, pp. 2514–2529. Churchill Livingstone, Philadelphia (2005)
44. WHO/EURO: Epidemic of sexually transmitted diseases in Eastern Europe. Report on a WHO meeting, Copenhagen, Denmark, 13–15 May 1996
45. Alary, M.: Epidemiology and control strategies. Can. J. Hum. Sexual **6**, 13–17 (1997)
46. Miller, W.C., Ford, C.A., Morris, M., Handcock, M.S., Schmitz, J.L., Hobbs, M.M., et al.: Prevalence of chlamydial and gonococcal infections among young adults in the United States. JAMA **291**(18), 2229–2236 (12 May 2004)
47. Fleming, D.T., Wasserheit, J.N.: From epidemiological synergy to public health policy and practice: the contribution of other sexually transmitted diseases to sexual transmission of HIV infection. Sex. Transm. Infect. **75**(1), 3–17 (Feb 1999)
48. Ford, K., Norris, A.E.: Urban Hispanic adolescents and young adults: Relationship of acculturation to sexual behavior. J. Sex Res. **29**, 189–205 (1993)
49. Weinstock, H., Berman, S., Cates Jr., W.: Sexually transmitted diseases among American youth: incidence and prevalence estimates, 2000. Perspect. Sex. Reprod. Health **36**(1), 6–10 (2004 Jan-Feb)
50. Datta, S.D., Sternberg, M., Johnson, R.E., Berman, S., Papp, J.R., McQuillan, G., et al.: Gonorrhea and chlamydia in the United States among persons 14 to 39 years of age, 1999 to 2002. Ann. Intern. Med. **147**(2), 89–96 (2007 Jul 17)
51. Workowski, K.A., Berman, S.M.: Sexually transmitted diseases treatment guidelines, 2006. MMWR Recomm. Rep. **55**(RR-11), 1–94 (2006 Aug 4)
52. Domantay-Apostol, G.P., Handog, E.B., Gabriel, M.T.: Syphilis: the international challenge of the great imitator. Dermatol. Clin. **26**(2), 191–202, v (Apr 2008)
53. Walker, D.G., Walker, G.J.: Forgotten but not gone: the continuing scourge of congenital syphilis. Lancet Infect. Dis. **2**(7), 432–436 (July 2002)
54. Golden, M.R., Marra, C.M., Holmes, K.K.: Update on syphilis: resurgence of an old problem. JAMA **290**(11), 1510–1514 (17 Sept 2003)
55. Gottlieb, S.L., Pope, V., Sternberg, M.R., McQuillan, G.M., Beltrami, J.F., Berman, S.M., et al.: Prevalence of syphilis seroreactivity in the United States: data from the National Health and Nutrition Examination Surveys (NHANES) 2001-2004. Sex. Transm. Dis. **35**(5), 507–511 (May 2008)
56. Ronald, A.R., Albritton, W.: Chancroid and Haemophilus ducreyi. In: Holmes, K.K., Sparling, P.F., Mardh, P., Lemon, S.M., Stamm, W.E., Plot, P., et al. (eds.) Sexually Transmitted Diseases, 3rd edn, pp. 515–523. McGraw-Hill, New York (1999)
57. Steen, R.: Eradicating chancroid. Bull. World Health Organ. **79**(9), 818–826 (2001)
58. Al-Tawfiq, J.A., Spinola, S.M.: Haemophilus ducreyi: clinical disease and pathogenesis. Curr. Opin. Infect. Dis. **15**(1), 43–47 (2002 Feb)
59. Mertz, K.J., Trees, D., Levine, W.C., Lewis, J.S., Litchfield, B., Pettus, K.S., et al.: Etiology of genital ulcers and prevalence of human immunodeficiency virus coinfection in 10 US cities. The Genital Ulcer Disease Surveillance Group. J. Infect. Dis. **178**(6), 1795–1798 (1998 Dec)
60. Hanenberg, R.S., Rojanapithayakorn, W., Kunasol, P., Sokal, D.C.: Impact of Thailand's HIV-control programme as indicated by the decline of sexually transmitted diseases. Lancet **344**(8917), 243–245 (23 July 1994)
61. Weiss, H.A., Thomas, S.L., Munabi, S.K., Hayes, R.J.: Male circumcision and risk of syphilis, chancroid, and genital herpes: a systematic review and meta-analysis. Sex. Transm. Infect. **82**(2), 101–109 (April 2006). discussion 10
62. O'Farrell, N.: Soap and water prophylaxis for limiting genital ulcer disease and HIV-1 infection in men in sub-Saharan Africa. Genitourin. Med. **69**(4), 297–300 (1993 Aug)
63. O'Farrell, N.: Donovanosis. Sex. Transm. Infect. **78**(6), 452–457 (Dec 2002)
64. O'Farrell, N.: Donovanosis. In: Holmes, K.K., Sparling, P.F., Mardh, P., Lemon, S.M., Stamm, W.E., Plot, P., et al. (eds.) Sexually Transmitted Diseases, 3rd edn, pp. 525–529. McGraw-Hill, New York (1999)
65. Bowden, F.J.: Donovanosis in Australia: going, going. Sex. Transm. Infect. **81**(5), 365–366 (Oct 2005)
66. WHO: Consensus report on STI, HIV and AIDS Epidemiology Papua New Guinea [cited] http://www.wpro.who.int/NR/rdonlyres/EEC64817-5D9F-4E72-9F7C-6014887E3483/0/Consensus_Report_PNG_2000.pdf (2000)
67. Simmons, A.: Clinical manifestations and treatment considerations of herpes simplex virus infection. J. Infect. Dis. **186**(suppl 1), S71–S77 (15 Oct 2002)

68. Freeman, E.E., Weiss, H.A., Glynn, J.R., Cross, P.L., Whitworth, J.A., Hayes, R.J.: Herpes simplex virus 2 infection increases HIV acquisition in men and women: systematic review and meta-analysis of longitudinal studies. AIDS **20**(1), 73–83 (2 Jan 2006)
69. Mertz, G.J., Benedetti, J., Ashley, R., Selke, S.A., Corey, L.: Risk factors for the sexual transmission of genital herpes. Ann. Intern. Med. **116**(3), 197–202 (1 Feb 1992)
70. Fleming, D.T., McQuillan, G.M., Johnson, R.E., Nahmias, A.J., Aral, S.O., Lee, F.K., et al.: Herpes simplex virus type 2 in the United States, 1976 to 1994. N. Engl. J. Med. **337**(16), 1105–1111 (16 Oct 1997)
71. Weiss, H.: Epidemiology of herpes simplex virus type 2 infection in the developing world. Herpes **11**(suppl 1), 24A–35A (Apr 2004)
72. Armstrong, G.L., Schillinger, J., Markowitz, L., Nahmias, A.J., Johnson, R.E., McQuillan, G.M., et al.: Incidence of herpes simplex virus type 2 infection in the United States. Am. J. Epidemiol. **153**(9), 912–920 (1 May 2001)
73. Malkin, J.E.: Epidemiology of genital herpes simplex virus infection in developed countries. Herpes **11**(suppl 1), 2A–23A (2004 Apr)
74. Fazel, N., Wilczynski, S., Lowe, L., Su, L.D.: Clinical, histopathologic, and molecular aspects of cutaneous human papillomavirus infections. Dermatol. Clin. **17**(3), 521–536, viii (July 1999)
75. Ferlay, J., Bray, F., et al.: GLOBCAN 2002: cancer incidence, mortality and prevalence worldwide. *IARC Cancer Base*, 2nd edn. IARC Press, Lyon (2004)
76. de Sanjose, S., Diaz, M., Castellsague, X., Clifford, G., Bruni, L., Munoz, N., et al.: Worldwide prevalence and genotype distribution of cervical human papillomavirus DNA in women with normal cytology: a meta-analysis. Lancet Infect. Dis. **7**(7), 453–459 (2007 Jul)
77. Munoz, N., Mendez, F., Posso, H., Molano, M., van den Brule, A.J., Ronderos, M., et al.: Incidence, duration, and determinants of cervical human papillomavirus infection in a cohort of Colombian women with normal cytological results. J. Infect. Dis. **190**(12), 2077–2087 (15 Dec 2004)
78. Dunne, E.F., Unger, E.R., Sternberg, M., McQuillan, G., Swan, D.C., Patel, S.S., et al.: Prevalence of HPV infection among females in the United States. JAMA **297**(8), 813–819 (28 Feb 2007)
79. Kahn, J.A., Lan, D., Kahn, R.S.: Sociodemographic factors associated with high-risk human papillomavirus infection. Obstet. Gynecol. **110**(1), 87–95 (July 2007)
80. Baldwin, S.B., Wallace, D.R., Papenfuss, M.R., Abrahamsen, M., Vaught, L.C., Kornegay, J.R., et al.: Human papillomavirus infection in men attending a sexually transmitted disease clinic. J. Infect. Dis. **187**(7), 1064–1070 (1 Apr 2003)
81. Castellsague, X., Bosch, F.X., Munoz, N., Meijer, C.J., Shah, K.V., de Sanjose, S., et al.: Male circumcision, penile human papillomavirus infection, and cervical cancer in female partners. N. Engl. J. Med. **346**(15), 1105–1112 (2002 Apr 11)
82. Clifford, G.M., Gallus, S., Herrero, R., Munoz, N., Snijders, P.J., Vaccarella, S., et al.: Worldwide distribution of human papillomavirus types in cytologically normal women in the International Agency for Research on Cancer HPV prevalence surveys: a pooled analysis. Lancet **366**(9490), 991–998 (17–23 Sept 2005)
83. Espinoza, L., Hall, H.I., Hardnett, F., Selik, R.M., Ling, Q., Lee, L.M.: Characteristics of persons with heterosexually acquired HIV infection, United States 1999-2004. Am. J. Publ. Health **97**(1), 144–149 (Jan 2007)
84. WHO/EM: Report on the intercountry workshop on STD prevalence study, Amman, Jordan, 12–15 Oct 1998
85. McNaghten, A.D., Hanson, D.L., Aponte, Z., Sullivan, P.S., Wolfe, M.I.: Gender disparity in HIV treatment and AIDS opportunistic illnesses (OI). XV International conference on AIDS, Bangkok, Thailand, July 2004
86. McKenna, M.T., Hu, X.: Recent trends in the incidence and morbidity that are associated with perinatal human immunodeficiency virus infection in the United States. Am. J. Obstet. Gynecol. **197**(suppl 3), S10–S16 (2007 Sep)
87. Over, M., Piot, P.: Human immunodeficiency virus infection and other sexually transmitted diseases in developing countries: public health importance and priorities for resource allocation. J. Infect. Dis. **174**(suppl 2), S162–S175 (Oct 1996)
88. Bourgeois, A., Henzel, D., Dibanga, G., Malonga-Mouelet, G., Peeters, M., Coulaud, J.P., et al.: Prospective evaluation of a flow chart using a risk assessment for the diagnosis of STDs in primary healthcare centres in Libreville, Gabon. Sex. Transm. Infect. **74**(suppl 1), S128–S132 (June 1998)
89. Jonsdottir, K., Geirsson, R.T., Steingrimsson, O., Olafsson, J.H., Stefansdottir, S.: Reduced prevalence of cervical Chlamydia infection among women requesting termination. Acta Obstet. Gynecol. Scand. **76**(5), 438–441 (1997 May)
90. Hader, S.L., Smith, D.K., Moore, J.S., Holmberg, S.D.: HIV infection in women in the United States: status at the Millennium. JAMA **285**(9), 1186–1192 (7 Mar 2001)
91. Prather, C., Fuller, T.R., King, W., Brown, M., Moering, M., Little, S., et al.: Diffusing an HIV prevention intervention for African American Women: integrating afrocentric components into the SISTA Diffusion Strategy. AIDS Educ. Prev. **18**(4 suppl A), 149–160 (Aug 2006)
92. Leigh, B.C., Stall, R.: Substance use and risky sexual behavior for exposure to HIV. Issues in methodology, interpretation, and prevention. Am. Psychol. **48**(10), 1035–1045 (Oct 1993)
93. McDavid, K., Li, J., Lee, L.M.: Racial and ethnic disparities in HIV diagnoses for women in the United States. J. Acq. Immun. Def. Synd. **42**(1), 101–107 (May 2006)
94. Truong, H.M., Kellogg, T., Klausner, J.D., Katz, M.H., Dilley, J., Knapper, K., et al.: Increases in sexually transmitted infections and sexual risk behaviour without a concurrent increase in HIV incidence among men who have sex with men in San Francisco: a suggestion of HIV serosorting? Sex. Transm. Infect. **82**(6), 461–466 (December 2006)
95. Millett, G., Malebranche, D., Mason, B., Spikes, P.: Focusing "down low": bisexual black men, HIV risk and heterosexual transmission. J. Natl. Med. Assoc. **97**(7 suppl), 52S–59S (July 2005)
96. Fullilove, R.E.: African Americans, Health Disparities and HIV/AIDS: Recommendations for Confronting the Epidemic in Black America. Columbia University, National Minority AIDS Council, New York (2006)
97. DeNavas-Walt, C., Proctor, B.D., Lee, C.H.: Income, poverty, and health insurance coverage in the United States: 2004. Current Population Reports, pp. 60–229. U.S. Government Printing Office, Washington (2005)

98. Valleroy, L.A., MacKellar, D.A., Behel, S.K., Secura, G.M.: Young men's survey. The bridge for HIV transmission to women from 23- to 29-year-old men who have sex with men in 6 U.S. cities. National HIV prevention conference, Atlanta, Georgia, July
99. MacKellar, D.A., Valleroy, L.A., Secura, G.M., Behel, S., Bingham, T., Celentano, D.D., et al.: Unrecognized HIV infection, risk behaviors, and perceptions of risk among young men who have sex with men: opportunities for advancing HIV prevention in the third decade of HIV/AIDS. J. Acq. Immun. Def. Synd. **38**(5), 603–614 (15 Apr 2005)
100. Connor, E.M., Sperling, R.S., Gelber, R., Kiselev, P., Scott, G., O'Sullivan, M.J., et al.: Reduction of maternal-infant transmission of human immunodeficiency virus type 1 with zidovudine treatment. Pediatric AIDS Clinical Trials Group Protocol 076 Study Group. N. Engl. J. Med. **331**(18), 1173–1180 (3 Nov 1994)
101. Cooper, E.R., Charurat, M., Mofenson, L., Hanson, I.C., Pitt, J., Diaz, C., et al.: Combination antiretroviral strategies for the treatment of pregnant HIV-1-infected women and prevention of perinatal HIV-1 transmission. J Acq Immun Def Synd **29**(5), 484–494 (15 Apr 2002)
102. CDC: HIV/AIDS surveillance report, vol. 18 [cited] http://www.cdc.gov/hiv/topics/surveillance/resources/reports/2006report/pdf/2006SurveillanceReport.pdf (2006)
103. Parkin, D.M., Bray, F., Ferlay, J., Pisani, P.: Estimating the world cancer burden: Globocan 2000. Int. J. Cancer **94**(2), 153–156 (15 Oct 2001)
104. McGlynn, K.A., Tsao, L., Hsing, A.W., Devesa, S.S., Fraumeni Jr., J.F.: International trends and patterns of primary liver cancer. Int. J. Cancer **94**(2), 290–296 (15 Oct 2001)
105. WHO: Hepatitis B: Fact sheet no. 204 (revised Oct 2000) [cited] http://www.who.int/mediacentre/factsheets/fs204/en/index.html (2000)
106. Hepatitis B vaccines: Releve epidemiologique hebdomadaire/Section d'hygiene du Secretariat de la Societe des Nations = Weekly epidemiological record/Health Section of the Secretariat of the League of Nations, 9;**79**(28):255–263 (July 2004)
107. Lavanchy, D.: Worldwide epidemiology of HBV infection, disease burden, and vaccine prevention. J. Clin. Virol. **34**(suppl 1), S1–S3 (2005 Dec)
108. Introduction of Hepatitis B vaccine into childhood immunization services: Management guidelines including information for health workers and parents [cited] http://www.who.int/vaccines-documents/DocsPDF01/www613.pdf (2001)
109. Disease burden from Hepatitis A, B, and C in the United States [cited] www.cdc.gov/ncidod/diseases/hepatitis/resource/PDFs/disease_burden.pdf
110. Wasley, A., Grytdal, S., Gallagher, K.: Surveillance for acute viral hepatitis–United States, 2006. MMWR Surveill. Summ. **57**(2), 1–24 (21 Mar 2008)
111. Smith, K.J., Yeager, J., Skelton, H.: Molluscum contagiosum: its clinical, histopathologic, and immunohistochemical spectrum. Int. J. Dermatol. **38**(9), 664–672 (1999 Sep)
112. Porter, C.D., Archard, L.C.: Characterisation by restriction mapping of three subtypes of molluscum contagiosum virus. J. Med. Virol. **38**(1), 1–6 (Sept 1992)
113. Shirodaria, P.V., Matthews, R.S.: Observations on the antibody rsponses in molluscum contagiosum. Br. J. Dermatol. **96**(1), 29–34 (Jan 1977)
114. Becker, T.M., Blount, J.H., Douglas, J., Judson, F.N.: Trends in molluscum contagiosum in the United States, 1966-1983. Sex. Transm. Dis. **13**(2), 88–92 (Apr–June 1986)
115. Lowy, D.R., Androphy, E.J.: Molluscum contagiosum. In: Freedberg, I.M., Eisen, A.Z., Wolff, K., Austen, K.F., Goldsmith, L.A., Katz, S.I. (eds.) Fitzpatrick's Dermatology in General Medicine, 6th edn. McGraw-Hill, New York (2003)
116. Strauss, R.M., Doyle, E.L., Mohsen, A.H., Green, S.T.: Successful treatment of molluscum contagiosum with topical imiquimod in a severely immunocompromised HIV-positive patient. Int. J. STD AIDS **12**(4), 264–266 (Apr 2001)
117. Schwartz, J.J., Myskowski, P.L.: Molluscum contagiosum in patients with human immunodeficiency virus infection. A review of twenty-seven patients. J. Am. Acad. Dermatol. **27**(4), 583–588 (Oct 1992)
118. Romiti, R., Ribeiro, A.P., Romiti, N.: Evaluation of the effectiveness of 5% potassium hydroxide for the treatment of molluscum contagiosum. Pediatr. Dermatol. **17**(6), 495 (Nov–Dec 2000)
119. Lee, B., Kang, H.Y.: Molluscum folliculitis after leg shaving. J. Am. Acad. Dermatol. **51**(3), 478–479 (Sept 2004)
120. National Guideline for the Management of Molluscum Contagiosum: Clinical Effectiveness Group (Association of Genitourinary Medicine and the Medical Society for the Study of Venereal Diseases). Sex Transm. Infect. **75**(suppl 1):S80–S81 (Aug 1999)
121. Buckley, R., Smith, K.: Topical imiquimod therapy for chronic giant molluscum contagiosum in a patient with advanced human immunodeficiency virus 1 disease. Arch. Dermatol. **135**(10), 1167–1169 (1999 Oct)
122. Petersen, C.S., Gerstoft, J.: Molluscum contagiosum in HIV-infected patients. Dermatology **184**(1), 19–21 (1992)
123. Picon, L., Vaillant, L., Duong, T., Lorette, G., Bacq, Y., Besnier, J.M., et al.: Cutaneous cryptococcosis resembling molluscum contagiosum: a first manifestation of AIDS. Acta Derm. Venereol. **69**(4), 365–367 (1989)
124. Cobbold, R.J., Macdonald, A.: Molluscum contagiosum as a sexually transmitted disease. Practitioner **204**(221), 416–419 (Mar 1970)
125. Billstein, S.A., Mattaliano Jr., V.J.: The "nuisance" sexually transmitted diseases: molluscum contagiosum, scabies, and crab lice. Med. Clin. N. Am. **74**(6), 1487–1505 (Nov 1990)
126. Leone, P.A.: Scabies and pediculosis pubis: an update of treatment regimens and general review. Clin. Infect. Dis. **44**(suppl 3), S153–S159 (1 Apr 2007)
127. Haag, M.L., Brozena, S.J., Fenske, N.A.: Attack of the scabies: what to do when an outbreak occurs. Geriatrics **48**(10), 45–46, 51–53 (Oct 1993)
128. Kolar, K.A., Rapini, R.P.: Crusted (Norwegian) scabies. Am. Fam. Physician **44**(4), 1317–1321 (1991 Oct)
129. Mathieu, M.E., Wilson, B.B.: Scabies. In: Mandell, G.L., Bennett, J.E., Dolin, R. (eds.) Principles and Practice of Infectious Diseases, 6th edn, pp. 3304–3307. Churchill Livingstone, London (2005)

130. Chosidow, O.: Clinical practices. Scabies. N. Engl J. Med. **354**(16), 1718–1727 (20 Apr 2006)
131. Mandell, G.L., Bennett, J.E., Dolin, R. (eds.): Principles and Practice of Infectious Diseases, 5th ed., pp. 2972–2973. Churchill Livingstone, London (2000)
132. Varela, J.A., Otero, L., Espinosa, E., Sanchez, C., Junquera, M.L., Vazquez, F.: Phthirus pubis in a sexually transmitted diseases unit: a study of 14 years. Sex. Transm. Dis. **30**(4), 292–296 (Apr 2003)
133. Manjunatha, N.P., Jayamanne, G.R., Desai, S.P., Moss, T.R., Lalik, J., Woodland, A.: Pediculosis pubis: presentation to ophthalmologist as pthriasis palpebrarum associated with corneal epithelial keratitis. Int. J. STD AIDS **17**(6), 424–426 (June 2006)
134. Orion, E., Matz, H., Wolf, R.: Ectoparasitic sexually transmitted diseases: scabies and pediculosis. Clin. Dermatol. **22**(6), 513–519 (Nov–Dec 2004)
135. Stone, S.P.: Scabies and pediculosis. In: Freedberg, I.M., Eisen, A.Z., Wolff, K., Austen, K.F., Goldsmith, L.A., Katz, S.I. (eds.) Fitzpatrick's Dermatology in General Medicine, 6th edn, pp. 2283–2289. McGraw-Hill, New York (2003)
136. Kralj, B., Kansky, A., Zgavec, B., Kraigher, A.: Scabies in Slovenia during the 1971-95 period. Acta Dermatoven APA **6**, 33–36 (1997)
137. Stork, J.: Scabies. Cesko-slovenska Dermatol. **74**, 28–33 (1999)
138. Kansky, A., Potocnik, M., Kraigher, A.: Scabies and venereal diseases in Slovenia. Acta Dermatoven APA **6**(suppl), 1–16 (1997)
139. Wendel, K., Rompalo, A.: Scabies and pediculosis pubis: an update of treatment regimens and general review. Clin. Infect. Dis. **35**(suppl 2), S146–S151 (15 Oct 2002)
140. Konstantinov, D., Stanoeva, L., Zaharijeva, L., Bitoljanu, V.: Epidemiological factors causing the present outbreak of scabies epidemic in the Socialist Republic of Macedonia. Acta Derm. Lug. **4**, 225–233 (1977)
141. Mimouni, D., Grotto, I., Haviv, J., Gdalevich, M., Huerta, M., Shpilberg, O.: Secular trends in the epidemiology of pediculosis capitis and pubis among Israeli soldiers: a 27-year follow-up. Int. J. Dermatol. **40**(10), 637–639 (Oct 2001)
142. Meinking, T.L., Burkhart, C.G., Burkhart, C.N.: Infestations. In: Bolognia, J.L., Jorizzo, J.L., Rapini, R.P. (eds.) Dermatology, pp. 1321–1332. Mosby, London (2003)
143. CDC: Ectoparasitic infections. Sexually transmitted diseases treatment guidelines 2002. Centers for Disease Control and Prevention. MMWR Recomm. Rep. **55**(RR-11), 79–80 (10 Aug 2002)
144. Armstrong, N.R., Wilson, J.D.: Did the "Brazilian" kill the pubic louse? Sex. Transm. Infect. **82**(3), 265–266 (2006 Jun)
145. CDC: Parasitic disease information: scabies fact sheet [cited] http://www.cdc.gov/ncidod/dpd/parasites/scabies/factsht_scabies.htm (2005)

Sexual Behavior and Psychological Aspects Associated with Sexually Transmitted Infections

3

Amber R. Gill, Parisa Ravanfar, Natalia Mendoza, and Stephen K. Tyring

Core Messages

- While the incidence of sexually transmitted infections (STIs) is largely dependent on the distribution and prevalence of infection in the population, it is also important to consider the behavior of an individual and his or her partner(s), as well as their psychological state.
- The term "sexual behavior" encompasses many components, including sexual experience and activity, age at sexual debut, current and lifetime number of sexual partners, frequency of sexual intercourse, consistency of sexual activity, mode of recruitment of sexual partners, duration of sexual relationships, and types of sexual practice.
- Some behaviors and practices that are associated with an increased risk of STIs include unprotected intercourse, receptive anal intercourse, having multiple and concurrent partners, and drug and alcohol use.
- Psychological factors, such as mood, mental health, and even personality types, may affect both risk of contracting STIs and presentation for and response to treatment.

A.R. Gill (✉)
School of Medicine, University of Texas Medical School, Houston, TX, USA
e-mail: amber.gill@uth.tmc.edu

P. Ravanfar
Center for Clinical Studies, Houston, TX, USA

N. Mendoza
Center for Clinical Studies, Houston, TX, USA and Universidad El Bosque, Bogota, Colombia

S.K. Tyring
Center for Clinical Studies, Houston, TX, USA and Department of Dermatology, The University of Texas Health Science Center, Houston, TX, USA

3.1 Introduction

The spread of sexually transmitted infections (STIs) is influenced by the distribution and prevalence of STIs in the population, as well as the behavior of an individual and his or her partner(s). Many social factors have been associated with increased risk of STIs and certain populations tend to have higher incidences of STIs, such as urban, low-income, minorities, and women. This may be due to the fact that socioeconomic factors help shape sexual behavior. The term "sexual behavior" involves many components: sexual experience and activity, age at sexual debut, current and lifetime number of sexual partners, frequency of sexual intercourse, consistency of sexual activity, mode of recruitment of sexual partners, duration of sexual relationships, and types of sexual practice [1]. It is likely that certain socioeconomic conditions modify sexual behavior. For example, people living in industrialized countries are more likely to use condoms, but are also more likely to report multiple sexual partners [2]. Low-income populations are more likely to have sex at a younger age, use condoms less often, and display other risky behaviors [2]. In addition, wealth and education have been shown to positively correlate with condom use [3].

G. Gross and S.K. Tyring (eds.), *Sexually Transmitted Infections and Sexually Transmitted Diseases*,
DOI: 10.1007/978-3-642-14663-3_3,

3.2 Age and Sexual Behavior

Sexuality is shaped by both biological and environmental cues. The display of sexual interest in adolescents is a function of the onset of puberty, as well as social influences surrounding them. The magnitude of influence peers have on adolescent sexuality varies across groups. Studies suggest the influence of peers is highest during the transition from childhood to early adolescence [4, 5]. Among racial groups, white females are likely to be influenced by their peers while peer influence is less significant among white males and black females [6]. However, a recent study in the Philippines found that having sexually active friends is associated with earlier sexual debut for both males and females [7]. It has also been noted that the kinds of peers adolescents mingle with determines the direction of the influence. Having peers with high-risk behavior is associated with earlier sexual debut and pregnancy, while the opposite is true of being connected with low-risk peers [8].

Sexual exploration among adolescents often occurs in a stepwise fashion with fondling and oral sex typically preceding vaginal intercourse [9]. By their late teens, most adolescents have had sexual intercourse [10]. On the other hand, only a small percentage of adolescents have engaged in anal sex [11].

There is a longstanding trend toward earlier sexual debut occurring worldwide [12]. While the gender gap is narrowing, males continue to have a younger age of sexual debut, as well as significantly more sexual partners than females [10]. Young age at first sexual intercourse has been associated with more lifetime partners, even after adjusting for more years of sexual activity, especially in men [13]. Sexual activity among adolescents also varies by race. For instance, a higher proportion of African Americans report sexual activity by their late teens [10]. African Americans also report more lifetime partners than white and Hispanic youth. Increased lifetime partner numbers can increase the probability of acquiring an STI. In one study, the number of sexual partners of heterosexual men could be predicted by hypermasculinity and sensation-seeking behavior [14]. However, if all partners are exclusively monogamous and uninfected, there is no risk of STI.

3.3 Various Aspects of Sexual Behavior

Most adults and adolescents report practicing “serial monogamy” with steady partners, but also identify “casual” sexual partners and “one-night stands” [15, 16]. Serial monogamous relationships lead to a highly segmented network with little chance for diffuse spread of STIs, while concurrent partnerships lead to a highly connected sexual network and an increased risk for spread of STIs [17, 18]. In serial monogamy, when an individual becomes infected, their past partners are not at risk because they are no longer in contact. However, when people have concurrent sexual partners who overlap in time, all partners are at risk. An individual’s practice of concurrency has been associated with higher prevalence of STIs, even after adjusting for total number of partners [17, 19]. In addition, individuals who have partners with concurrent partners, even if one individual is monogamous, are also at increased risk of acquiring an STI [18–20]. Concurrency affects not only the rate of spread, but also the total number of infected individuals [21]. Concurrency has been shown to play a fundamental role in the spread of chlamydia, gonorrhea, syphilis, and human immunodeficiency virus (HIV) [18, 21–23]. Concurrency has been reported more often by males than females [20].

The use of condoms and other barriers provides protection against transmission of many STIs, including HIV, especially in women [24]. For example, it has been shown that condom use during more than 25% of sex acts is associated with protection against HSV-2 acquisition for women but not for men [25]. In one study, about 40% of men and 22% of women reported using a condom during last sexual intercourse [26]. Condom use is more likely among those who are young and have never been married [26]. Adolescents who use a condom at sexual debut are more likely to continue to use them in subsequent sexual activities and have lower rates of STIs [27]. Among both adolescents and adults, condoms are more likely to be used among new or casual partners than in steady partnerships [23, 28]. This behavior suggests that individuals alter their protective and contraceptive methods depending on their assessment of risk associated with a sexual encounter. This is also the case among men who have sex with men (MSM). Interestingly, MSM who are HIV-positive are more likely to have unprotected anal sex with other men who are also seropositive than with men who are HIV-negative or whose serostatus is unknown, perhaps in an effort to reduce transmission [29].

Age is also a factor that affects sexual behavior and STI rates. Curable STIs, such as chlamydia and gonorrhea, are most prevalent among persons 15–24 years of age [30]. This population has frequent changes in partners and tends to choose partners in a similar age group. On the other hand, incurable STIs, such as HIV, will accumulate with years of exposure and thus be more prevalent among older populations.

The incidence of many STIs, including syphilis, gonorrhea, and chlamydia, is considerably higher in young women than in young men, not only because STIs are more efficiently transmitted from males to females [31], but also due to many behavioral factors. Women do not tend to have earlier sexual debut or more lifetime partners than men, but they do tend to have partners who are older and more likely to have an STI [32]. Power dynamics in heterosexual partnerships may also affect condom use and risk of contracting STIs. Women are less likely to ask their partners to wear a condom if they fear physical abuse or jeopardizing financial aid, thus increasing their risk for acquiring an STI [33]. In addition, treatment-seeking behavior is severely inhibited by stigma and shame associated with STIs [34]. Other barriers to treatment, especially for women, are financial dependency, being too busy caring for children, lack of symptoms or knowledge of symptoms, or limited access to health care [35].

The increasing incidence of STIs among the elderly may be attributed to many factors. For example, drugs which enhance sexual functioning, such as sildenafil citrate (Viagra®) and tadalafil (Cialis®), allow older adults to continue having sexual intercourse as they age [36]. In addition, postmenopausal women no longer fear getting pregnant and thus may be less likely to use a condom or other barrier to protect against STIs [37].

Unprotected receptive anal sex is associated with an increased risk for acquiring an STI, including HIV [38, 39]. For this reason, sex between men is a significant factor in the HIV and other STI epidemics. However, the risk associated with insertional anal intercourse is significantly less than receptive [38, 39]. Interestingly, some HIV-positive MSM report choosing lower-risk sexual positions to avoid disclosing their serostatus and to reduce the transmission of HIV [38]. There is also some evidence that HIV-negative MSM also use this sexual positioning strategy and practice unprotected insertional anal intercourse slightly more often than receptive, possibly to decrease their own risk of acquiring HIV [39]. Bisexuality contributes to the spread of HIV and other STIs from MSM to wider populations. Thus, the transmission of STIs and HIV among the heterosexual populations is likely through both vaginal and anal intercourse.

Special populations with high prevalence of STIs in the United States include sex workers, persons in detention centers, homeless persons, and those with traveling professions [40, 41]. The highest rates of STIs among male and female sex workers are among those who use illicit drugs, such as heroin, cocaine, and methamphetamine [41]. The increased risk for STIs in sex workers may be associated with an increased number of partners, riskier partners, and more unprotected sex [42, 43]. In addition, professions involving frequent travel and extended periods away from family, such as serving in the military and long haul trucking, are also associated with an increased risk of acquiring an STI [44–46]. These special populations can also contribute to linking populations that may otherwise be segregated. Efforts should be focused on these populations to control the spread of STIs.

Other behaviors that are associated with increased risk of STIs are drug and alcohol use. Alcohol and drug use among teens are associated with increased sexual activity (more often and with more partners), increased risk of pregnancy, decreased condom use, and increased risk for contracting an STI [47]. These substances may lower inhibitions and lead to risky sexual behavior. Other delinquent behaviors such as physical fighting and carrying weapons are also associated with increased sexual activity.

After adjusting for socioeconomic status and behavioral differences, there is still a racial disparity in STI prevalence across a wide range of pathogens [48, 49]. This is likely because people select sexual partners based on attributes such as age, sex, sexual preference, race/ethnicity, socioeconomic background, marital status, and geographic location and tend to choose partners similar to themselves. This tendency for assortative mixing leads to segregated sexual networks and is likely to blame for the persistent racial differences in STI rates in the United States [50]. However, sexual bridging by disassortative mixing helps spread infections between populations or sexual networks [51, 52].

3.4 Media and Sexual Behavior

Today's society is constantly exposed to sex in the media. Prominent sources of exposure are music, television, magazines, and the Internet. Studies suggest that the effects of media on teen sexuality may vary by sex and ethnicity. Exposure to suggestive content on TV may be associated with higher rates of sexual activity among adolescents [53]. This is unlikely a cause-and-effect type of relationship, but rather a function of parental monitoring. Subsequent studies found that girls who viewed sexual content on television had more sexual experience and less sexual empowerment than other girls, while few effects were noted in boys [54]. In another study, exposure to sexual content in any media form was related to earlier sexual debut among white, but not African American adolescents [55].

Recent data show that 90% of American adolescents have access to the Internet at home or at school [56, 57]. Teens spend much of their free time communicating with partners and potential partners on the Internet through email, chat rooms, or some form of instant messaging. A study of adolescents who were frequent chat room users found that the teens were intrigued by risk, likely to experiment with drugs and alcohol, and almost twice more likely to be sexually active than peers who were not frequent Internet users [58]. Another study reported that young adults who found partners via the Internet had a higher risk for acquiring STIs [59]. These studies suggest that frequent Internet users have riskier sexual behavior than adolescents who do not frequently use the Internet.

Adolescents in the United States have higher rates of pregnancy and STIs than teens in other developed countries like Canada, Great Britain, and Sweden, even though they share similar rates of sexual activity [60, 61]. Teen pregnancy rates are influenced by restricted access to and high costs of contraceptives and other reproductive health services, while the high STI rates are associated with more sexual partners and lower levels of condom use [60]. The lower rates of adverse sexual outcomes in Canada and European countries may be due to a more accepting social attitude toward teenage sexuality and greater access to contraceptives and condoms [61].

3.5 Psychological Perspectives of Sexual Behavior

Psychological factors, such as mood, mental health, and even personality types, may affect risk of contracting STIs, as well as presentation for and response to treatment.

For example, extroverts are more likely to have an earlier sexual debut than introverts. Extroversion is also associated with having sex more frequently, having a greater number of lifetime partners, and trying more sexual positions [62, 63]. From these data it seems that an outgoing personality may contribute to more risk-taking behavior. Contrary to this, though, assertive personality types are also more likely to use condoms [64, 65].

In addition, psychiatric disorders may affect sexual behavior. Patients who scored high on a neuroticism scale tended to report lower levels of sexual satisfaction, and significantly higher scores on excitement, nervousness, sexual hostility, sexual guilt, and sexual inhibition [63, 66]. Additionally, depressed and dysphoric moods are associated with decreased condom use [64, 65].

Several studies suggest that sexual, physical, or emotional abuse in childhood or as an adult can predict risky sexual behavior, increased risk of STIs, and mental health problems. In one study, African American adult rape victims were six times more likely to report more than ten lifetime partners and three times more likely to report not using condoms consistently [67]. In several studies using STI clinical attendees, abuse was significantly more prevalent in the STI sample than the non-STI sample, with the effects being stronger in females than males [68, 69]. In a psychiatric treatment sample, abused versus non-abused adolescents were more likely to report higher rates of STIs, less frequent condom use, and less impulse control [70]. In a study of Native American women, those who had been physically or emotionally abused as children were five times more likely to report having had an STI than the non-abused women [71]. In addition, minority women (African American and Hispanic) with an STI who reported a history of abuse reported more psychological distress than minority women with an STI who did not report abuse [72]. Sexual abuse is also associated with high-risk behaviors associated with STIs in the MSM population [73].

Family relations also influence teenage sexuality. Teens that live in less cohesive households, such as single-parent households, are more likely to have an earlier sexual debut, as well as teenage pregnancy [47, 74, 75]. In addition, a study of African American adolescent females found that even moderate psychological distress was associated with increased risk of STIs [76].

Psychological responses to STI diagnoses can also vary among patients. It has been estimated that 40% of patients attending STI clinics have been classified as having psychiatric problems on the basis of screening tests [77]. Patients with a history of psychotic illness are more likely to have abnormal psychological reactions to STI diagnoses. Patients also feel a varying degree of personal guilt associated with acquiring STIs, with women feeling more shame and isolation than men [78]. Reactions to HIV infection are often more extreme than other STIs because the fully developed disease is generally fatal and associated with stigmatization. Negative societal and interpersonal reactions to acquired immune deficiency syndrome (AIDS) may be internalized in those who are infected and lead to guilt and self-blame. HIV diagnosis is also associated with disbelief and denial, followed by depressed mood and social isolation [79]. Another study suggests that the psychological symptoms associated with HIV change as the disease progresses through different phases (asymptomatic, mild symptomatic, severe, and terminal) [80]. For example, mood states in the asymptomatic and mild symptomatic phase were characterized by anger, while the terminal phase brought on feelings of loneliness. Feelings of powerlessness and helplessness were expressed in all phases of HIV/AIDS. Some patients with STIs also develop psychosexual problems or sexual dysfunction secondary to pain from the infection or fear of infection, reinfection, or infection of others [77].

Certain psychological factors may also contribute to recurrence of STIs such as herpes simplex virus (HSV). In a study that compared people with HSV, gonorrhea, and a control group without STI, both the HSV and gonorrhea group reported significantly increased anxiety and other psychological complaints [81]. However, HSV is unique in that these negative psychological symptoms are associated with recurrence. HSV recurrence is more likely in patients who report negative life events, depression, low self-esteem, anxiety, anger, and social alienation [82]. In this way, HSV and the associated psychological consequences can become a repeating cycle of recurrence.

Still other patients refuse to see STI as an illness, but rather as a chance event, and do not alter their behavior accordingly. This attitude is more common among patients being diagnosed for the first time than in those with repeat STIs [83]. If a patient fails to acknowledge they have a disease, they may jeopardize their treatment by discontinuing medications when symptoms have resolved, or continue risky sexual behavior before their infection has been cleared, increasing the likelihood of transmission.

In addition, prophylactic and therapeutic treatments may lead to a false sense of security and behavioral disinhibition. In a recent study, MSM patients who perceived HIV infection as low in severity had a significantly increased likelihood of infection with STIs or HIV [84]. On the other hand, a high perceived severity of HIV infection seems to induce sexual behavior that protects against sexually transmitted diseases (STDs) and HIV infection [84]. In addition, the availability of highly active antiretroviral therapy (HAART) for the treatment of HIV/AIDS may lead to more risky sexual behavior among MSM. In support of this, a recent longitudinal study suggested an increased risk of STIs and HIV in MSM related to decreased perceived threat of HIV/AIDS since the availability of HAART [85]. Also, several studies have demonstrated that male circumcision reduces the risk of acquiring HIV by approximately 50% [86]. However, circumcision alone does not provide complete protection and this information should not give men a false sense of security.

In conclusion, while the incidence of STIs is largely dependent on the distribution and prevalence of infection in the population, it is also important to consider the behavior of an individual and his or her partner(s), as well as their psychological state. As always, it is important to counsel patients on safe sexual behavior in order to avoid contracting HIV and other STIs.

Take-Home Pearls

- The spread of STIs is influenced by the distribution and prevalence of STIs in the population, as well as the behavior of an individual and his or her partner(s).
- The term "sexual behavior" encompasses many components including sexual experience and activity, age at sexual debut, current and lifetime number of sexual partners, frequency of sexual intercourse, consistency of sexual activity, mode of recruitment of sexual partners, duration of sexual relationships, and types of sexual practice.
- It is likely that certain socioeconomic conditions modify sexual behavior.
- Sexuality is shaped by both biological and environmental cues.
- There is a longstanding trend toward earlier sexual debut occurring worldwide.
- Young age at first sexual intercourse has been associated with more lifetime partners, even after adjusting for more years of sexual activity.
- Most adults and adolescents report practicing "serial monogamy" with steady partners.
- Having multiple concurrent partners has been shown to play a fundamental role in the spread of chlamydia, gonorrhea, syphilis, and human immunodeficiency virus (HIV).
- Individuals alter their protective and contraceptive methods depending on their assessment of risk associated with a sexual encounter.
- Age affects sexual behavior and STI rates.
- Unprotected receptive anal sex is associated with an increased risk for acquiring an STI.
- Special populations with high prevalence of STIs in the United States include sex workers, persons in detention centers, homeless persons, and those with traveling professions.
- Exposure to suggestive content on TV may be associated with higher rates of sexual activity among adolescents.
- Psychological factors, such as mood, mental health, and even personality types, may affect both risk of contracting STIs and presentation for and response to treatment.
- Sexual, physical, or emotional abuse in childhood or as an adult may predict risky sexual behavior, increased risk of STIs, and mental health problems.

References

1. Aral, S.O., Cates Jr., W.: The multiple dimensions of sexual behavior as risk factor for sexually transmitted disease: the sexually experienced are not necessarily sexually active. Sex. Transm. Dis. **16**(4), 173–177 (1989)
2. Wellings, K., Collumbien, M., Slaymaker, E., et al.: Sexual behaviour in context: a global perspective. Lancet **368**(9548), 1706–1728 (2006)
3. Bloom, D., Mahal, A., Sevilla, J., River Path Associates: AIDS & economics. Commission on Macroeconomics and Health Working Paper Series (2001)
4. Brown, B.: Peer groups and peer cultures. In: Feldmann, S.S., Elliott, G.R. (eds.) At the Threshold: The Developing Adolescent, pp. 171–196. Harvard University Press, Cambridge (1990)
5. Berndt, T.J.: Developmental changes in conformity to peers and parents. Dev. Psychol. **15**, 608–616 (1979)
6. Bill, J.O., Udry, J.R.: The influence of male and female best friends on adolescent sexual behavior. Adolescence **20**, 21–32 (1985)
7. Upadhyay, U.D., Hindin, M.J.: Do perceptions of friends' behaviors affect age at first sex? Evidence from Cebu, Philippines. J. Adolesc. Health **39**, 570–577 (2006)
8. Bearman, P.S., Bruckner, H.: Power in numbers: peer effects on adolescent girls' sexual debut and pregnancy. National campaign to prevent teen pregnancy: research monographs, Washington (1999)
9. Carver, K., Joyner, K., Udry, J.R.: National estimates of adolescent romantic relationships. In: Florsheim, P. (ed.) Adolescent Romantic Relationships and Sexual Behavior: Theory, Research and Practical Implications, pp. 25–53. Lawrence Erlbaum Associates, Mahwah (2003)
10. Santelli, J.S., Lindberg, L.D., Abma, J., McNeely, C.S., Resnick, M.: Adolescent sexual behavior: estimates and trends from four nationally representative surveys. Fam. Plann. Perspect. **32**, 156–194 (2000)
11. Gates, G.J., Sonenstein, F.L.: Heterosexual genital sexual contact among adolescent males: 1988 and 1995. Fam. Plann. Perspect. **32**, 295–297, 304 (2000)
12. Friedman, H.L.: Changing patterns of adolescent sexual behavior: consequences for health and development. J. Adolesc. Health **13**, 345–350 (1992)
13. Kost, K., Forrest, J.D.: American women's sexual behavior and exposure to risk of sexually transmitted diseases. Fam. Plann. Perspect. **24**, 244–254 (1992)
14. Bogaert, A.F., Fisher, W.A.: Predictors of university men's number of sexual partners. J. Sex Res. **32**, 119–130 (1995)
15. Norris, A.E., Ford, K.: Sexual experiences and condom use of heterosexual, low-income African American and Hispanic youth practicing relative monogamy, serial monogamy, and nonmonogamy. Sex. Transm. Dis. **26**, 17–25 (1999)
16. Ellen, J.M., Cahn, S., Eyre, S.L., Boyer, C.B.: Types of adolescent sexual relationships and associated perceptions about condom use. J. Adolesc. Health **18**, 417–421 (1996)
17. Potterat, J., Zimmerman-Rogers, H., Muth, S., et al.: Chlamydia transmission: concurrency, reproduction number, and the epidemic trajectory. Am. J. Epidemiol. **150**(12), 1331–1339 (1999)
18. Koumans, E., Farely, T., Gibson, J.: Characteristics of persons with syphilis in areas of persisting syphilis in the United States: sustained transmission associated with concurrent partnerships. Sex. Transm. Dis. **28**, 497–503 (2001)

19. Rosenberg, M.D., Gurvey, J.E., Adler, N., Dunlop, M.B., Ellen, J.M.: Concurrent sex partners and risk for sexually transmitted diseases among adolescents. Sex. Transm. Dis. **26**(4), 208–212 (1999)
20. Manhart, L.E., Aral, S.O., Holmes, K.K., Foxman, B.: Sex partner concurrency: measurement, prevalence and correlates among urban 18-39 year olds. Sex. Transm. Dis. **29**(3), 133–143 (2002)
21. Kretzschmar, M., Morris, M.: Measures of concurrency in networks and the spread of infectious disease. Math. Biosci. **133**(2), 165–195 (1996)
22. SJ, G.A.C., Garnett, G.P.: The role of sexual partnership networks in the epidemiology of gonorrhea. Sex. Transm. Dis. **24**(1), 45–56 (1997)
23. Morris, M., Kretzschmar, M.: Concurrent partnerships and the spread of HIV. AIDS **11**(5), 641–648 (1997)
24. Weller, S.C., Davis, K.R.: Condom effectiveness in reducing heterosexual HIV transmission. Cochrane Database Syst. Rev. **1**, CD003255 (2002)
25. Wald, A., Langenberg, A.G., Link, K., Izu, A.E., Ashley, R., Warren, T., Tyring, S., Douglas Jr., J.M., Corey, L.: Effect of condoms on reducing the transmission of herpes simplex virus type 2 from men to women. JAMA **285**(24), 3100–3106 (27 June 2001)
26. Mosher, W.D., Chandra, A., Jones, J.: Sexual behavior and selected health measures: men and women 15-44 years of age, United States, 2002. Adv. Data **362**, 1–55 (2005)
27. Shafii, T., Stovel, K., Holmes, K.: Association between condom use at sexual debut and subsequent sexual trajectories: a longitudinal study using bio-markers. Am. J. Public Health **97**, 1090–1095 (2007)
28. DM, M.M., Artz, L.M., Hook, E.W.: Partner type and condom use. AIDS **14**(5), 537–546 (2000)
29. Parsons, J.T., Schrimshaw, E.W., Wolitski, R.J., et al.: Sexual harm reduction practices of HIV-seropositive gay and bisexual men: serosorting, strategic positioning, and withdrawal before ejaculation. AIDS **19**(Suppl 1), S13–S25 (2005)
30. Centers for Disease Control and Prevention: Sexually Transmitted Disease Surveillance, 2004. Department of Health and Human Services, Atlanta (2005)
31. Lycke, E., Lowhagen, G.-B., Hallhagen, G., et al.: The risk of transmission of genital *Chlamydia trachomatis* infection is less than that of genital *Neisseria gonorrhoeae* infection. Sex. Transm. Dis. **7**, 6–10 (1980)
32. Gragson, S., Nyamukapa, C.A., Garnett, G.P., et al.: Sexual mixing patterns and sex-differentials in teenage exposure to HIV infection in rural Zimbabwe. Lancet **359**, 1896–1903 (2002)
33. North, R.L.: Partner notification and the threat of domestic violence against women with HIV infection. N. Engl. J. Med. **329**(16), 1194–1196 (1993)
34. Fortenberry, J.D., McFarlane, M., Bleakley, A., et al.: Relationship of stigma and shame to gonorrhoea and HIV screening. Am. J. Public Health **92**(3), 378–381 (2002)
35. Voeten, H., O'Hara, H.B., Kusimba, J., et al.: Gender differences in health care seeking behavior for sexually transmitted diseases. Sex. Transm. Dis. **31**(5), 265–272 (2004)
36. Nusbaum, M.R.: Therapeutic options for patients returning to sexual activity. J. Am. Osteopath. Assoc. **104**(3 suppl 4), S2–S5 (March 2004). Review
37. Zablotsky, D., Kennedy, M.: Risk factors and HIV transmission to midlife and older women: knowledge, options, and the initiation of safer sexual practices. J. Acq. Immun. Def. Synd. **33**(suppl 2), S122–S130 (2003)
38. Van de Ven, P., Kippax, S., Crawford, J., et al.: In a minority of gay men, sexual risk practice indicates strategic positioning for perceived risk reduction rather than unbridled sex. AIDS Care **14**(4), 471–480 (2002)
39. Koblin, B.A., Husnik, M.J., Colfax, G., et al.: Risk factors for HIV infection among men who have sex with men. AIDS **20**(5), 731–739 (2006)
40. Aral, S.O., Ward, H.: Modern day influences on sexual behavior. Infect. Dis. Clin. N. Am. **19**(2), 297–309 (2005)
41. Ward, H., Aral, S.O.: Globalization, the sex industry and health. Sex. Transm. Infect. **82**, 345–347 (2006)
42. Haley, N., Roy, E., Leclerc, P., et al.: HIV risk profile of male street youth involved in survival sex. Sex. Transm. Infect. **80**, 526–530 (2004)
43. Weber, A.E., Boivin, J.F., Blais, L., et al.: HIV risk profile and prostitution among female street youths. J. Urban Health **79**, 525–535 (2002)
44. Bloom, D., Mahal, A., Rosenberg, L., Sevilla, J., Steven, D., Weston, M.: Asia's Economies and the Challenge of AIDS. Asian Development Bank, Manila (2004)
45. Mahal, A., Rao, B.: HIV/AIDS epidemic in India: an economic perspective. Indian J. Med. Res. **121**, 582–600 (2005)
46. Carswell, J.W., Lloyd, G., Howells, J.: Prevalence of HIV-1 in East-African lorry drivers. AIDS **3**(11), 759–761 (1989)
47. Kirby, D., Lepore, G., Ryan, J.: Sexual risk and protective factors: factors affecting teen sexual behavior, pregnancy, childbearing and sexually transmitted disease: Which are important? Which can you change? www.health.state.nm.us/phd/fp/Forms/risk%20 and%20protective%20factors Execsummary_kirby.pdf. Accessed 30 Mar 2009
48. Ellen, J., Kohn, R., Bolan, G., Shiboski, S., Krieger, N.: Socioeconomic differences in sexually transmitted disease rates among black and white adolescents, San Francisco, 1990 to 1992. Am. J. Public Health **85**, 1546–1548 (1995)
49. Ellen, J., Aral, S., Madger, L.: Do differences in sexual behaviors account for the racial/ethnic differences in adolescents' self-reported history of sexually transmitted disease? Sex. Transm. Dis. **25**, 125–129 (1998)
50. Laumann, E.O., Youm, Y.: Racial/ethnic group differences in the prevalence of sexually transmitted diseases in the United States: a network explanation. Sex. Transm. Dis. **26**(5), 250–261 (1999)
51. Laumann, E.O., Gagnon, J.H., Michael, R.T., Michaels, S.: The Social Organization of Sexuality. University of Chicago Press, Chicago (1994)
52. Rothenberg, R.B., Potterat, J.J.: Temporal and social aspects of gonorrhea transmission: the force of infectivity. Sex. Transm. Dis. **15**, 88–92 (1987)
53. Ashby, S.L., Arcari, C.M., Edmonson, B.M.: Television viewing and the risk of sexual initiation by young adolescents. Arch. Pediatr. Adolesc. Med. **160**, 375–380 (2006)
54. Tolman, D.L., Kim, J.L., Schooler, D., Sorsoli, C.L.: Rethinking the associations between television viewing and adolescent sexuality development: bringing gender into focus. J. Adolesc. Health **40**, 84 (2007)
55. Brown, J.D., L'Engle, K.L., Pardun, C.J., Guo, G., Kenneavy, K., Jackson, C.: Sexy media matter: exposure to sexual content in music, movies, television, and magazines predicts black and white adolescents' sexual behavior. Pediatrics **117**, 1018–1027 (2006)
56. Rideout, V., Roberts, D.F., Foehr, U.G.: Generation M: Media in the Lives of 8-18 Year Olds. Kaiser Family, Menlo Park (2005)

57. Stahl, C., Fritz, N.: Internet safety: adolescents' self report. J. Adolesc. Health **31**, 7–10 (2002)
58. Beebe, T.J., Asche, S.E., Harrison, P.A., Quinlan, K.B.: Heightened vulnerability increased risk-taking among adolescent chat room users: Results from a statewide school survey. J. Adolesc. Health **35**, 116–123 (2004)
59. McFarlane, M., Bull, S.S., Rietmeijer, C.A.: Young adults on the Internet: Risk behaviors for sexually transmitted diseases and HIV. J. Adolesc. Health **31**, 11–16 (2002)
60. Panchaud, C., Singh, S., Reivelson, D., Darroch, J.E.: Sexually transmitted diseases among adolescents in developed countries. Fam. Plann. Perspect. **32**(1), 24–32 (2000)
61. Darroch, J.E., Frost, J.J.: Differences in teenage pregnancy rates among five developed countries: the roles of sexual activity and contraceptive use. Fam. Plann. Perspect. **33**(5), 244–250 (2001)
62. Eysenck, H.J., Eysenck, S.B.G.: Manual of the EPI. London University Press, London (1964)
63. Eysenck, H.J.: Sex and Personality. Abacus, London (1978)
64. Ross, M.W.: Personality factors which differentiate homosexual men with positive and negative attitudes toward condom use. NY State J. Med. **88**, 626–628 (1988)
65. Ross, M.W.: Psychological determinants of increased condom use and safer sex in homosexual men: a longitudinal study. Int. J. STD AIDS **1**, 98–101 (1990)
66. Hart, G.: Sexual Maladjustment and Disease: An Introduction to Modern Venereology. Nelson-Hall, Chicago (1977)
67. Wingood, G.M., DiClemente, R.J.: Rape among African American women: sexual, psychological and social correlates predisposing survivors to risk of STD/HIV. J. Womens Health **7**, 77–84 (1998)
68. Pitzner, J.K., et al.: A history of abuse and negative life events in patients with a sexually transmitted disease and in a community sample. Child Abuse Negl. **24**, 715–731 (2000)
69. Petrak, J., et al.: The association between abuse in childhood and STD/HIC risk behaviours in female genitourinary medicine clinic attendees. Sex. Transm. Infect. **76**, 457–461 (2000)
70. Brown, L.K., et al.: Impact of sexual abuse on the HIV-risk-related behavior of adolescents in intensive psychiatric treatment. Am. J. Psychiat. **157**, 1413–1415 (2000)
71. Hobfoll, S.E., et al.: The impact of perceived child physical and sexual abuse history on Native American women's psychological well-being and AIDS risk. J. Consult. Clin. Psychol. **70**, 252–257 (2002)
72. Champion, J.D., et al.: Psychological distress among abused minority women with sexually transmitted diseases. J. Am. Acad. Nurse Pract. **14**, 316–324 (2002)
73. Bartholow, B.N.: Emotional, behavioral, and HIV risks associated with sexual abuse among adult homosexual and bisexual men. Child Abuse Negl. **18**, 747–761 (1994)
74. Whitbeck, L.B., Conger, R., Kao, M.-Y.: The influence of parental support, depressed affect, and peers on the sexual behaviors of adolescent girls. J. Fam. Issues **14**, 261–278 (1993)
75. Wu, L.L.: Effects of family instability, income, and income instability on the risk of a premarital birth. Am. Sociol. Rev. **61**, 386–406 (1996)
76. DiClemente, R.J., et al.: A prospective study of psychological distress and sexual risk behavior among black adolescent females. Pediatrics **108**, E85 (2001)
77. Catalan, J., Bradlet, M., Gallwey, J., Hawton, K.: Sexual dysfunction and psychiatric morbidity in patients attending a clinic for sexually transmitted diseases. Br. J. Psychiat. **138**, 292–296 (1981)
78. Pitts, M.K., et al.: Reactions to repeated STD infections: Psychosocial aspects and gender issues in Zimbabwe. Soc. Sci. Med. **40**, 1299–1304 (1995)
79. Faulstich, M.E.: Psychiatric aspects of AIDS. Am. J. Psychiat. **144**, 551–556 (1987)
80. Nilsson-Schonnesson, N.L., Ross, M.W.: Coping with HIV Infection: Psychological and Existential Responses in Gay Men. Kluwer/Plenum, New York (1999)
81. Stronks, D.L., Rijpma, S.E., Passchier, J., et al.: Psychological consequences of genital herpes: an exploratory study with a gonorrhea control group. Psychol. Rep. **73**, 395–400 (1993)
82. Longo, D., Koehn, K.: Psychosocial factors and recurrent genital herpes: a review of prediction and psychiatric treatment studies. Int. J. Psychiat. Med. **23**, 99–117 (1993)
83. Ross, M.W.: Illness behavior among patients attending a sexually transmitted disease clinic. Sex. Transm. Dis. **14**, 174–179 (1987)
84. van der Snoek, E.M., de Wit, J.B., Gotz, H.M., Mulder, P.G., Neumann, M.H., van der Meijden, W.I.: Incidence of sexually transmitted diseases and HIV infection in men who have sex with men related to knowledge, perceived susceptibility, and perceived severity of sexually transmitted diseases and HIV infection: Dutch MSM-Cohort Study. Sex. Transm. Dis. Mar. **33**(3), 193–198 (2006)
85. van der Snoek, E.M., de Wit, J.B., Mulder, P.G., van der Meijden, W.I.: Incidence of sexually transmitted diseases and HIV infection related to perceived HIV/AIDS threat since highly active antiretroviral therapy availability in men who have sex with men. Sex. Transm. Dis. **32**(3), 170–175 (Mar 2005)
86. Newell, M.L., Bärnighausen, T.: Male circumcision to cut HIV risk in the general population. Lancet **369**(9562), 617–619 (24 Feb 2007)

The Normal Genitalia – Structure and Physiology

4

Gunther Wennemuth and Walter Krause

4.1 Male Anatomy

4.1.1 Testis and Epididymis

4.1.1.1 Testis

The testis is comparable in size and shape to a plum. A normal testis has a volume of a mean 15 ml, being 5 cm in length and 3 cm in width. It is covered by three layers of connective tissue. The innermost layer is the tunica vasculosa, containing blood vessels. The tunica vasculosa is covered by the tunica albuginea, which is composed of dense connective tissue and the tunica vaginalis, which is part of the peritoneum, having descended during development of the testis. On the posterior apical part of the organ, blood vessels and nerves can enter through the mediastinum testis. The testicular tissue is made up of seminiferous tubules, convoluted ducts containing the stratified epithelium with different stages of spermatogenesis and spermiogenesis. In the most outer part of the seminiferous tubules (basal part), spermatogonia type A and type B are located on the basal membrane. Due to one mitotic and two subsequent meiotic divisions, cells of the spermatogenic series can be found with a different DNA content, namely primary (4n) and secondary spermatocytes (2n), spermatids (1n), and spermatozoa. The cells of the spermatogenic series are embedded in Sertoli cells reaching from the basal membrane to the lumen of the seminiferous tubules. Sertoli cells are important for controlling spermatogenesis and they produce androgen-binding protein. The seminiferous tubules are surrounded by myoid and fibroblast-like cells called peritubular cells. The areas between the tubules contain islands of the androgen-producing Leydig cells. The epididymis and the testis are connected by elongated tubules (efferent ductules), breaking through the tunica albuginea at the apical-posterior pole. Mature spermatozoa are transported through these efferent ductules into the epididymis, but infectious agents are also able to invade the testis in the opposite direction, causing orchitis. However, the main route of infection in the testis is that via the blood vessels (hematogenous). In contrast to the scrotum and the penis, the lymphatic drainage of the testis and the epididymis is not provided by inguinal or subinguinal lymph nodes. For these organs, the vessels run through the inguinal channel without passing any of the lymph nodes in this region. The first (regional) lymph nodes for the testis and the epididymis are located at the confluence of the testicular vein into the renal vein on the left side and the inferior cava vein on the right side (Figs. 4.1 and 4.2).

4.1.1.2 Epididymis

The epididymis is located posterior to the testis. The c-shaped organ is divided into three parts: caput, corpus, and cauda. The caput lies on top of the testis and meets the efferent ductule from the testis. They all merge into one single coiled duct called the epididymal duct, which is up to 6 m in length when unraveled.

G. Wennemuth (✉)
Department of Anatomy and Cell Biology, Saarland University, Building 61, 66424 Homburg, Saar, Germany
e-mail: gunther.wennemuth@uks.eu

W. Krause
Department Dermatology, and Allergology, Philipp University, Deutschhausstr. 9, 35033, Marburg, Germany
e-mail: krause@med.uni-marburg.de

G. Gross and S.K. Tyring (eds.), *Sexually Transmitted Infections and Sexually Transmitted Diseases*,
DOI: 10.1007/978-3-642-14663-3_4, © Springer-Verlag Berlin Heidelberg 2011

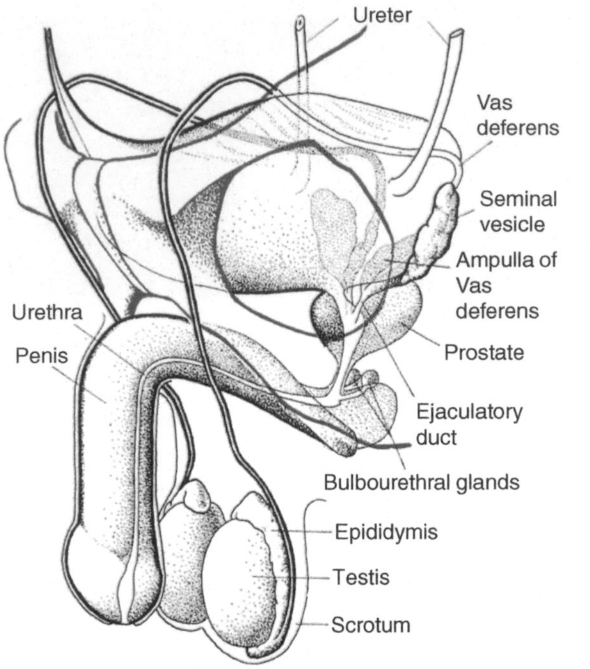

Fig. 4.1 Male genital tract (*black*) in relation to the pelvis (*red*) (Anatomie, Histologie, Entwicklungsgeschichte, makroskopische und mikroskopische Anatomie, Topographie, Theodor Heinrich Schiebler and Horst-Werner Korf, 2007, Springer, 10., vollständig überarbeitete Auflage)

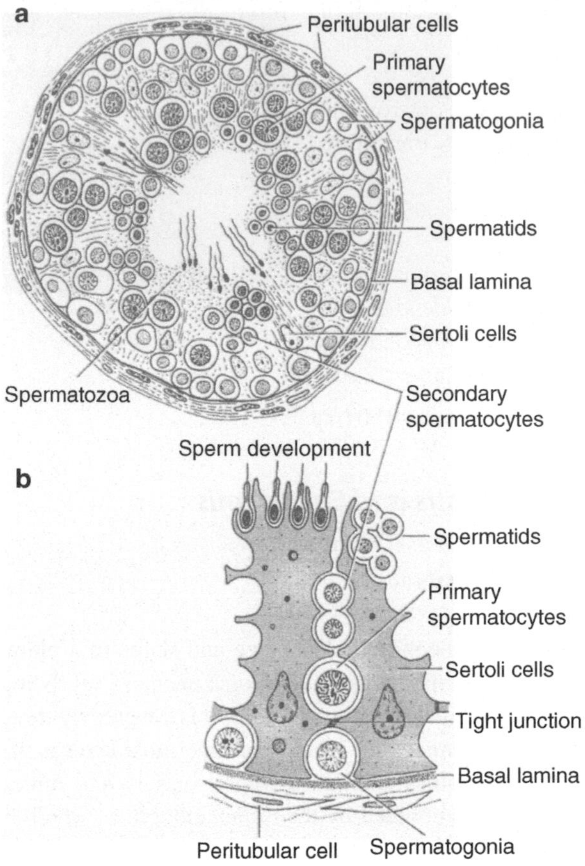

Fig. 4.2 Spermatogenesis. (**a**) Seminiferous tubule, overview. (**b**) Epithelia of seminiferous tubules (Anatomie, Histologie, Entwicklungsgeschichte, makroskopische und mikroskopische Anatomie, Topographie, Theodor Heinrich Schiebler and Horst-Werner Korf, 2007, Springer, 10., vollständig überarbeitete Auflage)

At the lower end (cauda epididymidis), the epididymal duct opens out into the vas deferens. The epididymal duct is lined by epithelium with two different cell types, columnar principal and short basal cells. The principal cells have oval nuclei in their basal part, the apical cell pole shows stereocilia. Their function is the secretion and absorption of fluid for continuous maturation during the passage of the spermatozoa through the epididymal duct, which can take up to 10 days. The passage of the immotile spermatozoa is ensured by peristalsis of smooth muscle cells, arranged in inner circular and outer longitudinal layers around the epididymal duct. At the cauda epididymidis, the spermatozoa have gained their motility and are further transported into the ductus deferens. Infectious agents may invade the epididymis in the opposite direction. An epidymitis is a typical disease resulting from sexually acquired infections with *Neisseria gonorrhoeae* and *Chlamydia trachomatis,* but also enterobacteria may cause inflammation, when the excreting ducts are disrupted.

4.1.1.3 Penis

Covered by a thin epidermis, the penis consists of three cylinder-shaped chambers that form the shaft; two corpora cavernosa and one corpus spongiosum. The corpora cavernosa are surrounded by dense connective tissue, the tunica albuginea, and they arise from the pelvic bone on each side with the penile crus to run parallel to the glans penis. The corpora cavernosa are connected to each other by small blood vessels. The corpus spongiosum contains the urethra and continues out into the glans penis. Connective tissue that covers all three corpora is called Buck's fascia and forms a tough membrane. The skin covering the penis is very expandable and mobile to allow erection.

Over the glans, the skin builds a double layer called foreskin (prepuce). The intact foreskin covers the glans completely; the secluded space enables infectious agents to destroy and invade the skin, thus facilitating sexually transmitted infections. Many studies show that the resection of the foreskin (circumcision) prevents the sexual transmission of HIV and other infections.

The dorsal artery of the penis is the final branch of the internal pudendal artery. It runs, together with the deep dorsal veins and nerves, along the dorsum penis to reach the glans. A second terminal branch of the internal pudendal arteria is the paired cavernosal artery that runs into the corpora cavernosa. Superficial and deep dorsal veins are separated by Buck's fascia. The glans penis and the corpora cavernosa release blood into the deep dorsal vein. The superficial dorsal vein receives blood from the prepuce and the penile skin. Vegetative innervation of the penis is responsible for erection and ejaculation. Sympathetic nerves from the lesser hypogastric plexus and parasympathetic fibers from sacral spinal segments reach the penis via the pudendal nerve. Nerve fibers running along the dorsum penis form the pudendal nerve. Through parasympathetic stimulation, vasodilatation and subsequent inflow of blood into the cavernous spaces as well as occlusion of the efferent veins occur and lead to erection. The lymphatic drainage of the penis and the scrotum is ensured by subinguinal lymph nodes and lymph nodes along the internal iliacal arteries. The scrotum is drained along inguinal lymph vessels and nodes.

4.1.1.4 Prostate

The prostate is located between the bladder and the pelvic floor and is a round-shaped structure with a weight of approximately 40 g. The prostatic part of the urethra is surrounded by prostatic tissue. The prostate is made up of three lobes and is divided into three zones: a peripheral, a transitional, and a central zone. The transitional zone surrounds the urethra directly above the ejaculatory ducts, coming from the seminal vesicle and the vas deferens. The central zone is located posterior to the transitional zone. The peripheral zone surrounds both the transitional zone and the central zone, in addition to the area found anterior to the urethra. The prostate gland consists of an epithelium, which is either pseudostratified or single layered and forms 40 to 50 branches of tubuloalveolar glands. The branches are divided by fibromuscular tissue arising from the capsule. The middle rectal, the internal pudendal, and the inferior vesical arteries release branches to the prostate. A venous plexus drains the blood into internal pudendal and inferior vesical vessels. The lymphatic drainage runs along the internal iliac vessels and they run toward their local lymph nodes of the same name. Other lymph nodes are sacral and obturator nodes.

The secretion of the prostate is slightly acidic and contains several proteins, mainly prostate specific antigen, glucose, acid phosphatase, fibrinolysin, and amylase. Irregular concrements called corpora amylacea are found in the lumen of the gland. The secretion is delivered into the posterior urethra and forms part of the seminal fluid (ejaculate), which is expulsed during ejaculation. Infectious agents may reach the prostate from the urethra in the opposite direction. The resulting prostatitis mainly affects the central and transitional zones.

4.1.1.5 Seminal Vesicle and Bulbourethral Glands

The seminal vesicle is a paired organ located laterally behind the bladder and in front of the rectum, separated by Denonvilliers' fascia. At their lower part, the seminal vesicles merge together with the vas deferens into the ejaculatory ducts. The blood vessels derive from or flow into the inferior vesical and middle rectal arteries or veins respectively. The gland tissue of the seminal vesicles consists of pseudostratified columnar epithelium, arranged in long tubular-shaped parts and attached by connective tissue containing circular and longitudinal smooth muscle cell layers. The secretion of the seminal vesicles accounts for most of the volume of the ejaculate and contains fructose as atypical secretory product. Infectious agents afflict the seminal vesicles mainly together with the prostate; glandulitis vesicalis is undistinguishable from prostatitis.

The bulbourethral glands (Cowper's glands) lubricate the urethra as a response to sexual arousal. In addition to galactose, the secretion contains sialic acid (Fig. 4.3).

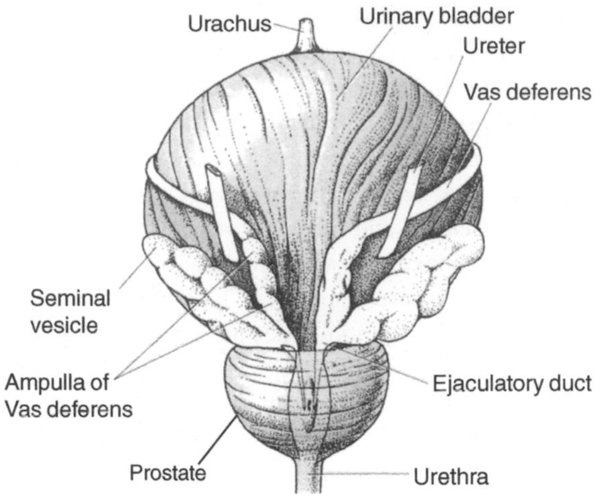

Fig. 4.3 Vas deferens, seminal vesicle and prostate in relation to the urinary bladder (view from dorsal) (Anatomie, Histologie, Entwicklungsgeschichte, makroskopische und mikroskopische Anatomie, Topographie, Theodor Heinrich Schiebler and Horst-Werner Korf, 2007, Springer, 10., vollständig überarbeitete Auflage)

4.2 Female Anatomy

4.2.1 Uterus

The uterus is a pear-shaped organ, approximately 7×5×2 cm in size. The upper part, located under the peritoneum, is called corpus uteri; the lower part reaches down to the vagina and is called cervix uteri. On the left and right sides, the corpus uteri continues into the uterine tube. A cavity between the corpus uteri and the posteriorly located colon is called the Douglas space. The bladder and the uterovesical space are located to the anterior of the corpus uteri. The uterus itself leans forward in relation to the vagina, which is called anteversion. An internal flexion of the uterus forms a concavity on the anterior side, the anteflexio. The conus-shaped cervix uteri ends with its external os, divided into anterior and posterior lips, in the vagina and with the internal os in the uterus. Along the endocervical canal, the cervical crypts function as glands, which produce the cervical mucus. The mucus undergoes cyclic changes with the menstrual cycle.

The cervix presents an open connection between the uterus and the vagina, which contains potentially infectious agents. The cervix mucus develops a special quality at the time of ovulation in order to allow a migration of spermatozoa which, however, also facilitates the permeation of infectious agents, partly attached to the spermatozoa. Passing the uterus and the uterine tubes, the agents also may reach the Douglas space (see above) and thus may cause "pelvic inflammatory disease."

The uterus has a strong blood supply. The uterine artery is a branch of the internal iliac artery, and the vessels of the right and left sides form many anastomoses. In addition, there are anastomoses with the ovarian artery and the vaginal artery. These arteries also supply blood to the vagina and the uterine tube. The veins run parallel to the arteries to reach the internal iliac vein. The microstructure of the uterus shows two areas: the endometrium and the myometrium. A layer of single columnar epithelial cells covers the endometrium. Deep retractions of the epithelium form the uterine glands, which change their secretion and shape during the menstrual cycle. Periodically, a part of the endometrium sloughs off under hormone's influence and is therefore called stratum functionalis, as opposed to the stratum basalis, which is responsible for the regeneration of the endometrium. At the cervix uteri there is a sharp change from the single columnar epithelium of the uterus to the multilayered epithelium of the vagina. Underneath the endometrium, a fibromuscular layer forms the myometrium. During pregnancy, hyperplasia of the smooth muscle cells of the myometrium permits the uterus to extend in size and shape. The lymphatic drainage of the uterus is assured along two different paths. The lymph vessels from the cervix reach the internal iliac lymph nodes, whereas the corpus uteri drains into lumbar lymphatic nodes.

4.2.2 Uterine Tubes

The infundibulum is the fimbriated part of the uterine tube close to the ovary. The next regions of the uterine tube (fallopian, oviduct) are ampulla, isthmus, and the connection to the uterus, the intramural part. The physiological place of fertilization is the ampulla. The mucosa is lined by ciliated and nonciliated (secretory) cells, which change under estrogen control. Underneath the mucosa, a lamina propria, a muscular layer, and a serosa form the wall of the uterine tube. Branches from the uterine and ovarian arteries supply blood to the Fallopian tube. The veins run parallel to the arterial vessels. Lymph

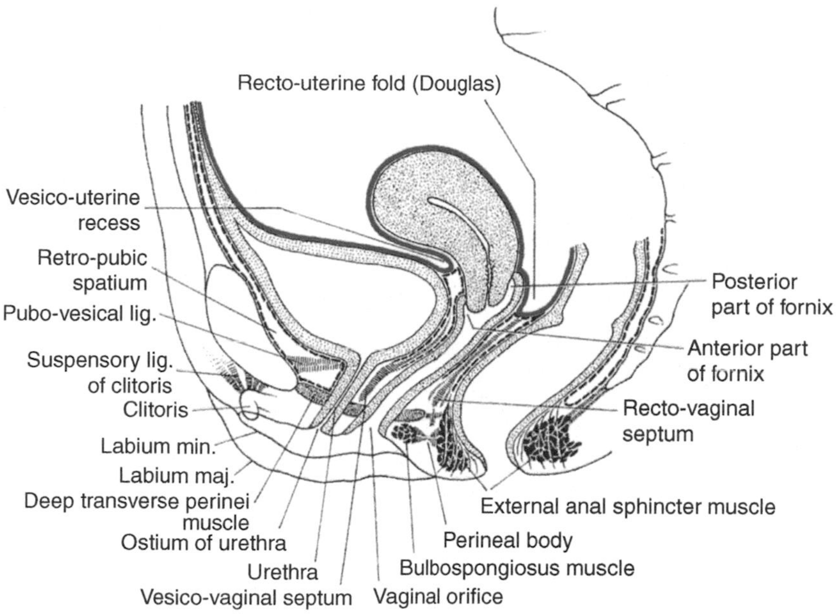

Fig. 4.4 Female pelvis in relation to the peritoneum (Anatomie, Histologie, Entwicklungsgeschichte, makroskopische und mikroskopische Anatomie, Topographie, Theodor Heinrich Schiebler and Horst-Werner Korf, 2007, Springer, 10., vollständig überarbeitete Auflage)

vessels and nodes of the uterine tube can be found along the aorta and the internal iliac vessels.

The endothelium of the tubes is highly vulnerable to inflammations caused by infectious agents, typically by *Neisseria gonorrhoeae* and *Chlamydia trachomatis*. The inflammations are usually combined with inflammations of the ovary and of the surrounding pelvic peritoneum ("pelvic inflammatory disease"). As a frequent consequence, partial or complete obstruction of the tubes and inhibition of tubal motility follow, which inhibit the transport of the oocyte. Infertility due to these pathologies is frequent. It may be overcome by in vitro fertilization (IVF) (Fig. 4.4).

4.2.3 Ovaries

The ovaries are intraperitoneal organs, located on the outer pelvic wall. As homologues to the testes, the ovaries contain the gametes called oocytes. The peritoneum expanding between the ovaries and the uterine tube is called mesosalpinx, between the ovaries and the uterus it is called mesometrium. The ovaries descend into the retroperitoneal space during their development. As a rudiment, they are connected to the suspensory ligament of the ovary in which the ovarian arteries run from the aorta to the ovaries. The veins first form several plexus to merge into the ovarian veins that run along the ovarian arteries. Finally, they merge into the renal vein on the left and into the vena cava inferior on the right side. The microstructure of the ovaries shows a cortex with the oocytes and follicles and a medulla with connective tissue, with an abundance of vessels and nerves. Different stages of oocyte development can be found in the cortex. The primordial follicles are single oocytes surrounded by a flat single-layered epithelium. After the single-layered epithelium becomes cuboid and a glycoprotein layer surrounds the oocyte (zona pellucida), the follicles are called primary follicles. Secondary follicles are defined as oocyte with an epithelium that forms multiple layers that differentiate in the theca interna and the theca externa. The mature follicle is called Graafian follicle and shows, in addition, a fluid-filled antrum with the oocyte and remnants of the theca (corona radiata) at its border (cumulus oophorus). During the process of ovulation, the Graafian follicle ruptures and releases the oocytes into the ampulla of the uterine tube. The lymphatic drainage of the ovary passes along lumbar vessel and lymph nodes (Fig.4.4).

4.2.4 Vagina

The vagina, 6–8 cm long and 2–3 cm wide, reaches from the labia minora to the uterus. The wall is made

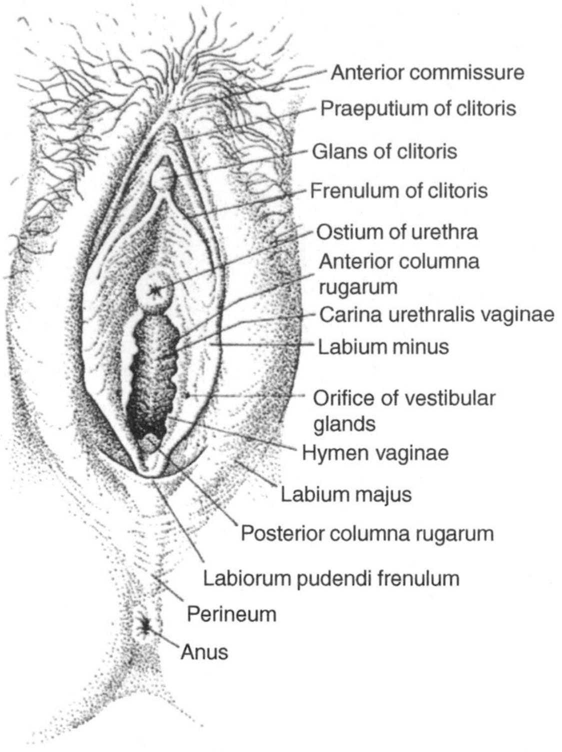

Fig. 4.5 Female external genital organs (vulva) (Anatomie, Histologie, Entwicklungsgeschichte, makroskopische und mikroskopische Anatomie, Topographie, Theodor Heinrich Schiebler and Horst-Werner Korf, 2007, Springer, 10., vollständig überarbeitete Auflage)

up of fibrous tissue and muscular layers, which are lined in the inner part by stratified nonkeratinized epithelium, which may be invaded by the papilloma virus, but is resistant to most sexually transmissible agents. The keratinocytes store large amounts of glycogen and change their characteristics along with the menstrual cycle. At the uterine cervix, the epithelium becomes single columnar. At a transformation zone, the distribution of the two epithelial types may vary with different endocrine conditions and throughout the menstrual cycle. Uterine, internal pudendal, and middle rectal arteries release blood vessels to the vagina. A lateral plexus is formed by the vaginal veins. The lymphatic drainage occurs through the internal and external iliac nodes and the superficial inguinal nodes (Fig. 4.5).

4.2.5 Female External Genital Organs (Vulva)

The old anatomical term "vulva" describes the visible external female genitalia, which include labia minora and majora, mons pubis, the clitoris, vestibule and vestibular bulb, and glands. The lateral boundaries of the pudendal cleft are formed by the labia majora with the labia minora in-between. In front of the pubic symphysis, connective tissue and fat form the mons pubis. The anterior ends of the labia majora border a cavity called vestibule that ends at the clitoris, the homologue to the penis. All parts of the vulva are covered with a thin epidermis, which is a keratinizing epithelium. They are often erroneously classified as mucous membranes. The orificium externum urethrae is located below the clitoris, where *Neisseria gonorrhoeae* and *Chlamydia trachomatis* may ingress. The greater vestibular glands, also called glands of Bartholin and corresponding to the male bulbourethral glands, open into the vestibule between the labia minora and the hymen, a thin fold of mucous membrane within the vaginal orifice. The lymph vessels of the vulva run through the inguinal channel where they reach their local lymph nodes (Fig. 4.6).

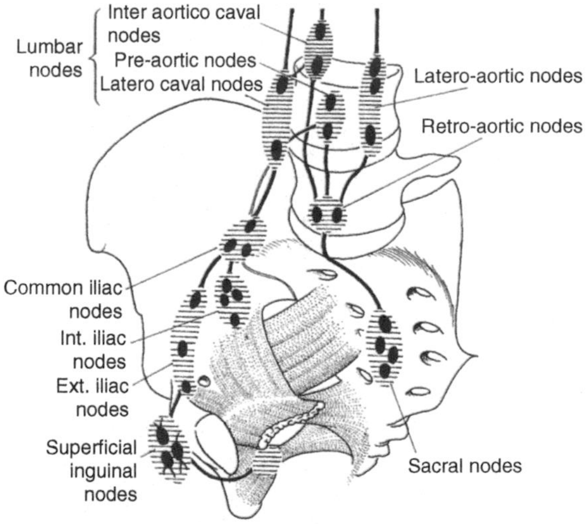

Fig. 4.6 Regional lymph nodes and lymph vessels in the subperitoneal tissue of the pelvis (Anatomie, Histologie, Entwicklungsgeschichte, makroskopische und mikroskopische Anatomie, Topographie, Theodor Heinrich Schiebler and Horst-Werner Korf, 2007, Springer, 10., vollständig überarbeitete Auflage)

Mucosal Immunity in Sexually Transmitted Infections

5

Anthony L. Cunningham, Suzanne M. Garland, Heather Donaghy, and Min Kim

Core Messages

- Vaccines and immunotherapies are urgently required for sexually transmitted diseases which are persistent and for which there is no cure.
- Progress in their rational development is limited by an incomplete understanding of the mechanisms of immune control of these STIs.
- For some STIs vaccine stimulation of just one immune modality has been sufficient, such as neutralizing antibody for human papillomavirus.
- However where there is little progress the complete spectrum of potential immune control mechanisms must be considered and explored, such as HIV, Herpes simplex and Chlamydial vaccines.
- This is leading to a focus on under investigated immune mechanisms, particularly mucosal innate immunity and adaptive cellular immunity.
- There have been major recent advances in understanding the importance of innate humoral mechanisms such as antimicrobial peptides, vaginal mucus, and cellular elements such as NK cells and macrophages in HIV, chlamydia and herpes simplex viral infection.
- Comparisons between gastrointestinal and genitourinary mucosal immune mechanisms reveal both distinct similarities and differences.

A.L. Cunningham (✉) and M. Kim
Centre for Virus Research, Westmead Millennium Institute, University of Sydney, Westmead, PO Box 412, Westmead, NSW 2145, Australia
e-mail: tony.cunningham@sydeny.edu.au; min.kim@sydeny.edu.au

S.M. Garland
Department of Microbiology and Infectious Diseases, Royal Women's Hospital, Department of Obstetrics and Gynecology, University of Melbourne, Murdoch Childrens Research Institute, Melbourne, Australia
e-mail: suzanne.garland@thewomens.org.au

H. Donaghy
Centre for Virus Research, Westmead Millennium Institute, Westmead, Australia
e-mail: heather.donaghy@sydeny.edu.au

5.1 General Overview

Sexually transmitted organisms invade both male and female genital tracts (MGT and FGT) and some also invade the gastrointestinal (GI) tract (e.g., HIV, herpes simplex virus [HSV]). The immune systems of the MGT and FGT are tightly regulated to allow reproductive functions but resist invasion by viruses, bacteria, fungi, and protozoa, while allowing the presence of beneficial commensal organisms in some sites.

There is a hierarchy of immune defenses, partly in order of evolutionary sophistication, which include physical barriers, innate immunity, humoral, and cellular immunity. Immune effectors may be locally produced or systemically derived with local homing/diffusion. There is a common mucosal immune system whereby induction of antibodies or other effectors in the respiratory or GI mucosa home to the genital mucosa but this is not as effective as locally induced immunity (e.g., for mucosal vaccines).

There are broad similarities between genital and GI tract mucosal immunity, especially as tolerance either to the enveloping fetus or food antigens/commensal bacteria, respectively, is required (see section below for discussion).

G. Gross and S.K. Tyring (eds.), *Sexually Transmitted Infections and Sexually Transmitted Diseases*,
DOI: 10.1007/978-3-642-14663-3_5, © Springer-Verlag Berlin Heidelberg 2011

In considering how to manipulate the immune system for development of new vaccines or immunotherapy for sexually transmitted infections (STIs), the emphasis is now on organisms which cannot be eradicated by antibiotics, viruses such as HIV, human papillomavirus (HPV), and HSV, and bacteria increasing in incidence such as *Chlamydia trachomatis*.

5.1.1 Male Genital Tract

The MGT consists of testes, efferent ducts, epididymis, ejaculatory ducts, ductus deferens, urethra, and penis. The posterior urethra is lined by transitional epithelium like the bladder and the anterior urethra by columnar epithelium. STI pathogens may infect via the penile skin or via the urethral opening. The penile skin consists of tough stratified squamous epithelium with a thick superficial protective stratum corneum. Beneath this layer, keratinocytes as well as resident better-recognized cells of the immune system such as Langerhans cells (LCs) and T lymphocytes are the next line of defense. In the foreskin the stratum corneum is thinner and the distribution of epidermal LC is denser [96]. Recently collections of T lymphocytes in pseudofollicles have been defined.

5.1.2 Female Genital Tract

The FGT is highly specialized into different compartments such as the sterile intrauterine cavity and fallopian tubes and the lower genital tract, consisting of the vagina, vulva, and ectocervix, colonized by complex diverse and dynamically changing commensal bacteria. All compartments are under tight control of sex hormones, which also control immune mechanisms. The vulva, vagina, and ectocervix are lined with tough stratified squamous epithelium with a thick stratum corneum over the labia majora, progressively thinning to be lost in the vagina. The thickness of the vaginal epithelium varies throughout the menstrual cycle, being thickest under estrogen control. Progestogens are used to artificially thin the vaginal mucosa in animal models of STIs [89]. The vaginal luminal pH is also under sex hormone control as estrogens increase mucosal glycogen, which is metabolized by *Lactobacillus* spp. that predominates in sexually active women. The endocervix and a variable proportion of the inner ectocervix around the endocervical os are composed of columnar epithelium interspersed with mucus-secreting ciliated cells which also contribute to antibacterial defences. The ectocervical transformation zone (TZ) at the junction of squamous and columnar epithelium is highly responsive to sex hormones and highly immunologically active being densely populated with antigen-presenting cells and T lymphocytes [121]. It is at the TZ that most cervical cancers arise. The endocervical mucus is a significant barrier to ascending infection from the vagina. It varies in viscosity and thus protects pathogen immobilization throughout the menstrual cycle, being least viscous at ovulation and absent during menstruation.

Commensal bacteria of numerous species (including *Lactobacilli*) adherent to vulval skin/mucosa and in the lumen of the vagina create a hostile environment for pathogens, e.g., glycogen metabolizing lactobacilli lower the pH to nonoptimal levels for pathogens.

5.2 Innate Immunity

The innate immune system is the evolutionarily primitive rapid response system to STIs. Innate responses can be classified as humoral, including interferons (IFNs), cytokines, chemokines, antimicrobial peptides, or cellular, consisting of macrophages, natural killer (NK) cells, or dendritic cells (DCs; myeloid and plasmacytoid). Myeloid dendritic cells (mDCs) bridge the innate and adaptive immune systems, demonstrating another feature of innate immunity, preparing the slower more specific adaptive immune responses which also possess memory to expedite more rapid response to second exposure with a given pathogen (Table 5.1).

Table 5.1 Innate immune mechanisms

Humoral	Type 1 interferons Cytokines Chemokines Natural antimicrobial peptides
Cellular	Macrophages NK cells pDCs (NK cells and $\gamma\delta$T cells)

5.2.1 Role of Epithelial Cells

The epithelium of the MGT and FGT is the first barrier to STIs and consists of immunoreactive epithelial cells and specialized resident immune cells. Both genital tract keratinocytes and cuboidal/columnar epithelial cells sense pathogen-associated molecular patterns (PAMPs) with surface and cytoplasmic pattern recognition receptors (PRRs). The Toll-like receptors (TLRs) are the best characterized of these PRRs. Both types of epithelial cells can synthesize antimicrobial peptides, including β-defensins, cytokines, and chemokines and in the presence of STIs induce inflammation, express major histocompatibility complex II (MHC II), and can even present microbial antigens to T cells, i.e., they are an integral part of the innate immune system.

5.2.2 Antimicrobial Peptides

The epithelium of the genital tract constitutively secretes various (natural) antimicrobial peptides, including the enzymes lactoferrin, lysozyme, cathelicidin, secretory leucocyte protease inhibitor (SLPI), surfactant protein A (SP-A), elafin, defensins (especially human β-defensin 2, hBD-2) and the cytokines, IL-1, IL-6, and TGF-β (Table 5.2, [25]). These proteins kill bacteria and restrict viral infection and also regulate macrophages and DCs. For example, SLPI and hBD-2 inhibit HSV and HIV infection and the latter activates macrophages and is chemotactic for DCs (reviewed in [72, 123]).

5.2.3 Pattern Recognition Receptors

Several families of PRRs, including the TLRs, cytoplasmic RIG-I-like receptors (RLRs) and NOD-like receptors (NLRs), in epithelial, endothelial, and innate immune cells recognize PAMPs to activate the innate immune system. These PAMPs may be proteins, lipids, carbohydrates, or nucleic acids in viruses, bacteria, fungi, and protozoa. TLRs 1, 2, 4, 5, 6, and 10 are expressed on the plasma membrane and TLRs 3 and 7–9 are on endosomal membranes of immune cells. TLRs 3, 7/8, and 9 recognize viral double-stranded RNA (dsRNA), single-stranded RNA (ssRNA), and CpG DNA, respectively, after acid proteolytic digestion of viruses in the endosome. TLRs 2 and 6 recognize some viral proteins and lipoproteins at the cell surface [69]. TLR1, 2, and 4–10 signaling occurs through an Myd88-dependent pathway and TLR3 signaling through an Myd88-independent pathway, resulting in either NF-κB nuclear translocation or interferon regulatory factor (IRF) activation and then either proinflammatory cytokine or IFN secretion. TLR signaling may also result in DC maturation and macrophage phagocytosis (Fig. 5.1).

RLRs include the cytoplasmic RNA helicase, RIG-I, and MDA5 and PKR. Most cell types recognize viral RNA through the RLRs RIG-I and MDA5 in the cytosol. The main ligand for RIG-I is ssRNA containing a 5'-triphosphate, generated by many viral RNA polymerases. It can also be activated by short fragments of dsRNA. However, MDA5 is the main cytoplasmic receptor for longer molecules of viral dsRNA and for poly-I:C [17].

Cytosolic NLRs provide a third reserve for response to PAMPs and also respond to damage-associated molecular patterns (DAMPs). Signaling may result in programmed cell death [152].

Table 5.2 Natural antimicrobial peptides

Peptide	Site of Production	Action
Secretory leukocyte Protease inhibitor (SLPI)	Upper and lower FGT	Blocks viral infection. Anti-inflammatory/antiproteolytic
Lactoferrin	Lower FGT Neutrophils	Blocks viral infection
Lysozyme	Lower FGT Neutrophils	Antiviral
Surfactant protein β-defensins	Upper and lower FGT	Blocks viral infection. Chemotactic for DCs and T cells

FGT female genital tract

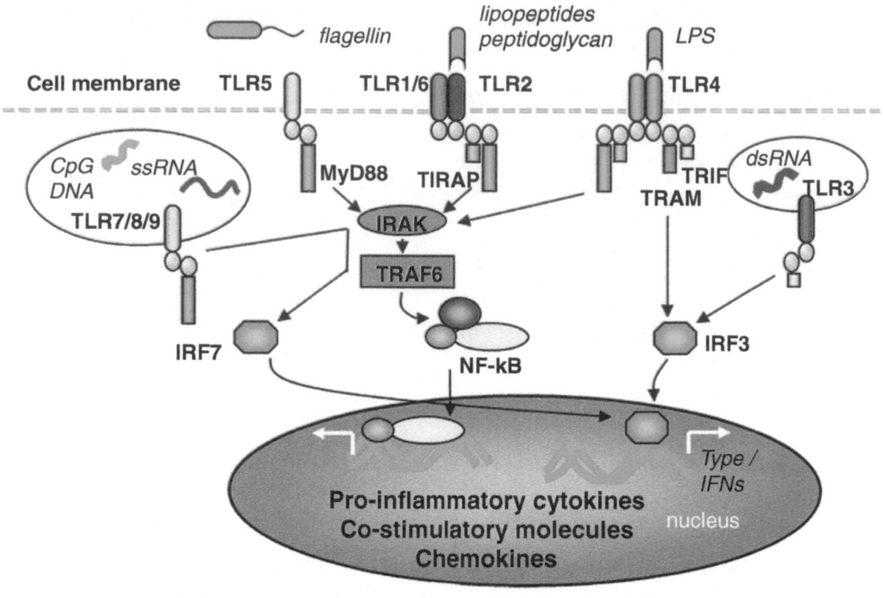

Fig. 5.1 TLR signaling pathways. The majority of TLRs signal via the MyD88 adaptor molecule. TLR-1 and TLR-6 form heterodimers with TLR-2 on the cell surface and ligand binding triggers the recruitment of MyD88 plus a second adaptor molecule, TIRAP, which associate with the TLR via their TIR domains. This sets off a signaling cascade that results in the activation of the transcription factor NF-κB and the production of pro-inflammatory cytokines, chemokines, and co-stimulatory molecules. TLR-5 and intracellular TLR-7, TLR-8, and TLR-9 signal via a similar MyD88-dependent pathway; however, the latter three may also induce activation of IRF-7, which in turn leads to the production of type I interferons. TLR-4 forms homodimers on the cell surface and may signal via the MyD88-dependent pathway, via TIRAP or may signal via an MyD88-independent pathway, through the adaptor molecules TRIF and TRAM, to activate IRF3 and the production of type I IFNs. Intracellular TLR3 is also capable of MyD88-independent signaling, associating directly with TRIF, for the production of type I interferons (From the Ph.D., thesis of Kerrie Sandgren, University of Sydney, 2008)

5.2.4 Macrophages

Macrophages in the genitourinary (GU) tract are replenished by monocytes emigrating from blood vessels (monocytes may also differentiate into DCs in inflammatory conditions). Macrophages actively phagocytose organisms, can kill infected cells, produce key proinflammatory cytokines such as IL-1, IL-6, and TNF-α, and present antigens to T cells, especially when surface MHC II is upregulated after activation by IFN-γ or TNF-α. However, the antigen-presenting function of macrophages is local as they do not migrate to local lymph nodes and also cannot prime naive T cells. In other mucosal sites such as gut, suppressor D1+ D7+ macrophages contribute to tolerance but D7+ effector macrophages appear to predominate in the cervix [2].

5.2.5 Natural Killer Cells

NK cells are a key component of innate immune defences, able to respond directly to pathogens or infected cells without prior sensitization. They are distributed throughout the body in primary and secondary lymphoid tissues, including intestinal and genital mucosa, and also throughout the uterus, cervix, and vagina. Human NK cells are divided into two subsets based on their surface density of CD56 molecules, which are $CD56^{bright}CD16^{dim/-}$ and $CD56^{dim}CD16^{+}$ subsets. The former produces abundant cytokines such as IFN-γ, GM-CSF, and TNF-α with low cytotoxicity, whereas the latter are more cytotoxic with low cytokine production [26, 62]. $CD56^{bright}$ NK cells also express MHC II and can present antigen [61]. In the upper FGT, the latter subset appears to dominate and NK cell density varies through the menstrual cycle, unlike the lower FGT [153]. CD56^{bright}CD16$^{dim/-}$ NK cells express homing markers for secondary lymphoid organs such as CCR7 and CD62L. NK cells can lyse target cells that have lost or express low amounts of MHC I molecules, especially cells infected by certain herpes viruses, including HSV. NK cells are sustained by IL-15 and activated by IL-12 and Type I IFNs [40].

5.2.6 Mucosal Dendritic Cells

DCs are heterogeneous, ubiquitous, and the most potent of antigen-presenting cells. They are classified as plasmacytoid dendritic cells (pDCs) or mDCs with the latter being either migratory or resident in lymphoid tissues [131]. Migratory DCs include LCs and interstitial DCs include dermal or lamina propria DCs in stratified squamous and cuboidal/columnar epithelium, respectively [64]. In mice there are five different types of DCs in mucosa/skin and at least a similar number in draining lymph nodes but not all these types have equivalents in humans as yet [131]. In the anogenital region they are distributed throughout the anogenital skin and mucosa including the vagina or ectocervix as well as the male foreskin. Recently, a distinct subset of langerin-expressing dermal DCs has been identified in mice following epithelial LCs knockout [21, 53, 122]. The human homolog is yet to be identified.

DCs express PRRs such as C-type lectin receptors (CLRs) and TLRs, to bind and capture pathogens and, through their signaling pathways, DCs bridge the innate and adaptive immune systems. The CLRs expressed by skin DCs differ by site: langerin by epidermal LCs and DC-SIGN and mannose receptor by dermal DCs. Epidermal LCs form a tight network with each other and with the surrounding keratinocytes via E-cadherin (Fig. 5.2). While sessile in the skin/mucosa, they are immature and highly endocytic, but after pathogen binding, they become mature, migratory, and downregulate endocytosis. LCs are characterized ultrastructurally by the presence of racket-shaped vesicles, Birbeck granules, which contain langerin endocytosed from the cell surface. They also express CD1a and Fc receptors for IgG, which enables them to take up pathogen-containing

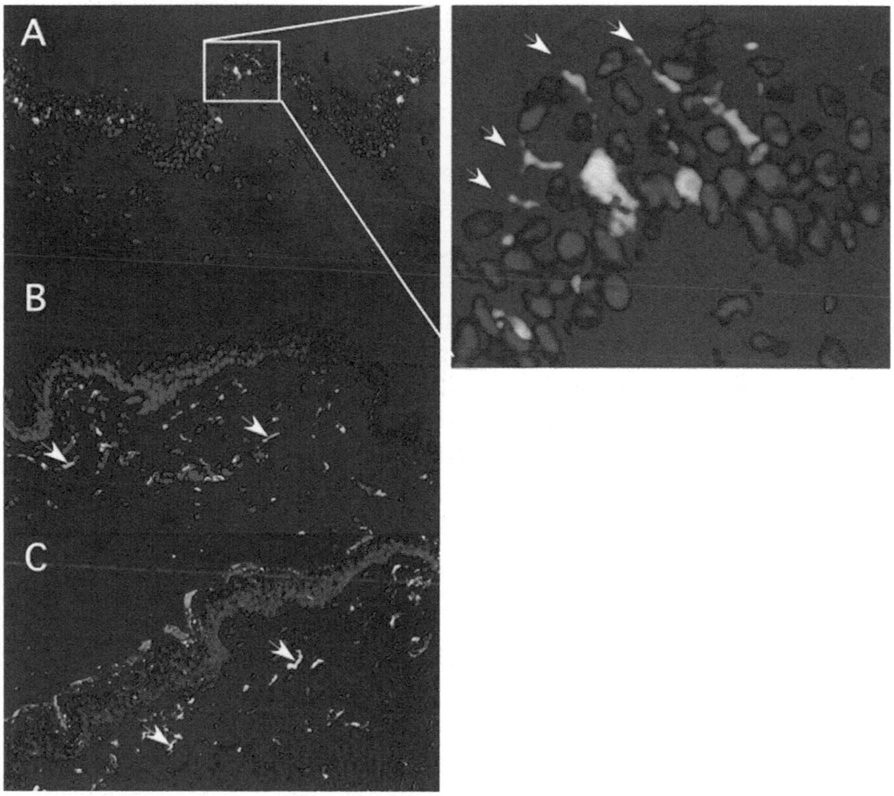

Fig. 5.2 Expression of CLRs on DC subsets in sections of skin. Cryostat sections of skin were stained with primary mAbs, then washed and stained with goat anti-mouse IgG. Cellular nuclei were detected by propidium iodide after immunofluorescent staining. Representative samples are shown. (**a**) Langerin staining on epidermal LCs. *Arrows* indicate langerin staining on LC cytoplasmic processes. (**b**) MR staining on dermal cells. (**c**) DC-SIGN staining on dermal cells. *Arrows* indicate representative MR$^+$ and DC-SIGN$^+$ cells. (**a–c**) Magnification: ×200. (**a**) Inset is magnified a further ×4 (Reproduced from [144]. With permission)

immune complexes [72]. Like other mDCs, LCs are able to bridge innate and adaptive immunity. They are able to interact directly with microorganisms at the periphery to produce effector cytokines or initiate or restimulate activation of T and B lymphocytes through antigen presentation. In some settings LCs may play an immunosuppressive rather than immunostimulatory role in certain inflammatory diseases of skin [27], with dermal DCs being immunostimulatory [73].

Migratory DCs such as LCs are in an immature, highly endocytic state while sessile in the skin/mucosa. However, after pathogen binding to TLRs and uptake, they become mature and migratory, downregulating their endocytic and antigen-processing capacity. Interestingly, maturation of myeloid DCs has recently been shown to freeze the capacity to process antigens through the MHC I but not the MHC II pathway, resulting in the preservation of capture and processed pathogen peptide epitopes on the migrating DCs [155].

Viruses infecting humans through skin or mucosa such as HIV, the herpesviruses, including HSV and varicella-zoster virus (VZV), poxviruses such as vaccinia virus and HPV interact with LCs (and other mucosal DCs) in different ways. Two opposing aspects to this virus–DC interaction need to be considered: infection of LCs by viruses and the immune responses of LCs to the infecting or captured virus.

5.2.7 Plasmacytoid Dendritic Cells (pDCs)

pDCs are important in both innate and adaptive immune responses. First, they produce IFN-α in response to stimulation with live or inactivated enveloped viruses, including HIV and HSV, to limit viral spread [43, 94, 128, 133]. Following viral interactions pDCs upregulate co-stimulatory molecules, which, coupled with cytokine secretion, allow them to present antigen and stimulate different T cells, including naive effector and regulatory T cells [44, 76, 80, 112].

5.3 Adaptive Immunity

The specific adaptive immune response usually follows initial innate immune mechanisms and also consists of humoral and cellular components.

5.3.1 Humoral Immunity

The role of systemic and mucosal antibody responses in preventing or clearing STIs is difficult to differentiate in many STIs. Both systemic and locally produced immunoglobulins (mainly IgG) are found in cervicovaginal secretions and semen. However, IgG dominates over IgA in these secretions, unlike the GI tract, because of the paucity of specialized inductive lympho–epithelial structures, such as Peyer's patches, although such tissue has recently been described in the ectocervical TZ [86]. Furthermore, mucosal immunization of the FGT produces much weaker local immunoglobulin responses than with intranasal, oral, or rectal immunization. The homing mechanisms of B lymphocytes to the genital tract mediating the latter responses are poorly defined but appear to differ from those to the GI tract, as the key homing receptor, MadCAM-1, is not expressed in the vascular endothelium of cervicovaginal mucosa [75]. Local responses to pathogens in the MGT also appear to be weak. The efficacy of systemic neutralizing IgG in controlling some cervicovaginal STIs is well shown by the recently successful phase 3 randomized controlled trials of a bivalent HPV16/18 L1 [118] and quadrivalent HPV6, 11, 16, and 18 prophylactic vaccines which utilize the outer coat protein (L1) formed as virus-like-particles (VLPs) and which when introduced systemically produce high titre, sustained levels of neutralizing antibodies several fold greater than that produced naturally [51, 118]. Another example is passive immunization of monkeys with systemic antibodies to simian immunodeficiency virus (SIV) against vaginal challenge with the virus [100].

5.3.2 Cell-Mediated Immunity

Until recently the classic paradigm was suggested to be that antigens from pathogens invading the epithelium were taken up by mucosal DCs, LCs in stratified squamous epithelium, and conveyed to draining lymph nodes where specific CD4, CD8, and B lymphocytes were generated and cycled back to the inflamed epithelium, guided by chemokine gradients. This was postulated to occur in both initial and

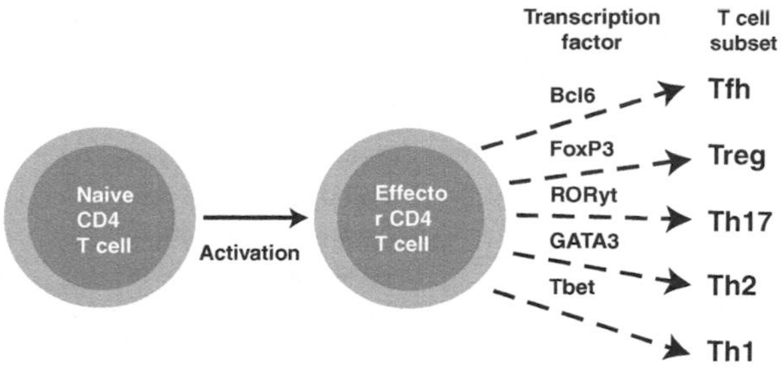

Fig. 5.3 T cell subsets which are regulated by transcription factors

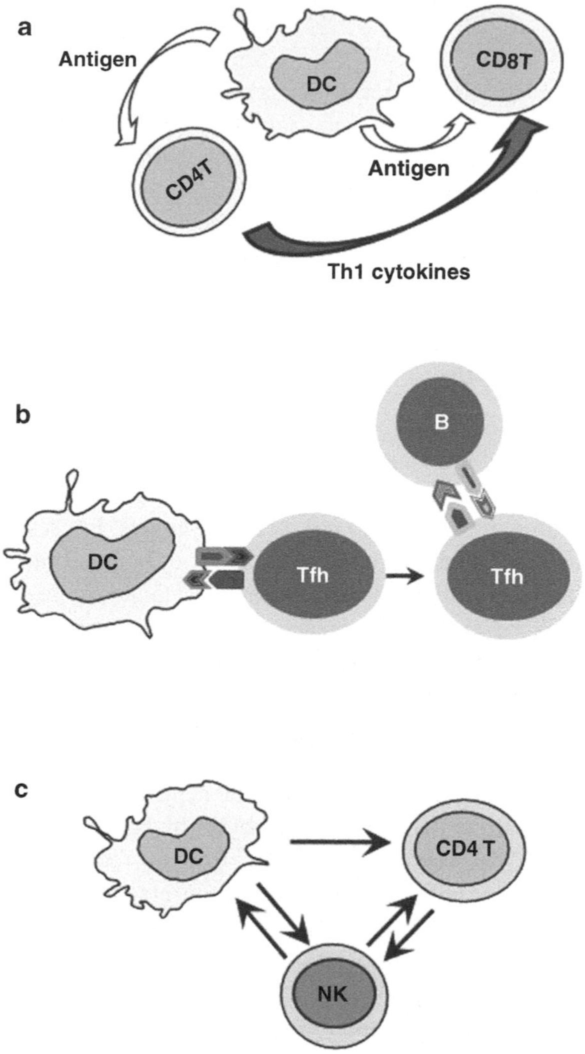

Fig. 5.4 Key interactions between DCs and lymphocytes. (**a**) DC interaction with CD4 and CD8 T lymphocytes. DCs can present antigens directly to CD8 or CD4 T lymphocytes in an MHC I or MHC II restricted fashion, respectively. However, for optimal CD8 T lymphocyte responses, CD4 T lymphocyte help byTh1 cytokines is usually required. (**b**) DC interaction with T cells and B cells in the lymph node. DCs and follicular helper T cells (Tfh) initially interact followed by Tfh-B lymphocyte interaction to provide optimal antibody responses to protein antigens. (**c**) DC interactions with NK cells and CD4 T lymphocytes. Recently it has become clear that there is "cross talk" between NK cells and CD4 T lymphocytes and also in a triad with DC, which leads to optimum CD4 T lymphocyte responses to antigens processed and presented by DCs

recurrent infections. As shown by the sections on HSV and HIV this paradigm is now being markedly modified. DC antigen uptake and transfer to T cells is much more complex involving cooperation of multiple subtypes of DCs. Generation of local memory T cells allows local interactions to occur rapidly with frequently recurring pathogens such as HSV.

Furthermore, a number of new subtypes of T cells have been defined (Fig. 5.3) which, according to the cytokine patterns, secreted different regulating transcription factors. Several are important in the mucosa, including Th17 and regulatory T cells.

Furthermore, multiple interactions between DCs and T cells and other cell types such as NK, NKT, and Tγδ cells are now known to modulate immune effector interactions against pathogens in the mucosa [114] (Fig. 5.4).

5.3.3 Comparison Between Genital and Gastrointestinal Tract Immunity

There are broad similarities between immune defences in these two sites. Gut and genital tract epithelial cells are immunologically reactive, producing antimicrobial peptides, cytokines, and chemokines and can present antigen. Commensal bacteria are present in both gut and MGT/lower FGT, although at lower concentrations and diversity in the latter. Both sites are now known to contain lymphoid aggregates (including Peyer's patches in gut) and similar complements of antigen-presenting and T lymphocytes, including activated memory cells. Differences include the greater density of organized lympho-epithelial tissue in the gut and ease of inducing local immunoglobulin and especially IgA responses in the GI tract. This has been reviewed recently by Shacklett et al. [130].

5.4 Specific Diseases

The following section on specific diseases provides examples of key persistent viral and chlamydial infections and diseases, which often cannot be completely eradicated by specific antivirals and are the subject of ongoing research for adequate vaccines or immunotherapy.

5.4.1 HIV

Mucosal immune mechanisms may be involved in the pathogenesis of HIV or the closely related SIV in four different ways: immune cells as targets for sexual transmission, barriers to or control over initial infection, control of chronic infection, and targets or mediators of immunodeficiency, especially inappropriate activation of T lymphocytes, macrophages, and pDCs. Although the first two have been extensively investigated in the genital tract, especially in SIV-macaque models, in the latter two the focus has been on the GI tract where most lymphoid tissue depletion occurs and activation of tissue T lymphocytes by bacterial endotoxin has been demonstrated. Recently comparative studies of immune control in chronic infection between genital and GI tracts have been initiated. Studies of genetic polymorphisms have provided clear indications of important immune mechanisms involved in progression to immunodeficiency, such as HLA-B57 and B27, but some of these also may play a role in the control of initial infection such as NK cell receptors and IL-10 polymorphisms [22].

5.4.1.1 Sexual Transmission of HIV and Infection of Immune Cells in the Genital Tract

During sexual transmission the highly heterogeneous quasi-species of HIV present in humoral or cellular components of male or female genital secretions is highly selected. Only CCR5 using variants are selected, usually only a single genotype except where inflammation is present. The cellular targets of activated and resting CD4 lymphocytes, macrophages, and DCs are abundant in the genital tract, especially where there is coinfection with ulcerating STIs such as HSV (see below). Prior infection with HSV-2 increases the risk of acquisition of HIV by three- to fourfold [47, 147].

There is now strong evidence supporting the role of LCs, the major HIV-infectable constitutive cell type in the anogenital stratified squamous epithelium, in HIV and SIV transmission [68, 108, 110] (Fig. 5.5). Vaginal SIV infection of Rhesus macaques resulted in infected LCs in the vaginal mucosa within a day of infection. After topical infection of human vaginal epithelial explants with HIV LCs and nonactivated T lymphocytes were the major cell types expressing HIV antigen in the mucosa. After emigration from the explants in doublets HIV antigen was concentrated at their contact region suggesting that LCs were transferring HIV to the CD4 lymphocytes [68]. GFP-labeled HIV is able to penetrate between the keratinocytes of the stratified squamous epithelium of human ectocervical epithelium to depths of 50 μm to be captured by LCs [67]. In a series of elegant studies in SIV-infected macaques Haase and Miller showed that SIV first appeared beneath the epithelium predominantly in resting CD4 lymphocytes (with a small proportion in activated CD4 lymphocytes), spreading through the submucosa in foci fuelled by immigrating CD4 lymphocytes over a period of 2–3 days, followed by spread to draining lymphocytes by the end of 1 week, and thereafter into the systemic circulation [92, 109]. Thus LCs probably preserve and transport HIV to CD4 lymphocytes in the submucosal lymphoid tissue (which are first infected) and thence to draining lymph nodes [68, 108, 158].

LCs are difficult to isolate from human tissues in sufficient amounts, so monocyte-derived DCs (MDDCs) have often been used as models to investigate interactions with HIV. Most of the HIV inoculum (>95%) is endocytosed and the remaining <5% (cis-) transferred directly to surface CD4 and CCR5 resulting in viral–cell membrane fusion and infection. Immature DCs and LCs express high levels of CCR5 but on maturation CCR5 is downregulated and CXCR4 upregulated, resulting in reduced infectability by CCR5 using (R5) HIV strains. Viral endocytosis leads to rapid acid-proteolytic degradation of HIV in the late endosome. In contrast, HIV entry via fusion leads to *de novo* productive infection. When DCs containing HIV contact activated or resting CD4 lymphocytes, HIV is rapidly transferred across a "viral synapse" to lymphocytes in two distinct phases: first

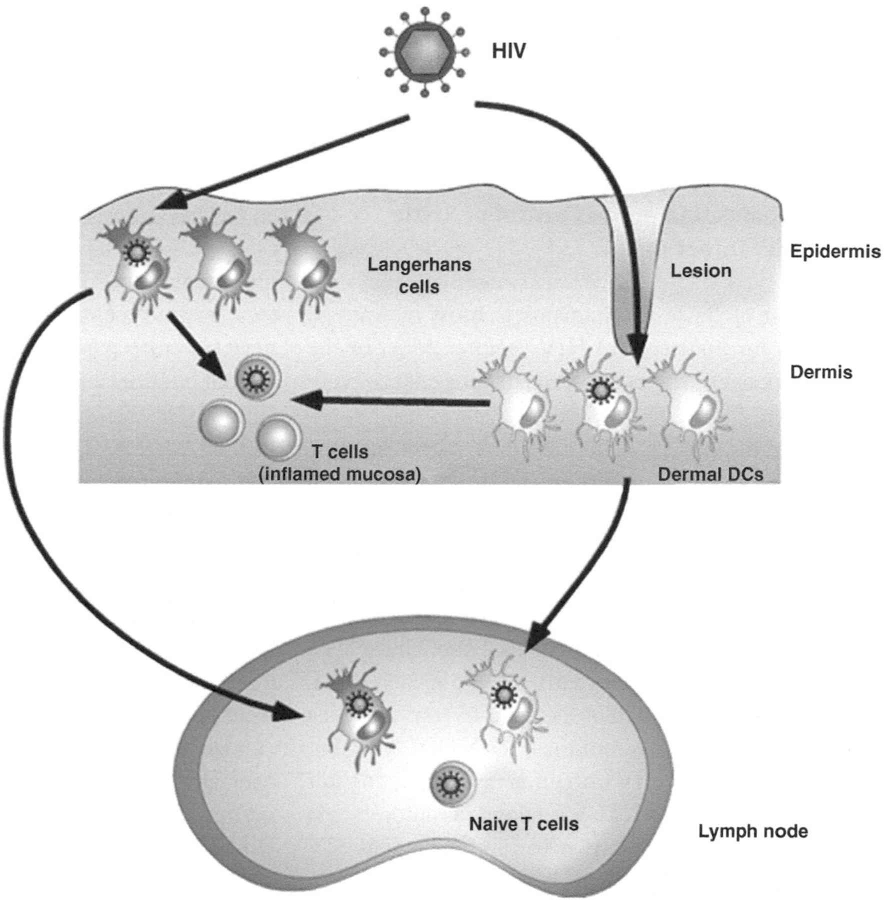

Fig. 5.5 HIV infection of Langerhans cells and/or dermal DCs that reside within an intact or breached mucosa. Infection of the DCs is likely to result in the transfer of virus to CD4+ T cells either locally in the dermis or within a distal lymph node (Reproduced from [151])

from surface accessible (s/a) vesicles and later from the cytosol [145]. The "viral synapse" is sealed and protected from antibody entry by interaction of adhesion molecules ICAM1 (CD54) and LFA1 respectively [45, 49, 58, 97]. CD4 and CCR5 are concentrated on the enclosed lymphocyte membrane. HIV-containing s/a vesicles are diverted to the contact region, fuse with the cell membrane, and expel their load of residual HIV into the synapse. Two-phase transfer has also been demonstrated in primary blood myeloid DCs [135]. In LCs the existence of these two stages is less clear. Several studies have demonstrated that de novo replication of R5 HIV in LCs is essential to their role in transmission [82, 125]. However, CD34+ -derived LC-like cells can also transmit HIV to T lymphocytes from s/a vesicles without infection [38]. The role of langerin on LCs after HIV capture and internalization into LC-specific vesicular organelle Birbeck granules for degradation (like MDDC endosomes) is controversial with one report that cis-transfer of HIV to CD4/CCR5 does not occur, differing from the DC-SIGN function on MDDCs [33] and another group reported evidence that langerin played no role in HIV transfer (although under their experimental conditions langerin is markedly downregulated [81]). This controversy about the relative roles of langerin and CD4/CCR5 in binding and entry of HIV into LCs is complicated by the utilization of mature LCs and low HIV inocula and variable read-outs and requires further clarification [28, 145].

HIV containing DCs may present viral antigen to specific CD4 lymphocytes activating and also transferring HIV to them, thus resulting in their death and perhaps explaining the selective depletion of HIV-specific CD4 lymphocytes [37, 93]. Recent studies from our laboratory and others show that HIV infection of DCs or LCs induces partial maturation and enhanced migration [63, 150]. The partial maturation is sufficient to enhance T lymphocyte stimulation and might also enhance DC–T cell contact and viral transfer, thus affecting both viral production and antiviral immunity.

5.4.1.2 Mucosal Immune Control of Acute HIV Infection

Elucidation of these mechanisms is most relevant to the search for a successful HIV vaccine. Most of the innate immune mechanisms have not been exhaustively investigated, partly because of the need to use expensive SIV-macaque models. However, there is now a major emphasis on exploring all mucosal immune mechanisms.

In innate immunity, physical barriers such as mucus are important in immobilizing HIV prior to entry. Antimicrobial peptides such as SLPI, lactoferrin, cathelicidin, and human β-defensins 2 and 3 have been shown to inhibit infection in vitro. Some, such as SLPI, also have immunomodulatory actions on the host immune cell. The β chemokines, RANTES, MIP-1α, and MIP-1β, block HIV infection by competing for binding to CCR5. RANTES analogs, as microbicide candidates, have been shown to inhibit vaginal SIV challenge in macaque models. Increased levels of these chemokines have been demonstrated in cervical washings from commercial sex workers who are frequently exposed to HIV via unprotected sex but remain uninfected. Blood pDCs secreting IFN-α are depleted during HIV infection and this appears to be at least partly due to viral infection [36, 137]. These cells also play a role in the genital tract as they have been shown to emigrate into the cervix after SIV infection of macaques [92]. IFN-α and IFN-β inhibit HIV replication at multiple points in its replication cycle. Once the virus enters cells there are also a number of intracellular HIV resistance factors, such as TRIM5α and APOBEC3G, which limit replication. Their specific role in the genital tract remains to be defined.

Among adaptive immune mechanisms the maximum focus has been on CD8 lymphocyte cytotoxicity because of evidence of control in SIV-macaque models and genetic studies indicating the importance of MHC I-restricted mechanisms in HIV immune control in humans. However, with the failure of trials aimed at these mechanisms investigation of other modalities has accelerated. In particular, recent studies of neutralizing antibodies have focused on the rare occurrence of broadly neutralizing antibodies which can be mimicked by monoclonals. It is well established now that the new variants emerging among the HIV quasispecies in vivo induce new type-specific neutralizing antibodies from which each subsequent new variant escapes. Mucosal IgA antibodies appear to be more important in the GI tract than in the genital tract; however, more recent evidence seems to challenge this view, and may partly be due to technical issues [4, 66]. Recent studies have demonstrated IgA-neutralizing antibody in the cervicovaginal fluids of HIV-infected women whereas IgA-binding antibodies appear to be low using conventional assays [66, 99]. The relative role of antibody-dependent cytotoxicity and neutralizing antibody also remains to be determined. Vaginal CD8 lymphocyte responses have been studied in SIV-macaque models where they are shown to remain very low until after the peak plasma viremia, suggesting there is "too little, too late" activity to control spread from the genital tract [126]. Nevertheless, in HIV-exposed uninfected women such CD8 responses have been detected in cervical cytobrush specimens, suggesting they may exert some early effect in such women [78].

During chronic HIV infection specific CD8 CTLs are present in the cervical mucosa and the similarity of their clonality and antigenic responses to those of blood CTLs has been examined, i.e., whether there is compartmentalization of such responses. Several groups have reported shared clonality and responses between cervix and blood CTLs [79, 113] and also GI CTLs [130], whereas another reported differences in antigenic specificities [59]; therefore, blood CTL responses are not necessarily predictive of those in the cervix. However, the magnitude of such responses did not correlate with reduced viral load in cervical secretions. Significantly there was a correlation between HIV presence in cervical secretions and levels of proinflammatory cytokines (TNF-α, Interleukins-1, 6, and 8), suggesting cervical inflammation might enhance local HIV shedding [59]. Regulatory T cells (Treg) have been detected in the mucosa of HIV-infected humans and SIV-infected macaques and have been postulated to mediate opposite effects of suppressing T lymphocyte control of HIV production or alternatively suppressing T lymphocyte activation.

A single study suggests a correlation with viral load [13], but this requires confirmation.

Recent work investigating progression to immunodeficiency in HIV-infected humans and also in SIV-infected macaques compared to nonprogressing SIV-infected old world monkeys (sooty mangabeys and African green monkeys) has demonstrated the importance of activation of immune cells, especially in depletion of CD4 lymphocytes. Activation also impairs function of macrophages and pDCs in blood and lymph node. In progressing SIV-infected macaques, there is selective loss of Th17 cells in the gut, microbial translocation across a damaged intestinal mucosa where epithelial cells are apoptotic, and activation (including increased CCR5 levels) and loss of CD4 lymphocytes. These features are absent in SIV-infected old world monkeys [136]. Parallels between activation of immune cells in GI and genital mucosa are expected in view of their other similarities in immune cell types, innate immune mechanisms, and colonization by commensal bacteria [130].

The foreskin appears to be a weak spot in the MGT as recent randomized controlled trials of male circumcision showed a 60% reduction in female to male transmission of HIV [8, 10, 55]. In male to female transmission, there is an overall decreased risk of HIV acquisition in partners of circumcised versus uncircumcised men [9, 56]. Male circumcision as a means of reducing HIV transmission is reviewed by Weiss [148].

5.4.2 Genital Herpes

HSV-1 and 2 are common human pathogens with worldwide distribution and are the etiological agents of the common cold sore and genital herpes respectively, although genital herpes caused by HSV-1 is increasing markedly, especially in adolescence. Usually HSV-1 or 2 initially infects oral or genital epidermal or mucosal tissues where it replicates and enters the cutaneous sensory axons. The virus is then transported along the axons of dorsal root ganglionic (DRG) sensory neurons in a retrograde direction to the neuronal cell body, where it establishes latent infection for the lifetime of the host. Periodic reactivation results in HSV-1 being transported back to nerve terminals, where it causes either recurrent clinical disease or asymptomatic viral shedding at the skin or mucous membranes of the same dermatome involved in the initial infection [127].

HSV-1 or 2 codes for structural and nonstructural viral proteins which are expressed as a temporal cascade of immediate early (IE), early (E), and late (L) proteins during viral replication. IE/E proteins are usually nonstructural (functional) and L proteins are usually structural. The herpes simplex virion has four components: an electron dense core containing the double-stranded DNA genome (152 kb), the capsid, the tegument, and an outer envelope containing glycoproteins [127]. The capsid encloses the DNA core and consists of six different viral proteins. The surrounding tegument contains at least 20 [101]. The envelope contains 11 different glycoproteins including gB and gD [101]. HSV-1 and 2 structural proteins show a high degree of serologic cross-reactivity. However, little is known about cross-reactive epitopes to T lymphocytes in HSV-1 and 2 structural and nonstructural proteins.

Innate and adaptive immune mechanisms operate at every level to control HSV: after entry infection in the skin/mucosa, at the DRG to control latency and reactivation, and then at the interface of sensory axons and mucosal epithelial cells to determine whether clinical disease or asymptomatic shedding occurs.

5.4.2.1 Innate Immunity

Antimicrobial peptides from cervicovaginal fluid such as lactoferrin and lysozyme inhibit HSV infection [132]. Type I IFNs (IFN-α and IFN-β), macrophages, NK cells, and $\gamma\delta$T cells all play a role in innate immunity to HSV [20, 24]. There is cross talk between NK cells, DCs, and T lymphocytes so that NK cells, like DCs, can bridge innate and adaptive immunity (Fig. 5.3c) [1, 112, 149]. In murine models, the protective role of IFN-α and IFN-β against HSV-1 infection has long been known. However, the relative importance, cell source, and mechanism of induction are somewhat confused in murine models and few data are available in humans. Early TLR-9-dependent production of IFN-α from plasmacytoid DCs soon after HSV-2 infection, followed by non-TLR-9 IFN-α and IFN-β production from several types was reported. The latter included conventional DCs, macrophages, and fibroblasts [124]. Older studies in humans claimed that IFN-β predominated in vesicle fluid (rather than IFN-α as previously reported [117]), and that keratinocytes cultured in vitro only produced IFN-β [142, 143].

These conflicting reports may reflect different sources of Type I IFNs such as IFN-β secreted by infected keratinocytes, IFN-α secreted by infiltrating pDCs, and probably macrophages. IFN-γ is secreted mainly by CD4 lymphocytes (and perhaps NK cells in herpetic lesions). All are present at high levels in the vesicle fluid of recurrent herpes simplex lesions [142, 143]. After axonal transmission from HSV-1-infected DRG neurons, both the number and size of viral cytopathic plaques in epidermal cells (ECs) were significantly reduced by addition of recombinant IFN-α and IFN-γ to ECs and the combination was at least additive [103]. Thus both IFN-α and IFN-γ can interfere with HSV-1 infection after axonal transmission and subsequent spread of HSV-1 in ECs by a direct antiviral effect.

Recently, TLRs have also been shown to be important mediators of innate immune responses in HSV infection in the genital tract and systemically. HSV-1 and 2 interact with both TLR-2 and 9 [41]. The interaction of HSV-1 and 2 with TLR-2 appears to be at the cell surface, whereas the interaction of HSV-2 with TLR-9 is via unmethylated CpGs in viral DNA within the endosomes, particularly of pDCs. This latter interaction is a potent stimulus to the production of IFN-α. Indeed, pDCs are the main producers of IFN-α from human blood mononuclear cells stimulated by the HSV antigen [94, 128, 133]. IFN-α production by pDCs also induces IFN-α production from NK cells, which, in turn, contributes to the Th1 adaptive immune response [111]. LCs express TLRs 1, 2, 3, 5, 6, and 10 [42]. The TLR repertoire of human dermal DCs is unknown but is likely to resemble MDDCs or CD34+ cell-derived DCs (TLRs 1, 2, 3, 4, 6, 8 and 10; [77]). A recent study reported a key role for TLR-3 in protection against HSV encephalitis in children which is supported by the potent protective effect of the TLR3-agonist poly-IC in murine models [157].

5.4.2.2 Adaptive Immunity

The cell-mediated immune response to HSV is of major importance in control and clearance of recurrent infection in recurrent oral or genital herpes.

Role of the Immune System in Maintenance of Latency and Prevention of Virus Reactivation in the Dorsal Root Ganglion

Immune control of neuronal latency or reactivation in the DRG is impossible to study in humans in vivo, so animal models of latency and reactivation have been developed. HSV latency in the DRG is maintained by noncytolytic CD8+ lymphocytes which secrete antiviral IFN-γ and granzyme B [83, 85]. CD4 T lymphocytes are also present in the DRG and may help maintain latency [83].

Immune Response to Human Recurrent Herpes in the Skin

In the skin the immunoreactive cells responsible for controlling the transmitted HSV include the normal constituents of the squamous epidermis, keratinocytes and LCs, and infiltrating cells. In particular, HSV-specific CD4 and CD8 T-lymphocytes play a central role in controlling primary and recurrent HSV infections in humans and primary disease in murine models. The increased severity and persistence of recurrent herpes as a presenting syndrome of AIDS reflects the key role of T cells, especially CD4 T cells [134]. Furthermore, there is a temporal sequence of cellular infiltration, first predominantly monocyte/macrophages and CD4 lymphocytes and later predominantly CD8 lymphocytes, as shown by immunohistochemistry and direct T-cell cloning from lesions biopsied serially. These infiltrating CD8 lymphocytes clear the HSV infection [32, 87] (Fig. 5.6).

HSV infection of keratinocytes in vitro and in vivo induces the secretion of a sequence of chemokines and cytokines, i.e., first IFN-β and β chemokines and then interleukin (IL)-12 followed by IL-1 and IL-6 [105]. The β chemokines attract monocytes, and CD4 and CD8 lymphocytes into lesions. IFN-γ and IL-12 may entrain Th1 patterns of cytokine response from HSV antigen-stimulated CD4 (and CD8) lymphocytes, especially IFN-γ. HSV-1/2 downregulate MHC I expression by keratinocytes via the viral protein ICP47 interaction with cellular translocator-associated proteins (TAP) in the endoplasmic reticulum. This is reversed by IFN-γ, mainly from infiltrating CD4 lymphocytes, thus allowing CD8 lymphocytes to recognize infected keratinocytes [31, 104]. IFN-γ

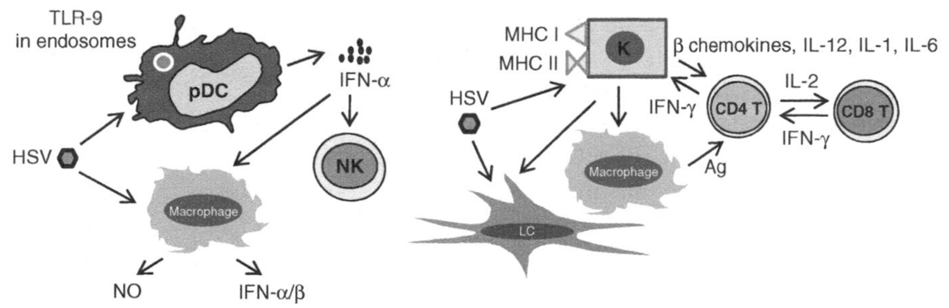

Fig. 5.6 Innate immune mechanisms induced by initial HSV infection. Role of LCs, keratinocytes (K), and T cells in connecting innate and adaptive immune control of recurrent herpes simplex. IFN, interferon; IL, interleukin; M, macrophage; MHC, major histocompatibility complex; NO, nitric oxide; pDCs, plasmacytoid dendritic cells; TLR, Toll-like receptor (Reproduced from [29])

also upregulate MHC class II expression on keratinocytes, allowing recognition by CD4 T lymphocytes. Thus Th1 rather than Th2 patterns of response are important for immune and vaccine control of HSV [106] reflected in a lower frequency of recurrent herpes with higher levels of IFN-γ produced by blood CD4 T lymphocytes [30, 107, 142]. Both CD4 and CD8 cytotoxic T lymphocytes (CTLs) have been isolated from genital lesions ex vivo and shown to have cytotoxic activity. Memory CD8 T lymphocytes can be induced to proliferate directly in (murine) skin without the requirement to migrate to the lymph nodes. This requires DC interactions with CD4 and CD8 T cells [146].

After lesion healing and loss of HSV DNA from skin biopsies, HSV-2-specific $CD8^+$ T lymphocytes persisted for more than 6 months at the dermal–epidermal junction, adjacent to peripheral nerve endings, and were accompanied by persistence of CD4 lymphocytes and myeloid DCs deeper in the dermis [161].

Homing and Infiltration of Monocytes and T Lymphocytes

The mechanisms responsible for the sequence of early infiltration of CD4 T lymphocytes and monocytes, and later of CD8 T lymphocytes, into herpetic lesions are unclear. E-selectin is upregulated on cutaneous venule endothelial cells in recurrent herpetic lesions, as expected in any inflammatory lesions [88]. This could be a result of secretion of IFN-β by keratinocytes and IFN-α from infiltrating pDCs [35] or, as the lesion progresses, by IFN-γ from $CD4^+$ T cells. In blood, HSV-2-specific CD4 and CD8 T cells express the E-selectin ligand and/or the similar cutaneous T cell-associated antigen at differing levels: 50–70% for CD8 T lymphocytes and 20% for CD4 T lymphocytes. However, HSV-2 stimulation of CD4 T lymphocytes markedly enhances their expression of these two antigens perhaps contributing to their earlier infiltration into herpes lesions [54].

Viral Antigens Recognized by T Lymphocytes

Which are the key immunogenic proteins within the HSV virion? Both human CD4 and CD8 T lymphocytes recognize IFN-γ stimulated, HSV-1-infected keratinocytes (as in lesions). Using Vaccinia virus recombinants expressing HSV-2 proteins and blood CD4 lymphocytes restimulated in vitro with inactivated HSV-2 (or 1) antigen almost all patients' cells recognized late HSV-1 or HSV-2 structural proteins, especially gD and gB, and also the major tegument protein VP16. This is consistent with earlier studies by Zarling et al., demonstrating gD can stimulate human CD4 T helper lymphocytes [156]. Parallel studies in mice have also showed CD4 T lymphocyte specificity for gD [142, 143].

Koelle et al. [87] cloned T cells out of recurrent herpes simplex lesions and reacted them against B cells infected with HSV-1, HSV-2, and recombinants of the two. In this system, several proteins from the tegument of the virus have been found to be important targets for type-specific immunity (HSV-2 but not HSV-1). The differing results may be complementary (i.e., HSV-1 and HSV-2 may have both cross-reactive and type-specific epitopes), but testing of these two systems in vivo is required.

Successful trials of gD2 immunization in mice and guinea pigs [16] preceded human trials of immunization with recombinant HSV-2 glycoprotein D (gD2) vaccine mixed with the adjuvants alum and deacylated monophosphoryl lipid A (dMPL). The latter were shown to substantially induce protection (>70%) against genital herpes disease in HSV-1 and 2 seronegative women in a consort setting but not in HSV-1 seropositive women, nor in any males at all irrespective of serostatus. Prior natural HSV-1 infection reduced development of HSV-2 genital herpes disease [139]. gD2 has also been shown to induce IFN-γ secretion from the peripheral blood mononuclear cells (PBMCs) of similarly immunized patients when stimulated in vitro [12].

In view of the importance of gD2 as an immunogen, the immunodominant gD2 peptides recognized by bulk human CD4 T lymphocytes in the majority of HSV-2 seropositive subjects were identified and their MHC II restriction defined. Such peptides were also recognized by HSV-1+ subjects [84].

Such studies provide an empirical basis for cross-reactive and possibly cross-protective epitopes between gD of HSV-1 and HSV-2 suspected from the vaccine studies. A vaccine effective against both genital HSV-1 and 2 infection and disease is required in view of the recent changing epidemiology in societies in the developed world, with more nuclear families, and thus the reduction in transmission of HSV-1 by the oral route as children, and also the increasing incidence of genital HSV-1 disease especially in adolescence [90].

In contrast, human CD8 T lymphocytes from HSV seropositive subjects recognized IE/E proteins and also a wide variety of other HSV proteins [11, 60, 104], showing considerable heterogeneity between subjects, rather than distinct immunodominance of single proteins. Both gB and ICP27 were also recognized by CD8 T lymphocytes in mice although the immunogenicity of individual proteins in mice and humans does not always correlate.

Although the above studies were conducted in humans with recurrent herpes simplex, the results correlate with human prophylactic vaccine studies where gD2 was shown to be partially protective in HSV-1/2 women in a consort setting, suggesting they will also be important in primary herpes infection [139].

The Role of Dendritic Cells in Innate and Adaptive Immunity to HSV

Mucocutaneous HSV infection is usually confined to the epidermal layer. Therefore, LCs are likely to be initially involved in initial HSV antigen uptake [141] as shown by older murine studies [138]. These studies showed that depletion of LCs from skin, after HSV-1 infection of mice via the footpad, led to increased HSV virulence [138]. In human recurrent herpes simplex, HSV structural antigens are present within LCs (L. Bosnjak et al., unpublished data). Involvement of dermal DCs in the upper region of the dermis has not been excluded [65]. In mice, recent studies have demonstrated that (CD103+) dermal DCs or resident CD8$^+$ DCs present HSV antigen to CD8 T lymphocytes cells in lymph nodes [5, 159]. The apparent paradox of initial HSV antigen uptake by LCs but presentation by another DC subtype may be explained by transfer of the antigens from one DC subtype to another (Fig. 5.7).

As immature human LCs are difficult to harvest, MDDCs have been used as a model. Immature MDDCs express the HSV receptors nectin-1, nectin-2, and herpesvirus entry mediator (HVEM) and can be infected productively with HSV-1 and HSV-2, which results in asynchronous downregulation of the key surface co-stimulatory molecules including CD40, CD80, and CD86 and maturation marker CD83 (and also CD54/ICAM-1), preventing proper maturation of the DCs [15, 35]. In contrast, exposure to UV-inactivated HSV results in their upregulation [103, 154]. Secretion of IL-12, the major Th1 cytokine, by DCs is also inhibited. As ICAM-1 provides potent co-stimulatory signals to CD4 and CD8 T lymphocytes, its downmodulation may inhibit anti-HSV immunity [34].

In most cell types, HSV is anti-apoptotic whereas in DCs, monocytes, and T lymphocytes, HSV-1/2 induces apoptosis via their IE/E proteins [15] despite encoding several anti-apoptotic gene products [6, 7, 48, 74, 91, 120, 160]. These apoptotic cells can then be phagocytosed by uninfected bystander cells, and the HSV antigens are then cross-presented to CD8+ lymphocytes [15], suggesting a mechanism for HSV antigen transfer between LCs and the other DC subtypes observed in murine models. Whether adjacent LCs or subjacent dermal DCs are such bystanders remains to be elucidated in human infection. Such a process would circumvent the HSV immunoevasive mechanisms of

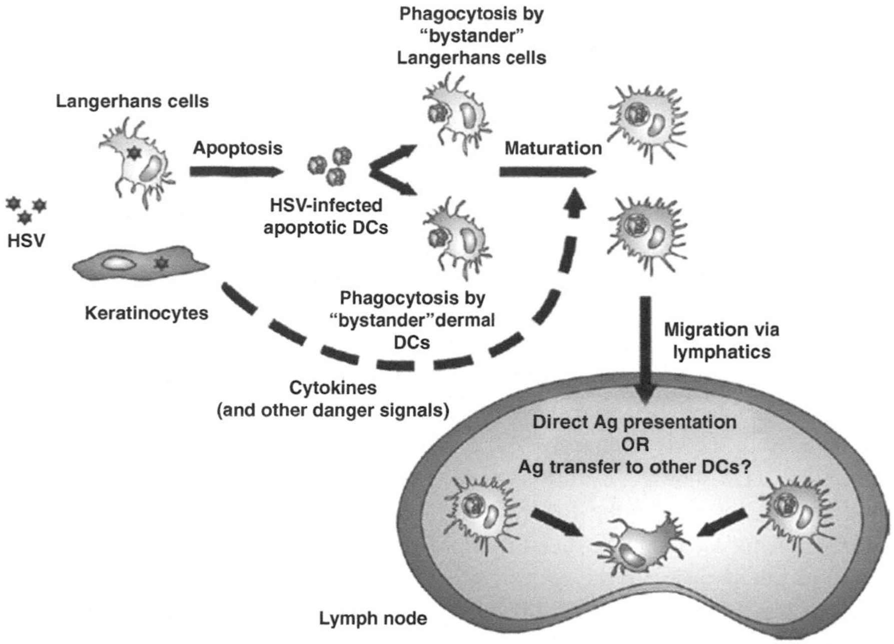

Fig. 5.7 Postulated interactions between HSV and DCs in the epidermis and transport of antigen to lymph node. HSV infection of epidermis LCs induces apoptosis followed by uptake by bystander LCs or dermal DCs moving into the area of inflammation. Cytokines/danger signals released from infected keratinocytes lead to maturation and migration of DCs to lymph nodes where they activate CD4 or CD8 T lymphocytes directly or via intermediate DCs (Reproduced from [14])

costimulatory molecule downregulation and apoptosis of DCs [102].

pDCs are not present in normal skin but recently they have been demonstrated to infiltrate herpes lesions [35]. The marked activation of pDCs by HSV suggests that they are important in vivo, as now demonstrated by their infiltration into the dermis and dermo–epidermal junction of recurrent herpes lesions. Here they appear to produce IFN-α as they are surrounded by cells producing IFN-stimulated proteins and they interact with activated CD4 and NK cells probably presenting antigen or via cytokines, respectively. In vitro pDCs can present HSV antigen to CD4 and CD8 lymphocytes [35]. Furthermore, pDC depletion of mice reduced recruitment of IFN-α secreting inflammatory cells to the site of infection [95].

5.4.3 Human Papillomavirus

The spectrum of disease in the genital tract caused by HPV ranges from asymptomatic to benign condylomata acuminata (genital warts), high- and low-grade dysplasias (only evident on magnification at colposcopy or by cytology on Pap-stained cervical cytology smears [as part of precancerous screening], or by histology of biopsy tissues), and is also known as intraepithelial neoplasia of the cervix, vagina, vulval, penile, or anal, as well as the invasive cancers of each of these anatomical sites. More recently, a proportion of oropharyngeal cancers, particularly tonsillar, have been found to be caused by HPV 16 [70].

HPV is a large group of noncultivatable, nonenveloped DNA viruses, with a proportion having specific tropism for the genital tract. Of these, some have a high risk for neoplasia (HPV 16 and 18, the most virulent types, collectively and consistently worldwide are the etiological agents of around 70% of cervical cancers), while others have low risk (HPV 6 and 11 cause around 90% of genital warts) [52]. Genital HPVs are extremely common, largely sexually transmitted, and it is estimated that up to 80% of the sexually active population have been exposed at some time. Cancer per se is a rare outcome therefore of an extremely common infection. However, worldwide cervical cancer is the second most common cancer in women, being the number one in many developing countries, where there are no functioning prevention programs such as Pap cytology.

HPV specifically infects keratinocytes in the stratified squamous epithelium of the lower FGT and penile skin, with complete virion production being intimately linked with the differentiation of squamous epithelium. While it was once believed that there was a continuum of effect from HPV infection from cervical intraepithelial neoplasia grade 1–3 (CIN 1–3), it is now realized that CIN 3 is the true precursor lesion to cancer, with CIN 1 just the viral cytopathic effect of infection (CIN 2 probably being a mix of 1 and 3).

Natural HPV infection induces a poor and slow local inflammatory response, with only 50% of subjects with detectable HPV DNA having a measurable neutralizing antibody response which can take many months to be seen. Of note, antibody responses are largely type-specific. Both the bivalent and HPV quadrivalent vaccine trials have shown prevention of infection, as well as disease (CIN, and for the quadrivalent vaccine, VIN, VAIN in females, and more recently AIN in males) for those recipients naive to the specific types covered by the vaccines [51, 52, 71, 119]. In addition, in prophylactic vaccine trials (but not in natural infection), there has been some cross protection shown for infection and disease to those genotypes that are phylogenetically related to the types covered by the vaccine [18].

In countries such as Australia where public health programs have embraced the HPV vaccine with high coverage and compliance, already a reduction in genital warts in young women less than 27 years of age is being seen [39].

Moreover, in a subset of individuals with previous infection from vaccine-related strains (HPV DNA negative, but antibody positive) there is reduced disease manifestations compare to placebo groups, likely reflecting immune memory with boosting of natural immunity [116]. In humans and animal models, regression of warts (clearance of HPV lesions) is associated with an active cell-mediated immune response, with CD4 lymphocyte infiltration and not necessarily with the presence of neutralizing antibody [115, 140]. This is exemplified clinically: those with acquired CD4 lymphocyte immunodeficiency such as in advanced HIV infection or organ transplantation, but not agammaglobulinemia, are predisposed to HPV disease, and are also recalcitrant to treatment and impaired clearance [46]. Nevertheless, prophylactic VLP-based vaccine studies have shown that high levels of neutralizing antibody can protect against infection by HPV (Fig. 5.8). Persistence of HPV16/18 infection occurs in about 2–5% of patients who are apparently immunocompetent and is a prerequisite for a development of the precursor lesions, the high-grade dysplasias. It takes >10 years and other mutagenic events for cancer to develop. HPVs are unique among many pathogens in showing multiple immunoevasive mechanisms. The major mechanism is avoidance of antigen presentation by lack of lysis of keratinocytes, expression of few proinflammatory signals, and lack of systemic spread. Others include downregulation of TLR-9 expression and MIP-3α by HPV 16 via E6 and E7, impairing viral DNA recognition and LC immigration, respectively. E5 also downregulates MHCI, thus impairing CD8 lymphocyte cytotoxicity. Current studies of mucosal immunity of HPVs are aimed at improving preventative vaccines for vulval and ectocervical HPV infections and for immunotherapy of cervical intraepithelial neoplasia or premalignant changes. The former depends on inducing high and persistent levels of neutralizing antibodies and the latter on cell-mediated immunity, especially against the viral oncogenes E6 and E7. Indeed in animal models transplanted tumors expressing E7 have been cured by E7-specific immunotherapies and are dependent on E7-specific cytotoxic CD8 T lymphocytes. In humans, cervical intraepithelial neoplasia increased numbers of activated CD8 T lymphocytes and bearing the cytotoxicity marker, T-cell intracellular antigen (TIA) and macrophages were demonstrated [3]. E6- and E7-specific immunotherapies in humans evoke similar responses but have shown limited disease efficacy so far.

It is highly likely that a proportion of HPV infections become latent infections (i.e., the virus can remain within basal epithelial cells either arrested or very slowly replicating, but undetectable by current DNA technology). This may well explain recurrences of disease in those not exposed to new partners or new infection.

Recent data show that male circumcision reduces the incidence of multiple high-risk HPV infections in HIV-negative and HIV-positive men [57, 129], as well as HPV infection and HPV-related disease in their female partners [23].

5.4.4 *Chlamydia trachomatis*

Chlamydia trachomatis is a small obligate intracellular bacterium which infects the MGT and FGT causing urethritis, cervicitis, endometritis, or pelvic inflammatory

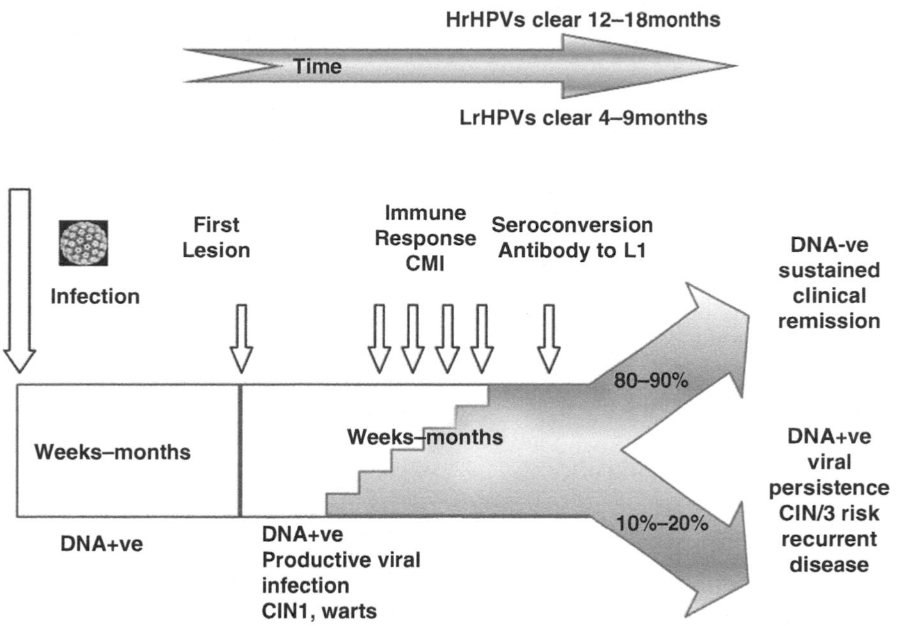

Fig. 5.8 The natural course of genital HPV infection. The incubation period after the initial infection is extremely variable (possibly as long as years) and may depend on viral dose. During this period, the virus cannot be detected. Then the lesions start to appear and HPV DNA can be detected. After a variable period of time, the cell-mediated response is mounted to clear infection and lesions. At this point, seroconversion occurs and antibodies are made to the L1 major capsid protein. On the whole, low-risk HPVs are cleared faster than high-risk HPVs. The infection then progresses in one of two ways, resulting in women with apparent sustained clinical remission who have no recurrent CIN or warts, and women with persistent or recurrent disease who are at risk of generating CIN 3. The second group of women have mounted an immune response, but it was insufficient. They may be seropositive, but they still have HPV DNA. Hr, high risk; Lr, low risk

disease, bartonolitis, proctitis, epidymo-orchitis. It is the commonest bacterial STI worldwide and most infections are asymptomatic and go unrecognized. In the FGT, chlamydia infect the endocervical columnar epithelial cells. The mouse model of infection with *Chlamydia muridarum* appears to closely mimic FGT infection and is useful for immunologic studies. *C. muridarum* and possibly *C. trachomatis* cell wall components interact with TLR-2 and, to a lesser extent, TLR-4 on DCs to stimulate IL-12 secretion and therefore a Th1 response. Infected epithelial cells also produce proinflammatory cytokines, including IL-6, 8, and 12, and TNF-α, and chemokines, including CCL-1 and CXCL-1, 10, and 16. Cell-mediated immunity is important in clearing chlamydial infection, especially the Th1 response; increased concentrations of monocytes, polymorphs, and CD4 and CD8 T lymphocytes are found at the site of infection and production of IFN-γ from CD4 and CD8 T lymphocytes, presumably after IL-12 stimulation from DCs and epithelial cells, correlates well with resolution. High titres of *C. trachomatis*-specific antibodies do not correlate with resolution of primary human infection. They appear to have only an ancillary role in clearing infection.

However, the high proinflammatory Th1 response also appears to result in immunopathologic consequences including tubal damage and infertility, especially following recurrent or persistent infection. Such responses also appear to correlate with increased local immigration of pDCs, enhanced local TNF-α and IFN-γ responses, and differential serologic "autoimmune" responses to heat shock proteins.

5.4.4.1 Implications for Vaccines and Immunotherapy

Further understanding of the mechanisms of mucosal immune control of the STIs discussed above should help in developing vaccines or, in the case of HPV where there are successful vaccines, immunotherapy. The initial goal may be to emulate successful immune control in individuals such as HIV elite controllers, or those who clear acute STIs, taking account of immunogenetic factors, but then it may be possible to further improve this optimal immune response. This may be facilitated by new generations of adjuvants or TLR agonists aimed at all or most of the relevant immune effector mechanisms, both innate and adaptive (Table 5.3). Thus the HPV16/18 L1-alum VLP vaccines from Merck and Glaxo Smithkline (GSK) with or without the adjuvant, deacyl monophosphoryl lipid A (dMPL, derived from the cell walls of bacteria), induces systemic neutralizing IgG antibody which protects against HPV16/18 infection and disease through transudation into the cervical (and vulval) mucosa. The adjuvant in the GSK vaccine stimulates follicular T helper lymphocytes to interact with B lymphocytes in lymph nodes. However, immunotherapy against established disease will require induction of CD8 T lymphocyte activity against E6/7 expressed in HPV-infected cells [46, 50].

For HSV-2, a vaccine candidate, Simplirix (from GSK), consisting of recombinant soluble glycoprotein D, which is widely recognized in human populations [104], and also dMPL showed partial efficacy of 73% in the prevention of genital herpes but only in women (not men) who were seronegative for both HSV-1 and HSV-2 add who were long-term consorts of partners with genital herpes [139]. The partial success of this vaccine candidate has been attributed to dMPL which is a TLR-4 agonist and induces Th1 patterns cytokine response, especially induction of IFN-γ, in guinea pig models and human phase 1 trials [16], as well as during the trial itself (L. R. Stanberry, A. L. Cunningham, S. L. Spruance et al., unpublished data). No induction of T cell cytotoxicity was demonstrated although neutralizing antibody was induced. Future improved vaccine candidates are needed and should probably aim at inducing innate immune and CD8 T cell responses.

Enormous effort is being invested in developing an HIV vaccine using similar principles. Recent candidates have either used hybrid vectors such as adenovirus type 5 (Merck) or canarypox expressing HIV proteins with immunodominant epitopes recognized by CD8 T lymphocytes such as gag, pol, or nef with or without additional immunogens such as DNA or recombinant gp120 often in a prime and then boost regime. Although as yet unsuccessful in major prevention of HIV infection and disease the hybrid vector vaccines have been shown to induce CD8 T lymphocyte responses (albeit at levels which are too narrow and low) and gp120 specific antibody-dependent cytotoxicity (ADCC) [19, 98]. Future vaccine attempts are aimed at inducing broad neutralizing antibodies and perhaps also innate immune mechanisms.

Acknowledgments Supported by: NHMRC Program Grant # 358399 NHMRC Project Grant # 632638, 408114.

The authors wish to thank Dr. Kerrie Sandgren, Dr. Stuart Turville, and Dr Margaret Stanley for providing figures and Denise Brown for clerical assistance.

Table 5.3 Correlation of key immune antiviral mechanisms and vaccine-induced immune modalities

Virus	Key Controlling Immune Mechanisms	Vaccine (candidate) Antigen	Adjuvant	Key Immune Modality Stimulated
HPV	IgG antibody transuding from the systemic system to the basal cells, as well as exuding into genital secretions	L1 virus-like particle	Alum (quadrivalent vaccine)	Systemic IgG antibody transcending into genital tract
			Alum + dMPL (bivalent vaccine)	Tfh cells
HSV-2	CD4 and CD8 T lymphocytes ? Neutralizing antibody	Glycoprotein D	Alum + dMPL	CD4 T lymphocytes Th1 response
HIV	? CD8 T lymphocytes ?? CD4 T lymphocytes ?? Neutralizing antibody ?? ADCC	Adenovirus(s) or canarypox vector + gag/pol/nef/ gp120		CD8 T lymphocytes ADCC

Take-Home Pearls

- Mucosal immunity to key STIs in the genitourinary tract have been less investigated than systemic immunity and requires future emphasis.
- There are marked differences in mucosal immune mechanisms between the sterile upper genitourinary tract and the lower genitourinary tract which is colonized by bacteria.
- Physical barriers, antimicrobial peptides pattern recognition receptors and the cellular elements macrophages, NK cells and dendritic cells are all important factors but differ in importance with different STIs.
- The uptake of viral pathogens by sessile dendritic cells within the genitourinary mucosa and their subsequent processing may differ markedly between pathogens and determine immune pathogenesis, e.g., for HIV and HSV.
- There are marked differences in the predominant immune effector mechanisms for different STIs, as confirmed by vaccine studies eg neutralizing antibody is of key importance in protection against human papillomavirus whereas CD4 and CD8 lymphocytes play a major role in HSV infection, especially where recurrent.
- Understanding the relative importance of immune control mechanisms for each STI is critical in rational approaches to development of systemic and mucosal vaccines and selection of adjuvants.
- Comparisons between systemic, gastrointestinal and genitourinary immune mechanisms should provide further insights, useful for development of vaccines and immunotherapies.

References

1. Adam, C., King, S., Allgeier, T., Braumuller, H., Luking, C., Mysliwietz, J., Kriegeskorte, A., Busch, D.H., Rocken, M., Mocikat, R.: DC-NK cell cross talk as a novel CD4+ T-cell-independent pathway for antitumor CTL induction. Blood **106**, 338–344 (2005)
2. Ahmed, S.M., Al-Doujaily, H., Johnson, M.A., Kitchen, V., Reid, W.M., Poulter, L.W.: Immunity in the female lower genital tract and the impact of HIV infection. Scand. J. Immunol. **54**, 225–238 (2001)
3. Ahmed, S.M., Al, H., Reid, W.M., Johnson, M.A., Poulter, L.W.: The cellular response associated with cervical intraepithelial neoplasia in HIV+ and HIV- subjects. Scand. J. Immunol. **56**, 204–211 (2002)
4. Alexander, R., Mestecky, J.: Neutralizing antibodies in mucosal secretions: IgG or IgA? Curr. HIV Res. **5**, 588–593 (2007)
5. Allan, R.S., Smith, C.M., Belz, G.T., van Lint, A.L., Wakim, L.M., Heath, W.R., Carbone, F.R.: Epidermal viral immunity induced by CD8alpha+ dendritic cells but not by Langerhans cells. Science **301**, 1925–1928 (2003)
6. Aubert, M., O'Toole, J., Blaho, J.A.: Induction and prevention of apoptosis in human HEp-2 cells by herpes simplex virus type 1. J. Virol. **73**, 10359–10370 (1999)
7. Aubert, M., Rice, S.A., Blaho, J.A.: Accumulation of herpes simplex virus type 1 early and leaky-late proteins correlates with apoptosis prevention in infected human HEp-2 cells. J. Virol. **75**, 1013–1030 (2001)
8. Auvert, B., Taljaard, D., Lagarde, E., Sobngwi-Tambekou, J., Sitta, R., Puren, A.: Randomized, controlled intervention trial of male circumcision for reduction of HIV infection risk: the ANRS 1265 trial. PLoS Med. **2**, e298 (2005)
9. Baeten, J.M., Donnell, D., Kapiga, S.H., Ronald, A., John-Stewart, G., Inambao, M., Manongi, R., Vwalika, B., Celum, C.: Male circumcision and risk of male-to-female HIV-1 transmission: a multinational prospective study in African HIV-1-serodiscordant couples. AIDS **24**, 737–744 (2010)
10. Bailey, R.C., Moses, S., Parker, C.B., Agot, K., Maclean, I., Krieger, J.N., Williams, C.F., Campbell, R.T., Ndinya-Achola, J.O.: Male circumcision for HIV prevention in young men in Kisumu, Kenya: a randomised controlled trial. Lancet **369**, 643–656 (2007)
11. Banks, T.A., Nair, S., Rouse, B.T.: Recognition by and in vitro induction of cytotoxic T lymphocytes against predicted epitopes of the immediate-early protein ICP27 of herpes simplex virus. J. Virol. **67**, 613–616 (1993)
12. Bastin, C., Hermand, P., Francotte, M., Garcon, N., Slaoui, M., Pala, P.: Synergistic association of adjuvants QS21 and MPL for induction of cytolytic T-lymphocytes and T-helper responses to recombinant protein antigens (abstract). In: 34th Interscience Conference on Antimicrobial Agents and Chemotherapy of the American Society for Microbiology, Washington DC (1994)
13. Boasso, A., Vaccari, M., Hryniewicz, A., Fuchs, D., Nacsa, J., Cecchinato, V., Andersson, J., Franchini, G., Shearer, G.M., Chougnet, C.: Regulatory T-cell markers, indoleamine 2, 3-dioxygenase, and virus levels in spleen and gut during progressive simian immunodeficiency virus infection. J. Virol. **81**, 11593–11603 (2007)
14. Bosnjak, L., Jones, C.A., Abendroth, A., Cunningham, A.L.: Dendritic cell biology in herpesvirus infections. Viral Immunol. **18**, 419–433 (2005)
15. Bosnjak, L., Miranda-Saksena, M., Koelle, D.M., Boadle, R.A., Jones, C.A., Cunningham, A.L.: Herpes simplex virus infection of human dendritic cells induces apoptosis and allows cross-presentation via uninfected dendritic cells. J. Immunol. **174**, 2220–2227 (2005)
16. Bourne, N., Bravo, F.J., Francotte, M., Bernstein, D.I., Myers, M.G., Slaoui, M., Stanberry, L.R.: Herpes simplex virus (HSV) type 2 glycoprotein D subunit vaccines and

protection against genital HSV-1 or HSV-2 disease in guinea pigs. J. Infect. Dis. **187**, 542–549 (2003)
17. Bowie, A.G., Unterholzner, L.: Viral evasion and subversion of pattern-recognition receptor signalling. Nat. Rev. Immunol. **8**, 911–922 (2008)
18. Brown, D.R., Kjaer, S.K., Sigurdsson, K., Iversen, O.E., Hernandez-Avila, M., Wheeler, C.M., Perez, G., Koutsky, L.A., Tay, E.H., Garcia, P., Ault, K.A., Garland, S.M., Leodolter, S., Olsson, S.E., Tang, G.W., Ferris, D.G., Paavonen, J., Steben, M., Bosch, F.X., Dillner, J., Joura, E.A., Kurman, R.J., Majewski, S., Munoz, N., Myers, E.R., Villa, L.L., Taddeo, F.J., Roberts, C., Tadesse, A., Bryan, J., Lupinacci, L.C., Giacoletti, K.E., Sings, H.L., James, M., Hesley, T.M., Barr, E.: The impact of quadrivalent human papillomavirus (HPV; types 6, 11, 16, and 18) L1 virus-like particle vaccine on infection and disease due to oncogenic nonvaccine HPV types in generally HPV-naive women aged 16-26 years. J. Infect. Dis. **199**, 926–935 (2009)
19. Buchbinder, S.P., Mehrotra, D.V., Duerr, A., Fitzgerald, D.W., Mogg, R., Li, D., Gilbert, P.B., Lama, J.R., Marmor, M., Del Rio, C., McElrath, M.J., Casimiro, D.R., Gottesdiener, K.M., Chodakewitz, J.A., Corey, L., Robertson, M.N.: Efficacy assessment of a cell-mediated immunity HIV-1 vaccine (the Step Study): a double-blind, randomised, placebo-controlled, test-of-concept trial. Lancet **372**, 1881–1893 (2008)
20. Bukowski, J.F., Welsh, R.M.: The role of natural killer cells and interferon in resistance to acute infection of mice with herpes simplex virus type 1. J. Immunol. **136**, 3481–3485 (1986)
21. Bursch, L.S., Wang, L., Igyarto, B., Kissenpfennig, A., Malissen, B., Kaplan, D.H., Hogquist, K.A.: Identification of a novel population of Langerin+ dendritic cells. J. Exp. Med. **204**, 3147–3156 (2007)
22. Carrington, M., Bontrop, R.E.: Effects of MHC class I on HIV/SIV disease in primates. AIDS **16**(Suppl 4), S105–S114 (2002)
23. Castellsague, X., Bosch, F.X., Munoz, N., Meijer, C.J., Shah, K.V., de Sanjose, S., Eluf-Neto, J., Ngelangel, C.A., Chichareon, S., Smith, J.S., Herrero, R., Moreno, V., Franceschi, S.: Male circumcision, penile human papillomavirus infection, and cervical cancer in female partners. N Engl J. Med. **346**, 1105–1112 (2002)
24. Cheng, H., Tumpey, T.M., Staats, H.F., van Rooijen, N., Oakes, J.E., Lausch, R.N.: Role of macrophages in restricting herpes simplex virus type 1 growth after ocular infection. Invest. Ophthalmol. Vis. Sci. **41**, 1402–1409 (2000)
25. Cole, A.M., Cole, A.L.: Antimicrobial polypeptides are key anti-HIV-1 effector molecules of cervicovaginal host defense. Am. J. Reprod. Immunol. **59**, 27–34 (2008)
26. Cooper, M.A., Fehniger, T.A., Caligiuri, M.A.: The biology of human natural killer-cell subsets. Trends Immunol. **22**, 633–640 (2001)
27. Cumberbatch, M., Singh, M., Dearman, R.J., Young, H.S., Kimber, I., Griffiths, C.E.: Impaired Langerhans cell migration in psoriasis. J. Exp. Med. **203**, 953–960 (2006)
28. Cunningham, A.L., Carbone, F., Geijtenbeek, T.B.: Langerhans cells and viral immunity. Eur. J. Immunol. **38**, 2377–2385 (2008)
29. Cunningham, A.L., Diefenbach, R.J., Miranda-Saksena, M., Bosnjak, L., Kim, M., Jones, C., Douglas, M.W.: The cycle of human herpes simplex virus infection: virus transport and immune control. J. Infect. Dis. **194**(Suppl 1), S11–S18 (2006)
30. Cunningham, A.L., Merigan, T.C.: Leu-3+ T cells produce gamma-interferon in patients with recurrent herpes labialis. J. Immunol. **132**, 197–202 (1984)
31. Cunningham, A.L., Nelson, P.A., Fathman, C.G., Merigan, T.C.: Interferon gamma production by herpes simplex virus antigen-specific T cell clones from patients with recurrent herpes labialis. J. Gen. Virol. **66**(Pt 2), 249–258 (1985)
32. Cunningham, A.L., Turner, R.R., Miller, A.C., Para, M.F., Merigan, T.C.: Evolution of recurrent herpes simplex lesions. An immunohistologic study. J. Clin. Invest. **75**, 226–233 (1985)
33. de Witte, L., Nabatov, A., Pion, M., Fluitsma, D., de Jong, M.A., de Gruijl, T., Piguet, V., van Kooyk, Y., Geijtenbeek, T.B.: Langerin is a natural barrier to HIV-1 transmission by Langerhans cells. Nat. Med. **13**, 367–371 (2007)
34. Deeths, M.J., Mescher, M.F.: ICAM-1 and B7-1 provide similar but distinct costimulation for CD8+ T cells, while CD4+ T cells are poorly costimulated by ICAM-1. Eur. J. Immunol. **29**, 45–53 (1999)
35. Donaghy, H., Bosnjak, L., Harman, A.N., Marsden, V., Tyring, S.K., Meng, T.C., Cunningham, A.L.: Role for plasmacytoid dendritic cells in the immune control of recurrent human herpes simplex virus infection. J. Virol. **83**, 1952–1961 (2009)
36. Donaghy, H., Pozniak, A., Gazzard, B., Qazi, N., Gilmour, J., Gotch, F., Patterson, S.: Loss of blood CD11c(+) myeloid and CD11c(-) plasmacytoid dendritic cells in patients with HIV-1 infection correlates with HIV-1 RNA virus load. Blood **98**, 2574–2576 (2001)
37. Douek, D.C., Brenchley, J.M., Betts, M.R., Ambrozak, D.R., Hill, B.J., Okamoto, Y., Casazza, J.P., Kuruppu, J., Kunstman, K., Wolinsky, S., Grossman, Z., Dybul, M., Oxenius, A., Price, D.A., Connors, M., Koup, R.A.: HIV preferentially infects HIV-specific CD4+ T cells. Nature **417**, 95–98 (2002)
38. Fahrbach, K.M., Barry, S.M., Ayehunie, S., Lamore, S., Klausner, M., Hope, T.J.: Activated CD34-derived Langerhans cells mediate transinfection with human immunodeficiency virus. J. Virol. **81**, 6858–6868 (2007)
39. Fairley, C.K., Hocking, J.S., Gurrin, L.C., Chen, M.Y., Donovan, B., Bradshaw, C.S.: Rapid decline in presentations of genital warts after the implementation of a national quadrivalent human papillomavirus vaccination programme for young women. Sex. Transm. Infect. **85**, 499–502 (2009)
40. Ferlazzo, G., Munz, C.: Dendritic cell interactions with NK cells from different tissues. J. Clin. Immunol. **29**, 265–273 (2009)
41. Finberg, R.W., Kurt-Jones, E.A.: Viruses and Toll-like receptors. Microbes Infect. **6**, 1356–1360 (2004)
42. Flacher, V., Bouschbacher, M., Verronese, E., Massacrier, C., Sisirak, V., Berthier-Vergnes, O., de Saint-Vis, B., Caux, C., Dezutter-Dambuyant, C., Lebecque, S., Valladeau, J.: Human Langerhans cells express a specific TLR profile and differentially respond to viruses and Gram-positive bacteria. J. Immunol. **177**, 7959–7967 (2006)
43. Fonteneau, J.F., Gilliet, M., Larsson, M., Dasilva, I., Munz, C., Liu, Y.J., Bhardwaj, N.: Activation of influenza virus-specific CD4+ and CD8+ T cells: a new role for

plasmacytoid dendritic cells in adaptive immunity. Blood **101**, 3520–3526 (2003)

44. Fonteneau, J.F., Larsson, M., Beignon, A.S., McKenna, K., Dasilva, I., Amara, A., Liu, Y.J., Lifson, J.D., Littman, D.R., Bhardwaj, N.: Human immunodeficiency virus type 1 activates plasmacytoid dendritic cells and concomitantly induces the bystander maturation of myeloid dendritic cells. J. Virol. **78**, 5223–5232 (2004)
45. Frank, I., Stossel, H., Gettie, A., Turville, S.G., Bess Jr., J.W., Lifson, J.D., Sivin, I., Romani, N., Robbiani, M.: A fusion inhibitor prevents spread of immunodeficiency viruses, but not activation of virus-specific T cells, by dendritic cells. J. Virol. **82**, 5329–5339 (2008)
46. Frazer, I.H.: Interaction of human papillomaviruses with the host immune system: a well evolved relationship. Virology **384**, 410–414 (2009)
47. Freeman, E.E., Weiss, H.A., Glynn, J.R., Cross, P.L., Whitworth, J.A., Hayes, R.J.: Herpes simplex virus 2 infection increases HIV acquisition in men and women: systematic review and meta-analysis of longitudinal studies. AIDS **20**, 73–83 (2006)
48. Galvan, V., Roizman, B.: Herpes simplex virus 1 induces and blocks apoptosis at multiple steps during infection and protects cells from exogenous inducers in a cell-type-dependent manner. Proc. Natl Acad. Sci. USA **95**, 3931–3936 (1998)
49. Ganesh, L., Leung, K., Lore, K., Levin, R., Panet, A., Schwartz, O., Koup, R.A., Nabel, G.J.: Infection of specific dendritic cells by CCR5-tropic human immunodeficiency virus type 1 promotes cell-mediated transmission of virus resistant to broadly neutralizing antibodies. J. Virol. **78**, 11980–11987 (2004)
50. Garland, S.M., Brotherton, J.M., Skinner, S.R., Pitts, M., Saville, M., Mola, G., Jones, R.W.: Human papillomavirus and cervical cancer in Australasia and Oceania: risk-factors, epidemiology and prevention. Vaccine **26**(Suppl 12), M80–M88 (2008)
51. Garland, S.M., Hernandez-Avila, M., Wheeler, C.M., Perez, G., Harper, D.M., Leodolter, S., Tang, G.W., Ferris, D.G., Steben, M., Bryan, J., Taddeo, F.J., Railkar, R., Esser, M.T., Sings, H.L., Nelson, M., Boslego, J., Sattler, C., Barr, E., Koutsky, L.A.: Quadrivalent vaccine against human papillomavirus to prevent anogenital diseases. N Engl J. Med. **356**, 1928–1943 (2007)
52. Garland, S.M., Steben, M., Sings, H.L., James, M., Lu, S., Railkar, R., Barr, E., Haupt, R.M., Joura, E.A.: Natural history of genital warts: analysis of the placebo arm of 2 randomized phase III trials of a quadrivalent human papillomavirus (types 6, 11, 16, and 18) vaccine. J. Infect. Dis. **199**, 805–814 (2009)
53. Ginhoux, F., Collin, M.P., Bogunovic, M., Abel, M., Leboeuf, M., Helft, J., Ochando, J., Kissenpfennig, A., Malissen, B., Grisotto, M., Snoeck, H., Randolph, G., Merad, M.: Blood-derived dermal langerin+ dendritic cells survey the skin in the steady state. J. Exp. Med. **204**, 3133–3146 (2007)
54. Gonzalez, J.C., Kwok, W.W., Wald, A., McClurkan, C.L., Huang, J., Koelle, D.M.: Expression of cutaneous lymphocyte-associated antigen and E-selectin ligand by circulating human memory CD4+ T lymphocytes specific for herpes simplex virus type 2. J. Infect. Dis. **191**, 243–254 (2005)
55. Gray, L., Churchill, M.J., Sterjovski, J., Witlox, K., Learmont, J.C., Sullivan, J.S., Wesselingh, S.L., Gabuzda, D., Cunningham, A.L., McPhee, D.A., Gorry, P.R.: Phenotype and envelope gene diversity of nef-deleted HIV-1 isolated from long-term survivors infected from a single source. Virol. J. **4**, 75 (2007)
56. Gray, R.H., Kiwanuka, N., Quinn, T.C., Sewankambo, N.K., Serwadda, D., Mangen, F.W., Lutalo, T., Nalugoda, F., Kelly, R., Meehan, M., Chen, M.Z., Li, C., Wawer, M.J.: Male circumcision and HIV acquisition and transmission: cohort studies in Rakai. Uganda. Rakai project team. AIDS **14**, 2371–2381 (2000)
57. Gray, R.H., Serwadda, D., Kong, X., Makumbi, F., Kigozi, G., Gravitt, P.E., Watya, S., Nalugoda, F., Ssempijja, V., Tobian, A.A., Kiwanuka, N., Moulton, L.H., Sewankambo, N.K., Reynolds, S.J., Quinn, T.C., Iga, B., Laeyendecker, O., Oliver, A.E., Wawer, M.J.: Male circumcision decreases acquisition and increases clearance of high-risk human papillomavirus in hiv-negative men: a randomized trial in Rakai, Uganda. J. Infect. Dis. **201**(10), 1455–1462 (2010)
58. Groot, F., Kuijpers, T.W., Berkhout, B., de Jong, E.C.: Dendritic cell-mediated HIV-1 transmission to T cells of LAD-1 patients is impaired due to the defect in LFA-1. Retrovirology **3**, 75 (2006)
59. Gumbi, P.P., Nkwanyana, N.N., Bere, A., Burgers, W.A., Gray, C.M., Williamson, A.L., Hoffman, M., Coetzee, D., Denny, L., Passmore, J.A.: Impact of mucosal inflammation on cervical human immunodeficiency virus (HIV-1)-specific CD8 T-cell responses in the female genital tract during chronic HIV infection. J. Virol. **82**, 8529–8536 (2008)
60. Hanke, T., Graham, F.L., Rosenthal, K.L., Johnson, D.C.: Identification of an immunodominant cytotoxic T-lymphocyte recognition site in glycoprotein B of herpes simplex virus by using recombinant adenovirus vectors and synthetic peptides. J. Virol. **65**, 1177–1186 (1991)
61. Hanna, J., Gonen-Gross, T., Fitchett, J., Rowe, T., Daniels, M., Arnon, T.I., Gazit, R., Joseph, A., Schjetne, K.W., Steinle, A., Porgador, A., Mevorach, D., Goldman-Wohl, D., Yagel, S., LaBarre, M.J., Buckner, J.H., Mandelboim, O.: Novel APC-like properties of human NK cells directly regulate T cell activation. J. Clin. Invest. **114**, 1612–1623 (2004)
62. Hanna, J., Mandelboim, O.: When killers become helpers. Trends Immunol. **28**, 201–206 (2007)
63. Harman, A.N., Wilkinson, J., Bye, C.R., Bosnjak, L., Stern, J.L., Nicholle, M., Lai, J., Cunningham, A.L.: HIV induces maturation of monocyte-derived dendritic cells and Langerhans cells. J. Immunol. **177**, 7103–7113 (2006)
64. Hart, D.N.: Dendritic cells: unique leukocyte populations which control the primary immune response. Blood **90**, 3245–3287 (1997)
65. Hengel, H., Lindner, M., Wagner, H., Heeg, K.: Frequency of herpes simplex virus-specific murine cytotoxic T lymphocyte precursors in mitogen- and antigen-driven primary in vitro T cell responses. J. Immunol. **139**, 4196–4202 (1987)
66. Hirbod, T., Broliden, K.: Mucosal immune responses in the genital tract of HIV-1-exposed uninfected women. J. Intern. Med. **262**, 44–58 (2007)
67. Hladik, F., Hope, T.J.: HIV infection of the genital mucosa in women. Curr. HIV/AIDS Rep. **6**, 20–28 (2009)

68. Hladik, F., Sakchalathorn, P., Ballweber, L., Lentz, G., Fialkow, M., Eschenbach, D., McElrath, M.J.: Initial events in establishing vaginal entry and infection by human immunodeficiency virus type-1. Immunity **26**, 257–270 (2007)
69. Honda, K., Takaoka, A., Taniguchi, T.: Type I interferon [corrected] gene induction by the interferon regulatory factor family of transcription factors. Immunity **25**, 349–360 (2006)
70. Hong, A.M., Grulich, A.E., Jones, D., Lee, C.S., Garland, S.M., Dobbins, T.A., Clark, J.R., Harnett, G.B., Milross, C.G., O'Brien, C.J., Rose, B.R.: Squamous cell carcinoma of the oropharynx in Australian males induced by human papillomavirus vaccine targets. Vaccine **28**, 3269–3272 (2010)
71. II, F.: Quadrivalent vaccine against human papillomavirus to prevent high-grade cervical lesions. N Engl J. Med. **356**, 1915–1927 (2007)
72. Iijima, N., Thompson, J.M., Iwasaki, A.: Dendritic cells and macrophages in the genitourinary tract. Mucosal Immunol. **1**, 451–459 (2008)
73. Iwasaki, A.: The importance of CD11b+ dendritic cells in CD4+ T cell activation in vivo: with help from interleukin 1. J. Exp. Med. **198**, 185–190 (2003)
74. Jerome, K.R., Fox, R., Chen, Z., Sears, A.E., Lee, H., Corey, L.: Herpes simplex virus inhibits apoptosis through the action of two genes, Us5 and Us3. J. Virol. **73**, 8950–8957 (1999)
75. Johansson, E.L., Rudin, A., Wassen, L., Holmgren, J.: Distribution of lymphocytes and adhesion molecules in human cervix and vagina. Immunology **96**, 272–277 (1999)
76. Kadowaki, N., Antonenko, S., Lau, J.Y., Liu, Y.J.: Natural interferon alpha/beta-producing cells link innate and adaptive immunity. J. Exp. Med. **192**, 219–226 (2000)
77. Kadowaki, N., Ho, S., Antonenko, S., Waal Malefyt, R., Kastelein, R.A., Bazan, F., Liu, Y.J.: Subsets of human dendritic cell precursors express different toll-like receptors and respond to different microbial antigens. J. Exp. Med. **194**, 863–870 (2001)
78. Kaul, R., Plummer, F.A., Kimani, J., Dong, T., Kiama, P., Rostron, T., Njagi, E., MacDonald, K.S., Bwayo, J.J., McMichael, A.J., Rowland-Jones, S.L.: HIV-1-specific mucosal CD8+ lymphocyte responses in the cervix of HIV-1-resistant prostitutes in Nairobi. J. Immunol. **164**, 1602–1611 (2000)
79. Kaul, R., Thottingal, P., Kimani, J., Kiama, P., Waigwa, C.W., Bwayo, J.J., Plummer, F.A., Rowland-Jones, S.L.: Quantitative ex vivo analysis of functional virus-specific CD8 T lymphocytes in the blood and genital tract of HIV-infected women. AIDS **17**, 1139–1144 (2003)
80. Kawamura, K., Kadowaki, N., Kitawaki, T., Uchiyama, T.: Virus-stimulated plasmacytoid dendritic cells induce CD4+ cytotoxic regulatory T cells. Blood **107**, 1031–1038 (2006)
81. Kawamura, T., Bruse, S.E., Abraha, A., Sugaya, M., Hartley, O., Offord, R.E., Arts, E.J., Zimmerman, P.A., Blauvelt, A.: PSC-RANTES blocks R5 human immunodeficiency virus infection of Langerhans cells isolated from individuals with a variety of CCR5 diplotypes. J. Virol. **78**, 7602–7609 (2004)
82. Kawamura, T., Koyanagi, Y., Nakamura, Y., Ogawa, Y., Yamashita, A., Iwamoto, T., Ito, M., Blauvelt, A., Shimada, S.: Significant virus replication in Langerhans cells following application of HIV to abraded skin: relevance to occupational transmission of HIV. J. Immunol. **180**, 3297–3304 (2008)
83. Khanna, K.M., Lepisto, A.J., Decman, V., Hendricks, R.L.: Immune control of herpes simplex virus during latency. Curr. Opin. Immunol. **16**, 463–469 (2004)
84. Kim, M., Taylor, J., Sidney, J., Mikloska, Z., Bodsworth, N., Lagios, K., Dunckley, H., Byth-Wilson, K., Denis, M., Finlayson, R., Khanna, R., Sette, A., Cunningham, A.L.: Immunodominant epitopes in herpes simplex virus type 2 glycoprotein D are recognized by CD4 lymphocytes from both HSV-1 and HSV-2 seropositive subjects. J. Immunol. **181**, 6604–6615 (2008)
85. Knickelbein, J.E., Khanna, K.M., Yee, M.B., Baty, C.J., Kinchington, P.R., Hendricks, R.L.: Noncytotoxic lytic granule-mediated CD8+ T cell inhibition of HSV-1 reactivation from neuronal latency. Science **322**, 268–271 (2008)
86. Kobayashi, A., Darragh, T., Herndier, B., Anastos, K., Minkoff, H., Cohen, M., Young, M., Levine, A., Grant, L.A., Hyun, W., Weinberg, V., Greenblatt, R., Smith-McCune, K.: Lymphoid follicles are generated in high-grade cervical dysplasia and have differing characteristics depending on HIV status. Am. J. Pathol. **160**, 151–164 (2002)
87. Koelle, D.M., Frank, J.M., Johnson, M.L., Kwok, W.W.: Recognition of herpes simplex virus type 2 tegument proteins by CD4 T cells infiltrating human genital herpes lesions. J. Virol. **72**, 7476–7483 (1998)
88. Koelle, D.M., Liu, Z., McClurkan, C.M., Topp, M.S., Riddell, S.R., Pamer, E.G., Johnson, A.S., Wald, A., Corey, L.: Expression of cutaneous lymphocyte-associated antigen by CD8(+) T cells specific for a skin-tropic virus. J. Clin. Invest. **110**, 537–548 (2002)
89. Lackner, A.A., Veazey, R.S.: Current concepts in AIDS pathogenesis: insights from the SIV/macaque model. Annu. Rev. Med. **58**, 461–476 (2007)
90. Lafferty, W.E.: The changing epidemiology of HSV-1 and HSV-2 and implications for serological testing. Herpes **9**, 51–55 (2002)
91. Langelier, Y., Bergeron, S., Chabaud, S., Lippens, J., Guilbault, C., Sasseville, A.M., Denis, S., Mosser, D.D., Massie, B.: The R1 subunit of herpes simplex virus ribonucleotide reductase protects cells against apoptosis at, or upstream of, caspase-8 activation. J. Gen. Virol. **83**, 2779–2789 (2002)
92. Li, Q., Skinner, P.J., Ha, S.J., Duan, L., Mattila, T.L., Hage, A., White, C., Barber, D.L., O'Mara, L., Southern, P.J., Reilly, C.S., Carlis, J.V., Miller, C.J., Ahmed, R., Haase, A.T.: Visualizing antigen-specific and infected cells in situ predicts outcomes in early viral infection. Science **323**, 1726–1729 (2009)
93. Lore, K., Smed-Sorensen, A., Vasudevan, J., Mascola, J.R., Koup, R.A.: Myeloid and plasmacytoid dendritic cells transfer HIV-1 preferentially to antigen-specific CD4+ T cells. J. Exp. Med. **201**, 2023–2033 (2005)
94. Lund, J., Sato, A., Akira, S., Medzhitov, R., Iwasaki, A.: Toll-like receptor 9-mediated recognition of Herpes simplex virus-2 by plasmacytoid dendritic cells. J. Exp. Med. **198**, 513–520 (2003)
95. Lund, J.M., Linehan, M.M., Iijima, N., Iwasaki, A.: Cutting Edge: Plasmacytoid dendritic cells provide innate immune protection against mucosal viral infection in situ. J. Immunol. **177**, 7510–7514 (2006)

96. McCoombe, S.G., Short, R.V.: Potential HIV-1 target cells in the human penis. AIDS **20**, 1491–1495 (2006)
97. McDonald, D., Wu, L., Bohks, S.M., KewalRamani, V.N., Unutmaz, D., Hope, T.J.: Recruitment of HIV and its receptors to dendritic cell-T cell junctions. Science **300**, 1295–1297 (2003)
98. McElrath, M.J., De Rosa, S.C., Moodie, Z., Dubey, S., Kierstead, L., Janes, H., Defawe, O.D., Carter, D.K., Hural, J., Akondy, R., Buchbinder, S.P., Robertson, M.N., Mehrotra, D.V., Self, S.G., Corey, L., Shiver, J.W., Casimiro, D.R.: HIV-1 vaccine-induced immunity in the test-of-concept Step Study: a case-cohort analysis. Lancet **372**, 1894–1905 (2008)
99. Mestecky, J., Jackson, S., Moldoveanu, Z., Nesbit, L.R., Kulhavy, R., Prince, S.J., Sabbaj, S., Mulligan, M.J., Goepfert, P.A.: Paucity of antigen-specific IgA responses in sera and external secretions of HIV-type 1-infected individuals. AIDS Res. Hum. Retroviruses **20**, 972–988 (2004)
100. Mestecky, J., Raska, M., Novak, J., Alexander, R.C., Moldoveanu, Z.: Antibody-mediated protection and the mucosal immune system of the genital tract: relevance to vaccine design. J. Reprod. Immunol. **85**(1), 81–85 (2010)
101. Mettenleiter, T.C.: Intriguing interplay between viral proteins during herpesvirus assembly or: the herpesvirus assembly puzzle. Vet. Microbiol. **113**, 163–169 (2006)
102. Mikloska, Z., Bosnjak, L., Cunningham, A.L.: Immature monocyte-derived dendritic cells are productively infected with herpes simplex virus type 1. J. Virol. **75**, 5958–5964 (2001)
103. Mikloska, Z., Cunningham, A.L.: Alpha and gamma interferons inhibit herpes simplex virus type 1 infection and spread in epidermal cells after axonal transmission. J. Virol. **75**, 11821–11826 (2001)
104. Mikloska, Z., Cunningham, A.L.: Herpes simplex virus type 1 glycoproteins gB, gC and gD are major targets for CD4 T-lymphocyte cytotoxicity in HLA-DR expressing human epidermal keratinocytes. J. Gen. Virol. **79**(Pt 2), 353–361 (1998)
105. Mikloska, Z., Danis, V.A., Adams, S., Lloyd, A.R., Adrian, D.L., Cunningham, A.L.: In vivo production of cytokines and beta (C-C) chemokines in human recurrent herpes simplex lesions–do herpes simplex virus-infected keratinocytes contribute to their production? J. Infect. Dis. **177**, 827–838 (1998)
106. Mikloska, Z., Ruckholdt, M., Ghadiminejad, I., Dunckley, H., Denis, M., Cunningham, A.L.: Monophosphoryl lipid A and QS21 increase CD8 T lymphocyte cytotoxicity to herpes simplex virus-2 infected cell proteins 4 and 27 through IFN-gamma and IL-12 production. J. Immunol. **164**, 5167–5176 (2000)
107. Mikloska, Z., Sanna, P.P., Cunningham, A.L.: Neutralizing antibodies inhibit axonal spread of herpes simplex virus type 1 to epidermal cells in vitro. J. Virol. **73**, 5934–5944 (1999)
108. Miller, C.J., Hu, J.: T cell-tropic simian immunodeficiency virus (SIV) and simian-human immunodeficiency viruses are readily transmitted by vaginal inoculation of rhesus macaques, and Langerhans' cells of the female genital tract are infected with SIV. J. Infect. Dis. **179**(Suppl 3), S413–S417 (1999)
109. Miller, C.J., Li, Q., Abel, K., Kim, E.Y., Ma, Z.M., Wietgrefe, S., La Franco-Scheuch, L., Compton, L., Duan, L., Shore, M.D., Zupancic, M., Busch, M., Carlis, J., Wolinsky, S., Haase, A.T.: Propagation and dissemination of infection after vaginal transmission of simian immunodeficiency virus. J. Virol. **79**, 9217–9227 (2005)
110. Miller, C.J., Vogel, P., Alexander, N.J., Dandekar, S., Hendrickx, A.G., Marx, P.A.: Pathology and localization of simian immunodeficiency virus in the reproductive tract of chronically infected male rhesus macaques. Lab. Invest. **70**, 255–262 (1994)
111. Morandi, B., Bougras, G., Muller, W.A., Ferlazzo, G., Munz, C.: NK cells of human secondary lymphoid tissues enhance T cell polarization via IFN-gamma secretion. Eur. J. Immunol. **36**, 2394–2400 (2006)
112. Moretta, L., Ferlazzo, G., Bottino, C., Vitale, M., Pende, D., Mingari, M.C., Moretta, A.: Effector and regulatory events during natural killer-dendritic cell interactions. Immunol. Rev. **214**, 219–228 (2006)
113. Musey, L., Ding, Y., Cao, J., Lee, J., Galloway, C., Yuen, A., Jerome, K.R., McElrath, M.J.: Ontogeny and specificities of mucosal and blood human immunodeficiency virus type 1-specific CD8(+) cytotoxic T lymphocytes. J. Virol. **77**, 291–300 (2003)
114. O'Shea, J.J., Paul, W.E.: Mechanisms underlying lineage commitment and plasticity of helper CD4+ T cells. Science **327**, 1098–1102 (2010)
115. Olsson, S.E., Kjaer, S.K., Sigurdsson, K., Iversen, O.E., Hernandez-Avila, M., Wheeler, C.M., Perez, G., Brown, D.R., Koutsky, L.A., Tay, E.H., Garcia, P., Ault, K.A., Garland, S.M., Leodolter, S., Tang, G.W., Ferris, D.G., Paavonen, J., Lehtinen, M., Steben, M., Bosch, F.X., Dillner, J., Joura. E.A., Majewski S, Munoz N, Myers ER, Villa LL, Taddeo FJ, Roberts C, Tadesse A, Bryan, J., Maansson, R., Vuocolo. S., Hesley, T.M., Saah, A., Barr, E., Haupt, R.M.: Evaluation of quadrivalent HPV 6/11/16/18 vaccine efficacy against cervical and anogenital disease in subjects with serological evidence of prior vaccine type HPV infection. Hum. Vaccin. **5**, 696–704 (2009)
116. Olsson, S.E., Villa, L.L., Costa, R.L., Petta, C.A., Andrade, R.P., Malm, C., Iversen, O.E., Hoye, J., Steinwall, M., Riis-Johannessen, G., Andersson-Ellstrom, A., Elfgren, K., von Krogh, G., Lehtinen, M., Paavonen, J., Tamms, G.M., Giacoletti, K., Lupinacci, L., Esser, M.T., Vuocolo, S.C., Saah, A.J., Barr, E.: Induction of immune memory following administration of a prophylactic quadrivalent human papillomavirus (HPV) types 6/11/16/18 L1 virus-like particle (VLP) vaccine. Vaccine **25**, 4931–4939 (2007)
117. Overall Jr., J.C., Spruance, S.L., Green, J.A.: Viral-induced leukocyte interferon in vesicle fluid from lesions of recurrent herpes labialis. J. Infect. Dis. **143**, 543–547 (1981)
118. Paavonen, J., Jenkins, D., Bosch, F.X., Naud, P., Salmeron, J., Wheeler, C.M., Chow, S.N., Apter, D.L., Kitchener, H.C., Castellsague, X., de Carvalho, N.S., Skinner, S.R., Harper, D.M., Hedrick, J.A., Jaisamrarn, U., Limson, G.A., Dionne, M., Quint, W., Spiessens, B., Peeters, P., Struyf, F., Wieting, S.L., Lehtinen, M.O., Dubin, G.: Efficacy of a prophylactic adjuvanted bivalent L1 virus-like-particle vaccine against infection with human papillomavirus types 16 and 18 in young women: an interim analysis of a phase III

double-blind, randomised controlled trial. Lancet **369**, 2161–2170 (2007)

119. Paavonen, J., Naud, P., Salmeron, J., Wheeler, C.M., Chow, S.N., Apter, D., Kitchener, H., Castellsague, X., Teixeira, J.C., Skinner, S.R., Hedrick, J., Jaisamrarn, U., Limson, G., Garland, S., Szarewski, A., Romanowski, B., Aoki, F.Y., Schwarz, T.F., Poppe, W.A., Bosch, F.X., Jenkins, D., Hardt, K., Zahaf, T., Descamps, D., Struyf, F., Lehtinen, M., Dubin, G., Greenacre, M.: Efficacy of human papillomavirus (HPV)-16/18 AS04-adjuvanted vaccine against cervical infection and precancer caused by oncogenic HPV types (PATRICIA): final analysis of a double-blind, randomised study in young women. Lancet **374**, 301–314 (2009)
120. Perkins, D., Pereira, E.F., Aurelian, L.: The herpes simplex virus type 2 R1 protein kinase (ICP10 PK) functions as a dominant regulator of apoptosis in hippocampal neurons involving activation of the ERK survival pathway and upregulation of the antiapoptotic protein Bag-1. J. Virol. **77**, 1292–1305 (2003)
121. Poppe, W.A., Drijkoningen, M., Ide, P.S., Lauweryns, J.M., Van Assche, F.A.: Lymphocytes and dendritic cells in the normal uterine cervix. An immunohistochemical study. Eur. J. Obstet. Gynecol. Reprod. Biol. **81**, 277–282 (1998)
122. Poulin, L.F., Henri, S., de Bovis, B., Devilard, E., Kissenpfennig, A., Malissen, B.: The dermis contains langerin+ dendritic cells that develop and function independently of epidermal Langerhans cells. J. Exp. Med. **204**, 3119–3131 (2007)
123. Quayle, A.J.: The innate and early immune response to pathogen challenge in the female genital tract and the pivotal role of epithelial cells. J. Reprod. Immunol. **57**, 61–79 (2002)
124. Rasmussen, S.B., Sorensen, L.N., Malmgaard, L., Ank, N., Baines, J.D., Chen, Z.J., Paludan, S.R.: Type I interferon production during herpes simplex virus infection is controlled by cell-type-specific viral recognition through Toll-like receptor 9, the mitochondrial antiviral signaling protein pathway, and novel recognition systems. J. Virol. **81**, 13315–13324 (2007)
125. Reece, J.C., Handley, A.J., Anstee, E.J., Morrison, W.A., Crowe, S.M., Cameron, P.U.: HIV-1 selection by epidermal dendritic cells during transmission across human skin. J. Exp. Med. **187**, 1623–1631 (1998)
126. Reynolds, M.R., Rakasz, E., Skinner, P.J., White, C., Abel, K., Ma, Z.M., Compton, L., Napoe, G., Wilson, N., Miller, C.J., Haase, A., Watkins, D.I.: CD8+ T-lymphocyte response to major immunodominant epitopes after vaginal exposure to simian immunodeficiency virus: too late and too little. J. Virol. **79**, 9228–9235 (2005)
127. Roizman, B., Knipe, D.M., Whitley, R.: Herpes simplex viruses. In: Knipe, D.M., Howley, P.M., Griffin, D.E., Lamb, R.A., Martin, M.A., Roizman, B., Straus, S.E. (eds.) Field's Virology, 5th edn, pp. 2501–2601. Lippincott Williams & Wilkins, New York (2007)
128. Sato, A., Linehan, M.M., Iwasaki, A.: Dual recognition of herpes simplex viruses by TLR2 and TLR9 in dendritic cells. Proc. Natl Acad. Sci. USA **103**, 17343–17348 (2006)
129. Serwadda, D., Wawer, M.J., Makumbi, F., Kong, X., Kigozi, G., Gravitt, P., Watya, S., Nalugoda, F., Ssempijja, V., Tobian, A.A., Kiwanuka, N., Moulton, L.H., Sewankambo, N.K., Reynolds, S.J., Quinn, T.C., Oliver, A.E., Iga, B., Laeyendecker, O., Gray, R.H.: Circumcision of HIV-infected men: effects on high-risk human papillomavirus infections in a randomized trial in Rakai. Uganda. J. Infect. Dis. **201**(10), 1463–1469 (2010)
130. Shacklett, B.L.: Cell-mediated immunity to HIV in the female reproductive tract. J. Reprod. Immunol. **83**, 190–195 (2009)
131. Shortman, K., Liu, Y.J.: Mouse and human dendritic cell subtypes. Nat. Rev.Immunol. **2**, 151–161 (2002)
132. Shust, G.F., Cho, S., Kim, M., Madan, R.P., Guzman, E.M., Pollack, M., Epstein, J., Cohen, H.W., Keller, M.J., Herold, B.C.: Female genital tract secretions inhibit herpes simplex virus infection: correlation with soluble mucosal immune mediators and impact of hormonal contraception. Am. J. Reprod. Immunol. **63**, 110–119 (2010)
133. Siegal, F.P., Kadowaki, N., Shodell, M., Fitzgerald-Bocarsly, P.A., Shah, K., Ho, S., Antonenko, S., Liu, Y.J.: The nature of the principal type 1 interferon-producing cells in human blood. Science **284**, 1835–1837 (1999)
134. Siegal, F.P., Lopez, C., Hammer, G.S., Brown, A.E., Kornfeld, S.J., Gold, J., Hassett, J., Hirschman, S.Z., Cunningham-Rundles, C., Adelsberg, B.R., et al.: Severe acquired immunodeficiency in male homosexuals, manifested by chronic perianal ulcerative herpes simplex lesions. N Engl J. Med. **305**, 1439–1444 (1981)
135. Smed-Sorensen, A., Lore, K., Vasudevan, J., Louder, M.K., Andersson, J., Mascola, J.R., Spetz, A.L., Koup, R.A.: Differential susceptibility to human immunodeficiency virus type 1 infection of myeloid and plasmacytoid dendritic cells. J. Virol. **79**, 8861–8869 (2005)
136. Sodora, D.L., Allan, J.S., Apetrei, C., Brenchley, J.M., Douek, D.C., Else, J.G., Estes, J.D., Hahn, B.H., Hirsch, V.M., Kaur, A., Kirchhoff, F., Muller-Trutwin, M., Pandrea, I., Schmitz, J.E., Silvestri, G.: Toward an AIDS vaccine: lessons from natural simian immunodeficiency virus infections of African nonhuman primate hosts. Nat. Med. **15**, 861–865 (2009)
137. Soumelis, V., Scott, I., Gheyas, F., Bouhour, D., Cozon, G., Cotte, L., Huang, L., Levy, J.A., Liu, Y.J.: Depletion of circulating natural type 1 interferon-producing cells in HIV-infected AIDS patients. Blood **98**, 906–912 (2001)
138. Sprecher, E., Becker, Y.: Detection of IL-1 beta, TNF-alpha, and IL-6 gene transcription by the polymerase chain reaction in keratinocytes, Langerhans cells and peritoneal exudate cells during infection with herpes simplex virus-1. Arch. Virol. **126**, 253–269 (1992)
139. Stanberry, L.R., Spruance, S.L., Cunningham, A.L., Bernstein, D.I., Mindel, A., Sacks, S., Tyring, S., Aoki, F.Y., Slaoui, M., Denis, M., Vandepapeliere, P., Dubin, G.: Glycoprotein-D-adjuvant vaccine to prevent genital herpes. N Engl J. Med. **347**, 1652–1661 (2002)
140. Stanley, M.: Immune responses to human papillomavirus. Vaccine **24**(Suppl 1), S16–S22 (2006)
141. Stingl, G., Tamaki, K., Katz, S.I.: Origin and function of epidermal Langerhans cells. Immunol. Rev. **53**, 149–174 (1980)
142. Torseth, J.W., Merigan, T.C.: Significance of local gamma interferon in recurrent herpes simplex infection. J. Infect. Dis. **153**, 979–984 (1986)
143. Torseth, J.W., Nickoloff, B.J., Basham, T.Y., Merigan, T.C.: Beta interferon produced by keratinocytes in human

cutaneous infection with herpes simplex virus. J. Infect. Dis. **155**, 641–648 (1987)

144. Turville, S.G., Cameron, P.U., Handley, A., Lin, G., Pohlmann, S., Doms, R.W., Cunningham, A.L.: Diversity of receptors binding HIV on dendritic cell subsets. Nat. Immunol. **3**, 975–983 (2002)
145. Turville, S.G., Santos, J.J., Frank, I., Cameron, P.U., Wilkinson, J., Miranda-Saksena, M., Dable, J., Stossel, H., Romani, N., Piatak Jr., M., Lifson, J.D., Pope, M., Cunningham, A.L.: Immunodeficiency virus uptake, turnover, and 2-phase transfer in human dendritic cells. Blood **103**, 2170–2179 (2004)
146. Wakim, L.M., Waithman, J., van Rooijen, N., Heath, W.R., Carbone, F.R.: Dendritic cell-induced memory T cell activation in nonlymphoid tissues. Science **319**, 198–202 (2008)
147. Wald, A.: Synergistic interactions between herpes simplex virus type-2 and human immunodeficiency virus epidemics. Herpes **11**, 70–76 (2004)
148. Weiss, H.A.: Male circumcision as a preventive measure against HIV and other sexually transmitted diseases. Curr. Opin. Infect. Dis. **20**, 66–72 (2007)
149. Wendt, K., Wilk, E., Buyny, S., Buer, J., Schmidt, R.E., Jacobs, R.: Gene and protein characteristics reflect functional diversity of CD56dim and CD56bright NK cells. J. Leukoc. Biol. **80**, 1529–1541 (2006)
150. Wilflingseder, D., Mullauer, B., Schramek, H., Banki, Z., Pruenster, M., Dierich, M.P., Stoiber, H.: HIV-1-induced migration of monocyte-derived dendritic cells is associated with differential activation of MAPK pathways. J. Immunol. **173**, 7497–7505 (2004)
151. Wilkinson, J., Cunningham, A.L.: Mucosal transmission of HIV-1: first stop dendritic cells. Curr. Drug Targets **7**, 1563–1569 (2006)
152. Williams, A., Flavell, R.A., Eisenbarth, S.C.: The role of NOD-like receptors in shaping adaptive immunity. Curr. Opin. Immunol. **22**, 34–40 (2010)
153. Wira, C.R., Fahey, J.V., Sentman, C.L., Pioli, P.A., Shen, L.: Innate and adaptive immunity in female genital tract: cellular responses and interactions. Immunol. Rev. **206**, 306–335 (2005)
154. Xiang, J., Huang, H., Liu, Y.: A new dynamic model of CD8+ T effector cell responses via CD4+ T helper-antigen-presenting cells. J. Immunol. **174**, 7497–7505 (2005)
155. Young, L.J., Wilson, N.S., Schnorrer, P., Mount, A., Lundie, R.J., La Gruta, N.L., Crabb, B.S., Belz, G.T., Heath, W.R., Villadangos, J.A.: Dendritic cell preactivation impairs MHC class II presentation of vaccines and endogenous viral antigens. Proc. Natl Acad. Sci. USA **104**, 17753–17758 (2007)
156. Zarling, J.M., Moran, P.A., Lasky, L.A., Moss, B.: Herpes simplex virus (HSV)-specific human T-cell clones recognize HSV glycoprotein D expressed by a recombinant vaccinia virus. J. Virol. **59**, 506–509 (1986)
157. Zhang, S.Y., Jouanguy, E., Sancho-Shimizu, V., von Bernuth, H., Yang, K., Abel, L., Picard, C., Puel, A., Casanova, J.L.: Human Toll-like receptor-dependent induction of interferons in protective immunity to viruses. Immunol. Rev. **220**, 225–236 (2007)
158. Zhang, Z., Schuler, T., Zupancic, M., Wietgrefe, S., Staskus, K.A., Reimann, K.A., Reinhart, T.A., Rogan, M., Cavert, W., Miller, C.J., Veazey, R.S., Notermans, D., Little, S., Danner, S.A., Richman, D.D., Havlir, D., Wong, J., Jordan, H.L., Schacker, T.W., Racz, P., Tenner-Racz, K., Letvin, N.L., Wolinsky, S., Haase, A.T.: Sexual transmission and propagation of SIV and HIV in resting and activated CD4+ T cells. Science **286**, 1353–1357 (1999)
159. Zhao, X., Deak, E., Soderberg, K., Linehan, M., Spezzano, D., Zhu, J., Knipe, D.M., Iwasaki, A.: Vaginal submucosal dendritic cells, but not Langerhans cells, induce protective Th1 responses to herpes simplex virus-2. J. Exp. Med. **197**, 153–162 (2003)
160. Zhou, G., Roizman, B.: The domains of glycoprotein D required to block apoptosis depend on whether glycoprotein D is present in the virions carrying herpes simplex virus 1 genome lacking the gene encoding the glycoprotein. J. Virol. **75**, 6166–6172 (2001)
161. Zhu, J., Hladik, F., Woodward, A., Klock, A., Peng, T., Johnston, C., Remington, M., Magaret, A., Koelle, D.M., Wald, A., Corey, L.: Persistence of HIV-1 receptor-positive cells after HSV-2 reactivation is a potential mechanism for increased HIV-1 acquisition. Nat. Med. **15**, 886–892 (2009)

Part II

Bacterial Infections

Biology of *Neisseria gonorrhoeae* and the Clinical Picture of Infection

6

Catherine A. Ison

Core Messages

- Gonorrhoea is the second most common sexually transmitted infection; 62 million cases were reported by the World Health Organisation in 2001.
- The burden of infection is in young women and sequelae can occur and include pelvic inflammatory disease resulting in ectopic pregnancy and infertility.
- Molecular testing using nucleic acid amplification tests (NAATs) is now known to detect more infection than culture for *Neisseria gonorrhoeae*, including in extra-genital sites.
- Isolation of *Neisseria gonorrhoeae*, the causative agent of gonorrhoea remains essential to provide a viable organism to detect emerging resistance.
- Emerging decreased susceptibility to the third generation extended spectrum cephalosporins is a threat to the treatment of gonorrhoea, as alternative therapies are lacking.

6.1 Introduction

Neisseria gonorrhoeae is an obligate human pathogen, which colonises primarily the mucosa of the lower anogenital tract, resulting in uncomplicated gonococcal infection (UGI). The organism can ascend to the normally sterile upper genital tract and cause complicated gonococcal infection (CGI) but this is relatively uncommon and is a consequence of undetected or poorly treated UGI. Invasion into the blood to cause disseminated gonococcal infection (DGI) can occur but is rare. Gonorrhoea is considered unequivocally a sexually transmitted infection (STI) and as such has been used as a marker of sexual activity. Gonorrhoea, together with other STIs, facilitates human immunodeficiency virus (HIV) transmission and hence effective treatment plays an important role in HIV prevention strategies.

6.2 Pathogenesis

Gonococcal infection occurs when the organism attaches to the mucosal surface, invades the epithelium and establishes itself in the lamina propria or sub-epithelial space. *N. gonorrhoeae* is a highly adapted organism and can acquire nutrients from its host and has developed mechanisms to evade the immune response. Once infection is established gonococcal antigens will elicit an inflammatory response resulting in infiltration of polymorphs, which manifests as a discharge.

For colonisation to be successful the organism must first avoid removal by urine in men and cervical secretions in women, by attaching to the epithelial cell

C.A. Ison
Sexually Transmitted Bacteria Reference Laboratory,
Health Protection Agency Centre for Infections,
61 Colindale Avenue, London, NW9 5EQ, UK
e-mail: catherine.ison@hpa.org.uk

G. Gross and S.K. Tyring (eds.), *Sexually Transmitted Infections and Sexually Transmitted Diseases*,
DOI: 10.1007/978-3-642-14663-3_6, © Springer-Verlag Berlin Heidelberg 2011

surface. Pili, hydrophobic surface appendages, are the primary mediators of attachment and overcome the electrostatic forces between the host and bacterial cell and then attach by specific receptors. *N. gonorrhoeae* produce type VI pili [31] which attach to CD46, a member of the complement resistance proteins [24], which is the host cell receptor. The Opa proteins, a family of 11 proteins, are secondary mediators but lipooligosaccharide (LOS) and the gonococcal porin, Por, have also been implicated in adhesion to the cell surface. Opa proteins confer a tight attachment to the epithelial cell, recognising one of two classes of cellular receptors, the heparan sulfate proteoglycans and distinct carcinoembryonic antigens (CD66). Once successfully attached, invasion and transcytosis through the epithelial cell is initiated by the Opa proteins [33] [20] but has also been associated with LOS [49] and the major outer membrane protein, Por [30], whose major function is as a channel for essential nutrients. Once colonisation is established in the sub-epithelial layer, cytokines are induced, including tumour necrosis factor-α, that initiate an inflammatory response or may lead to the induction of apoptosis and loss of epithelial cells. In order for the organism to invade and cause systemic infection it needs to be able to resist the bactericidal activity of normal human serum which it achieves by sialylation of the LOS, rather than expression of a capsule as found in *Neisseria meningitidis*.

N. gonorrhoeae need to acquire iron to survive and maintain the infection and, unlike other organisms which produce siderophores to chelate iron from the environment, *N. gonorrhoeae* have evolved mechanisms to acquire iron directly from human transferrin and lactoferrin [1]. It is postulated that in the absence of sufficient iron, transcription of transferrin and lactoferrin receptors and transferring binding proteins is induced in the organism. These receptors interact with human transferrin and lactoferrin and iron is removed and transported across the bacterial cell membrane into the periplasmic space. During this process there is a transient association with iron-binding proteins and then iron is transported across the cytoplasmic membrane. Other essential nutrients are transported through the porin, which is a polymer of the outer membrane proteins Por and Rmp.

N. gonorrhoeae does not elicit a protective immune response and this is attributed to its ability to control and change the expression of its major outer membrane antigens which enables the organism to appear novel to the host. This plays an important role in pathogenesis as it acts to prolong infections, prevent immunity to reinfection and to change the functional properties of the organism.

6.3 Epidemiology

The World Health Organisation estimated the global burden of gonorrhoea in 1999 to be 62 million new cases [60], although this is considered an underestimate because of under-reporting due to high levels of asymptomatic infection and the lack of good surveillance systems in some countries. Gonorrhoea in the twentieth century showed peaks around both world wars followed by a decline resulting from the introduction of penicillin in the 1950s. However, in the period 1960–1970 there was a substantial increase in many industrialised countries that has been attributed to the introduction of the contraceptive pill and increase in promiscuity [9, 21]. In the early 1980s the use of effective therapy, good diagnostics and contact tracing began to reduce the prevalence of gonorrhoea but a considerably more dramatic decline followed with the advent of acquired immunodeficiency syndrome (AIDS), the first fatal STI and the subsequent changes in sexual behaviour [35]. In countries such as the UK and the USA the number of cases was lowest in 1995–1997, with 12,000 cases reported in 1995 in the UK and 392,848 cases in the USA. A similar picture was seen across most of Europe [17]. In the developing world the prevalence of gonorrhoea is higher than in most industrialised countries because of the lack of resources for effective therapy and good diagnostics. However, although good prevalence estimates are lacking, recent surveillance data suggest that there may have been a decline in the decade prior to 2008 [55].

Gonorrhoea is found in core groups of individuals, usually concentrated in inner cities often in areas of low socio-economic status [63] [46]. Individuals in core groups often have a higher rate of partner change, more concurrent sexual partners and/or shorter periods between consecutive sexual partnerships compared to the general population. High prevalence of infection can be perpetuated within the core group by assortative (like with like) sexual mixing patterns [10]. Core groups that are important for gonorrhoea include female sex workers, ethnic minorities and men who have sex with men (MSM). In common with other STIs, the burden of infection in many countries is found among young adults; women between 16 and 19 years of age are particularly at risk.

The amount of gonorrhoea found outside core groups is largely unknown. Unlike chlamydial infection, which in the UK has been found to be widespread in the population in approximately 10% of sexually active young people under 25 years of age, gonorrhoea is believed to be a very low prevalence in the general population because infection is symptomatic in most men who would therefore seek treatment. However, there is very little evidence to support or dispute this assumption, and although emerging reports suggest that asymptomatic gonorrhoea can be found by opportunistic screening [28, 42, 51], the levels are variable and considerably lower than those for chlamydia [27].

Gonorrhoea is transmitted during sexual intercourse, with the chance of acquisition from an infected man to a women being estimated at 50–60% and from an infected women to an uninfected man at 20%. Gonorrhoea does occur in children and colonisation can occur in the vulval–vaginal area as this is lined with columnar epithelia in the pre-pubertal girls. Infection is most likely to have resulted from sexual activity but there are multiple reports of non-sexual transmission and the likelihood of this is difficult to exclude.

6.4 Clinical Presentation

6.4.1 Uncomplicated Gonococcal Infection

The primary site of infection is the urethra in men and the endocervix in women because *N. gonorrhoeae* attaches preferentially to columnar epithelium and not to squamous epithelia as found in the vagina. Infection does occur in the rectum and oropharynx, mostly in MSM or individuals who practice anal and/or oral intercourse. Urethral or rectal infection in women may reflect contamination with, or secondary colonisation from, cervical secretion.

In men symptoms of urethral discharge or dysuria occur in the majority of infected individuals, over 90%, and the discharge is classically described as purulent but can be scanty and clear [22]. Symptoms appear within 3–7 days following exposure, although recent evidence suggests that this interval has lengthened increasing the chance of transmission before diagnosis and treatment. Asymptomatic urethral infection is found in a minority of men in most populations but is an important reservoir for transmission. Rectal infection can be symptomatic in approximately 18–30% of men whereas pharyngeal infection seldom presents with symptoms.

In women symptoms may present as a vaginal discharge, due to increased exudate from the cervix, but at least 50% of infections are asymptomatic and are diagnosed as sexual contacts of infected partners or by screening in either specialised sexual health or gynaecological clinics. Rectal infections are only symptomatic in a small number of women and pharyngeal infection is asymptomatic, as in men, and usually detected by screening individuals at risk. Local infection of Bartholin's or Skene's glands can occur but is uncommon.

6.4.2 Complicated Gonococcal Infection

Complicated infection occurs when the organism ascends to the upper genital tract, the epididymis and testis in men and the endometrium, fallopian tubes or the pelvic peritoneum in women resulting in pelvic inflammatory disease (PID). Complicated infection is believed to occur if the primary infection is inadequately treated or left untreated and is therefore more common in women than in men, because of the higher rate of asymptomatic infection in women. PID presents as acute pelvic pain and has the serious sequelae of infertility or ectopic pregnancy. The chance of infertility increases with each subsequent episode of gonococcal PID. However, in Europe, PID is more commonly caused by *Chlamydia trachomatis* than by *N. gonorrhoeae* and gonococcal PID is relatively uncommon. In other parts of the world, where resources for diagnosis and effective treatment are not always available, gonococcal PID is more common. Complications of PID include ovarian abscesses, pelvic peritonitis and peri-hepatitis (Fitz–Hugh–Curtis syndrome, inflammation of Glisson's capsule of the liver) [22].

6.4.3 Disseminated Gonococcal Infection

DGI, where *N. gonorrhoeae* invades into the bloodstream following a primary mucosal infection and causes a systemic infection, is a distinct entity rather than a complication of an untreated infection. DGI is more common in women than men and this may be associated with the ability of the organism to invade during menstruation when the cervix is more friable. DGI is rare in most countries but in the 1970s was associated with certain nutritionally requiring strains of *N. gonorrhoeae*, which were highly sensitive to penicillin, and several small clusters were reported in western USA and Sweden. Individuals with deficiencies in the late complement components are more susceptible to systemic infection with both *N. gonorrhoeae* and *N. meningitidis*. DGI often presents as arthritis, commonly in the knee or ankle joint, with or without septicaemia, and a rash. It can be difficult to isolate *N. gonorrhoeae* from the aspirate and so diagnosis is often confirmed by the presence of an anogenital or pharyngeal infection. Molecular detection of *N. gonorrhoeae* from the aspirate can be successful in some instances.

6.4.4 Eye Infections

Gonococcal infection can be acquired by neonates during delivery through the birth canal of infected mothers (Ophthalmia neonatorum) and occasionally occurs in adults probably by self-inoculation. Infection of the conjunctiva and oedema of the lid are followed by a purulent exudate. Corneal scarring and perforation can result without prompt diagnosis and treatment.

6.4.5 Gonorrhoea in Children

Gonorrhoea in young girls can present as a vulvovaginitis as the epithelium of the lower genital tract is immature and not keratinised. In girls aged less than 13 years gonorrhoea is a marker of sexual abuse and care should be taken to obtain appropriate specimens.

6.5 Diagnosis

6.5.1 Presumptive Diagnosis

Microscopy to detect the presence of intracellular Gram-negative diplococci is used for the presumptive diagnosis of gonorrhoea in primary care settings worldwide. Direct microscopy is a simple, inexpensive and rapid means of identifying potentially infected patients to enable treatment to be administered immediately and hence prevent further transmission of infection.

The sensitivity using urethral smears from symptomatic men is 95% or greater (Fig. 6.1) although it is considerably less in asymptomatic men. In women the sensitivity is also lower (30–50%) and probably reflects the smaller number of organisms found particularly in asymptomatic individuals and the presence of contaminating normal flora from the vagina (Fig. 6.2). It is no longer routine practice to take blind rectal smears for microscopy, as the sensitivity is low due to the large number of bacteria found in the rectum, many of which would be Gram-negative cocci. Microscopy is most useful for specimens from the rectum if there is evidence of infection and if exudates are obtained through a proctoscope. There is no value in using microscopy for pharyngeal specimens due to the large numbers of commensal Neisseriae found at this site.

In some resource-poor settings where Gram stains are not available smears are stained by methylene blue, which has a similar sensitivity to the Gram stain but

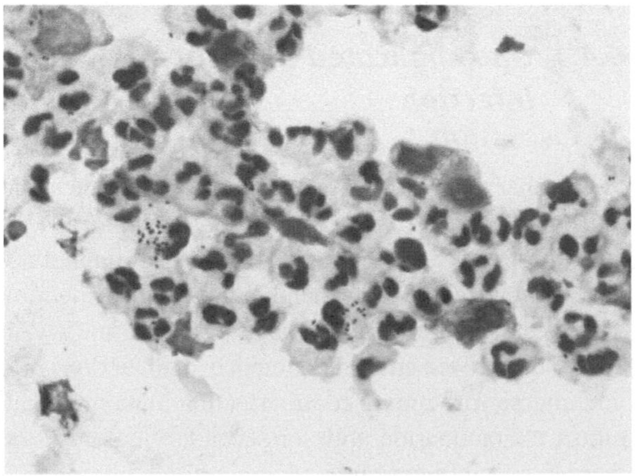

Fig. 6.1 Gram-stained urethral smear from a symptomatic man showing intracellular gram-negative diplococci

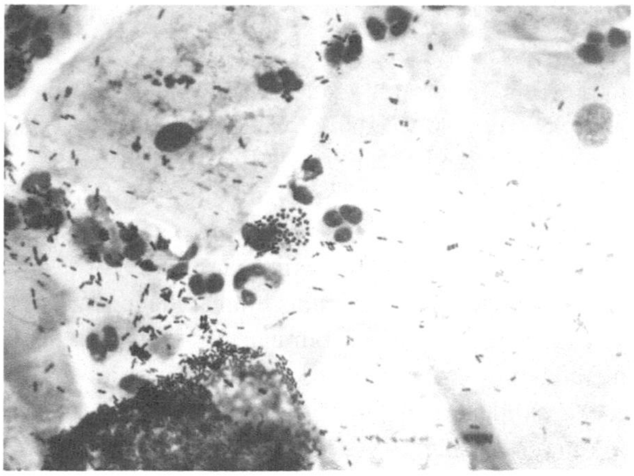

Fig. 6.2 Gram-stained cervical smear showing intracellular gram-negative diplococci and mixed vaginal flora

lacks specificity, as it is not possible to confirm the presence of Gram-negative diplococci. Despite the many advances in detection methods for gonorrhoea, microscopy for Gram-negative diplococci remains a very valuable tool and in some settings is the only method available. In these instances there is the obvious disadvantage that at least 50% of women will remain undiagnosed but it does allow those with a positive smear to receive appropriate treatment immediately.

The specificity of the Gram-stained smear with urethral and endo-cervical smears is high with trained personnel. The presence of extracellular Gram-negative diplococci when there is no evidence of intracellular organisms does pose a clinical challenge. Extracellular organisms do not fulfill the diagnostic criteria but in some instances clinical judgment may result in offering the patient treatment.

6.5.2 Isolation

Isolation of the infecting organism has been the mainstay of the laboratory diagnosis of infectious disease for many decades. However, the development of highly sensitive, specific and rapid methods has revolutionised the approach to confirming the cause of an infection. The use of culture remained the method of choice for gonorrhoea for considerably longer than many other infections, but in recent years commercially available tests that provide accurate and rapid detection with non-invasively taken samples are being used to supplement or replace culture methods. However, there is a continuing need to maintain culture to provide viable organisms to detect emerging resistance and for medico-legal purposes.

N. gonorrhoeae is a fastidious organism and hence requires an enriched medium for growth. Media such as Thayer-Martin or modified New York City or equivalents consist of GC agar base, which is rich in peptones and starch, supplemented with a source of iron and growth factors, usually lysed horse blood, or serum-free supplements such as Vitox or IsoVitaleX, although haemoglobin can be used. The addition of antimicrobial and antifungal agents to prevent overgrowth of normal flora is recommended particularly for use with endocervical and rectal specimens. A cocktail containing vancomycin or lincomycin, to inhibit Gram-positive organisms, colistin and trimethoprim, to inhibit other Gram-negative organisms, and nystatin or amphotericin, to inhibit yeasts, is widely used and available commercially. Vancomycin-sensitive strains do occur but lincomycin is less inhibitory and overgrowth can occur, particularly from normal flora found in rectal specimens such as *Proteus* spp.

N. gonorrhoeae colonise mucosal surfaces and therefore require warm, moist conditions for optimal growth; high humidity (>90%) with 5–7% carbon dioxide at 36°C, for a minimum of 48 h before being discarded as negative.

The sensitivity of isolation of *N. gonorrhoeae* as a diagnostic tool can be variable and is dependent on good specimen collection, and transportation to the laboratory in addition to an appropriate isolation procedure. Specimens can be collected either with cotton-tipped swab or a plastic disposable loop. In many clinics the specimen is inoculated directly onto the gonococcal isolation medium and then incubated immediately until transported to the laboratory. An alternative approach, particularly if the laboratory is a significant distance from the clinic, is for a swab to be placed in transport medium such as Amie's or Stuart's before sending to the laboratory. If swabs in transport medium need to be stored prior to transfer then they should be stored in the refrigerator as the principle of transport medium is that the organisms are held in a minimal medium designed to retard growth, and prevent autolysis, and this is best achieved at a reduced temperature. The swab should be used to inoculate gonococcal culture medium within 48 h to achieve acceptable retrieval of *N. gonorrhoeae*, after that time some bacterial loss will occur. Many consider direct inoculation the method of choice but there is little evidence base to support this assumption and transport swabs are an acceptable alternative when the situation necessitates their use. Commercial isolation medium that can be inoculated, incubated overnight and then transported by post or courier such as Jembec and Transgrow are available.

6.5.3 Identification

Colonies that grow on specialised gonococcal medium that are Gram-negative cocci and give a positive oxidase test (presence of cytochrome c oxidase) can be presumptively identified as *N. gonorrhoeae*. In some parts of the world where there are not sufficient resources further identification may not be performed but in most industrialised countries it is still standard practice to undertake further testing to confirm the identity as *N. gonorrhoeae* by eliminating *N. meningitidis*, *Neisseria lactamica* and *Neisseria cinerea*.

Two approaches can be used: biochemical tests to provide a full speciation and immunological testing to specifically confirm the identity of *N. gonorrhoeae*. Biochemical identification is now usually achieved using commercial kits that detect preformed enzymes to give a result within 4 h. These kits include testing for utilisation of carbohydrates, which has historically been the gold standard for identification of *N. gonorrhoeae* but also include aminopeptidases, which aid the differentiation between *N. gonorrhoeae* and *N. meningitidis*. A suspension of a pure growth of *N. gonorrhoeae* is inoculated into a series of cupules containing individual substrates and following incubation each cupule is scored and a profile obtained which is interpreted using the manufacturer's manual website. These kits are particularly useful for laboratories those only encounter gonococcal isolates infrequently. Commercial products that test the production of aminopeptidases alone should be used with caution as gonococcal isolates that lack proline iminopeptidase [3], normally indicative of *N. gonorrhoeae*, have been identified in many countries [5, 57].

Immunological reagents that confirm the identification of *N. gonorrhoeae* but do not provide a speciation of isolates are useful for laboratories that regularly isolate *N. gonorrhoeae*. All the reagents available are based on a mixture of monoclonal antibodies to the major outer membrane protein, Por. The most commonly used reagents that utilise the antibodies are linked to staphylococcal protein A (Phadebact) and fluorescein (Microtrak), and reagents linked to latex particles are also available. The advantages of these reagents is that they can usually be performed directly from the primary isolation plate and provide a rapid result. These reagents are often used as a first-line approach to identification, which is followed by testing all negative results using biochemical identification.

Molecular identification can be achieved using methods primarily described for detection of gonorrhoea. While molecular identification is currently used in reference laboratories, it has the potential to be the method of choice for identification in future years.

6.5.4 Molecular Detection

The use of the isolation and identification of *N. gonorrhoeae* has remained the gold standard of the diagnosis of gonorrhoea until recent years because earlier attempts at antigen or molecular detection were unsuccessful. This has largely been due to the difficulty in targeting an antigen or nucleic acid sequence specific to *N. gonorrhoeae*, hence resulting in large numbers of false positives. However, the isolation of *N. gonorrhoeae*, which can have a high sensitivity and specificity, is intolerant of problems with transportation or isolation methods resulting in a reduced sensitivity and there are reports of sensitivities as low as 60%. Nucleic acid amplification tests (NAATs) have a greater tolerance to inadequacies in specimen collection or storage and in some cases can be stored at room temperature for several days or many weeks once frozen and are therefore more applicable in different settings. The greater tolerance is important as more individuals are increasingly tested or screened for gonorrhoea in a variety of different settings, from specialised sexual health clinics to primary care and this has helped drive a change towards molecular detection using NAAT in recent years. In many settings where a high throughput of patients is desirable or there are no facilities for obtaining invasive specimens NAATS facilitate the use of non-invasive specimens such as urine and self-taken vaginal swabs. It should be noted that urine is not the optimal specimen for the detection of *N. gonorrhoeae* in women [12].

The commercially available kits are now considerably more robust than they were previously and have a high sensitivity and specificity and offer dual detection of *N. gonorrhoeae* and *C. trachomatis*. Commercial kits currently available use different methods of nucleic acid amplification including polymerase chain reaction (PCR), strand displacement amplification (SDA), transcription-mediated amplification (TMA) and real-time PCR (RT-PCR), and target different genes. These kits are Conformité Européenne (CE)-marked and Food and Drug Administration (FDA)-approved for a variety of genital specimen types and they are widely used. A number of in-house tests have been reported and those targeting the pseudo *por*A and *opa* gene are particularly useful [59]. Care should be taken when using any assay that targets the *cpp*B gene, as this gene is not present in all gonococci and is occasionally found in strains of *N. meningitidis*.

The use of NAATs for extra-genital specimens, rectal and pharyngeal, has been controversial because none of the NAATS are licensed or approved for specimens from these sites for *N. gonorrhoeae* or *C. trachomatis*. There is now increasing evidence that NAATs have a superior sensitivity [4] when compared to culture and are now the method of choice [2]. The possibility of cross-reaction with genes in the closely related commensal Neisseria remains [39] and it is recommended that all positives from these sites should be confirmed using a different target [59].

All commercially available NAATs have a high sensitivity and specificity but the positive predictive value of a test will be dependent on the prevalence. Gonorrhoea differs from chlamydial infection in this regard, in that the prevalence of chlamydial infection is reported as high as 10% in young people under the age of 25 years whereas the prevalence of gonorrhoea is considerably lower and often unknown. It is recommended that the testing algorithm for any specimen type for the detection of *N. gonorrhoeae* should have a positive predictive value of greater than 90% [59] and in many populations this will require the use of a supplementary test. In some countries it is standard practice to repeat any positive result using the same specimen and the same target. This checks both the reproducibility of the result and the testing process but is considered unnecessary by many and is not recommended by some guidelines.

6.5.5 Point of Care Tests

Microscopy itself is the current best point of care testing (POCT) or near patient tests available for gonorrhoea. It is simple and rapid to perform and gives a result within 30 min which can be used to guide treatment. Lateral flow-based POCTs that are available for *C. trachomatis* have been lacking for the diagnosis of gonorrhoea because of the difficulty in finding an antigen specific to *N. gonorrhoeae*, the problem faced by earlier laboratory antigen detection tests. The next generation of these tests will be nucleic acid-based and given the success of NAATs there is potential that these may be successful. The question remains for which population these would be most useful for a low prevalence infection, and it would seem sensible to use them in genito-urinary medicine (GUM) clinics, at least in the first instance, where quality assurance can be monitored and surveillance data obtained.

6.6 Mechanisms of Antimicrobial Resistance

N. gonorrhoeae are inherently susceptible to antimicrobial agents but have an extraordinary ability to acquire and develop resistance. Sulphonamides were initially used to treat gonorrhoea, but resistance emerged rapidly, and was followed by penicillin during the 1940s using very small doses, as the organism was highly susceptible to this new agent. Unfortunately, *N. gonorrhoeae* became progressively less susceptible over the next 5 decades and was treated by increasing the dosage. Resistance emerged first in 1976 [6, 41] by the acquisition of a plasmid, probably from *Haemophilus* spp., that encoded for the TEM-1 type penicillinase, and then in 1985 by accumulation of multiple chromosomal mutations.

6.6.1 Penicillin

Enzyme-mediated resistance to penicillin was carried out initially on a plasmid of either 4.4 Megadaltons (MD) or 3.2 MD which were found in gonococci isolated in the Far East and Africa, respectively. These plasmids required the presence of a conjugative plasmid of 24.5 MD, which was already found in some gonococci, to transfer between gonococci and eventually spread worldwide [43]. Subsequently a number of plasmids of differing sizes were described but these caused more localised outbreaks and all the plasmids were found to carry the complete TEM-1 gene with varying deletions in the non-functional part of the gene [37]. Penicillinase-producing *N. gonorrhoeae* (PPNG) exhibit high-level resistance whereas chromosomally resistant *N. gonorrhoeae* (CMRNG) exhibit low-level resistance with less chance of therapeutic failure. Chromosomal resistance results from the additive effect of multiple mutations, which have probably been selected by the use of a single agent over many years. The mutations of *pen*A, *mtr* and *pen*B were believed to be responsible for chromosomal resistance to penicillin [50], although it was noted that it was not possible to produce the same levels of resistance in laboratory experiments as was found in clinical isolates. A further two mutations, *pon*A and *pen*C, were described more recently [45] and together they effect the permeability of the cell wall acting as a barrier to the penicillin and exhibit full resistance.

6.6.2 Spectinomycin

Spectinomycin, a macrolide, replaced penicillin in areas where penicillin was no longer effective for a short time. It was not an ideal agent as it was delivered by injection, often causing pain for the patient and one-step high-level resistance did emerge in areas of high usage [7, 16].

6.6.3 Ciprofloxacin

Ciprofloxacin, a fluoroquinolone, administered orally, to which *N. gonorrhoeae* were exquisitely sensitive, became the agent of choice in the 1990s. Initially dosage of 250 mg was recommended, with anecdotal reports of usage of 125 mg. However, resistance emerged, probably as the result of misuse of the earlier quinolones in areas such as the Western Pacific Region, and a 500 mg dose was recommended by most guidelines. Other quinolones such as ofloxacin were sometimes used as alternatives. Resistance occurred in a stepwise manner over a few years by the selection of strains carrying mutations first in the DNA gyrase, *gyr*A, and then in the topoisomerase IV gene, *par*C [8]. High-level resistance to ciprofloxacin is now common and is predominantly the result of multiple mutations in the quinolone-resistance-determining region (QRDR) of the *gyr*A and *par*C, but mutations in *gyr*B and *mtr* may also contribute [25, 54].

6.6.4 Cephalosporins

The choice of the next antimicrobial agent for gonorrhoea was limited, but the third-generation cephalosporins offered a very effective alternative. Only ceftriaxone, the injectable agent, and cefixime, the oral agent, had efficacy data for gonorrhoea to support their choice, creating problems of availability, mainly of cefixime, in some countries leading to the use of other oral agents such as ceftibuten and cefpodoxime. Ceftriaxone is the most active with the longest half-life and was initially recommended at a 125 mg dose by the Centers for Disease Control and Prevention (CDC) guidelines but is now recommended at the 250 mg dose by most guidelines and therapeutic failure is still not reported. Cefixime is used at a dose of 400 mg, and has been the preferred choice for many because it is given as a single oral dose. However, therapeutic failure with cefixime and ceftibuten has been reported in Japan. Ceftriaxone remains active and increased usage at a 1 g dose has been reported [62]. However, drifts in susceptibility to ceftriaxone reported in US and UK surveillance programmes are a concern that therapeutic failure is inevitable.

The mechanism of resistance to cefixime appears to be predominantly related to the *pen*A mosaic gene, probably acquired from commensal neisseriae, with contribution from *mtr* and *por*B1 (*pen*B). In contrast, these latter mutations, which are involved in penicillin resistance, seem to be more important in decreased susceptibility to ceftriaxone than the *pen*A mosaic.

6.6.5 Tetracycline

Tetracycline has not been recommended as a first-line agent for gonorrhoea but has been used in countries where it was inexpensive and available and there were no resources for more effective agents. Low-level tetracycline resistance is due to the same mutations that result in penicillin resistance but the effect on therapy is largely undocumented. Plasmid-mediated, high-level tetracycline resistance was first described in 1985 due to the insertion of the *tet*M determinant into the 24.5 MD conjugative plasmid [32]. The resulting plasmid of 25.2 MD, unlike penicillinase plasmids, can mobilise itself between gonococci and other bacteria including those found in the genital tract and hence spread rapidly [26]. This plasmid can also be mobilised into PPNG resulting in strains exhibiting high-level resistance to both penicillin and tetracycline.

6.6.6 Azithromycin

Azithromycin has activity against a number of STIs, including *N. gonorrhoeae*, *C. trachomatis* and *Treponema pallidum*, but is most commonly used for chlamydial infections, at a 1 g dose. It is not recommended as a first-line treatment for gonorrhoea but can be used as an alternative treatment at a 2 g dose, which is reported to cause gastrointestinal problems in some patients. Azithromycin belongs to the Macrolide-Lincosamide-Streptogramnin class of antibiotics and inhibits protein synthesis by binding to the 23S rRNA component of the 50S ribosome. Low-level resistance (minimum inhibitory concentration (MIC) 1–4 mg/L) has been recognised for some time and has been attributed to alteration in the target site of the 23S rRNA, due to mutation [34] or enzymatic modification by methylases, encoded by the *erm*B and *erm*F genes [44]. Efflux pumps, which actively transport antibiotics out of the cell, are reported to play a role, of which the MtrCDE-encoded efflux, regulated by the MtrR repressor mutation, is the best characterised [13, 64]. However, other efflux pumps are known to be associated with azithromycin resistance in gonococci including the MacA-MacB system [47] and that encoded by the *mef* gene [29]. High-level resistance to azithromycin (MIC>256 mg/L) has only been reported in Europe since 2004 [11, 40, 52] but had previously been found in Argentina [18]. Recent evidence has shown that high-level resistance to azithromycin results from a single-point mutation in the peptidyltransferase region of domain V of the 23S rRNA gene (Chisholm et al., personal communication). Treatment for gonorrhoea is unlikely to be the selective pressure for high-level resistance but is more likely to have resulted from the widespread use of azithromycin for chlamydial infection and the inadvertent treatment of undetected concomitant gonococcal infections.

6.7 Susceptibility Testing

The treatment for gonorrhoea is often given on the basis of clinical presentation or to a contact of a known case, before the outcome of the diagnostic tests is known. The aim is to provide effective therapy to the patient on the first clinic visit, if possible, and to prevent further transmission of the infection. National and international guidelines are produced to inform therapeutic choice, and surveillance programmes inform these. However, there is still a need to test the susceptibility of the infecting organism for individual patient management to ensure that therapy will be successful, particularly at this time when therapeutic failure to the third-generation cephalosporins is emerging. The aim of susceptibility testing is to categorise strains into susceptible, intermediate or decreased susceptibility and resistant, which predict the chance of therapeutic failure, with susceptible predicting a less than 5% and resistant a greater than 15% chance of failure. When interpreting the patient's response to therapy it should be remembered that the in vitro result is only an indicator and therapeutic failure can also occur because of non-compliance with treatment or reinfection.

6.7.1 Choice of Method

For individual patient management the method of choice in most laboratories is disc diffusion whereas agar dilution is used for surveillance purposes. Epsilometer tests are an alternative method where the MIC can easily be obtained on a single isolate and can be applicable for both patient management and surveillance programmes. Susceptibility testing of *N. gonorrhoeae* can be a challenge as it is a fastidious organism requiring an enriched medium, which may affect the activity of certain antimicrobial agents, and different strains can vary in their growth rate, making interpretation difficult.

6.7.2 Disc Diffusion

Disc diffusion is the most variable of the methods used, but is the most convenient for many clinical microbiology laboratories. A number of recommended methods are described by the National Committee for Clinical Laboratory Standards, now called the Clinical Laboratory Standards Institute (CSLI), the World Health Organisation (1989) and the British Society of Antimicrobial Chemotherapy among others, which differ largely in medium used and concentration of antibiotic in the disc. Despite its difficulties disc diffusion can give useful results if used with a good panel of control strains.

6.7.3 Epsilometer Tests

Epsilometer tests (Etests) offer an alternative method for laboratories, either clinical or reference, that wish to determine the MIC of a single or few strains. The Etest consists of a strip impregnated with antimicrobial agent at varying concentrations, which is placed directly onto a seeded lawn of the test strain. After incubation overnight a zone of inhibition is seen, similar to disc diffusion, and the MIC is indicated where the ellipse crosses the strip. This approach has been increasingly popular and useful in recent years but remains an expensive option and not applicable to large numbers of isolates.

6.7.4 Agar Dilution

Agar dilution is used extensively for surveillance purposes, but again choice of culture medium remains the main difference with GC agar base recommended by the CSLI guidelines and sensitivity base agars used by other surveillance programmes, such as Isosensitest and Diagnostic Sensitivity Agar. The antimicrobial agents are incorporated into the agar base using doubling dilutions and then inoculated with suspensions of the gonococcal strains to deliver a concentration of 10^4 colony-forming units, often using a multipoint inoculator. After incubation for 24 h the growth is scored and the MIC determined as the dilution that completely inhibits growth. The differences in the medium used again can affect the MIC and historically has resulted in two breakpoints for penicillin resistance: ≥ 2 mg/L for GC agar and ≥ 1 mg/L for sensitivity base agars. Appropriate breakpoints to categorise strains into susceptible or resistant can be determined using control strains, and an extended WHO panel, which has been extensively characterised, is now available [56]. Agar dilution is the most efficient method of testing large numbers of isolates but the end point can be difficult to determine when testing agents which are highly active, such as the third-generation cephalosporins. Agar dilution, using either a full range of concentrations or one or two concentrations to give a break point, can be used to screen for potentially resistant isolates and then confirmed using the Etest.

6.7.5 Molecular Detection of Antimicrobial Resistance

A viable organism is required to determine susceptibility and will always be required to detect emerging resistance. The use of molecular methods for diagnosis has raised the desire to also detect resistance in this manner, and while this is technically possible, it can only be performed if the gene/mutation associated with resistance is known. Techniques are well described that detect the penicillinase and tetracycline plasmids and divide them into different types, which is useful for epidemiological purposes. Molecular detection of ciprofloxacin resistance has been more problematic in that resistance is associated with multiple mutations in the QRDR of the *gyr*A and *par*C and, although some changes are very common, it has not been possible to find mutations that are found in all resistant strains, and it is therefore useful as a marker of resistance. In an era where third-generation cephalosporins are being widely used, and the mechanism for resistance is not yet fully known, it is questionable whether molecular detection of resistance is a good use of resources, at least for patient management.

6.8 Surveillance of Antimicrobial Resistance

Surveillance of antimicrobial-resistant gonorrhoea has always been important to determine trends of resistance, monitor drifts in susceptibility and detect the emergence of resistance because *N. gonorrhoeae* has been particularly adept at evading control measures using antimicrobial therapy. The current therapy with third-generation cephalosporins is likely to remain effective for only a limited time and it is of paramount importance that surveillance programmes provide timely information, as there is little or no choice for new alternative treatments. The greatest challenge, as molecular detection becomes widely used, is to continue to collect a representative sample that enables surveillance programmes to produce meaningful data. It may become necessary to set up sentinel sites to collect extra specimens to provide gonococcal isolates for testing or, as is current practice in some countries, to maintain culture as a diagnostic tool for patients with signs and symptoms of gonorrhoea or for patients with a positive NAAT, from whom samples are taken when recalled and before treatment.

6.8.1 Surveillance Programmes

Surveillance programmes have sometimes been difficult to establish because of the resources required but there are now many active programmes including the well-established programmes in the USA [48], Canada [15], Australia [53], the Western Pacific Region [61], the Netherlands [58], and England and Wales [38], as well as many others that have provided longitudinal data which are useful to show temporal changes. The WHO initiated a global antimicrobial surveillance programme (GASP) in 1990 but this was only active in the Americas and the Caribbean and the Western Pacific Region. The potential threat to the control of gonorrhoea by the emergence of resistance to the cephalosporins has rejuvenated attempts to coordinate approaches to address the threat worldwide.

Surveillance programmes aim to produce comparable data that will allow monitoring of global trends. Attempts to produce a common methodology have failed and recent data from the European programme show that if good internal and external quality assurance programmes are maintained and strains are compared in categories of susceptibility, then differences in methodology can be overcome [23].

6.8.2 Trends in Resistance

It is recommended that first-line treatment for gonorrhoea should be at least 95% successful, or a change in treatment regimen should be considered. Monitoring trends to determine when this level is exceeded has been the prime focus for surveillance programmes. This was exemplified by changes in national guidelines for the management of gonorrhoea as increasing resistance to ciprofloxacin over time was demonstrated in national programmes in the USA (Gonococcal Isolate Surveillance Programme [GISP]) and in England and Wales (Gonococcal Resistance to Antimicrobial Surveillance Programme).

6.8.3 Risk Factors

The collection of demographic, epidemiological and behavioural data in combination with the gonococcal isolate has provided the most detailed enhanced surveillance data on patients with gonorrhoea in countries such as England and Wales [14], in addition to highlighting a higher prevalence of ciprofloxacin-resistant gonorrhoea in MSM compared to heterosexuals [19]. In the USA, quinolone resistance was initially restricted to MSM and ciprofloxacin was retained for therapy for heterosexuals until 2008 when the prevalence of resistance detected by GISP indicated that the first-line treatment should be changed to a third-generation cephalosporin. Conversely, in Ontario, Canada and quinolone-resistant gonorrhoea was associated with heterosexual men [36].

6.9 Conclusion

N. gonorrhoeae is a highly versatile organism and continues to evade the immune response, causing repeated infections, and to develop or acquire resistance to therapeutic agents. Prevention measures have concentrated on the identification of infected individuals, provision of good diagnostic tests and timely and effective treatment, in the absence of a gonococcal vaccine. The treatment of gonorrhoea has reached a critical point in that resistance continues to evolve and new or alternative therapies are lacking. The need to continue to provide effective therapy will challenge our current approach of single-dose therapy for the treatment of gonorrhoea and the use of multiple doses, dual therapy or even cycling of antimicrobial agents will need to be considered.

Take-Home Pearls

- Gonorrhoea is caused by the bacterium *Neisseria gonorrhoeae*.
- *N. gonorrhoeae* is an obligate human pathogen and primarily causes infection in the lower genital tract.
- Complicated gonococcal infection of the upper genital tract can result from undetected or inadequately treated infection and result in serious sequelae.
- Gonorrhoea is found among core groups of individuals primarily in inner cities or areas of low socio-economic status.
- Is found disproportionally in certain ethnic groups, men who have sex with men (MSM), young people and those with high rate of partner change.
- Gonococcal infection facilitates HIV transmission.
- Presumptive diagnosis by microscopy for the detection on intra-cellular Gram negative cocci is used universally for symptomatic patients.
- Historically, isolation and identification of *N. gonorrhoeae* has been considered the gold standard for confirmation of the diagnosis of gonorrhoea.
- Nucleic acid amplification tests are now known to detect more positive cases than culture for confirmation of the diagnosis of gonorrhoea.
- *N. gonorrhoeae* is adept at acquiring or selecting resistance to therapeutic agents.
- A viable culture is required to detect emerging resistance.
- Third generation extended spectrum cephalosporins are the current treatment of choice.
- Surveillance programme inform national and international guidelines.

References

1. Alcorn, T.M., Cohen, M.S.: Gonococcal pathogenesis: adaptation and immune evasion in the human host. Curr Opin Infect Dis **7**, 310–316 (1994)
2. Alexander, S.: The challenges of detecting gonorrhoea and chlamydia in rectal and pharyngeal sites: could we, should we, be doing more? Sex Transm Infect **85**, 159–160 (2009)
3. Alexander, S., Ison, C.: Evaluation of commercial kits for the identification of *Neisseria gonorrhoeae*. J Med Microbiol **54**, 827–831 (2005)
4. Alexander, S., Ison, C., Parry, J., et al.: Self-taken pharyngeal and rectal swabs are appropriate for the detection of *Chlamydia trachomatis* and *Neisseria gonorrhoeae* in asymptomatic men who have sex with men. Sex. Transm. Infect. **84**, 488–492 (2008)
5. Alexander, S., Martin, I.M., Fenton, K., et al.: The prevalence of proline iminopeptidase negative *Neisseria gonorrhoeae* throughout England and Wales. Sex. Transm. Infect. **82**, 280–282 (2006)
6. Ashford, W.A., Golash, R.G., Hemming, V.G.: Penicillinase-producing *Neisseria gonorrhoeae*. Lancet **2**, 657–658 (1976)
7. Ashford, W.A., Potts, D.W., Adams, H.J., et al.: Spectinomycin-resistant penicillinase-producing *Neisseria gonorrhoeae*. Lancet **2**, 1035–1037 (1981)
8. Belland, R.J., Morrison, S.G., Ison, C., et al.: *Neisseria gonorrhoeae* acquires mutations in analogous regions of *gyr*A and *par*C in fluoroquinolone-resistant isolates. Mol. Microbiol. **14**, 371–380 (1994)
9. CDC: Trends in Reportable Sexually Transmitted Diseases in the United States, 2006 – National Surveillance Data for Chlamydia, Gonorrhea and Syphilis, pp. 1–7. Centers for Disease Control and Prevention (2007)
10. Chen, M.I., Ghani, A.C., Edmunds, J.: Mind the gap: the role of time between sex with two consecutive partners on the transmission dynamics of gonorrhea. Sex. Transm. Dis. **35**, 435–444 (2008)
11. Chisholm, S.A., Neal, T.J., Alawattegama, A.B., et al.: Emergence of high-level azithromycin resistance in *Neisseria gonorrhoeae* in England and Wales. J. Antimicrob. Chemother. **64**, 353–358 (2009)
12. Cook, R.L., Hutchison, S.L., Ostergaard, L., et al.: Systematic review: noninvasive testing for *Chlamydia trachomatis* and *Neisseria gonorrhoeae*. Ann. Intern. Med. **142**, 914–925 (2005)
13. Cousin Jr., S.L., Whittington, W.L., Roberts, M.C.: Acquired macrolide resistance genes and the 1 bp deletion in the mtrR promoter in *Neisseria gonorrhoeae*. J. Antimicrob. Chemother. **51**, 131–133 (2003)
14. Delpech, V., Martin, I.M., Hughes, G., et al.: Epidemiology and clinical presentation of gonorrhoea in England and Wales: findings from the gonococcal resistance to antimicrobials surveillance programme 2001–2006. Sex. Transm. Infect. **85**, 317–321 (2009)
15. Dillon, J.R.: National microbiological surveillance of the susceptibility of gonococccal isolates to antimicrobial agents. Can. J. Infect. Dis. **3**, 202–206 (1992)
16. Easmon, C.S., Ison, C.A., Bellinger, C.M., et al.: Emergence of resistance after spectinomycin treatment for gonorrhoea due to beta-lactamase producing strain of *Neisseria gonorrhoeae*. Br. Med. J. (Clin. Res. Ed.) **284**, 1604–1605 (1982)
17. Fenton, K.A., Lowndes, C.M.: Recent trends in the epidemiology of sexually transmitted infections in the European Union. Sex. Transm. Infect. **80**, 255–263 (2004)
18. Galarza, P.G., Alcala, B., Salcedo, C., et al.: Emergence of high level azithromycin-resistant *Neisseria gonorrhoeae* strain isolated in Argentina. Sex. Transm. Dis. **36**, 787–788 (2009)

19. GRASP Steering Group: The Gonococcal Resistance to Antimicrobials Surveillance Programme (GRASP) Year 2008 Report. Health Protection Agency, London (2009)
20. Hauck, C.R., Meyer, T.F.: 'Small' talk: Opa proteins as mediators of Neisseria-host-cell communication. Curr. Opin. Microbiol. **6**, 43–49 (2003)
21. Hughes, G., Brady, A.R., Catchpole, M.A., et al.: Characteristics of those who repeatedly acquire sexually transmitted infections: a retrospective cohort study of attendees at three urban sexually transmitted disease clinics in England. Sex. Transm. Dis. **28**, 379–386 (2001)
22. Ison, C., Martin, D.: Gonorrhea. Atlas of Sexually Transmitted Diseases and AIDS, pp. 109–139 (2003)
23. Ison, C.A., Martin, I.M., Lowndes, C.M., et al.: Comparability of laboratory diagnosis and antimicrobial susceptibility testing of *Neisseria gonorrhoeae* from reference laboratories in Western Europe. J. Antimicrob. Chemother. **58**, 580–586 (2006)
24. Kallstrom, H., Liszewski, M.K., Atkinson, J.P., et al.: Membrane cofactor protein (MCP or CD46) is a cellular pilus receptor for pathogenic *Neisseria*. Mol. Microbiol. **25**, 639–647 (1997)
25. Knapp, J.S., Fox, K.K., Trees, D.L., et al.: Fluoroquinolone resistance in *Neisseria gonorrhoeae*. Emerg. Infect. Dis. **3**, 33–39 (1997)
26. Knapp, J.S., Johnson, S.R., Zenilman, J.M., et al.: High-level tetracycline resistance resulting from TetM in strains of *Neisseria* spp., Kingella denitrificans, and Eikenella corrodens. Antimicrob. Agents Chemother. **32**, 765–767 (1988)
27. LaMontagne, D.S., Fenton, K.A., Pimenta, J.M., et al.: Using chlamydia positivity to estimate prevalence: evidence from the Chlamydia Screening Pilot in England. Int. J. STD AIDS **16**, 323–327 (2005)
28. Lavelle, S.J., Jones, K.E., Mallinson, H., et al.: Finding, confirming, and managing gonorrhoea in a population screened for chlamydia using the Gen-Probe Aptima Combo2 assay. Sex. Transm. Infect. **82**, 221–224 (2006)
29. Luna, V.A., Cousin Jr., S., Whittington, W.L., et al.: Identification of the conjugative mef gene in clinical Acinetobacter junii and *Neisseria gonorrhoeae* isolates. Antimicrob. Agents Chemother. **44**, 2503–2506 (2000)
30. Massari, P., Ram, S., Macleod, H., et al.: The role of porins in neisserial pathogenesis and immunity. Trends Microbiol. **11**, 87–93 (2003)
31. Merz, A.J., So, M.: Interactions of pathogenic neisseriae with epithelial cell membranes. Annu. Rev. Cell Dev. Biol. **16**, 423–457 (2000)
32. Morse, S.A., Johnson, S.R., Biddle, J.W., et al.: High-level tetracycline resistance in *Neisseria gonorrhoeae* is result of acquisition of streptococcal *tet*M determinant. Antimicrob. Agents Chemother. **30**, 664–670 (1986)
33. Naumann, M., Rudel, T., Meyer, T.F.: Host cell interactions and signalling with *Neisseria gonorrhoeae*. Curr. Opin. Microbiol. **2**, 62–70 (1999)
34. Ng, L.K., Martin, I., Liu, G., et al.: Mutation in 23S rRNA associated with macrolide resistance in *Neisseria gonorrhoeae*. Antimicrob. Agents Chemother. **46**, 3020–3025 (2002)
35. Nicoll, A., Hughes, G., Donnelly, M., et al.: Assessing the impact of national anti-HIV sexual health campaigns: trends in the transmission of HIV and other sexually transmitted infections in England. Sex. Transm. Infect. **77**, 242–247 (2001)
36. Ota, K.V., Jamieson, F., Fisman, D.N., et al.: Prevalence of and risk factors for quinolone-resistant *Neisseria gonorrhoeae* infection in Ontario. CMAJ **180**, 287–290 (2009)
37. Pagotto, F., Aman, A.T., Ng, L.K., et al.: Sequence analysis of the family of penicillinase-producing plasmids of *Neisseria gonorrhoeae*. Plasmid **43**, 24–34 (2000)
38. Paine, T.C., Fenton, K.A., Herring, A., et al.: GRASP: a new national sentinel surveillance initiative for monitoring gonococcal antimicrobial resistance in England and Wales. Sex. Transm. Infect. **77**, 398–401 (2001)
39. Palmer, H.M., Mallinson, H., Wood, R.L., et al.: Evaluation of the specificities of five DNA amplification methods for the detection of *Neisseria gonorrhoeae*. J. Clin. Microbiol. **41**, 835–837 (2003)
40. Palmer, H.M., Young, H., Winter, A., et al.: Emergence and spread of azithromycin-resistant *Neisseria gonorrhoeae* in Scotland. J. Antimicrob. Chemother. **62**, 490–494 (2008)
41. Phillips, I.: Beta-lactamase-producing, penicillin-resistant gonococcus. Lancet **2**, 656–657 (1976)
42. Rao, G.G., Bacon, L., Evans, J., et al.: Prevalence of *Neisseria gonorrhoeae* infection in young subjects attending community clinics in South London. Sex. Transm. Infect. **84**, 117–121 (2008)
43. Roberts, M.C.: Plasmids of *Neisseria gonorrhoeae* and other *Neisseria* species. Clin. Microbiol. Rev. **2**(suppl), S18–S23 (1989)
44. Roberts, M.C., Chung, W.O., Roe, D., et al.: Erythromycin-resistant *Neisseria gonorrhoeae* and oral commensal *Neisseria* spp. carry known rRNA methylase genes. Antimicrob. Agents Chemother. **43**, 1367–1372 (1999)
45. Ropp, P.A., Hu, M., Olesky, M., et al.: Mutations in ponA, the gene encoding penicillin-binding protein 1, and a novel locus, penC, are required for high-level chromosomally mediated penicillin resistance in *Neisseria gonorrhoeae*. Antimicrob. Agents Chemother. **46**, 769–777 (2002)
46. Rothenberg, R.B.: The geography of gonorrhea. Empirical demonstration of core group transmission. Am. J. Epidemiol. **117**, 688–694 (1983)
47. Rouquette-Loughlin, C.E., Balthazar, J.T., Shafer, M.: Characterization of the MacA-MacB efflux system in *Neisseria gonorrhoeae*. J. Antimicrob. Chemother. **56**, 856–860 (2005)
48. Schwarcz, S.K., Zenilman, J.M., Schnell, D., et al.: National surveillance of antimicrobial resistance in *Neisseria gonorrhoeae*. The Gonococcal Isolate Surveillance Project. JAMA **264**, 1413–1417 (1990)
49. Song, W., Ma, L., Chen, R., et al.: Role of lipooligosaccharide in Opa-independent invasion of *Neisseria gonorrhoeae* into human epithelial cells. J. Exp. Med. **191**, 949–960 (2000)
50. Sparling, P.F., Sarubbi Jr., F.A., Blackman, E.: Inheritance of low-level resistance to penicillin, tetracycline, and chloramphenicol in *Neisseria gonorrhoeae*. J. Bacteriol. **124**, 740–749 (1975)
51. Stanley, B., Todd, A.: Testing for *Neisseria gonorrhoeae* by nucleic acid amplification testing of chlamydia samples using Roche Cobas Amplicor in a rural area in the north of England does not find more gonorrhoea in primary care. Sex. Transm. Infect. **81**, 518 (2005)
52. Starnino, S., Stefanelli, P., *Neisseria gonorrhoeae* Italian Study Group: Azithromycin-resistant *Neisseria gonorrhoeae* strains recently isolated in Italy. J. Antimicrob. Chemother. **63**, 1200–1204 (2009)

53. Australian Gonococcal Surveillance Programme, Tapsall, J.: Annual report of the Australian Gonococcal Surveillance Programme, 2008. Commun. Dis. Intell. **33**, 268–274 (2009)
54. Trees, D.L., Sandul, A.L., Neal, S.W., et al.: Molecular epidemiology of *Neisseria gonorrhoeae* exhibiting decreased susceptibility and resistance to ciprofloxacin in Hawaii, 1991–1999. Sex. Transm. Dis. **28**, 309–314 (2001)
55. Trotter, C., Hughes, G., Ison, C.: Epidemiology in the Vaccine Era. Neisseria Molecular Mechanisms of Pathogenesis, pp. 227–243. (2010)
56. Unemo, M., Fasth, O., Fredlund, H., et al.: Phenotypic and genetic characterization of the 2008 WHO *Neisseria gonorrhoeae* reference strain panel intended for global quality assurance and quality control of gonococcal antimicrobial resistance surveillance for public health purposes. J. Antimicrob. Chemother. **63**, 1142–1151 (2009)
57. Unemo, M., Palmer, H.M., Blackmore, T., et al.: Global transmission of prolyliminopeptidase-negative *Neisseria gonorrhoeae* strains: implications for changes in diagnostic strategies. Sex. Transm. Infect. **83**, 47–51 (2007)
58. van de Laar, M.J., van Duynhoven, Y.T., Dessens, M., et al.: Surveillance of antibiotic resistance in *Neisseria gonorrhoeae* in The Netherlands, 1977–95. Genitourin. Med. **73**, 510–517 (1997)
59. Whiley, D.M., Garland, S.M., Harnett, G., et al.: Exploring 'best practice' for nucleic acid detection of *Neisseria gonorrhoeae*. Sex. Health **5**, 17–23 (2008)
60. WHO: Global prevalence and incidence of selected curable sexually transmitted infections: overview and estimates WHO/HIV-AIDS/2001.02,WHO/CDS/CSR/EDC/2001.10, pp. 1–43. WHO, Geneva (2001)
61. WHO: Surveillance of antibiotic resistance in *Neisseria gonorrhoeae* in the WHO Western Pacific Region, 2006. Commun. Dis. Intell. **32**, 48–51 (2008)
62. Workowski, K.A., Berman, S.M., Douglas, JM, Jr.: Emerging antimicrobial resistance in *Neisseria gonorrhoeae*: urgent need to strengthen prevention strategies. Ann. Intern. Med. **148**, 606–613 (2008)
63. Yorke, J.A., Hethcote, H.W., Nold, A.: Dynamics and control of the transmission of gonorrhea. Sex. Transm. Dis. **5**, 51–56 (1978)
64. Zarantonelli, L., Borthagaray, G., Lee, E.H., et al.: Decreased azithromycin susceptibility of *Neisseria gonorrhoeae* due to mtrR mutations. Antimicrob. Agents Chemother. **43**, 2468–2472 (1999)

Biology of Chlamydiae

7

Jürgen Rödel and Eberhard Straube

Core Messages

- Chlamydiae are bacteria that are highly adapted to an intracellular life cycle in eukaryotic host cells.
- Host cell functions are specifically modulated by chlamydial proteins or products that are translocated from the bacteria into the host cell cytosol.
- *Chlamydia trachomatis* has evolved effective strategies to interfere with cellular immune responses and establish acute as well as chronic infections of susceptible mucous membranes.
- Persistent infections are characterized by atypical and non-replicative forms of the pathogen.

7.1 Introduction

The *Chlamydiales* are bacteria that live within the cells of vertebrates and amoebae, while similar particles have been reported in invertebrate species including coelenterates, arthropods, and mollusks. Chlamydiae are small nonmotile Gram-negative bacteria with a biphasic development cycle. They are not cultivable in media free of living eukaryotic cells. Many chlamydiae coexist in an apparently asymptomatic state within hosts that probably act as a natural reservoir for them. The first detailed description of chlamydiae came from Halberstaedter and von Provazek [1] who inoculated trachoma scrapings from a man to orangutans that developed inclusion conjunctivitis. By means of Giemsa stain inclusion bodies containing reticulate bodies as well as elementary bodies were visible and could be exactly drawn. This was a triumph of observational science as the 0.3 μm elementary bodies were only just a little above the resolution limit of the conventional light microscope at that time. Halberstaedter and von Provazek called the newly discovered pathogen *Chlamydozoa* (Greek: χλαμνς, mantle) because elementary bodies were embedded in a blue-stained matrix. These authors found *Chlamydozoa* also in newborns suffering from non-gonorrhoic blennorrhoea [2]. Bedson et al. [3] found *Chlamydozoa*-like organisms in a case of ornithosis. These organisms were called *Bedsonia* and were accounted to the viruses for a while. At the same time Miyagawa isolated *Chlamydozoa*-like organisms from a woman suffering from lymphogranuloma venereum and called them *Miyagawanella*. Later on this group was called psittacosis-lymphogranuloma-trachoma (PLT) group or pathogens causing trachoma or inclusion conjunctivitis (TRIC). The name *Chlamydia* was proposed by Jones et al. in 1945 [4]. In 1965 a *Chlamydia*-like organism called TW-183 could be isolated from the conjunctiva of a control child in a trachoma vaccine study in Taiwan. A similar strain called AR-39 could be isolated in 1983 from a University of Washington student with pharyngitis. Since these strains were different from *Chlamydia trachomatis* they were assumed to be *Chlamydia psittaci* and called TWAR. Detailed investigations showed

J. Rödel (✉) and E. Straube
Institute of Medical Microbiology,
Friedrich Schiller University, Jena, Germany
e-mail: juergen.roedel@med.uni-jena.de;
eberhard.straube@med.uni-jena.de

G. Gross and S.K. Tyring (eds.), *Sexually Transmitted Infections and Sexually Transmitted Diseases*,
DOI: 10.1007/978-3-642-14663-3_7, © Springer-Verlag Berlin Heidelberg 2011

that TWAR strains share the genus *Chlamydia* but are different from *C. psittaci*. Therefore, the new species *Chlamydia pneumoniae* was proposed by Grayston et al. in 1989 [5].

7.2 Taxonomy of Chlamydiae

Chlamydiae belong to a very old family and are adapted early in phylogeny to a parasitic intracellular life in host cells. Despite chlamydiae having a long existence, only few pathogenic species are known so far. Analyses of the 16SrRNA- as well as 23SrRNA-gene led to a revised taxonomy of the order *Chlamydiales* proposed primarily by Everett and coworkers [6]. Since that time, *Chlamydiales* is a fast-growing order of bacteria specific for different hosts. The adaptation to the intracellular life led to a reduction in the genome of chlamydiae. While an extracellular bacterium like *Pseudomonas aeruginosa* has a genome size of about 6.3 million base pairs *C. trachomatis* has a chromosome containing only about 1.1 million base pairs and some plasmids with unknown function.

The Family I: *Chlamydiaceae* of the order *Chlamydiales* contain some well-known human pathogens like *C. trachomatis*, *C. pneumoniae*, and *C. psittaci*. Other mainly animal pathogens are accidentally found as a cause of a severe infection in man, e.g., *Chlamydophila abortus*. Even members of Family II to IV of *Chlamydiales* may contain human pathogens, e.g., *Simkania negevensis*, which is found in respiratory infections (Fig. 7.1).

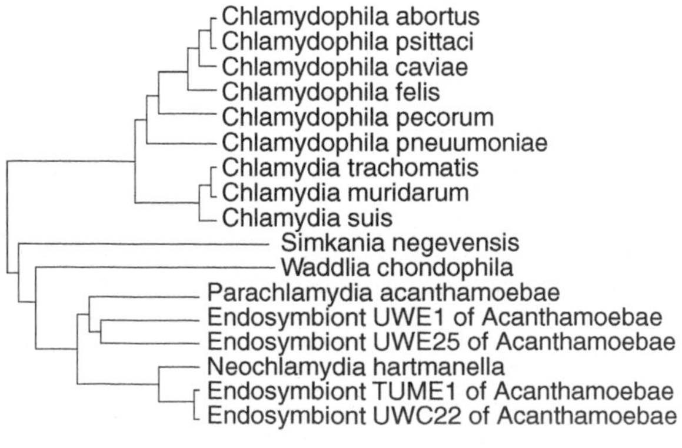

Fig. 7.1 Current taxonomic structure of the *Chlamydiales* [7]

7.2.1 *Chlamydia trachomatis*

C. trachomatis causes the most common bacterial sexually transmitted disease worldwide, with around 90 million cases each year, which is treatable by antibiotic drugs. Usually, the disease is acquired by young people starting their sexual activities. Because of the lack of symptoms, especially in women, and the tendency to develop persistent infections of the uterus as well as adnexae, *C. trachomatis* is a common cause of tubal-factor infertility in women.

As well as sexually transmitted disease, it causes eye infection, trachoma, or follicular keratoconjunctivitis. Since trachoma is the leading infectious cause of blindness worldwide and affects hundreds of millions of people, primarily in poor and rural regions, the Johns Hopkins University has received a $10 million grant from the Bill & Melinda Gates Foundation to lead a consortium that will study ways to improve the treatment of trachoma and to accelerate progress toward the goal of eliminating the disease.

Another sexually transmitted disease caused by *C. trachomatis* strains with high invasivity is lymphogranuloma venereum (LGV, lymphogranuloma inguinale or Nicolas-Durand-Favre disease). LGV was known for a long period as a tropical disease. Some years ago, the disease entered the industrial countries of Europe and North America transmitted by HIV-positive men who have sex with men.

These very different infections are caused by strains of *C. trachomatis* that are very similar to one another genetically. Strains can be divided by antibodies against the variable moieties of the major outer membrane protein (MOMP) or outer membrane protein 1 (OMP1) into serotypes. Currently 18 serovars are divided: A, B, Ba, and C causing trachoma; D through K including Da and Ia causing the most common bacterial sexually transmitted infection, in some cases conjunctivitis, and rarely pneumonia in newborns; and L1, L2, L2a, and L3 causing LGV.

7.3 Life Cycle of Chlamydiae

The life cycle of chlamydiae is divided into an extracellular and an intracellular part (Fig. 7.2). The extracellular part is represented by elementary bodies.

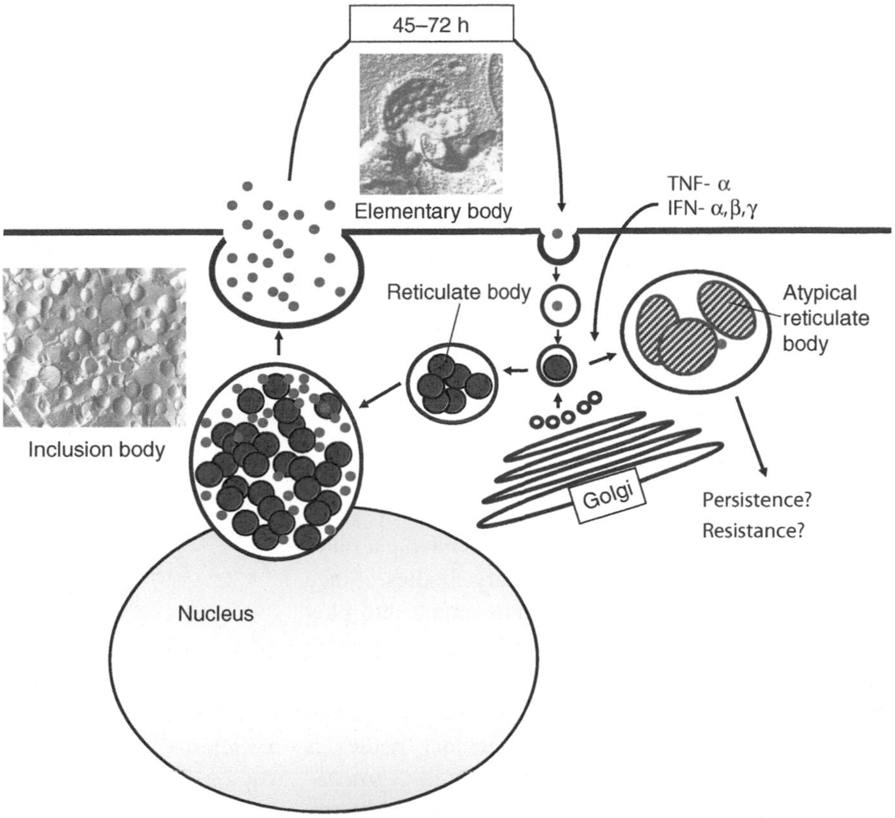

Fig. 7.2 Life cycle of *Chlamydia trachomatis*

They are small, round, or occasionally pear-shaped electron-dense structures and have a size of about 0.3 μm. Elementary bodies are highly infective for epithelial cells which uptake these bodies by a kind of endocytosis. Within the endosome *Chlamydiae* form reticulate bodies that are metabolically active bacteria. Reticulate bodies have a size of about 1 μm and multiply strictly in the intracellular part. These endosomes are called inclusion bodies. In case of multiple infection of a host cell *Chlamydiae* bearing endosomes show the tendency of confluence. After about 45–72 h the inclusion bodies can contain thousands of bacterial cells (Fig. 7.3). At this time reticulate bodies form in a process of condensation new elementary bodies which get released by rupture of the host cell or by exocytosis.

While the replication of *Chlamydia* in cell cultures is well defined, the life cycle in a host or patient is influenced by cytokines, interferons, and defense mechanisms that lead to modulation of the cycle.

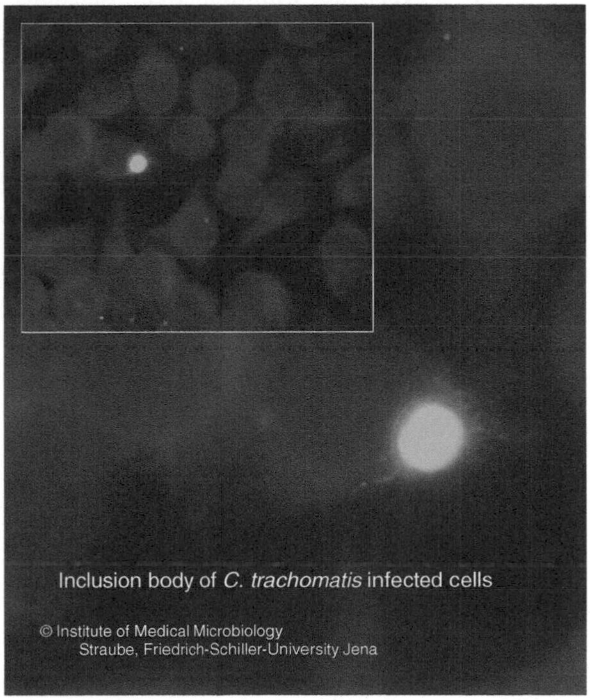

Inclusion body of C. trachomatis infected cells
© Institute of Medical Microbiology
Straube, Friedrich-Schiller-University Jena

Fig. 7.3 Inclusion body of *Chlamydia trachomatis* in BGM cells after 72 h (Straube)

7.3.1 Elementary Body

The elementary body (EB) is the infectious stage of *Chlamydia* whose function is to permit chlamydial entrance in the host cell. It is a spore-like body which enables *Chlamydia* to survive in a non-supportive environment outside the host cell. There are differences of environmental resistance in different *Chlamydia* species. Elementary bodies of *C. psittaci* seem to be the most resistant (Fig. 7.4).

7.3.2 Attachment

Formerly, the MOMP was described as having a function in the adhesion of elementary bodies. Since MOMP is a porin, secreted proteins come into play for the adhesion process. The polymorphic protein pmpD is one of these proteins believed to have an adhesive function [8]. The most probable candidate to be an adhesin of *Chlamydia* elementary bodies is OmcB. OmcB plays a role as an adhesin in *C. trachomatis*. The OmcB protein is a cysteine-rich outer membrane polypeptide with important functional, structural, and immunogenic properties [9]. OmcB binds to glycosaminoglycan of the host cells. Beside this, protein disulfide isomerase (PDI), a component of the estrogen receptor complex, is associated with *C. trachomatis* elementary bodies attached to human endometrial epithelial cells. The attachment and infectivity of *C. trachomatis* are dramatically enhanced in estrogen-dominant primary human endometrial epithelial cells. Productive entry into host cells of EB is dependent on reduction of EB disulfide-cross-linked outer membrane proteins at the host cell surface, and PDI is closely associated with adherent EB [10]. Additionally, sulfated polyanions like heparin inhibit substantially the adhesion of elementary bodies because they serve as receptors [11].

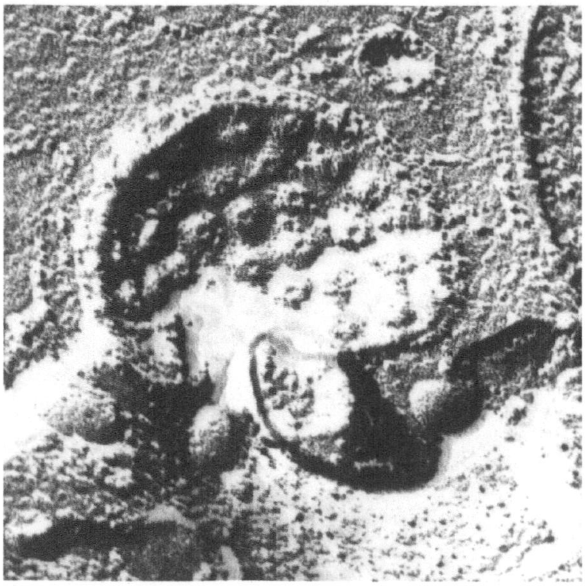

Fig. 7.4 Electron micrograph of the freeze fractured surface of an elementary body (J. Rödel)

7.3.3 Entry

Chlamydia elementary bodies attach to the host cell near the base of microvilli, from which site they are actively endocytosed by the host cell in tight endocytic vesicles. *C. trachomatis* enter host cells via polyene (nystatin or filipin) disruptible, cholesterol-rich, lipid raft domains characterized by insolubility in cold Triton X100 detergent. These domains form caveolae in association with the host protein caveolin 1 and 2 respectively [12].

Entry of *C. trachomatis* elementary bodies also induces the induction of microvilli and is accompanied by tyrosine-dependent phosphorylation of host cell proteins [13]. Up to 4 h post infection there is only occasional co-localization of the tyrosine phosphorylated proteins with endocytosed elementary bodies. *C. trachomatis* attachment to cells induces the secretion of the elementary body-associated protein translocated actin-recruiting protein (TARP). TARP crosses the plasma membrane probably by means of a type III secretion apparatus where it is immediately phosphorylated at tyrosine residues by unknown host kinases. The Rac GTPase is also activated, resulting in WAVE2 and Arp2/3-dependent recruitment of actin to the sites of *Chlamydia* attachment. TARP participates directly in chlamydial invasion activating the Rac-dependent signaling cascade to recruit actin. TARP seems to be signaling to the actin cytoskeleton remodeling machinery by which *C. trachomatis* invades non-phagocytic cells [14]. So TARP might be a marker for a productive infection with *C. trachomatis*.

Shortly after entry into host cells, *C. trachomatis* elementary bodies move to the peri-Golgi region of the cell that corresponds to the microtubule-organizing center. The Golgi apparatus is the intracellular organelle responsible for much of the vesicular/membrane trafficking in the host cell. Clearly the growing chlamydial vacuole must intercept this membrane traffic somehow, in order to enlarge the inclusion membrane. Endocytosed elementary bodies begin to acquire sphingomyelin from vesicles exocytosed from the Golgi within 2 h of infection, in an energy-dependent process. Sphingomyelin acquisition and the translocation of *C. trachomatis* vacuoles to the Golgi region are blocked by inhibitors of chlamydial gene transcription or translation [15], indicating that chlamydiae actively and rapidly modify the host cell response to their invasion. Within the family *Chlamydiaceae* there is a variety of different entry mechanisms and there are probably also different host cell-determined entry routes which depend on the cell surface membrane receptors that are displayed and their links to the underlying cell transport machinery.

7.3.4 Reticulate Body

The reticulate bodies represent the stage of intracellular replication in the chlamydial developmental cycle. Reticulate bodies have a diameter of about 1 μm and are fragile, pleomorphic, and not infectious. Therefore they are hardly available for experimental investigations. Reticulate bodies are metabolically active, so their cytoplasm is rich in ribosomes, which are required for protein synthesis. Their nucleic acid appears diffuse and fibrillar. The bacterial cell wall of reticulate bodies is covered with projections and rosettes. These projections can be seen extending from the chlamydial surface into the inclusion membrane representing the type III secretion machine that functions as an injectisome that crosses the chlamydial outer membrane and the inclusion membrane, thereby allowing the translocation of bacterial effector proteins. The chlamydial genome contains all genes necessary to encode proteins to carry out peptidoglycan synthesis, assembly, and degradation. However, peptidoglycan is not found in reticulate bodies in a significant amount. Although *Chlamydiae* do not accumulate peptidoglycan, there is metabolic evidence that peptidoglycan synthesis occurs. The production of infectious elementary bodies is highly sensitive to inhibitors of PG synthesis, including β-lactam antibiotics, and D-cycloserine. Treatment of infected cells with these agents inhibits cell division and leads to the formation of large, aberrant reticulate bodies that cannot differentiate to elementary bodies and might be a cause for persisting infection.

7.3.5 Regulation of the Replication Cycle

During its developmental cycle chlamydiae translocate effector proteins into the host cell cytosol to modulate cellular functions (Valdivia, 2008). Chlamydial species code for a type III secretion (TTS) apparatus which is well known from other bacteria [16]. A group of TTS-dependent proteins are the inclusion membrane proteins (Inc) that share a hydrophobic motif and are incorporated into the inclusion membrane, thereby residing at the interface of the inclusion to the host cell cytoplasm. Inc proteins participate in the recruitment of RhabGTPases, which are involved in the regulation of membrane and organelle trafficking. IncA plays a role in the homotypic fusion of chlamydial inclusions in an infected cell and IncG binds 14-3-3β and phosphor-BAD, thereby contributing to the modulation of host cell signaling pathways involved in mitogen-activated protein kinase (MAPK) regulation and apoptosis [17]. Another important chlamydial effector protein which is TTS-independent is the chlamydial protease-like activity factor (CPAF). CPAF shares a type II secretion signal and is secreted into the inclusion before being translocated into the host cell cytosol [18]. The identification of chlamydial virulence factors that are intracellularly produced and secreted by chlamydiae has a fundamental impact on the understanding of the interaction of chlamydiae with their host cells.

7.3.6 Release of Chlamydiae from the Host Cell

After a replication cycle of approximately 2 days, the chlamydial reticulate bodies reorganize into new infectious elementary bodies that are released from the cells by two pathways: lysis and extrusion [19]. Lysis is a destructive release mode resulting from the sequential rupture of inclusions and host cell membranes. Release by extrusion is characterized by the formation of a membranous protrusion in which a chlamydial inclusion containing elementary bodies is packaged. The extrusion release pathway involves actin polymerization.

7.4 The Fate of the Infected Cell: Interference of Chlamydial Infection with Host Cell Death Pathways

As an intracellular pathogen *Chlamydia* has evolved strategies to interfere with host cell death pathways to maintain the intracellular environment for replication as well as persistence. In general, apoptosis can be induced via two pathways: the death-receptor-mediated apoptotic pathway is characterized by the activation of initiator caspase 8 that directly activates effector caspase 3; the alternative pathway involves a mitochondrial amplification step with the release of cytochrome c. In consequence, a complex with apoptotic protease-activating factor 1 (APAF1) and caspase 9, designated as apoptosome, is formed. The apoptosome activates caspase 3 and other effector molecules. The release of cytochrome c from mitochondria is driven by the pro-apoptotic BH3-only proteins which activate factors of the Bax/Bak family. Bax proteins directly affect the integrity of mitochondrial membranes, thereby inducing cytochrome c release [20, 21]. As shown in many studies *Chlamydia* clearly inhibits chemically and spontaneously induced apoptotic cell death [21, 22]. In infected epithelial cells stimulated with apoptosis inducers the release of cytochrome c from mitochondria is completely blocked and no activation of caspase 3 occurs [22]. The potent antiapoptotic activity of *Chlamydia* is due to a broad proteolytic cleavage of BH3-only protein family members by the chlamydial protease CPAF, which is secreted from the bacteria into the host cell cytosol [23].

Despite an antiapoptotic effect chlamydial infection causes massive stress to the host cell and cytopathic changes resulting in host cell lysis during productive infection. Host cell death induced by *C. trachomatis* is caspase-independent and may rather represent a necrotic-like cell death [21, 24].

During apoptosis, effector caspase 3 cleaves poly (ADP-ribose) polymerase 1 (PARP-1), a nuclear repair enzyme which binds to DNA strand breaks and catalyzes the synthesis of ADP-ribose polymers from NAD, into two characteristic fragments. In *C. trachomatis*-infected cells PARP-1 is also degraded but into fragments that do not correspond to those generated during apoptosis [25]. The cleavage of PARP-1 is catalyzed by the chlamydial protease CPAF and it has been suggested that CPAF is a major factor of chlamydia cytopathicity [25, 26]. Cell death upon infection may be a defense mechanism of the cell restricting chlamydial replication but it may also promote the spread of infection. The induction of a caspase-independent cell death by *C. trachomatis* provides an explanation for infection-induced epithelial damage and inflammation.

7.5 Immunology

Since chlamydiae multiply only within an endosomal compartment of the host cell, there are limited possibilities for immune competent cells of the host to make contact with *Chlamydia* antigens.

First, there is an antigen contact: when *Chlamydia* elementary bodies enter mucous membranes or get released by infected cells they present several outer antigens at the surface, which might be of importance in pathogenicity, e.g., the MOMP or ompA [27], porin B (ompB), polymorphic membrane proteins (pmps) [28], cysteine-rich outer membrane complex proteins (OmcA, OmcB), macrophage infectivity potentiator (MIP), and chlamydial lipopolysaccharide (LPS). Besides these antigens elementary bodies may present some other immunogenic proteins with so far unknown functions.

Second, antigens might be available for the immune system, when *Chlamydia* enclosed in an endosome-like inclusion body form metabolically active bacteria which replicate and have cross talk with the host cell by means of antigens that might be presented by the host cell to the immune system like heat shock proteins and others (see Sects. 7.3.4., 7.3.5., 7.4, and 7.5.1).

MOMP: It is called major outer membrane protein, since it takes about 60% of the protein mass of elementary bodies. This protein is porin with 40 kDa encoded by the ompA gene. It is both structurally and immunologically the dominant protein in the chlamydial outer membrane complex. It has also conserved four variable moieties which enable the typing of *C. trachomatis* strains by means of antibodies specific to the variable parts of the antigen. The MOMP gene shows comparable variations in sequence. Consequently, these variable sequences are specific for genotypes of *C. trachomatis* corresponding to serotypes. MOMP is immunodominant, especially at the VS3 region, and generates host antibodies which are protective against infection.

ompB: This protein is expressed in the outer membrane complex at low levels throughout the developmental cycle and is surface-exposed. It is species-specific, since it has only 59.3% identity to ompB of *C. pneumoniae* [29]. PorB probably serves to get dicarboxylic acids across the outer membrane of *Chlamydia*. Antibodies against ompB have protective capacity.

OmcA, OmcB: These two cysteine-rich proteins are genus-specific and mainly present on the surface of elementary bodies [30].

pmps: *C. trachomatis* has nine genes coding these proteins. There are two gene clusters of pmpA, pmpB, pmpC, and pmpE, pmpF, pmpG, pmpH respectively. To these clusters pmpI is associated whereas pmpD is separated. PmpD is believed to function as an adhesive factor. The pmps are common in *Chlamydiaceae,* but species-specific [31].

MIP: The macrophage infectivity potentiator is a bacterial lipoprotein, exposed at the surface of elementary bodies. Native MIP is able to induce TNF-alpha and IL-8 secretion in the host. The pro-inflammatory activity of MIP is dependent from the lipid moiety of the protein. MIP-stimulated pathways appear to involve TLR2/TLR1/TLR6 with the help of CD14 but not TLR4 [32].

LPS: As a common feature of the outer envelope of Gram-negative bacteria lipopolysaccharide is a major surface component also in *C. trachomatis* [33]. LPS in *C. trachomatis* consists of lipid A and 3-deoxy-d-manno-octulosonic acid (Kdo) like a rough enterobacterial LPS and is common for all *Chlamydiae* [34]. The LPS of *C. trachomatis* has spermicidal activity. Chlamydial LPS shows only weak endotoxic activity in terms of lethality, fever production, or Schwartzman reactivity but it is active in B cell mitogenicity and in the induction of prostaglandin E2 from host cells [35].

7.5.1 Mucosal Immunology

The immune response to *C. trachomatis* represents a complex network in which innate immune cells, B cells, and T cells act in concert, and it can be assumed that a highly regulated balance between different T and B cell subsets decides whether an infection is cleared or develops into a prolonged infection ascending the upper genital tract.

During genital infection, the mucosa provides the first line of defense against pathogens and the shedding of the endometrial epithelium during the estrus cycle can limit the spread of chlamydial infection. Epithelial cells are the primary host cells for *C. trachomatis* and they are capable of initiating the innate immune response. Infected epithelial cells release interleukin 1 α (IL-1α), which in turn stimulates the production of chemokines, such as IL-8 [36]. The activation of the cytokine and chemokine response of infected epithelial cells obviously plays an important role in the recruitment of immune cells (natural killer (NK) cells, neutrophils, macrophages, and dendritic cells) to the site of infection. Furthermore IL-1α produced by *Chlamydia*-infected epithelial cells downregulates the synthesis of interstitial collagens by fibroblasts, which may also facilitate cell migration in the affected tissues [37]. Recruited immune cells produce inflammatory and immune-modulatory cytokines. One of these factors, tumor necrosis factor α (TNF-α), can directly restrict the growth of *Chlamydia* inside its host cells but may also represent an important mediator promoting tissue pathology. The innate cytokine and chemokine response is activated following recognition of pathogen-associated molecular patterns (PAMP) by toll-like receptors (TLRs). Although chlamydial LPS and Hsp60 are recognized by TLR4, intact organisms stimulate innate immune cells predominantly through TLR2 [38]. As professional antigen-presenting cells dendritic cells provides a link between innate and adaptive immunity.

The presence of B cell-produced *Chlamydia*-specific antibodies has been proposed to mediate protective immunity; however, during primary infection B cells are not sufficient to eliminate the pathogen, as shown in models using B cell-deficient mice. On the other hand, it can be proposed that B and CD4 T cells act in synergy and B cells may play an important role in the memory response [39].

Specific antibodies can neutralize the infectivity of chlamydiae but are ineffective when the pathogen exists in the stage of intracellular replication. At this stage the recognition of infected cells by T cells becomes the critical step. CD4 T cells recognize antigens that are processed within the lysosomal compartments of cells and the resulting peptides are presented by major histocompatibility class II (MHC-II) molecules on the cell surface. Because *Chlamydiae* avoid the lysosomal maturation of their inclusion (endosome) in epithelial cells, antigen presentation via the MHC-II pathway may be restricted to professional antigen-presenting cells, e.g., dendritic cells. CD8 T cells recognize antigens that gain access to the cytosol. Such antigens are processed by the proteasome and the resulting peptides are presented by MHC-I molecules. Although chlamydiae exist within an endosomal inclusion, they secrete several proteins into the cytosol of the infected host cell and some of them are incorporated in the inclusion membrane but possess domains that extend *into* the cytosol. Since MHC-I molecules are expressed on virtually all nucleated cells and epithelial cells are the primary target cells of *C. trachomatis*, it becomes clear that the recognition of infected cells by specific CD8 T cells is important for an effective immune response. Indeed both specific CD4 and CD8 T cells are not only activated during human genital infection but have also been found to contribute to the clearance of *Chlamydia* infection in mice, as shown in gene knockout models [39].

The genital mucosa lacks an organized lymphoid element and *Chlamydia*-specific T cells are activated and proliferate in the iliac lymph nodes that drain antigens from the genital tract. Proliferation of specific T cells is initiated after several days of primary infection. In general, the types of activated CD4 T cell subsets depend on the nature of infection and the innate cytokine and chemokine expression. Th1 cells are the major source of IFN-γ, the most important cytokine inhibiting intracellular replication of chlamydiae, and are crucial for a protective immunity against *C. trachomatis*. In contrast, Th2 cells produce IL-4, IL-5, IL-10, and IL-13, cytokines that are not protective [39]. A strong activation of Th2 cells during chlamydial infection may increase the bacterial load and promote the development of chronic infection by suppressing a potent Th1-dominated immune response. *Chlamydia*-specific CD8 T cells also produce IFN- γ. The lysis of infected cells by CD8 T cells has been demonstrated ex vivo but may be restricted to the presentation of antigens by non-classical MHC-I molecules (CD1 a-d; HLA-E, -F, and -G). CD8 T cells restricted to classical MHC-I molecules (HLA-A, B, and C) only produce IFN- γ but do not kill target cells [40].

7.6 Pathogenic Mechanisms Induced by *Chlamydia trachomatis*

Despite a local inflammation, *C. trachomatis* infections often remain subclinical and in most persons a normal immune response occurs, resulting in a clearance of the pathogen. However, a subset of patients get ascending infection associated with PID, endosalpingeal damage and tubal infertility in women. The outcome of a chlamydial infection might be determined by differences in virulence factors between serovars or single strains. Although it has been reported that persistent infection occurs more often among serovars D and E, there is no clear evidence that the course of infection is strain-specific or determined by the *C. trachomatis* serovar. Diseases caused by *Chlamydia* are immunopathologically mediated and it can be considered that host immune factors determine the outcome and course of an infection. Antibodies and T cells that are reactive against chlamydial Hsp60 are characteristic for the immune response in infected patients, and it has been hypothesized that a molecular mimicry to human Hsp60 might lead to autoimmunity, which is responsible for serious complications of chlamydial infections. However, because of inconsistent results of several studies there is no clear evidence that Hsp60 or another protein acts as an autoantigen [41, 42]. Another hypothesis on the immunopathogenesis of diseases caused by *C. trachomatis* argues for a delayed hypersensitivity that might occur on the basis of Th1 or Th2 cells. At present the most convincing concept suggests that an inadequate Th1 response in a subset of infected persons may result in long-lasting infection, continuous production of inflammatory cytokines, such as IL-1, TNF-α, and IL-6, and subsequently in ongoing tissue destruction associated with fibrotic remodeling [39, 41]. Genetic variations in host genes may be determinants of the inter-patient variability of the infection outcome. Immunogenetic studies investigating single-nucleotide polymorphisms (SNPs) and multiple variations in immunologically important genes, such as TLRs, will provide further insight into the pathogenic role of host immune factors in chlamydial infections [38].

Chlamydia-infected host cells not only secrete inflammatory cytokines and chemokines but also factors that are involved in tissue remodeling processes. Monocytes and macrophages respond to the infection by an increased expression of matrix metalloproteinase 9 (MMP-9), whereas *Chlamydia*-infected smooth muscle cells and fibroblasts produce the interstitial collagenase MMP-1 and MMP-3 [43, 44]. The induction of MMPs by chlamydiae may be responsible for an increased matrix turnover. Infected host cells also produce mediators regulating the proliferation of mesenchymal cells, such as basic fibroblast growth factor (bFGF) and connective tissue growth factor (CTGF); however, mechanisms of tissue-remodeling processes during chlamydial infections are poorly understood at present [45, 46].

In some studies a role of *C. trachomatis* as a cofactor of human papillomavirus in the development of cervical neoplasia has been proposed but it remains unclear whether this may be due to the stimulation of epithelial cell proliferation [47, 48]. On one hand, chlamydiae can activate proliferative signals in epithelial cells via activation of the glucocorticoid receptor or the early growth response gene 1; on the other hand, the infection of epithelial cells in culture has been reported to result in an inhibition of cytokinesis or induction of a non-apoptotic cell death (Gencay et al., 2004) [24, 49]. Effects of intracellularly persisting chlamydiae on the proliferative activity of host cells are unknown.

7.7 The Cell as *Chlamydia's* Hideout: Persistence and Chronic Disease

Chronic chlamydial infection of the upper genital tract can lead to severe sequelae such as tubal infertility. Chronic inflammation and scarring may be caused either by repeated infections or due to persistence of the pathogen.

Intracellular persistence is characterized by the ability of chlamydiae to convert from normal reticulate bodies into atypical forms that do not redifferentiate into elementary bodies. In cell culture persistent chlamydiae can be induced by stimulation of infected cells with IFN-γ or TNF-α, suggesting that during infection a Th1-driven IFN-γ response may not only inhibit chlamydial replication but also lead to the generation of atypical chlamydial forms that can persist [50]. A strong and rapid induction of an appropriate innate and specific immune response orchestrated by the production of high levels of IFN-γ may be essential for the elimination of the pathogen during the acute phase of the infection whereas a low ratio of IFN-γ to inhibitory cytokines such as IL-10 may favor the development of persistent infection.

The most important mechanism underlying the IFN-γ-mediated alteration of chlamydial growth is the induction of indoleamine 2,3-dioxygenase (IDO), which catalyzes the catabolism of intracellular tryptophan. Inclusions in IFN-γ-treated cells contain only small numbers of enlarged pleomorphic chlamydial forms [51, 52]. When IFN-γ is removed from the culture medium these persistent forms are reactivated and can convert to elementary bodies, suggesting that alterations in the IFN-γ levels during natural infection may promote persistence or reactivation of the pathogen [52]. IFN-γ can also inhibit chlamydial growth and differentiation by the induction of iNOS and iron depletion; however, iNOS-dependent mechanisms have been described in mouse but not human cells [53]. Interestingly, antibiotics added to infected cells at subinhibitory concentrations promote the development of persistent forms, indicating that an inadequate antibiotic treatment in vivo may result in chronic infection [54].

The genome of genital *C. trachomatis* serotypes encodes a tryptophansynthase operon which shows a frame shift mutation in ocular trachoma serotypes. Tryptophansynthase catalyzes the synthesis of tryptophan by an alternative biochemical pathway from indole, which is normally not present in the tissues but can be produced by bacteria of the genital flora [55]. Because indole is IDO-insensitive, the ability of genital chlamydia strains to synthesize tryptophan from this component may allow the pathogen to replicate even in the presence of IFN-γ-induced IDO, thereby promoting the establishment of ascending infections and chronic inflammation.

Several chlamydial genes up- or down-regulated upon conversion to atypical persistent forms have been identified but the precise mechanisms of differential gene expression that drive chlamydiae into persistence are not yet understood. In cell cultures treated with IFN-γ, chlamydiae up-regulate the expression of hsp60 genes but produce only low amounts of OMP-1 (MOMP) [52]. Furthermore, the expression of cytokinesis-associated genes but not of DNA synthesis genes is suppressed in persistent reticulate bodies [56].

Until now, most evidence that in vitro findings on persistent chlamydiae reflect real in vivo situations comes from reactive arthritis (ReA), a sequelae of genital *C. trachomatis* infections occurring in about 3% of the patients. First, aberrant *Chlamydia* reticulate bodies could be found by immune electron microscopy in synovial tissue of ReA patients although the pathogen cannot be isolated in culture from such samples [57]. Second, as shown by RT-PCR these chlamydiae are viable and express Hsp60 but not MOMP mRNA [58]. Synovial fibroblasts isolated from rats, infected with *C. trachomatis* ex vivo, and injected into rat knee joints induce synovitis with cartilage erosion [59]. ReA is associated with HLA-B27 which obviously represents a risk factor for a chronic cause of the disease [60]. The most favored hypothesis of this association is the arthritogenic peptide theory which suggests that a HLA-B27-restricted T-cell response characterizes the intraarticular inflammatory response [61]. Interestingly, HLA-B27-positive patients develop lower levels of IFN-γ in the synovial fluid than HLA-B27-negative patients, which might promote a chronic course of an intraarticular chlamydial infection [62].

7.8 Vaccine Development

A vaccine against *C. trachomatis* would reduce the significant financial burden associated with the treatment and management of *Chlamydia*-induced sequelae such as PID, ectopic pregnancy, and infertility. The major problem in the development of a vaccine providing long-lasting immunity is based on the intracellular nature of the pathogen with its unique replication cycle and the critical balance of Th1, Th2, cytotoxic T, and B cells deciding on the clearance or persistence of chlamydiae [63]. Furthermore, natural infections do not result in a significant immunity against re-infection. Most subunit vaccines generated for tests in animal models have been focused on MOMP. Although recombinant MOMP can elicit neutralizing antibodies and specific T cells, protection after immunization is rather poor. Regarding the intracellular life cycle of *C. trachomatis,* a vaccine should activate immune cells that can recognize intracellular chlamydiae and therefore also include antigens that are expressed by reticulate bodies during chlamydial replication and presented to T cells by the host cells. The inclusion membrane-associated proteins CrpA (cysteine-rich protein A) and Cap1 (class I accessible protein 1), which contain *C. trachomatis*-specific T-cell epitopes, have been proposed as potential vaccine candidates besides OMPs or Hsp60 [39].

Take-Home Pearls

- *Chlamydia* has a biphasic replication cycle that includes the infectious elementary bodies and intracellular forms called reticulate bodies that multiply within an inclusion body in the host cell.
- *C. trachomatis* inhibits the apoptosis of the host cell during its replication cycle.
- The chlamydial protease CPAF which is translocated by the bacteria from the inclusion into the host cell cytosol cleaves and inactivates host cell proteins involved in the regulation of apoptosis and MHC antigen presentation pathways.
- IFN-γ, subinhibitory concentrations of antibiotics, and nutrient deprivation can induce the transformation of chlamydial reticulate bodies into atypical persistent forms that probably play an important role in the establishment of persistent infection and disease.
- An effective immune response against *C. trachomatis* is characterized by a strong and rapid activation of CD4 Th1 lymphocytes as well as CD8 T lymphocytes.
- Vaccines that might provide protective immunity against *C. trachomatis* infection should include antigens that induce a sufficient cellular immune response.

References

1. Halberstaedter, L., von Provazek, S.: Über Zelleinschlüsse pasitärer Natur beim Trachom. Arbeiten aus dem Kaiserlichen Gesundheitsamte **26**, 44–47 (1907)
2. Halberstaedter, L., von Provazek, S.: Über Chlamydozoenbefunde bei Blennorroea neon. non gonorrhoica. Berliner Klinische Wochenschrift 41 (1909)

3. Bedson, S.P., Western, G.T., Simpson, S.L.: Observations on the aetiology of psittacosis. Lancet **1**, 235–246 (1930)
4. Jones, H., Rake, G., Stearns, B.: Studies on lymphogranuloma venereum. III. The action of the sulfonamides on the agent of lymphogranuloma venereum. J Infect Dis **76**, 55–69 (1945)
5. Grayston, J.T., Kuo, C.C., Campbell, L.A., Wang, S.P.: *Chlamydia pneumoniae* sp. nov. lbr *Chlamydia* strain TWAR. Int J Syst Bacteriol **39**, 88–90 (1989)
6. Everett, K.D.E., Bush, R.M., Andersen, A.A.: Emended description of the order *Chlamydiales*, proposal of *Parachlamydiaceae* fam. nov. and *Simkaniaceae* fam. nov., each containing one monotypic genus, revised taxonomy of the family *Chlamydiaceae*, including a new genus and five new species, and standards for the identification of organisms. Int J Syst Evol Bacteriol **49**, 415–440 (1999)
7. Horn, M., Wagner, M., Muller, K.D., Schmid, E.N., Fritsche, T.R., Schleifer, K.H., Michel, R.: *Neochlamydia hartmannellae* gen. nov., sp. nov. (Parachlamydiaceae), an endoparasite of the amoeba *Hartmannella vermiformis*. Microbiol UK **146**, 1231–1239 (2000)
8. Wehrl, W., Wehrl, W., Brinkmann, V., Jungblut, P.R., Meyer, T.F., Szczepek, A.J.: From the inside out--processing of the Chlamydial autotransporter PmpD and its role in bacterial adhesion and activation of human host cells. Molec Microbiol **51**, 319–334 (2004)
9. Fadel, S., Eley, A.: Chlamydia trachomatis OmcB protein is a surface-exposed glycosaminoglycan-dependent adhesin. J Med Microbiol **56**, 15–22 (2007)
10. Davis, C.H., Raulston, J.E., Wyrick, P.B.: Protein disulfide isomerase, a component of the estrogen receptor complex, is associated with Chlamydia trachomatis serovar E attached to human endometrial epithelial cells. Infect Immun **70**, 413–418 (2002)
11. Herold, B.C., Siston, A., Bremer, J., Kirkpatrick, R., Wilbanks, G., Fugedi, P., Peto, C., Cooper, M.: Sulfated carbohydrate compounds prevent microbial adherence by sexually transmitted disease pathogens. Antimicrob Agents Chemother **41**, 2776–2780 (1997)
12. Stuart, E.S., Webley, W.C., Norkin, L.C.: Lipid rafts, caveolae, caveolin-1, and entry by Chlamydiae into host cells. Exp Cell Res **287**(1), 67–78 (2003)
13. Birkelund, S., Johnsen, H., Christiansen, G.: *Chlamydia trachomatis* serovar L2 induces tyrosine phosphorylation during uptake by HeLa cells. Infect Immun **62**, 4900–4908 (1994)
14. Lane, B.J., Mutchler, C., Al Khodor, S., Grieshaber, S.S., Carabeo, R.A.: Chlamydial entry involves TARP binding of guanine nucleotide exchange factors. PLoS Pathog Mar **4**(3), e1000014 (2008)
15. Scidmore, M.A., Fischer, E.R., Hackstadt, T.: Sphingolipids and glycoproteins are differentially trafficked to the *C. trachomatis* inclusion. J Cell Biol **134**, 363–374 (1996)
16. Peters, J., Wilson, D.P., Myers, G., Timms, P., Bavoil, P.M.: Type III secretion à la Chlamydia. Trends Microbiol **15**, 241–251 (2007)
17. Betts, H.J., Wolf, K., Fields, K.A.: Effector protein modulation of host cells: examples in the *Chlamydia* spp. Arsenal Curr Opin Microbiol **12**, 81–87 (2009)
18. Zhong, G., Fan, P., Ji, H., Dong, F., Huang, Y.: Identification of a chlamydial protease-like activity factor responsible for the degradation of host transcription factors. J Exp Med **193**, 935–942 (2001)
19. Hybiske, K., Stephens, R.S.: Mechanisms of host cell exit by the intracellular bacterium *Chlamydia*. Proc Natl Acad Sci USA **104**, 11430–11435 (2007)
20. Fink, S.L., Cookson, B.T.: Apoptosis, pyroptosis, and necrosis: mechanistic description of dead and dying eukaryotic cells. Infect Immun **73**, 1907–1916 (2005)
21. Ying, S., Pettengill, M., Ojcius, D.M., Häcker, G.: Host cell survival and death during *Chlamydia* infection. Curr Immunol Rev **3**, 31–40 (2007)
22. Fan, T., Lu, H., Hu, H., Shi, L., McClarty, G.A., Nance, D.M., et al.: Inhibition of apoptosis in *Chlamydia*-infected cells: blockade of mitochondrial cytochrome *c* release and caspase activation. J Exp Med **187**, 487–496 (1998)
23. Pirbhai, M., Dong, F., Zhong, Y., Pan, K.Z., Zhong, G.: The secreted protease factor CPAF is responsible for degrading pro-apoptotic BH3-only proteins in *Chlamydia trachomatis*-infected cells. J Biol Chem **281**, 31495–31501 (2006)
24. Ying, S., Fischer, S.F., Pettengill, M., Conte, D., Paschen, S.A., Ojcius, D.M., Häcker, G.: Characterization of Host Cell Death Induced by *Chlamydia trachomatis*. Infect Immun **74**, 6057–6066 (2006)
25. Yu, H., Schwarzer, K., Förster, M., Kniemeyer, O., Forsbach-Birk, V., Straube, E., Rödel, J. Role of high-mobility group box 1 protein and poly(ADP-ribose) polymerase 1 degradation in Chlamydia trachomatis-induced cytopathicity. Infect Immun **78**, 3288–3297 (2010)
26. Paschen, S.A., Christian, J.G., Vier, J., Schmidt, F., Walch, A., Ojcius, D.M., Häcker, G.: Cytopathicity of *Chlamydia* is largely reproduced by expression of a single chlamydial protease. J Cell Biol **182**, 117–127 (2008)
27. Hatch, T.P., Vance Jr., D.W., Al-Hossainey, E.: Identification of a major envelope protein in Chlamydia spp. J Bacteriol **146**, 426–431 (1981)
28. Stephens, R.S., Kalman, S., Lammel, C., et al.: Genome sequence of an obligate intracellular pathogen of humans: *Chlamydia trachomatis*. Science **282**, 754–759 (1998)
29. Stephens, R.S., Lammel, C.J.: Chlamydia outer membrane protein discovery using genomics. Curr Opin Microbiol **4**, 16–20 (2001)
30. Sardinia, L.M., Segal, E., Ganem, D.: Developmental regulation of the cysteine-rich outer-membrane proteins of murine Chlamydia trachomatis. J Gen Microbiol **134**, 997–1004 (1988)
31. Crane, D.D., Carlson, J.H., Fischer, E.R., BavoiTan Cl, P., Hsia, R.C., Tan, C., Kuo, C.C., Caldwell, H.D.: Chlamydia trachomatis polymorphic membrane protein D is a species-common pan-neutralizing antigen. Proc Natl Acad Sci USA **103**, 1894–1899 (2006)
32. Bas, S., Neff, L., Vuillet, M., Spenato, U., Seya, T., Matsumoto, M., Gabay, C.: The proinflammatory cytokine response to Chlamydia trachomatis elementary bodies in human macrophages is partly mediated by a lipoprotein, the macrophage infectivity potentiator, through TLR2/TLR1/TLR6 and CD14. J Immunol **180**, 1158–1168 (2008)
33. Rund, S., Lindner, B., Brade, H., Holst, O.: Structural analysis of the lipopolysaccharide from Chlamydia trachomatis serotype L2. J Biol Chem **274**, 16819–16824 (1999)
34. Fadel, S., Eley, A.: Is lipopolysaccharide a factor in infectivity of Chlamydia trachomatis? J Med Microbiol **57**, 261–266 (2008)

35. Brade, L., Nurminen, M., Makela, P.H., Brade, H.: Antigenic properties of *Chlamydia trachomatis* lipopolysaccharide. Infect Immun **48**, 569–572 (1985)
36. Buchholz, K.R., Stephens, R.S.: Activation of the host cell proinflammatory interleukin-8 response by *Chlamydia trachomatis*. Cell Microbiol **8**, 1768–1779 (2006)
37. Baumert, J., Schmidt, K.H., Eitner, A., Straube, E., Rödel, J.: Host cell cytokines induced by *Chlamydia pneumoniae* decrease the expression of interstitial collagens and fibronectin in fibroblasts. Infect Immun **77**, 867–876 (2009)
38. den Hartog, J.E., Morré, S.A., Land, S.A.: *Chlamydia trachomatis*-associated tubal factor subfertility: immunogenetic aspects and serological screening. Hum Reprod Update **12**, 719–730 (2006)
39. Roan, N.R., Starnbach, M.N.: Immune-mediated control of *Chlamydia* infection. Cell Microbiol **10**, 9–19 (2008)
40. Gervassi, A.L., Probst, P., Stamm, W.E., Marrazzo, J., Grabstein, K.H., Alderson, M.R.: Functional characterization of class Ia- and Non-class Ia-restricted *Chlamydia*-reactive $CD8^+$ T cell responses in humans. J Immunol **171**, 4278–4286 (2003)
41. Stephens, R.S.: The cellular paradigm of chlamydial pathogenesis. Trends Microbiol **11**, 44–51 (2003)
42. Yi, Y., Yang, X., Brunham, R.C.: Autoimmunity to heat shock protein 60 and antigen-specific production of interleukin-10. Infect Immun **65**, 1669–1674 (1997)
43. Imtiaz, M.T., Distelhorst, J.T., Schripsema, J.H., Sigar, I.M., Kasimos, J.N., Lacy, S.R., Ramsey, K.H.: A role for matrix metalloproteinase-9 in pathogenesis of urogenital *Chlamydia muridarum* infection in mice. Microbes Infect **9**, 1561–1566 (2007)
44. Rödel, J., Prochnau, D., Prager, K., Pentcheva, E., Hartmann, M., Straube, E.: Increased production of matrix metalloproteinases 1 and 3 by smooth muscle cells upon infection with *Chlamydia pneumoniae*. FEMS Immunol Med Microbiol **38**, 159–164 (2003)
45. Peters, J., Hess, S., Endlich, K., Thalmann, J., Holzberg, D., Kracht, M., et al.: Silencing or permanent activation: host-cell response in models of persistent *Chlamydia pneumoniae* infection. Cell Microbiol **7**, 1099–1108 (2005)
46. Rödel, J., Woytas, M., Groh, A., Schmidt, K.H., Hartmann, M., Lehmann, M., Straube, E.: Production of basic fibroblast growth factor and interleukin 6 by human smooth muscle cells following infection with *Chlamydia pneumoniae*. Infect Immun **68**, 3635–3641 (2000)
47. Lehmann, M., Groh, A., Rödel, J., Nindl, I., Straube, E.: Detection of *Chlamydia trachomatis* DNA in cervical samples with regard to infection by human papillomavirus. J Infect **38**, 12–17 (1999)
48. Simonetti, A.C., melo, J.H., de Souza, P.R., Bruneska, D., de Lima Filho, J.L.: Immunological's host profile for HPV and *Chlamydia trachomatis*, a cervical cancer cofactor. Microbes Infect **11**, 435–442 (2009)
49. Greene, W., Xiao, Y., Huang, Y., McClarty, G., Zhong, G.: *Chlamydia*-infected cells continue to undergo mitosis and resist induction of apoptosis. Infect Immun **72**, 451–460 (2004)
50. Hogan, R.J., Mathews, S.A., Mukhopadhyay, S., Summersgill, J.T., Timms, P.: Chlamydial persistence: beyond the biphasic paradigm. Infect Immun **72**, 1843–1855 (2004)
51. Beatty, W.L., Belanger, T.A., Desai, A.A., Morrison, R.P., Byrne, G.I.: Tryptophan depletion as a mechanism of gamma interferon-mediated chlamydial persistence. Infect Immun **62**, 3705–3711 (1994)
52. Beatty, W.L., Byrne, G.I., Morrison, R.P.: Morphologic and antigenic characterization of interferon γ-mediated persistent *Chlamydia trachomatis* infection in vitro. Proc Natl Acad Sci USA **90**, 3998–4002 (1993)
53. Rothfuchs, A.G., Gigliotti, D., Palmblad, K., Andersson, U., Wigzell, H., Rottenberg, M.E.: IFN-alpha beta-dependent, IFN-gamma secretion by bone marrow-derived macrophages controls an intracellular bacterial infection. J Immunol **167**, 6453–6461 (2001)
54. Gieffers, J., Rupp, J., Gebert, A., Solbach, W., Klinger, M.: First-choice antibiotics at subinhibitory concentrations induce persistence of *Chlamydia pneumoniae*. Antimicrob Agents Chemother **48**, 1402–1405 (2004)
55. Caldwell, H.D., Wood, H., Crane, D., Bailey, R., Jones, R.B., Mabey, D., et al.: Polymorphisms in *Chlamydia trachomatis* tryptophan synthase genes differentiate between genital and ocular isolates. J Clin Invest **111**, 1757–1769 (2003)
56. Byrne, G.I., Ouellette, S.P., Wang, Z., Rao, J.P., Lu, L., Beatty, W.L., Hudson, A.P.: *Chlamydia pneumoniae* expresses gene required for DNA replication but not cytokinesis during persistent infection of Hep-2 cells. Infect Immun **69**, 5423–5429 (2001)
57. Nanagara, R., Li, F., Beutler, A.M., Hudson, A.P., Schumacher Jr., H.R.: Alterations of *Chlamydia trachomatis* biologic behavior in synovial membranes: suppression of surface antigen production in reactive arthritis and Reiter's syndrome. Arthritis Rheum **38**, 1410–1417 (1995)
58. Gérard, H.C., Branigan, P.J., Schumacher Jr., H.R., Hudson, A.P.: Synovial *Chlamydia trachomatis* in patients with reactive arthritis/Reiter's syndrome are viable but show aberrant gene expression. J Rheumatol **25**, 734–742 (1998)
59. Inman, R.D., Chiu, B.: Synoviocyte-packaged *Chlamydia trachomatis* induces a chronic aseptic arthritis. J Clin Invest **102**, 1776–1782 (1998)
60. Colmegna, I., Cuchacovich, R., Espinoza, L.R.: HLA-B27-associated reactive arthritis: pathogenetic and clinical considerations. Clin Microbiol Rev **17**, 348–369 (2004)
61. Zeidler, H., Kuipers, J., Köhler, L.: *Chlamydia*-induced arthritis. Curr Opin Rheumatol **16**, 380–392 (2004)
62. Bas, S., Kvien, T.K., Buchs, N., Fulpius, T., Gabay, C.: Lower level of synovial fluid interferon-γ in HLA-B27-positive than in HLA-B27-negative patients with Chlamydia trachomatis reactive arthritis. Rheumatology **42**, 461–467 (2003)
63. Igietseme, J., Eko, F., He, Q., Bandea, C., Lubitz, W., Carcia-Sastre, A., Black, C.: Delivery of *Chlamydia* vaccines. Expert Opin Drug Deliv **2**, 549–562 (2005)
64. Miyagawa, Y.: Studies on the characteristics of Miyagawanella lymphogranulomatis. Jpn J Exp Med **26**, 157–159 (1956)
65. Valdivia, R.H.: *Chlamydia* effector proteins and new insights into chlamydial cellular microbiology. Curr Opin Microbiol **11**, 53–59 (2009)
66. Follmann, F., Olsen, A.W., Jensen, K.T., Hansen, P.R., Andersen, P., Theisen, M.: Antigenic profiling of a *Chlamydia trachomatis* gene-expression library. J Infect Dis **197**, 897–905 (2008)
67. Gencay, M.M., Tamm, M., Glanville, A., Perruchoud, A.P., Roth, M.: *Chlamydia pneumoniae* activates epithelial cell proliferation via NF-kappaB and the glucocorticoid receptor. Infect Immun **71**, 5814–5822 (2004)

8 *Chlamydia trachomatis* Infections in Women and Men

Jorma Paavonen

Core Messages

- *Chlamydia trachomatis* is an important genital pathogen and the most common bacterial cause of sexually transmitted infections.
- Most clinical manifestations of *C. trachomatis* genital infections are silent and the majority of chlamydial infections are asymptomatic.
- Symptomatic chlamydial infections only represent the tip of the iceberg.
- Screening for chlamydial infections remains important in the secondary prevention.
- Genital chlamydial infections are strikingly common in young populations with risk-taking sexual behavior.
- Natural history of chlamydial infection is not well understood.
- Nucleic acid amplification tests are highly sensitive and specific.
- Urine-based screening tests have comparable sensitivity and specificity to cervical and urethral specimens. Vulvar and vaginal swabs and self-sampling also perform well.
- A new genetic variant of *C. trachomatis* was discovered in Sweden in 2006. So far, there is little evidence that this new variant has spread outside Sweden or other Scandinavian countries.
- Azithromycin is the best single-dose agent for treatment of chlamydial infections.
- Screening programs remain important in limiting the upper genital tract complications of chlamydial infection.
- Despite increased screening activity *C. trachomatis* rates are on the rise in many countries in Europe.
- Previous estimates of *C. trachomatis* complication rates have been based on selected high-risk populations and case-control studies and may have been overestimated. More recent revised estimates are based on population registry networks.

8.1 Introduction

Chlamydia trachomatis (*C. trachomatis*) is an important genital pathogen and the most common bacterial cause of sexually transmitted infections (STI). Chlamydial infections of the genital tract are highly prevalent globally. *C. trachomatis* is a true obligate intracellular pathogen that has a unique growth cycle distinguished from all other microorganisms. Because of this slow growth cycle, chlamydial diseases tend to be chronic in nature. The clinical spectrum of *C. trachomatis* infections is extensive. Selected highlights of the evolution and development of understanding of *C. trachomatis* infections are shown in Table 8.1. Most clinical manifestations of *C. trachomatis* genital infections are silent and the majority of chlamydial infections are in fact asymptomatic. Therefore, symptomatic

J. Paavonen
Department of Obstetrics and Gynecology, Helsinki University Central Hospital, Haartmaninkatu 2, 00290 Helsinki, Finland
e-mail: jorma.paavonen@hus.fi

G. Gross and S.K. Tyring (eds.), *Sexually Transmitted Infections and Sexually Transmitted Diseases*,
DOI: 10.1007/978-3-642-14663-3_8,

Table 8.1 Selected highlights

1950s
• First isolation from genital tract
1960s
• Cell culture developed
1970s
• Wide spectrum of clinical manifestations described
• Early prevalence data
1980s
• Rapid tests (DFA, EIA, slide tests) emerged
• National surveillance systems
• Major role of chlamydia in tubal factor infertility and adverse pregnancy outcome
1990s
• Most women and men with chlamydial infection are asymptomatic
• NAATs
– First void urine (FVU) testing
– Self-sampling (vulva, vagina)
• Single-dose therapy
• Patient-delivered partner therapy
• Guidelines for screening
2000s
• Reported case rates are on the rise again
• Self-sampling and FVU testing emerge
– Gynecologic examination not necessary
• Home sampling – a new innovation
– Better compliance
• Rescreening of Chlamydia-positive individuals
– Core group with high risk for reinfection
• Discovery of mutant Chlamydia!
– Chlamydia strikes back!

chlamydial infections only represent the tip of the iceberg. Screening for chlamydial infections remains important in the secondary prevention. *C. trachomatis* vaccine development has proven difficult because of the complex antigenic structure and limited knowledge of protective antigens. Chlamydial infections of the genital tract are primarily caused by serovars D, E, F, G, H, I, J, and K. However, not much is known of specific virulence factors of different *C. trachomatis* serovars.

8.2 Epidemiology

Genital chlamydial infections are strikingly common in young populations with risk-taking sexual behavior. Sexually active individuals 24 years of age or younger including adolescents are at increased risk for chlamydial infection. In addition to sexual activity and age, other risk factors for chlamydial infection include history of chlamydial or other STI, new or multiple sexual partners, inconsistent condom use, and exchanging sex for money or drugs. Risk factors for pregnant women are the same as for non-pregnant women. Prevalence varies widely among populations both in men and women. WHO estimates that almost 100 million new cases of genital chlamydia infections occur worldwide. The baseline prevalence among 15–26 year old women is approximately 4% based on screening of approximately 40,000 women enrolled in HPV vaccination efficacy trials in 14 countries in 4 continents. Prevalence rates in selected high-risk populations are much higher. Guidelines for screening for chlamydial infection have been developed and implemented in many countries.

8.2.1 Infections in Women

In women, genital chlamydial infection may result in urethritis, cervicitis, pelvic inflammatory disease, infertility, ectopic pregnancy, and chronic pelvic pain. Chlamydial infection during pregnancy is related to adverse pregnancy outcome including miscarriage, preterm premature rupture of membranes, preterm labor, and low birth weight. Chlamydial infection during pregnancy may also lead to neonatal chlamydial infections including conjunctivitis or pneumonia or both.

8.2.2 Infections in Men

Chlamydia infections in men include urethral infection (nongonococcal urethritis, NGU), epididymitis and proctitis particularly in homosexual men. *C. trachomatis* is one of the microorganisms which can trigger reactive arthritis or Reiter's syndrome among those genetically susceptible.

8.3 Natural History

Natural history of chlamydial infection is not well understood since most chlamydial infections are asymptomatic. Past chlamydial infection does not protect against recurrent infections by the same or different serovars. In the absence of antimicrobial therapy, *C. trachomatis* infections typically last for many months or even years, but these infections can also undergo spontaneous clearance. This is clearly immune mediated. There is a fine balance between protective immunity and immune-associated disease pathogenesis which characterizes the deleterious host response to chlamydia infection. A better understanding of immune response is an important research priority from the point of view of *C. trachomatis* vaccine development which is a major challenge.

8.3.1 Clinical Manifestations in Women

8.3.1.1 Cervical Infection

Chlamydial infection of the cervix leads to mucopurulent cervicitis (MPC). Characteristic features are mucopurulent endocervical discharge, edema and induced mucosal bleeding (Fig. 8.1). Colposcopically, immature squamous metaplasia and hypertrophic ectopy are characteristic features of chlamydial cervicitis. Cytologic manifestations include increased number of PMNs, metaplastic cell atypia and endocervical cell atypia. One can suspect cervicitis based on increased number of PMNs on vaginal wet mount or gram-stained cervical smears. Unfortunately, none of the clinical findings are specific to *C. trachomatis*, and in fact majority of women with chlamydial infection show no abnormal signs. Therefore, clinical recognition of chlamydial cervicitis very much depends on a high index of suspicion and a careful clinical examination. Key findings suggestive of chlamydial infection should be recognized and those are edema and hypertrophy of cervical

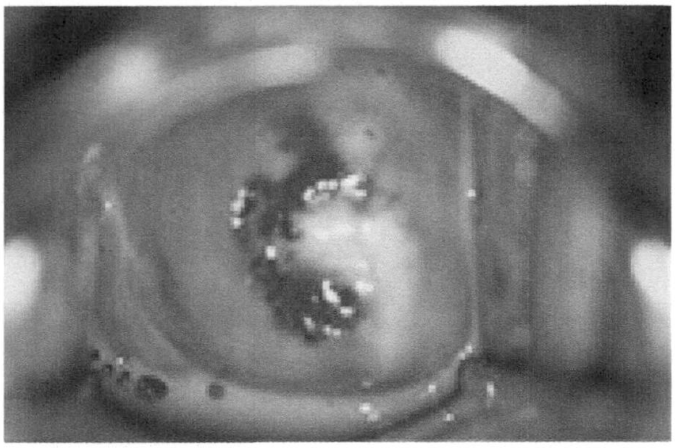

Fig. 8.1 Mucopurulent cervicitis. Note mucopurulent discharge, erythema and edema

ectopy, easily induced endocervical mucosal bleeding and of course, mucopurulent discharge.

8.3.1.2 Urethral Infection

At least 50% of women with chlamydial cervicitis also have chlamydial urethral infection. *C. trachomatis* has been linked to acute urethral syndrome with pyuria and no bacteriuria. Again, often times chlamydial urethritis may be minimally symptomatic.

8.3.1.3 Pelvic Inflammatory Disease

Chlamydial MPC can cause ascending infection into the upper genital tract. Chlamydial endometritis has been well described as a distinct disease entity. Endometritis can cause metrorrhagia. Endometrial aspiration biopsy shows increased number of plasma cells, i.e. plasma cell endometritis. Clinical diagnosis of endometritis is difficult, since pelvic examination usually shows no specific findings and chlamydial endometritis can be minimally symptomatic. Again, high index of suspicion augments in the diagnosis of chlamydial endometritis. Particularly, spotting or metrorrhagia in sexually active young women on oral contraceptives may suggest chlamydial endometritis. Natural history of chlamydial endometritis is not well understood. However, most likely, this condition may lead to acute salpingitis with more severe symptoms such as lower abdominal pain (Fig. 8.2). *C. trachomatis* was first isolated from fallopian tube specimens in

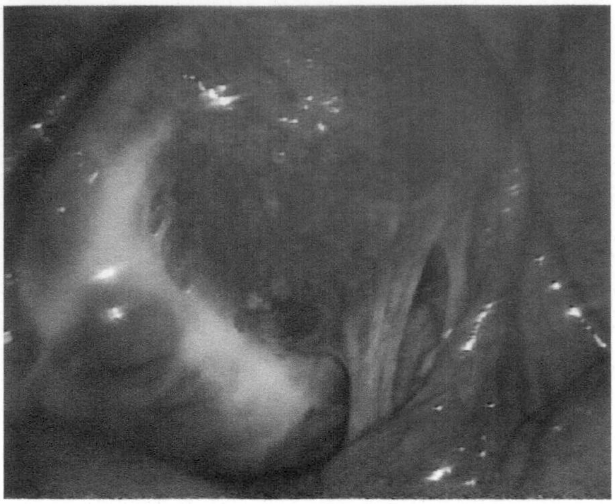

Fig. 8.2 Laparoscopic view of pelvic inflammatory disease. Note purulent discharge, occluded Fallopian tubes, and tubo-ovarian adhesions

1977. Subsequently, multiple studies have confirmed that *C. trachomatis* indeed can cause salpingitis followed by tubal scarring and tubal factor infertility or increased risk for tubal pregnancy. PID was epidemic in the 1970s and 1980s. However, inpatient PID has become a rare disease. Reported cases of PID have decreased. Obvious explanation increased *C. trachomatis* screening activity. Screening programs have already been implemented in many countries. Also, oral contraceptives are more commonly used and oral contraceptive use seems to decrease the risk for ascending chlamydial infection. Also, contact tracing efforts decrease the risk for recurrent chlamydial infection. Population-based studies suggest that the overall prevalence of chlamydial infections has been steadily decreasing, at least based on prevalence rates of *C. trachomatis* antibodies in young age groups. Although *C. trachomatis* infection is still highly prevalent in selected populations, reproductive health consequences seem not to reflect this at population level.

8.3.1.4 Perihepatitis

Sometimes, chlamydial PID can cause upper abdominal infection which manifests as perihepatitis, i.e. right upper quadrant pain. Perihepatitis should be suspected in young sexually active women who develop right upper quadrant pain associated with general symptoms such as fever, nausea and increased C-reactive protein concentration.

8.3.2 Clinical Manifestations in Men

8.3.2.1 Urethral Infection

Chlamydial urethritis in men, also known as nongonococcal urethritis, is the male counterpart of MPC in women. NGU is extremely common among male patients seen in STD clinics, since it is more often symptomatic than MPC in women and easier to diagnose. Chlamydial urethritis is less often symptomatic than gonococcal urethritis. The diagnosis is usually based on the number of PMNs on urethral smear gram stain or the presence of pyuria in first void urine.

8.3.2.2 Epididymitis

Acute epididymitis is a rare complication of chlamydial NGU and certainly less common than PID in women with chlamydial MPC. At least two thirds of epididymitis cases in young sexually active men are attributable to *C. trachomatis*

8.3.2.3 Proctitis

Lymphogranuloma venereum (LGV) serovars of *C. trachomatis* cause proctitis. However, also non-LGV serovars can infect rectal mucosa particularly among homosexual men. Clinical, proctoscopic, cytologic, and histopathologic manifestations of chlamydial proctitis have been described. Typically, the findings mimic those associated with chlamydial MPC in women.

8.3.2.4 Reiter's Syndrome

Reiter's syndrome is characterized by the presence of urethritis, conjunctivitis, arthritis, and typical mucocutaneous lesions. Reiter's syndrome can be caused by *C. trachomatis* among individuals with class 1 HLA-B27 haplotype. *C. trachomatis* as well as other infections such as salmonellosis, shigellosis, yersinia, and campylobacter enteric infections can all trigger Reiter's syndrome. Most patients with Reiter's syndrome are men.

8.4 Diagnosis

All men and women suspected of having *C. trachomatis* genital infection must have specific diagnostic testing. This is because the diagnosis is difficult to establish on clinical findings alone. Although so-called syndromic diagnosis and treatment, that is, empiric treatment without testing, is perhaps an acceptable strategy, in settings where costs or other circumstances prohibit laboratory testing, specific diagnostic testing should be mandatory if affordable. Furthermore, unrecognized *C. trachomatis* infections should be identified by appropriate screening of asymptomatic men and women in high-risk groups such as STD clinics, family planning clinics, adolescents clinics, and student health clinics.

An important development in chlamydial diagnostic testing has been the introduction of automated methods for the detection of amplified *C. trachomatis* DNA or RNA for which cervical, urethral, urine, or vulvar or vaginal self sampling can be used. These amplification tests are highly sensitive and specific. PCR-based assays are most commonly used. Nucleic acid amplification tests (NAATs) are recommended for screening for chlamydial infection in both men and women. Urine-based screening tests have comparable sensitivity and specificity to cervical and urethral specimens. Vulvar and vaginal swabs and self-sampling also perform well. Therefore, gynecologic examination is not necessary for *C. trachomatis* screening in women.

A new genetic variant of *C. trachomatis* was discovered in Sweden in 2006. This variant had a 377 base pair deletion in the plasmid which was a target for NAATs and therefore was not detected by these tests. So far, there is little evidence that this new variant has spread outside Sweden or other Scandinavian countries. Subsequently, NAATs have been modified so that this variant can be detected.

Diagnosis of *C. trachomatis* infections will be presented in detail in another chapter. Selected clinical aspects of diagnosis in clinical practice are briefly presented here.

8.4.1 Microscopy

Direct light microscopy of vaginal wet mount can be valuable to suspect chlamydial infection. Increased white cells on vaginal wet mount or cervical gram stain suggest that specific testing for *C. trachomatis* must be performed. On the other hand, lack of white cells and presence of lactobacilli have a high negative predictive value of *C. trachomatis*. A simple algorithm of vaginal wet mount as a bedside test is useful in clinical practice (Table 8.2).

8.4.2 Culture

C. trachomatis is an intracellular pathogen and requires a cell culture system for propagation in the laboratory. Cell culture was the gold standard test for the detection of *C. trachomatis* for several years, but has now been replaced by more sensitive molecular techniques.

Table 8.2 Differential diagnosis of vaginal infections and interpretation of vaginal wet mount findings

	Normal	Yeast	BV	Trichomonas	DIV (aerobic vaginitis)	Atrophic vaginitis
Etiology	–	Candida	Anaerobic bacteria	*T. vaginalis*	Virulent aerobic bacteria (GBS, *E. coli*)	Estrogen deficiency
Wet mount	Lactobacilli dominate	Mycelia, yeast cells	Clue cells	Mobile trichomonas, leukocytes ++	Parabasal cells, leukocytes +++, heavy bacterial flora, no clue cells	Parabasal cells, variable amount of leukocytes
Vaginal discharge	Whitish, nonhomogenous	Curdy or watery	Grey, homogenous	Purulent, heavy, with bubbles	Purulent, yellow, heavy	Scanty, bloody
KOH-test	(–)	(–)	(+)	(+/–)	(-)	(+/–)
pH	<4.7	<4.7	≥4.7	≥4.7	Variable	≥4.7

8.4.3 Antigen Detection

Rapid antigen detection assays by EIA also suffered from low sensitivity and have been replaced by molecular techniques.

8.4.4 Nucleic Acid Detection

Several different types of NAAT technologies are now commercially available for *C. trachomatis*. These methods have excellent sensitivity and high specificity and have replaced all other diagnostic tests in microbiology laboratories. NAATs perform well on all genital samples. Home sampling based on home sampling kits decreases compliance problems, decreases the prevalence of *C. trachomatis* infections and also decreases the risk for complications such as PID.

8.4.5 Antibody Detection by Serology

The MIF test for chlamydial antibody has been extensively used in population-based studies of associations of *C. trachomatis* with several clinical syndromes, such as PID, adverse pregnancy outcome, tubal factor infertility and others. MIF test is extremely cumbersome and observer dependent and not useful for the diagnosis of chlamydial genital infections in clinical practice. The only exception is the diagnosis of lymphogranuloma venereum (LGV) proctitis caused by LGV serovars of *C. trachomatis*.

8.4.6 Diagnostic Test Performance

Important parameters for diagnostic test performance are sensitivity (ability of test to identify people who are truly positive), specificity (ability of test to identify people who are truly negative), positive predictive value (PPV; probability of a positive test being true positive), negative predictive value (probability of a negative test being true negative), false positive (true negative specimens that test positive), false negative (true positive specimens that test negative), and accuracy (percentage of correct results obtained by test compared to results of reference standard). Sensitivity is the measure of test efficiency in detecting the infection and specificity is the measure of a test's efficiency in ruling out an infection. Predictive values are meaningful in evaluating test performances in specific populations. Predictive values vary significantly with the prevalence of infection. As the prevalence of the infection decreases, PPV decreases leading to more false positive test results. When the prevalence is low, even small decrease in test specificity will result in a large decrease in PPV. Test reproducibility is another important parameter although less of a problem with automated techniques. Quality assurance measures in clinical laboratories are increasingly important with implementation of new diagnostic tests.

8.5 Therapy

Azithromycin with a half-life of 5–7 days and excellent intracellular and tissue penetration is the best single-dose agent for treatment of chlamydial infection in men and women. Single-dose therapy is particularly important in less compliant patients such as adolescents or asymptomatic men and women with chlamydial infection. Directly observed single-dose therapy maximizes compliance. Single-dose azithromycin or doxycycline 100 mg bid for 7 days are equally effective approaching 100%. Other antimicrobials effective against *C. trachomatis* include erythromycin, lymecycline, trimethoprim-sulfadiazine, minocycline, ofloxacin, and rifampicin among others. Expedited treatment of sex partners through patient-delivered partner therapy reduces rates of persistent or recurrent chlamydial infection.

8.6 Prevention

C. trachomatis is the most common bacterial STI. Screening programs remain important in limiting the complications of chlamydial infection. Antimicrobial treatment of infected individuals helps to reduce transmission by shortening the average duration of infection. In the absence of antimicrobial therapy, *C. trachomatis* infection typically last for many months, but may undergo spontaneous clearance which seems to be immune mediated.

Prevention of *C. trachomatis* infection could be primary, secondary or tertiary. Primary prevention by education and behavioral change has not proven effective. Primary prevention by vaccination is problematic since development of a vaccine against *C. trachomatis* remains a challenge. This results from poor understanding or the regulation of the immune response in the genital tract and limited knowledge of protective *C. trachomatis* antigens inducing protective immune responses. Thus, better definition of human immune response correlates of *C. trachomatis* protective immunity and disease pathogenesis remain an important research priority. Clearly, search for a vaccine with protective and not harmful effects is a complex task.

Secondary prevention with early detection of asymptomatic infection by screening is the most powerful prevention effort, since prevalence of *C. trachomatis* among asymptomatic women is strikingly high in many populations. For instance, prevalence of *C. trachomatis* infection was in the range of 5.1–5.5% among approximately 40,000 15- to 26-year-old women enrolled in phase 3 HPV vaccination trials during 2002–2005 in 4 continents. *C. trachomatis* infection certainly fills the prerequisites for disease prevention by screening. However, despite emerging screening recommendation and increasing screening activity reported *C. trachomatis* case rates are on the rise in many countries in Europe. For instance, in Finland, there has been 60% increase of *C. trachomatis* infections during the past 10 years. There is already major frustration with opportunistic screening programs, implementation of management guidelines and contact tracing efforts. Opportunistic screening activity may benefit individuals, but seems to have little public health benefit based on the reported chlamydia rates. Nevertheless, truly population-based data may differ from reported infection rates which is explained by so-called core group hypothesis. This means that early detection and effective treatment may lead to poor or short antibody response leaving individuals susceptible to reinfection. High reinfection rates have recently been reported from England, United States and Canada. However, population-based seroepidemiologic studies have provided surprising findings: *C. trachomatis* seroprevalence rates have decreased during the past 20 years in Finland suggesting that truly population-based data may differ from data based on reported *C. trachomatis* infection rates. Furthermore, if the primary objective is to improve reproductive health, good news are emerging. Inpatients PID has become a rare disease, ectopic pregnancy rates are decreasing and the proportion of tubal factor infertility of all infertility is decreasing. Previous estimates of *C. trachomatis* complication rates have been based on selected high-risk populations and mostly, case-control studies subject to major biases. More recent revised estimates are based on population registry networks which are more reliable and can be validated. These revised lower estimates may have an impact on health gains and cost savings obtained by extensive *C. trachomatis* screening programs.

Undoubtedly, current screening programs are an important step toward limiting the complications of chlamydial infection although these programs are likely to have more individual than public health benefit. More research on the efficacy and effectiveness of *C. trachomatis* screening programs are needed and the question still remains: Are we doing enough?

Acknowledgment The author's work is in part supported by the European Commission within the Sixth Framework Programme through the EpiGenChlamydia project (contract no. LSHG-CT-2007-037637). See www.EpiGenChlamydia.eu for more details.

Further Reading

Aral, S.O., Fenton, K.A., Holmes, K.K.: Sexually transmitted disease in the USA. Temporal trends. Sex. Transm. Infect. **83**, 257–266 (2007)

Batteiger, B.E., Tu, W., Ofner, S., Van Der Pol, B., Stothard, D., Orr, D.P., Katz, B.P., Fortenberry, J.D.: Repeated *Chlamydia trachomatis* genital infections in adolescent women. J. Infect. Dis. **201**, 42–51 (2010)

Bjartling, C., Osser, S., Johnsson, A., Persson, K.: Clinical manifestaitons and epidemiology of the new genetic variant of *Chlamydia trachomatis*. Sex. Transm. Dis. **36**, 529–535 (2009)

Brunham, R.C., Pourbohloul, B., Mak, S., White, R., Rekart, M.L.: The unexpected impact of a *Chlmaydia trachomatis* infection control program on susceptibility to reinfection. J. Infect. Dis. **192**, 1836–1844 (2005)

Brunham, R.C., Rey-Ladino, J.: Immunology of Chlamydia infection: implications for a *Chlamydia trachomatis* vaccine. Nature **5**, 149–161 (2005)

Fung, M., Scott, K.C., Kent, C.K., et al.: Chlamydial and gonococcal reinfection among men: a systematic review of data to evaluate the need for retesting. Sex. Transm. Infect. **83**, 304–309 (2007)

Golden, M.R., Whittington, W.L.H., Handsfield, H.H., et al.: Effect of expedited treatment of sex partners on recurrent or persistent gonohhrea or chlamydial infection. N Engl J. Med. **352**, 676–685 (2005)

Guipers, J., Gaidos, C.A., Peeling, R.W.: Principals of laboratory diagnosis of STI's. In: Holmes, K.K., et al. (eds.) Sexually Transmitted Disease, 4th edn. McGraw-Hill, New York (2008). Chapter 52, p. 937

Haggerty, C.L., Ness, R.B.: Diagnosis and treatment of pelvic inflammatory disease. Women's Health **4**, 383–397 (2008)

Judlin, P.: Current concepts in managing pelvic inflammatory disease. Curr. Opin. Infect. Dis. **23**, 83–87 (2010)

Kamwendo, F., Forslin, L., Bodin, L., et al.: Epidemiology of ectopic pregnancy during a 28 year period and the role of pelvic inflammatory disease. Sex. Transm. Infect. **76**, 28–32 (2000)

LaMontagne, D.S., Baster, K., Emmett, L., et al.: Incidence and reinfection rates of genital chlamydial infection among women aged 16-24 years attending general practice, family planning and genitourinary medicine clinics in England: a prospective cohort study by the Chlamydia Recall Study Advisory Group. Sex. Transm. Infect. **83**, 292–303 (2007)

Low, N., Egger, M., Sterne, J.A.C., Harbord, R.M., Ibrahim, F., Lindblom, B., Herrmann, B.: Incidence of severe reproductive tract complications associated with diagnosed genital chlamydial infection: the Uppsala Women's Cohort Study. Sex. transm. Infect. **82**, 212–218 (2006)

Miller, W.C.: Screening for chlamydial infection: are we doing enough? Lancet **365**, 456–458 (2005)

Ostergaard, L., Andersen, B., Moller, J.K., et al.: Home sampling versus conventional swab sampling for screening of *Chlamydia trachomatis* in women: a cluster-randomized 1-year follow-up study. Clin. Infect. Dis. **31**, 951–957 (2000)

Scholes, D., Stergachis, A., Heidrich, F.E., et al.: Prevention of pelvic inflammatory disease by screening of cervical chlamydial infection. N Engl J. Med. **334**, 1362–1366 (1996)

Stamm, W.E.: Chlamydia trachomatis infections of the adult. In: Holmes, K.K., et al. (eds.) Sexually Transmitted Disease, 4th edn. McGraw-Hill, New York (2008). Chapter 32, p. 575

van der Snoek, E.M., Ossewaarde, J.M., van der Meijden, W.I., et al.: The use of serological titres of IgA and IgG in (early) discrimination between rectal infection with non-lymphogranuloma venereum and lymphogranuloma venereum serovaras of *Chlamydia trachomatis*. Sex. Transm. Infect. **83**, 330–334 (2007)

van Valkengoed, I.G.M., Morre, S.A., van den Brule, A.J.C., Meijer, C.J.L.M., Bouter, L.M., Boeke, A.J.P.: Overestimation of comlication rates in evaluations of *Chlamydia trachomatis* screening programmes – implications for cost-effectiveness analyses. Int. J. Epidemiol. **33**, 416–425 (2004)

Wallace, L.A., Scoular, A., Hart, G., Reid, M., Wilson, P., Goldberg, D.J.: What is the excess risk of infertility in women after genital chlamydia infection? A systematic review of the evidence. Sex. Transm. Infect. **84**, 171–175 (2008)

Chlamydia trachomatis: Diagnostic Procedures

9

Angelika Stary and Georg Stary

Core Messages

- Molecular biological technologies provide a high sensitivity and specificity for chlamydia diagnosis and are now considered to be the gold standard method for detection of *Chlamydia trachomatis*.
- Nucleic acid amplification technologies enable chlamydia diagnosis from invasive and noninvasive specimens in both men and women.
- The high number of asymptomatic infection and severe sequela in adolescents indicates the importance of chlamydia screening in young men and women by testing urine or vaginal samples.

9.1 Introduction

Infections with *Chlamydia trachomatis* (CT) are currently the most frequently reported sexually transmitted bacterial diseases in the world. In the United States, a total of 1,030,911 cases of CT infections (of which 22% are men) were reported to the Centers for Disease Control and Prevention (CDC) in 2006 (www.cdc.gov). The lower rate of CT infection in men reflects the lack of systematic screening of asymptomatic men and an under-reporting number of cases.

Signs or symptoms of CT infections in men include urethral discharge, burning sensation when urinating, and (rarely) swollen testicles. The infection can sometimes spread to the epididymis (epididymitis), causing pain, fever, and rarely sterility. Both symptomatic and asymptomatic men can transmit the microorganisms to female partners. Chlamydial infections in women vary from an asymptomatic self-limiting infection to a severe illness with serious long-term complications such as pelvic inflammatory disease, chronic pelvic pain, tubal infertility, and ectopic pregnancy. It has been demonstrated that 70–80% of women and up to 50% of men infected with CT do not experience any clinical symptoms and are an unrecognized large reservoir of infected persons, capable of transmitting the infection to their partner or to newborns during perinatal exposure [1, 2]. The high number of asymptomatic cases and severe sequelae show the importance of screening as an appropriate intervention to control infections in both men and women.

9.2 Diagnostic Methods

Most common measures of reliability of diagnostic test performance are sensitivity, specificity, and predictive values, and perfect tests would give no false positive or false negative results. Chlamydia culture was established in the 1970s and relies on the growth or nongrowth of genital pathogens, giving a high grade of specificity but seldom a sensitivity of 100% (Fig. 9.1). Culture for CT has been the gold standard method for chlamydia diagnosis as the method to

A. Stary (✉)
Outpatients Centre for Infectious Venerodermatological Diseases, Vienna, Austria
e-mail: angelika.stary@meduniwien.ac.at

G. Stary
Department of Dermatology, Division of Immunology, Allergy, and Infectious Diseases, General Hospital, University of Vienna, Vienna, Austria

G. Gross and S.K. Tyring (eds.), *Sexually Transmitted Infections and Sexually Transmitted Diseases*,
DOI: 10.1007/978-3-642-14663-3_9, © Springer-Verlag Berlin Heidelberg 2011

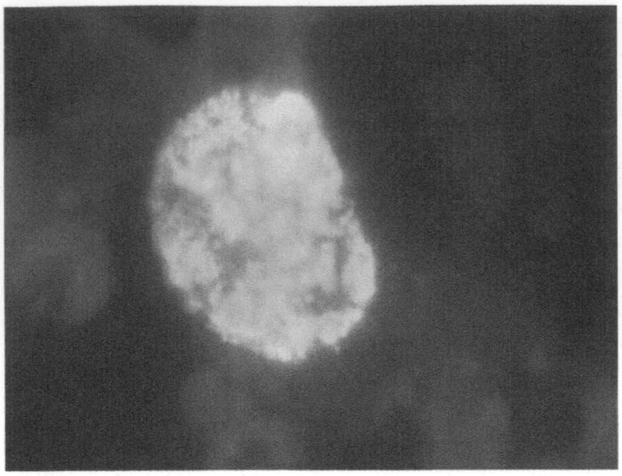

Fig. 9.1 Immunofluorescent staining of an inclusion body of McCoy cells infected with *Chlamydia trachomatis*

compare with for all other alternative technologies. However, the sensitivity of chlamydia culture differs worldwide between 50% and 80% and is dependent on the possibility of the laboratory to establish a high-quality cell culture, on the specimen collection, transport and storage conditions, and the expertise of the technical assistant. Further technological advantages were based on the visual observation of elementary bodies by direct immunofluorescence or other staining methods for the detection of antigens of the pathogens. Direct immunofluorescence assays (DFA) utilize a fluorescein-tagged monoclonal antibody which is specific for the presence of CT and allows visualizing the quality of the cell smear. A main disadvantage of this technology is the limited number of specimens to be tested and the need of an expert microscopist. Enzyme-linked immunosorbent assays (ELISA) have the advantage of time- and cost-effectiveness, but results are based on a cut-off value, leading to a possible decrease of sensitivity and specificity.

9.3 Nucleic Acid Amplification Tests (NAATs)

The most recent and important advance in the field of diagnosis of chlamydia infections during the last 20 years is the development of nucleic acid amplification tests (NAATs), which have been shown to be more accurate than any other diagnostic methods for various genital pathogens and lead to a better insight in the epidemiology and clinical importance for infections in both men and women. Especially for CT, NAATs enable the detection of small amounts of chlamydial nucleic acids and transcripts in genital as well as in noninvasive specimens such as first void urine (FVU) and introital swabs of the vulvovaginal area. This is an important approach for screening possibilities in individuals with and without symptoms at risk for being infected with CT. Using noninvasive methods in men and in women provides a better access to screening programs for asymptomatic persons in sexually transmitted disease (STD) risk groups. In addition, a further advantage of nucleic acid amplification tests may be the fact that pooling of specimens in a low prevalence setting adds to reduced costs and a better cost/benefit ratio.

Commercially available NAATs provide laboratories with powerful tools with particular impact in the detection of genital chlamydial and gonococcal infections, and enzyme immunoassays and immunofluorescence techniques, used for many years for routine diagnosis of genital chlamydial infections, are now more and more substituted by NAATs (Table 9.1). Similar to the performance of chlamydial diagnosis, the codetection of a genital infection with *Neisseria gonorrhoeae* (GC) is possible and has shown a high sensitivity and specificity using NAATs on both male and female specimens. Limitations of NAATs may still be the high costs of the performance in laboratories. Furthermore, problems with inhibition of amplification and contamination under certain conditions may lead to reduced reproducibility of positive and negative results. Collection, transport, and storage of samples are of importance and may influence the results even when using amplification techniques.

The amplification tests focusing on the diagnosis of lower genital tract infection have long been restricted to two commercially available techniques: the Amplicor PCR, a DNA target amplification test for the diagnosis of CT, and the ligase chain reaction (LCR), a DNA probe amplification assay for the diagnosis of both CT and GC. In one of the first urine studies in symptomatic and asymptomatic women, the sensitivity and specificity of the LCR assay with FVU samples compared with an expanded gold standard were 93.8% and 99.9%, respectively [3]. In this study, the LCR assay of readily obtained urine samples showed a

Table 9.1 Commercially available NAATs for CT diagnosis

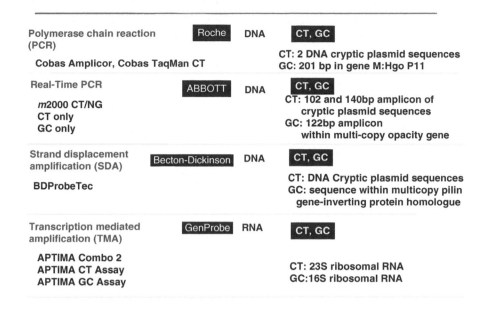

Polymerase chain reaction (PCR) **Cobas Amplicor, Cobas TaqMan CT**	Roche	**DNA**	**CT, GC**	**CT: 2 DNA cryptic plasmid sequences** **GC: 201 bp in gene M:Hgo P11**
Real-Time PCR ***m*2000 CT/NG** **CT only** **GC only**	ABBOTT	**DNA**	**CT, GC**	**CT: 102 and 140bp amplicon of cryptic plasmid sequences** **GC: 122bp amplicon within multi-copy opacity gene**
Strand displacement amplification (SDA) **BDProbeTec**	Becton-Dickinson	**DNA**	**CT, GC**	**CT: DNA Cryptic plasmid sequences** **GC: sequence within multicopy pilin gene-inverting protein homologue**
Transcription mediated amplification (TMA) **APTIMA Combo 2** **APTIMA CT Assay** **APTIMA GC Assay**	GenProbe	**RNA**	**CT, GC**	**CT: 23S ribosomal RNA** **GC:16S ribosomal RNA**

detection rate for infected women almost 30% greater than that of endocervical swab culture. In asymptomatic male recruits the Amplicor polymerase chain reaction (PCR) and LCR were compared with the enzyme immunoassay (EIA) using urine samples for the detection of genital chlamydial infections [4]. Both amplification assays were performed with a high sensitivity of 93% when using frozen urine while the EIA showed a detection rate of only 37%. This comparison study demonstrated that urine as a noninvasive sample can only be recommended when NAATs are used as diagnostic methods. However, in 1996, the Amplicor PCR for CT was compared with other diagnostic methods such as culture and Gen Probe by testing cervical and urine samples and showed sensitivity similar but not higher than chlamydial culture [5]. Since several years, the LCR was taken off the market.

During the last 10 years, the quality of the NAATs has been improved and the number has increased. The COBAS Amplicor CT/NG assay (Roche Diagnostics Corporation, Indianapolis, IN, USA) uses PCR technology to amplify the target DNA located on the cryptic plasmid. Approximately 96 samples can be tested in one shift and is Food and Drug Administration (FDA)-approved for cervical, urethral, urine samples, and liquid cytology medium. The assay includes a measure for inhibition and indicates the inhibition of amplification in case of a negative reaction. Due to the recent emergence of a new variant strain of CT (nvCT) which has a 377 base-pair deletion in the target DNA on the cryptic plasmid, a second target located on the major outer membrane protein was included in the test system in order not to miss these infections.

The BDProbeTec ET chlamydia and gonorrhea assay (BD Diagnostic Systems, Sparks, MD, USA), a thermophilic strand displacement amplification assay, has been approved for practical use for the diagnosis of chlamydial as well as gonococcal infections and offers real-time amplification and detection [6, 7]. The amplification target is a 100 base-pair fragment of the 75 kb cryptic plasmid for CT (which is not located in the deletion region of the nvCT) and 103 base-pair target region located within the pilin gene for GC. In the first phase, the target generation step creates the structure that feeds into the second phase, which is the exponential amplification, using two primers and two bumpers as well as a detector probe. This amplification is based on the simultaneous amplification and detection of target DNA by the use of amplification primers along with a fluorescein-labeled detector probe for the fluorescent energy transfer (ET) measurement. The analytical sensitivity or limit of detection was shown to be 0.4 inclusion-forming units. The advantage of DNA amplification using strand displacement amplification is that isothermal amplification does not need expensive thermal cycling equipment and that post-amplification sample manipulation for detection is not needed. This assay can be used for urine as well as genital swabs for testing both CT and GC simultaneously. The sample-processing method for urine employs an inhibitor removal system that can easily be added at the collection site. Multicenter evaluation of the ProbeTec system for simultaneous detection of chlamydial and gonococcal infections in both men and women demonstrated a high sensitivity of about 90% for cervical and urethral swabs and about 80–85% in the urine of asymptomatic individuals [7].

In addition to DNA amplification, detection of CT RNA in clinical specimens was shown to be as successful as the DNA detection by PCR in cervical scrapings as well as in urine samples [8]. The 16S rRNA appeared to be the most sensitive RNA target for amplification. An internal control was developed for some of these systems to detect false negative results due to improper sample preparation or amplification inhibition. The AMP CT assay was a commercially available first-generation transcription-mediated amplification (TMA) test and was recommended as an alternative NAAT for both genital and urine samples in men and women [9, 10]. The APTIMA Combo 2 (AC2) assay (Gen-Probe, Inc., San Diego, CA, USA) is a second-generation NAAT that utilizes target capture, TMA, and dual kinetic assay technologies to resolve the issues associated with first-generation amplification (Fig. 9.2). This assay qualitatively detects CT and GC ribosomal RNA (rRNA) in endocervical and urethral swab specimens as well as in urine samples from symptomatic and asymptomatic individuals and is also FDA-approved for vaginal samples. After the chemical release of the rRNA targets, these molecules are isolated from urine or swab samples by the use of capture oligomers, which contain complementary sequences to specific regions of the target molecules and hybridize at higher temperature of 62°C. The target capture is followed by target amplification similar to the TMA assay. Specific regions of the 23S rRNA for CT and the 16S rRNA for GC are amplified via DNA intermediates and are detected by chemoluminescence.

The RealTime CT/NG (ABBOTT Moleculardiagnostics, ABBOTT Park, IL, USA) is the most recently developed and FDA-approved NAAT for chlamydial and gonococcal diagnosis. It is based on the PCR for the qualitative detection of the CT plasmid DNA including the nvCT and is recommended for diagnosis of CT and GC using invasive and noninvasive specimens (Fig. 9.3). The RealTime CT/NG runs on the Abbott m2000 system (m2000sp for sample preparation and m2000rt).

The AC2 and the ProbeTec assay have both shown reliable performance for the diagnosis of CT and GC in men in urethral swab and FVU specimens. Urethral swabs do not represent a convenient collection method for large-scale screening of men for CT and GC infections because the sample needs to be collected by a

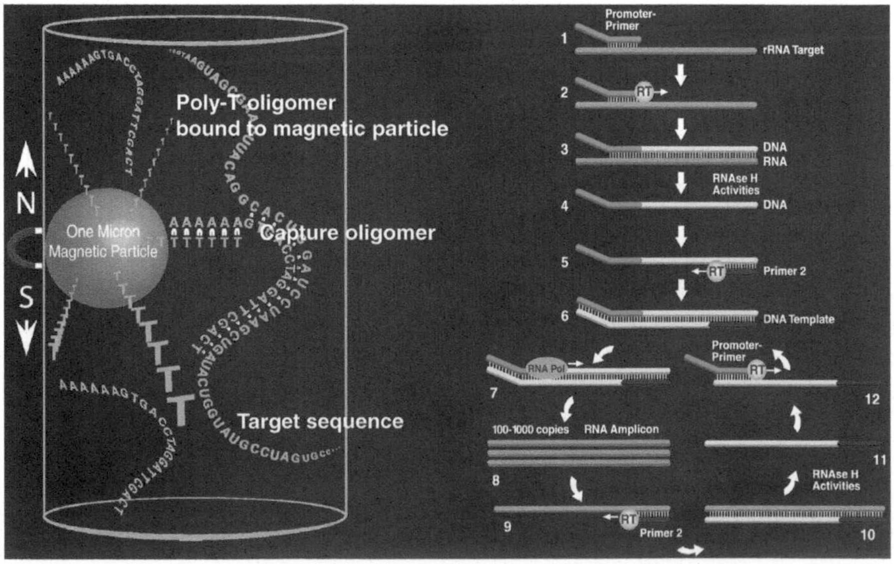

Fig. 9.2 Transcription-mediated amplification (TMA)

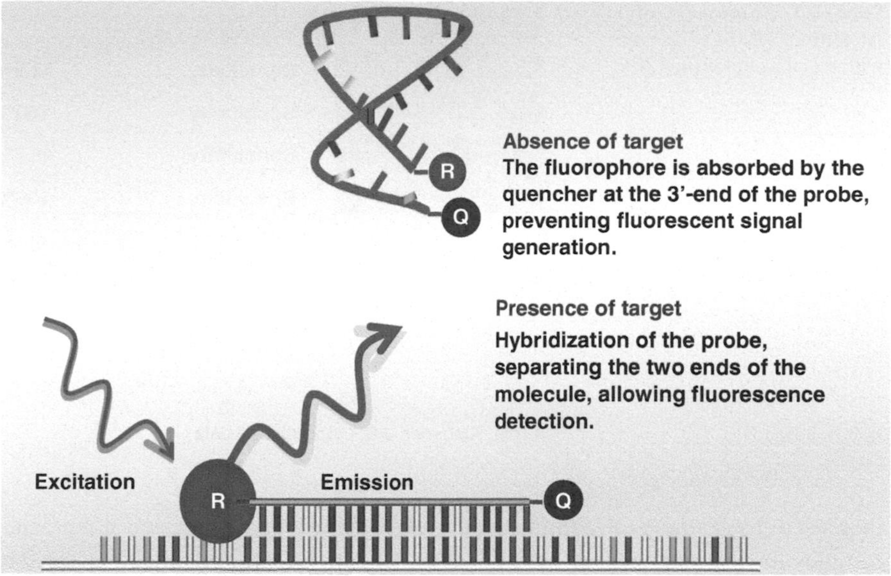

Absence of target
The fluorophore is absorbed by the quencher at the 3'-end of the probe, preventing fluorescent signal generation.
R
Q
Presence of target
Hybridization of the probe, separating the two ends of the molecule, allowing fluorescence detection.
Excitation
Emission
R
Q

Fig. 9.3 Single-stranded linear probe design Abbott M2000rt

health-care professional, and sample collection is invasive, uncomfortable, and not well accepted by the subjects. Thus, the specimen of choice for screening asymptomatic men is FVU since it can be easily self-collected by the subject and is noninvasive. Urine is the only self-collected noninvasive specimen currently FDA-cleared. FVU has been shown to yield similar sensitivity and specificity to traditional urethral swabs in AC2, ProbeTec, and APTIMA assays. Also penile swabs can be recommended as an alternative noninvasive specimen type if a high sensitivity NAAT such as the AC2 assay is used and instructions for collection are provided, but are not FDA-approved.

In women, two types of self-collected noninvasive specimens, urine and vulvovaginal swabs, have demonstrated a high detection rate for CT using NAATs in several studies and vaginal swabs are now FDA-cleared in the AC2 assay for testing women [11–14]. One disadvantage of the FVU specimen is that sample variability may occur because a midstream rather than a first catch urine may be collected, or excess volume may be collected. This results in diluted samples with low concentrations of bacteria that can result in a decreased NAAT sensitivity. It has been shown that in artificially diluted specimens tested with PCR, ProbeTec, and AC2, the highest sensitivity was provided by the AC2 assay for both cervical and urine specimens.

9.4 Practical Advances of NAA Assays for Diagnosis of Chlamydial Infections

The advantage of the high sensitivity of NAATs is their ability to detect organisms with a low target concentration, which often occurs in genital samples of asymptomatic individuals and their contact persons without signs of inflammation. A low number of organisms may also be observed at atypical infection sites such as rectal or pharyngeal regions, where amplification tests are recommended as the preferable diagnostic techniques to all other methods (Table 9.2). Furthermore, the detection of nonviable organisms offers the opportunity to detect specific nucleic acids in noninvasive specimens. In contrast to NAATs, urine is not an appropriate sample for chlamydial diagnosis by cell culture, as it gives a sensitivity of only up to 30% [15]. In a comparison study using vulval smears obtained from the introital area the sensitivity of culture on vulval swabs was only 22.2%, similar to data from urine [11]. Several comparison studies have indicated that vulval or vaginal specimens and even patient-obtained vaginal swabs serve as a suitable alternative to noninvasive urine testing for detection of CT. Screening abilities are even

Table 9.2 Performance of APTIMA COMBO 2® assay with rectal samples ($n = 205$)

		Culture	AC2
GC (17 pos)	Sensitivity	52.9%	100%
	Specificity	100%	98.9%
CT(13pos)	Sensitivity	46.2%	100%
	Specificity	100%	97.9%

CT	Culture	AC2	SDA	PCR
Sens%	46	100	85	85
Spec%	100	97.9	99.5	100

From: Klausner, J.D. (unpublished data)

increased by using self-administered vulvovaginal samples for the diagnosis of both CT and GC, which permit testing without a speculum examination within few hours and even without clinical inspection.

9.5 Screening for CT

Several comparison studies confirm that selective screening in asymptomatic women, which has been suggested many years ago, has become more realistic with the use of NAATs [16, 17]. The utility of screening for *C. trachomatis* by using urine samples by different NAATs has already been evaluated in a community-based screening program among teenagers in school-based clinics and community-based youth organizations in Seattle and in other areas and communities [18]. A study was performed as a site-specific activity of community-based organizations to screen high-risk populations for sexually transmitted infections (STIs) [19]. In addition to institutional settings such as drug treatment centers and shelters, bars and stores were also used as "user-friendly" neighborhood settings. This project was effective in promoting early detection and treatment of high-risk individuals with the highest concentration of infections at shelters and residence facilities.

Since chlamydia transmission can occur from the infected mother to the newborn, screening for CT is recommended in pregnant women. Several studies were performed to evaluate whether the sensitivity and specificity of NAATs is different in the urine of pregnant and nonpregnant women. In a comparison study using FVU tested by LCR a sensitivity of 88.6% with no difference between both groups was reported [20, 21].

Screening programs are only effective if infected persons are successfully notified and brought to treatment. This is important if field-treatment services are generally not available and positive individuals have to seek care from a health-care provider. Especially for asymptomatic persons a delay to obtain adequate treatment may occur despite notification efforts. Almost one fourth of individuals with STD-related symptoms may have a delayed treatment care over 1 month. Although commercially available amplifying techniques with high sensitivities and specificities are able to improve the number of treated patients, delays of several days between the time of specimen collection and patients' return are common and may lead to a percentage of patients failing to return for counseling and treatment in a reasonable time. Calculation was performed comparing the use of NAATs for the detection of a chlamydial infection with an onsite EIA technique with a lower sensitivity but offering an immediate result for the patient during the first visit [22]. In settings where the return rate is less than 65%, the use of NAATs did not contribute significantly to the detection and treatment of chlamydial infections among women compared with onsite testing with a point-of-care test system. Processing time, patient flow, patient acceptance, patient management, and real-time trials of rapid tests have to be considered in the choice of diagnostic procedure for infected individuals.

9.6 Problems of NAATs for Chlamydial Diagnosis

Reproducibility of NAATs is already high but still shows room for improvement. A low copy number already under the detection limit of PCR was discussed as one of the reproducibility problems when testing asymptomatic men and women [23–25]. However, since the internal control for inhibition has been included, the performance pattern of Amplicor and COBAS Amplicor has been improved. The occurrence of a false negative result for NAATs in an infected individual may be due to different reasons. Beside the inability of the test to detect a low number of nucleic acids, improper sample collection, transportation, specimen preparation, or the presence of inhibitors may cause false results. The quality of endocervical specimens is still relevant for the outcome of an amplifying assay and inadequate samples may be the reason that in some comparison studies the sensitivities for genital samples are lower than for urine [26]. Considering the influence of transport on the sensitivity of NAATs, it may be important to maintain a cold chain for sample processing.

A further reason for a false negative outcome of the test, especially on urine samples, may be the presence of substances inhibiting amplification [27, 28]. In contrast to genital samples urine samples are more often inhibited when tested by NAATs. Urinary structures associated with inhibition and removal of inhibitory activity were described in pregnant and nonpregnant women in different NAATs from 2.6% up to 7.5% due to different chemical substances. For PCR Amplicor, inhibitors were observed in 19% of cervical specimens, and could be reduced by heat treatment at 95°C, freeze-thawing, by a tenfold dilution of the samples, and at a higher degree by combined methods. Roche COBAS Amplicor-automated PCR methodology and the ProbeTec technology have included an optional internal control.

Recent observations have demonstrated that the target sequence used in the NAAT for chlamydia detection is of major importance. A new problem for chlamydia diagnosis was realized in Sweden, when a new strain variant was detected in 2006 (nvCT). It was described in Southwest Sweden (County Halland) in 13% of all detected cases. This strain has a 377 base-pair deletion in the cryptic plasmid and therefore escaped chlamydia detection for those commercial tests using targeting in this region (Figs. 9.4 and 9.5). This had a major influence on the epidemiology of CT in Sweden and indicates the importance for active monitoring of test accuracy, epidemiological surveillance, and the use of several test systems at the national level. Both test systems, the COBAS Amplicor and the ABBOTT 2000, have already included a second target for CT amplification and are able to detect nvCT strains.

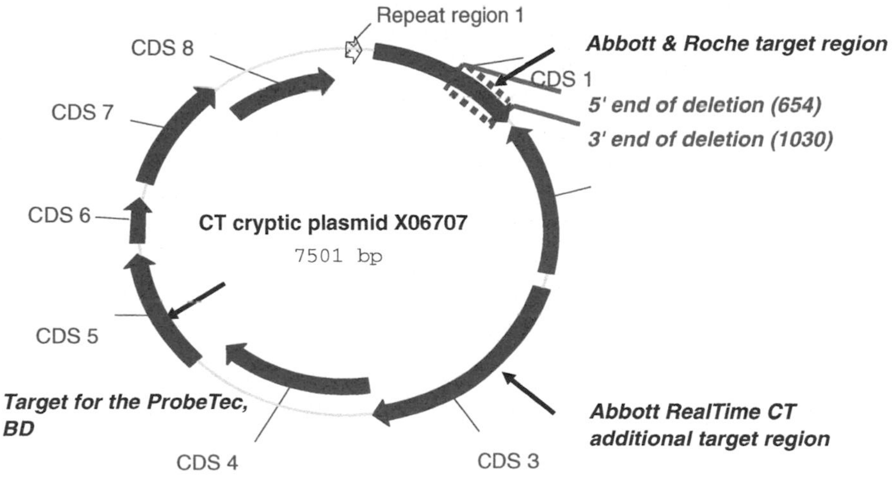

Fig. 9.4 nvCT cryptic plasmid

Fig. 9.5 Swedish mutant CT

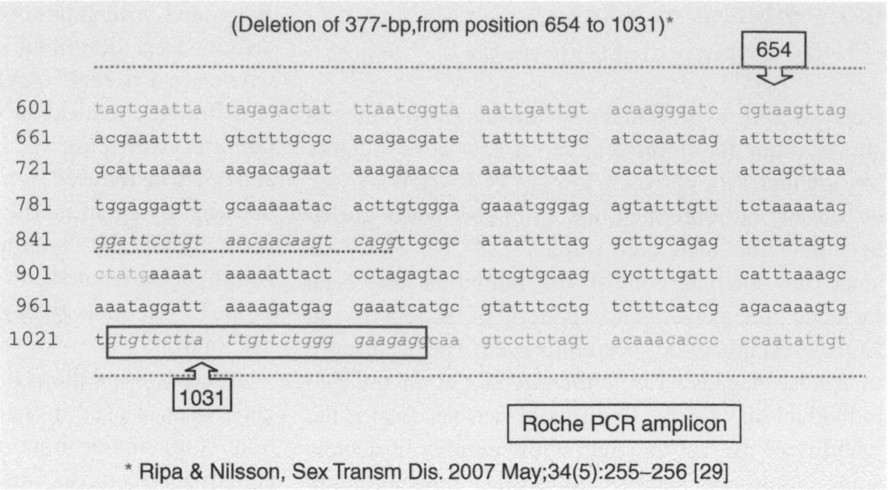

9.7 Conclusion

NAATs represent a major improvement over previous methods for STI diagnosis. They are capable of detecting small amounts of nucleic acids in genital and noninvasive specimens and facilitate the performance of screening programs in asymptomatic individuals. It is important to be aware of limitations of amplification techniques and variations of commercially available NAATs.

Take-Home Pearls

- The most important advance in the field of chlamydia diagnosis is the development of nucleic acid amplification tests (NAATs).
- NAATs can be used for chlamydia screening purposes in asymptomatic individuals.
- Several NAATs are already available for chlamydia diagnosis.
- The target sequence used for chlamydia detection in different NAATs is of major importance since a new variant of the organism with a deletion of base pairs in the cryptic plasmid has been detected in Sweden.

References

1. Schachter, J., Stoner, E., Moncada, J.: Screening for chlamydial infections in women attending family planning clinics. West. J. Med. **138**, 375–379 (1983)
2. Stamm, W., Cole, B.: Asymptomatic urethritis in men. Sex. Transm. Dis. **13**, 163–165 (1986)
3. Lee, H.H., Chernesky, M., Schachter, J., et al.: Diagnosis of *Chlamydia trachomatis* genitourinary infection in women by ligase chain reaction assay of urine. Lancet **345**, 213–216 (1995)
4. Stary, A., Tomazic-Allen, S., Choueiri, B., et al.: Comparison of DNA amplification methods for the detection of *Chlamydia trachomatis* in first-void urine from asymptomatic military recruits. Sex. Transm. Dis. **23**, 97–102 (1996)
5. Pasternack, R., et al.: Detection of *Chlamydia trachomatis* infections in women by Amplicor PCR: Comparison of diagnostic performance with urine and cervical specimens. J. Clin. Microbiol. **334**, 995–998 (1996)
6. Van Dyck, E., Ieven, M., Pattyn, S., et al.: Detection of *Chlamydia trachomatis* and *Neisseria gonorrhoeae* by enzyme immunoassay, culture, and three nucleic acid amplification tests. J. Clin. Microbiol. **39**, 1751–1756 (2001)
7. Van der Pol, B., Ferrero, D.V., Buck-Barrington, L., et al.: Multicenter evaluation of the BDProbeTec ET system for detection of *Chlamydia trachomatis* and *Neisseria gonorrhoeae* in urine specimens, female endocervical swabs, and male urethral swabs. J. Clin. Microbiol. **39**, 1008–1016 (2001)
8. Morre, S.A., Sillekens, P., Jacobs, M.V., et al.: RNA amplification by nucleic acid sequence-based amplification with an internal standard enables reliable detection of *Chlamydia trachomatis* in cervical scrapings and urine samples. J. Clin. Microbiol. **34**, 3108–3114 (1996)
9. Ferrero, D.V., Meyers, H.N., Schultz, D.E., Willis, S.A.: Performance of the Gen-Probe Amplified *Chlamydia trachomatis* assay in detecting *Chlamydia trachomatis* in

endocervical and urine specimens from women and urethral and urine specimens from men attending sexually transmitted disease and family planning clinics. J. Clin. Microbiol. **36**, 3230–3233 (1998)

10. Stary, A., Schuh, E., Kerschbaumer, M., et al.: Performance of transcription-mediated amplification and ligase chain reaction assays for detection of chlamydial infection in urogenital samples obtained by invasive and noninvasive methods. J. Clin. Microbiol. **36**, 2666–2670 (1998)
11. Stary, A., Najim, B., Lee, H.H.: Vulval swabs as alternative specimens for ligase chain reaction detection of genital chlamydial infection in women. J. Clin. Microbiol. **35**, 836–838 (1997)
12. Pasternack, R., Vourinen, P., Pitkäjärvi, T., et al.: Comparison of manual amplicor PCR, Cobas Amplicor PCR, and LCR Assays for detection of *Chlamydia trachomatis* infection in women by using urine specimens. J. Clin. Microbiol. **35**, 402–405 (1997)
13. Hook, E.W., Smith, K., Mullen, C., et al.: Diagnosis of genitourinary Chlamydia trachomatis infections using the ligase chain reaction on patient-obtained vaginal swabs. J. Clin. Microbiol. **35**, 2133–2135 (1997)
14. Hook III, E.W., Ching, S.F., Stephens, J., et al.: Diagnosis of *Neisseria gonorrhoeae* infections in women by using the ligase chain reaction on patient-obtained vaginal swabs. J. Clin. Microbiol. **35**, 2129–2132 (1997)
15. Smith, T.F., Weed, L.A.: Comparison of urethral swabs, urine, and urinary sediment for the isolation of Chlamydia. J. Clin. Microbiol. **2**, 111–123 (1975)
16. Handsfield, H.H., Jasman, L.L., Roberts, P.L., et al.: Criterias for selective screening for *Chlamydia trachomatis* infection in women attending family planning clinics. JAMA **255**, 1730–1734 (1986)
17. Marrazzo, J.M., Whittington, W.L.H., Celum, C.L., Handsfield, H.H., et al.: Urine-based screening for *Chlamydia trachomatis* in men attending sexually transmitted disease clinics. Sex. Transm. Dis. **28**, 219–225 (2001)
18. Marrazzo, J.M., White, C.L., Krekeler, B., et al.: Community-based urine screening for *Chlamydia trachomatis* with a ligase chain reaction assays. Ann. Intern. Med. **127**, 796–803 (1997)
19. Jones, C.A., Knaup, R.C., Hayes, M., Stoner, B.P.: Urine screening for gonococcal and chlamydial infections at community-based organizations in a high-morbidity area. Sex. Transm. Dis. **27**, 146–151 (2000)
20. Gaydos, C.A., Howell, M.R., Quinn, T., et al.: Use of ligase chain reaction with urine versus cervical culture for detection of *Chlamydia trachomatis* in an asymptomatic military population of pregnant and nonpregnant females attending Papanicoulaou smear clinics. J. Clin. Microbiol. **36**, 1300–1304 (1998)
21. Jensen, I.P., Thorsen, P., Møller, B.R.: Sensitivity of ligase chain reaction assay of urine from pregnant women for Chlamydia trachomatis. Lancet **349**, 329–330 (1997)
22. Gift, T.L., Pate, M.S., Hook III, E.W., Kassler, W.J.: The rapid test paradox: when fewer cases detected lead to more cases treated. Sex. Transm. Dis. **26**, 232–240 (1999)
23. Toye, B., Peeling, R.W., Yessamine, P., Claman, P., Gemmill, I.: Diagnosis of infection in asymptomatic men and women by PCR assay. J. Clin. Microbiol. **34**, 1396–1400 (1996)
24. Peterson, E.M., Darrow, V., Blanding, J., et al.: Reproducibility problems with the Ampliocr PCR *Chlamydia trachomatis* test. J. Clin. Microbiol. **35**, 957–959 (1997)
25. Gronowsky, A.M., Copper, S., Baorto, D., Murray, P.R.: Reproducibility problems with the Abbott Laboratories LCR assay for *Chlamydia trachomatis* and *Neisseria gonorrhoeae*. J. Clin. Microbiol. **38**, 2416–2418 (2000)
26. Welsh, L.A., Quinn, T., Gaydos, C.A.: Influence of endocervical specimen adequacy on PCR and direct fluorescent-antibody staining for detection of *Chlamydia trachomatis* infection. J. Clin. Microbiol. **35**, 3078–3081 (1997)
27. Mahony, J., Chong, S., Jang, D., et al.: Urine specimens from pregnant and nonpregnant women inhibitory to amplification of *Chlamydia trachomatis* nucleic acid by PCR, ligase chain reaction, and transcription mediated amplification: identification of urinary substances associated with inhibition and removal of inhibitory activity. J. Clin. Microbiol. **36**, 3122–3126 (1998)
28. Chernesky, M., Jang, D., Luinstra, K., Chong, S., Smieja, M., Cai, W., Hayhoe, B., Portillo, E., Macritchie, C., Main, C., Ewert, R.: High analytical sensitivity and low rates of inhibition may contribute to detection of Chlamydia trachomatis in significantly more women by the APTIMA Combo 2 assay. J. Clin. Microbiol. **44**, 400–405 (2006)
29. Ripa, T., Nilsson, P.A.: A Chlamydia trachomatis strain with a 377-bp deletion in the cryptic plasmid causing false-negative nucleic acid amplification tests. Sex. Transm. Dis. **34**, 257 (2007)

Lymphogranuloma Venereum

10

Omar Lupi, Janaína Ribeiro, Paula Chicralla, and Carlos Jose Martins

Core Messages

› LGV is primarily an infection of lymphatics and lymph nodes. *Chlamydia trachomatis* is the bacteria responsible for LGV. It gains entrance through breaks in the skin, or it can cross the epithelial cell layer of mucous membranes. The organism travels from the site of inoculation down the lymphatic channels to multiply within mononuclear phagocytes of the lymph nodes it passes. LGV may begin as a self-limited painless genital ulcer that occurs at the contact site 3-12 days after infection. Women rarely notice a primary infection because the initial ulceration where the organism penetrates the mucosal layer is often located out of sight, in the vaginal wall. In men fewer than 1/3 of those infected notice the first signs of LGV. This primary stage heals in a few days. Late manifestations include unilateral (in 2/3 of cases) lymphadenitis and lymphangitis, often with tender inguinal and/or femoral lymphadenopathy because of the drainage pathway for their likely infected areas. Fistulas mainly affect the penis, urethra, vagina, uterus, or rectum. Also, surrounding edema often occurs, rectal or other strictures and scarring. Systemic spread may occur possible results are arthritis, pneumonitis, hepatitis, or perihepatitis.

10.1 Introduction

Members of the order *Chlamydiales* are obligate intracellular gram-negative bacteria. The order *Chlamydiales* has one family, the *Chlamydiaceae*, containing one genus, *Chlamydia*, and three species pathogenic to humans: *Chlamydia trachomatis, C. psittaci, and C. pneumoniae* [1].

C. trachomatis is a strictly human pathogen, with a tropism for the genital and conjunctival epithelia. *C. trachomatis* consists of 19 different serovars [2]. Types A, B, Ba and C infect mainly the conjunctiva and are associated with endemic trachoma; serovars D, Da, E, F, G, Ga, H, I, Ia, J, and K are predominantly isolated from the urogenital tract and are associated with sexually transmitted diseases (STDs), Reiter's syndrome, inclusion conjunctivitis or neonatal pneumonitis in infants born to infected mothers. Serovars L1, L2, L2a, and L3 can be found in the inguinal lymph nodes and are associated with lymphogranuloma venereum (LGV). The *C. trachomatis* genome sequence revealed an organism with a high coding ratio and a small genome (1,042 Kb) with 895 annotated genes [3].

LGV is an uncommon STD with transient genital lesions followed by significant regional lymphadenopathy and systemic manifestations. LGV may progress to late fibrosis and tissue destruction in untreated cases.

O. Lupi (✉)
Dermatology Department, Universidade Federal do Estado do Rio de Janeiro (UniRio) and Policlinica Geral do Rio de Janeiro (PGRJ) and
Immunology Department, Universidade Federal do Rio de Janeiro (UFRJ), Rio de Janeiro, Brazil
e-mail: omarlupi@globo.com

J. Ribeiro, P. Chicralla, and C.J. Martins
Dermatology Department, Universidade Federal do Estado do, Rio de Janeiro, Brazil

G. Gross and S.K. Tyring (eds.), *Sexually Transmitted Infections and Sexually Transmitted Diseases*,
DOI: 10.1007/978-3-642-14663-3_10, © Springer-Verlag Berlin Heidelberg 2011

10.2 Epidemiology

C. trachomatis has the highest prevalence among young men and women. It is the most common STD in Western countries [4]. Worldwide, 89 million cases are estimated to occur each year [5]. Infection with this agent can be asymptomatic in up to 80% of women. Left undetected and untreated, *Chlamydia* can ascend the upper genital tract, causing inflammation and scarring in both female and the male reproductive tracts. In women, it is responsible for urethritis, cervicitis, pelvic inflammatory disease, and sequelae, such as infertility and ectopic pregnancy. In men, it can cause arthritis and epididymitis, which can result in urethral obstructions and decreased fertility in some cases. Neonates may present conjunctivitis and pneumonia.

The disease is almost always transmitted by sexual contact. Transmission has been attributed largely to asymptomatic female carriers. The main age of onset is 25 years, but the disease can be seen in any age group and it is endemic in areas at Africa, Asia, South America, and the Caribbean; it accounts for 2–10% of genital ulcer disease in India and Africa. Highest prevalence was found in young single male patients of low socioeconomic and educational status. Prostitutes and male homosexuals used to have a major role in the transmission of the disease.

However, recent outbreaks [6] in MSM (men who have sex with men) have been occurred in industrialized countries [7, 8] starting in the Netherlands in 2003, with reports of cases in Belgium [9], France [10], Germany [11], Sweden, the UK [12], Italy, Switzerland [13], Spain [14], Austria [15], Australia, the USA, and Canada [16, 17]. These outbreaks among MSM are related to a high-risk behavior for STIs (sexual transmitted illness), to a high HIV prevalence and also to participation in casual sex gatherings, sex parties, sex toy use, and "fisting."

10.3 Clinical Manifestations

The clinical course of LGV is classically divided into three stages [18].

10.3.1 Primary Lesion

The incubation period is extremely variable but has been estimated to be between 1 and 2 weeks. This transient primary lesion usually appears as a vesicle, small erosion, or an exulcerated area that lasts for 2–3 days (Fig. 10.1) [19]. The site of primary lesion is usually around the genitals but may be anal, rectal, or oral, mainly in male homosexuals.

10.3.2 Secondary Lesions, Lymphadenitis or Bubo

LGV is primarily a disease of the lymphatic system that progresses to lymphangitis. Adenopathy represents the most important objective element of the clinical exam and is unilateral in 60% of these cases (Fig. 10.2). It usually occurs 2–4 weeks after onset of the primary lesion. In its earlier stages, the adenopathy syndrome consists of painful inflammation and infection of the inguinal and/or femoral lymph nodes (Figs. 10.2 and 10.3). In women, the deep pelvic nodes may also be involved. After several days, they become matted, with a firm lobulated swelling not attached to the deep tissues. The overlying skin is often slightly reddened and edematous, but it later may become thickened and develop a purple hue (Fig. 10.1). In a

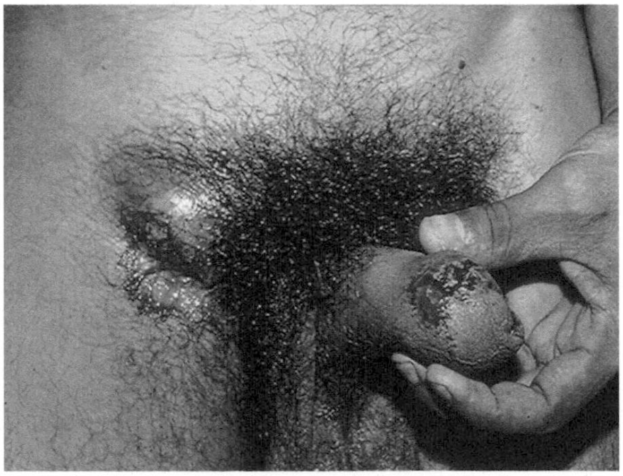

Fig. 10.1 LGV chancre and adenopathy

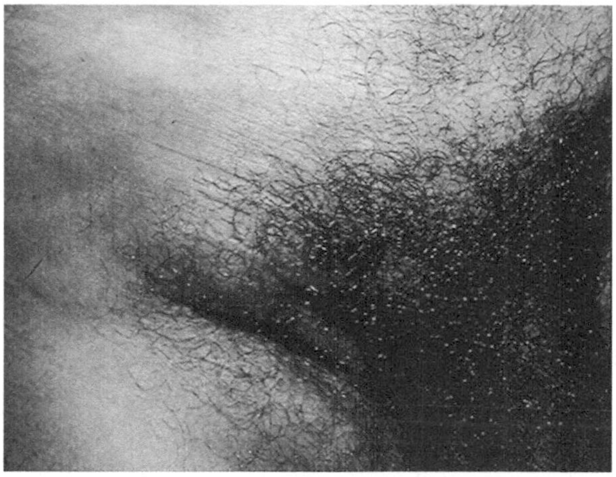

Fig. 10.2 LGV massive regional lymphadenopathy

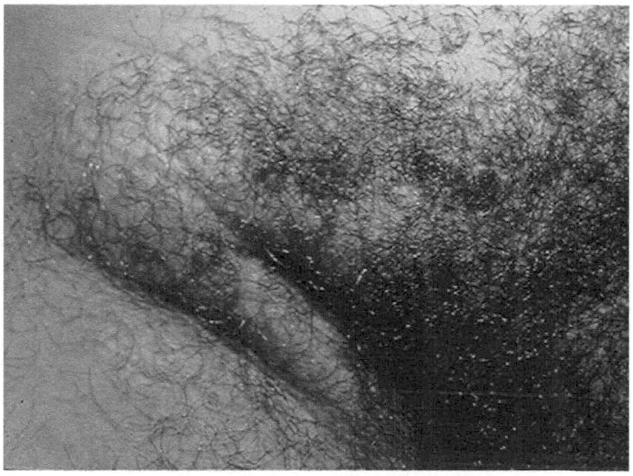

Fig. 10.3 Groove sign

short time, the lymph nodes become tender and fluctuant and are referred to as buboes. In the natural evolution of LGV, the nodes may undergo necrosis and spontaneous fistula tracts may develop. These nodes may also become fluctuant and rupture in 30% of patients. Although most buboes eventually heal without complications, some may progress to develop chronic sinus formation. The emergence of many fistulous orifices explains the comparison made with "watering-can." There may be fever and chills during this stage of LGV, associated with other nonspecific systemic symptoms such as headache, nausea, anorexia, and myalgia) [20].

10.3.3 Tertiary Stage or the Genito-Anorectal Syndrome

This stage does not necessarily follow the lymphadenopathy. It involves a series of conditions, resulting from progressive spread of the disease with destruction of tissue in the involved areas, including proctitis, genital edema (Fig. 10.4) acute proctocolitis mimicking Crohn's disease, fistulae, strictures, and chronic granulomatous disfiguring condition of the vulva (esthiomene). The lymph nodes rupture, causing hemorrhage and friability of the anorectal mucosa, with rectitis, tenesmus, mucosanguineous rectal discharge, and constipation. Later, as healing occurs, there is formation of strictures, fistulas, and abscesses with destruction of anal and rectal structures. In addition, there can also be observed gastrointestinal disturbance such as bleeding and rectum or colon inflammation, which in general, clinicians would not consider LGV as a cause of gastrointestinal illness [21].

10.3.4 Long-Term Complications

The destruction of lymph nodes may result in elephantiasis of the vulva or penis and scrotum. It represents late manifestations, which are rare today [22]. An association with rectal cancer has been reported. The esthiomenic syndrome, composed by vulvar ulceration

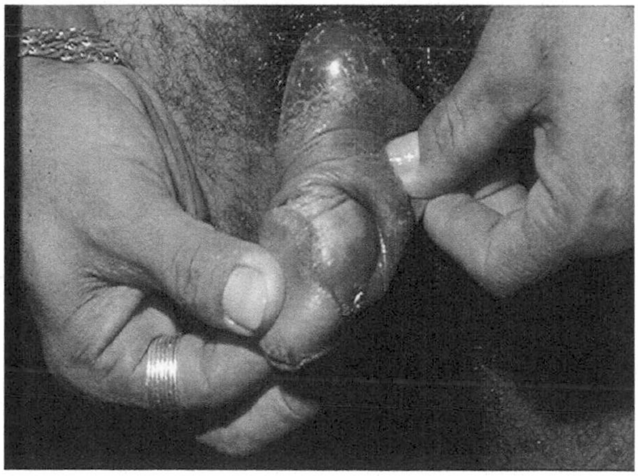

Fig. 10.4 Genital edema following LGV

followed by sclerosis and tegumentar hypertrophy, can occur in patients with LGV.

Significant burden of LGV among MSM in industrialized countries [23] is associated with unprotected anal intercourse, multiple partners, having sex with HIV seropositives [24], sex toy use, and the most implicated factor, in some series, the enhancement of "fisting" activity, once to do so, their practicers make an enema use before anal intercourse, which breaks the mucosal barrier by irrigation. Enema use seems to play a key role in transmission of LGV proctitis [25] and needs further investigation.

These clusters of cases show an initial connection with the Netherlands (Rotterdam-2003, the first new outbreak), all of them were related to L2b serovar [23], the same detected in anal swabs collected in San Francisco in at least 1981 [26, 27].

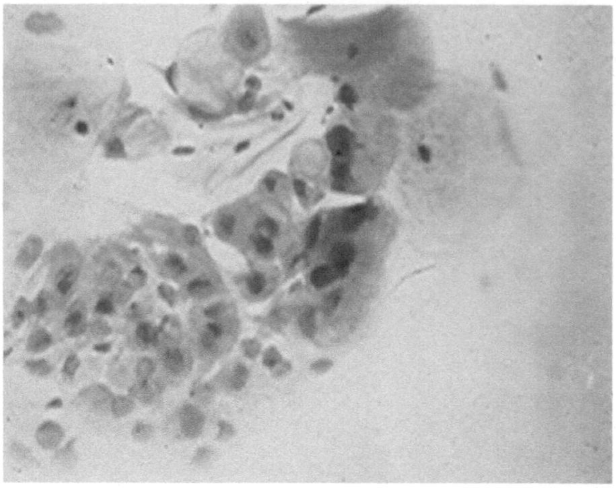

Fig. 10.5 *Chlamydia trachomatis*. Elementary bodies stained (Papanicolaou stain)

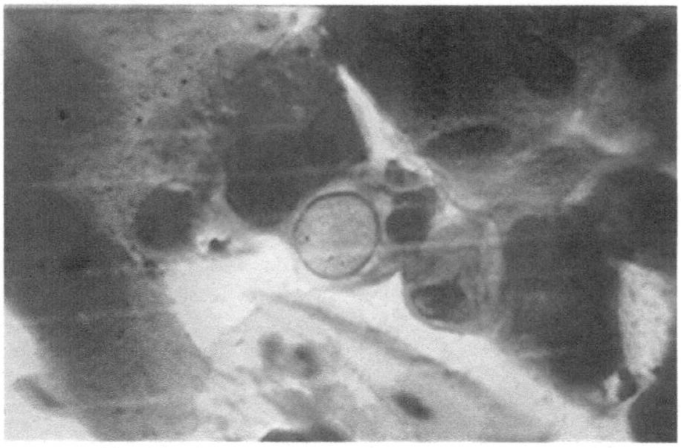

Fig. 10.6 *Chlamydia trachomatis*. Intracellular corpuscles of Gamma-Miyagawa (Papanicolaou stain)

10.4 LGV Infection Among HIV Patients

No studies have been performed on patients with concomitant HIV infection and LGV, and remarkably little anecdotal evidence regarding clinical features and treatment has been published. HIV appears to have no effect on the clinical presentation of the disease.

10.5 Diagnosis

LGV can be suspected on positive *Chlamydia* serology, isolation of *Chlamydia trachomatis* from the infected site. Samples must contain cellular material, which is obtained for direct bacteriological exam and culture from affected lymph nodes by aspiration from fluctuant lymph nodes/buboes, from the ulcer base exudates, or from rectal tissue. Staining of the smear (Giemsa or fuchsin) reveals the intracellular corpuscles of Gamma-Miyagawa, which occur in some chlamydial infections (Figs. 10.5 and 10.6).

The culture on cycloheximide-treated McCoy cells of material from suspected LGV lesion is labor intensive, expensive, and of restricted availability. Its sensitivity is 75–85% at best, and often closer to 50% in the case of the bubo aspirate.

A complement fixation test, using group-specific antigens, is typically positive within 2 weeks of the onset of disease. A titer of greater than or equal to 1:16, in the presence of a compatible clinical syndrome, is suggestive of LGV. Titers greater than 1:64 are considered diagnostic of LGV [28]. Serial samples with a 15-day interval frequently show a fourfold increment in titer in the acute stage of the disease. Indirect immunofluorescence represents a sensitive method but is not widely available. Antibody titers do not necessarily correspond with disease activity and may not decline after treatment [29]. Microimmunofluorescence test is the only serological means of distinguishing between different serotypes of *C. trachomatis* and is therefore the diagnostic test of choice.

ELISA is considered a convenient and objective method, suitable for ulcer scrapes or bubo aspirates. Sensitivity is lower than other methods (75–80%) and should be confirmed by another method. Monoclonal antibodies are an extremely sensitive method and have high specification in the diagnosis of the LGV, capable of preventing serological cross-reactivity among the causative, and other serotypes of C. *trachomatis.*

Detection of nucleic acid is done by DNA amplification techniques such as the ligase chain reaction (LCR) or polymerase chain reaction (PCR) [30]; these methods are becoming established for routine testing.

More recently, a Nested Real Time-PCR [31] was successfully demonstrated for the genotype-specific typing of C. *trachomatis* strains that cause STDs.

10.6 Differential Diagnosis

Chancroid, syphilis, donovanosis, herpes simplex, cutaneous leishmaniasis, ganglionar tuberculosis, cat-scratch disease, and Hodgkin's disease. Late manifestations must be distinguished from neoplastic skin disease, filariasis, rectal cancer, inflammatory bowel disease, and hidradenitis suppurativa [32].

10.7 Treatment

No controlled double-blind treatment trials have been published on LGV [33]. The low incidence of the disease, its complex presentation, and its natural history have precluded any rigorous evaluation of management. Early treatment is important to reduce the chronic phase. Prolonged treatment (at least 3 weeks) is the norm.

Antibiotics

According to CDC 2006 [34]:
First choice: Doxycycline: 100 mg p.o. every 12 h, for 3 weeks.
Second choice: -Erythromycin: 500 mg every 6 h, for 3 weeks and Azithromycin 1 g orally once a week for 3 weeks.
Other treatments have been used with good results:

- Tetracyclines: 500 mg p.o. every 6 h, during 2–4 weeks.
- Sulfadiazine: 500 mg p.o. every 6 h, during 2–3 weeks.
- Sulfisoxazole: beginning dose of 4 g p.o. and then 2 g during 2–3 weeks.

The activity of azithromycin against *C trachomatis* suggests that it may be effective, but clinical data on its use are lacking.

After an initial course of treatment, patients should be seen at least every 3 months for 1 year. Retreatment should be given if there is clinical evidence of relapse. Sexual contacts should be treated similarly.

Pregnant and lactating women should be treated with the erythromycin (non-estolate) regimen; however, one new treatment strategy is the use of Azithromycin as a primary, rather than alternative, medication for pregnant women; but no published data are available regarding its safety and efficacy.

People who have had sexual contacts with a patient who has LGV within the 60 days before onset of the patient's symptoms should be examined, tested for urethral or cervical chlamydial infection, and treated empirically as follows: Azithromycin 1 g PO in a single dose OR Doxycycline 100 mg PO bid 7 days. Should test result positive, treat as recommended for any cases.

The CDC recommends the same treatments for LGV in HIV-negative and HIV-positive patients, with the note that these patients may not respond as well to therapy and prolonged treatment may be required [35, 36].

Tense and fluctuant nodules should be aspirated, rather than incised and drained. Dilation and partial amputation of the rectum are measures occasionally indicated to correct rectal stricture. Vulvectomy and colostomy are seldom necessary.

10.8 Follow-up and Prognosis

Patients should be followed clinically until signs and symptoms have resolved. This may occur within 3–6 weeks. However, there is also evidence of spontaneous remission in 8 weeks. Tests of cure should be performed at 3–4 weeks after completion of effective treatment to avoid false positive due to the presence of nonviable organisms, especially if using NAAT (nucleic acid amplification).

The prognosis is excellent for acute infections treated with appropriate antibiotics. The late disease becomes rare each day, but severe lymphatic involvement is frequently irreversible. Malignant transformation of the genital lesions of elephantiasis and anorectal syndrome, more common in females, is considered exceptional.

HIV appears not to change LGV clinical presentation, but it can have a longer duration course.

Coinfections with HIV and other STIs should always have to be considered.

10.9 Synonyms

Nicolas-Favre-Durand; Tropical bubo; Climatic bubo; d'emblé bubo; Scrofulous bubo; Subacute inguinal lymphogranulomatosis; Inguinal lymphogranuloma [32].

Take-Home Pearls

- In developed nations, it was considered rare before 2003. However, a recent outbreak in the Netherlands among men who have sex with men has led to an increase of LGV in Europe and the United States. A majority of these patients are HIV co-infected.
- Soon after the initial Dutch report, national and international health authorities launched warning initiatives and multiple LGV cases were identified in several more European countries (Belgium, France, the UK, Germany, Sweden, Italy and Switzerland) and the US and Canada. All cases reported in Amsterdam and France and a considerable percentage of LGV infections in the UK and Germany were caused by a newly discovered Chlamydia variant, L2b, a.k.a the Amsterdam variant.
- Erythema nodosum occurs in 10% of cases
- Genital elephantiasis or esthiomene, which is the dramatic end-result of lymphatic obstruction, which may occur because of the strictures themselves, or fistulas. This is usually seen in females, may ulcerate and often occurs 1-20 years after primary infection.

References

1. Cevenini, R., Donati, M., Sambri, V.: *Chlamydia trachomatis* – the agent. Best Pract. Res. Clin. Obstet. Gynaecol. **16**, 761–773 (2002)
2. Jensen, K.T., Petersen, L., Falk, S., Iversen, P., Andersen, P., Theisen, M., Krogh, A.: Novel overlapping coding sequences in Chlamydia trachomatis. FEMS Microbiol. Lett. **265**(1), 106–117 (2006)
3. Mayaud, P. National guideline for the management of lymphogranuloma venereum. Clinical Effectiveness Group (Association of Genitourinary Medicine and the Medical Society for the Study of Venereal Diseases) Sex Transm Inf **35**(4): 243–251 (1999)
4. Stamm, W.E.: *Chlamydia trachomatis* infections: progress and problems. J. Infect. Dis. **179**(Suppl 2), S380–S383 (1999)
5. Koedijk, F.D., de Boer, I.M., de Vries, H.J., Thiesbrummel, H.F., van der Sande, M.A.: An ongoing outbreak of lymphogranuloma venereum in the Netherlands, 2006–2007. Euro Surveill. 2007 Apr 19
6. Dougan, S., Evans, B.G., Elford, J.: Sexually transmitted infections in Western Europe among HIV-positive men who have sex with men. Am. Sex. Transm. Dis. Assoc. **34**(10), 783–790 (2007)
7. Blank, S., Schillinger, J.A., Harbatkin, D.: Lymphogranuloma venereum in the industrialized world. Lancet **365**, 1607–1608 (2005)
8. Vandenbruaene, M., Ostyn B, Crucitti T, De Schrijver K, Sasse A, Sergeant M, Van Dyck E, Van Esbroeck M, Moerman F. Lymphogranuloma venereum outbreak in men who have sex with men (MSM) in Belgium, January 2004 to July 2005. Euro Surveill. 2005 Sep 29
9. Herida, M., Barbeyrac, B., Sednaoui, P., Scieux, C., Lemarchand, N., et al.: Rectal lymphogranuloma venereum surveillance in France 2004–2005. Euro Surveill. **11**(9), 155–156 (2006)
10. Halioua, B., Bohbot, J.M., Monfort, L., Nassar, N., Barbeyrac, B., Monsonego, J., Sednaoui, P.: Ano-rectal lymphogranuloma venereum: 22 cases reported in a Sexually Transmited Infections center in Paris. Eur. J. Dermatol. **16**(2), 177–180 (2006). Clinical report
11. Bremer, V., Meyer, T., Marcus, U., Hamouda, O.: Lymphogranuloma venereum emerging in men who have sex with men in Germany. Euro Surveill. **11**(9), 152–154 (2006)
12. Jebbari, H., Alexander, S., Ward, H., Evans, B., Solomou, M., Thornton, A., Dean, G., White, J., French, P., Ison, C., UK LGV Incident Group.: Update on lymphogranuloma venereum in the United Kingdom. Sex. Transm. Infect. 2007 Jul
13. Liassine N, Caulfield A, Ory G, Restellini A, de Barbeyrac B, Sitavanc R, Descombes MC, Luescher D. First confirmed case of lymphogranuloma venereum (LGV) in Switzerland. Euro Surveill; **10**(7):E050714.4 (2005)
14. Vall Mayans M, Sanz Colomo B, Ossewaarde JM. First case of LGV confirmed in Barcelona. Euro Surveill; **10**(2): E050203.2 (2005)
15. Stary G, Meyer T, Bangert C, Kohrgruber N, Gmeinhart B, Kirnbauer R, Jantschitsch C, Rieger A, Stary A, Geusau A. New Chlamydia trachomatis L2 Strains Identified in a Recent Outbreak of Lymphogranuloma Venereum in Vienna, Austria. Sex Transm Dis; **35**(4):377–82 (2008)
16. Kropp RY, Wong T; Canadian LGV Working Group. Emergence of lymphogranuloma venereum in Canada. CMAJ, **172**(13):1674–6 (2005)
17. Brown, T.J., Yen-Moore, A., Tyring, S.K.: An overview of sexually transmitted diseases. Part I. J. Am. Acad. Dermatol. (1999)

18. Neves RG, Lupi O. Lymphogranuloma venereum In: Sexually transmitted diseases. Borchardt KA, Noble MA, eds. CRC Press LLC (1997) pages 117–130
19. Tinmouth, J., Rachlis, A., Wesson, T., Hsieh, E.: Lymphogranuloma venereum in North America: case reports and an update for astroenterologists. Clin. Gastroenterol. Hepatol. **4**(4), 469–473 (2006)
20. van de Laar, M.J.: The emergence of LGV in Western Europe: what do we know, what can we do? Euro Surveill. 2006 Sep
21. Dougan, S., Evans, B.G., Elford, J.: Sexually transmitted infections in Western Europe among HIV-positive men who have sex with men. Sex. Transm. Dis. **34**(10), 783–790 (2007)
22. Haugstvedt, A., Thorvaldsen, J., Halsos, A.M.: Tidsskr Nor Laegeforen. Lymphogranuloma venerum as ulcerous proctitis in men who have sex with men – Norwegian 2007 Aug 23
23. Tinmouth J, Rachlis A, Wesson T, Hsieh E. Lymphogranuloma venereum in North America: case reports and an update for gastroenterologists. Clin Gastroenterol Hepatol. Clin Gastroenterol Hepatol, (4):469–73 (2006)
24. Spaargaren, J., Schachter, J., Moncada, J., de Vries, H.J.C., Fennema, H.S.A., et al.: Slow epidemic of Lymphogranuloma venereum L2b Strain. Emerging infectious diseases www.cdc.gov/eid vol. 11, No. 11, November 2005
25. van de Laar, M.J.W., Koedijk, F.D.H., Gotz, H.M., de Vries, H.J.C.: A slow epidemic of LGV in the Netherlands in 2004 and 2005. Euro Surveill. 2006
26. Siedner, M.J., Pandori, M., Leon, S.R., Espinosa, B.J., Hall, E.R., Caceres, C., Coates, T.J., Klausner, J.D., NIMH Collaborative HIV/STD Prevention Trial Group: Facilitating lymphogranuloma venereum surveillance with the use of real time polymerase chain reaction. Int J STD AIDS. **18**, 506–507 (2007)
27. Jalal, H., Stephen, H., Alexander, S., Carne, C., Sonnex, C.: Development of real-time PCR assays for genotyping of *Chlamydia trachomati*. J. Clin. Micobiol. **45**(8), 2649–2653 (2007)
28. Lupi, O., Joffe, R., Neves, R.G.: Chlamydial Infection. In: Tyring, S., Lupi, O., Hengge, U. (eds.) Tropical Dermatology. Elsevier (2005)
29. Centers for Disease Control and Prevention Sexually transmitted diseases treatment guidelines. MMWR. http://www.cdc.gov/mmwr/preview/mmwrhtml/rr5511a1.htm (Aug 4 2006)
30. Rosen, T., Brown, T.J.: Cutaneous manifestations of STDs. Med. Clin. North Am. **82**(5), 1081–1104 (1998)
31. Czelusta, A., Yen-Moore, A., Van der Straten, M., Carrasco, D., Tyring, S.K.: An overview of sexually transmitted diseases. Part III. Sexually transmitted diseases in HIV-infected patients. J. Am. Acad. Dermatol. **43**(3), 409–432 (2000)
32. Guaschino, S., de Seta, F.: Update on *Chlamydia trachomatis*. Ann. NY Acad. Sci. **900**, 293–300 (2000)

Biology and Natural History of Syphilis

11

Attila Horváth

Core Messages

- Syphilis continues to have great public health importance because it increases the risk of human immunodeficiency virus (HIV) infection significantly; furthermore, statistical studies suggest that there are no chances of eradicating it in the foreseeable future.
- The *T. pallidum* Genome Sequencing Project also confirmed what had already been suggested by ongoing experimental efforts: this bacterium is a fastidious, microaerophilic, obligate parasite of humans.
- *T. pallidum* derives most essential macromolecules from the host, using interconversion pathways to generate others.
- The course of untreated syphilis consists of intermittent stages with sequential symptomatic and asymptomatic (latency) periods. This regular choreography, however, may be disturbed if the immunological competence of the host organism is severely compromised (HIV infection) by inappropriately administered prevention or antimicrobial therapy for another disease.
- Much progress has been made during the past 2 decades in the following areas:

1. Identification of *T. pallidum* polypeptides; production of recombinant DNA reagents and monoclonal antibodies for their study, characterization of certain subsets (flagellins and membrane-associated lipoproteins), determination of their structural locations and functional activities.
2. Isolation and characterization of the outer membrane and cytoplasmic membrane of *T. pallidum*, identification of their associated proteins, and determination of the role of the outer-membrane proteins in immunity.
3. Elucidation of important metabolic and biosynthetic pathways and associated enzymes in *T. pallidum*, and their relationship with the unusual physiology of the organism; continued study of the induction of antibody and cellular responses to *T. pallidum* proteins and the potential for immunoprotection; and clarification of the roles of toxins, secreted enzymes, adhesins, or other factors in the pathogenesis of *T. pallidum*.

11.1 Introduction

The epidemiological significance of what was a dreaded disease in the years before World War II has diminished considerably. The introduction of effective penicillin therapy in the 1940s, improvements in diagnosis (serodiagnosis), as well as targeted and efficiently organized epidemiological work were equally important contributory factors. These developments notwithstanding, syphilis continues to have great

A. Horváth
Levendula u.19, Budapest 1124, Hungary
e-mail: aurelius@bor.sote.hu, horvathagy@yahoo.com

G. Gross and S.K. Tyring (eds.), *Sexually Transmitted Infections and Sexually Transmitted Diseases*,
DOI: 10.1007/978-3-642-14663-3_11,

public health importance because it increases the risk of HIV infection significantly; furthermore, statistical studies suggest that there are no chances of eradicating it in the foreseeable future.

The infection may be transmitted through sexual intercourse or blood (*syphilis d'emblée*). However, infection through blood occurs extremely rarely these days, due to the careful control of blood preparations for therapeutic purposes. *Treponema pallidum* may be transmitted to the fetus via the placenta (*congenital syphilis*) [41, 42].

T. pallidum subsp. *pallidum* is one of the few bacteria that are pathogenic to humans and have not been cultured continuously in vitro. It is propagated by intratesticular infection of rabbits for research and diagnostic purposes. Long thought to be an obligate anaerobe, *T. pallidum* is now known to be a microaerophilic organism.

With the absence of biosynthetic pathways, it is suspected that *T. pallidum* derives most essential macromolecules from the host, using interconversion pathways to generate others.

The course of untreated syphilis consists of intermittent stages with sequential symptomatic and asymptomatic (latency) periods. This regular choreography, however, may be disturbed if the immunological competence of the host organism is severely compromised (HIV infection) by inappropriately administered prevention or antimicrobial therapy for another disease. These may modify or change the time of presentation and character of symptoms and signs (*syphilis decapitata*).

Despite research efforts, some chapters in the scenario of the natural course of syphilis, the molecular biological details of its pathomechanism are not fully understood, although the sequentiation in 1997 of the genome of *T. pallidum* subsp. *pallidum* yielded many new pieces of information.

11.2 Biology of *T. Pallidum* subsp. *pallidum*, the Etiological Agent of Syphilis

T. pallidum is one of a small group of treponemes, members of the "corkscrew-shaped," motile, prokaryotic bacteria with a flexible, helically coiled cell wall, phylum Spirochaetes, which are pathogenic for human beings.

This group of bacteria was reclassified in 1984 as *T. pallidum* subsp. *pallidum*, which was first discovered as the etiological agent of syphilis in 1905 [58], as *T. pallidum* subsp. *endemicum* causing bejel (endemic syphilis), and as *T. pallidum* subsp. *pertenue* (yaws). These organisms are virtually identical in terms of morphology, DNA homology which is >95% [15, 39], and protein composition, although they exhibit different patterns of pathogenesis in humans. They can be also differentiated from each other by the clinical manifestations of their respective diseases and, in part, epidemiological characteristics of infections, and more recently, by genetic differences [8]. *Treponema carateum* (*pinta*) and related organism, *Treponema paraluiscuniculi* (venereal spirochetosis of rabbits), are believed to be separate species [62].

T. pallidum subsp. *pallidum* measures between 6 and 15 μm (usually 10–13 μm) in length and between 0.10 and 0.18 μm in width, which is below the level of resolution, and is therefore not visible by light microscopy without silver staining. It has tapered ends with 6 to 14 spiral coils between them. When fixed for histological analysis the spirals seem to have a wavelike configuration.

In clinical practice, dark-field microscopy is used to study a wet preparation; this technique reveals rotatory motion with flexion and back-and-forth squiggle that are said to be characteristic of the virulent treponemes. This form of motion is suggested to facilitate penetration of *T. pallidum* through tissue. The spiral-shaped body of *T. pallidum* is surrounded by a cytoplasmic membrane, which is enclosed by a loosely associated outer membrane. A thin layer of peptidoglycan between the membranes provides structural stability. Endoflagella, organelles that allow for the characteristic corkscrew motility of *T. pallidum*, are located in the periplasmic space [27].

Electron microscopy can be used in special clinical problems and investigative research work.

T. pallidum subsp. *pallidum* is an unusual bacterium in terms of its structure, physiology, and host–parasite interactions. All of these features are related, either directly or indirectly, to its proteins, which are responsible for most of its functional activities.

Over the past 25 years, there has been very intensive research on polipeptides of *T. pallidum*. Considerable progress was made during this time in the characterization of *T. pallidum*'s components according to their antigenic, structural, and functional roles. This was rendered possible by the development of new, sophisticated methods: electrophoretic techniques (SDS-PAGE-dodecyl sulfate-polyacrylamide gel electrophoresis, crossed immunoelectrophoresis, and 2DGE-two-dimensional gel electrophoresis), DNA and hybridoma technologies and recombinant DNA techniques [59, 66].

A recommended nomenclature has been developed to aid in the identification of *T. pallidum* polypeptides. The format consists of the prefix TpN (for *T. pallidum* Nichols, the reference strain) followed by a consensus Mr (relative molecular mass, based on SDS-PAGE results), and, if necessary, a letter to distinguish between polypeptides with similar Mrs. The corresponding gene can be indicated by lowercase italics; for example, the TpN47 is expressed by the gene *tpn47*.

There is practical classification of isolated *T. pallidum*'s polypeptides depending on localization: flagellar proteins, outer and cytoplasmic membrane proteins (lipoproteins, other membrane-associated proteins), other *T. pallidum* polypeptides (cytoplasmic filaments, penicillin-binding proteins, and extracellular proteins).

The complete genome sequence has also greatly enhanced our knowledge of the protein components of *T. pallidum* in 1998 [18]. The *T. pallidum* genome, known to be small, was confirmed by the Genome Sequencing Project to be 1.14 Mb and to encode 1,041 predicted protein coding sequences [18]. The genomes of many bacteria are several times larger.

The *T. pallidum* Genome Sequencing Project also confirmed what had already been suggested by ongoing experimental research, that this bacterium is a fastidious, microaerophilic, obligate parasite of humans.

T. pallidum cannot be cultured in vitro; however, it is only propagated by intratesticular infection of rabbits for research and diagnostic purposes. That is probably why the studies of this bacterium are restricted. The study of metabolism, toxin production, and antigenic composition has been hindered and has also made it difficult to examine the induction of immunity. In 1981 and 1982 some studies defined the growth conditions of *T. pallidum* better and enabled limited replication of these organisms (up to 25-fold increases over an initial treponemal inoculum). The medium must contain cells (a line of rabbit epithelial cells was used with greatest success) [26]. The optimal temperature is 34–35°C, and growth seems to be best in the presence of 3–5% O_2 and 5% CO_2 in H_2; thus, the traditional suggestion that *T. pallidum* is an obligate anaerobe is mistaken, and *T. pallidum* subsp. *pallidum* is now known to be a microaerophilic organism [10, 26].

Under these in vitro conditions, the replication time, or in other words the generation time of *T. pallidum*, is similar to that reported in vivo, and is unusually slow, taking about 30–33 h [10, 36]. The main course of this sluggish replication rate is the lack of a tricarboxylic acid cycle and an electron transport chain. *T. pallidum* depends upon glycolysis as the sole pathway for the synthesis of adenosine triphosphate (ATP). This pathway is not so effective, much less ATP-synthesized from glycolysis. Low energy production is not the only factor that inhibits *T. pallidum* replication. Because of a lack of enzymes such as catalase and oxidase that detoxify reactive oxygen species the in vitro survival of *T. pallidum* is prolonged by low oxygen concentrations.

It is propagated by serial intratesticular passage in rabbits. Most laboratory studies were conducted using the rabbit-passaged Nichols-type strain of *T. pallidum*, which was isolated from the cerebrospinal fluid of a patient with secondary syphilis in 1912 [44].

T. pallidum has a striking lack of metabolic capabilities; it is able to carry out glycolysis [18, 45] but lacks tricarboxylic acid cycle enzymes and an electron transport chain [18], as mentioned above. There are no pathways for the use of alternative carbon sources for energy and for "de novo" synthesis of enzyme cofactors and nucleotides, it is also out of amino acid and fatty acid synthesis pathways, whereas interestingly *T. pallidum* does carry enzymes for the interconversion of amino acids and fatty acids.

With this absence of biosynthetic pathways, it is suspected that *T. pallidum* derives most essential macromolecules from the host, using interconversion pathways to generate others. To take up macromolecules from the host environment, specific transporters may be utilized by *T. pallidum*. Homologs of transporters for a variety of amino acids are found in the *T. pallidum* genome. The lipoprotein TpN32 is homologous to a member of the newly identified methionine uptake transporter family in *Escherichia coli* [71], and the methionine-binding properties of TpN32 were recently described [12], suggesting that these are part of a methionine transport system in *T. pallidum*. Six *T. pallidum* transporters have specificity for cations. The most extensively studied of these is the ATP-binding cassette (ABC) transporter encoded by the *tro* operon.

TroA (alternatively termed TROMP1), the cation-binding protein of the Tro complex, binds zinc and manganese, trace metals that may be required for enzyme function in *T. pallidum*[11, 24].

Carbon utilization studies demonstrated that ribose is not degraded by *T. pallidum* [45] and its inability to utilize galactose as a carbon source. It was suggested that the RbsAC homolog may function to transport other sugars because *T. pallidum* may utilize MglABC as a glucose transporter [11].

Because the *T. pallidum* genome encodes no known homologs to porin proteins, it is unclear how nutrients are moved across the outer membrane into the periplasmic space. A recent study suggests that Tp0453, a putative outer membrane protein, may perturb the outer membrane by insertion into its inner leaflet, allowing nonselective diffusion of nutrients into the periplasm [5].

One of most important goals of the *T. pallidum* Genome Sequencing Project was to identify possible virulence factors. It is true that the *T. pallidum* genome sequence does not reveal any classical virulence factors that could account for syphilis signs and symptoms. *T. pallidum* lacks lipopolysaccharide (LPS) [18], an endotoxin found in the outer membranes of many Gram-negative bacteria that causes fever and inflammation.

However, *T. pallidum* does produce a number of lipoproteins which may induce the expression of inflammatory mediators via toll-like receptor 2 (TLR2) recognition [5, 34]. Many Gram-negative pathogens utilize type III secretion systems to insert virulence-related proteins into the cytoplasm of host cells. *T. pallidum* lacks homologs for the recognized type III components [18]. Cytolytic enzymes or other cytotoxins have not been shown to play a role in syphilis pathogenesis. The cytopathic effect of treponemes on cells in culture requires extraordinarily high numbers of bacteria [17].

Genes for several other oxygen-protective enzymes have been identified in the *T. pallidum* genome. Neelaredoxin (Tp0823) is hypothesized to convert superoxide to peroxide, which is then reduced to water by hydroperoxide reductase C (Tp0509). Each of these enzymes is regenerated by other *T. pallidum* proteins [23].

In addition to its sensitivity to oxygen, *T. pallidum* may have a limited stress response. The typical heat shock response regulated by $\sigma 32$ is lacking [18, 65], possibly reflecting the sensitivity of the organism to growth temperature [14]. At least one *T. pallidum* enzyme is unstable at normal body temperature [4], suggesting that the heat lability of enzymes may also contribute to the slow growth of the organism. It is clear that *T. pallidum* has limited heat tolerance; this, along with oxygen sensitivity and possibly other as-yet-unrecognized factors, may hinder the replication of *T. pallidum* both in vivo and in vitro.

The limited heat tolerance of *T. pallidum* was well known earlier. Heat therapy for late neurosyphilis was introduced in 1918 by the Julius Wagner von Jauregg [69]. Later, he was awarded the Nobel Prize in Medicine. His therapy regimen consisted of inoculating patients with malaria-infected blood and, after 10 to 12 febrile episodes, treating them with quinine. The induced high temperatures presumably killed *T. pallidum* in the central nervous system (CNS). Doctors reported high percentages of complete or partial remission of general paresis symptoms, although the rate of lethal complications was about 10%.

T. pallidum subsp. *pallidum* has been called a "stealth pathogen" because it has a remarkable aptitude to evade the humoral and cellular immune responses in infected hosts, which was formerly attributed to the presence of an outer coat comprising the host's serum proteins and/or mucopolysaccharides. Evidence indicates that the immuno-evasiveness of this bacterium is largely the result of its unusual molecular structure. Based upon ultrastructural, biochemical, and molecular data, it is believed that the *T. pallidum* outer membrane contains a paucity of poorly immunogenic transmembrane proteins ("rare outer membrane proteins") and that its highly immunogenic proteins are lipoproteins anchored predominantly to the periplasmic leaflet of the cytoplasmic membrane.

Some organisms survive in infected hosts despite the presence of strongly reactive antibodies directed against a number of *T. pallidum* proteins [1, 46] and activated T cells and macrophages in lesions. Researchers noted that antibodies in serum from infected animals did not readily bind to intact treponemes [48] and only those treponemes that had been physically disrupted reacted with anti-*T. pallidum* antiserum, leading them to propose that the surface of *T. pallidum* in nonantigenic.

Furthermore, in experiments involving the interaction of *T. pallidum*-specific antibodies with viable organisms – agglutination, neutralization, and opsonization – organisms must be incubated with antibodies for unusually long periods before effects are observed. These observations suggest that there are few antigenic targets on the surface of the organisms, causing the binding and aggregation of antibodies to proceed slowly.

Visualized by freeze-fracture electron microscopy (EM) *T. pallidum* was shown to have only rare integral proteins in its outer membrane [50, 70]. These studies confirmed the paucity of integral outer membrane proteins in *T. pallidum*. This is the reason the pathogen is able to escape immune detection, and that has inspired researchers to call T. pallidum "the stealth pathogen" [57].

Many techniques have been used to explore the identity of *T. pallidum* outer membrane proteins (various detergents, separation of membranes with acid, or density gradient ultracentrifugation of organisms lysed in a hypotonic solution). Several of these, including TpN47, were initially identified as surface-exposed proteins, and much effort was devoted to confirming their location [28]. However, further studies indicated that these proteins are not surface-exposed but are more likely to be anchored in the inner membrane with portions extending into the periplasm [6, 19, 67].

The *T. pallidum* outer membrane is easily damaged by these procedures [9, 49]. Most bacteria with a double membrane have a peptidoglycan layer that is linked to the outer membrane by lipoprotein molecules; but in *T. pallidum*, peptidoglycan is thought to be associated with the more abundant inner membrane proteins. Additionally, *T. pallidum* lacks LPS, a molecule that lends structural stability to bacterial outer membranes.

11.3 Natural History of Untreated Syphilis

T. pallidum's only known natural host is the human. It is able to invade and survive in different tissues and organs; in spite of this, it has a lack of metabolic capabilities, sensitivity to oxygen, and decreased viability in an environment warmer than body temperature (see above). The detection of *T. pallidum* in the cerebrospinal fluid (CSF) of the greatest proportion of patients with early syphilis, as well as the disseminated clinical manifestations of secondary, tertiary, and congenital syphilis, goes to show that the organism has highly invasive capabilities. Dissemination is not only widespread, it is very rapid. *T. pallidum* enters the bloodstream within minutes of intratesticular or intradermal inoculation and organisms applied to mucosa are found in deeper tissues within hours [10, 38].

Syphilis is a chronic, systemic infection with many kinds of symptoms. It is acquired by direct contact, usually sexual, with active primary or secondary lesions. Studies have shown that 16–30% of individuals who have had sexual contact with a syphilis-infected person in the preceding 30 days become infected, and in some cases the transmission rates may be much higher [60]. Infection also occurs when organisms cross the placenta to infect the fetus in a pregnant woman.

Syphilis is a multistage disease with diverse and wide-ranging manifestations, having an accurate choreography. The distinct stages of syphilis were first described in detail by Philippe Ricord in the mid-1800s [51]. The natural course of syphilis, including its individual stages and clinical features, has been identified in three large comparative studies conducted at the turn of the first half of the 20th century. A common feature of these studies was that one group of patients was not treated, which raised ethical concerns. It is true, however, that no definitive treatment was available for syphilis at the time.

The first of the three large prospective studies of patients was conducted in Oslo from 1890 to 1910 by Boeck, and subsequently followed up retrospectively by Bruusgaard and later by Gjestland et al. Boeck was concerned that therapy available – mercurial – might be more toxic than the disease itself [19].

In 1932, a second study of the natural history of ostensibly untreated syphilis was undertaken by the US Public Health Service in Macon County, Alabama, which is generally known as the "Tuskegee study." It has been challenged in recent years on ethical grounds because written informed consent was never obtained from the involved patients; furthermore, patients were misled into participating by giving them the impression that they were receiving treatment. Because the study was limited to black males, some have chosen to view the study as essentially racist.

A third significant study of the natural course of syphilis was conducted by Paul Rosahn. It was based entirely on a cross-sectional review of all autopsies conducted at Yale University School of Medicine from

1917 to 1941; among almost 4,000 persons over 20 years of age at death, 9.7% had clinical, laboratory, or autopsy evidence of syphilis. About half of the patients had not been treated. Overall, 51% of syphilitic patients had specific lesions at autopsy. Among clinically diagnosed patients about 30% developed late syphilitic lesions of syphilis. This experiment was very similar to the Oslo study. About 20% of patients died because of syphilis. Among 77 patients with untreated syphilis with late anatomic lesions at autopsy, 83% of lesions were cardiovascular, 7.6% were neurological, and 8.5% were gummas. Many patients had been suffering from multiple, combined symptoms [30].

The stages of untreated syphilis can be classified as follows: primary syphilis (chancre, regional lymphadenopathy), secondary syphilis (disseminated maculo-papular eruption, generalized lymphadenopathy), latent syphilis (recurrence of secondary syphilis symptoms), and tertiary syphilis (gummas, cardiovascular syphilis and late neurological symptoms). A schematic diagram of untreated syphilis is shown in Fig. 11.1.

11.3.1 Primary Syphilis

The primary stage is initiated when *T. pallidum* penetrates epidermal microabrasions or intact mucous membranes, resulting in a single chancre at the site of inoculation, with a moderate regional lymphadenopathy. Classically, neurological complications of syphilis have been associated with tertiary disease, but studies have demonstrated that penetration of the CNS by *T. pallidum* occurs during earlier stages of disease. About 40% of early syphilis patients and 25% of individuals with latent infection meet at least one of the diagnostic criteria for neurosyphilis [40].

The chancre usually becomes indurated and will progress to ulceration but typically is not purulent. Polymorphonuclear lymphocytes (PMNs) are seen in very early acquired and experimentally induced syphilis lesions [7]. These infiltrations are transient and the number of PMNs is low relative to that seen in other acute bacterial infections. That presumably is why primary chancre is not purulent. Apart from PMNs T cells and macrophages are found in human primary chancres.

In heterosexual men, primary chancres most commonly occur on the penis. Among MSM 32–36% have primary chancres in other sites, including the rectum, anal canal, and oral cavity.

In women, the primary chancre usually occurs on the labia or cervix. Because the chancre is painless and may be located in an inconspicuous anatomical site, diagnosis of syphilis in women and MSM is sometimes delayed until secondary syphilis manifestations become apparent. Sometimes the clinical evaluation is not easy due to the fact that the appearance of primary chancres in some individuals does not fit the classic description. In immunocompromised, HIV-infected patients nonindurated lesions with irregular borders have been observed. These chancres often are multiple, and painful especially in the anal area [55].

The primary chancre develops an average of 3 weeks after exposure; the incubation period ranges between 10 and 90 days. Based on intradermal inoculation of human volunteers with graded doses of *T. pallidum*, the 50% infectious dose is estimated to be 57 organisms [37]. Lesions develop more rapidly when the inoculum size is larger. The generation time of *T. pallidum* is unusually slow. Inoculation studies determined that *T. pallidum* doubles every 30–33 h in vivo. Several biological factors may contribute to *T. pallidum*'s sluggish replication rate (see above).

T. pallidum quickly gains access to deeper tissues and the bloodstream, probably by traversing the junctions between endothelial cells [38, 53]. The characteristic form of *T. pallidum* motion is thought to facilitate penetration of *spirochetes* through tissue.

T. pallidum has been shown to induce the production of matrix metalloproteinase-1 (MMP-1) in dermal cells. MMP-1 is involved in breaking down collagen, which may help *T. pallidum* to penetrate tissues. The presence of a pathogen signals inflammatory and immune cells to migrate from the bloodstream to the site of infection. An early step in this homing mechanism is the expression of cell adhesion molecules on capillary endothelial cells, promoting the leakage of serous fluids and the migration of leukocytes out of blood vessels into infected tissues. Virulent *T. pallidum* induces cultured endothelial cells to express the adhesion molecules ICAM-1, VCAM-1, and E-selectin. These are also activated by the 47-kDa *T. pallidum* lipoprotein TpN47 but not by heat-killed *T. pallidum* or the nonpathogenic treponeme (*T. phagedenis*), suggesting that endothelial cell activation is a pathogen-specific, active process mediated by specific *T. pallidum* molecules [31]. Preincubation with virulent *T. pallidum* organisms increases the ability of endothelial

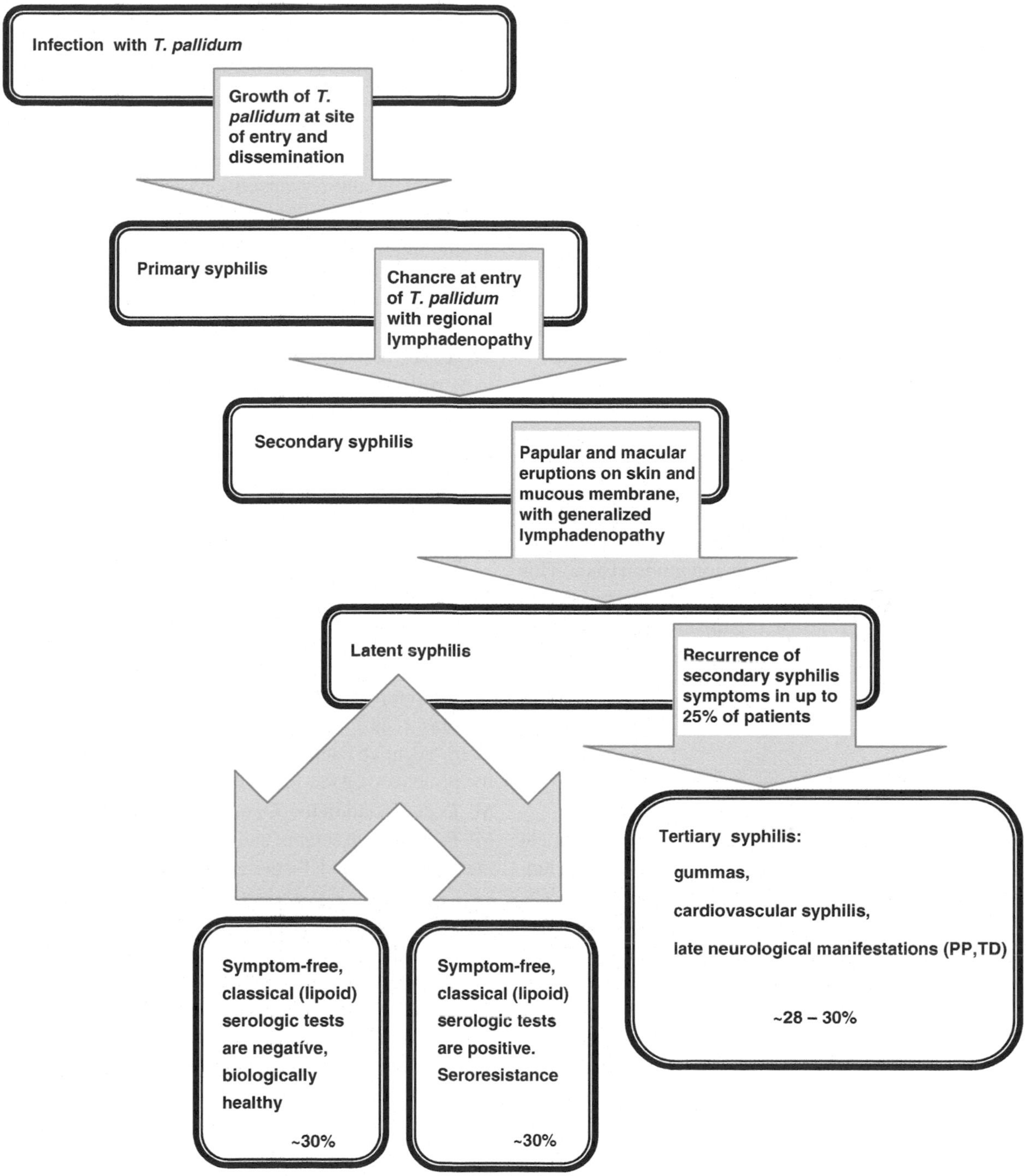

Fig. 11.1 Natural history of untreated syphilis

cells to bind to lymphocytes [52], and this binding is blocked by antibodies against the cell adhesion molecules, supporting a functional role for ICAM-1, VCAM-1, and E-selectin expression in the inflammation caused by *T. pallidum* infection [31].

The primary chancre heals spontaneously within 4–6 weeks, but may still be discernible in about 15% of patients at the onset of secondary syphilis. HIV-infected individuals are reported to be two to three times more likely to have concurrent primary and secondary disease than HIV-uninfected individuals.

11.3.2 Secondary Syphilis

In syphilis, the chancre represents a localized, primary infection from which the organism disseminates.

The "virulence factors" of *T. pallidum*, which result in extreme invasiveness, rapid attachment to cell surfaces, and penetration of endothelial junctions and tissue layers are motility, attachment, and chemotaxis.

11.3.2.1 Motility

Motility is a virulence factor for many bacterial pathogens. *T. pallidum* is a highly motile organism that propels itself by rotating around its longitudinal axis. This corkscrew-like motility is common to other spirochetes and allows this group of organisms to swim easily through gel-like materials that hinder most other flagellated organisms.

11.3.2.2 Attachment

The first step in *T. pallidum* invasion is the attachment of organisms to a wide variety of host cell types including epithelial, fibroblast-like, and endothelial cells [32, 68]. A reduction in attachment occurs when either bacterial or eukaryotic cells in culture are not viable. Organisms are also able to adhere to isolated capillary, kidney, and abdominal wall tissues ex vivo. Microscopic examination of *T. pallidum* associated with cell cultures reveals that large numbers of organisms attach to cells by one or the other end. Some researchers have speculated that specialized *T. pallidum* adhesins are located at the tips of the organisms, but treponemes have also been observed to be attached to host cells along their length [16, 64]. It has been speculated that initial attachment can occur at multiple sites along the length of the bacterium but that the active motility of the attached treponemes serves to cause the bacterial adhesin molecules to migrate through the somewhat fluid outer membrane toward the tips, in a "capping" phenomenon. The number of treponemes that can attach to each host cell appears to be limited [25]. This limitation of binding may occur because all of the receptors on the host cell are occupied, implying a specific adhesin–ligand interaction; integrins have been implicated as host cell receptors for *T. pallidum* [31]. The nonpathogenic treponemal species (*T. phagedenis*, *T. refringens*, and *T. vincentii*), heat-killed *T. pallidum*, and nonmotile *T. pallidum* after 22–23 h of incubation at 37°C do not adhere to cultured cells, indicating that attachment is specific to pathogenic treponemes. Immune rabbit or human serum prevents the adherence of viable *T. pallidum* organisms to cell cultures, suggesting that specific surface antigens of *T. pallidum* may mediate attachment to host cells [63].

11.3.2.3 Chemotaxis

Motile bacteria depend upon chemotactic responses to move toward favorable environments and away from hostile environments. The dissemination of motile bacterial pathogens in tissues may be facilitated by chemotaxis. Methyl-accepting chemotaxis transmembrane proteins (MCPs) and cytoplasmic chemotaxis proteins (Che) comprise the chemotaxis system of Gram-negative bacteria, and *T. pallidum* has homologs for proteins of each of these systems. Four genes for MCPs are found in the *T. pallidum* genome [18,21,22]. MCPs sense attractants and repellents in the environment; glucose and histidine are molecules that may have affinity for *T. pallidum* MCPs. Two operons in the *T. pallidum* genome contain genes for the Che response regulators [18, 20].

Secondary syphilis, which occurs in roughly one-fourth of all untreated syphilis cases, results from the multiplication of disseminated *T. pallidum* and formation of lesions at multiple sites in the skin and internal organs, despite the presence of a significant antibody response. The diverse manifestations of human syphilis also demonstrate the invasiveness of *T. pallidum*.

T. pallidum has been detected directly in tissues and fluids far from the initial site of infection. Using polymerase chain reaction (PCR) and infectivity testing, *T. pallidum* is routinely found in the CSF of individuals with early and latent syphilis [35, 40]. *T. pallidum* has been detected decades after initial infection in tertiary gummatous lesions of the skin by silver staining and immunofluorescence microscopy, and by PCR.

The treponemes proliferate in the chancre and are carried via lymphatics to the bloodstream, from which they disseminate throughout the body. The time at which the secondary lesions make their appearance basically depends on two factors: the virulence of the treponeme and the systemic response of the host. Pathologically the cutaneous lesions of secondary syphilis can be regarded as local reactions induced in highly susceptible tissue by metastatic accumulations of treponemes. The tendency for the skin to be the most extensively involved of all organs may reflect the slightly lower temperature. The temperature of outer skin surface is optimal for *T. pallidum*.

The generalized lymphadenopathy that results from the passage of treponemes through satellite glands or buboes of the primary chancre into the lymphatic channels sets the stage for subsequent events in untreated individuals. Contrasted with the regional involvement seen in primary syphilis, early secondary syphilis involves all lymphatic structures. The lymphadenopathy is typically without any relationship to cutaneously involved areas. Lymphatic involvement usually runs an indolent course similar to that seen with the primary or secondary stage. There is a tendency for the nodes to become compact and painless for weeks or months prior to spontaneous resolution.

Neurologic manifestations that appear in early syphilis have received increased attention, especially because of the relationship with concurrent HIV infection. Before the occurrence of HIV infection, abnormalities in the CSF – increased white blood cell counts, elevated protein level, a positive Venereal Disease Research Laboratory (VDRL) test, or the presence of viable *T. pallidum* organisms – were detected in up to 40% of patients with secondary syphilis in the absence of neurologic abnormalities [3, 13]. However, no more than 1–2% of patients with secondary syphilis were found to have symptoms (meningismus, meningitis, headaches, mental changes, ocular palsy, deafness, or nystagmus, internuclear ophthalmoplegia, and signs of spinal cord or nerve disorder). Before the penicillin era they nearly always occurred in subjects who had received inadequate therapy for syphilis. It is important to note, however, that at this stage the symptoms are reversible with treatment. The frequency and the severity of neurologic involvement in secondary syphilis are greatly increased in patients with HIV infection [29].

Lesions of secondary syphilis result from the hematogenous dissemination of treponemes from syphilitic chancres. Secondary-stage lesions generally appear 4–10 weeks after the initial appearance of primary lesions.

Malignant syphilis (lues maligna), wherein disseminated lesions resemble primary chancres, is rare. HIV infections have often been identified as host factors that contribute to this unusual manifestation of syphilis [29, 54].

The initial finding in disseminated syphilis (secondary syphilis) is a macular rash that is often overlooked. A few days later, a symmetric papular eruption appears, involving the entire trunk and the extremities, including the palms of the hands and the soles of the feet. They are generally scaly, although they may be smooth, follicular, or rarely, pustular. Mucosal lesions are also quite common and characteristic of secondary syphilis. Alopecia also occurs in untreated cases, reflecting involvement of hair follicles.

Concurrent with the appearance of secondary lesions, about 10% of patients develop condylomata lata. These enlarged lesions, appearing in warm and moist areas including the perineum and anus, are highly infectious. Localized inflammation of the oral cavity, tongue, and genital mucous membranes can cause mucous patches [2].

A detailed description of secondary syphilis can be found in the review by Baughn and Musher [2]. Sore throat, muscle aches, malaise, and weight loss are examples of variable systemic symptoms of secondary syphilis. Generalized nontender lymphadenopathy occurs in up to 85% of cases.

Infrequently, secondary syphilis can be accompanied by gastric and renal involvement and hepatitis [2]. *T. pallidum* has been found in liver biopsy samples taken from patients with secondary syphilis while glomerulonephritis resulting from immunoglobulin–treponeme antigen complexes deposited in the glomeruli appears to cause kidney damage [13, 33, 47]. Nephrosis syndrome may also be present.

11.3.3 Latent Syphilis

The clinical manifestations of secondary syphilis resolve within 3 months – even in untreated patients; seropositivity, however, persists. The subsequent stage of "latent syphilis" can be divided into the two periods of early and late latent syphilis. The transition between the early and the late latent period is continuous, during which infected but untreated patients are symptom-free for a longer or shorter period. By this time, the characteristic, granulomatous immune reaction has evolved gradually in the host – it is intended to surround and isolate invading pathogens (demarcation).

During the period of early latency (lasting 12–18 months after the infection), the typical symptoms of secondary syphilis may recur in approximately 25% of cases [19]. Changes occurring in host defenses against *T. pallidum* are reflected also by the characteristics of symptoms. Compared to the symptoms seen in the secondary period, recent skin manifestations decrease in numbers, skin lesions emerge in groups, and individual lesions become larger as well as assume a distinctive appearance (syphilis corymbiformis) occasionally. Histological evaluation of these lesions reveals tissue components typical of tertiary syphilis already. Previously, this stage was identified as the "transitional" period.

The patient may be still infective during the early latent stage. Untreated syphilis is considered communicable for 2 years after the infection.

Late in the latent stage of syphilis, clinical manifestations are lacking, but serological tests are still positive; however, the intensity of serological reactions decreases gradually. This holds true for lipid tests only; the *Treponema* immobilization test (TIT) yields consistently positive results.

The pathogen may occasionally persist in the bloodstream, although in small numbers, and can cause vertical infection (transmission from the mother to the fetus), but this occurs only infrequently [61]. At this stage, the infection is no longer communicable by sexual intercourse. Owing to the safe contemporary practices for handling blood products, the transfusion of donor blood drawn during this stage carries no risk.

The onset of the manifestations of the late tertiary stage heralds the end of late latent syphilis.

11.3.4 Tertiary Syphilis

Fortunately, opportunities for studying the symptoms of tertiary syphilis are extremely uncommon nowadays. Introduced during the middle of the last century, penicillin therapy has proven unequivocally successful; it prevents the evolution of symptoms effectively and regardless of the stage of the infection. During retrospective studies conducted in the pre-antibiotic era, the manifestations of late syphilis were observed in approximately one-third of infected patients; these symptoms appeared 15–30 years after the infection. Within the tissues, *T. pallidum* is present in smaller numbers and isolated by a granulomatous tissue reaction – accordingly, the pathogen interferes with certain functions.

The patient is noninfective; *T. pallidum* is not detectable in the blood and body fluids. The clinical symptoms result from various forms of dysfunction, corresponding to the location of the granulomatous reaction launched by the host in defense against the pathogen.

Skin manifestations are the earliest symptoms of tertiary syphilis. Infrequently, these may occur as early as during the fourth year after the infection; however, appearance beyond a decade is more usual. Skin lesions evolve in approximately 15% of untreated patients: cutaneous nodules and syphilitic gummas in the subcutis and deeper tissues are benign lesions, unless their destructive effect involves vital organs. Therefore, this stage is reasonably termed as "late benign syphilis."

Cardiovascular manifestations occur within 10–15 years of the infection. The most typical lesion is granulomatous inflammation of the tunica media of the ascending aorta. This syphilitic aortitis follows a symptom-free course in the majority of patients. The proportion of symptomatic patients – afflicted by the consequences of aortic valve insufficiency, stenosis of coronary ostia, and dissecting aortic aneurysm – is as low as 10%. Before the introduction of penicillin therapy, these complications were fatal in syphilitic patients [56].

The third cluster of symptoms comprises late neurological manifestations. Meningeal-vascular syphilis with personality changes and dizziness may evolve 8–10 years after the infection. Later, these are accompanied by focal symptoms, corresponding to the localization of the small arteries involved. A prerequisite to the appearance of these symptoms is previous invasion of the CNS by *T. pallidum*, during the early stage of the disease.

"Late parenchymatous syphilis" is the last to evolve. The typical symptoms (paresis, severe personality changes, memory impairment, and hallucinations) occur 20–30 years after the initial infection. Involvement of the spinal cord causes tabes dorsalis, characterized by sensory ataxia in the lower extremities, accompanied by gastric pain and paroxysms of vomiting. The clinical picture is supplemented by optic nerve injury in 10–15% of cases [65].

Take-Home Pearls

- The *T. pallidum* Genome Sequencing Project also confirmed what had already been suggested by ongoing experimental efforts; this bacterium is a fastidious, microaerophilic, obligate parasite of humans.
- *Treponema pallidum* subsp. *pallidum* has been called a "stealth pathogen" because of its remarkable aptitude to evade the humoral and cellular immune responses in the infected host. Evidence indicates that the immuno-evasiveness of this bacterium is largely the result of its unusual molecular structure; the *T. pallidum* outer membrane (OM) contains a paucity of poorly immunogenic transmembrane proteins, its highly immunogenic proteins are lipoproteins anchored predominantly to the periplasmic leaflet of the cytoplasmic membrane.
- There is no efficient vaccine.
- The course of untreated syphilis consists of intermittent stages with sequential symptomatic and asymptomatic (latency) periods. This regular choreography, however, may be disturbed if the immunological competence of the host organism is severely compromised (HIV-infection), or by inappropriately administered prevention or antimicrobial therapy for another disease.

References

1. Baker-Zander, S.A., Hook III, E.W., Bonin, P., Handsfield, H.H., Lukehart, S.A.: Antigens of *Treponema pallidum* recognized by IgG and IgM antibodies during syphilis in humans. J. Infect. Dis. **151**, 264–272 (1985)
2. Baughn, R.E., Musher, D.M.: Secondary syphilitic lesions. Clin. Microbiol. Rev. **18**, 205–216 (2005)
3. Bauer, T.J., Price, E.V., Cutler, J.C.: Spinal fluid examinations among patients with primary or secondary syphilis. Am. J. Syph. **36**, 309–318 (1952)
4. Benoit, S., Posey, J.E., Chenoweth, M.R., Gherardini, F.C.: *Treponema pallidum* 3-phosphoglycerate mutase is a heat-labile enzyme that may limit the maximum growth temperature for the spirochete. J. Bacteriol. **183**, 4702–4708 (2001)
5. Blanco, D.R., Champion, C.I., Miller, J.N., Lovett, M.A.: Antigenic and structural characterization of *Treponema pallidum* (Nichols strain) endoflagella. Infect. Immun. **56**, 168–175 (1988)
6. Blanco, D.R., Champion, C.I., Exner, M.M., Shang, E.S., Skare, J.T., Hancock, R.E., Miller, J.N., Lovett, M.A.: Recombinant *Treponema pallidum* rare outer membrane protein 1 (Tromp1) expressed in *Escherichia coli* has porin activity and surface antigenic exposure. J. Bacteriol. **178**, 6685–6692 (1996)
7. Bos, J.D., Hamerlinck, F., Cormane, R.H.: Immunoglobulin-bearing polymorphonuclear leucocytes in primary syphilis. Br. J. Vener. Dis. **56**, 218–220 (1980)
8. Centurion-Lara, A., Castro, C., Castillo, R., Shaffer, J.M., Van Voorhis, W.C., Lukehart, S.A.: The flanking region sequences of the 15-kDa lipoprotein gene differentiate pathogenic treponemes. J. Infect. Dis. **177**, 1036–1040 (1998)
9. Cox, D.L., Chang, P., McDowall, A.W., Radolf, J.D.: The outer membrane, not a coat of host proteins, limits antigenicity of virulent *Treponema pallidum*. Infect. Immun. **60**, 1076–1083 (1992)
10. Cumberland, M.C., Turner, T.B.: The rate of mutiplicatio of *Treponema pallidum* in normal and immune rabbits. Am.J.Syph. Gonorrhea Vener. Dis. **33**, 201 (1949)
11. Deka, R.K., Lee, Y.H., Hagman, K.E., Shevchenko, D., Lingwood, C.A., Hasemann, C.A., Norgard, M.V., Radolf, J.D.: Physicochemical evidence that *Treponema pallidum* TroA is a zinc-containing metalloprotein that lacks porin-like structure. J. Bacteriol. **181**, 4420–4423 (1999)
12. Deka, R.K., Neil, L., Hagman, K.E., Machius, M., Tomchick, D.R., Brautigam, C.A., Norgard, M.V.: Structural evidence that the 32-kilodalton lipoprotein (Tp32) of Treponema pallidum is an L-methionine-binding protein. J. Biol. Chem. **279**, 55644–55650 (2004)
13. Feher, J., Somogyi, T., Timmer, M., Jozsa, L.: Early syphilitic hepatitis. Lancet **ii**, 896–899 (1975)
14. Fieldsteel, A.H., et al.: Cultivation of virulent *Treponema pallidum* in tissue culture. Infect. Immun. **32**, 908 (1981)
15. Fieldsteel, A.H.: Genetics. In: Schell, R.F., Musher, D.M. (eds.) Pathogenesis and Immunology of Treponemal Infection, pp. 39–54. Dekker, New York (1983)
16. Fitzgerald, T.J., Johnson, R.C., Miller, J.N., Sykes, J.A.: Characterization of the attachment of *Treponema pallidum* (Nichols strain) to cultured mammalian cells and the potential relationship of attachment to pathogenicity. Infect. Immun. **18**, 467–478 (1977)
17. Fitzgerald, T.J., Repesh, L.A., Oakes, S.G.: Morphological destruction of cultured cells by the attachment of *Treponema pallidum*. Br. J. Vener. Dis. **58**, 1–11 (1982). 104
18. Fraser, C.M., Norris, S.J., Weinstock, G.M., White, O., Sutton, G.G., Dodson, R., Gwinn, M., Hickey, E.K., Clayton, R., Ketchum, K.A., Sodergren, E., Hardham, J.M., McLeod, M.P., Salzberg, S., Peterson, J., Khalak, H., Richardson, D., Howell, J.K., Chidambaram, M., Utterback, T., McDonald, L., Artiach, P., Bowman, C., Cotton, M.D., Fujii, C., Garland, S., Hatch, B., Horst, K., Roberts, K., Sandusky, M., Weidman, J., Smith, H.O., Venter, J.C.: Complete genome sequence of Treponema *pallidum*, the syphilis spirochete. Science **281**(5375), 324–325 (1998)
19. Gjestland T.: The Oslo study of untreated syphilis: an epidemiologic investigation of the natural course of syphilitic inection based on a restudy of the Boeck-Bruusgaard material. Acta. Derm. Venereal **35**(I Suppl [Stockh]34):1 (1955)
20. Greene, S.R., Stamm, L.V., Hardham, J.M., Young, N.R., Frye, J.G.: Identification, sequences, and expression of *Treponema pallidum* chemotaxis genes. DNA Seq. **7**, 267–284 (1997)

21. Greene, S.R., Stamm, L.V.: Molecular characterization of *Treponema pallidum mcp2*, a putative chemotaxis protein gene. Infect. Immun. **66**, 2999–3002 (1998)
22. Hagman, K.E., Porcella, S.F., Popova, T.G., Norgard, M.V.: Evidence for a methyl-accepting chemotaxis protein gene (*mcp1*) that encodes a putative sensory transducer in virulent *Treponema pallidum*. Infect. Immun. **65**, 1701–1709 (1997)
23. Hazlett, K.R., Cox, D.L., Sikkink, R.A., Auch'ere, F., Rusnak, F., Radolf, J.D.: Contribution of neelaredoxin to oxygen tolerance by *Treponema pallidum*. Methods Enzymol. **353**, 140–156 (2002)
24. Hazlett, K.R., Rusnak, F., Kehres, D.G., Bearden, S.W., La Vake, C.J., La Vake, M.E., Maguire, M.E., Perry, R.D., Radolf, J.D.: The *Treponema pallidum tro* operon encodes a multiple metal transporter, a zinc-dependent transcriptional repressor, and a semi-autonomously expressed phosphoglycerate mutase. J. Biol. Chem. **278**, 20687–20694 (2003)
25. Hayes, N.S., Muse, K.E., Collier, A.M., Baseman, J.B.: Parasitism by virulent *reponema pallidum* of host cell surfaces. Infect. Immun. **17**, 174–186 (1977)
26. Jenkin, H.: Cultivation of treponemes. In: Schell, R.F., Musher, D.M. (eds.) Pathogenesis and Immunology of Treponemal Infection. Dekker, New York (1982)
27. Jepsen, O.B., Hougen, K.H., Birch-Andersen, A.: Electron microscopy of *Treponema pallidum* Nichols. Acta Pathol. Microbiol. Scand. **74**, 241–258 (1968)
28. Jones, S.A., Marchitto, K.S., Miller, J.N., Norgard, M.V.: Monoclonal antibody with hemagglutination, immobilization, and neutralization activities defines an immunodominant, 47, 000 mol wt, surface-exposed immunogen of Treponema pallidum (Nichols). J. Exp. Med. **160**, 1404–1420 (1984)
29. Kumar, B., Muralidhar, S.: Malignant syphilis: a review. AIDS Patient Care STDs **12**, 921–925 (1998)
30. La Fond, R.E., Lukehart, S.A.: Biological Basis of Syphilis. Clin. Microbiol. Rev. **19**, 29–49 (2006)
31. Lee, K.H., Choi, H.J., Lee, M.G., Lee, J.B.: Virulent *Treponema pallidum* 47 kDa antigen regulates the expression of cell adhesion molecules and binding of T-lymphocytes to cultured human dermal microvascular endothelial cells. Yonsei Med. J. **41**, 623–633 (2000)
32. Lee, J.H., Choi, H.J., Jung, J., Lee, M.G., Lee, J.B., Lee, K.H.: Receptors for *Treponema pallidum* attachment to the surface and matrix proteins of cultured human dermal microvascular endothelial cells. Yonsei Med. J. **44**, 371–378 (2003)
33. Lee, R.V., Thornton, G.F., Conn, H.O.: Liver disease associated with secondary syphilis. N Engl J. Med. **284**, 1423–1425 (1971)
34. Lien, E., Sellati, T.J., Yoshimura, A., Flo, T.H., Rawadi, G., Finberg, R.W., Carroll, J.D., Espevik, T., Ingalls, R.R., Radolf, J.D., Golenbock, D.T.: Toll-like receptor 2 functions as a pattern recognition receptor for diverse bacterial products. J. Biol. Chem. **274**, 33419–33425 (1999)
35. Lukehart, S.A., Hook III, E.W., Baker-Zander, S.A., Collier, A.C., Critchlow, C.W., Handsfield, H.H.: Invasion of the central nervous system by *Treponema pallidum*: implications for diagnosis and treatment. Ann. Intern. Med. **109**, 855–862 (1988)
36. Magnuson, H.J., Eagle, H., Fleischmann, R.: The minimal infectious inoculum of *Spirochaeta pallida* (Nichols strain), and a consideration of its rate of multiplication in vivo. Am. J. Syph. Gonorrhea Vener. Dis. **32**, 1–18 (1948)
37. Magnuson, H.J., Thomas, E.W., Olansky, S., Kaplan, B.I., DeMello, L., Cutler, J.C.: Inoculation syphilis in human volunteers. Medicine **35**, 33–82 (1956)
38. Mahoney, J.F., Bryant, K.K.: The time element in the penetration of the genital mucosa of the rabbit by the *Treponema pallidum*. J. Vener. Dis. Inf. **15**, 1–5 (1934)
39. Maio, R.M., Fieldsteel, A.H.: Genetic relationship between *Treponema pallidum* and *Treponema pertenue*, two noncultivable human pathogens. J. Bacteriol. **141**, 427–429 (1980)
40. Marra, C.M., Maxwell, C.L., Smith, S.L., Lukehart, S.A., Rompalo, A.M., Eaton, M., Stoner, B.P., Augenbraun, M., Barker, D.E., Corbett, J.J., Zajackowski, M., Raines, C., Nerad, J., Kee, R., Barnett, S.H.: Cerebrospinal fluid abnormalities in patients with syphilis: association with clinical and laboratory features. J. Infect. Dis. **189**, 369–376 (2004)
41. Mascola, L., Pelosi, R., Blount, J.H., Alexander, C.E., Cates Jr., W.: Congenital syphilis revisited. Am. J. Dis. Child. **139**, 575–580 (1985)
42. Metzger, M., Hardy Jr., P.H., Nell, E.E.: Influence of lysozyme upon the treponeme immobilization reaction. Am. J. Hyg. **73**, 236–244 (1961)
43. Mullick, C.J., Liappis, A.P., Benator, D.A., Roberts, A.D., Parenti, D.M., Simon, G.L.: Syphilitic hepatitis in HIV-infected patients: a report of 7 cases and review of the literature. Clin. Infect. Dis. **39**, 100–105 (2004)
44. Nichols, H.J., Hough, W.H.: Demonstration of *Spirochaeta pallida* in the cerebrospinal fluid. JAMA **60**, 108 (1913)
45. Nichols, J.C., Baseman, J.B.: Carbon sources utilized by virulent *Treponema pallidum*. Infect. Immun. **12**, 1044–1050 (1975)
46. Norris, S.J., Sell, S.: Antigenic complexity of *Treponema pallidum*: antigenicity and surface localization of major polypeptides. J. Immunol. **133**, 2686–2692 (1984)
47. O'Regan, S., Fong, J.S., de Chadarevian, J.P., Rishikof, J.R., Drummond, K.N.: Treponemal antigens in congenital and acquired syphilitic nephritis: demonstration by immunofluorescence studies. Ann. Intern. Med. **85**, 325–327 (1976)
48. Penn, C.W., Rhodes, J.G.: Surface-associated antigens of *Treponema pallidum* concealed by an inert outer layer. Immunology **46**, 9–16 (1982)
49. Purcell, B.K., Chamberlain, N.R., Goldberg, M.S., Andrews, L.P., Robinson, E.J., Norgard, M.V., Radolf, J.D.: Molecular cloning and characterization of the 15-kilodalton major immunogen of *Treponema pallidum*. Infect. Immun. **57**, 3708–3714 (1989)
50. Radolf, J.D., Norgard, M.V., Schulz, W.W.: Outer membrane ultrastructure explains the limited antigenicity of virulent *Treponema pallidum*. Proc. Natl Acad. Sci. USA **86**, 2051–2055 (1989)
51. Ricord, P.: A Practical Treatise on Venereal Diseases. Rouvier et le Bouvier, Paris (1838)
52. Riley, B.S., Oppenheimer-Marks, N., Hansen, E.J., Radolf, J.D., Norgard, M.V.: Virulent *Treponema pallidum* activates human vascular endothelial cells. J. Infect. Dis. **165**, 484–493 (1992)
53. Riley, B.S., Oppenheimer-Marks, N., Radolf, J.D., Norgard, M.V.: Virulent *Treponema pallidum* promotes adhesion of leukocytes to human vascular endothelial cells. Infect. Immun. **62**, 4622–4625 (1994)

54. Romero-Jimenez, M.J., Suarez, L.I., Fajardo, P.J.M., Baron, F.B.: Malignant syphilis in patient with human immunodeficiency virus (HIV); case report and literature review. Ann. Med. Intern. **20**, 373–376 (2003)
55. Rompalo, A.M., Joesoef, M.R., O'Donnell, J.A., Augenbraun, M., Brady, W., Radolf, J.D., Johnson, R., Rolfs, R.T.: Clinical manifestations of early syphilis by HIV status and gender: results of the syphilis and HIV study. Sex. Transm. Dis. **28**, 158–165 (2001)
56. Rosahn, P.D.: Autopsy studies in syphilis. J. Vener. Dis. Inf. **649**, 1–67 (1947)
57. Salazar, J.C., Hazlett, K.R., Radolf, J.D.: The immune response to infection with *Treponema pallidum*, the stealth pathogen. Microbes Infect. **4**, 1133–1140 (2002)
58. Schaudinn, F.N.: Vorlaufiger bericht über das vorkommen von spirochaeten in syphilitischen krankheitsprodukten und bei papillomen. Arbeiten K. Gesundheits **22**, 527–534 (1905)
59. Schouls, L.M.: Recombinant DNA technology in syphilis research. In: Wright, D.J.M., Archard, L. (eds.) Molecular Biology of Sexually Transmitted Diseases. Chapman & Hall, London (1992)
60. Schroeter, A.L., Turner, R.H., Lucas, J.B., Brown, W.J.: Therapy for incubating syphilis. Effectiveness of gonorrhea treatment. JAMA **218**, 711–713 (1971)
61. Sheffield, J.S., Sanchez, P.J., Morris, G., Maberry, M., Zeray, F., McIntire, D.D., and Wendel Jr., G.D.: Congenital syphilis after maternal treatment for syphilis during pregnancy. Am. J. Obstet. Gynecol. **186**, 569–573 (2002)
62. Smibert, R.M.: Genus III: *Treponema* Schaudinn 1905, 1728AL. In: Kreig, N.R., Holt, J.G. (eds.) Bergey's Manual of Systematic Bacteriology, vol. 1, pp. 49–57. Williams & Wilkins, Baltimore (1984)
63. van der Sluis, J.J., Koehorst, J.A., Boer, A.M.: Factors that inhibit adherence of *Treponema pallidum* (Nichols strain) to a human fibroblastic cell line: development in serum of patients with syphilis. Genitourin. Med. **63**, 71–76 (1987)
64. Stamm, L.V., Hodinka, R.L., Wyrick, P.B., Bassford Jr., P.J.: Changes in the cell surface properties of *Treponema pallidum* that occur during in vitro incubation of freshly extracted organisms. Infect. Immun. **55**, 2255–2261 (1987)
65. Stamm, L.V., Gherardini, F.C., Parrish, E.A., Moomaw, C.R.: Heat shock response of spirochetes. Infect. Immun. **59**, 1572–1575 (1991)
66. Strugnell, R., Cockayne, A., Penn, C.W.: Molecular and antigenic analysis of treponemes. Crit. Rev. Microbiol. **17**, 231–250 (1990)
67. Swancutt, M.A., Riley, B.S., Radolf, J.D., Norgard, M.V.: Molecular characterization of the pathogen-specific, 34-kilodalton membrane immunogen of *Treponema pallidum*. Infect. Immun. **57**, 3314–3323 (1989)
68. Thomas, D.D., Navab, M., Haake, D.A., Fogelman, A.M., Miller, J.N., Lovett, M.A.: *Treponema pallidum* invades intercellular junctions of endothelial cell monolayers. Proc. Natl Acad. Sci. USA **85**, 3608–3612 (1988)
69. Wagner von Jauregg, J.: Uber die Einwirkung der Malaria auf die progressive Paralyse. Psychiatr. Neurol. Wochenschr. **20**, 132 (1918)
70. Walker, E.M., Zampighi, G.A., Blanco, D.R., Miller, J.N., Lovett, M.A.: Demonstration of rare protein in the outer membrane of *Treponema pallidum* susp. Pallidum by freez-fracture analysis. J. Bacteriol. **171**, 5005–5011 (1989)
71. Zhang, Z., Feige, J.N., Chang, A.B., Anderson, I.J., Brodianski, V.M., Vitreschak, A.G., Gelfand, M.S., Saier Jr., M.H.: A transporter of *Escherichia coli* specific for L- and D-methionine is the prototype for a new family within the ABC superfamily. Arch. Microbiol. **180**, 88–100 (2003)

Laboratory Diagnosis of Syphilis

12

H.-J. Hagedorn

Core Messages

- Dark field microscopy (DFM) is the only test that allows immediate diagnosis, treatment, and partner notification, thereby preventing further transmission.
- A highly positive IgM titer indicates, independently from the value of IgG or TPHA titer, an active infection and the need for treatment. A low IgM titer, in combination with a high IgG or TPHA titer, is consistent with a latent or chronic treponemal infection. A negative IgM test, in combination with a high positive IgG or TPHA titer and a positive nontreponemal test, is consistent with an active infection as well.
- A reinfection and endogenous reactivation cannot be differentiated by serological methods.
- However, the posttherapeutic kinetics of the lipid antibodies and analogous of the specific IgM antibodies can be very variable. The longer the time interval between infection and start of treatment, the slower is the decline of the antibody titers.
- Therefore, for safety reasons it is recommended to treat pregnant women with an uncertain anamnesis according to the course of infection and/or adequate therapy, especially if the treponema IgG titers are high, e.g., the TPHA titer is ≥1:5.000 and/or the nontreponemal test is positive.
- In order to assess the relevance of treponemal and lipid antibody findings in the serum of the newborn, it is necessary to test serum samples from the mother and the newborn in parallel using quantitative methods.
- The detection of an intrathecal IgG antibody synthesis does not imply the diagnosis of active neurosyphilis since it remains detectable for years, and in many patients for life, even after adequate therapy. For assessment of disease activity, nonspecific parameters such as pleocytosis with predominant lymphocytes, total CSF protein, and the function of the blood–cerebrospinal fluid (CSF) barrier must be considered.
- Due to the variety of clinical symptoms and the long-lasting asymptomatic periods during the course of the disease, laboratory tests, in particular serological tests, are very important for the confirmation and/or exclusion of syphilis. Methods for the direct visualization of the causative pathogen *Treponema pallidum* subsp. *pallidum*, mostly by dark field examination from exudates of lesions are very helpful for the correct diagnosis of the early seronegative stage of primary syphilis. In addition, histology, immunohistochemistry, and DNA amplification techniques can be used for the differential diagnosis of atypical skin and tissue manifestations.

H.-J. Hagedorn
Department of Clinical Microbiology and Immunology,
Labor Krone, Siemensstr. 40, D-32105 Bad Salzuflen,
Germany
e-mail: hagedorn@laborkrone.de

G. Gross and S.K. Tyring (eds.), *Sexually Transmitted Infections and Sexually Transmitted Diseases*,
DOI: 10.1007/978-3-642-14663-3_12,

12.1 Direct Detection of *T. pallidum*

Specimen collection. Specimens collected from active epidermal and mucosal lesions of primary, secondary, and early congenital syphilis are most useful. Moist lesions (e.g., chancres, condylomata lata, or mucous patches) tend to contain high concentration of treponemes. A suspected syphilitic lesion should be cleansed with saline using a gauze swab, dried and abraded with a dry gauze swab. Clear serous fluid free of erythrocytes should be squeezed and material collected using a sterile bacteriological loop. For dark field microscopy (DFM) material has to be transferred to a glass slide and covered immediately with a coverslip; for examination by direct immunofluorescence assay (DFA) the material on the glass slide has to be air-dried.

Skin biopsies and tissue specimens for histology and demonstration of treponemes by silver staining methods or immunohistochemistry should be fixed in a formaldehyde solution and later paraffin embedded. Examination of 2–4 μm thick sections of the fixed, embedded material is recommended [1–3]. For polymerase chain reaction (PCR) testing untreated fresh or snap-frozen biopsy samples is preferred [4]. But PCR can also be performed from the formaldehyde-fixed paraffin-embedded sections [4, 5].

Dark field microscopy (DFM). The sample should be examined immediately with a dark field microscope using a 400× magnification for the presence of mobile treponemes. The detection limit is ca. 1×10^5 organisms/mL [6]. The technique should be restricted to experienced persons, since the differentiation between *T. pallidum* and treponemes commonly occurring on mucous membranes, e.g., *Treponema denticola*, is not always easy. The test is not recommended for samples from the oral cavity. The sensitivity and specificity of DFM approaches are 80–95% and 77–100%, respectively, depending on the preselection of cases investigated in different studies [3, 7–12]. Furthermore, DFM is the only test that allows immediate diagnosis, treatment, and partner notification, thereby preventing further transmission [6].

Direct immunofluorescence assay (DFA). The air-dried samples or tissue sections on slides are coated with monoclonal fluorescein isothiocyanate (FITC)-conjugated antibodies to *T. pallidum*. The appearance of green treponemes in the fluorescence microscope at a wavelength of 480 nm is specific for *T. pallidum*.

The DFA has sensitivity and specificity that are comparable to that of DFM. The technique is more time-consuming and cannot be performed on site but can be used if a direct examination by DFM is not realizable. The main advantage is the possibility to examine materials potentially contaminated with other saprophytic treponemes, e.g., from the oral cavity or the intestinum [3, 7, 9, 11, 12].

Rabbit infectivity testing (RIT). Efforts to cultivate *T. pallidum* in vitro have been largely unsuccessful. The pathogen is readily cultivated by animal inoculation. Any source of material can be used for inoculation of rabbits. The RIT is highly sensitive and theoretically able to detect a single viable organism. Therefore, the RIT is the gold standard for measuring the sensitivity of methods, such as the PCR. However, the RIT is expensive and requires 3–6 months to be completed. This method is impractical for routine clinical use and is restricted to special research units [3, 9, 11].

Nucleic acid amplification techniques (NAATs). The detection of *T. pallidum* using NAATs like the PCR is in principle possible from any material, e.g., blood, cerebrospinal fluid (CSF), swabs, punctates, tissue biopsies, and amniotic fluid [3, 8, 9, 13]. The PCR assays demonstrate specificity of 95–98% for pathogenic treponemes and can be used for oral and rectal samples as well. The detection limit is reported as low as 1–65 organisms. The sensitivity depends on the clinical samples investigated in different studies. Sensitivity of PCR is superior to microscopy and reaches up to 95% in primary syphilis and 80% in secondary syphilis [10]. In tissue fluids from neonates (amniotic fluid, neonatal sera, or CSF) the overall sensitivity was 78% in comparison to the RIT [9]. The introduction of PCR as an additional method for the examination of problem patients is under discussion.

Detection of *T. pallidum* in tissue sections. The traditional method for detecting spirochetes in tissue sections is through silver staining using either the Warthin-Starry technique or the more sensitive Dieterle staining method or the Steiner modification of the Dieterle technique [2, 5, 14]. Marked background artifacts are, thus, commonplace, as the silver stain also highlights melanin granules and reticulin fibers, making it difficult to visualize the organisms. In skin biopsies the detection rate of *T. pallidum* by silver staining methods varies from 33% to 71% [2]. Comparative studies demonstrate that the sensitivity of immunohistochemical staining of tissue sections using a polyclonal antitreponemal antibody is superior to the silver staining methods [1, 2, 5, 14]. PCR testing is at least as sensitive as immunohistochemistry for the detection of *T. pallidum* in formalin-fixed, paraffin-embedded skin biopsies or frozen tissue samples [4, 5, 15]. Therefore, if a treponemal infection is suspected from histological findings or clinical aspects silver staining is no longer recommended for testing tissue samples since immunohistochemistry and PCR are more sensitive and reliable methods for the detection of *T. pallidum*.

12.2 Serologic Tests

The serologic tests for syphilis can be divided into two groups: nontreponemal and treponemal. Both groups have distinctive characteristics and are used for different purposes. But the findings are complementary and for the final assessment of the sample status of an individual patient results from both test groups have to be taken into consideration.

Specimen collection. Serum is the specimen of choice for both nontreponemal and treponemal tests. For plasma samples the same tests can be used except for the Venereal Disease Research Laboratory (VDRL) test, because the sample has to be heated up to 56°C before this test is performed. CSF can be tested with all methods as well. If congenital syphilis is suspected, serum samples from the mother and the newborn should be used. Cord blood is not recommended [3, 8, 13].

Nontreponemal tests. Principle: quantitative detection of anti-lipid IgG and IgM antibodies by means of precipitation or complement fixation.

The tests use a tissue lipid, called cardiolipin, complexed with lecithin and cholesterol as antigen [3]. The lipid antigen is a component of the mitochondrial membrane of mammalian and plant cells as well as of the cell wall of treponemes. The origin of the anti-lipid antibodies in the patient's serum has not yet been elucidated. It is presumed that they represent immune reactions to products of inflammation-induced cellular destruction. The occurrence of these antibodies is characteristic of an active treponemal infection but is not a proof for a specific immune response [3, 8, 13].

The reference test is the VDRL. In this test the antigen is added to serial dilutions of heat-inactivated serum. In the presence of anti-lipid antibodies flocculation of the crystalline antigen ensues. The results are read under a microscope or a magnification mirror. Alternatively, the rapid plasma reagin (RPR) test is used often. The RPR antigen is a variation of the VDRL antigen containing charcoal microparticles to facilitate the reading of the results. In contrast to the VDRL there is no need for heat pretreatment of the samples and the test can be used for testing of serum as well as of plasma. The test is carried out on cards. The results are read macroscopically. The titer values are comparable to those of the VDRL test. The cardiolipin complement fixation (cardiolipin CF) test demonstrates a higher sensitivity than the VDRL and RPR tests, but is not often used because of the expenditure of the work [3, 8, 9, 16].

Anti-lipid antibodies occur 4–6 weeks post infection, reaching the maximum concentration during the second stage of the disease, and decline again during latency. After a successful treatment of syphilis, in most cases the nontreponemal test becomes nonreactive during a follow-up. False positive reactions are associated with different bacterial and viral infections, autoimmune diseases, and malignancies [3, 8, 9, 11, 13].

Treponemal tests. These tests detect specific antibodies against *T. pallidum* but cannot differentiate between syphilis and the nonvenereal treponematoses (Yaws, Bejel, Pinta), because the antigen structures of all these pathogens are almost identical.

Treponema pallidum hemagglutination assay (TPHA), Treponema pallidum particle agglutination assay (TPPA), Treponema pallidum latex agglutination assay (TPLA). Principle: indirect (hem- or particle-) agglutination. Ultrasonicated antigens or detergent extracts of *T. pallidum* (Nichols strain) are fixed on erythrocytes, gelatine, bentonite, or latex particles. In the presence of homologous antibodies a macroscopically recognizable agglutination occurs. Because TPHA and TPPA are comparable according to the qualitative and quantitative results, the term TPHA is used as a synonym for both tests in the following text.

The agglutination assays react with IgM and IgG antibodies simultaneously. They are able to detect specific antibodies from the third week post infection and in most cases remain positive lifelong, even after adequate antibiotic therapy. False positive results occur rarely. The clinical sensitivity of the tests is in the range of 96–99%. A quantification of the test results (titers or index values) is recommended [8, 9, 11, 13, 17].

Treponema pallidum enzyme-linked immunosorbent assay (ELISA). Principle: competitive antibody assay using detergent extract of *T. pallidum*, or indirect assays using a mixture of recombinant antigens from *T. pallidum*, e.g., the antigens tp15, tp17, and tp47 [18]. After incubation with the patient samples, human antibodies bound to the treponemal antigens are detected by enzyme-labeled anti-human antibodies. Different ELISA modifications allow the simultaneous qualitative determination of IgG and IgM antibodies (polyvalent ELISA) or the separate quantitative determination of IgG or IgM antibodies. The main advantage of the ELISA technology is the possibility of automatization and standardization of the test procedure. The sensitivity and specificity of polyvalent ELISA screening assays are generally comparable to that of agglutination assays, e.g., the TPHA [3, 8, 9, 13, 19].

Fluorescent treponema antibody absorption test (FTA-ABS). Principle: indirect immunofluorescence assay. Treponemes of the pathogenic Nichols strain are fixed on slides. The specificity of the test results is ensured by a 1:5 predilution of the patient's sample using a sorbent (extract of a culture from non-pathogenic *Treponema phagedenis*, Reiter strain), in order to remove cross-reacting treponemal antibodies. After incubation of the preabsorbed samples on the slides and washing steps in order to remove unbound material, antibodies attached to the surface of the test antigen will be detected by FITC-labeled antihuman antibodies. The assay simultaneously detects IgG and IgM antibodies. The results are usually expressed qualitatively as reactive, minimal reactive or borderline, nonreactive or atypical [9]. Using test modifications, a differentiated determination of IgG and IgM antibodies as well as a quantification of the results in titers is possible. The FTA-ABS assay converts from the beginning of the third week post infection. This test is considered as the most sensitive assay for the detection of treponemal antibodies in the earliest stage of the disease with a mean sensitivity of 84% (70–100%) in primary syphilis, whereas the sensitivity in later stages is >99%. The mean specificity of the assay is 97% (94–100%). The quality and reliability of FTA-ABS results depend on a consequent quality management of this multicomponent assay as well as the specific experience of the investigator. False positive test results are mostly observed in samples containing a high concentration of antibodies to *Borrelia burgdorferi* [3, 8, 9, 11, 13].

IgM fluorescent treponema antibody assay (19S-IgM-FTA or 19S-IgM-FTA-ABS test). Principle: demonstration of IgM treponema-specific antibodies by the FTA-ABS test procedure after separation of the IgM fraction of serum by ultracentrifugation, column chromatography, or nowadays in the routine laboratory mostly by pretreatment of the samples with an anti-IgG serum (RF absorbent). IgM antibodies can be detected by using a μ-chain-specific FITC-conjugated antiserum instead of a polyvalent antiserum [8].

The 19S-IgM-FTA-ABS test is the reference assay for the determination of treponeme-specific IgM antibodies. The specificity is close to 100%. The findings can be recorded quantitatively (titer). The sensitivity is high in all active stages of the disease, but a negative result does not rule out an active or persisting asymptomatic infection, especially in late latent syphilis, in the tertiary stage of syphilis, or in case of reinfection or reactivation. After adequate antibiotic treatment positive findings should return to negativity analogous to the lipoid antibody kinetics [8, 13, 16, 17]. A problem is the inadequate standardization of the test procedure as demonstrated by external quality control surveys in Germany [20].

T. pallidum immunoblot (Tp IB), T. pallidum line assay (Tp LIA). Principle: in case of immunoblot tests *T. pallidum* proteins are separated by sodium dodecyl sulfate (SDS) polyacrylamide gel electrophoresis (SDS-PAGE) and transferred to nitrocellulose stripes; in case of line assays purified antigens or recombinant antigens are sprayed on nitrocellulose stripes. The stripes are commercially available and can be used for the determination of IgG or IgM antibodies with appropriate enzyme-labeled antisera.

The nomenclature of the proteins of the Nichols *T. pallidum* subsp. *pallidum* reference strain separated by SDS-PAGE is well defined. It includes 16 proteins with a molecular mass of 190–15.5 kDa. For the Tp IB/Tp LIA only those with molecular masses of 47, 17, and 15.5 kDa are considered diagnostically significant because of their *T. pallidum* specificity [3]. In addition, further antigens like the less specific 44.5 kDa TmpA antigen are integrated in the tests of most manufacturers. The clinical specificity of the IgG and IgM blot tests is >99%. The IgG IB/LIA demonstrates a sensitivity of >99% in all stages of the infection except the very early primary syphilis. The reactivity with IgM antibodies is excellent in primary, secondary, and early latent syphilis. In chronic infections (late latency, stage III) and in case of reinfection the sensitivity of the 19S-IgM-FTA is superior to the IB/LIA [8, 9, 13, 17].

12.3 Standard Procedure for the Serodiagnosis of Syphilis

If syphilis is clinically suspected or a recent or past treponemal infection has to be ruled out for other reasons (e.g., blood donors, organ tissue donors, pregnancy, risk groups for sexually transmitted infection (STI)), a stepwise diagnostic approach is recommended [3, 8, 13, 16, 17, 19, 21]: first a treponemal screening assay has to be carried out. Useful for screening purposes are the TPHA/TPPA or assays with a comparable sensitivity, e.g., ELISA or TPLA. In case of a negative result there is no serological evidence for a recent or past treponemal infection, except a very early stage of infection prior to seroconversion. If acute syphilis is still suspected, the screening assay should be repeated after 1–2 weeks and if necessary more than once in 2-weekly intervals.

Positive, nonspecific, or undetermined findings of the screening assay have to be reexamined by a different treponemal test as a confirmatory test. The FTA-ABS is accepted worldwide for this purpose. Alternatively, the IgG-FTA-ABS test, the IgG-specific immunoblot, in case of a TPHA/TPPA screening the IgG ELISA, and vice versa in case of an ELISA screening the TPHA/TPPA can be used [19]. Demonstration of antibodies in the screening as well as in the confirmatory tests is accepted as a proof of the presence of treponemal antibodies in the sample but not as an indication of an active infection. Therefore, the next diagnostic step is to assess the probable disease activity and the need for specific therapy by the quantitative determination of lipoidal antibodies (VDRL, RPR, cardiolipin CF) and *T. pallidum*-specific IgM antibodies (19S-IgM-FTA, IgM ELISA, IgM IB/LIA). In untreated patients a positive nontreponemal and/or positive specific IgM antibody test are indications for antibiotic treatment [3, 8, 9, 13, 16, 17].

12.4 Interpretation of Serological Findings

All laboratory findings have to be interpreted in regard to the anamnesis of the patient including the course of infection, former therapy, and the actual clinical questioning.

Specific treponemal IgM antibodies can be detected as early as 2–3 weeks post infection. Lipoidal antibodies occur a little later and can be normally demonstrated after 4–6 weeks. The treponemal IgM antibodies and the nontreponemal antibodies reach the maximum concentrations during the second stage of syphilis and decline slowly afterward. In prolonged persisting infections the IgM titer can drop under the detection limit of the IgM assay, whereas nontreponemal antibodies still remain positive. Treponemal IgG antibodies appear only a few days after the specific IgM antibodies and reach the maximum titers during the secondary stage of syphilis as well. In untreated cases the IgG antibody titer remains at high level. In the routine laboratory the TPHA titer is often used for the interpretation of the results instead of the IgG titer, because in persisting infections with a low positive or negative IgM test, the reactivity of the screening assay is due to the IgG antibody concentration.

A high positive IgM titer indicates, independently from the value of IgG or TPHA titer, an active infection and the need for treatment. A low IgM titer, in combination with a high IgG or TPHA titer, is consistent with a latent or chronic treponemal infection. A negative IgM test, in combination with a high positive IgG or TPHA titer and a positive nontreponemal test, is consistent with an active infection as well.

A reinfection and endogenous reactivation cannot be differentiated by serological methods. The humoral immune response corresponds to IgG booster effect. Generally there is a strong increase of the IgG, the TPHA, and the lipoidal antibody titers, but the specific IgM antibody response is very variable and can remain negative, or turn delayed positive in comparison to the lipoidal antibodies or can show high titers from the beginning [8, 17].

12.5 Follow-Up of Antibody Kinetics After Treatment

Because antibody titers can increase during the course of antibiotic therapy, it is necessary to determine again the titers of the tests as reference level 2–4 weeks later. Thereafter the tests should be repeated in 3-month intervals during the first year [17]. Whether the observation period has to be extended for more than 1 year depends on the individual course of the posttherapeutic antibody kinetics. Irrespective of this, a continuous monitoring in risk groups (e.g., men who have sex with men (MSM)) has to be taken into consideration.

Generally it is sufficient to verify the success of the treatment by quantitative cardiolipin antibody tests. In addition, the monitoring of specific IgM antibodies can be used depending on the initial findings. At least a three- to fourfold decline of the nontreponemal antibody titer within 1 year is considered as indicative for a successful therapy. However, the posttherapeutic kinetics of the lipid antibodies and analogous of the specific IgM antibodies can be very variable. The longer the time interval between infection and start of treatment, the slower is the decline of the antibody titers. After treatment of a first illness episode of syphilis in the primary, secondary, or early latent stage the lipid and IgM antibodies reconvert to negativity often within few months, at the most within 2 years. On the other hand, after a treatment of late latent syphilis, tertiary syphilis, or a reinfection a very slow decline or even a persistence of the antibodies over years is possible. If during the observation period there is a rise of the lipid and/or specific IgM antibody titers, a treatment failure or a reinfection has to be considered [8, 9, 11, 17, 22].

The quantitative monitoring of the TPHA titer or a comparable quantitative screening assay is recommended as well. After treatment of a first infection with *T. pallidum* the TPHA titer declines continuously over the years or persists at low titer levels. If the antibiotic therapy was initiated very early during the course of the disease, a reconversion of treponemal tests to negativity can be observed in some cases as well [23]. After treatment of a reinfection the antibody titers of the TPHA and other treponemal tests persist due to the booster effect at a high positive level or decline very slowly over the years [8, 11, 22].

12.6 Syphilis Serology and Pregnancy

The diagnostic procedure and the interpretation of the laboratory findings are corresponding to the principles mentioned before. A positive specific IgM antibody test is usually an indication for therapy. It is important to be aware that a negative IgM test does not rule out an active or persistent syphilitic infection. In late latency there are often found strongly reacting screening assays, elevated lipid antibody titers but negative or not significant IgM findings. Therefore, for safety reasons it is recommended to treat pregnant women with an uncertain anamnesis according to the course of infection and/or adequate therapy, specially if the treponema IgG titers are high, e.g., the TPHA titer is ≥1:5.000 and/or the nontreponemal test is positive [21, 24].

12.7 Diagnosis of Congenital Syphilis

The diagnosis of congenital syphilis depends on a combination of physical, radiographic, serologic findings and efforts to demonstrate the pathogen directly. The diagnosis is proven when it is possible to identify *T. pallidum* by microscopy, PCR, or RIT in specimens from lesions, placenta, umbilical cord, plasma, CSF, or autopsy material [9, 11, 25].

In order to assess the relevance of treponemal and lipid antibody findings in the serum of the newborn, it is necessary to test serum samples from the mother and the newborn in parallel using quantitative methods. IgG antibodies from the mother can cross the placenta and can be detected in the serum of the child. These maternal antibodies are eliminated within a half-life of ca. 21 days [26]. Depending on the initial antibody titer, the syphilis tests in a noninfected child decline continuously and reconvert to negative within some months, at the latest during the first year of life. Indications for a congenital infection are positive IgM antibody findings using the 19S IgM-FTA-ABS test, IgM EIA, or IgM IB/LIA; demonstration of lipid IgM antibodies by immunoblot, in comparison to the mother's; higher antibody titers in the child; different patterns in immunoblots from mother and child; or persistence of antibodies during the first year of life. In addition (with no other cause), an elevated cell count or protein level in the CSF can be indicative as well [11, 13, 17, 25].

12.8 Diagnosis of Neurosyphilis

Because *T. pallidum* reaches all organs via hematogenous spread, neurosyphilis is not an isolated infection of the central nervous system (CNS). Therefore, a negative treponemal screening test in the serum is sufficient for excluding this condition. To confirm CNS involvement, however, concurrent examination of serum and CSF samples obtained on the same day is mandatory. The most important diagnostic criterion is the demonstration of a local specific antibody synthesis within the CNS [8, 13, 17, 27, 28]. A precise analysis of whether *T. pallidum*-specific antibodies in the CSF originated in the serum or the CNS can be done easily by calculation of the ITpA-index [8, 27, 28]:

$$\text{ITpA - index} = \frac{\text{TPHA - titer (CSF)}}{\text{Total IgG (CSF)}} \times \frac{\text{Total IgG (serum)}}{\text{TPHA - titer (serum)}}$$

If the antibodies in the CSF have been derived from the serum the index reveals a ratio of 0.5–2.0. Index values in the range >2–3 are classified as equivocal and no valid conclusion can be deducted from the findings. In case of a local synthesis of treponemal antibodies this value increases to >3.0, supporting the diagnosis of a recent or a former treponemal CNS infection. The detection of an intrathecal IgG antibody synthesis does not imply the diagnosis of active neurosyphilis since it remains detectable for years, and in many patients for life, even after adequate therapy [27, 29]. For assessment of disease activity, nonspecific parameters such as pleocytosis predominantly with lymphocytes, total CSF protein and the function of the blood–CSF barrier must be considered [9, 11, 30, 31]. In addition, the demonstration of lipoidal and/or specific IgM antibodies within the CSF supports the diagnosis of an active CNS infection. In the early stage of CNS involvement during secondary syphilis the serologic CSF findings can be very discrete or normal, whereas nonspecific signs of inflammation can be observed or a direct detection of the pathogen by PCR or RIT is possible [9, 11, 31].

Take-Home Pearls

- The method of choice for the laboratory diagnosis of syphilis is the demonstration of antibodies using a stepwise diagnostic approach consisting of a screening assay, a confirmatory test, and methods for the assessment of the probable disease activity and the need for specific therapy.
- All laboratory findings have to be interpreted in regard to the anamnesis of the patient including the course of infection, former therapy, and the actual clinical questioning.
- Because specific antibodies persist lifelong even after adequate therapy of syphilis in most cases, a reactive treponema antibody assay alone is no proof for the need of antibiotic treatment.

References

1. Engelkens, H.J.H., ten Kate, F.J.W., Judanarso, J., Vuzevski, V.D., van Lier, J.B.H.J., Godschalk, J.C.J., van der Sluis, J.J., Stolz, E.: The localisation of treponema and characterisation of the inflammatory infiltrate in skin biopsies from patients with primary or secondary syphilis, or early infectious yaws. Genitourin. Med. **69**, 102–107 (1993)
2. Hoang, M.P., High, W.A., Molberg, K.H.: Secondary syphilis: a histologic and immunohistochemical evaluation. J. Cutan. Pathol. **31**, 595–599 (2004)
3. Norris, S.J., Pope, V., Johnson, R.E., Larsen, S.A.: *Treponema* and other human host-associated spirochetes. In: Murray, P.R., Baron, E.J., Jorgensen, J.H., Pfaller, M.A., Yolken, R.H. (eds.) Manual of clinical microbiology, 8th edn, pp. 955–971. ASM, Washington, D.C. (2003)
4. Buffet, M., Grange, P.A., Gerhardt, P., Carlotti, A., Calvez, V., Bianchi, A., Dupin, N.: Diagnosing *Treponema pallidum* in secondary syphilis by PCR and immunohistochemistry. J. Invest. Dermatol. **127**, 2345–2350 (2007)
5. Behrhof, W., Springer, E., Bräuninger, W., Kirkpatrick, C.J., Weber, A.: PCR testing for *Treponema pallidum* in paraffin-embedded skin biopsy specimens: test design and impact on the diagnosis of syphilis. J. Clin. Pathol. **61**, 390–395 (2008)
6. Lautenschlager, S.: Cutaneous manifestations of syphilis. Am. J. Clin. Dermatol. **7**, 291–304 (2006)
7. Cummings, M.C., Lukehart, S.A., Marra, C., Smith, B.L., Shaffer, J., Demeo, L., Castro, C., McCormack, W.M.: Comparison of methods for the detection of *Treponema pallidum* in lesions of early syphilis. Sex. Transm. Dis. **23**, 366–369 (1996)
8. Hagedorn, H.-J., Müller, F.: Syphilis. In: Thomas, L. (ed.) Labor und Diagnose, 6th edn, pp. 1629–1638. TH-Books, Frankfurt/Main (2005)
9. Larsen, S.A., Steiner, B.M., Rudolph, A.H.: Laboratory diagnosis and interpretation of tests for syphilis. Clin. Microbiol. Rev. **8**, 1–21 (1995)
10. Palmer, H.M., Higgins, S.P., Herrig, A.J., Kingston, M.A.: Use of PCR in the diagnosis of early syphilis in the United Kingdom. Sex. Transm. Infect. **79**, 479–483 (2003)
11. Singh, A.E., Romanowski, B.: Syphilis: review with emphasis on clinical, epidemiologic, and some biologic features. Clin. Microbiol. Rev. **12**, 187–209 (1999)
12. Wheeler, H.L., Agarwal, S., Goh, B.T.: Dark ground microscopy and treponemal serological tests in the diagnosis of early syphilis. Sex. Transm. Infect. **80**, 411–414 (2004)
13. Hagedorn, H.-J.: Syphilis. In: Mauch, H., Lütticken, R. (eds.) Qualitätsstandards in der mikrobiologisch-infektiologischen Diagostik. Urban & Schwarzenberg, München **16**, 1–39 in Hagedom (2001)
14. Anemüller, W., Bräuninger, W., Krahl, D., Turzynski, A., Rose, C.: Primäraffekt am Finger unter dem Bild einer chronischen Paronychie. Hautarzt **59**, 499–502 (2008)
15. Zoechling, N., Schluepen, E.M., Soyer, H.P., Kerl, H., Volkenandt, M.: Molecular detection of *Treponema pallidum* in secondary and tertiary syphilis. Br. J. Dermatol. **136**, 683–686 (1997)
16. Bundesgesundheitsamt: Richtlinie 1979 für die Serodiagnose der Syphilis. Bundesgesundheitsbl **22**, 471–474 (1979)
17. Schöfer, H., Brockmeyer, N.H., Hagedorn, H.-J., Hamouda, O., Handrick, W., Krause, W., Marcus, U., Münstermann, D.,

Petry, K.U., Prange, H., Potthoff, A., Gross, G.: Syphilis. Guidelines of the German Sexually Transmitted Diseases Society for diagnosis and therapy of syphilis. J. Dtsch. Dermatol. Ges. **4**, 160–177 (2006)
18. Norris, S.J., Treponema pallidum research group: Polypeptides of *Treponema pallidum*: progress towards understanding their structural, functional and immunologic roles. Microbiol. Rev. **57**, 750–779 (1993)
19. Goh, B.T., van Vorst Vader, P.C.: European guideline for the management of syphilis. Int. J. STD AIDS **12**(Suppl 3), 14–26 (2001)
20. Mueller, I., Brade, V., Hagedorn, H.-J., Straube, E., Schoerner, C., Frosch, M., Hlobil, H., Stanek, G., Hunfeld, K.-P.: Is serological testing a reliable tool in laboratory diagnosis of syphilis? Meta-analysis of eight external quality control surveys performed by the German infection serology proficiency testing program. J. Clin. Microbiol. **44**, 1335–1341 (2006)
21. Robert Koch-Institut: Praktische Empfehlungen zur Serodiagnostik der Syphilis. Epidemiol. Bull. **25**, 191–192 (2003)
22. Fiumara, N.J.: Reinfection primary, secondary, and latent syphilis. Sex. Transm. Dis. **7**, 111–115 (1980)
23. Romanowski, B., Sutherland, R., Fick, G.H., Mooney, D., Love, E.J.: Serologic response to treatment of infectious syphilis. Ann. Intern. Med. **114**, 1005–1009 (1991)
24. Enders, M., Knaub, I., Gohl, M., Pieper, I., Bialek, C., Hagedorn, H.-J.: Konnatale Syphilis trotz Mutterschaftsvorsorge? Eine Evaluierung von 14 Fällen. Z. Geburtshilfe Neonatol. **210**, 141–146 (2006)
25. Sanchez, P.J., Wendel, G.D., Grimprel, E., Goldberg, M., Hall, M., Arencibia-Mireles, O., Radolf, J.D., Norgard, M.V.: Evaluation of molecular methodologies and rabbit infectivity testing for the diagnosis of congenital syphilis and neonatal central nervous system invasion by *Treponema pallidum*. J Infect Dis **148**, 148–157 (1993)
26. Hagedorn, H.-J., Kraminer, A., Wiegel, U.: Prophylaxe und Diagnostik der Syphilis connata aus immunologischer Sicht. Dtsch. Med. Wochenschr. **108**, 142–145 (1983)
27. Prange, H.: Neurosyphilis. In: Prange, H. (ed.) Infektionskrankheiten des ZNS, pp. 237–250. Chapman & Hall, Weinheim (1995)
28. Prange, H.W., Moskophidis, M., Schipper, H.I., Mueller, F.: Relationship between neurological features and intrathecal synthesis of IgG antibodies in untreated and treated human syphilis. J. Neurol. **230**, 241–250 (1983)
29. Oschmann, P.: Neurosyphilis. In: Wildemann, B., Oschmann, P., Reiber, H. (eds.) Neurologische Labordiagnostik, pp. 137–139. Georg Thieme, Stuttgart/New York (2006)
30. Rolfs, R.T., Joesoef, M.R., Hendershot, E.F., Rompalo, A.M., Augenbraun, M.H., Chiu, M., Bolan, G., Johnson, S.C., French, P., Steen, E., Radolf, J.D., Larsen, S.: A randomized trial of enhanced therapy for early syphilis in patients with and without human immunodeficiency virus infection. The syphilis and HIV study group. N. Engl. J. Med. **337**, 307–314 (1997)
31. Tramont, E.C.: *Treponema pallidum* (syphilis). In: Mandell, G.L., Bennett, J.E., Dolin, R. (eds.) Principles and practice of infectious diseases, 6th edn, pp. 2769–2785. Elsevier Churchill Livingstone, Philadelphia (2005)

Early and Late Syphilis

13

Helmut Schöfer

Core Messages

- *Primary syphilis* is a genital ulcer disease. The leading signs and symptoms are painless and indurated ulcers and regional lymph nodes.
- *Secondary syphilis* is marked by non-itching exanthema with involvement of the palms and the soles of the feet.
- *Bacteremia* in secondary syphilis leads to general symptoms and generalized lymphadenopathy.
- *Plasma cells* in skin histopathology: think of syphilis!
- *Herxheimer's reaction* may begin within a few hours after the first penicillin dose and can be confused with a severe drug reaction.
- A single oral dose of corticosteroids is very effective to prevent Herxheimer's reaction.
- In secondary, latent, and late syphilis neurosyphilis has to be excluded.
- *Early neurosyphilis* is more frequent in human immunodeficiency virus (HIV)-infected patients with syphilis.
- *HIV infection* may alter the clinical symptoms and serological parameters of early and late syphilis.
- Tertiary, quaternary, and congenital syphilis are rare diseases in developed countries.
- *Tertiary syphilis* is hyperergic and is marked by granulomatous syphilids and gummas.
- *Quaternary syphilis* is hyperergic/anergic and is mainly a neurological disease (tabes dorsalis, progressive paralysis).

13.1 Introduction

Syphilis is a chronic systemic disease with four clinical stages and several periods of latency (see Table 13.1 and Chap. 11). For diagnostic, epidemiologic, and therapeutic reasons, it is also classified into early and late syphilis. High titers of cardiolipin and specific IgM antibodies, which are characteristic for early syphilis, decrease in the late state. Infectivity is high in primary and secondary syphilis with moist, ulcerating lesions, but very low (or missing) in late-state disease, with asymptomatic latency or granulomatous lesions with very few treponemas in tertiary syphilis. Concerning treatment, it is presumed that *T. pallidum* has an even longer lifecycle in late syphilis compared to early syphilis. Therefore, antibiotic treatment has to be given longer than 2 weeks in late syphilis. Although this concept has never been proved by experimental investigations, it has been kept to date. Early syphilis subsumes primary, secondary, and early latent syphilis. Late syphilis is defined as untreated syphilis more than 1 year after infection or any untreated syphilis of unknown duration.

H. Schöfer
Department of Dermatology and Venerology, University Hospital, Johann W. Goethe University, Theodor-Stern-Kai 7, 60590 Frankfurt, Germany
e-mail: schoefer@em.uni-frankfurt.de

G. Gross and S.K. Tyring (eds.), *Sexually Transmitted Infections and Sexually Transmitted Diseases*,
DOI: 10.1007/978-3-642-14663-3_13, © Springer-Verlag Berlin Heidelberg 2011

Table 13.1 Stages and variants of clinical syphilis

Early syphilis	
Primary syphilis	Localized infection (primary chancre and lymphadenopathy) at the site of inoculation
Secondary syphilis	*T. pallidum* bacteremia with skin rash (syphilid), mucocutaneous lesions, lymphadenopathy, general symptoms
Early latent syphilis	Seropositivity without clinical symptoms Serological parameters diagnostic for active disease (IgM antibodies, high cardiolipin antibody titers) Infection acquired within the preceding 12 months
Late syphilis	
Late latent syphilis	Seropositivity without clinical symptoms Serological parameters diagnostic for active disease (IgM antibodies, low cardiolipin antibody titers) Infection of unknown duration (or >1 year)
Tertiary syphilis	Hyperergy → Spontaneous cure → Syphilids (tuberoserpigineous, tuberonodular rash), gumma → Neurosyphilis → Cardiovascular syphilis (aneurysm, etc.)
Quaternary[a] syphilis (meta syphilis)	Hypergy/anergy → Tabes dorsalis, progressive paralysis
Neurosyphilis (clinical symptoms in stages II–IV)	Asymptomatic/symptomatic meningovascular syphilis, basilar meningitis with cranial nerve palsy and pupillary abnormalities (Argyll-Robertson pupil), cerebral gumma, progressive paralysis, tabes dorsalis
Syphilis connata	Syphilis connata praecox Syphilis connata tarda (>2 years), stigmas

[a]Some authors regard quaternary syphilis as a part of tertiary syphilis, but in contrast to tertiary syphilis it is a hypererg disease. A high number of treponemas are directly involved in severe destructive inflammation of the spinal cord (tabes dorsalis) and the brain (progressive paralysis)

13.1.1 Early Syphilis

13.1.1.1 Primary Syphilis

Symptomatic syphilis starts about 3 weeks (range 9–90 days) after infection with *T. pallidum*. The typical initial (primary) lesion is a single brown-red papule of varying size (0.5–1.5 cm in diameter) which tends to erode within a few days, resulting in a primary ulcer (chancre). The primary chancre is located at the former contact site to moist infectious lesions of a sexual partner, which in 95% of all cases is in the genitoanal area. In men it is frequently found on the penis (especially on the glans and around the coronary sulcus, Fig. 13.1) and the scrotum, and in women on the vulva, cervix, fourchette, or perineum. Perianal and intraanal chancres are particularly common in men who have sex with men (MSM). About 5% of all primary chancres are found in extragenital locations [4], mostly on the patients lips (Fig. 13.2) or in the oral cavity, but very rarely on "normal" skin (e.g., fingers, toes, around the nipples). These lesions, not being expected to be sexually transmitted at first glance, have a broad spectrum of differential diagnoses and are frequently misdiagnosed. Although a painless, indurated primary ulceration might be the leading sign eczematous surroundings can mimic to be contact dermatitis, fungal infection, etc.

The typical primary chancre is painless and has characteristic indurated boarders, which led to the term hard chancre or ulcus durum (in contrast to the soft boarders of ulcus molle, which is a synonym for chancroid). Most chancres are single lesions with a round or oval shape and a clean red surface which may be covered by a yellowish or grey exudate. The surrounding tissue may be indurated or edematous. Multiple chancres occur in case of simultaneous or consecutive infection of several sites before activation of the immune system. As described by Chapel [5] in a series

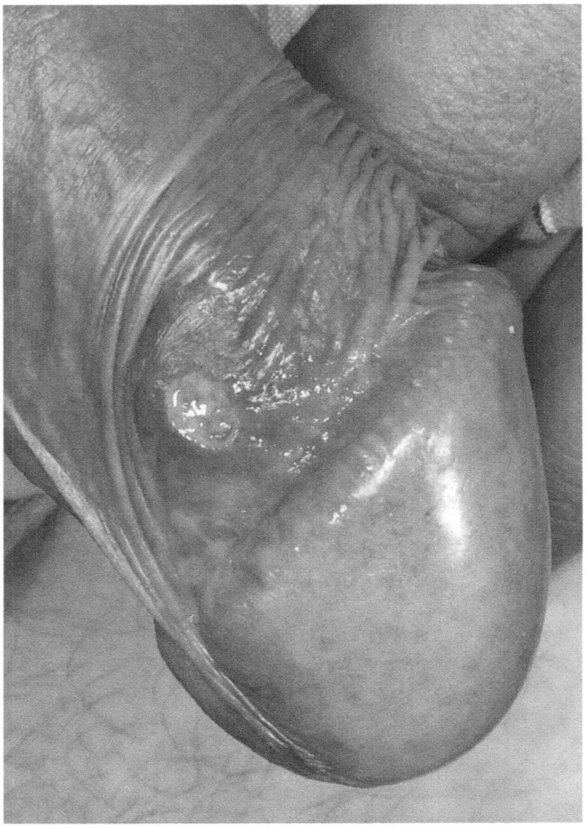

Fig. 13.1 Primary syphilis. Painless genital primary chancre

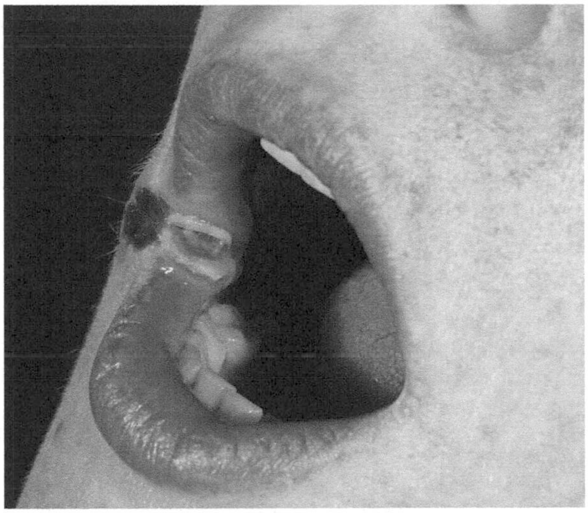

Fig. 13.2 Primary syphilis. Painless labial primary chancre

of 64 primary chancres, the typical single lesion with indurated margins is not as frequent as mentioned in most textbooks. Chapel found multiple primary chancres in 46% and in 8% the margins were soft and the shape of the lesions was irregular. This was confirmed by clinical investigations on genital ulcer disease (GUD), which resulted in the recommendation to perform specific diagnostic tests for syphilis, chancroid, and herpes simplex virus to confirm the clinical diagnosis.

T. pallidum spreads from the primary lesion via lymphatic vessels to the regional lymph nodes, causing an asymptomatic uni- or bilateral lymphadenopathy. The lymph nodes are indurated, relocatable, and the skin is neither erythematous nor fixed to the lymph nodes. They might disappear with the spontaneous regression of the primary chancre (after 3–8 weeks) or persist until secondary syphilis occurs after another 4–6 weeks. Table 13.2 summarizes the clinical differential diagnoses of primary, secondary, and tertiary syphilis lesions.

To diagnose primary syphilis, dark-field microscopy, direct immune fluorescence tests, and polymerase chain reaction (PCR) tests for *T. pallidum* are appropriate [7] (for details see Chap. 12). Histopathology is not specific, but swelling and proliferation of endothelium cells as well as perivascular infiltrates with lymphocytes and plasma cells are suggestive of treponemal infections. On staining with silver stain (e.g., Warthin-Starry stain) or immunohistochemistry with specific monoclonal antibodies [3, 14] spirochetes can be detected in the epidermis and around the dermal capillaries. Seroconversion starts about 3 weeks after infection (simultaneously with the manifestation of the primary chancre) with the occurrence of specific IgM antibodies (ELISA, 19sIgM-test, Western Blot). Specific IgG antibodies occur 4–6 weeks after infection and finally about 1 week later serology is completed by the appearance of cardiolipin antibodies (for details see Chap. 12).

Special clinical and diagnostic features of primary syphilis are seen in some, but not all, patients with human immunodeficiency virus (HIV) coinfection or other forms of immunodeficiency. Early seroconversion and occurrence of multiple primary lesions, persisting primary, and painful anal chancres as well as unreliable serologic tests are discussed in detail in Chap. 15.

In numerous patients primary syphilis is neither diagnosed nor treated due to different reasons: primary chancres are not painful and are mostly located in a

Table 13.2 Clinical differential diagnosis of syphilis

Primary chancre	*Genital/anal:* Herpes simplex genitalis, traumatic wounds, chancroid, lymphogranuloma venereum, ulcera of secondary and tertiary syphilis, erosive balanitis, tuberculosis cutis, malignant tumors (e.g., squamous cell carcinoma) *Oral/perioral:* Furuncle, giant aphthae, ulcerating herpes simplex, cytomegalovirus (CMV) ulceration, pyoderma vegetans, keratoacanthoma, lip cancer
Secondary syphilis	*Exanthema:* Drug eruptions, viral exanthema (e.g., measles, rubella), vasculitis, pityriasis lichenoides chronica, lichen generalisatus, exathematic psoriasis, disseminated Kaposi's sarcoma *Genital/anal/intertriginous (condylomata lata):* Genital warts (human papillomavirus [HPV]), Bowen's disease, bowenoid papulosis, squamous cell carcinoma *Oral cavity:* Angina tonsillaris (sore throat), diphtheria, aphthae, Plaut's angina, perlèche *Capillitium:* Alopecia areata/diffusa, impetigo contagiosa
Tertiary syphilis	*Tuberoserpiginous, tuberosquamous syphilids:* Cutaneous tuberculosis, cutaneous sarcoidosis, tinea, erythema necrolyticum migrans, cutaneous histoplasmosis, mycosis fungoides *Gummas:* Furuncle, carbuncle, abscesses, septic metastasis, panniculitis, actinomycosis, Bazin's disease, tuberculosis cutis colliquativa, lupus erythematodes profundus

anogenital area. Therefore, some patients just being ashamed or unaware of an infectious disease hesitate for a considerable time to see a physician. As the primary lesion tends to heal spontaneously within 4–6 weeks, these patients misbelieve that they have overcome the disease. In other patients, the primary chancre is clinically misdiagnosed (see Table 13.2) or is hidden under the foreskin, in the vagina, or in the anal canal and is not detected unless the patient has a very careful physical examination. All symptoms of primary syphilis disappear spontaneously; the patient seems to be in good health but remains infected and enters a period of latency (50%) or progresses directly to secondary syphilis (50%) [16].

Primary syphilis is one possible cause of GUD [23]. The syphilitic chancre must be differentiated from ulcerations by herpes simplex viruses, *Haemophilus ducreyi*, traumatic ulcerations, etc. (see Table 13.2). Peri- and intraanal chancres may cause pain or rectal bleeding and thus have to be differentiated from acute or chronic anal fissures, hemorrhoids and anal tumors (Fig. 13.3, [9]).

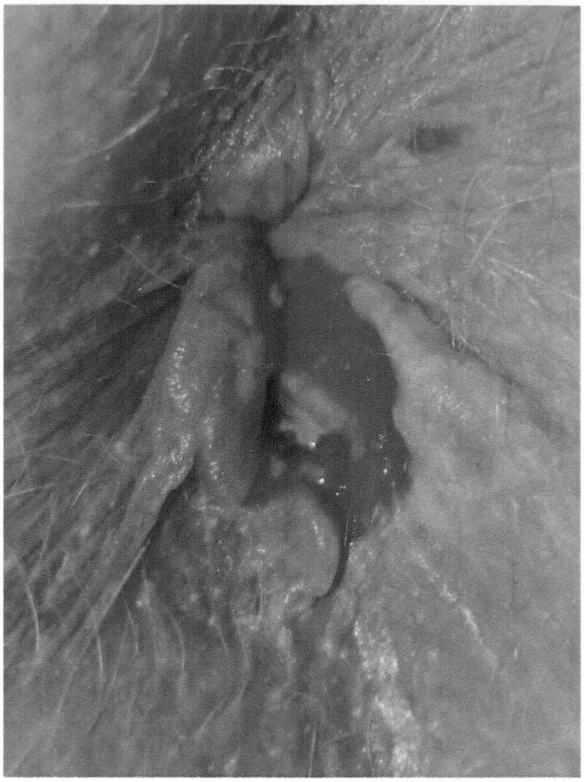

Fig. 13.3 Primary syphilis. Painful anal primary chancre

13.1.1.2 Secondary Syphilis

Secondary syphilis is characterized by *T. pallidum* bacteremia, which begins between 7 and 12 weeks after infection. From a status of good health, the patients now develop a spectrum of clinical signs and symptoms, which show a large variety concerning manifestation and severity from individual to individual [1, 6, 13]. In this stage, the primary chancre and the associated regional lymphadenopathy have regressed spontaneously and completely in about 70–80% of all patients [10, 20].

Associated general symptoms are fatigue, weakness, lack of appetite, slightly raised temperatures, sore throat, pain accentuated at nighttime (headache, myalgia, arthralgia), and a generalized lymphadenopathy (enlarged, nontender, relocatable lymph nodes) in 85% of all patients [6]. Only a few patients suffer from treponemal hepatitis, or glomerulonephritis (kidney damage by immuno-complexes), but about 5% develop symptoms of early neurosyphilis (meningitis, iridocyclitis with vision impairment). Treponemal infection may also be the cause of associated deafness, periosteitis, arthritis, bursitis, phlebitis, and periphlebitis. Although more than 80% of all patients suffer from skin or mucosal membrane symptoms, general symptoms might be completely lacking.

The extremely broad spectrum of skin and mucosal membrane symptoms seen in patients with secondary syphilis had inspired some authors to name syphilis "the great imitator" or "the clown" of dermatology.

The first visible lesions of secondary syphilis are pale reddish macules with a diameter of 0.5–1.5 cm on the patient's body and limbs. This eruption, called the macular rash of secondary syphilis or roseola syphilitica (Fig. 13.4), is asymptomatic. Not clearly demarcated, discrete macules are found on the patient's palms of the hands, soles of the feet, and forehead. Because this rash is transient (1–2 weeks only), and not itching, it is frequently not noticed by the patient.

The transient macular rash may change into or be followed by a symmetric, nonpruritic eruption, which involves more or less the entire body, including palms of the hands and soles of the feet (Figs. 13.5 and 13.6), face and capillitium. The rash usually is composed of reddish-brown, coppery or slightly livid macules and papules (50–70%), but also might be follicular or pseudovesicular, lichenoid, papulosquamous (like guttate psoriasis), corymbiform (Fig. 13.7), or ulcerating

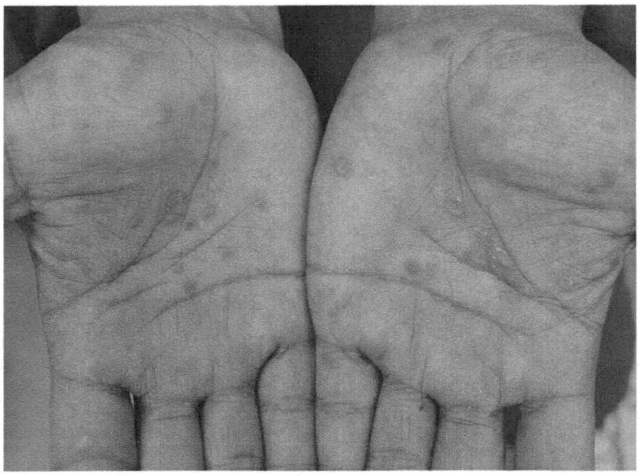

Fig. 13.5 Secondary syphilis. Palmar syphilid

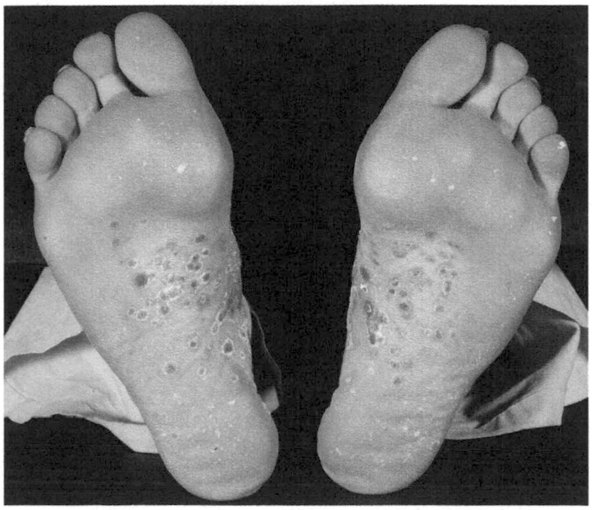

Fig. 13.6 Secondary syphilis. Plantar syphilid

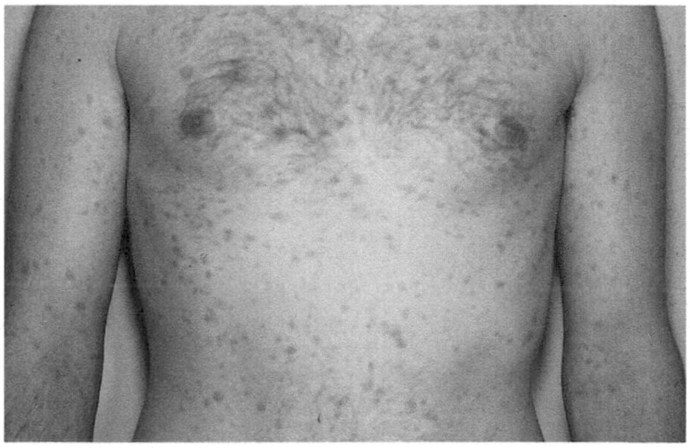

Fig. 13.4 Secondary syphilis. Macular rash (asymptomatic, non-itching)

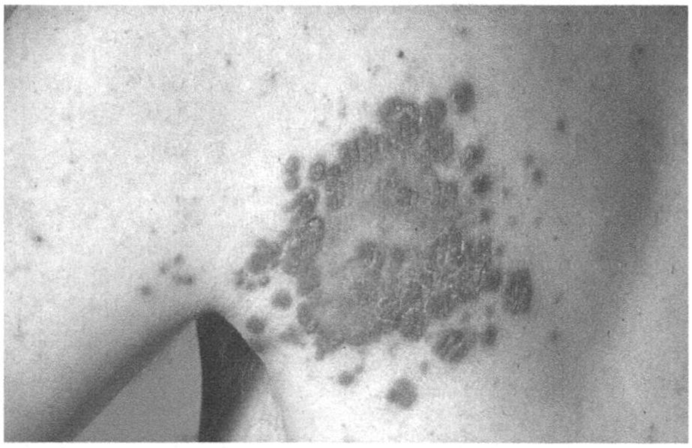

Fig. 13.7 Secondary syphilis. Corymbiform syphilid

but not vesicular, bullous or urticarial [1, 2, 13]. The ulcerating form can be associated with severe general symptoms (weakness, malaise, high fever) and the flat ulcers can be covered by typical, rupia-like crusts (malignant syphilis [8] Figs. 13.8 and 13.9).

Lack of itching and involvement of palms and soles are the cardinal symptoms of the rashes of secondary syphilis (syphilids), which may last for several weeks up to 1 year. About 20% of all patients have at least one relapse after spontaneous resolution of the rash.

In about 10% of all patients erythematous papular lesions in moist intertriginous areas progress to condylomata lata, which are very infective, plaquelike sometimes granulomatous vegetations [6]. Condylomata lata are predominantly found in the genitoanal region (Fig. 13.10), but sometimes multiple moist and highly infective lesions occur in other intertriginous areas too (between the toes and fingers, axillary, and in the umbilical region [15, 24]). Especially genital and

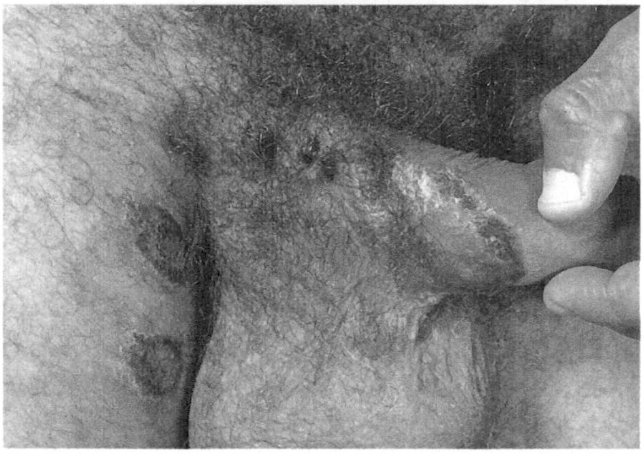

Fig. 13.8 Secondary syphilis. Ulcerating lesions of malignant syphilis

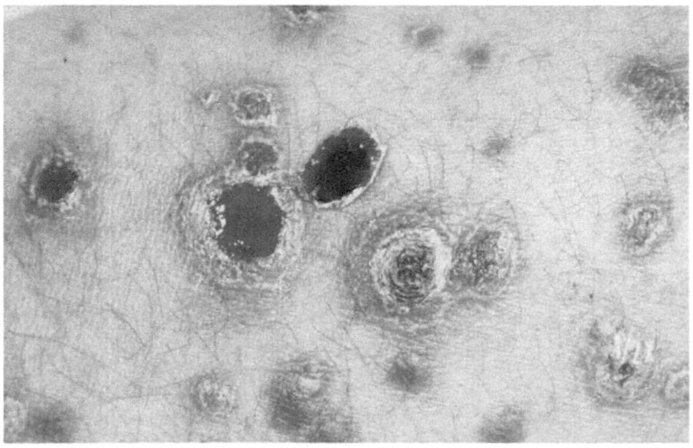

Fig. 13.9 Secondary syphilis. Crusted lesions of malignant syphilis: Rupia syphilitica

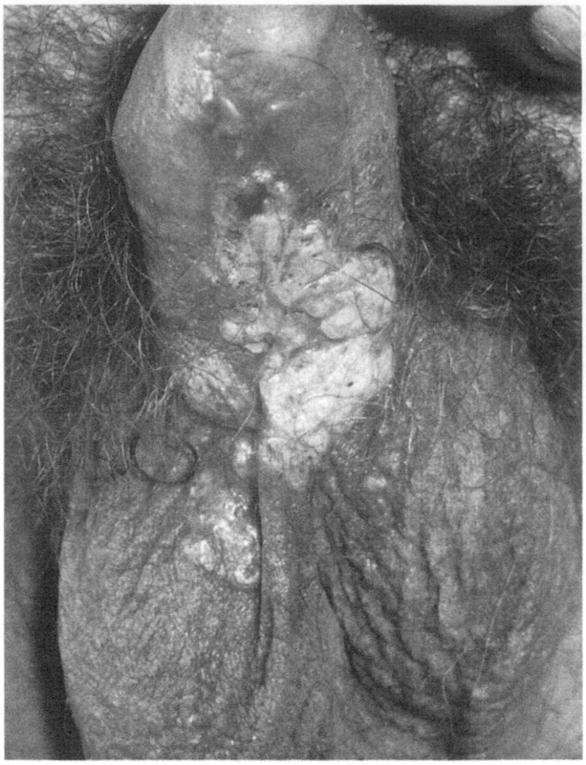

Fig. 13.10 Secondary syphilis. Genital condylomata lata

perianal condylomata lata are sometimes difficult to differentiate clinically from HPV-induced genital warts (condylomata acuminata). If there is any doubt, syphilis serology must be performed.

Scalp involvement in secondary syphilis leads to diffuse, irregular papular lesions and a typical patchy type of hair loss, which is best described as "moth-eaten" alopecia (Fig. 13.11) or alopecia specifica. Recently Nam-Cha et al. [21] demonstrated that hair loss in syphilis patients is due to a direct spirochetal infection of the hair follicle. Syphilitic alopecia is found in 4–11% of all patients [13].

The involvement of the oral mucous membranes starts with patchy erythemas on the soft and hard palate, and the buccal mucosa. These lesions progress to slightly papular mucous patches with macerated (Fig. 13.12) sometimes opalescent surfaces (plaques opalines). On the tongue infiltration and maceration may cause tender swollen lesions, covered with a gray or white exudate (plaques lisses, Fig. 13.13). Typical mucous patches show oval or serpiginous shapes, and in case of ulceration severe pain may occur.

Another very significant symptom of secondary syphilis is angina (angina specifica, syphilitic tonsillitis,

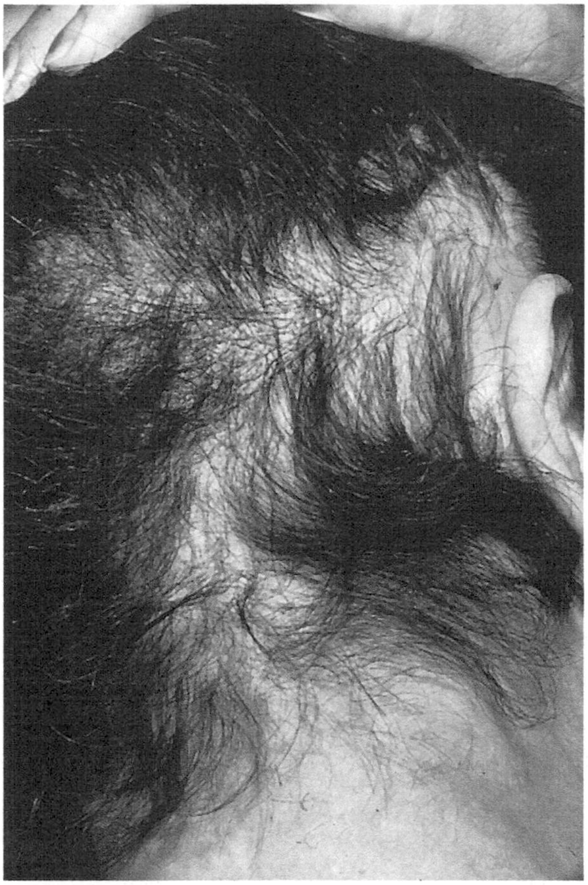

Fig. 13.11 Secondary syphilis. "Moth-eaten" alopecia diffusa specifica

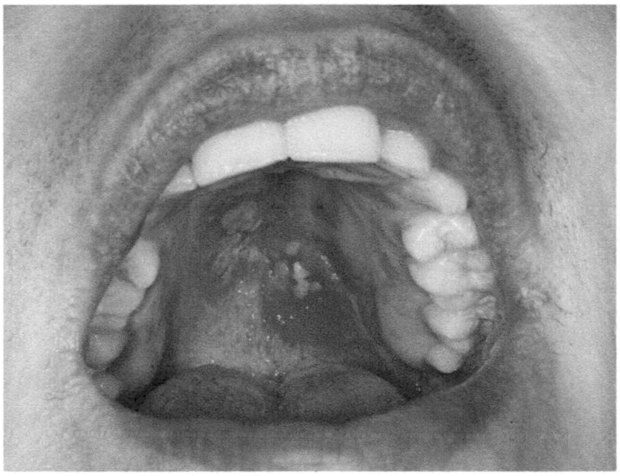

Fig. 13.12 Secondary syphilis. Mucosal plaques

Fig. 13.14), which is part of the syphilitic polyscleradenitis (i.e., a treponemal infection of the lymphadnoid tissues). Associated with a hoarse voice there is pharyngitis, and a firm swelling of both tonsils which are erythematous or covered by a grayish exudate. Swallowing usually is painful, but in contrast to other infections of the tonsils fever is absent [11, 22].

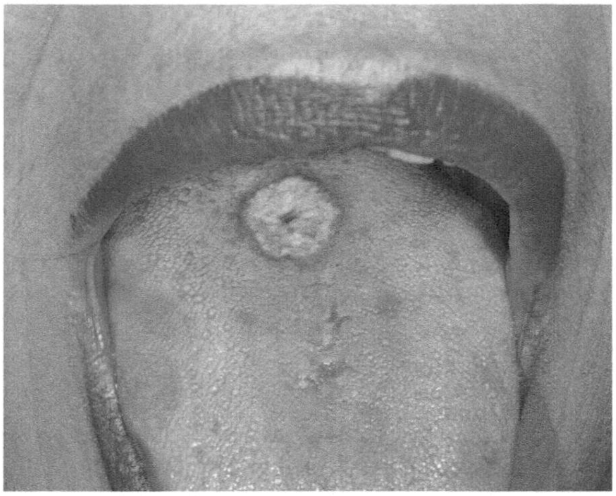

Fig. 13.13 Secondary syphilis. Mucosal plaques, plaques lisses

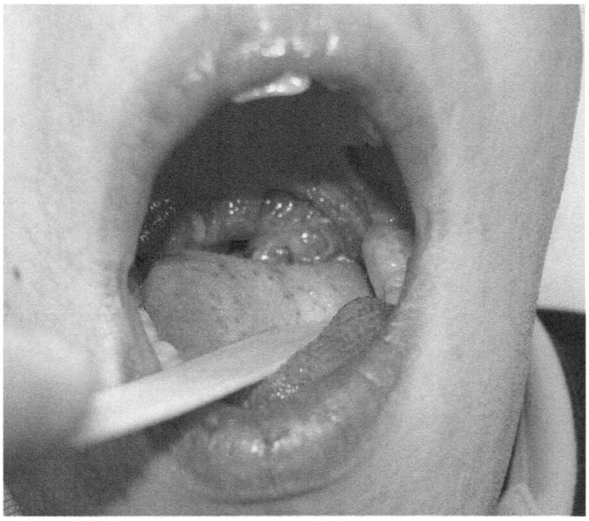

Fig. 13.14 Secondary syphilis. Angina specifica

In the late stage of secondary syphilis, general clinical symptoms decrease and the initially symmetric rashes change to grouped lesions (corymbiform syphilids, Fig. 13.7). After spontaneous regression, syphilitic rashes heal without scars but have a tendency to develop longlasting postinflammatory hyper- or depigmentations (leukoderma syphiliticum). In typical cases leucoderma is accentuated as small patches around the patient's neck, termed "Venus' collar" or "Necklace of Venus."

A small number of patients (including patients with immunodeficiency, HIV infection, history of syphilis, or MSM) suffer from malignant syphilis (ulceronodular cutaneous syphilis) [26]. This clinical variant is characterized by violent ulcerations of the skin and the oral mucosa combined with severe general symptoms (fever, fatigue, anemic pallor, weight loss, but no lymphadenopathy). Usually the number of skin ulcerations is low, but the oral mucosa is frequently involved with destructive ulcerations of the tonsils, the uvula, and the soft palate. The skin lesions develop from small red papules which rapidly ulcerate from the center (Fig. 13.8). The initial punched-out aspect of these superficial ulcerations with soft boarders is soon hidden under scaly crusts, which resemble the shells of oysters (rupia syphilitica, Fig. 13.9). Among 60 HIV-infected patients with active syphilis malignant syphilis was diagnosed in 4 cases (7%) [25]. This is about 50 times more frequent than in the pre-AIDS era, when malignant syphilis was only diagnosed in 0.12% of all cases [17]. All clinical symptoms of secondary syphilis are likely to disappear after a clinical course with several recurrences within a period of 4–12 months (or longer).

Normally, syphilis now proceeds to a second phase of longlasting latency without any clinical signs or symptoms. In some rare cases nodular or ulcerating lesions of secondary syphilis, which clinically resemble cutaneous gummas, can persist and be the first clinical sign of an early progression to tertiary syphilis (syphilis tertiaria praecox). Histopathology shows granulomatous infiltrates in these lesions which seem to be more frequent in HIV-infected patients.

Jarisch–Herxheimer Reaction

In patients with early syphilis, carrying a high load of *T. pallidum*, an acute febrile reaction might be provoked by the initial dose of any effective antibiotic therapy. Bacterial toxins are able to cause general symptoms like fatigue, weakness, headache, and myalgia, which usually occur within the first 24 h of treatment. In addition a preexisting skin rash might worsen or a new rash might occur. The patient should be informed about the possibility and course of this reaction prior to the first injection. In addition, clinicians have to consider Jarisch-Herxheimer reaction as an important differential diagnosis of anaphylactic reactions against antibiotics. To avoid Herxheimer reaction we give a single dose of corticosteroids 1 h before starting syphilis treatment (1 mg prednisolone equivalent/kg bodyweight PO or IV).

13.1.1.3 Early Latent Syphilis

Latent syphilis within the first year after infection is characterized by the lack of any clinical signs and symptoms and (in typical cases) serological parameters indicative for active syphilis (high titres in non-treponemal and treponemal tests, including positive IgM tests). The diagnosis of latent syphilis is made by serological parameters only (for details see Chap. 12).

13.1.2 Late Syphilis

If the patient's history reveals that the time of infection or the start of clinical symptoms of primary or secondary syphilis has passed more than 12 months syphilis is termed as late syphilis. In addition, any patient whose history does not exclude that he has syphilis longer than 1 year, per definition is a patient with late syphilis.

13.1.2.1 Late Latent Syphilis

Early latent syphilis proceeds seamlessly into late latent syphilis. There are still no clinical signs and symptoms but from then on treponemal cardiolipin antibodies (rapid plasma regain [RPR], Venereal Disease Research Laboratory [VDRL], etc.) slowly decline and residual low or even negative titres are found (for details see Chap. 12). The individual outcome of late latent syphilis is uncertain. There is a 72% chance of spontaneous healing for all untreated patients, the remaining 28% patients will proceed to tertiary syphilis (after 3–10 years) or to quaternary syphilis (after 3 or 4 decades) [10].

13.1.2.2 Tertiary Syphilis

The late cutaneous, cardiovascular, and neurological stages of syphilis today are rare diseases compared to the preantibiotic era. Due to the introduction of penicillin and the reduced virulence of the treponemas only 28% of untreated patients proceed to late clinical stages. Tertiary syphilis is characterized by hypererg reactions against few spirochetes, which have survived in different tissues. In typical cases the clinical symptoms begin 3–5 (10) years after secondary syphilis. Severe or even lethal courses are possible, especially when the cardiovascular system (mesaortitis syphilitica, aneurysms) is involved or gummas occur in parenchymatous organs and the brain.

Skin lesions are either from cutaneous (tuberous syphilids) or subcutaneous origin (gummas) and show asymmetric, grouped nodules. The lesions are not infectious, heal spontaneously, and leave scars. Tuberoserpiginous syphilids with arciform papules, hyper- or depigmented areas of atrophy, scarring in the center and progression at the margins are typical, but ulceration, crusts, and scaling might be found too (Fig. 13.15).

Histopathology reveals tuberculid-like granulomas with inflammatory reactions, epitheloid cells, plasma cells, lymphocytes, multinuclear giant cells, and central necrosis. Differential diagnoses include mycosis fungoides, lupus vulgaris, sarcoidosis, and other diseases with granulomas. Low numbers of treponemas are found with very sensitive methods [12], but gummas and tuberous syphilids are not supposed to be infective lesions.

Gummas begin with small, firm, subcutaneous nodules that grow and invade the dermis. The lesions present with livid or red-brown discoloration of the overlying skin and are generally localized on the scalp, forehead, neck, oral and nasal cavity, tonsils, lips, and the genitoanal region. After several weeks, central necrosis leads to fluctuation and perforation (Fig. 13.16). The resulting ulcerations are still firm along the margins, of reniform shape, and have a considerable potency of tissue destruction. Even bones

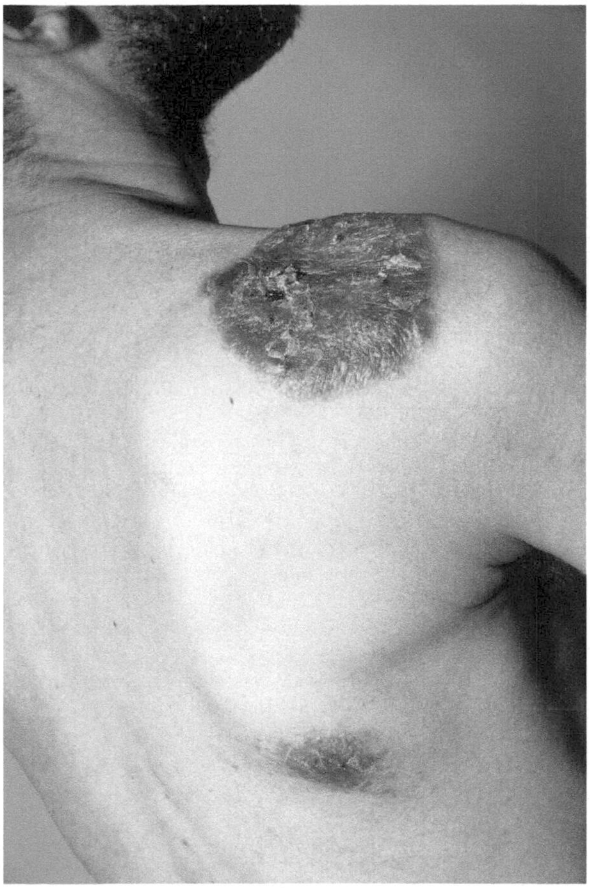

Fig. 13.15 Tertiary syphilis. Tuberosquamous syphilid

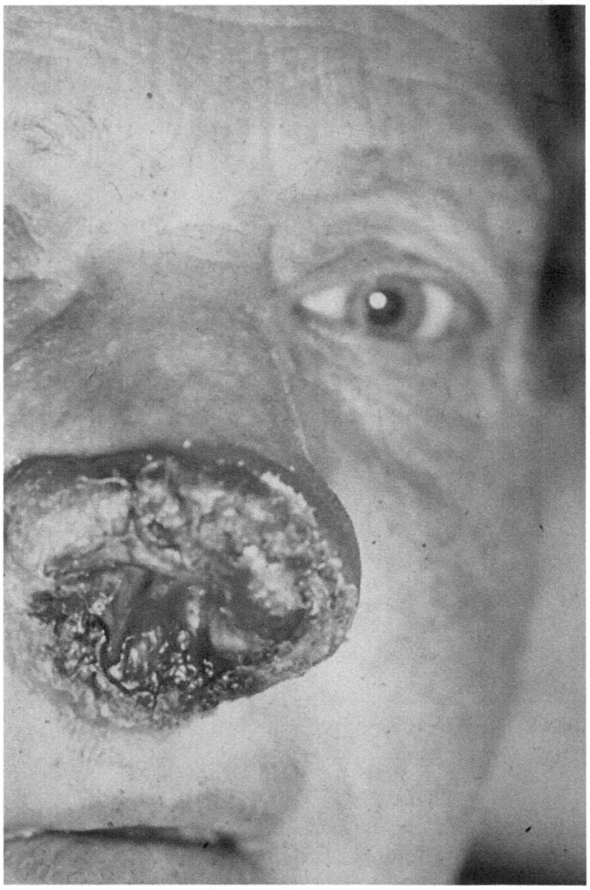

Fig. 13.16 Tertiary syphilis. Gumma of the nose

and muscles may be involved and destroyed. Differential diagnosis includes any kind of chronic ulcerating nodules, e.g., tuberculosis cutis colliquativa, lupus erythematosus profundus, phagedenic ulcers, and panniculitis. Parenchymatous lesions, especially of the brain, liver, and lungs, may occur. In addition, the eyes (Argyll-Robertson sign, nervus opticus atrophy, etc.), ears (deafness), heart and blood vessels (aneurysms), and bones may be affected.

Gummas owe their name to the gum-like secretion which can be drawn from these ulcerations with a platinum loop. They are preferably located in the median of the body (nose, palate, tongue), and heal with deep scars.

Early manifestations of tertiary syphilis, even comorbidity with late secondary syphilis, and the occurrence of cerebral gummas were reported from HIV-infected patients [27] (for details see Chap. 15).

13.1.2.3 Quaternary Syphilis (Metasyphilis)

Some authors regard quaternary syphilis as a part of tertiary syphilis, but in contrast to tuberous syphilids and gummas in tertiary syphilis, which are characterized as hyperergic lesions with very rare spirochetes, quaternary syphilis is a anergic disease. A high number of spirochetes are directly involved in severe destructive inflammation of the spinal cord (tabes dorsalis) and the cortex of the brain (progressive paralysis). These fatal types of parenchymatous syphilis occur in about 4% (tabes dorsalis 3%, progressive paralysis 1%) of all untreated syphilis patients 10–30 years after infection. Both destructive and degenerative neurologic diseases have been combined to coin the term "metasyphilis" before their infective nature had been detected. Now there is evidence that treponema are directly involved [18, 19] (for details see Chap. 14).

Tabes dorsalis is characterized by inflammatory degeneration of the posterior spinal cord with spinal ataxia, lancinating pain, loss of reflexes, tonic pupil (Argyll-Robertson sign), and optical nerve atrophy.

Progressive paralysis results from massive invasion of treponemas into the central nervous system (CNS) decades after the beginning of syphilis. The gradual destruction of the cortex of the brain leads to loss of memory, lalopathy, and personality disorder, finally resulting in severe dementia, paresis, seizures, and death.

(For more details about these severe neurological diseases see Chap. 14).

Take-Home Pearls

> Uncertain clinical symptoms in the twenty-first century? Think of syphilis!
> For the clinician, syphilis is still the "great imitator"!
> Syphilis has several periods of latency; serology is mandatory to diagnose latent syphilis.
> Neurosyphilis is found in early syphilis too. Benzathine benzylpenicillin does not cure neurosyphilis.
> Is your patient too old to have syphilis? Think of recreational drugs and dating opportunities via the Internet (early syphilis) and decades of latent disease (late syphilis)!
> Fighting syphilis (and other sexually transmitted infections) is very effective in reducing HIV transmission.

References

1. Baughn, R.E., Musher, D.M.: Secondary syphilitic lesions. Clin. Microbiol. Rev. **18**, 205–216 (2005)
2. Brown, T.J., Yen-Moore, A., Tyring, S.K.: An overview of sexually transmitted diseases. Part. 1. (Syphilis). J. Am. Acad. Dermatol. **41**, 511–529 (1999)
3. Buffet, M., Grange, P.A., Gerhardt, P., et al.: Diagnosing *Treponema pallidum* in secondary syphilis by PCR and immunohistochemistry. J. Invest. Dermatol. **127**, 2345–2350 (2007)
4. Buntin, D.M., Rosen, T., Lesher, J.L., et al.: Sexually transmitted diseases: bacterial infections. J. Am. Acad. Dermatol. **25**, 287–299 (1991)
5. Chapel, T.A.: The variability of syphilitic chancres. Sex. Transm. Dis. **5**, 68–70 (1978)
6. Chapel, T.A.: The signs and symptoms of secondary syphilis. Sex. Transm. Dis. **7**, 161–164 (1980)
7. Cummings, M.C., Lukehart, S.A., Marra, C., et al.: Comparison of methods for the detection of treponema pallidum in lesions of early syphilis. Sex. Transm. Dis. **23**, 366–369 (1996)
8. D'Amico, R., Zalusky, R.: A case of lues maligna in a patient with acquired immunodeficiency syndrome (AIDS). Scand. J. Infect. Dis. **37**, 697–700 (2005)

9. Drusin, L.M., Singer, C., Valenti, A.J., Armstrong, D.: Infectious syphilis mimicking neoplastic disease. Arch. Intern. Med. **137**, 156–160 (1977)
10. Gjestland, T.: The Oslo study of untreated syphilis. Acta Derm. Venereol. **35**, 1 (1955)
11. Hamlyn, E., Marriott, D., Gallagher, R.M.: Secondary syphilis presenting as tonsillitis in three patients. J. Laryngol. Otol. **120**, 602–604 (2006)
12. Handsfield, H.H., Lukehart, S.A., Sell, S., et al.: Demonstration of Treponema pallidum in a cutaneous gumma by indirect immunofluorescence. Arch. Dermatol. **119**, 677–680 (1983)
13. Hira, S.K., Patel, J.S., Bhat, S.G., et al.: Clinical manifestations of secondary syphilis. Int. J. Dermatol. **26**, 103–107 (1987)
14. Hoang, M.P., High, W.A., Molberg, K.H.: Secondary syphilis: a histologic and immunohistochemical evaluation. J. Cutan. Pathol. **31**, 595–599 (2004)
15. Hua, H., Zhu, X., Yang, L., et al.: Multiple condylomata lata: a case report. Int. J. Dermatol. **47**, 56–58 (2008)
16. Hutchinson, C.M., Hook 3rd, E.W.: Syphilis in adults. Med. Clin. N. Am. **74**, 1389–1416 (1990)
17. Kampmier, R.H.: Essentials of Syphiology, p. 148. J.B. Lippincott, Philadelphia (1943)
18. Lukehart, S.A., Hook, E.W., Kaker-Zander, S.A., et al.: Invasion of the central nervous system by *Treponema pallidum*: implications for diagnosis and treatment. Ann. Intern. Med. **109**, 855–862 (1988)
19. Marra, C.M.: Neurosyphilis. Curr. Neurol. Neurosci. Rep. **4**, 435–440 (2004)
20. Mindel, A., Tovey, S.J., Timmins, D.J., Williams, P.: Primary and secondary syphilis, 20 years´ experience. 2. Clinical features. Genitourin. Med. **65**, 1–3 (1989)
21. Nam-Cha, S.H., Guhl, G., Fernandez-Pena, P., Fraga, J.: Alopecia syphilitica with detection of Treponema pallidum in the hair follicle. J. Cutan. Pathol. **34**(suppl 1), 37–40 (2007)
22. Oddó, D., Carrasco, G., Capdeville, F., Ayala, M.F.: Syphilitic tonsillitis presenting as an ulcerated tonsillar tumor with ipsilateral lymphadenopathy. Ann. Diagn. Pathol. **11**, 353–357 (2007)
23. Rosen, T., Brown, T.J.: Genital ulcers. Evaluation and treatment. Dermatol. Clin. **16**, 673–85 (1998)
24. Rosen, T., Hwong, H.: Pedal interdigital condylomata lata: a rare sign of secondary syphilis. Sex. Transm. Dis. **28**, 184–186 (2001)
25. Schöfer, H., Imhof, M., Thoma-Greber, E., et al.: Active syphilis in HIV infection: a multicentre retrospective survey. The German AIDS Study Group (GASG). Genitourin. Med. **72**, 176–181 (1996)
26. Shulkin, D., Tripoli, L., Abell, E.: Lues maligna in a patient with human immunodeficiency virus infection. Am. J. Med. **85**, 425–427 (1988)
27. Weinert, L.S., Scheffel, R.S., Zoratto, G., et al.: Cerebral syphilitic gumma in HIV-infected patients: case report and review. Int. J. STD AIDS **19**, 62–64 (2008)

Neurosyphilis

14

Hilmar W. Prange

14.1 Introduction

The clinical problem of neurosyphilis lies in the fact that younger doctors are no longer familiar with this condition and do not take it into consideration in their differential diagnoses. Regular testing for syphilis reactions in the blood has been abandoned, but the incidence of syphilitic infections appears to be on the incline in many countries. As a result, the recognition of syphilitic complications takes place tardily and therefore the remission of symptoms after treatment remains incomplete.

14.2 Epidemiology

According to the World Health Organization (WHO) global estimates, over 12 million cases of syphilis exist worldwide. For Germany, the Robert Koch Institute Berlin reported in 2006 an incidence of 3,147 cases annually, corresponding to 3.8/100,000 inhabitants [30]. This number is higher in cities and metropolis than in provincial regions. Thus, the number of new infections rose in Hamburg, Germany, to 7.5/100,000; in Berlin to 16.8/100,000; in Murmansk, Russia, to 132/100,000; and, based on older reports, in St. Petersburg to 300/100,000. The principal risk group consists of males between the age of 25 and 40. Homosexuals and heterosexual drug addicts form prominent subgroups.

Because most of the infected people are treated with antibiotics during the early stage, at present the prevalence of neurosyphilis is low. In untreated cases neurosyphilis evolves with a time lag of up to 2 decades after the infection. The epidemiological curve of neurosyphilis is therefore not in parallel with new infections. As demonstrated in earlier studies on the natural course of syphilis, only 5–10% of treponema-infected patients develop central nervous system (CNS) syndromes in the tertiary stage. It is as yet unclear why the majority of untreated patients are spared CNS complications while only a few contract one of the various neurosyphilis manifestations, namely general paresis, tabes dorsalis, or meningovascular neurosyphilis. Surveys conducted between the 1950s and 1970s revealed that the incidence of neurosyphilis is lower by a factor of 0.07 than that of new infections. By calculation, the present incidence level for Germany could attain 0.15 to 0.20 cases of neurosyphilis per 100,000 inhabitants. Principally, coinfection of syphilis and HIV is not infrequent, resulting in a special disposition to treponemal CNS involvement.

14.3 Definition

There is a controversy over how to define neurosyphilis. The Centers for Disease Control and Prevention (CDC, Atlanta, USA) perpetuated the cerebrospinal fluid (CSF) criteria by Bracero et al. (1979) and Burke and Schaberg (1985) proceeding from the assumption that neurosyphilis is present when a positive Venereal Disease Research Laboratory (VDRL) test and an increased count of white blood cells (WBCs) in CSF exist [1–3]. However, sensitivity of CSF-VDRL merely amounts to 30–78% depending on the manifestation

H.W. Prange
Neurologische Universitätsklinik Göttingen,
Konrad-Adenauer Str. 42, Niedersachsen 37075,
Göttingen, Germany
e-mail: hilmarprange@gmx.de

G. Gross and S.K. Tyring (eds.), *Sexually Transmitted Infections and Sexually Transmitted Diseases*,
DOI: 10.1007/978-3-642-14663-3_14, © Springer-Verlag Berlin Heidelberg 2011

form of syphilitic CNS involvement. Moreover, pleocytosis may be missing in cases of tabes dorsalis and meningovascular neurosyphilis. Therefore, we suggest a definition which is founded on clinical symptomatology, course of disease, serologic tests, and analysis of the CSF. According to this definition, neurosyphilis is *probable* when positive treponemal reactions in serum and two of the following three criteria are present [11]:

1. Neurologic and/or psychiatric symptomatology with chronic progressive course and phases of partial remission or deterioration.
2. Abnormal CSF findings with mixed cellular or mononuclear pleocytosis, blood/brain barrier dysfunction (total protein >500 mg/l, CSF/serum quotient of albumin $>7.8\times10^{-3}$), and/or IgG-dominated immunoreaction in CSF (including oligoclonal IgG bands).
3. Positive effect of antibiotic therapy consisting of improvement of symptoms and signs and/or CSF abnormalities.

Neurosyphilis is *proven* when a de novo synthesis of antitreponemal antibodies is present in the CNS, substantiated by an antibody index like ITpA index (see below).

14.4 Symptomatology

Syphilis is a multistage complaint with variable organ manifestations induced by *Treponema pallidum*, as mentioned above. Treponemal invasion of the CNS may take place in all stages after infection. Interestingly, some authors found that one-third of the patients who develop secondary syphilis show abnormal CSF findings such as moderate pleocytosis, mild hypoglycorrhachia, and a slight rise in total protein [15]. Patients may be asymptomatic, complaining only of headaches or signs of meningitis.

The most typical CNS manifestation of the primosecondary stage is acute syphilitic meningitis. Patients complain of holocephalic headaches (mostly slight), nausea, and stiff necks. At times, the condition is complicated by cranial nerve alterations, predominantly the nerves II, III, VII, and VIII. Patients are usually afebrile. Laboratory indicators of systemic inflammation such as increased sedimentation rate, C-reactive protein, or procalcitonin are mostly absent, as are intrathecally produced antibodies against *T. pallidum*. In rare cases hydrocephalus or spinal cord lesions evolve.

In the late latent stage, there are some asymptomatic patients who show signs of a slight CNS involvement detected by imaging procedures, evoked potentials, lumbar puncture (and CSF analysis) or neuroophthalmologic and neurootologic examinations. The term "asymptomatic neurosyphilis" dates back to the early 1920s [20]. At that time, it was found that patients in whom CNS abnormalities of early syphilis persisted over the whole phase of latency were at risk of developing a full-blown neurosyphilis later on [21]. Typical of these patients were slight abnormalities of the CSF, e.g., low pleocytosis, de novo IgG synthesis, and increased protein.

The Oslo study of the natural course of untreated syphilis revealed that 5–10% of the patients develop manifestations of neurosyphilis during the stage of the late latency which lasts between 2 years and 2 decades [4]. Such organ manifestations meet the definition of tertiary syphilis.

"Classic" CNS syndromes of tertiary syphilis are meningovascular (syphilis cerebrospinalis), paretic (general paresis), and tabetic (tabes dorsalis) neurosyphilis. These clinical syndromes may overlap, e.g., appearing as taboparesis. Rare manifestations of CNS syphilis in the late latency or tertiary stage are cerebral gumma, syphilitic amyotrophy, spastic spinal paralysis, and cervical hyperplastic pachymeningitis.

Meningovascular neurosyphilis manifests itself about 4–7 years after the primary stage. The inflammatory process occurs subacutely in meningeal and vascular tissues of the CNS, in some cases mainly in the cerebral part, in others in the spinal part of the neuraxis. The manifestations of meningovascular neurosyphilis are highly variable; therefore Hutchinson (1863) called this form "the great imitator" [12]. Early symptoms are impaired vision (50%), vertigo (35%), mono- or hemiparesis with stroke-like onset (20%), and headache (20%), as well gait disturbances, hearing deficits, and behavioral deviations (20% each). In the further course of disease, typical symptom combinations develop, such as dysfunctions of the brain stem and cranial nerves (25%), hemisyndromes including homonymous anopia (20%), impairment of acoustic and vestibular functions (13%), meningitic symptoms (10%), spinal syndromes (10%), epileptic fits (8%), or organic brain syndromes (8%). Without therapy the conditions progress, resulting in severe defect syndromes.

While in meningovascular neurosyphilis mainly mesenchymal structures of the CNS (vascular and

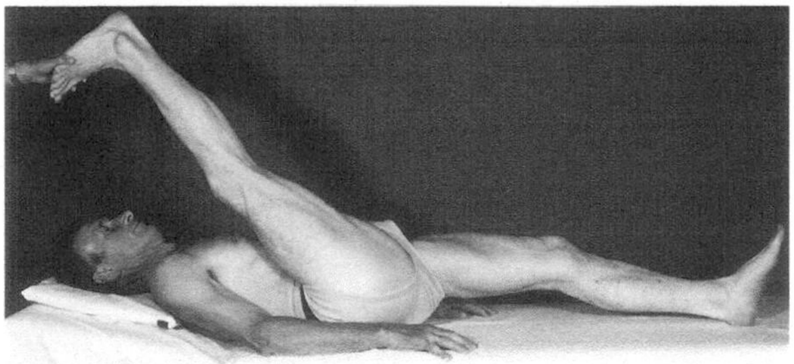

Fig. 14.1 Hyperflexibility of the hip joints in a patient with tabetic neurosyphilis, treated 5 years ago

meningeal tissue) are damaged, tabetic and paretic neurosyphilis (so-called parenchymatous neurosyphilis) are characterized by diffuse, progressive, and irreversible neuronal degeneration.

Tabetic neurosyphilis evolves as a chronic dorsal radiculopathy and manifests as a well-defined syndrome, characterized by episodic lightning pains, absence of ankle and knee reflexes, abnormal pupils, hyperflexibility of the hip joints (Fig. 14.1), gait disturbances, atonic bladder, and optic atrophy. The most frequent initial symptoms in 26 of our patients were lightning pains (54%), impairment of vision (27%), gait ataxia (27%), gastric and visceral crises often resulting in laparotomy (15%), paresthesias (15%), vertigo (15%), and behavioral abnormalities (5%).

Paretic neurosyphilis (general paresis) is basically a chronic (meningo-)encephalitis with very slow progress in most cases. The reason for the latter may be the treponemal lack of lipopolysaccharides and a natural shutdown of the vigorous early immune system response after clearance of most of the pathogens in the latent stage. The illness evolves over 10–20 years after primary infection. Initially, there are complaints of headache and vertigo, slight behavioral changes, subtle deteriorations of cognitive functions, and dysarthria. As the illness progresses, organic brain syndrome with confusion or psychotic episodes, abnormal pupils, tremor of tongue and hands, and epileptic fits develop. Some patients present with manic or paranoid ideas, like the philosopher Friedrich Nietzsche and the composer Robert Schumann, but this comprises the minority of the patients with general paresis. In the final stage speech decay and quadriparesis as well as loss of bowel and bladder control occur. If untreated, general paresis is fatal within 3–5 years. The administration of penicillin in advanced cases may stop the inflammation in the brain, but the cerebral functions will not be restored.

14.5 Diagnostic Procedures

In the primosecondary syphilis, *T. pallidum* can be detected in exudates taken from lesions and also occasionally in CSF with fluorescent or dark-field microscopy. Since cultivation of *T. pallidum* is not possible, great expectations were ascribed to polymerase chain reaction (PCR) in the early 1990s [10]. However, it became apparent that PCR is not a sensitive enough method for diagnosing late stages of syphilis [9]. Thus, serologic tests have remained the cornerstone of the diagnosis of secondary and tertiary syphilis (Fig. 14.2).

In suspected neurosyphilis the pathway of diagnostic procedures is as follows:

1. After anamnestic exploration and clinical examination, specific serological tests are to be carried out; first TPHA (or TPPA) test as searching reaction and then FTA-ABS test as confirming reaction.
2. When these tests are positive, the process activity will be estimated by an unspecific reagin test like VDRL or cardiolipin complement fixation reaction (cardiolipin CFR) or by an IgM test which is available as 19 S-(IgM)FTA-Abs test or *T. pallidum* IgM ELISA.
3. When treponemal infection is proven and there are any suspicions of CNS involvement, lumbar puncture is mandatory. Analysis of CSF includes cell count ($n<5$ c/μl), total protein ($n<500$ mg/l), CSF/serum quotient of albumin ($n<7.8\times10^{-3}$), CSF/serum quotient of IgG, IgM, and IgA (normal range related to albumin quotient [27]), and isoelectric focusing with search for oligoclonal IgG bands as the most sensitive criterion of de novo IgG synthesis in CNS (Fig. 14.3).

The CSF sample is additionally used for quantitative antitreponemal antibody testing. For this purpose, *T. pallidum* particle agglutination assay (TPPA) or *T. pallidum* hemagglutination assay (TPHA) test is best suited; an alternative method is the *T. pallidum* enzyme-linked immunosorbent assay (ELISA). Quantitative CSF values were measured in parallel with those of the serum to form the CSF/serum quotient, which is divided by the CSF/serum quotient of IgG resulting in

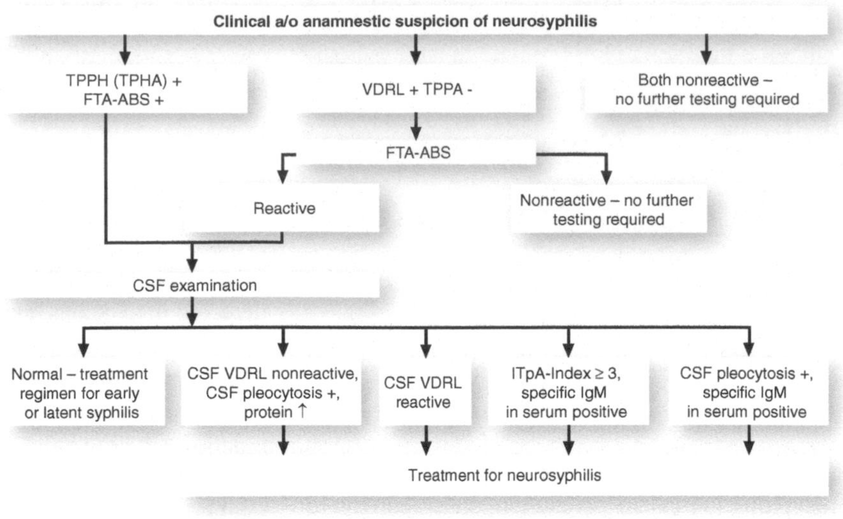

Fig. 14.2 Laboratory diagnosis in cases of suspected CNS syphilis

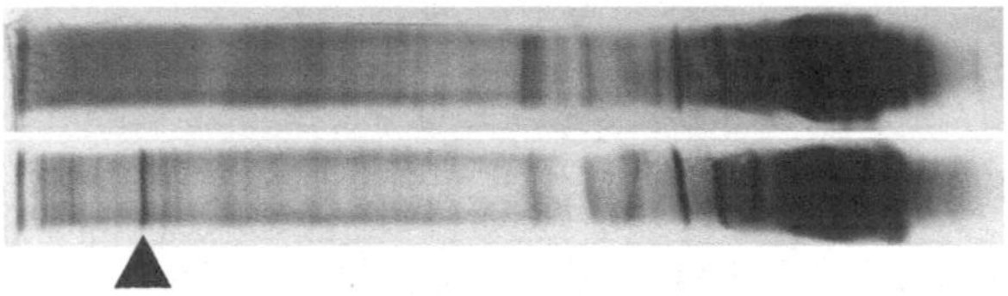

Fig. 14.3 Oligoclonal IgG band (lower track) in the CSF in a patient with meningovascular neurosyphilis; upper track serum without specific bands

the ITpA index. Because TPHA (TPPA) recognizes IgG antibodies in the first line, this index is a measure for the intrathecal synthesis of antitreponemal IgG antibodies. Their presence verifies syphilitic CNS involvement, but does not permit any statement as to the process activity.

$$\text{ITpA index} = \frac{\text{TPHA titre}_{\text{CSF}} \times \text{IgG}_{\text{serum}}}{\text{TPHA titre}_{\text{serum}} \times \text{IgG}_{\text{CSF}}}$$

(ITpA index = intrathecal produced *T. pallidum* antibody index: index of 1 is normal, 2 is suspect, and 3 is definitively pathological; [24, 25]).

4. Activity of the CNS manifestation is confirmed when CSF pleocytosis, positive IgM antibodies to *T. pallidum* in serum, positive cardiolipin reaction in serum, and clinical deterioration are present. Normalization of pleocytosis after therapy takes some weeks. Disappearance of IgM and cardiolipin antibodies takes months, and in some cases even longer than a year.
5. In order to realize the extent of CNS derangement, functional test and imaging procedures are necessary depending on the clinical manifestations of neurosyphilis. These include:

(a) Electrophysiological techniques like electroencephalogram (EEG), visually evoked potentials (VEP), early acoustically evoked brainstem potentials (AEP), somatosensory evoked potentials (SSEP), and in special cases conduction measurements on peripheral nerves.
(b) Imaging examinations with computer-assisted tomography (CAT) and/or magnetic resonance imaging (MRI), and in special cases native X-ray examinations of the thorax, lumbar spine, or ankle joint.
(c) Ultrasonic examination of the abdomen (exclusion of an aortic aneurysm) and Doppler sonography of the brain vessels.
(d) Neuropsychological testing to record cognitive deficits in patients with paralytic neurosyphilis.
(e) Urodynamic examination in patients with tabetic neurosyphilis and other spinal manifestations accompanied by bladder disorders.

Differential diagnostic considerations should include multiple sclerosis, other chronic inflammatory CNS diseases (e.g., neuroborreliosis, herpetic CNS involvement,

Behcet's disease), diabetic complications of the nervous system, and porphyria.

14.6 Pathogenetic Considerations

Over the last 25 years it has become apparent that *T. pallidum* has a certain neurotropism for CNS and peripheral nerves. Electron microscopy of the syphilic primary lesions revealed that treponemes enter peripheral nerve endings around the ulcer early after infection [31]. They can invade the CNS even in the primary stage, frequently inducing an inflammatory reaction there [16]. CNS invasion was thought to take place only by hematogenous propagation, but early presence of treponemes in peripheral nerves may point to an axonal transport as an alternative route to central nervous structures. Moreover, treponemes were detected in CSF samples taken from patients with primary syphilis whose CSF was otherwise normal.

During the secondary stage, about one-third of the examined patients showed pleocytosis and/or increased protein in CSF; de novo IgG synthesis was detected in 15–20% of the CSF samples. The majority of the patients were asymptomatic or complained of mild headaches [15]. Obviously, treponemes invade the CNS during the secondary stage in many patients. The microorganisms apparently disappear spontaneously even without special therapy. The underlying immunological mechanisms have not been clarified to date. Individuals in whom treponema persist in CNS are at special risk of developing neurosyphilis, unless they have received specific or inadvertently effective antibiotic therapy. In the framework of the inflammatory reaction, lymphocytes and other mononuclear cells infiltrate the meninges and cranial nerves. When small meningeal and parenchymatous vessels are involved, an endothelial proliferation ensues and may induce vascular occlusions causing ischemic necroses in the cerebral and spinal parenchyma. In the case that the proliferatory inflammation continues, chronic meningitis, vasculitis, neuronal loss, spinal damage, and/or ependymal granulation around the cerebral ventricles will result.

Clinical observations of syphilitic patients with HIV coinfection revealed that treponemal CNS invasion may take place even during the stage of late latency, which so far was presumed not to be infectious. For many decades, it has been a subject of debate whether or not antibiotic treatment can completely eradicate treponemes at this progressed stage of the disease. The aforementioned observations underline the fundamental necessity of long-term controls after treatment.

14.7 Treatment

14.7.1 Pharmacological Aspects

Clinical experiences over the last 50 years have shown that *T. pallidum* is susceptible to penicillin, other beta-lactams, tetracyclines, and macrolides. Because the microorganism cannot be cultivated by standard microbiological procedures, it was difficult to determine the susceptibility of *T. pallidum* to the respective antibiotics. Factors governing therapeutic efficacy of bacterial agents against a microorganism include:

1. Concentration, which can be achieved at the focus of infection.
2. Replication time of *T. pallidum* in the involved tissue.
3. Support of the tissue defense mechanisms at the site of infection.

Data obtained by in vitro and in vivo studies revealed that serum penicillin concentrations of 0.1 mg/ml are the most treponemocidal, but lower levels will also result in a cure when given for longer periods [28]. In a basic article composed on behalf of the WHO, Idsoe et al. (1972) stated that a serum penicillin concentration exceeding 0.0018 mg/ml (according to 0.03 IU/ml) for 7–10 days without interruption for more than 24–30 h is the standard therapeutic goal for early syphilis [13]. Later on, the therapeutic level of 0.018 mg/ml was extended to include CSF in cases of neurosyphilis. In pharmacokinetic studies, some authors could show that the standard dosage recommended for the treatment of early syphilis as well as syphilic CNS complications (e.g., 2.4 mio IU procaine penicillin G per day combined with 4×500 mg probenecid) was insufficient to achieve such CSF concentrations. This was possible only with doses as high as 20–30 mio IU penicillin G per day in three to six single doses [8, 19, 33].

Another point to be considered is *T. pallidum*'s slow replication, which in vitro can take up to 30–33 h. Treponemal cell division may be much slower in humans, especially during the latent period or tertiary syphilis. As most antibiotics act only during active microbial metabolism, prolonged treatment is thought to be necessary.

A third significant factor in the efficacy of antibacterial chemotherapy is the as yet obscure role of the defense mechanisms in the CNS. While in early stages of syphilis the local defense of the host is characterized by predominating T-helper/inducer cell infiltrates within the lesions, in later stages the lesions prevalently show T-suppressor cells which are presumed to cause a natural shutdown of the vigorous early immune system response [6]. Additionally, *T. pallidum* is thought to employ special strategies to elude tissue defense mechanisms, e.g., masking with substances derived from the host. This precondition justifies the necessity of high-dose systemic antibiotics to eradicate the pathogen.

In vitro concentrations which immobilize 50% of the treponemes are 0.002 μg/ml, 0.07 μg/ml, and 0.01 μg/ml for penicillin G, amoxicillin, and ceftriaxone, respectively [14]. These concentrations ought to be exceeded in vivo by a factor of 10. Doses of ceftriaxone of 2 g/day (initial 4 g/day) are suited to achieve corresponding CSF concentrations [22]. Because the efficacy of this compound against neurosyphilis was confirmed in a clinical study [18], it is an attractive alternative to penicillin G. Advantages of ceftriaxone are its long half-life (only one dose daily) and its ability to sufficiently penetrate the CNS, although its antitreponemal activity is probably not better than that of high-dose penicillin. Chloramphenicol and doxycycline have also been administered to small groups of patients suffering from neurosyphilis; however, definite recommendations cannot yet be made [5, 26].

14.8 Clinical Recommendations

The current recommendations of the CDC for the treatment of neurosyphilis are aqueous crystalline penicillin G, 3–4 mio IU every 4 h (18–24 mio IU/day) for 10–14 days [3]. In some European clinics, administration of 3×10 or 5×5 mio IU/day is usual. Its efficacy is comparable to the regimen recommended by the CDC [29]. Procaine penicillin G 2.4 (as well 4.8) mio IU/day by intramuscular injection, plus probenecid 500 mg orally four times daily for 10–14 days, may fail to reach treponemocidal levels in CSF [8]. In contrast to the CDC we therefore do not recommend this regimen.

A therapeutic alternative constitutes of ceftriaxone 2 g i.v. once daily with an initial dose of 4 g given for 10–14 days. The regimens using high-dose penicillin G or ceftriaxone are suggested in patients with CNS symptoms as well as those with pathologic CSF findings, irrespective of the stage of syphilis.

As a third-line therapy, doxycycline can be administered to individuals who are allergic to beta-lactam antibiotics. The recommended dose is 2×200 mg/day orally for 4 weeks [5]. Doxycycline is contraindicated during pregnancy and breastfeeding.

In the past, some clinics used chloramphenicol in patients with neurosyphilis. As the efficacy of this compound has not been tested in controlled studies, it should be given only in special cases in which the aforementioned antibiotics are contraindicated.

14.9 Symptomatic Therapy

Paretic neurosyphilis frequently manifests as epileptic fits (up to 38%), psychotic episodes (54%), and headaches (27%) [23]. Epileptic fits and states should be treated according to the general guidelines for anticonvulsive therapy. First-choice drugs in complex focal seizures are still carbamazepine and lamotrigine. Promising alternatives are levetiracetam and zonisamide. Psychotic episodes associated with massive agitation or excitation may require neuroleptics (haloperidol, olanzapine, melperone). Headaches can be treated, if at all necessary, by paracetamol or Voltaren-potassium.

Attacks of lightning pain and gastric crises in tabetic patients should be treated with potent analgesics, but lightning pains often are unresponsive to "classic" analgesic. In such cases a tentative therapy of carbamazepine (or pregabalin), amitryptiline, and flupirtine (or an opioid) in combination can be attempted. In patients with meningovascular neurosyphilis cerebral ischemia has to be treated according to the guidelines for strokes. Hydrocephalus, a rare complication of neurosyphilis, sometimes requires ventricular shunting. Syphilitic polyradiculitis can be managed like

Guillain-Barré syndrome. The use of corticosteroids (only along with antibiotics) for neurosyphilis must be considered experimental.

14.10 Evaluation of the Therapeutic Effect

After successful treatment the CSF pleocytosis will fade within a few weeks or months, and *T. pallidum*-specific IgM antibodies in serum will disappear within 6–12 months. In exceptional cases it may take 2–3 years for the 19 S-(IgM)FTA-ABS test to become negative. The reappearance of specific serum IgM antibodies after chemotherapy points to reinfection or relapse. After effective therapy, the quantitative results of the reagin tests (VDRL, cardiolipin complement-fixation reaction (CFR)) should decrease fourfold in 3 months and no longer be positive after 1 year. Intrathecally produced IgG (increased IgG index; oligoclonal bands) may persist for years; the IgG index declines exponentially. The ITpA index ≥ 3 should not be used as a parameter for therapy response since it may be unchanged for long periods of time in spite of effective treatment. Patients who have positive reagin tests (VDRL, cardiolipin CFR) in serum should be checked serologically every 6 months until they are negative.

Lumbar puncture and CSF analysis should be repeated every 6 months until the cell count is normal. Treatment failure is recognizable by clinical progression, increased titers of reagin tests by two or more dilutions, and the failure of CNS pleocytosis to resolve.

Jarisch-Herxheimer reaction (convulsions, worsening of neurological signs, etc.) seldom occurs in neurosyphilis (1–2%). According to some authors [32], this reaction can be mitigated by meptazinol.

14.11 Neurosyphilis and HIV Infection

Syphilitic patients coinfected with HIV seem to show an accelerated and more aggressive course of both treponemal and retroviral infection [9]. Moreover, there is evidence that coexistent HIV infection can impair the response of patients with early syphilis to benzathine penicillin G [10]. Observations (ours and [7]) that meningovascular neurosyphilis can develop after antibiotic chemotherapy of early syphilis suggest that neurosyphilis may be a more common complication of syphilis in HIV patients. Retrospective studies suggest that the procaine penicillin G regimen recommended by CDC for neurosyphilis fails in 23–60% of HIV-infected patients [18].

Coinfection of syphilis and HIV may pose problems of discrimination between a syphilitic and an HIV origin of CNS symptoms. Both infections may cause cognitive deficits and neurological abnormalities as well as CSF pleocytosis, higher immunoglobulin production rates, and/or increased CSF protein concentrations. The CSF-VDRL test (in Germany less common) is sensitive in only 70% of the HIV infected. Consequently, a negative result does not exclude a syphilitic CNS involvement. Conversely, false positive reagin tests may occur in earlier stages of the HIV infection, probably due to polyclonal B-cell activation [10]. The CSF-PCR for *T. pallidum* has also been shown to be of limited usefulness for diagnosing neurosyphilis in HIV-infected individuals [17]. These circumstances substantiate a certain diagnostic dilemma in HIV and *T. pallidum* coinfected patients who exhibit CNS symptoms and pathologic CSF findings. Theoretically, the determination of intrathecal antibody synthesis against the two pathogens could resolve this dilemma and make it feasible to discriminate among syphilitic, HIV, and a simultaneously syphilitic and HIV related origin of the inflammatory CNS process. We have shown in our laboratory for more than two decades that this procedure is practicable.

As to the therapy of coinfected individuals, we recommend high-dose penicillin G (30 mio IU/day in three doses) or ceftriaxone (initial 4 g/day, then 2 g/day) for 2 weeks. The need for careful follow-up after treatment is imperative. In case of doubt, a retreatment should be carried out.

Take-Home Messages

- As a result of the rarity of neurosyphilis, it is often recognized too late, the more so as the serologic screening tests were abandoned in clinical routines.
- The diagnosis of neurosyphilis is founded on clinical symptomatology, serologic tests

(TPPH and FTA-ABS test), and analysis of the CSF, which reveals indications of a chronic inflammatory CNS process including an intrathecal IgG-dominant immunoglobulin production.

- Syphilitic CNS involvement is proven when an *intrathecal synthesis* of syphilis-specific antibody takes place, i.e., ITpA index ≥ 3
- Criteria of process activity are: (a) presence of *T. pallidum*-specific IgM antibodies and/or positive reagin tests (VDRL, cardiolipin CFR) *in blood*, and (b) CSF pleocytosis and alteration of the blood–brain barrier with elevated protein *in CSF*.
- Successful chemotherapy leads to: (a) normalization of pleocytosis within a few weeks or months, (b) disappearance of specific IgM antibodies in serum within 6–12 months or longer (19 S-(IgM)FTA-ABS test becomes negative) and decreasing titers of the reagin tests, (c) exponential reduction of (unspecific) intrathecal IgG production over the years, and (d) termination of the disease's clinical progress.
- First-choice therapy is now as before high-dose penicillin G intravenously. Ceftriaxone also is sufficient for treating neurosyphilis; an advantage of this compound is that the therapy can be continued outpatient.

References

1. Bracero, I., Wormser, G.P., Bottone, E.J.: Serologic tests for syphilis: a guide to interpretation in various states of disease. Mt. Sinai J. Med. **46**, 289–292 (1979)
2. Burke, J.M., Schaberg, D.R.: Neurosyphilis in the antibiotic era. Neurology **35**, 1368–1371 (1985)
3. Centers for Disease Control and Prevention: Sexually transmitted disease treatment guidelines. MMWR Morb. Mortal Wkly Rep. **55**, 40–43 (2006)
4. Clark, E.G., Danbolt, N.: The Oslo study of the natural history of untreated syphilis. J. Chron. Dis. **2**, 311–344 (1955)
5. Clinical Effectiveness Group: UK national guidelines for the management of late syphilis. http://www.bashh.org/guidelins.asp (2002).
6. Engelkens, H.J.H., ten Kate, F.J.W., Judanarso, J., et al.: The localisation of treponemes and characterisation of the inflammatory infiltrate in skin biopsies from patients with primary or secondary syphilis, or early infectious yaws. Genitourin. Med. (England) **69**, 102–107 (1993)
7. Fox, P.A., Hawkin, D.A., Dawson, D.: Dementia following an acute presentation of meningovascular neurosyphilis in an HIV-1 positive patient. AIDS **14**, 2062–2063 (2000)
8. Goh, B., Smith, G.W., Samarasinghe, L., et al.: Penicillin concentrations in serum and cerebrospinal fluid after intramuscular injection of aqueous procaine penicillin 0.6 MU with and without probenecid. Br. J. Vener. Dis. **60**, 371–373 (1984)
9. Gordon, S.M., Eaton, M.E., George, R., et al.: The response of symptomatic neurosyphilis to high-dose intravenous penicillin G in patients with HIV infection. N Engl. J. Med. **331**, 1469–1473 (1994)
10. Hook, E.W., Marra, C.: Acquired syphilis in adults. N Engl. J. Med. **326**, 1060–1069 (1992)
11. Hooshmand, H., Escobar, M.R., Kopf, S.W.: Neurosyphilis. A study of 241 patients. JAMA **219**, 726–729 (1972)
12. Hutchinson, J.: Disease of the Eye and Ear Consequent upon Inherited Syphilis. Churchill, London (1863)
13. Idsøe, O., Guthe, T., Willcox, R.R.: Penicillin in the treatment of syphilis. The experience of three decades. Bull. World Health Organ. **47**(Suppl), 1–68 (1972)
14. Korting, H.C., Walther, G., Riethmüller, U., et al.: Comparative in vivo susceptibility of *Treponema pallidum* to ceftizoxime, ceftriaxone and penicillin G. Chemotherapy **32**, 352–355 (1986)
15. Löwhagen, G.B., Andersen, M., Blomstrand, C., et al.: Central nervous system involvement in early syphilis. Acta Derm. Venereol. (Stockholm) **63**, 409–417 (1983)
16. Lukehart, S.A., Hook, E.W., Baker-Zander, S.A., et al.: Invasion of the central nervous system by *Treponema pallidum*. Ann. Intern. Med. **109**, 855–862 (1988)
17. Marra, C.M., Gary, D.W., Kuypers, J. et al.: Diagnosis of neurosyphilis in patients infected with human immunodeficiency virus type 1. J. Infect. Dis. **174**, 219–221 (1996)
18. Marra, C.M., Boutin, P., McArthur, J.C., et al.: A pilot study evaluating ceftriaxone and penicillin G as treatment agents for neurosyphilis in human immunodeficiency virus-infected individuals. Clin. Infect. Dis. **30**, 540–544 (2000)
19. Mohr, J.A., Griffiths, W., Jackson, R., et al.: Neurosyphilis and penicillin levels in cerebrospinal fluid. JAMA **236**, 2208–2209 (1976)
20. Moore, J.E., Faupel, M.: Asymptomatic neurosyphilis. A comparison of early and late asymptomatic neurosyphilis. Arch. Dermatol. Syph. **18**, 99–108 (1928)
21. Moore, J.E., Hopkins, H.H.: Asymptomatic neurosyphilis. VI. The prognosis of early and late asymptomatic neurosyphilis. JAMA **95**, 1637–1641 (1930)
22. Nau, R., Prange, H.W., Muth, P., et al.: Passage of cefotaxime and ceftriaxone into the cerebrospinal fluid of patients with uninflamed meninges. Antimicrob. Agents Chemother. **27**, 1518–1524 (1993)
23. Prange, H.: Neurosyphilis. VCH Verlag, Weinheim (1987)
24. Prange, H.W., Moskophidis, M., Schipper, H., et al.: Relationship between neurological features and intrathecal synthesis of IgG antibodies to *Treponema pallidum*. J. Neurol. **230**, 241–252 (1983)
25. Prange, H.W., Bobis-Seidenschwanz, I.: Zur Evaluierung serologischer Aktivitätskriterien bei Neurosyphilis. Verh. Dtsch. Ges. Neurol. **8**, 789–791 (1994/95)
26. Quinn, T.C., Bender, B.: Sexually transmitted diseases. In: Harvey, A.M., Johns, R.J. (eds.) The Principles and Practice of Medicine, 22nd edn, pp. 661–663. Appleton & Lange, Norwalk (1988)

27. Reiber, H., Lange, P.: Quantification of virus-specific antibodies in cerebrospinal fluid and serum. Clin. Chem. **37**, 1153–1160 (1991)
28. Rein, M.: Treatment of neurosyphilis. JAMA **246**, 2613–2614 (1981)
29. Robert-Koch-Institut: Syphilis in Deutschland. Neurosyphilis – Fallbericht, Bedeutung, Diagnostik und Prävention. Epidemiol. Bull. **5**, 35–36 (2002)
30. Robert-Koch-Institut: Syphilis in Deutschland. Berichtsmonat Juli. Epidemiol. Bull. **29**, 257 (2007)
31. Secher, L., Weismann, K., Kobayshi, T.: *Treponema pallidum* in peripheral nerve tissue of syphilitic chancre. Acta Derm. Veneral. (Stockholm) **62**, 407–411 (1982)
32. Silberstein, P., Lawrence, R., Pryor, D., et al.: A case of neurosyphilis with florid Jarisch-Herxheimer reaction. J. Clin. Neurosci. **9**, 689–690 (2002)
33. Volles, E., Ritter, G.: Zur Penicillin-Behandlung der Neurolues unter pharmakokinetischem Aspekt. Z. Neurol. **206**, 235–242 (1974)

Syphilis and HIV

15

Natalia Mendoza, Adriana Motta, Brenda L. Pellicane, Parisa Ravanfar, and Stephen K. Tyring

Core Messages

- Syphilis incidence has increased since HIV has become a chronic disease due to the antiretroviral therapy.
- Genital ulcers increase the transmission of HIV.
- Patients with HIV are at an increased risk for syphilis.
- Neurosyphilis is more common in HIV positive patients, therefore early recognition of syphilis is mandatory in order to prevent neurologic complications.
- Clinical manifestations of syphilis in an HIV infected patient may vary. Skin exam, including the adnexa of the skin, anogenital area, and oral mucosa should be performed. An examination for lymphadenopathy and for neurological symptoms must also be completed.
- Early diagnosis and treatment of syphilis may reduce the incidence especially in the HIV population.

N. Mendoza (✉)
Center for Clinical Studies, Universidad El Bosque, Bogota, Colombia
e-mail: nmendoza@ccstexas.com

A. Motta
Dermatology Department, Universidad El Bosque, Carrera 7 B Bis No. 132 – 11, Bogota, Colombia
e-mail: motticas@gmail.com

B.L. Pellicane, P. Ravanfar, and S.K. Tyring
Dermatology Department, Center for Clinical Studies, University of Texas, 6655 Travis suite 100, Houston, TX 77030, USA
e-mail: Bbartlett@ccstexas.com; pravanfar@ccstexas.com; styring@ccstexas.com

15.1 Introduction

Syphilis is a fascinating and challenging disease because of its variable clinical presentation and course. Its history is colorful and full of controversy. The discovery of penicillin and the public health efforts made to reduce transmission brought down its rate significantly; however, syphilis resurged in the 1990s along with one of the most important pandemic diseases, human immunodeficiency virus (HIV).

15.2 Epidemiology

Syphilis and HIV have played an important role in public health. These two infections overlap, interact, and share significant characteristics. They are both sexually transmitted with the potential for vertical infection from the mother to the fetus and are substantial health problems worldwide [1].

Syphilis incidence peaked in the 1940s in the United States; however, health interventions such as contact tracing, case finding, and the use of penicillin significantly decreased this incidence [2]. In the 1980s the incidence increased primarily among heterosexuals and African Americans. The increase was in part attributed to high-risk activities such as the use of IV drugs and the involvement in the sexual industry [3].

After the HIV pandemic period in the 1990s, the rates for sexually transmitted diseases decreased in Western countries, reaching the lowest rates for syphilis and gonorrhea, especially in the United States and in some of the European countries. The decrease in infection rates during the last decade of the twentieth century was related to the high anti-immunodeficiency

G. Gross and S.K. Tyring (eds.), *Sexually Transmitted Infections and Sexually Transmitted Diseases*,
DOI: 10.1007/978-3-642-14663-3_15,

syndrome (AIDS) mortality rate. Data suggest that per every 20 AIDS deaths in a population of 100,000, the primary and secondary syphilis rate decreased between 7% and 12%. In addition, during 1990 and 1995, the increase in AIDS mortality was related to a one-third decrease in the syphilis rate between men [4].

The lowest incidence of syphilis was reached in 2000 during the early HIV campaigns. Between 1990 and 2000, the primary and secondary syphilis rate in the United States decreased by 90%, from 2.34 per 100,000 people to 2.12 per 100,000 [4,5]. Some of these changes were attributed to population-wide behavioral modifications in response to AIDS campaigns [5]. However, since 1995, some outbreaks related to major metropolitan areas and to HIV-infected men who have sex with men (MSM) were reported in the Soviet Union, followed by the United States and other Western countries [6]. This became a reality for the United States soon after 2000. The age group with the highest rate of infection consisted of men aged 33–44 years, exceeding the rates in 20–24-year-olds [7]. The 2003 rate signaled the third consecutive year of increase in the overall rate; it was 19% higher than the rate in 2002, reflecting a 62% increase in men and a 53% decrease in women [5].

A disproportionate increase in the MSM population was noticed in western Europe (Denmark, France, Germany, Ireland, Spain, Switzerland, and the United Kingdom). Dougan et al. reviewed all of the published literature between 1996 and 2006 which included HIV patients on treatment with highly active antiretroviral therapy (HAART). The authors found that the prevalence of HIV in the communities of MSM increased from 5% to 18% between 2000 and 2004. The HIV prevalence between the MSM populations with a diagnosis of syphilis varied from 14% to 59%, with a mean of 42%. The most affected European cities were Paris, London, and Dublin [8]. Depending on the geographic location, the rate of coinfection with HIV and syphilis in MSM ranged from 30% to 60% [1,8].

The resurgence of syphilis has occurred around the world. Some have suggested that advances in the treatment of HIV have led to lax behaviors among MSM. Another factor to consider is biologic, since the syphilitic ulcer can facilitate HIV transmission [9]. Some authors have suggested that syphilis could increase the viral load in men with HIV and decrease the CD4 count [10].

Specifically in the United States, the lowest syphilis rate was in the twentieth century, in part due to the national program to eradicate syphilis. Unfortunately, since 2001 the primary and secondary rates have increased 12% per 100,000 and the incidence has increased from 2.1 in 2000 to 2.7 in 2004. [11] The infection is 5.2 times more common in men, [12] with 4.2 cases per 100,000 men versus 0.8 cases per 100,000 women, in 2003.

It has been estimated that 16% of all patients and 28% of all men infected with syphilis are coinfected with HIV in the United States. [13] Some studies have shown that one of the most important risk factors for syphilis is having HIV infection (odds ratio (OR) 7.3). Others factors include the use of methamphetamines and/or sildenafil citrate (OR 6.2), a strong gay community affiliation, and sexual partners who met through Internet communications [14].

Considering this new syphilitic "outbreak" and altered epidemiology, the current knowledge of HIV and syphilis coinfection for practitioners becomes essential.

15.3 Natural History and Clinical Manifestations

Syphilis is a highly infectious sexually transmitted disease (STD) caused by *Treponema pallidum*. [15] It is a systemic disease characterized by symptomatic periods alternating with periods of clinical latency, which results in a wide variety of clinical presentations [2]. Classically, syphilis infection has been divided into primary, secondary, latent, and tertiary stages.

The clinical manifestations of syphilis in HIV patients can be very similar to those seen in an otherwise healthy host; however, coinfection with these two organisms may also alter the symptoms and signs, the progression of the disease, and the risk of progressing to the tertiary stage [16].

In an immunocompetent host, primary syphilis is characterized by the presence of a chancre which develops 2–6 weeks after exposure to *T. Pallidum*, and is associated with localized lymphadenopathy. This chancre is a unique, firm, usually painless, nonpurulent, indurated, round ulcer located in the inoculation area. It initially presents as a small papule that ulcerates very rapidly.

Genital ulcers primarily increase the transmission of HIV for two reasons: the loss of the epidermal barrier and local inflammation [17]. Some studies report that syphilis increases viral replication, viral shedding, and the viral load in the seminal fluid in HIV patients [18,19]. In addition, a transient decrease in CD4 T cell counts and increase in the HIV viral load have been demonstrated in chronically infected HIV patients [20,21]. Syphilis has been estimated to increase HIV transmission two to ninefold and HIV acquisition two to fourfold [22].

In HIV-positive patients, primary syphilis can present with multiple ulcers that are similar to herpetic lesions (soft chancre) [23,24]. These lesions are deeper, persist longer, [25] may leave a scar upon healing, and may lead to perforations in the prepuce or labia majora [26]. Some authors have described the presence of a chancre (primary syphilis) and clinical manifestations of secondary syphilis simultaneously [16,24]. In these patients coinfected with HIV, the lesions may be localized in the mouth [27] and pharynx due to oral sex [12]. The distribution of syphilis ulcers in homosexuals has been reported as 12.5% in the oral mucosa and 20% in the anus and rectum; however, the involvement of lymph nodes is not clinically evident since the paraaortic lymph nodes are affected [28]. The duration of the lesions may vary from 30 to 90 days [2].

Secondary syphilis presents after hematogenous dissemination from the chancre has occurred, usually 4–10 weeks after appearance of the primary chancre in the immunocompetent patient. It usually manifests as mucocutaneous lesions with systemic symptoms. However, 75% of coinfected HIV patients present with secondary syphilis while the chancre is still present. Systemic symptoms include fever, anorexia, muscle pain, depression, arthritis, and weight loss [29]. Mucocutaneous lesions typically present as generalized, nonpruritic, symmetric, oval, violaceous, pink or coppery brown macules varying in size from 1 to 20 mm with involvement of the palms and soles [29] (Figs 15.1 and 15.2), which tend to disappear within 2 weeks. Papules and lichenoid lesions can be present in 50–80% of the cases, and some individuals may have painful palmoplantar keratoderma (resembling psoriasis) and osteitis [2]. The scalp may be involved, resulting in alopecia; the eyebrows and beard area can be affected as well. Oral lesions present as small to medium-sized, highly contagious, grayish ulcers localized to the tongue, labia, and oral mucosa [12] (Fig. 15.3). Raised papules and plaques, known as latum condylomata lata, can be present on the perineum, external genitalia, or inguinal area (Fig. 15.4) [29].

Malignant syphilis is a rare, aggressive, ulcerating form of secondary syphilis occurring more frequently

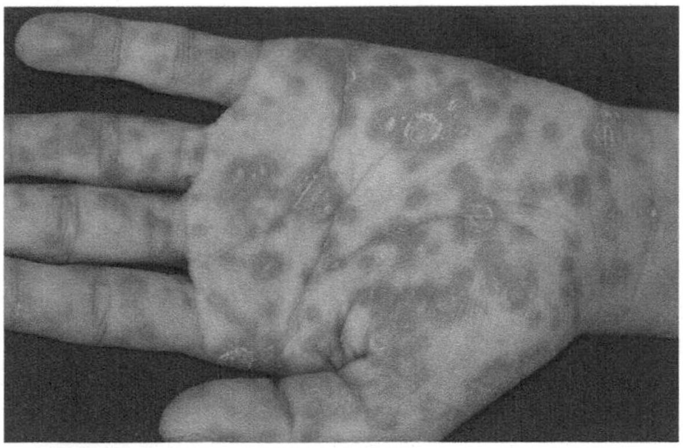

Fig. 15.1 Oval, violaceous, pink or coppery brown macules involving the palms. Secondary syphilis

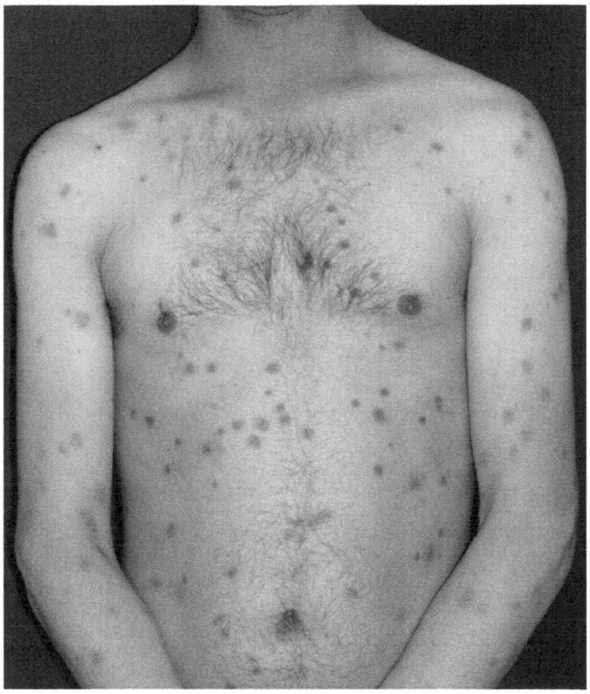

Fig. 15.2 Oval, violaceous, pink or coppery brown macules involving the trunk. Secondary syphilis

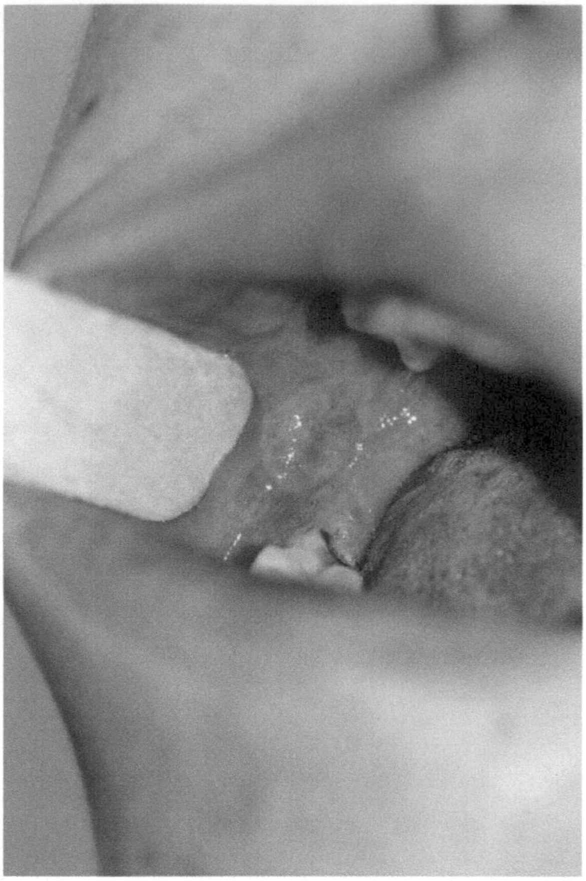

Fig. 15.3 Medium sized grayish ulcers localized to the oral mucosa

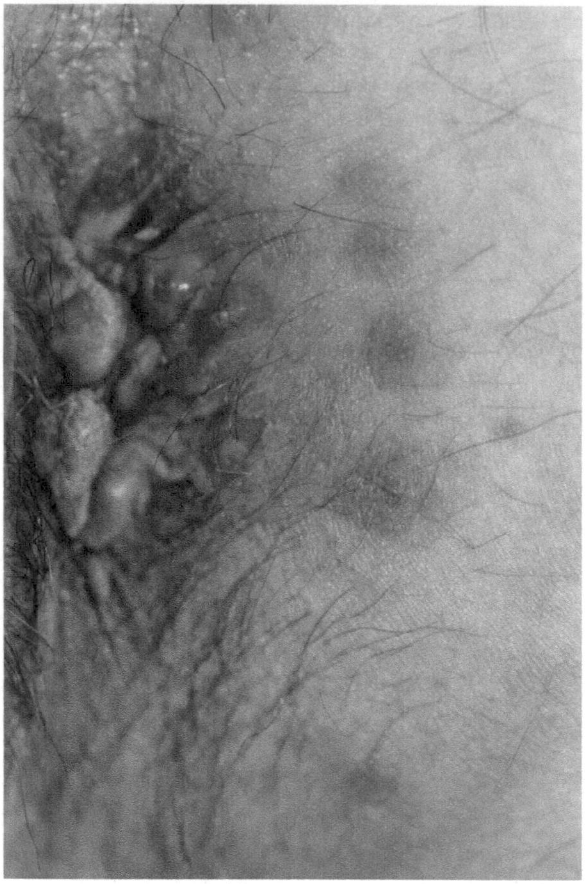

Fig. 15.4 Condyloma latum

in HIV-coinfected patients. It is characterized by crusted, ulcerative nodules that grow rapidly. These lesions localize to the face and inferior extremities (Fig. 15.5); however, the oral and nasal mucosa can be involved as well. Systemic symptoms are common and include vomiting, diarrhea, hepatomegaly, splenomegaly, and lymphadenopathy [2,30]. This type of syphilis must be differentiated from mycosis fungoides and lymphomatoid papulosis [30].

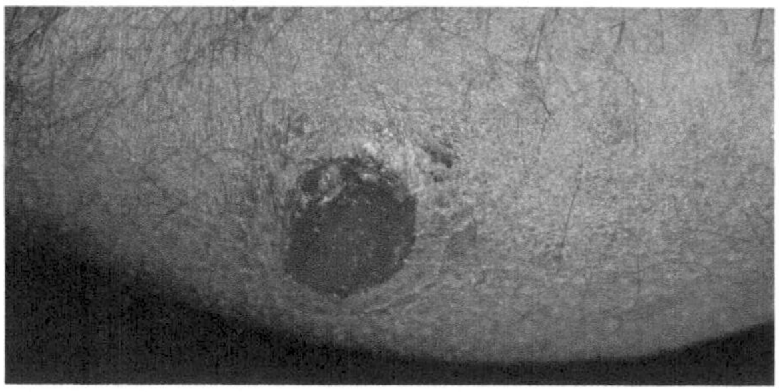

Fig. 15.5 Malignant syphilis

15.3.1 Ocular Syphilis

Ocular involvement has been reported with primary and secondary syphilis; in the primary stage the chancre is localized on the eyelids and conjunctiva and resolves spontaneously. During the secondary stage, unilateral anterior and posterior granulomatous uveitis can be seen. Other manifestations include episcleritis, blepharitis, conjunctivitis, iris nodules, neuroretinitis, and vasculitis. During the tertiary stage the pupils are compromised and do not react to light. In HIV patients, ocular involvement is increased and the retina is frequently affected, manifesting as retinal detachment and acute necrosis. Patients with such presentations should always be evaluated for neurosyphilis [31]. In patients with ocular syphilis or tertiary syphilis, lumbar punctures must be done every 3 months to evaluate their response to therapy [31].

15.3.2 Latent Syphilis

Latent syphilis is an asymptomatic period, in which diagnosis can be only made by serologic testing. Latent syphilis has been divided into an early phase (less than 12 months) and a late phase (≥12 months). It appears that during this period the patient is not contagious. Twenty-five percent of patients with latent syphilis will develop tertiary syphilis [32].

15.3.3 Tertiary Syphilis

Tertiary syphilis is characterized by long-term complications of the infection. This stage is considered noninfectious [32]. Tertiary syphilis can manifest in three main forms: benign, cardiovascular, and neurosyphilis.

The benign form is characterized by gummas, which are granulomatous-like indolent lesions; gummas vary in size from millimeters to large masses and are located primarily in the skin, liver, and bone, but can affect any organ. They manifest approximately 15 years after infection [32,33]. Mucocutaneous gummas can be disfiguring and destructive (palate or nasal septum) [27]; however, gummas are still a rare clinical manifestation [1]. In the HIV era the most common gummas described are visceral, especially cerebral [34].

Cardiovascular syphilis is characterized by asymptomatic ascending aortitis resulting in aortic regurgitation, aortic aneurysm, and coronary stenosis; it is caused by damage to the vasa vasorum, where *T. pallidum* resides. [1] Cardiovascular syphilis remains rare since the introduction of penicillin. Interestingly, coinfection with HIV has not increased its rate of occurrence [35].

15.3.4 Neurosyphilis

Treponemal invasion of the CSF occurs in approximately 25% of patients infected with syphilis. Most cases, including HIV-positive and HIV-negative patients, will have spontaneous resolution with or without treatment [36].

Neurosyphilis may occur at any stage of the disease and has been divided into early and late neurosyphilis to facilitate a better understanding. Early neurosyphilis is characterized by the compromise of the meninges and associated blood vessels, leading to meningovascular disease including strokes, meningitis, seizures, acute and subacute myelopathy, brainstem or cranial nerve alterations, and vestibular and optic disease. [2] Late neurosyphilis tends to affect the spinal cord parenchyma and brain presenting as dementia, tabes dorsalis, sensory ataxia, general paresis, and/or bladder and bowel dysfunction [2].

It has been reported in the literature that neurosyphilis can occur earlier and more frequently in HIV patients (11-fold) than in those subjects who are not coinfected with HIV [37]. In addition, neurosyphilis can develop in HIV-infected patients despite receipt of the conventional treatment for syphilis. While clinical manifestations vary, the most common include meningeal compromise, cranial nerve palsies, dysarthria, and ocular disease. Lesions tend to recur more often in HIV patients [37].

Katz et al. (1993) compared HIV-infected patients with those who were HIV-negative and found that neurosyphilis occurred earlier (younger patients) in HIV-infected patients and presented with more secondary symptoms such as fever, malaise, skin lesions, lymphadenopathy, and headache. Syphilitic meningitis and ocular involvement were also more common in the HIV population. The CSF of HIV-positive patients had higher protein and lower glucose levels [38].

Several reports describe the accelerated progression through the syphilitic stages in HIV patients [16,29]. The interactions between HIV and syphilis have been gaining more and more attention due to the rapid progression from primary syphilis to neurosyphilis, which is directly correlated with the level of immunosuppression and similarly the level of HIV/AIDS disease [16].

15.4 Diagnosis

Diagnosing syphilis requires taking a detailed medical history including risk assessment for STDs with an emphasis on symptoms related to dermatological, neurological, ocular, auditory, and vestibular manifestations. A complete skin exam, including the adnexa of the skin, anogenital area, and oral mucosa should be performed. An examination for lymphadenopathy and for neurological symptoms must also be completed [2]. The diagnosis of syphilis is confirmed by serologic tests and by the visualization of the treponema using dark field microscopy (not appropriate for oral and rectal samples due to the presence of other spirochetes) [39]. However, serologic tests usually do not become positive until after the clinical manifestations have been present for at least 3 weeks. Direct fluorescent antibodies and polymerase chain reaction (PCR) can be used, especially when the symptoms and the serologic tests are discordant [1].

Dark field microscopy is the only test that allows for immediate diagnosis. The sample must be taken from the lesions, avoiding blood, and read very quickly by an experienced person [2]. The spirochete is identified by its shape and movement [39]. Direct immunofluorescence allows for distinguishing of *T. pallidum* from other nonpathogenic treponema. PCR has a 95–97% specificity and a 91–95% sensitivity; however, due to a high cost, it is not commonly used [39]. Some cases require performing a skin biopsy to visualize the bacteria using a Warthin Starry stain.

The most common nonspecific treponema tests used are the rapid plasma reagin (RPR) and the Venereal Disease Research Laboratory (VDRL). The specific tests include fluorescent treponemic antibody absorption (FTA-ABS), microhemagglutination test for antibodies to *T. pallidum* (MHA-TP) and *T. pallidum* particle agglutination assay (TPPA).

For the majority of the HIV population coinfected with syphilis, laboratory tests can be interpreted as they would be in an immunocompetent host; however, atypical serologic results can occur (false negatives, delayed titer responses) [16]. If the serology tests are negative, then skin biopsy, dark field microscopy, or PCR testing would be necessary to confirm the diagnosis. Serology tests may remain positive despite an appropriate treatment after 1 year in 18% of the coinfected population but in only 5% of the non-HIV-infected population. [40] Some studies report cases of seronegativity and return of titers to nonreactive as immunosuppression advances [1,41].

Neurosyphilis diagnosis is based on clinical symptoms, signs, serology, and CSF tests. Its diagnosis is difficult in most of the patients but is even more difficult in HIV-infected patients. A CSF-VDRL, increased CSF protein, or CSF pleocytosis (>5 white blood cells/uL) is considered positive; however, HIV infection alone is associated with CSF pleocytosis and increased proteins making the diagnosis more difficult [16].

15.4.1 Pathology

Skin biopsy is recommended in discordant cases. Depending on the stage of the syphilis infection the skin histological findings will vary. Plasma cell-rich infiltrate within the dermis is the classic finding seen in primary and secondary syphilis. In secondary syphilis, the epidermal changes include acanthosis and spongiosis. The infiltrate compromises the superficial and deep perivascular dermis. Some authors have described lichenoid, granulomatous and neutrophil-rich patterns [8].

15.5 Treatment

15.5.1 Primary and Secondary Syphilis

The CDC guidelines for treatment of primary, secondary, tertiary, and early latent syphilis (less than 1 year) in HIV patients are very similar compared to those of HIV-negative patients. The recommended treatment is benzathine penicillin G administered parenterally, 2.4 million units IM in a single dose. Other specialists recommend penicillin G administered at 1-week intervals for 3 weeks in addition to the regular doses, especially in those patients with CSF abnormalities.

15.5.2 Latent Syphilis

Patients with latent syphilis of unknown duration and a normal CSF examination can be treated with benzathine penicillin G at weekly doses of 2.4 million units for 3 weeks. The patients must be evaluated both clinically and serologically at 6, 12, 18, and 24 months after therapy. If the titers do not decline fourfold during the first 12–24 months, the CSF must be reexamined and treatment readministrated.

For cases of late and tertiary syphilis without neurosyphilis a total dose of 7.2 million units of benzathine penicillin is recommended.

15.5.3 Tertiary Syphilis

Tertiary syphilis refers to cardiovascular and gumma syphilis. Tertiary syphilis does not always include neurosyphilis. The recommended treatment regimen is benzathine penicillin G 7.2 million units totally administered as three doses of 2.4 million units IM weekly for a total of 3 weeks. Patients who have cardiovascular syphilis are occasionally treated in the same manner as those with neurosyphilis.

15.5.4 Neurosyphilis

The recommended treatment for neurosyphilis is with aqueous crystalline penicillin G 18–24 million units per day, administrated as 3–4 million units IV every 4 h or continuous infusion for 10–14 days. CSF examinations should be repeated every 6 months if pleocytosis was initially present; additionally VDRL must be closely followed and both test results should normalize within 2 years.

In the case of treatment failure, the patient must be treated with aqueous crystalline penicillin G followed by three weekly doses of benzathine penicillin. If a reduction in titer is not obtained after the second treatment the patient should not be re-treated unless there is clinical evidence of reinfection or signs of the disease.

15.5.5 Pregnancy and HIV Coinfection

There is no sufficient evidence to determine optimal penicillin regimens in pregnancy; therefore, the same doses should be used as in nonpregnant patients.

15.5.6 Penicillin Allergy

There are few data supporting the use of alternative treatments to penicillin. Some therapies used in nonpregnant, penicillin-allergic patients include doxycycline (100 mg orally twice daily for 14 days), tetracycline (500 mg four times daily for 14 days), ceftriaxone (1 g daily either IM or IV for 8–10 days), and azithromycin (single oral dose 2 g) without complete success [32–34,42]. These therapies have not been well studied in patients coinfected with HIV [43,44].

For patients who may not be compliant with medication and/or treatment follow-up should be desensitized and treated with benzathine penicillin.

15.5.7 Jarisch-Herxheimer Reaction

Within 24 h after any therapy for syphilis, the patients can develop a Jarisch-Herxheimer reaction, an acute febrile reaction associated with myalgia, headache, fever, chills, and exacerbation of the skin lesions. It is produced as the result of the release of dead spirochete bacteria after the initial treatment. Patients should be aware of the possibility of developing this reaction [45].

15.5.8 Treatment Follow-up

Patients must be evaluated for treatment failure at 3, 6, 9, 12, and 24 months after initial therapy. Treatment failure is considered when the signs and symptoms persist or recur in patients who have a fourfold increase in their nontreponemal test titer. In these cases, patients are managed similar to non-HIV-infected patients. CSF and re-treatment is considered in patients whose nontreponemal tests do not decrease (fourfold) within 6–12 months of therapy. The majority of specialists treat treatment failure with benzathine penicillin G, three doses of 2.4 million units IM at weekly intervals (if CSF examinations are normal).

15.6 Conclusion

The incidence of syphilis is increasing again, especially in association with the HIV pandemic. The clinical manifestations in most of the cases remain the same; however, the lesions are more aggressive, the coexistence of primary and secondary syphilis is more frequent, and the progression to neurosyphilis is faster. The diagnosis can be confusing due to false negatives serologies, but must be suspected when clinical lesions are present. All patients presenting with syphilis manifestations must be tested for HIV and HIV-positive patients must be continually tested for syphilis since it is known that the syphilis infection increases the transmission of HIV. Patients coinfected with HIV and syphilis may experience reactivation, a greater risk of neurological complications, and increased therapeutic failure.

Take-Home Pearls

- Consider syphilis as a diagnosis in HIV positive patients with atypical skin lesions with or without systemic symptoms.
- Primary syphilis can be silent in HIV positive patients. Secondary syphilis may present as the first manifestation.
- Neurosyphilis is more common in HIV infected patients. Serology and cerebrospinal fluid tests are recommended in all HIV positive patients.

References

1. Stevenson, J., Heath, M.: Syphilis and HIV infection: an update. Dermatol. Clin. **24**(4), 497–507 (2006). vi
2. Zetola, N.M., Engelman, J., Jensen, T.P., Klausner, J.D.: Syphilis in the United States: an update for clinicians with an emphasis on HIV coinfection. Mayo Clin. Proc. **82**(9), 1091–1102 (2007)
3. Buckley, H.B.: Syphilis: a review and update of this 'new' infection of the '90s. Nurse Pract. **25**(8), 9–32 (1992)
4. Chesson, H.W., Dee, T.S., Aral, S.O.: AIDS mortality may have contributed to the decline in syphilis rates in the United States in the 1990s. Sex. Transm. Dis. **30**(5), 419–424 (2003)
5. Lautenschlager, S.: Cutaneous manifestations of syphilis: recognition and management. Am. J. Clin. Dermatol. **7**(5), 291–304 (2006)
6. Nicoll, A., Hamers, F.F.: Are trends in HIV, gonorrhoea, and syphilis worsening in western Europe? BMJ (Clinical research ed) **324**(7349), 1324–1327 (2002)
7. Peterman, T.A., Heffelfinger, J.D., Swint, E.B., Groseclose, S.L.: The changing epidemiology of syphilis. Sex. Transm. Dis. **32**(10 Suppl), S4–S10 (2005)
8. Couturier, E., Michel, A., Janier, M., Dupin, N., Semaille, C.: Syphilis surveillance in France, 2000–2003. Euro Surveill. **9**(12), 8–10 (2004)
9. Rottingen, J.A., Cameron, D.W., Garnett, G.P.: A systematic review of the epidemiologic interactions between classic sexually transmitted diseases and HIV: how much really is known? Sex. Transm. Dis. **28**(10), 579–597 (2001)
10. Buchacz, K., Patel, P., Taylor, M., et al.: Syphilis increases HIV viral load and decreases CD4 cell counts in HIV-infected patients with new syphilis infections. AIDS (London, England) **18**(15), 2075–2079 (2004)
11. Zeltser, R., Kurban, A.K.: Syphilis. Clin. Dermatol. **22**(6), 461–468 (2004)
12. Scott, C.M., Flint, S.R.: Oral syphilis–re-emergence of an old disease with oral manifestations. Int. J. Oral Maxillofac. Surg. **34**(1), 58–63 (2005)
13. Trends in primary and secondary syphilis and HIV infections in men who have sex with men–San Francisco and Los Angeles, California, 1998–2002. MMWR Morb. Mortal Wkly. Rep. **53**(26), 575–578 (2004)
14. Wong, W., Chaw, J.K., Kent, C.K., Klausner, J.D.: Risk factors for early syphilis among gay and bisexual men seen in an STD clinic: San Francisco, 2002–2003. Sex. Transm. Dis. **32**(7), 458–463 (2005)
15. Garnett, G.P., Aral, S.O., Hoyle, D.V., Cates Jr., W., Anderson, R.M.: The natural history of syphilis. Implications for the transmission dynamics and control of infection. Sex. Transm. Dis. **24**(4), 185–200 (1997)
16. Czelusta, A., Yen-Moore, A., Van der Straten, M., Carrasco, D., Tyring, S.K.: An overview of sexually transmitted diseases. Part III. Sexually transmitted diseases in HIV-infected patients. J. Am. Acad. Dermatol. **43**(3), 409–432 (2000). quiz 33–6
17. Baeten, J.M., Overbaugh, J.: Measuring the infectiousness of persons with HIV-1: opportunities for preventing sexual HIV-1 transmission. Curr. HIV Res. **1**(1), 69–86 (2003)
18. Quinn, T.C., Wawer, M.J., Sewankambo, N., et al.: Viral load and heterosexual transmission of human immunodeficiency virus type 1. Rakai project study group. N Engl J. Med. **342**(13), 921–929 (2000)
19. Dyer, J.R., Eron, J.J., Hoffman, I.F., et al.: Association of CD4 cell depletion and elevated blood and seminal plasma human immunodeficiency virus type 1 (HIV-1) RNA concentrations with genital ulcer disease in HIV-1-infected men in Malawi. J. Infect. Dis. **177**(1), 224–227 (1998)
20. Mehta, S.D., Ghanem, K.G., Rompalo, A.M., Erbelding, E.J.: HIV seroconversion among public sexually transmitted disease clinic patients: analysis of risks to facilitate early identification. J. Acquir. Immune Defic. syndr. (1999) **42**(1), 116–122 (2006)
21. Fleming, D.T., Wasserheit, J.N.: From epidemiological synergy to public health policy and practice: the contribution of other sexually transmitted diseases to sexual transmission of HIV infection. Sex. Transm. Infect. **75**(1), 3–17 (1999)
22. Chesson, H.W., Pinkerton, S.D., Voigt, R., Counts, G.W.: HIV infections and associated costs attributable to syphilis coinfection among African Americans. Am. J. Public Health **93**(6), 943–948 (2003)
23. Hutchinson, C.M., Hook 3rd, E.W., Shepherd, M., Verley, J., Rompalo, A.M.: Altered clinical presentation of early syphilis in patients with human immunodeficiency virus infection. Ann. Intern. Med. **121**(2), 94–100 (1994)
24. Rompalo, A.M., Joesoef, M.R., O'Donnell, J.A., et al.: Clinical manifestations of early syphilis by HIV status and

gender: results of the syphilis and HIV study. Sex. Transm. Dis. **28**(3), 158–165 (2001)
25. Rompalo, A.M., Lawlor, J., Seaman, P., Quinn, T.C., Zenilman, J.M., Hook 3rd, E.W.: Modification of syphilitic genital ulcer manifestations by coexistent HIV infection. Sex. Transm. Dis. **28**(8), 448–454 (2001)
26. Inamadar, A.C., Palit, A.: Perforating chancre: any cause-effect relation with HIV infection? Sex. Transm. Infect. **79**(3), 262 (2003)
27. Little, J.W.: Syphilis: an update. Oral Surg. Oral Med. Oral Pathol. Oral Radiol. Endod. **100**(1), 3–9 (2005)
28. Hourihan, M., Wheeler, H., Houghton, R., Goh, B.T.: Lessons from the syphilis outbreak in homosexual men in east London. Sex. Transm. Infect. **80**(6), 509–511 (2004)
29. Angus, J., Langan, S.M., Stanway, A., Leach, I.H., Littlewood, S.M., English, J.S.: The many faces of secondary syphilis: a re-emergence of an old disease. Clin. Exp. Dermatol. **31**(5), 741–745 (2006)
30. D'Amico, R., Zalusky, R.: A case of lues maligna in a patient with acquired immunodeficiency syndrome (AIDS). Scand. J. Infect. Dis. **37**(9), 697–700 (2005)
31. Primary and secondary syphilis among men who have sex with men–New York City, 2001. MMWR Morb. Mortal Wkly Rep. **51**(38):853–856 (2002)
32. Kent, M.E., Romanelli, F.: Reexamining syphilis: an update on epidemiology, clinical manifestations, and management. Ann. Pharmacother. **42**(2), 226–236 (2008)
33. Dourmishev, L.A., Dourmishev, A.L.: Syphilis: uncommon presentations in adults. Clin. Dermatol. **23**(6), 555–564 (2005)
34. Regal, L., Demaerel, P., Dubois, B.: Cerebral syphilitic gumma in a human immunodeficiency virus-positive patient. Arch. Neurol. **62**(8), 1310–1311 (2005)
35. Bleeker-Rovers, C.P., van der Ven, A.J., Zomer, B., et al.: F-18-fluorodeoxyglucose positron emission tomography for visualization of lipodystrophy in HIV-infected patients. AIDS (London, England) **18**(18), 2430–2432 (2004)
36. Marra, C.M., Gary, D.W., Kuypers, J., Jacobson, M.A.: Diagnosis of neurosyphilis in patients infected with human immunodeficiency virus type 1. J. Infect. Dis. **174**(1), 219–221 (1996)
37. Wohrl, S., Geusau, A.: Clinical update: syphilis in adults. Lancet **369**(9577), 1912–1914 (2007)
38. Katz, D.A., Berger, J.R., Duncan, R.C.: Neurosyphilis. A comparative study of the effects of infection with human immunodeficiency virus. Arch. Neurol. **50**(3), 243–249 (1993)
39. Wheeler, H.L., Agarwal, S., Goh, B.T.: Dark ground microscopy and treponemal serological tests in the diagnosis of early syphilis. Sex. Transm. Infect. **80**(5), 411–414 (2004)
40. Malone, J.L., Wallace, M.R., Hendrick, B.B., et al.: Syphilis and neurosyphilis in a human immunodeficiency virus type-1 seropositive population: evidence for frequent serologic relapse after therapy. Am. J. Med. **99**(1), 55–63 (1995)
41. Radolf, J.D., Kaplan, R.P.: Unusual manifestations of secondary syphilis and abnormal humoral immune response to Treponema pallidum antigens in a homosexual man with asymptomatic human immunodeficiency virus infection. J. Am. Acad. Dermatol. **18**(2 Pt 2), 423–428 (1988)
42. Dowell, M.E., Ross, P.G., Musher, D.M., Cate, T.R., Baughn, R.E.: Response of latent syphilis or neurosyphilis to ceftriaxone therapy in persons infected with human immunodeficiency virus. Am. J. Med. **93**(5), 481–488 (1992)
43. Ghanem, K.G., Erbelding, E.J., Cheng, W.W., Rompalo, A.M.: Doxycycline compared with benzathine penicillin for the treatment of early syphilis. Clin. Infect. Dis. **42**(6), e45–e49 (2006)
44. Smith, N.H., Musher, D.M., Huang, D.B., et al.: Response of HIV-infected patients with asymptomatic syphilis to intensive intramuscular therapy with ceftriaxone or procaine penicillin. Int. J. STD AIDS **15**(5), 328–332 (2004)
45. Lynn, W.A., Lightman, S.: Syphilis and HIV: a dangerous combination. Lancet Infect. Dis. **4**(7), 456–466 (2004)

Chancroid

16

Thais Harumi Sakuma, Daniel Dal'Asta Coimbra, and Omar Lupi

Core Messages

- Chancroid is caused by the gram negative bacteria *Haemophilus ducreyi*.
- The disease is found mainly in developing countries. Most people in the U.S. and Europe diagnosed with chancroid have traveled outside the country to areas where the disease is known to occur frequently.
- Uncircumcised men are at much higher risk than circumcised men for getting chancroid from an infected partner. Chancroid is a risk factor for the HIV virus.

16.1 Introduction

Chancroid is one of the classical genital ulcerative diseases (GUDs). It is caused by the Gram-negative coccobacillus *Haemophilus ducreyi* and its principal mode of transmission is sexual intercourse. Chancroid is a public health problem because *H. ducreyi* and the human immunodeficiency virus (HIV) facilitate each other's transmission. Therefore, it is assumed that chancroid is one of the factors responsible for the rapid spread of HIV in the endemic countries, e.g., African countries [1].

T.H. Sakuma (✉) and D.D. Coimbra
Dermatology Department, Universidade Federal do Estado do, Rio de Janeiro, Brazil

O. Lupi
Dermatology Department, Universidade Federal do Estado do Rio de Janeiro (UniRio) and Policlinica Geral do Rio de Janeiro (PGRJ), Immunology Section, Universidade Federal do Rio de Janeiro (UFRJ), Rio de Janeiro, Brazil
e-mail: omarlupi@globo.com

16.2 History

Bassereau and Ricord, in France, first distinguished the soft from the indurated (syphilitic) chancre in 1852. Ducreyi, a bacteriologist at the University of Naples, identified the causative organism of chancroid in 1889 [2].

16.3 Epidemiology

It is estimated that over seven million cases of chancroid occur each year [3]. However, misdiagnosis and underreporting make accurate predictions of the prevalence difficult [4].

Chancroid is still common in many of the world's underdeveloped regions, such as areas of Africa, Asia, Latin America and the Caribbean [3, 5]. More recently, chancroid prevalence has declined markedly in countries such as China, the Philippines, Senegal, and Thailand. Occasional outbreaks of the disease have been reported from the USA and Europe, among the communities with high-risk behavior. In the USA, since 1987, reported cases of chancroid declined steadily until 2006, when 33 cases of the disease were reported [5–7].

Chancroid is an important cofactor in the transmission of HIV. Its ulcers contain increased CD4 positive lymphocytes, induced by *H. ducreyi* cellular immune response, that act as primary targets of HIV. In fact, chancroid is a common infection in all 18 countries where the

G. Gross and S.K. Tyring (eds.), *Sexually Transmitted Infections and Sexually Transmitted Diseases*,
DOI: 10.1007/978-3-642-14663-3_16,

adult human immunodeficiency virus prevalence surpasses 8% of the population [2, 8, 9]. It is also known that the disruption of mucosal integrity acts as a portal of entry for the virus and that *H. ducreyi* increases CCR-5 receptor expression on macrophages, thus increasing the susceptibility of these cells to HIV invasion. Studies also demonstrated that HIV-positive patients with GUD had higher rates of HIV-1 shedding into the genital tract than those without ulcer disease, and that there is increased fluid viral concentration in men with GUD [8].

The disease occurs more frequently in men than in women. In some countries, the male to female rates range from 3:1 to 25:1. Women may represent asymptomatic carriers of the organism as they may have internal vaginal and cervical ulcers that are painless, and they may not seek medical attention as often as men. In an experimental model of *Haemophilus ducreyi* infection, women inoculated with *H. ducreyi* resolved their initial lesions more frequently than males without progressing to the pustular stage of the disease. The mechanism that underlies this gender difference is not known at the moment, but studies show no direct effect of gonadal hormones on bacterial growth in vitro. The population subgroups more affected are sex workers and subjects with poor hygiene, and the age group of 18–45 years is the most vulnerable. Studies indicate that circumcised men are at lower risk of chancroid [1, 10, 11].

16.4 Pathogenesis and Etiology

Chancroid is an infectious disease caused by the Gram-negative, unencapsulated, facultative anaerobic bacillus *Haemophilus ducreyi* [7, 12].

H. ducreyi is a strict human pathogen and naturally infects genital and nongenital skin, mucosal surfaces, and regional lymph nodes. The disease is largely disseminated through sexual intercourse with an infected individual. The organism enters the skin and/or mucous membrane of the new host through microabrasions received during sexual intercourse, and colonizes extracellularly. PMN and macrophages recruited by the innate immune response quickly surround the bacteria in micropustules but are unable to clear the organism. The continued presence of the bacteria causes the evolution from the pustular to the ulcerative stage of the disease, when *H. ducreyi* can be found within a granulocytic infiltrate, colocalizing with neutrophils and fibrin. Then, it continues to replicate in the ulcer and prevent clearance, presumably by evading phagocytosis [13, 14].

Natural chancroid infection does not protect against subsequent infection. This way, the study of chancroid pathogenesis has led to the identification of a number of *H. ducreyi* virulence factors that may be potential candidates for vaccine development:

1. LspA1 and LspA2: *H. ducreyi* genes whose encoded proteins inhibit the phagocytic activity of granulocyte and macrophage-like cell lines [15], facilitating its ability to initiate disease and to progress to pustule formation in humans [1, 16].
2. DsrA (Ducreyi serum resistance A): member of a family of multifunctional outer membrane proteins; is involved in resistance to killing by serum complement [7], is the major factor involved in FN binding by *H. ducreyi*, and has been shown to bind to human keratinocytes [12].
3. MOMP (Major outer membrane protein): involved in serum resistance [17]and may have a minor role in FN binding [15].
4. NcaA (Necessary for collagen adhesion A): mediates type 1 collagen binding by *H. ducreyi* [18].
5. GroEL heat shock protein: responsible for the attachment of *H. ducreyi* to carbohydrate receptors, representing a potential bacterial adhesin [14].
6. flp (fimbria-like protein): products secreted by this locus are involved in the attachment to human foreskin fibroblasts [10, 14].
7. DltA (Ducreyi lectin A): may recognize glycosylated receptors on host cells and plays a role in adhesion of *H. ducreyi* to host tissues [19], and also contributes to serum resistance [17].
8. LOS (lipooligosaccharide): adherence of the bacteria to keratinocytes and human foreskin fibroblasts [20].
9. OmpP2A and OmpP2B: are proteins that exhibit porin activity. Porins not only facilitate nutrient acquisition and provide membrane stability, but also have been shown to act as virulence determinants [3].
10. FtpA(fine tangled pili): help in adherence to the host cell [5].
11. HgbA (hemoglobin-binding protein): iron acquisition [21].
12. Cu,Zn-SOD (Cu, Zn-superoxide dismutase): iron acquisition [21] and detoxification [22], has the ability to scavenge the superoxide radical produced in the respiratory burst of neutrophils [21].
13. Hemolysin: lyses keratinocytes, fibroblasts, macrophages, T cells, and B cells [22].

14. CDT (cytolethal distending toxin): causes arrest of epithelial cells in G2, and induces B-cell and T-cell apoptosis [22].
15. PAL (peptidoglycan-associated lipoprotein): major lipoprotein of *H. ducreyi* that links the outer membrane to peptidoglycan [22].

16.5 Clinical Features

The incubation period for chancroid is short and varies between 3 and 7 days, rarely more than 10 days, with no prodromal symptoms. This may be longer with preexisting HIV infection [8].

Small erythematous papules arise at each site of inoculation and evolve into pustules in 2–3 days. After a few days to 2 weeks, the pustules evolve into a painful, deep ulceration. The ulcer is typically dirty, rounded or oval, tender, nonindurated and soft, with ragged edges. Its base is covered by a gray or yellow necrotic, foul-smelling exudate, that frequently bleeds when scraped (Fig. 16.1). Autoinoculation from the primary lesion may lead to the development of satellite and/or "kissing ulcers" on apposing skin surfaces [1, 8, 13, 23, 24].

In males, lesions are most commonly found on the prepuce, frenulum, and glans. In females, the fourchette, labia, vestibule, clitoris, vaginal wall, cervix, and perianal area may be involved.

Painful inguinal adenitis occurs in 30–60% of patients and is more common in men. The adenitis, usually unilateral and ipsilateral to the ulcer, develops within 1–2 weeks after its appearance and may have progression to a suppurative bubo in 25% of patients [24].

In patients with both chancroid and HIV, the size of the ulcer is unaffected, but the number of ulcers at initial presentation is greater than in HIV-seronegative patients, with longer ulcer duration as well [8, 24].

Untreated ulcers may persist for 1–3 months, but it may eventually heal. *H. ducreyi* infection has never been reported to become systemic, but extragenital lesions do occur and are thought to be due to autoinoculation. Infection on hands, eyelids, lips, breasts, and on oral mucosa have been reported [1, 8, 15].

Several clinical variants have been identified [25, 26]:

1. Dwarf chancroid: a small, superficial, relatively painless ulcer.
2. Giant chancroid: a large granulomatous ulcer at the site of a ruptured inguinal bubo, extending beyond its margins.

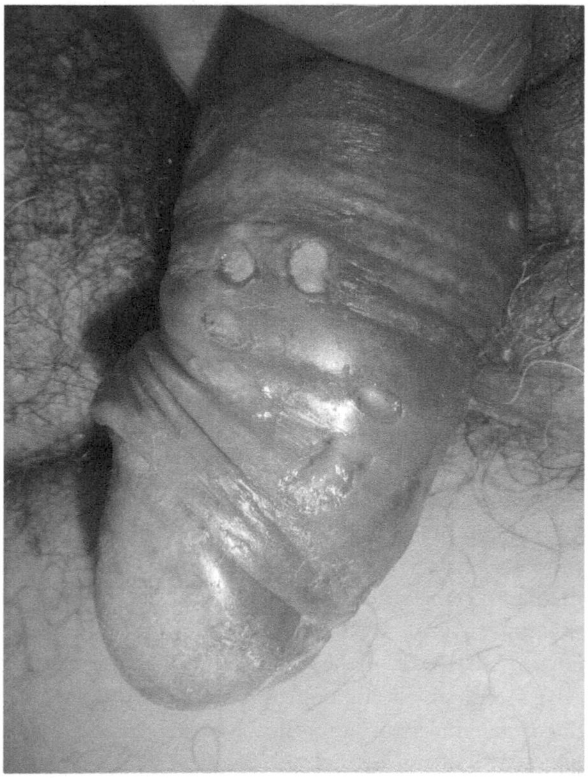

Fig. 16.1 Small, rounded, dirty, and nonindurated genital ulcers due to chancroid (Courtesy Jose Augusto Nery, M.D., Ph.D.)

3. Follicular chancroid: essentially seen in women in association with hair follicles of the labia majora and pubis, initial appearance as a follicular pustule, later resulting in a classic ulcer at the site.
4. Transient chancroid (French: *chancre mou volant*): very superficial ulcers, which may soon heal, followed by a typical inguinal bubo.
5. Serpiginous chancroid: multiple ulcers coalesce, spreading by extension and autoinoculation.
6. Phagedenic chancroid (*ulcus molle gangrenosum*): caused by superinfection with fusospirochetoses. The ulceration causes extensive destruction of the genitalia.
7. Papular chancroid (*ulcus molle elevatum*): a granulomatous ulcerated papule that might resemble donovanosis or condyloma-latum.
8. Mixed chancroid: nonindurated, tender ulcers of chancroid together with an indurated, nontender ulcer of syphilis with an incubation period of 10–90 days.

16.6 Diagnosis

The diagnosis of chancroid is based on a history of sexual intercourse and development of painful genital ulcers following the incubation period associated with tender inguinal lymphadenopathy or suppurative adenopathy and also in the following diagnostic tests [27]:

Gram stain of the ulcer exudate may demonstrate short, plump, Gram-negative rods in the classic "school of fish" appearance; however, *H. ducreyi* is difficult to demonstrate in Gram smears and frequently the material has polymicrobial contamination. Sensitivity ranges from 5% to 63% and specificity from 51% to 99% [28] (Fig. 16.2).

Culture is the best diagnostic method widely available to most laboratories, though, it is difficult to grow *H. ducreyi* in vitro. Using the optimal combination media, it is about 80% sensitive. The material is obtained from a swab that has been taken from the edge or the base of the ulcer, after flushing the area with sterile physiological saline [28]. *H. ducreyi* produce characteristic tan-yellow colonies that are self adherent and can be "nudged" intact over the surface of the agar. Culture of pus aspirate from bubo inguinal buboes is also possible, but less sensitive [28–30] (Fig. 16.3).

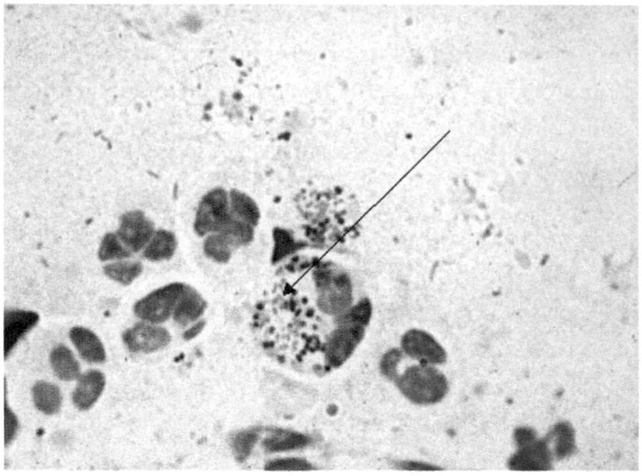

Fig. 16.2 Gram stain of the ulcer exudate demonstrates Gram-negative *coccobacilli* in clusters, in the classic "school of fish" appearance (Courtesy Luiz Jorge Fagundes, M.D., Ph.D. and Fátima Morais)

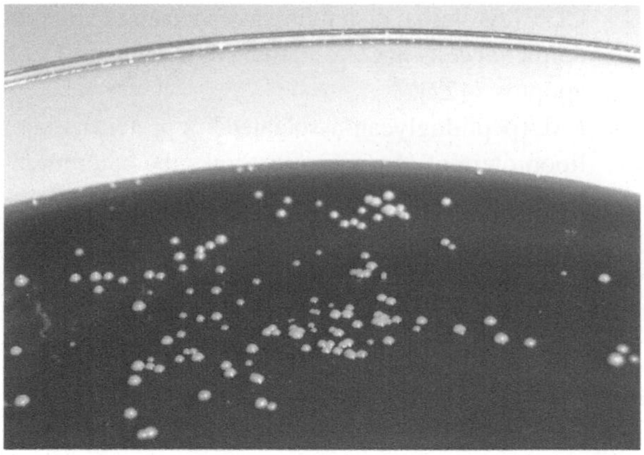

Fig. 16.3 *H. ducreyi* characteristic tan-yellow colonies (Courtesy Emerson Cavassin)

Polymerase chain reaction (PCR) testing is the diagnostic test with greatest sensibility and specificity and is considered the gold-standard test for diagnosis, but it is expensive and no FDA-cleared PCR test for *H. ducreyi* is available in the USA [31].

Serological tests have been useful for epidemiological studies but have limited value as a diagnostic test, especially in areas where chancroid is endemic. Humoral immune response in patients infected with *H. ducreyi* is often cross-reactive with other *Haemophilus* species, may last a long time after the infection has resolved [28, 29].

Direct immunofluorescent testing for *H. ducreyi* antigen detection of ulcer material using specific monoclonal antibody appears to be useful. Sensitivity and specificity to detect *H. ducreyi* lipooligosaccharide (LOS) using an LOS-specific monoclonal antibody are 89–100% and 63–81% respectively. However, it is not currently commercially available [28].

When investigating GUD that is believed to be due to *H. ducreyi*, herpes simplex virus (culture or antigen test), syphilis (syphilis serology, dark field examination, direct immunofluorescence test), and HIV testing should also be performed. Patients should be retested for HIV and syphilis 3 months after the diagnosis of chancroid, if the initial test results were negative [29, 31].

16.7 Differential Diagnosis

Disease	Incubation	Genital Ulceration	Adenopathy	Etiology	Diagnosis
Syphilis	30–90 days	Round or oval, sharply defined, regular, indurated borders, nontender, with smooth, brownish-red base,	Rubbery, movable, nontender, nonsuppurative, painless, uni or bilateral	*Treponema pallidum*	Dark-field examination, serologic testing for antibodies
Herpes simplex	2–7 days	Small but grouped vesicular lesions that ulcerate. Very painful	Tender, painful, bilateral	Herpes simplex virus (HSV) 2 and, less commonly, HSV 1	Tzanck smear, Papanicolaou staining method, culture, HSV antigen detection, HSV DNA detection by PCR
Donovanosis	2 weeks to 3 months	Large spreading, exuberant ulcers, with bright-red granulating surface (ulcero-vegetative)	True adenopathy is rare. Subcutaneous nodule may be mistaken for lymph nodes (pseudobubo)	Calymmatobacterium granulomatis	Wright's or Giemsa's stain from a fresh biopsy permits the demonstration of Donovan bodies
Lymphogranuloma venereum	3–30 days	Soft, erythematous, painless erosion that heals spontaneously	Nodes that coalesce to form a firm, elongated, unilateral, immovable mass. The fistulization may form multiple openings	*Chlamydia trachomatis*, serologic varieties L1, L2, L3	Culture, Complement fixation test (titer 1:64, or greater) PCR DNA

Superinfected traumatic lesions and noninfectious causes of genital ulceration, such as Crohn's disease or Behçet's syndrome, must be considered in the differential diagnosis.

16.8 Pathology

Histopathology is a complement to the diagnosis. The tissue below the floor of the ulcer can be arbitrarily divided into three zones. The more superficial zone consists of necrotic tissues and an inflammatory infiltrate. The broad midzone contains the new blood vessels with patchy proliferative changes on the one hand and degenerative changes on the other. The deeper zone shows a chronic inflammatory infiltrate of plasma cells and lymphocytes.

16.9 Treatment

Specific and prompt treatment of chancroid is imperative to lower the transmission rates in endemic countries and to prevent outbreaks. The patients should be oriented to avoid unprotected sexual intercourse during the treatment. See in the table below recommended treatment regimens for chancroid from the World Health Organization (WHO), and the Centers for Disease Control and Prevention (CDC) [2, 3, 31]

Antibiotic	Dose	Duration	Route	Recommending Body
Azithromycin	1 g	Single dose	Oral	WHO, CDC
Ceftriaxone	250 mg	Single dose	IM	WHO, CDC
Ciprofloxacin	500 mg two times daily	3 days	Oral	WHO, CDC
Erythromycin base	500 mg three times daily	7 days	Oral	CDC
Erythromycin base	500 mg four times daily	7 days	Oral	WHO

Ciprofloxacin is contraindicated for pregnant and lactating women. The safety and efficacy of azithromycin for pregnant and lactating women have not been established

Amoxycillin/clavulanate, tetracyclines, and penicillins are no longer recommended because of resistance of *H. ducreyi* to this antibiotic. In patients with concomitant *H. ducreyi* and HIV infection, a longer course of therapy and close monitoring are mandatory. As a group, these patients are more likely to experience treatment failure and to have ulcers that heal more slowly. Some specialists prefer the erythromycin 7-day regimen for treating HIV-infected patients [31, 32].

If treatment is successful, ulcers usually improve symptomatically within 3 days and objectively within 7 days after therapy. The time required for complete healing depends on the size of the ulcer; large ones might require more than 2 weeks [31]. A test of cure for chancroid is not necessary. If clinical manifestations persist after therapy, a chancroid culture should be performed to determine if the strain of *H. ducreyi* is resistant to the antimicrobial prescribed [29].

Fluctuant lymph nodes might require needle aspiration or incision and drainage [31]. If not treated, chancroid can complicate with rupture of buboes and subsequent scarring and/or chronic sinus tract drainage. Phimosis and balanoposthitis may also occur. It is important to emphasize to the patient to avoid high-risk sexual activities, such as unprotected sexual intercourse or sexual intercourse with high-risk partners.

Sex partners of patients should be examined and treated; regardless of whether symptoms of the disease are present, if they had sexual contact with the patient during the 10 days preceding the patient's onset of symptoms [31].

16.10 Synonyms

Chancroid; Soft chancre; *Ulcus molle*; Soft ulcer; Dwarf chancre; Transient chancroid; Phagedenic chancroid; Follicular chancroid; Papular chancroid; Giant chancroid.

Take-Home Pearls

- Within 1 day - 2 weeks after getting chancroid, a patient will notice a small papule in the genitals that becomes an within a day of its appearance. The ulcer:
- Ranges in size from 1/8 inch to 2 inches across
- Is painful and soft
- Has sharply defined borders
- Has irregular or ragged borders
- Has a base that is covered with a gray or yellowish-gray exudate
- Has a base that bleeds easily if banged or scraped
- About half of infected men have only a single ulcer. Women often have 4 or more ulcers. The ulcers appear in specific locations.
- Common locations in men are:
- Foreskin (prepuce)
- Coronal sulcus and urethral meatus
- Shaft of the penis
- Glans and scrotum

References

1. Bong, C.T.H., Bauer, M.E., Spinola, S.M.: *Haemophilus ducreyi*: clinical features, epidemiology, and prospects for disease control. Microbes Infect. **4**, 1141–1148 (2002)
2. Steen, R.: Eradicating Chancroid. Bull. World Health Organ. **79**, 818–826 (2001)
3. Prather, D.T., Bains, M., Hancock, R.E.W., Filiatrault, M.J., Campagnari, A.A.: Differential expression of porins OmpP2A and OmpP2B of *Haemophilus ducreyi*. Infect. Immun. **72**, 6271–6278 (2004)
4. White, C.D., Leduc, I., Olsen, B., Jeter, C., Harris, C., Elkins, C.: *Haemophilus ducreyi* outer membrane determinants, including DsrA, define two clonal populations. Infect. Immun. **73**, 2387–2399 (2005)

5. Inamadar, A.C., Palit, A.: Chancroid: an update. Indian J. Dermatol. Venereol. Leprol. **68**, 5–9 (2002)
6. http://www.cdc.gov/std/stats/other.htm
7. Cole, L.E., Kawula, T.H., Toffer, K.L., Elkins, C.: The *Haemophilus ducreyi* serum resistance antigen DsrA confers attachment to human keratinocytes. Infect. Immun. **70**, 6158–6165 (2002)
8. Mohammed, T.T., Olumide, Y.M.: Chancroid and human immunodeficiency virus infection – a review. Int. J. Dermatol. **47**, 1–8 (2008)
9. Lewis, D.A.: Chancroid: clinical manifestations, diagnosis, and management. Sex. Transm. Infect. **79**, 68–71 (2003)
10. Spinola, S.M., Fortney, K.R., Katz, B.P., Latimer, J.L., Mock, J.R., Vakevainen, M., Hansen, E.J.: *Haemophilus ducreyi* requires an intact *flp* gene cluster for virulence in humans. Infect. Immun. **71**, 7178–7182 (2003)
11. Weiss, H.A., Thomas, S.L., Munabi, S.K., Hayes, R.J.: Male circumcision and risk of syphilis, chancroid, and genital herpes: a systematic review and meta-analysis. Sex. Transm. Infect. **82**, 101–110 (2006)
12. Leduc, I., White, C.D., Nepluev, I., Throm, R.E., Spinola, S.M., Elkins, C.: The outer membrane protein DsrA is the major fibronectin-binding determinant of *Haemophilus ducreyi*. Infect. Immun. **76**, 1608–1616 (2008)
13. Bauer, M.E., Townsend, C.A., Ronald, A.R., Spinola, S.M.: Localization of *Haemophilus ducreyi* in naturally acquired chancroidal ulcers. Microbes Infect. **8**, 2465–2468 (2006)
14. Pantzar, M., Teneberg, S., Lagergard, T.: Binding of *Haemophilus ducreyi* to carbohydrate receptors is mediated by the 58.5-kDa GroEL heat shock protein. Microbes Infect. **8**, 2452–2458 (2006)
15. Vakevainen, M., Greenberg, S., Hansen, E.J.: Inhibition of phagocytosis by *Haemophilus ducreyi* requires expression of the LspA1 and LspA2 proteins. Infect. Immun. **71**, 5994–6003 (2003)
16. Janowicz, D.M., Fortney, K.R., Katz, B.P., Latimer, J.L., Deng, K., Hansen, E.J., Spinola, S.M.: Expression of the LspA1 and LspA2 proteins by *Haemophilus ducreyi* is required for virulence in human volunteers. Infect. Immun. **72**, 4528–4533 (2004)
17. Leduc, I., Richards, P., Davis, C., Schilling, B., Elkins, C.: A novel lectin DltA, is required for expression of a full serum resistance phenotype in *Haemophilus ducreyi*. Infect. Immun. **72**, 3418–3428 (2004)
18. Fulcher, R.A., Cole, L.E., Janowicz, D.M., Toffer, K.L., Fortney, K.R., Katz, B.P., Orndorff, P.E., Spinola, S.M., Kawula, T.H.: Expression of *Haemophilus ducreyi* collagen binding outer membrane protein NcaA is required for virulence in swine and human challenge models of chancroid. Infect. Immun. **74**, 2651–2658 (2006)
19. Janowicz, D., Leduc, I., Fortney, K.R., Katz, B.P., Elkins, C., Spinola, S.M.: A DltA mutant of *Haemophilus ducreyi* is partially attenuated in its ability to cause pustules in human volunteers. Infect. Immun. **74**, 1394–1397 (2006)
20. Post, D.M.B., Mungur, R., Gibson, B.W., Munson Jr., R.S.: Identification of a novel sialic acid transporter in *Haemophilus ducreyi*. Infect. Immun. **73**, 6727–6735 (2005)
21. Post, D.M.B., Gibson, B.W.: Proposed second class of *Haemophilus ducreyi* strains show altered protein and lipooligosaccharide profiles. Proteomics **7**, 3131–3142 (2007)
22. Al-Tawfiq, J.A., Spinola, S.M.: Haemophilus ducreyi: clinical disease and pathogenesis. Curr. Opin. Infect. Dis. **15**, 43–47 (2002)
23. Humphreys, T.L., Li, L., Li, X., Janowicz, D.M., Fortney, K.R., Zhao, Q., Li, W., McClintick, J., Katz, B.P., Wilkes, D.S., Edenberg, H.J., Spinola, S.M.: Dysregulated immune profiles for skin and dendritic cells are associated with increased host susceptibility to *Haemophilus ducreyi* infection in human volunteers. Infect. Immun. **75**, 5686–5697 (2007)
24. Wu, J.J., Huang, D.B., Pang, K.R., Tyring, S.K.: Selected sexually transmitted diseases and their relationship to HIV. Clin. Dermatol. **22**, 499–508 (2004)
25. Sehgal, V.N., Srivastava, G.: Chancroid: contemporary appraisal. Int. J. Dermatol. **42**, 182–190 (2003)
26. Bauer, M.E., Goheen, M.P., Townsend, C.A., Spinola, S.M.: Haemophilus ducreyi associates with phagocytes, collagen, and fibrin and remains extracellular throughout infection of human volunteers. Infect. Immun. **69**, 2549–2557 (2001)
27. Lewis, D.A.: Diagnostic tests for chancroid. Sex. Transm. Infect. **76**, 137–141 (2000)
28. Alfa, M.: The laboratory diagnosis of *Haemophilus ducreyi*. Can. J. Infect. Dis. Med. Microbiol. **16**, 31–34 (2005)
29. Lewis, D.A., Ison, C.A.: Chancroid. Sex. Transm. Infect. **82**, 19–20 (2006)
30. Kaimal, S., Thappa, D.M.: Methods of specimen collection for the diagnosis of STIs. Indian J. Dermatol. Venereol. Leprol. **73**, 129–132 (2007)
31. Centers for Disease Control and Prevention: Sexually transmitted diseases guidelines. MMWR **55**, 14–16 (2006)
32. World Health Organization. Treatment of specific infections. Guidelines for the management of sexually transmitted infections, p. 46 (2003)

Donovanosis

17

Omar Lupi, Paula Chicralla, and Carlos José Martins

Core Messages

› Granuloma inguinale is a *bacterial disease* characterized by *ulcerative* genital *lesions* that is *endemic* in many less developed regions. The disease often goes untreated because of the scarcity of medical treatment in the countries in which it is found. In addition, the painless *genital* ulcers can be mistaken for *syphilis*. The ulcers ultimately progress to destruction of internal and external tissue, with extensive leakage of *mucus* and *blood* from the highly *vascular* lesions. The destructive nature of donovanosis also increases the risk of *superinfection* by other *pathogenic* microbes.

17.1 Introduction

Donovanosis is an indolent, progressive, ulcerative, granulomatous skin disease caused by *Calymmatobacterium granulomatis*, formerly known as *Donovania granulomatis*. It mainly assails the skin and subcutaneous cell tissue of the genital and perianal areas and inguinal region, implicating with less frequency other regions of the skin, mucosa, or even the internal organs.

It is probably spread by both homosexual and heterosexual venereal contact and by nonvenereal means as well. Untreated, it exhibits no tendency to go into spontaneous remission and in later stages may be severely debilitating.

Many denominations were proposed for this disease: inguinal granuloma, venereum granuloma, tropicum granuloma, pudendi tropicum granuloma, contagious granuloma, ulcerating granuloma, sclerosing granuloma, chronic venereum ulcer, and granuloma donovani.

17.2 History

Donovanosis was described for the first time in 1882 by McLeod, in Madras, India, who named it serpiginous ulcer. Many other names have been suggested, but aside from granuloma inguinale, only the term *donovanosis* persists.

In 1905, Donovan demonstrated the causative agent of the disease, and considered it in the protozoa group. He described the bipolar-staining, intracellular inclusions in macrophages from lesion exudate (termed *Donovan bodies*) [1].

O. Lupi (✉)
Dermatology Department, Universidade Federal do Estado do Rio de Janeiro (UniRio) and Policlinica Geral do Rio de Janeiro (PGRJ), Immunology Section, Universidade Federal do Rio de Janeiro (UFRJ), Rio de Janeiro, Brazil
e-mail: omarlupi@globo.com

P. Chicralla and C.J. Martins
Dermatology Department, Universidade Federal do Estado do, Rio de Janeiro, Brazil

G. Gross and S.K. Tyring (eds.), *Sexually Transmitted Infections and Sexually Transmitted Diseases*,
DOI: 10.1007/978-3-642-14663-3_17,

In a very well-established work, Aragão and Vianna published in 1913 their conclusions about the etiological agent, also proposing the name *Calymmatobacterium granulomatis* [2].

During this century, the microorganism received other names, such as *Donovania granulomatis* and *Klebsiella granulomatis*, despite the research of Brazilians Aragão and Vianna [2]. After detailed bacteriological, clinical, and therapeutic studies, the bacteria was called *Calymmatobacterium granulomatis* [3].

Anderson, in 1943, established the bacterial nature of Donovan´s bodies, when he cultivated the microorganism in the vitelline embryonic yolk sac. Requirements for growth on artificial media were established in 1959.

In 1950, Marmell and Santora proposed the term Donovanosis, in homage to Donovan.

17.3 Epidemiology

Sporadic cases of donovanosis occur worldwide with recent reports from developed countries such as Canada, Sweden, Italy, France, and Japan. Endemic foci are usually seen only in tropical and subtropical environments, such as New Guinea, Brazil, central Australia, the Caribbean, and parts of India [1, 3, 4].

The sexually transmitted nature of donovanosis is controversial, seeming to be, by clinical and epidemiological observations, that it is not only transmitted by sexual intercourse. Strong arguments indicate the importance of sexual contact: The lesions are more frequent in the genital or anal region; the disease is more frequent in the sexually active group, and the anal localization of the disease in male homosexuals [5–8]. The possibility of nonvenereal transmission is suggested by the occurrence of disease in sexually inactive children, the infrequency of infection in partners repeatedly exposed to open lesions, and the infrequency of infection in sexually active people (e.g., prostitutes) in some endemic areas [3, 5, 6, 9].

Sehgal [7] published a donovanosis case, which he considers an example of nonvenereal transmission in adults since the lesions were restricted to arms, face, and neck, without any evidence of lesions on the genital, inguinal, or oral regions.

Some authors such as Jardim [10] affirm that the contact with bearers of donovanosis does not always result in infection in a normal person, and that the skin, healthy or scraped, does not seem to enhance the transmission of the disease. The author also points out that the experiences with infection are only positive when pieces from the sick tissue or pus aspirated from pseudobuboes were implanted or inoculated on subcutaneous tissue of human volunteers.

It seems clear, however, that donovanosis is one of a class of diseases causing genital ulceration that may predispose persons to the transmission of HIV.

Although many authors affirm that the disease attacks more individuals of the male sex, the tendency today is to consider that it affects both men and women. Some authors, such as Lal, Lynchg and Kubersky [11–13], observed more cases among men, while Bhagwandeen [4] and Ribeiro [14] reported that the majority of their cases belonged to the female sex.

Other authors refer that the disease is more frequent among male homosexuals.

As for the age, all of them say that the absolute majority of the cases assailed young adults (20–40 years old), which constitutes the age rate that presents greater sexual activity.

However, the reports of the disease in children and aged people are rare, Banerjee [3] observed the disease in a 6-month-old child, and Ribeiro published a case of a 94-old-year patient with donovanosis [14].

17.4 Pathogenesis and Etiology

The causative agent is formerly termed *Donovania granulomatis*. It is a gram-negative rod, sometimes coccobacilli, measuring 0.5–1.5 μ wide by 1.0–2.0 μ long, presenting round extremities. They are steadfast and have a polysaccharide and fibrous capsule.

They appear isolated or form bunches in the interior of big mononuclear macrophages (corpuscles of Donovan), being found also in extracellular space. The cellular wall is gram negative, similar to the *Klebsiella*'s wall, although, it has not yet demonstrated any correlation to this bacteria.

It has been demonstrated in fecal flora, and there is evidence by electron microscopy that it may share bacteriophage with *Enterobacteriaceae*.

The microorganism stains with great intensity in the extremities than in the center, varying from deep blue to black, and its capsule, red. They can be stained by Giemsa, Leishman, or Wright.

Antibody against the organism may be detected by the complement-fixation test, though the test has little diagnostic value. Circulating antibody, which does not affect the relentless course of untreated disease, has raised the possibility that a defect in cell-mediated immunity may predispose the patient to clinical illness, as is the case in the other diseases caused by intracellular organisms (e.g., leprosy and tuberculosis) [12, 15].

17.5 Clinical Features

The incubation period is poorly defined and may range from 2 weeks to 3 months. According to Jardim et al. [16] the period is 2 weeks to 1 month; Greenblat and Torpin [8], 42–50 days; Lal and Nicholas [12], 3 days to 6 months. Experimental human inoculation has produced lesions after latency of 21 days.

The disease begins as single or multiple subcutaneous nodules, which erode through the skin, producing very well-defined ulceration that grows slowly and bleeds readily on contact (Fig. 17.1). From this point, the manifestations are directly linked to the tissue responses of the host, originating localized or extensive forms and, may even be visceral lesions through hematogenic dissemination. The subcutaneous nodule, if large enough, may be mistaken for a lymph node, giving rise to the term *pseudobubo*. True adenopathy or general symptoms are rare.

The bottom of the lesion is soft and beefy red (Fig. 17.2). The edges are irregular, elevated, well defined, and indurated. In recent lesions, the bottom is filled with serobloody secretion, while in old lesions, the surface of the lesions becomes granulated and the secretion is seropurulent and has a fetid odor [16].

In men, the penis, scrotum, and glans are the most common sites of primary lesions; in females, the labia minora, vulva, vagina, cervix and pubis.

In most of the cases of donovanosis registered in literature, localization is restricted to cutaneous areas and mucosa of the genitalia and anal, perianal, and inguinal regions, where the lesion generally initiates as

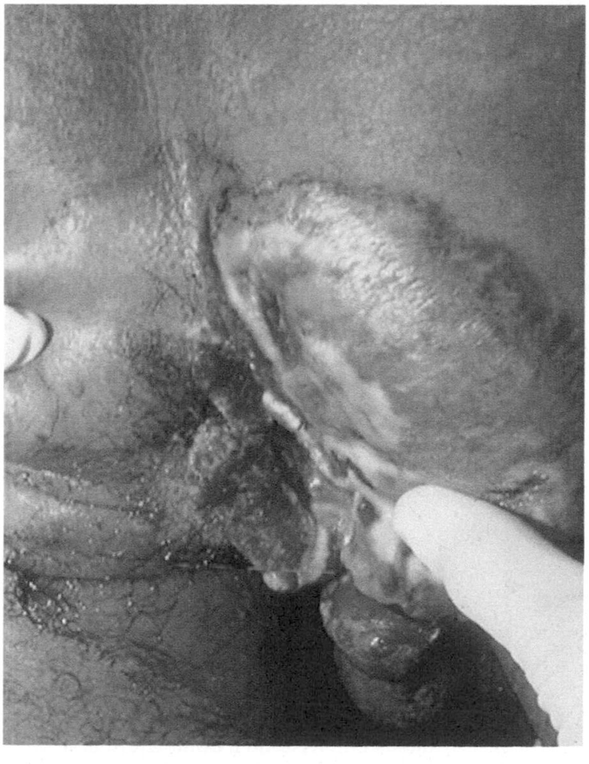

Fig. 17.1 Very well-defined ulceration that grows slowly and bleeds readily on contact

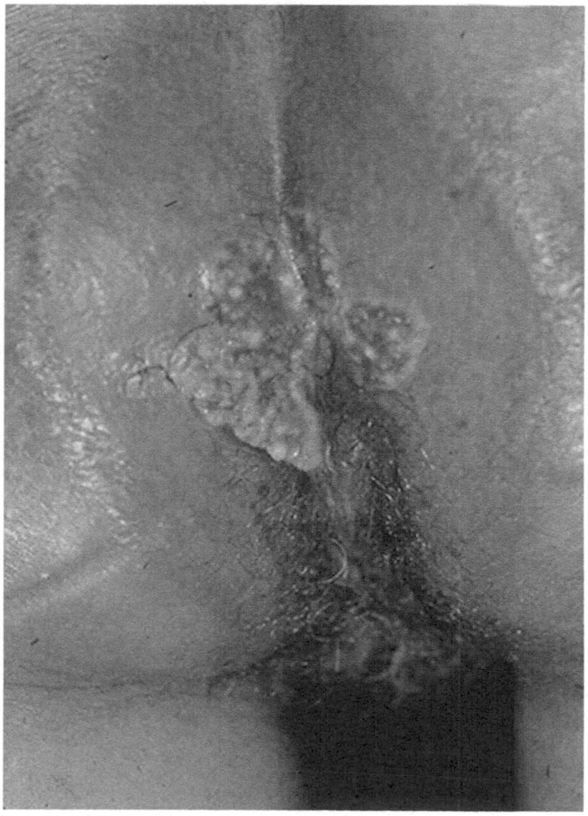

Fig. 17.2 The bottom of the lesion is soft and beefy red

a small papule or painless nodule that ulcerates and grows as it develops (Figs. 17.1, 17.2 and 17.3). Through autoinoculation, satellite lesions emerge and join, reaching great areas [16].

The lesion can be presented as a vegetating mass or tends to form fibrous or keloid tissues, sometimes leading to deformity of the genitalia, paraphimosis, or elephantiasis (Figs. 17.4 and 17.5).

Superinfection with fusospirochetal organisms may give rise to necrotic lesions with massive tissue

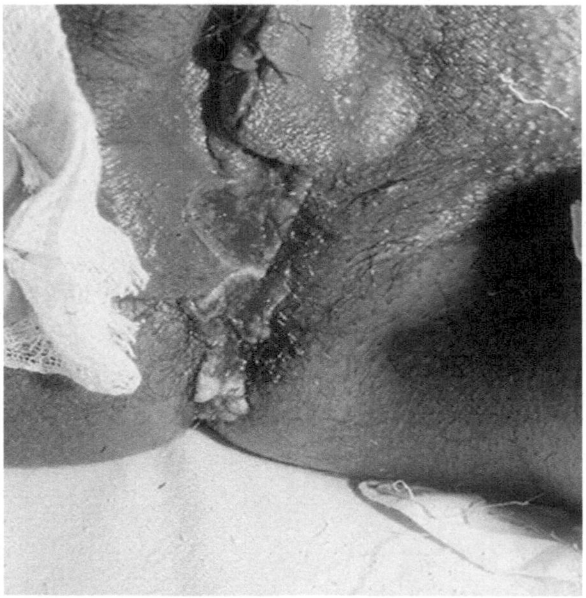

Fig. 17.3 Perianal lesions in a pregnant woman

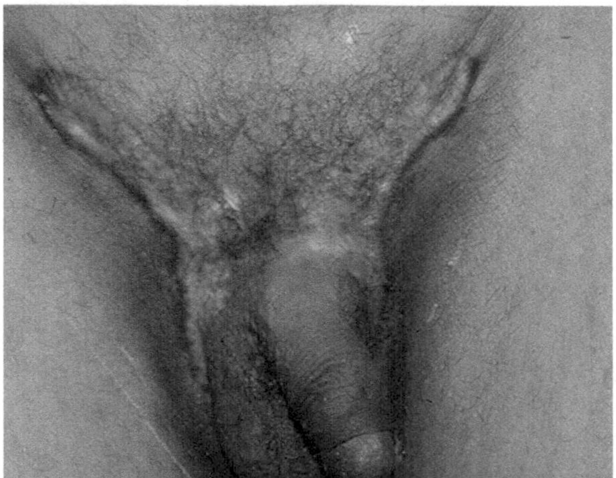

Fig. 17.4 Genital keloids secondary to donovanosis

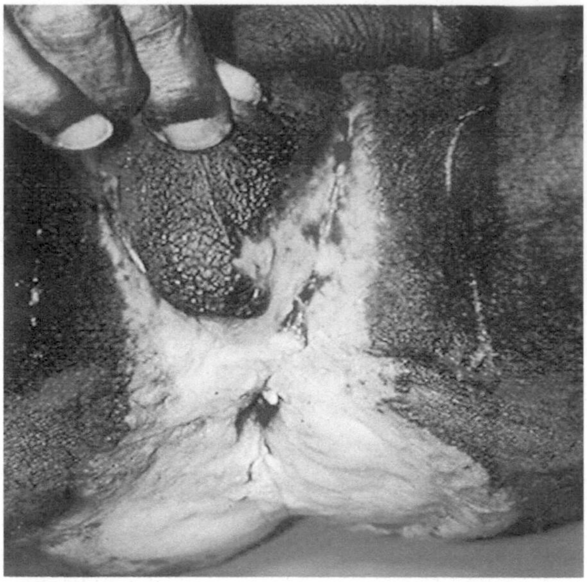

Fig. 17.5 Genital and perianal scars secondary to donovanosis

destruction, similar to the situation in so-called phagedenic chancroid.

The extragenital donovanosis represents a casualty in 3–6% of cases, with occasional systemic involvement, notably in the gastrointestinal tract and bone, including the bony orbit and orbital skin. Almost all of them proceed from endemic areas.

The localization of the disease out of the anogenital site can be explained by the following: hematogenous dissemination to organs, such as the liver, lungs, bones, and spleen; continuity or contiguity to adjacent pelvic organs; lymphatic dissemination; autoinoculation.

Jardim et al. proposed a clinical classification [16]:

- Genitals and perigenitals
  1. Ulcerous
  2. With hypertrophic edges
  3. With plane edges
  4. Ulcerovegetating
  5. Vegetating
  6. Elephantiasic
- Extragenital
- Systemic

In HIV-positive patients and mainly in patients with AIDS, donovanosis can assume a completely abnormal clinical development. This situation can complicate both diagnosis and treatment [1, 5, 6, 8, 10, 12, 15, 16].

17.6 Patient Evaluation, Diagnosis and Differential Diagnosis

The clinical diagnosis of donovanosis, based on history and appearance, may be fairly accurate in endemic areas. The correct diagnosis can be performed if appropriately selected laboratorial techniques are used to confirm the presumptive clinical aspects.

The organism is difficult to cultivate and demands special growth nutrients and factors for its development. It can be cultivated in vivo in the chick embryonic yolk sac and in vitro in culture means enriched with egg yolk. It is always arduous, expensive, and of low reproducibility.

Laboratory diagnosis requires a crush or touch preparation stained with Wright or Giemsa stain from a punch biopsy specimen.

The most adequate clinical material are fragments of subsuperficial tissue of an active granulation area. It is suggested to collect five to six tissue samples of different areas, radially, right below the edges of the lesions. The biopsy should be obtained before cleaning the lesion and removing necrotic tissue with saline solution and sterilized gauze, to finish contamination. Scrapings from the base of the lesion or exudate aspirated from pseudobuboes can also be used. The diagnostic Donovan bodies are seen as deeply staining, bipolar, safety pin-shaped rods in the cytoplasm of macrophages [16, 17].

Many pathologies can be clinically assimilated to donovanosis: primary syphilis, chancroid, lymphogranuloma venereum, neoplasia, condyloma acuminatum, leishmaniasis, deep mycosis, cutaneous tuberculosis, atypical mycobacteriosis, and cutaneous amebiasis. The differentiation can be obtained through demonstration of the specific casual agent or histopathological examination [12, 15].

17.7 Pathology

The biopsy must be done, preferentially on the edge of the lesion, where the pathological modifications are more substantial.

The coloration usually made by hematoxylin eosin is not ideal for demonstration of Donovan´s bodies in the interior of histiocytes or macrophages.

Histologically, the skin exhibits a massive cellular reaction, predominantly polymorphonuclear, with occasional plasma cells and, rarely, lymphocytes. The marginal epithelium demonstrates acanthosis, elongation of rete pegs, and pseudoepitheliomatous hyperplasia. These latter changes are highly suggestive of early malignancy and squamous cell carcinoma. Hypertrophic and cicatricial forms demonstrate the appropriate increase in fibrous tissue. Typically, large mononuclear cells containing numerous cytoplasmic inclusions (Donovan bodies) are scattered throughout the lesions. These are considered to be diagnostic of donovanosis and are often best demonstrated with special stains, such as Giemsa stain, Delafield hematoxylin, Dieterle silver stain, and the Warthin-Starry stain.

The differential histological diagnosis can be done with rhinoscleroma, histoplasmosis, leishmaniasis, and squamous cells carcinoma [12, 15–17].

17.8 Treatment

There is a varied therapeutic arsenal for the treatment of donovanosis. The medications can be used alone or in associations:

- Streptomycin 1 g/day, IM, 20–30 days.
- Sulfamethoxazole 800 mg + trimethoprim 160 mg, 12/12 h, orally, 20–30 days.
- Tetracycline 500 mg, 6/6 h, orally, 30–60 days.
- Doxycycline 100 mg, 12/12 h, orally, 30–60 days.
- Erythromycin 500 mg, 6/6 h, orally, 30–60 days.
- Chloramphenicol 500 mg, 6/6 h, orally, 15 days.
- Thiamphenicol 500 mg, 8/8 h, orally, 15–20 days.
- Gentamycin 30 mg, 12/12 h, IM, 15 days.
- Ampicillin 500 mg, 6/6 h, orally, 20–30 days.
- Amoxicillin 500 mg, 8/8 h, orally, 20–30 days.
- Lincomycin 500 mg, 6/6 h, orally, 20–30 days.

With the recent emergence of new macrolides, drugs of low toxicity which are very well tolerated, mainly Azithromycin which has excellent permanency on the tissues, are being tested. The therapeutic results were encouraging.

Response may be monitored by clinical appearance and serial biopsy specimens examined for persistent presence of Donovan bodies. In early cases, prognosis for complete healing is good. In late cases, irreparable tissue destruction may have supervened and radical surgery may be required [12, 15].

Take-Home Pearls

- In contrast to *syphilitic* ulcers, inguinal *lymphadenopathy* is generally absent.
- Tissue *biopsy* and *Wright-Giemsa stain* is used to aid in the diagnosis.
- The presence of Donovan bodies in the tissue sample confirms donovanosis. Donovan bodies are rod-shaped, oval organisms that can be seen in the *cytoplasm* of *mononuclear phagocytes* or *histiocytes* in tissue samples from patients with granuloma inguinale. They appear deep purple when stained with *Wright's stain*. These *intracellular inclusions* are the encapsulated gram-negative rods of the causative organisms.

References

1. Donovan, R.F.: Ulcerating granuloma of the pudenda. Int. Med. Gaz. **40**, 414 (1905)
2. Aragão, H.D., Viana G. Pesquisas sobre o granuloma venéreo, Mem. do Instituto Oswaldo Cruz, p 45., (1912–1913)
3. Banerjee, K.: Donovanosis in a child of six months. J. Indian Med. Assoc. **59**, 293 (1972)
4. Bhagwandeen, B.S.: Granuloma venereum (granuloma inguinale) in Zambia. East Afr. Med. J. **54**(11), 637–642 (1977)
5. Golberg, J.: Studies on granuloma inguinale. Isolation of bacterium from faeces of a patient with granuloma inguinale. Brit. J. Vener. Dis. **38**, 99–102 (1962)
6. Golberg, J.: Studies on granuloma inguinale. Some epidemiological considerations of the disease. Brit. J. Vener. Dis. **40**, 140–145 (1964)
7. Sehgal, V.N., Shyam, P., et al.: Donovanosis current concepts. Int. J. Dermatol. **25**(1), 8–16 (1986)
8. Greenblat, R.B., Torpin, R.: Experimental and clinical granuloma inguinale. JAMA **113**(12), 1109–1116 (1939)
9. Hart, G.: Psychological and social aspects of venereal disease in Papua New Guinea. Br. J. Vener. Dis. **50**, 453 (1974)
10. Jardim, M.L.: Donovanose em pacientes portadores de AIDS. An. Bras. Dermatol. **65**(4), 175–177 (1990)
11. Kuberski, T.: Granuloma inguinale (donovanosis). Sex Transm. Dis. **7**, 29–36 (1980)
12. Lal, S., Nicholas, C.: Epidemiological and clinical features in 165 cases of granuloma inguinale. Br. J. Vener. Dis. **46**, 461 (1970)
13. Lynchg, P.J.: Sexually transmitted disease: Granuloma inguinale, lymphogranuloma venerium, chancroid and infectious syphilis. Clin. Obst. Gynecol. **21**(4), 2 (1978)
14. Ribeiro, J.: Granuloma inguinale. Practioner **209**, 628–630 (1972)
15. Passos, M.R.L., et al.: Donovanosis. In: Kenneth, A.B., Noble, M.A. (eds.) Sexually Transmitted Diseases – Epidemiology, Pathology, Diagnosis and Treatment, pp. 103–116 (1997)
16. Jardim, M.L., Spinelli, L., Lupi, O. Donovanosis (Granuloma Inguinale). In: Tyring, S., Lupi, O., Hengge, U. (eds.). Tropical Dermatology, Chapter 26. Elsevier (2005)
17. Rothenberg, R.B.: Granuloma inguinale. In: Freedberg, I.M., Eisen, A.Z., et al. (eds.) Fitzpatrick´s – Dermatology in General Medicine, 5th edn, pp. 2595–2598 (1999)

Genital Mycoplasma Infection

18

Natalia Mendoza, Parisa Ravanfar, Anita K. Shetty, Brenda L. Pellicane, Rosella Creed, Sara Goel, and Stephen K. Tyring

Core Messages

- *M. hominis* and *Ureaplasma urealyticum* (Ureaplasmas) are two of the most frequent microorganisms isolated from the genitourinary tract.
- *Mycoplasma genitalium* has recently been detected and associated with pelvic inflammatory disease (PID) in women.
- An association between *M. genitalium* and persistent or recurrent urethritis has been described.

N. Mendoza (✉)
Universidad El Bosque, Center for Clinical Studies, Travis Street, Suite 100, Bogota, Colombia
e-mail: nmendoza@ccstexas.com

P. Ravanfar, A.K. Shetty, B.L. Pellicane, R. Creed, and S.K. Tyring
Center for Clinical Studies, University of Texas, Health Science Center, 6655 Travis Street, Suite 100, Houston, TX 77030, USA
e-mail: pravanfar@ccstexas.com; styring@ccstexas.com

S. Goel
D.O. PGY 2 Physical Medicine and Rehabilitation, Baylor College of Medicine, Houston, TX, USA
e-mail: sgoel@westernu.edu

18.1 Introduction

Mycoplasmas/ureaplasmas are the smallest free-living known organisms known. They are characterized by a tri-layer outer membrane and a total lack of a cell wall [1, 2], which make these organisms insensitive to β-lactam antibiotics.

The lack of genes involved in amino acid synthesis makes mycoplasma totally dependent on the exogenous supply of amino acids [3], which in part explains the difficulties with in vitro cultivation of this microorganism.

Mycoplasmas exhibit organ and tissue specificity. *M. pneumoniae* is usually found in the respiratory tract, and *M. genitalium* is primarily found in the urogenital tract [3]. The main mechanism involved in this tropism is the presence of specific cytoadhesins. The virulence factors of mycoplasmas include the mildly toxic metabolic products (hydrogen peroxide and superoxide radicals), organelles which allow the mycoplasma to adhere to the host target cells, and their intracellular location which protects them from the effects of the host immune system and antibiotics [4, 5].

The mechanism of cell entry is still unclear. Some studies have described that following the contact of *M. pneumonia* with human lung fibroblasts, the membrane develops pockets resembling clathrin-coated pits, suggesting that the microorganism enters the cell by a site-directed, receptor-mediated event resembling cell entry by *Chlamydia* [3, 6]. Once the mycoplasma is inside the cell's cytoplasm, it resides and replicates intracellularly [3, 7].

It is theorized that most of the clinical manifestations of mycoplasma infection are primarily due to the inflammatory response, rather than the direct toxic effect of the mycoplasma cell components [3].

G. Gross and S.K. Tyring (eds.), *Sexually Transmitted Infections and Sexually Transmitted Diseases*,
DOI: 10.1007/978-3-642-14663-3_18, © Springer-Verlag Berlin Heidelberg 2011

In humans, 16 species have been identified, six of which colonize the genitourinary tract (*M. hominis, U. urelyticum, M. primatum, M. genitalium, M. spermatophilum, M. penetrans*) [3, 8]. *M. primatum* (detected in rectal specimens from homosexual men) and *M. spermatophilum* have not been associated with pathologic disease. *M. penetrans* has been isolated from the urine of homosexual men who are HIV(+) [9]. *M. hominis* and *Ureaplasma urealyticum* (Ureaplasmas) are two of the most frequent microorganisms isolated from the genitourinary tract, and *Mycoplasma genitalium* has recently been detected and associated with pelvic inflammatory disease (PID) in women [8].

18.2 Epidemiology

The group of pathogens identified as early as 1898, generally known as "genital mycoplasmas," represents a species frequently found in the lower genitourinary tracts of healthy men and women who are sexually active, and is responsible for many common infections. The most prevalent genital mycoplasmas are *M. hominis, M. genitalium,* and *U. urealyticum.* In evaluating the role of these organisms in human disease, their high prevalence among healthy people must be taken into account.

Genital mycoplasmas are generally found in sexually active, adolescent and adult, women and men. Only approximately 10% of prepubertal females and even fewer prepubertal males are colonized with ureaplasmas. After puberty, colonization occurs mainly as a result of sexual activity, depending on frequency of sexual relations and the number of sexual partners. A recent study showed that physicians were able to isolate *M. hominis* in approximately 16% of women with multiple life partners, versus 2% in women with no sexual history. These patients were classified as carriers.

18.3 Clinical Manifestations

18.3.1 Nongonococcal Urethritis (NGU)

Although mycoplasmas have been associated with NGU for more than 40 years, there is still much debate as to their role in this condition. NGU is the most common sexually transmitted disease in men [3] and although *U. urealyticum* has been implicated as its primary cause, it is unclear exactly what proportion of NGU is due to this microorganism. Studies have shown that the initial inoculation of *U. urealyticum* into the urethra causes disease, while subsequent invasions result in colonization without disease [3].

As expected, the incidence of *M. genitalium* infection in men with NGU is usually greater than in those without the disease [1, 10–12]. The identification of *M. genitalium* as a causative agent in NGU occurred after 1993 as a result of the development of the polymerase chain reaction (PCR) [3, 13]. Many studies support the role of *M. genitalium* as the etiology of NGU, independent of *C. trachomatis. M. genitalium* is an important cause of NGU constituting 13–45% of *C. trachomatis*–negative NGU cases [1, 3].

There is a correlation between the amount of inflammation as well as the type of microorganisms and the grade of urethritis. A high-grade urethritis is defined as >10 polymorphonuclear neutrophils (PMNs) cells per high-power microscopic field. *M. genitalium* has been strongly correlated with a high-grade urethritis (PMNs) [3, 14]. Some authors have noted the association between *M. genitalium* and persistent or recurrent urethritis [3, 14, 15, 16].

18.3.2 Bacterial Vaginosis

Bacterial vaginosis (BV) is believed to be caused by a synergistic mixture of microorganisms. Genital mycoplasmas are one of the major etiological agents for bacterial vaginosis [3]. Both *M. hominis* and *U. urealyticum* have been associated with BV, causing 58–76% [3] and 62–92% of cases, respectively [3, 17–19].

18.3.3 Cervicitis

The connection between *M. genitalium* and cervicitis has been suggested [3, 20–22]; however, the role of mycoplasma is still controversial. The presence of *M. genitalium* is significantly greater in *C. trachiomatis*–negative women with symptomatic genital infections than in asymptomatic women [3, 23–25].

18.3.4 Pelvic Inflammatory Disease

Pelvic inflammatory disease (PID) is common in women of childbearing age and is diagnosed in approximately 8% of US women and 15% of Swedish women [26, 27]. It has a polymicrobial etiology and up to 70% of PID cases have an unidentified etiology while one-third to one-half are due to *C. trachomatis* and/or *Neisseria gonorrhoeae* [28, 29].

Cervicitis is a common antecedent of PID since PID typically occurs as microorganisms ascend from the lower genital tract and infect the uterus, fallopian tubes, and ovaries through the cervical os, [30]. The PEACH study of women with clinically suspected PID found that *M. genitalium* was as prevalent as *C. trachomatis* and *N. gonorrhoeae,* highlighting its importance as a pathogen in the female genital tract [31]. Further studies are necessary among high-risk populations to demonstrate causality.

18.3.5 Reproductive Morbidity Associated with Mycoplasma genitalium

Major reproductive and gynecologic sequelae result from PID. The most common sequelae are infertility, ectopic pregnancy, recurrent PID, and chronic pelvic pain [32].

Like *C. trachomatis*, *M. genitalium* is most often asymptomatic, known as silent PID. *M. genitalium* antibodies have been found more frequently among women with tubal-factor infertility compared to women with nontubal-factor infertility [33]; however, there is inconsistent data to prove causality [34].

Larger prospective studies are needed to better understand the possible reproductive or gynecologic sequelae of *M. genitalium* as a pathogen in upper-genital-tract infections.

18.4 Diagnosis

M. genitalium is difficult to diagnose; it is fastidious and difficult to culture; several weeks to months are required to culture the organism [35]. Detection of *M. genitalium* often requires PCR technology [8, 30, 36]. PCR detects *M. genitalium* in women with PID with rates ranging from 14% to 16% [29, 37], but it is often negative among healthy nonpregnant women and those without endometritis [37]. Recently nucleic acid amplification tests (NAATs) have been used to conduct diagnostic studies (not commercially available) [35].

An optimal specimen is necessary for the correct diagnosis since the results may vary depending on the sample taken. It is recommended that more than one specimen be taken in addition to a urine specimen and a cervical swab [26].

Sexual transmission of *M. genitalium* has been implicated by the high concordance of PCR positivity within sexual dyads [30].

18.5 Treatment

Management of mycoplasma infections depends upon the clinical suspicion of the possible involvement of this microorganism [8]. Some authors consider the presence of *M. hominis*, ureaplasmas, or *M. genitalium* as insufficient for treatment. However, treatment for mycoplasma should be considered in symptomatic cases or in those that do not respond to the initial treatment.

Mycoplasmas lack a cell wall and are therefore resistant to cell-wall-inhibiting antibiotics such as penicillin and cephalosporins, as well as tetracycline and levofloxacin [3, 38].

Macrolides, especially azithromycin, are among the best treatments for *M. genitalium,* with cures between 85% with one single dose of 1 g, and 95% with one initial dose of 500 mg on day one followed by 250 mg daily for 4 days [39, 40]. Patients with treatment failure after azithromycin have been successfully treated with moxifloxacin 400 mg daily for 10 days [41].

Tetracyclines are effective against some strains of *M. hominis* but have a high incidence of resistance [42]. Approximately 10% of the ureaplasmas are resistant to tetracyclines [42]. Clindamycin is the treatment of choice for pregnant patients [8].

U. urealyticum has been shown to be highly sensitive to doxycycline, erythromycin, clarithromycin, and moxifloxacin; *M. hominis* is extremely sensitive to clindamycin and highly sensitive to moxifloxacin [8].

18.6 Conclusions

Mycoplasmas are found in the genital tract of men and women at considerably high rates. *M. genitalium* has been considered a potential cause of sexually transmitted urethritis in men, especially those with persistent or recurrent urethritis.

The high rate of treatment failure among women with PID testing positive for *M. genitalium* establishes the need for antibiotic treatment that covers for this microorganism. The role of screening for infection is currently unknown. The testing and treatment of symptomatic individuals infected with *M. genitalium* are recommended, but limited by the lack of commercially suitable tests.

Evidence-based data is still needed for further diagnosis, treatment, and management guidelines.

Take-Home Pearls

- *M. genitalium* is often asymptomatic but can cause cervicitis, PID and bacterial vaginosis.
- *M. genitalium* is difficult to diagnose. An optimal specimen is necessary for the correct diagnosis since the results may vary depending on the sample taken.
- Treatment for mycoplasma should be considered in those PID, bacterial vaginosis and cervicitis cases that do not respond to conventional treatment.

References

1. Jensen, J.S.: Mycoplasma genitalium: the aetiological agent of urethritis and other sexually transmitted diseases. J. Eur. Acad. Dermatol. Venereol. **18**(1), 1–11 (2004)
2. Razin, S., Yogev, D., Naot, Y.: Molecular biology and pathogenicity of mycoplasmas. Microbiol. Mol. Biol. Rev. **62**, 1094–1156 (1998)
3. Uuskula, A., Kohl, P.K.: Genital mycoplasmas, including Mycoplasma genitalium, as sexually transmitted agents. Int. J. STD AIDS **13**(2), 79–85 (2002)
4. Burgos, R., Pich, O.Q., Ferrer-Navarro, M., Baseman, J.B., Querol, E., Pinol, J.: Mycoplasma genitalium P140 and P110 cytadhesins are reciprocally stabilized and required for cell adhesion and terminal-organelle development. J. Bacteriol. **188**(24), 8627–8637 (2006)
5. Burgos, R., Pich, O.Q., Querol, E., Pinol, J.: Functional analysis of the Mycoplasma genitalium MG312 protein reveals a specific requirement of the MG312 N-terminal domain for gliding motility. J. Bacteriol. **189**(19), 7014–7023 (2007)
6. Mernaugh, G.R., Dallo, S.F., Holt, S.C., Baseman, J.B.: Properties of adhering and nonadhering populations of Mycoplasma genitalium. Clin. Infect. Dis. **17**(Suppl 1), S69–S78 (1993)
7. Dallo, S.F., Baseman, J.B.: Intracellular DNA replication and long-term survival of pathogenic mycoplasmas. Microb. Pathog. **29**(5), 301–309 (2000)
8. Taylor-Robinson, D.: The role of mycoplasmas in pregnancy outcome. Best Pract. Res. **21**(3), 425–438 (2007)
9. Blanchard, A., Hamrick, W., Duffy, L., Baldus, K., Cassell, G.H.: Use of the polymerase chain reaction for detection of Mycoplasma fermentans and Mycoplasma genitalium in the urogenital tract and amniotic fluid. Clin. Infect. Dis. **17**(Suppl 1), S272–S279 (1993)
10. Ishihara, S., Yasuda, M., Ito, S., Maeda, S., Deguchi, T.: Mycoplasma genitalium urethritis in men. Int. J. Antimicrob. Agents **24**(Suppl 1), S23–S27 (2004)
11. Maeda, S., Deguchi, T., Ishiko, H., et al.: Detection of Mycoplasma genitalium, Mycoplasma hominis, Ureaplasma parvum (biovar 1) and Ureaplasma urealyticum (biovar 2) in patients with non-gonococcal urethritis using polymerase chain reaction-microtiter plate hybridization. Int. J. Urol. **11**(9), 750–754 (2004)
12. Wikstrom, A., Jensen, J.S.: Mycoplasma genitalium: a common cause of persistent urethritis among men treated with doxycycline. Sex. Transm. Infect. **82**(4), 276–279 (2006)
13. Baseman, J.B., Tully, J.G.: Mycoplasmas: sophisticated, reemerging, and burdened by their notoriety. Emerg. Infect. Dis. **3**(1), 21–32 (1997)
14. Bjornelius, E., Lidbrink, P., Jensen, J.S.: Mycoplasma genitalium in non-gonococcal urethritis–a study in Swedish male STD patients. Int. J. STD AIDS **11**(5), 292–296 (2000)
15. Taylor-Robinson, D.: Mycoplasma genitalium – an up-date. Int. J. STD AIDS **13**(3), 145–151 (2002)
16. Totten, P.A., Schwartz, M.A., Sjostrom, K.E., et al.: Association of Mycoplasma genitalium with nongonococcal urethritis in heterosexual men. J. Infect. Dis. **183**(2), 269–276 (2001)
17. Keane, F.E., Thomas, B.J., Whitaker, L., Renton, A., Taylor-Robinson, D.: An association between non-gonococcal urethritis and bacterial vaginosis and the implications for patients and their sexual partners. Genitourin. Med. **73**(5), 373–377 (1997)
18. Keane, F.E., Thomas, B.J., Gilroy, C.B., Renton, A., Taylor-Robinson, D.: The association of Mycoplasma hominis, Ureaplasma urealyticum and Mycoplasma genitalium with bacterial vaginosis: observations on heterosexual women and their male partners. Int. J. STD AIDS **11**(6), 356–360 (2000)
19. Hill, G.B.: The microbiology of bacterial vaginosis. Am. J. Obstet. Gynecol. **169**(2 Pt 2), 450–454 (1993)
20. Falk, L., Fredlund, H., Jensen, J.S.: Signs and symptoms of urethritis and cervicitis among women with or without Mycoplasma genitalium or Chlamydia trachomatis infection. Sex. Transm. Infect. **81**(1), 73–78 (2005)

21. Manhart, L.E., Critchlow, C.W., Holmes, K.K., et al.: Mucopurulent cervicitis and Mycoplasma genitalium. J. Infect. Dis. **187**(4), 650–657 (2003)
22. Pepin, J., Labbe, A.C., Khonde, N., et al.: Mycoplasma genitalium: an organism commonly associated with cervicitis among west African sex workers. Sex. Transm. Infect. **81**(1), 67–72 (2005)
23. Uno, M., Deguchi, T., Komeda, H., et al.: Mycoplasma genitalium in the cervices of Japanese women. Sex. Transm. Dis. **24**(5), 284–286 (1997)
24. Perez, G., Skurnick, J.H., Denny, T.N., et al.: Herpes simplex type II and Mycoplasma genitalium as risk factors for heterosexual HIV transmission: report from the heterosexual HIV transmission study. Int. J. Infect. Dis. **3**(1), 5–11 (1998)
25. Palmer, H.M., Gilroy, C.B., Claydon, E.J., Taylor-Robinson, D.: Detection of Mycoplasma genitalium in the genitourinary tract of women by the polymerase chain reaction. Int. J. STD AIDS **2**(4), 261–263 (1991)
26. Jensen, J.S., Bjornelius, E., Dohn, B., Lidbrink, P.: Comparison of first void urine and urogenital swab specimens for detection of Mycoplasma genitalium and Chlamydia trachomatis by polymerase chain reaction in patients attending a sexually transmitted disease clinic. Sex. Transm. Dis. **31**(8), 499–507 (2004)
27. Stephen, E.H., Chandra, A.: Declining estimates of infertility in the United States: 1982–2002. Fertil. Steril. **86**(3), 516–523 (2006)
28. Ness, R.B., Soper, D.E., Holley, R.L., et al.: Effectiveness of inpatient and outpatient treatment strategies for women with pelvic inflammatory disease: results from the Pelvic Inflammatory Disease Evaluation and Clinical Health (PEACH) randomized trial. Am. J. Obstet. Gynecol. **186**(5), 929–937 (2002)
29. Simms, I., Eastick, K., Mallinson, H., et al.: Associations between Mycoplasma genitalium, Chlamydia trachomatis and pelvic inflammatory disease. J. Clin. Pathol. **56**(8), 616–618 (2003)
30. Haggerty, C.L.: Evidence for a role of Mycoplasma genitalium in pelvic inflammatory disease. Curr. Opin. Infect. Dis. **21**(1), 65–69 (2008)
31. Haggerty, C.L., Totten, P.A., Astete, S.G., Ness, R.B.: Mycoplasma genitalium among women with nongonococcal, nonchlamydial pelvic inflammatory disease. Infect. Dis. Obstet. Gynecol. **2006**, 30184 (2006)
32. Westrom, L., Joesoef, R., Reynolds, G., Hagdu, A., Thompson, S.E.: Pelvic inflammatory disease and fertility. A cohort study of 1,844 women with laparoscopically verified disease and 657 control women with normal laparoscopic results. Sex. Transm. Dis. **19**(4), 185–192 (1992)
33. Cluasen, H.F., Fedder, J., Drasbek, M., et al.: Serological investigation of Mycoplasma genitalium in infertile women. Hum. Reprod. **16**, 1866–1874 (2001)
34. Haggerty, C.L., Ness, R.B., Amortegui, A., et al.: Endometritis does not predict reproductive morbidity after pelvic inflammatory disease. Am. J. Obstet. Gynecol. **188**(1), 141–148 (2003)
35. Ross, J.D., Jensen, J.S.: Mycoplasma genitalium as a sexually transmitted infection: implications for screening, testing, and treatment. Sex. Transm. Infect. **82**(4), 269–271 (2006)
36. Yoshida, T., Maeda, S., Deguchi, T., Miyazawa, T., Ishiko, H.: Rapid detection of Mycoplasma genitalium, Mycoplasma hominis, Ureaplasma parvum, and Ureaplasma urealyticum organisms in genitourinary samples by PCR-microtiter plate hybridization assay. J. Clin. Microbiol. **41**(5), 1850–1855 (2003)
37. Cohen, C.R., Manhart, L.E., Bukusi, E.A., et al.: Association between Mycoplasma genitalium and acute endometritis. Lancet **359**(9308), 765–766 (2002)
38. Goulet, M., Dular, R., Tully, J.G., Billowes, G., Kasatiya, S.: Isolation of Mycoplasma pneumoniae from the human urogenital tract. J. Clin. Microbiol. **33**(11), 2823–2825 (1995)
39. Bjarnelius, E.A.C., Bojs, G., et al.: Mycoplasma genitalium: when to test and treat. Present status in Scandinavia. In: 15th Biennial meeting of the International Society for Sexually Transmited Diseases Research, Otawa (2003)
40. Mroczkowski, T.F.M.L., Nsuami, M., et al.: A randomized comparison of azithromycin and doxycycline for the treatment of Mycoplasma genitalium positive urethritis in men. In: ISSTDR Conference, 2005
41. Bradshaw, C.S.T.S., Read, T.R., et al.: Mycoplasma genitalium, herpes simplex viruses and adenoviruses in non-genitalium urethritis. In: 16th Biennal meeting of the International Society for Sexually Transmitted Diseases Research, Amsterdam (2005)
42. Taylor-Robinson, D., Bebear, C.: Antibiotic susceptibilities of mycoplasmas and treatment of mycoplasmal infections. J. Antimicrob. Chemother. **40**(5), 622–630 (1997)

19 Bacterial Vaginosis

A. Rubins

Core Messages

> Bacterial vaginosis is a common vaginal disorder, especially in women of childbearing age. Pathogenesis is multifactorial involving *Gardnerella vaginalis* and other anaerobes. Diagnosis is clinical and by finding "clue cells" in vaginal microscopy. Therapy is antibacterial.

Bacterial vaginosis (BV) is a clinical syndrome of dysbiosis of the vaginal flora with reduction in H_2O_2-producing *Lactobacillus* by polymicrobial flora such as *Gardnerella vaginalis, Mobiluncus curtisii*, and/or *M. mulieris*, other anaerobic bacteria and *Mycoplasma hominis*. The etiology of BV is not well understood. Frequency of BV is increased with multiple sex partners, but rare cases are seen in virgins. Treatment of male sex partners is not helpful [1,2].

19.1 Epidemiology

BV is most common in women of childbearing age. It has been diagnosed in 17–20% of women seeking gynecologic care in family practice or student health care settings. The prevalence increases considerably in symptomatic women attending STI clinics, reaching 24–37%. BV has been observed in 16–29% of pregnant women. *Gardnerella vaginalis* has been found in 10–31% of virgin adolescent girls, but is significantly more frequent among sexually active women, reaching a prevalence of 50–60% in some high-risk populations [3,4]. Evaluation of epidemiologic factors has revealed few clues about the cause of BV. Use of intrauterine devices and douching was found to be more common in women with BV. BV is significantly more common among African-American and sexually active women including lesbians [5].

19.2 Pathogenesis and Pathology

The cause of BV is unknown. Microscopic examination shows no polymorphonuclear cells, sparse lactobacilli, and numerous coccobacillary forms on vaginal epithelial cells. Cultures are not indicated. *Gardnerella vaginalis* rods and *Mobiluncus species* occur in association with other anaerobic and partially anaerobic microorganisms. *Gardnerella vaginalis* is a tiny wood-like rod. Mobiluncus species are semicircular concave-shaped rods of various size and thickness. Both agents possess an important specificity – they, together with the existing microflora, concentrate on the epithelial cell surface, forming the so-called clue cells (Fig. 19.1). These are the cells by whose presence one can determine bacterial vaginosis in native and stained samples. In BV cases, the changes occur in vaginal ecosystem: normal *Lactobacillus* morphotype microflora is substituted by anaerobic microorganisms. The proportion between aerobic and anaerobic microorganisms changes in favor of anaerobic, pH of the normal vaginal secretion rises above 4.5. Microorganisms per 1 g tissues increase by 100 times

A. Rubins
Dermatovenerology, Faculty of Medicine,
University of Latvia, 19 Raina Boulevard, Riga,
LV 1586, Latvia
e-mail: arubins@apollo.lv

G. Gross and S.K. Tyring (eds.), *Sexually Transmitted Infections and Sexually Transmitted Diseases*,
DOI: 10.1007/978-3-642-14663-3_19, © Springer-Verlag Berlin Heidelberg 2011

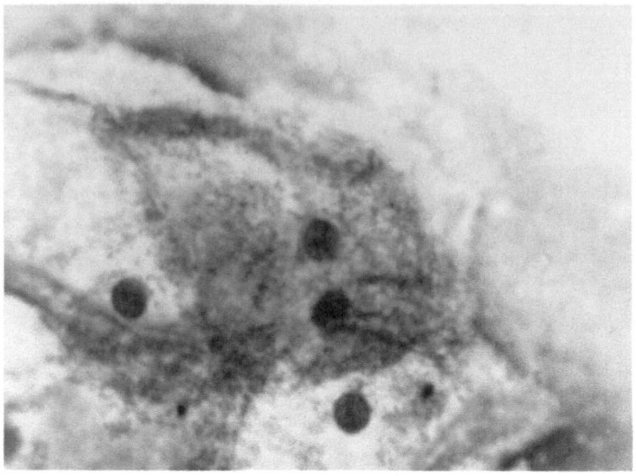

Fig. 19.1 Clue cells

Table 19.1 Comparison of vaginal ecosystem

Normal Vagina	Bacterial Vaginosis
H_2O_2 producing *Lactobacillus* are dominating	H_2O_2 producing *Lactobacillus* are less than 30%
Ratio of anaerobic microorganisms to aerobic 2–5:1	Ratio of anaerobic microorganisms to aerobic 100–1,000:1
Presence of *Gardnerella vaginalis* <40%	Presence of *Gardnerella vaginalis* >90%
Presence of *Mobiluncus* 0–5%	Presence of *Mobiluncus* 50–70%
Presence of *Mycoplasma hominis* in 15–30% sexually active females	Presence of *Mycoplasma hominis* in 60–75% of sexually active females

(Table 19.1). *G. vaginalis* could be found also in male urinary pathways. Since the inflammation reaction in BV case is practically absent, BV microflora in mucosa of male and female urinary pathways usually do not cause symptoms [6, 7].

19.3 Clinical Features

As many as 50% of women with bacterial vaginosis may be asymptomatic. An abnormal malodorous vaginal discharge, often described as fishy, that is infrequently profuse and often appears after unprotected coitus, is usually described. Pruritus, dysuria, and dyspareunia are rare. Examination reveals a nonviscous, grayish-white adherent discharge.

Bacterial vaginosis has been considered to be largely of nuisance value only. There is now considerable evidence of serious obstetric and gynecologic complications of bacterial vaginosis, including asymptomatic bacterial vaginosis diagnosed by Gram stain. Obstetric complications include chorioamnionitis, preterm delivery, prematurity, and postpartum fever [8]. Gynecologic sequelae are postabortion fever, posthysterectomy fever, vaginal cuff infection, and chronic mast cell endometritis [9]. A more recent association is reported between untreated bacterial vaginosis and cervical inflammation and low-grade dysplasia [10]. Bacterial vaginosis is a risk factor for HIV infection (Table 19.2), [11].

The Amsel criteria for diagnosis of bacterial vaginosis*:

1. Thin, white/gray discharge, coating the vagina and vestibule.
2. Clue cells (vaginal epithelial cells heavily coated with bacteria) present in the discharge.
3. Release of a fishy odor on adding 10% potassium hydroxide to the discharge.
4. pH of vaginal fluid greater than 4.5.

*Three of these criteria must be present to confirm the diagnosis [12].

19.4 Management

Poor efficacy has been observed with triple sulfa creams, erythromycin, tetracycline, acetic acid gel, and povidone-iodine vaginal douches.

The most successful oral therapy remains metronidazole. Most studies using multiple divided dose regimens of 800–1,200 mg/day for 1 week achieved clinical cure rates in excess of 90% immediately and of approximately 80% at 4 weeks. Although single-dose therapy with 2 g metronidazole achieves comparable immediate clinical response rates, higher recurrence rates have been reported. The beneficial effect of metronidazole results predominantly from its antianaerobic activity and because *G. vaginalis* is susceptible to the hydroxymetabolites of metronidazole. Although *Mycoplasma hominis* is resistant to metronidazole, the organisms are usually not detected at follow-up visits of successfully treated

Table 19.2 Diagnostic features of bacterial vaginosis, candida vaginitis, and trichomonas vaginalis

		Normal	Bacterial Vaginosis	Candida Vaginitis	Trichomonas Vaginalis
Symptoms		None or physiologic leucorrhea	Malodorous moderate discharges	Vulvar pruritus, soreness, increased discharge, dysuria, dyspareunia	Profuse purulent discharge, offensive odor, pruritus, and dyspareunia
Discharge	*Amount*	Variable, scant to moderate	Moderate	Scant to moderate	Profuse
	Color	Clear or white	White/gray	White	Yellow
	Consistency	Floccular nonhomogenous	Homogenous, uniformly coating walls	Clumped but variable	Homogenous
	"Bubbles"	Absent	Present	Absent	Present
	Appearance of vulva and vagina	Normal	No inflammation	Introital and vulvar erythema, edema and occasional pustules, vaginal erythema	Erythema and swelling of vulvar and vaginal epithelium (strawberry cervix)
	pH of vaginal fluid	<4.5	>4.5	<4.5	5.0–6.0
	Amine test (10%) potassium hydroxide	Negative	Positive	Negative	Occasionally present
	Saline microscopy	Normal epithelial cell, lactobacilli predominant	Clue cells, coccobacillary flora predominant, absence of leucocytes, motile curved rods	Normal flora, blastospores (yeast) 40–50%	PMNs +++, motile trichomonads (80–90%, no clue cells, abnormal flora)
10% potassium hydroxide microscopy		Negative	Negative (except in mixed infections)	Positive (60–90%)	

patients. Similarly, *Mobiluncus curtisii* is resistant to metronidazole but usually disappears after therapy.

Topical therapy with 2% clindamycin cream once daily for 7 days, clindamycin ovules for 3 days, or metronidazole gel 0.75% administered daily for 5 days have been shown to be as effective as oral metronidazole, without any of the side effects of the latter.

In the past, asymptomatic bacterial vaginosis was not treated, especially because patients often improve spontaneously over several months. However, the growing evidence linking asymptomatic bacterial vaginosis with numerous obstetric and gynecologic upper tract complications has caused reassessment of this policy, especially with additional convenient topical therapies. Asymptomatic bacterial vaginosis should be treated before pregnancy, in women with cervical abnormalities and before elective gynecologic surgery. Routine screening for and treatment of asymptomatic bacterial vaginosis in pregnancy remains controversial, pending the outcome of studies proving that therapy of bacterial vaginosis reduces preterm delivery and prematurity.

Despite indirect evidence of sexual transmission, no study has documented reduced recurrence rates of bacterial vaginosis in women whose partners have been treated with a variety of regimens, including metronidazole. Accordingly, most clinicians do not routinely treat male partners [13].

After therapy with oral metronidazole, approximately 30% of patients initially responding, experience recurrence of symptoms within 3 months. Reasons for recurrence are unclear, including the possibility of reinfection, but recurrence more likely reflects vaginal relapse, with failure to eradicate the offending organisms and reestablish the normal protective *Lactobacillus* spp. dominant vaginal flora. Management of bacterial vaginosis relapse includes oral or vaginal metronidazole, or topical clindamycin, usually prescribed for 14 days. Maintenance antibiotic regimens have been disappointing and new experimental approaches include exogenous *Lactobacillus* spp. recolonization using selected bacteria-containing suppositories [14].

19.5 Prevention

Because the pathogenesis of bacterial vaginosis is obscure, preventive measures have not been forthcoming. Although not typically sexually transmitted, barrier contraception may reduce occurrence and avoiding douching is recommended [15].

Take-Home Pearls

- Bacterial vaginosis is a common vaginal disorder.
- *Gardnerella vaginalis* and other anaerobes are involved in pathogenesis.
- Malodorous vaginal discharge is a characteristic clinical sign.
- Diagnosis is based on finding "clue cells" in vaginal secretions.
- Therapy is mainly antibacterial.
- Lactobacillar supplements can be preventive.

References

1. Allsworth, J.E., Peipert, J.F.: Prevalence of bacterial vaginosis: 2001–2004 National Health and Nutrition Examination Survey data. Obstet. Gynecol. **109**, 114–120 (2007)
2. Smart, S., Singal, A., Mindel, A.: Social and sexual risk factors for bacterial vaginosis. Sex. Transm. Infect. **80**, 58–62 (2004)
3. Yen, S., Shafer, M.A., Moncada, J., et al.: Bacterial vaginosis in sexually experienced and non-sexually experienced young women entering the military. Obstet. Gynecol. **102**, 927–933 (2003)
4. Bump, R.C., Buesching, W.J.: Bacterial vaginosis in virginal and sexually active adolescent females: evidence against exclusive sexual transmission. Am. J. Obstet. Gynecol. **158**, 935–939 (1988)
5. Avonts, D., Sercu, M., Heyerick, P., et al.: Incidence of uncomplicated genital infections in women using oral contraception or an intrauterine device: a prospective study. Sex. Transm. Dis. **17**, 23–29 (1990)
6. Hawes, S.E., Hillier, S.L., Benedetti, J., et al.: Hydrogen peroxide-producing lactobacilli and acquisition of vaginal infections. J. Infect. Dis. **174**, 1058–1063 (1996)
7. Nilsson, U., Hellberg, D., Shoubnikova, M., et al.: Sexual behavior risk factors associated with bacterial vaginosis. Sex. Transm. Dis. **24**, 241–246 (1997)
8. Hillier, S.L., Nugent, R.P., Eschenbach, D.A., et al.: Association between bacterial vaginosis and preterm delivery of a low-birth-weight infant: the vaginal infections and prematurity study group. N Engl J. Med. **333**, 1737–1742 (1995)
9. Meis, P.J., Goldenberg, R.L., Mercer, B., et al.: The preterm prediction study: significance of vaginal infections: National Institute of Child Health and Human Development Maternal-Fetal Medicine Units Network. Am. J. Obstet. Gynecol. **173**, 1231–1235 (1995)
10. Larsson, P., Platz-Christensen, J.J., Thejls, H., et al.: Incidence of pelvic inflammatory disease after first trimester legal abortion in women with bacterial vaginosis after treatment with metronidazole: A double-blind, randomized study. Am. J. Obstet. Gynecol. **166**, 100–103 (1992)
11. Spiegel, C.A.: Bacterial vaginosis. Clin. Microbial Rev. **4**, 485–502 (1991)
12. Amsel, R., Totten, P.A., Spiegel, C.A., et al.: Nonspecific vaginitis: diagnostic criteria and microbial and epidemiologic associations. Am. J. Med. **74**, 14–22 (1983)
13. Koumans, E.H., Markowitz, L.E., Hogan, V.: Indications for therapy and treatment recommendations for bacterial vaginosis in nonpregnant women: a synthesis of data. Clin. Infect. Dis. **35**(Suppl 2), S152–S172 (2002)
14. Workowski KA, Berman SM: For the Centers for Disease Control and Prevention. Sexually transmitted diseases treatment guidelines, 2006 [Published correction appears in MMWR Recomm Rep 2006;55:997]. MMWR Recomm. Rep. 2006;55(RR-11):1–94. www.cdc.gov/mmwr/PDF/rr/rr5511.pdf. Accessed 8 March 2007
15. Koumans, E.H., Kendrick, J.: CDC bacterial vaginosis working group. Preventing adverse sequelae of bacterial vaginosis: a public health program and research agenda. Sex. Transm. Dis. **28**, 292–297 (2001)

Part III

Viral Infections

20 Biology of Sexually Transmitted Herpes Viruses

H.W. Doerr, Lutz G. Gürtler, and M.W. Wittek

Core Message

> There are five human herpesviruses that are transmitted by intercourse and by other routes of intimate contact: Herpes simplex virus type 1 (HSV-1) and type 2 (HSV-2), cytomegalovirus (HCMV), Kaposi's sarcoma-associated herpesvirus (KSHV or HHV-8), and Epstein-Barr virus (EBV). Among them only HSV-2 and less frequently HSV-1 cause primary and recurrent genital disease (herpes genitalis). Intrapartum, the newborn may be infected and suffer from a life-threatening herpes neonatorum generalisatus. Sexually transmitted and ascending HCMV may prenatally infect and damage the fetus in utero, usually in the second and third trimester of pregnancy or intrapartum. Occult damages of the brain may lead to mental retardation. HHV-8 and EBV are (also) sexually transmitted and are responsible for oncologic diseases (lymphomas etc.) and other disorders of the lymphatic systems. For EBV infection, sexually transmission is of minor relevance. Herpesvirus infections persist –life-long by establishing a proviral latency in distinct body cells and by special immune escape mechanisms. 90, 80, 50, 20 and <1% of young adults in Europe have acquired EBV, HSV-1, HCMV, HSV-2, and HHV-8 infections. They are reactivated and spread during deficiency of the cell-mediated immunity causing opportunistic, partially life-threatening infectious diseases. Vaccination is not currently available, but antivirals can be successfully applied against HSV and HCMV. HHV-8 (and EBV) infection is stopped by natural or therapeutic immunoreconstitution. Laboratory diagnosis is fully developed with all kinds of virus (antigen/ nucleic acid) and antibody detection.

20.1 Introduction and Taxonomy

To date, five herpesvirus species that are sexually transmitted between humans have been identified:

1. Herpes simplex virus type 1 (HSV-1) = herpesvirus hominis 1 (HHV-1).
2. Herpes simplex virus type 2 (HSV-2) = herpesvirus hominis 2 (HHV-2).
3. Human cytomegalovirus (HCMV) = herpesvirus hominis 4 (HHV-4).
4. Kaposi's sarcoma-associated herpesvirus (HHV-8) = herpesvirus hominis 8 (HHV-8).
5. Epstein–Barr Virus (EBV) = herpesvirus hominis 5 (HHV-5).

EBV can be transmitted by sexual contact, in around 10% of sexually active subjects it is found in high-titer secretions [1]. Since this virus is usually transmitted by saliva and smear infection, it is not further discussed in this contribution.

H.W. Doerr (✉) and M.W. Wittek
Institute for Medical Virology at the hospital of the Johann Wolfgang Goethe-University, Paul-Ehrlich-Str. 40, 60596 Frankfurt, Germany
e-mail: h.w.doerr@em.uni-frankfurt.de

L.G. Gürtler
Max von Pettenkofer Institute of the University München, Pettenkofer Str 9A, 80336 München, Germany
e-mail: lutzg.guertler@vodafone.de

G. Gross and S.K. Tyring (eds.), *Sexually Transmitted Infections and Sexually Transmitted Diseases*,
DOI: 10.1007/978-3-642-14663-3_20,

The other herpesviruses, which are established in humans, are varicella zoster virus (VZV = herpesvirus hominis 3) and herpesviruses hominis 6 and 7. The human and numerous animal herpesviruses comprise the taxonomic family of herpesviridae. This family is divided into three subfamilies: alpha-, beta- and gamma-herpesvirinae, each of which consists of several genera. HSV-1 and HSV-2 belong to the genus *Simplexvirus* of alpha-herpesvirinae, HCMV to the genus *Cytomegalovirus* of beta-herpesvirinae, HHV-8 and EBV to the genus *Rhadinovirus* of gamma-herpesvirinae. Although modern genetic analysis has revised taxonomy, traditional biologic criteria have been preserved.

Alpha-herpesvirinae are characterized by rapid replication in vivo and in vitro and a variable host range, while beta-herpesvirinae reveal a slow replication cycle and a restricted host range. Gamma-herpesvirinae are lymphotropic and macrophagotropic. Alpha-herpesvirus replication is hampered by acyclovir and derivates while for beta-herpesvirus ganciclovir has to be used. Each herpesvirus establishes a life-long persistent infection, which gets latent in distinct body cells, from which recurrent reactivation of productive and cell lytic infections take place. Among the sexually transmitted herpesviruses, only HSV infection causes genital lesions: HSV-2 infection is more frequent and severe than HSV-1, which is found in up to 30% of herpes genitalis cases.

20.2 Structure of Herpesviruses

Human herpesviruses are spherical particles with a diameter of 180–220 nm, depending on the shape of outer envelope (Fig. 20.1). In the center of the virus, the genome is embedded in a proteinaceous core resembling a spindle. The genome consists of a linear double-stranded (ds)DNA, which harbors more than 170 genes. Molecular weight (MW) of herpesviral DNA ranges from 125 kbp (VZV) to 235 kbp (HCMV). The dsDNA strand is divided into two parts of unique base-pair sequences, the longer (Ul) and the shorter (Us), which are interrupted and flanked by short internal, respectively terminal reiterative sequences. HHV-8 DNA lacks the Us part of the genome compared to HSV-1. The genes (and gene products) are designated as, for example, Ul 57, Us 30, etc. The numeration of genes differs between the single herpesvirus species in terms of their function. About 35 genes are conserved among all herpesviruses and are designated as HSV homolog. Up to 100 additional genes have been identified in the different herpesviruses. The genes code for structural elements of the virus and for nonstructural functions (nonstructural (NS) genes). The DNA–core complex is embedded in an icosaeder-derived capsid, which is composed by 162 nearly identical proteinaceous units, called capsomeres. Each capsomere consists of several polypeptides (viral proteins/VP), but one of them is the main brick, e.g., VP5 in HSV. Between capsid and outer envelope, there is a loosely formed layer of phosphorylated proteins (pp). Some of them are enzymes with regulating functions, e.g., in HCMV the pp65 (UL 83), which acts as proteinkinase. In this "tegument" surrounding the viral capsid, cellular and viral mRNA molecules have been detected without known function. The viral envelope is derived from the cell nucleus and other inner lipid membranes of the infected cell spiked with a couple of virus DNA-coded glycoproteins (gB–gN). Some of them, mainly gB, serve as antireceptors for adsorption to cell membrane receptors (mainly heparan sulfate), which initiate the first step of infection.

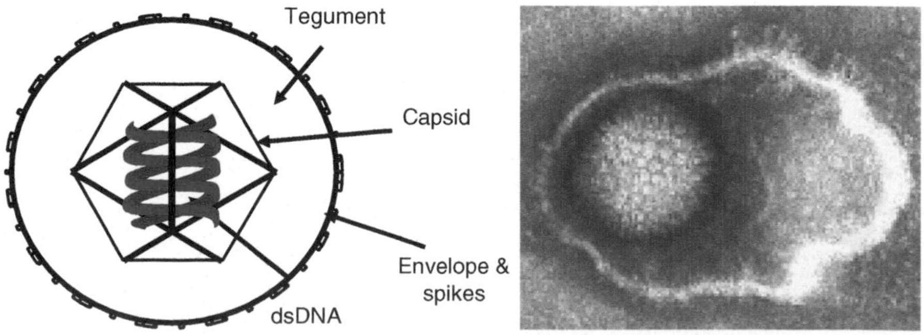

Fig. 20.1 Structure of human herpesvirus

By the use of neutralizing antibodies, serotypes of herpesvirus species have been established basically, but not completely correlating to genotypes, which are defined by nucleic acid sequences of gB and gN genes [2, 4, 5].

20.3 Replication Cycle of Herpesvirus

After receptor-mediated virus adsorption to the membrane of target cells, viral envelope and membrane undergo fusion. The inner particles, i.e., capsid and surrounding tegument, are released into the cytoplasm and transported to the cell nucleus via the tubules of endoplasmic reticulum. Entering the nucleus, tegument and capsid are dissolved, releasing proteins and the dsDNA, which is circularized to a closed ring. DNA transcription proceeds in cascades: It is slowly started by cellular RNA polymerase II by the help of transactivating tegument proteins (alpha-TIF of HSV, pp71 of HCMV) and produces immediate early mRNA molecules, which are exported from the nucleus. They are spliced and are translated via the cytoplasmatic ribosomes to IE proteins (antigens/IEA). These proteins are retransported into the nucleus and exert cis- and transactive signals to the viral and cellular genome. IE proteins are the main switch of ongoing viral DNA transcription (ICP0 of HSV; IE1, IE2 of HCMV). They activate the promoters of genes coding for (delayed) EA molecules, which are expressed in a similar way. In case of HCMV, cell nuclear transcription factor kappa B (NFkB) is involved in this signaling. Important EAs are enzymes for the viral DNA synthesis and polymerization; those kinases and polymerases are targets of antiviral drugs. In the third cascade of viral gene transcription, "late" mRNA molecules and corresponding LA proteins are produced. After retransportation into the nucleus, these proteins are composed of the new capsid, into which the progeny DNA transcribed in the mode of "rolling circle" is packaged. Tegumentation and envelopment of capsids is proceeded at the nuclear and other inner cell membranes, in which a lot of virus-coded proteins and glycoproteins have been inserted, in a "budding" process. The reliability of herpesviral reproduction process is low. Only 1 of 1,000 new virus particles is correctly and completely composed to be an infectious "virion" and released.

20.4 Latency and Reactivation of Herpesvirus Infection

The most characteristic feature of herpesviral infection is the establishment of latency, which is best studied in HSV. Latent infection is defined as persistency of viral DNA in special target cells, in which LA genes are not transcribed. No viral structure proteins are produced. In the state of latency, up to 100 copies of circularized herpesvirus DNA remain in the cell nucleus as parachromosomal episomes. The sites of HSV latency are sensoric neurons, preferentially in the trigeminal (HSV-1) and sacral spine ganglia (HSV-2 and 1). HCMV and HHV-8 establish latent infection in blood and tissue mononuclear cells, especially in (pro) monocytes, respectively in precursors of lymphocytes. Latent HHV-8 infection is also detected in all HHV-8-associated tumor cells, as angiosarcoma and lymphoma. Although a lot of scientific research has been done, basic mechanisms are still not completely understood. Obviously, cells being primarily nonpermissive for productive infection like neurons harbor certain factors, which interfere with signals necessary for initiation of viral DNA transcription. In case of HSV, only a unique latency-associated mRNA transcript (LAT) can be detected. It is supposed that this mRNA, which reveals an anti-sense orientation to IE gene carrying DNA segment, blocks the main switch of herpesviral DNA transcription (ICP0). The blockage is obviously supported by cytokines of CD8 lymphocytes, since decrease of herpesvirus-specific CD8 cells moves the balance of latent to lytic infection. The blockage of herpesviral gene transcription is furthermore resolved by hormonal signals (e.g., epinephrine). Reactivation to productive and cell lytic infection of herpesviruses is provoked by exogenous (trauma, UV light) and endogenous stress factors (menstruation). In case of HCMV, an important stimulator of reactivation is, e.g., bacterial sepsis, which induces elevated plasma level of TNF alpha stimulating the activity of NFkB. The mechanisms of HHV-8 latency and reactivation are similar to those of EBV, the other human gamma-herpesvirus, but much less investigated. Productive infection of HHV-8 and subsequent antibody stimulation is – like VZV – even more closely correlated to the function of cell-mediated immunity than of the other human herpesviruses [2, 4].

20.5 Herpesvirus Transmission and Epidemiology

Besides VZV, herpesviruses are transmitted by contact to infectious oral or genital body fluids resulting in a biphasic kinetic of infection spread in mankind. Obviously, HSV, HCMV, and HHV-8 infectivity is associated both with free virions and with cells (leukocytes), since infection cannot be prevented by immunoglobulins (in contrast to VZV). Leukocyte-depleted blood units are nearly free of herpesvirus infectivity. The first rise of incidence is due to maternal–infantile contacts (saliva), and the second one due to juvenile sexual activity. Every infection persists life-long and stimulates antibody production. So, serum surveys are informative on herpesvirus carriers (Figs. 20.2–20.4) [3]. The rate of young immunocompetent adults seropositive for HSV-1 is approximately 80%, for HCMV 50%, for HSV-2 it is 20%, and around 1% for HHV-8 in Europe and North America. In southern parts of the world (countries of the Mediterranean and Africa) and in HIV carriers, the rates are much higher (up to 30% for HHV-8 and more than 90% for the other herpesviruses). Herpesvirus can be traced by genotyping. Two clades of HSV-2 (A and B) were recently described on DNA sequence data of the envelope glycoproteins E, G and I [5].

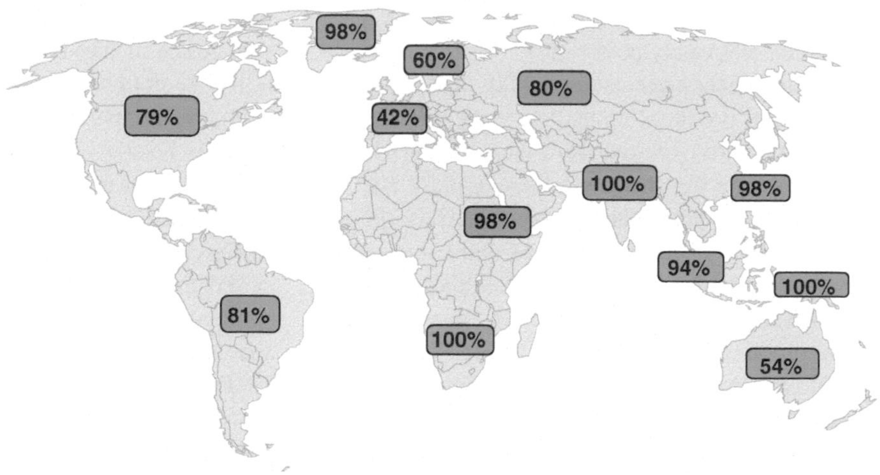

Fig. 20.2 Reported seroprevalence of HCMV

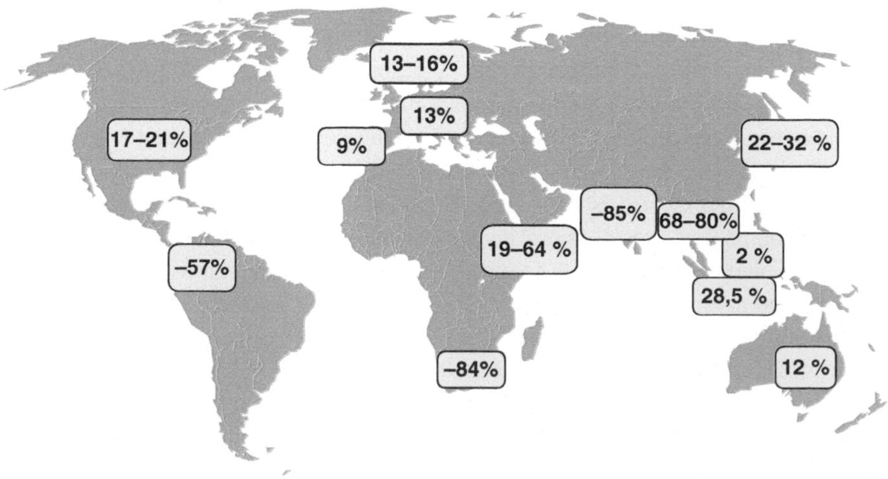

Fig. 20.3 Reported seroprevalence of HSV-2

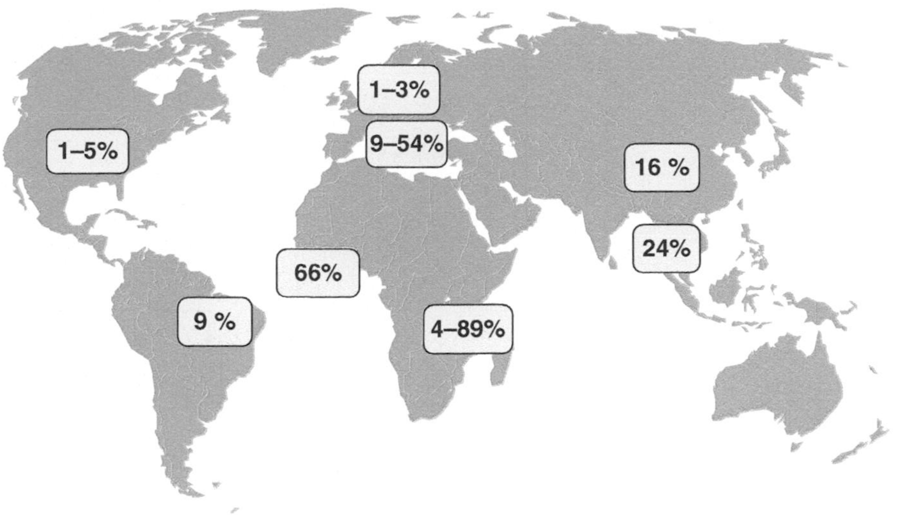

Fig. 20.4 Reported seroprevalence of HHV-8

20.6 Course of Sexual HSV Infection

Sexually transmitted HSV infection may lead to severe herpes genitalis. Such cases are due to HSV-2, while genital HSV-1 infections are less severe. However, the true manifestation rate is unknown, since patients present only with more painful lesions such as ulcers. Many people who are exposed to sexual HSV contact have previously had oral infection (usually HSV-1). However, seropositivity does not prevent subsequent genital infection, but may reduce virus replication and result in a milder clinical course, especially with genital HSV-1 infection. After mucocutaneous acquisition, HSV replicates in larger quantities and is excreted, more than 10^6 HSV-2 particles/mL inoculum, for a time interval up to 3 weeks. Lower virus shedding is detected in asymptomatic cases. Though a short viremic period is frequent, systemic complications like aseptic meningitis are uncommon. Mucocutaneous virus replication is stopped by cell-mediated immunoreactions, but the virus is not eliminated. The virus enters the axonal termini of sensory neurons and is retrogradely transported to the nucleus of cell body in the paravertebral (dorsal root) ganglion of the sacral spine, where a latent infection is permanently established (Fig. 20.5). Its reactivation is frequently recurrent. However, only a fraction of virus shedders develop signs of disease; vice versa, a silent primary infection may later on present clinically apparent recurrences. As mentioned above, exogenous and endogenous stress factors stimulate recurrences though the presence of fully working humoral and cellular immunity. However, loss of cell-mediated immune functions prevents intermediate healing and increases the rate of recurrency. This is in distinct opposition to VZV, where cell-mediated immunity, mainly based on the function of CD8 lymphocytes, is strictly correlated to (at least clinical) latency, so that herpes zoster is usually seen only in elder people as a unique event, as far as immunocompetence is preserved. Primary, clinically apparent type-2 HSV infections usually present larger virus shedding than recurrent, asymptomatic, or type-1 infections. So, infectivity is especially dangerous in cases of primary herpes genitalis caused by HSV-2. This has to be kept in mind, when a pregnant woman suffers from herpes genitalis at the time point of birth. In this case, the risk of a newborn to acquire a generalized, life-threatening herpes generalisatus is very high. Preexisting antibodies transferred from the mother to the child via placenta are not protective.

During life, the statistical frequency of herpes recurrences decreases. This may be due to hormonal changes, especially in females, and "burning out" of latent infected neurons, which are more permissive for reactivation and destroyable by cell-lytic infection [3].

20.7 Course of Sexual HCMV Infection

Free virions or virus-carrying leukocytes are transmitted via intercourse and establish infection. Serum antibodies of the recipient confer only restricted protection.

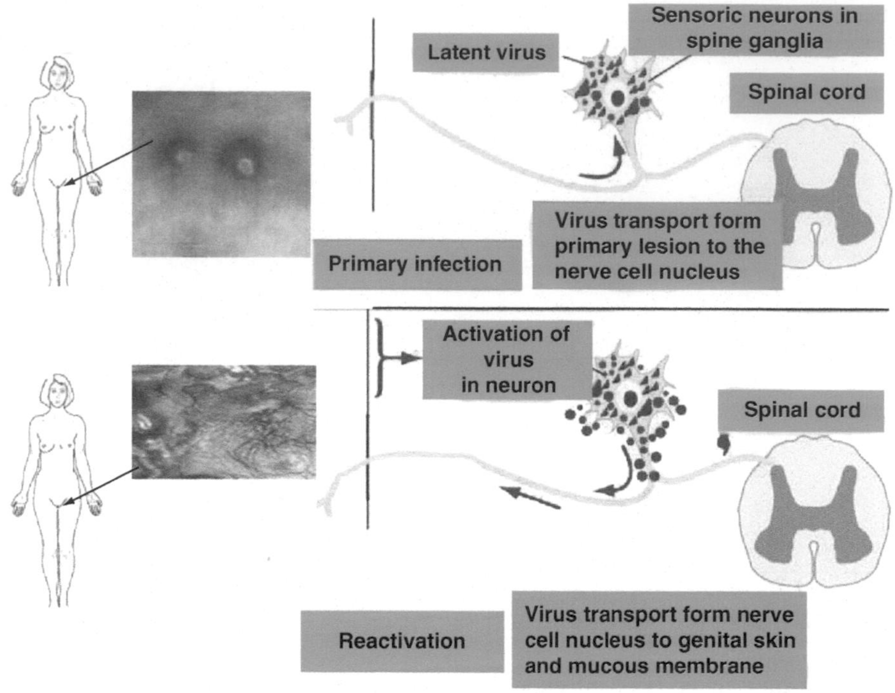

Fig. 20.5 Schematic scheme of HSV-2 primary infection and reactivation

The virus is spread in the body either by viremia or within the genital tract. In blood HCMV is associated with leukocytes. Between them and other cells the virus can be transmitted via direct contact and cell fusion, which causes the typical cytomegalic inclusion "disease" (usually only a histological finding). Important target cells of infection are the endothelium of blood vessels. All visceral organs and preferentially epithelial cells can be infected, furthermore cells of the lymphatic system, sometimes causing an infectious mononucleosis-like disease, although this is rare in immunocompetent humans.

While prenatal HSV transmission from the pregnant woman to the fetus is rare, HCMV is a common agent both of prenatal and perinatal vertical infection of infants. It is assumed, that about 0.1–0.5% of all newborns in the developed countries shed the virus in the urine. Ten times more siblings are infected in their early postnatal life by close contact to the mother (via saliva, breast milk, urine). Because of a physiological decrease of immunity during pregnancy, seropositive females shed HCMV in urine in increasing rates up to birth. In other regions of the world, the rates are much higher. The risk of vertical virus transmission is considered 30% in case of primary infection, but is still present during a secondary infection or recurrence. In one third of vertical infections, the fetus is affected and injured, preferentially in the central nervous system. The risk of damage is statistically reduced in case of recurrence; nevertheless it may be up to lethal in the individual infant. As mentioned above, sites of HCMV latency are precursors of monocytes and other blood mononuclear cells. Recurrences are frequent, but asymptomatic in the immunocompetent host. This frequency induces significant humoral and cellular booster immune reactions. Nearly 3% of all seropositive humans have (low) IgM antibody levels, and up to 10% of all CD8 lymphocytes are directed against HCMV epitopes [4].

20.8 Course of Sexual HHV-8 Infection

HHV-8 was detected in AIDS patients presenting angiosarcoma, first clinically described by the dermatologist Kaposi. The tumor was rare in Europe and North America, but well known in Africa and Mediterranean countries. This herpesvirus hominis No.8 was first recovered from lymphocytes, both B and T cells, later on in the tumor cells, where the virus persists in a latent state, i.e., only in form of proviral DNA detectable as parachromosomal episome in the cell nucleus. In state of latency, viral DNA is replicated by cellular enzymes like cell DNA. The viral genome is generally considered as transforming (oncogenic) agent, aggressively growing but tumor only develops if immunosurveillance decreases. By immune reconstitution, HHV-8-associated tumors vanish, if not too much outgrown or disseminated. Further HHV-8-associated diseases are body-caved lymphomas (Castleman's disease) and myelopathies caused by infiltration of transformed lymphocytes to the nervous system. Obviously, latency of HHV-8 infection is under control of cell-mediated immunity (CMI). If number of specific CD4 cells, in part Th1 cells, decreases, productive virus infection is reactivated causing a plasma viremia, which can be diagnosed by PCR technology as "viral load." In those cases also sexual secretions, in part ejaculate, shed virions. So the spread of HHV-8 was associated closely with the HIV epidemic. The virus, formerly not present in developed countries, spread in the same risk groups, especially in promiscuous male homosexuals. Like other herpesviruses, HHV-8 is also transmitted by saliva, i.e., via oral contact. The risk of smear infection is low, but it depends on human behavior [5].

Take-Home Pearls

> Five human herpesviruses are sexually transmitted. Only HSV-2 and less frequently HSV-1 cause (primary and recurrent) genital disease. Intrapartum transmitted infection may cause lethal herpes neonatorum generalisatus. The genital tract ascending (and blood-borne recurrent) HCMV infection may damage the fetus in utero or intra partum. These infectious diseases can be successfully treated by antiviral, if applied on time. EBV is the classic agent of infectious mononucleosis and other lymphatic disorders. Transmission by intercourse is of minor relevance. HHV-8 is a rare infection in the northern hemisphere and has been widely known as opportunistic infections during AIDS and other immunologic disorders. Although Kaposi's sarcoma is the source of the original designation for HHV-8, i.e. HHV-8, the virus is also linked to Castleman's disease.

References

1. Embom, M., Strand, A., Falk, K.I., Linde, A.: Detection of Epstein-Barr Virus, but not human herpesvirus 8, DNA in cervical secretions from Swedish women by real-time polymerase chain reaction. Sex. Transmis. Dis. **28**, 300–306 (2001)
2. Greene, W., Kuhne, K., Chen, J., Zhou, F., Lei, X., Gao, S.J.: Molecular biology of HHV-8 in relation to AIDS-associated oncogenesis. Cancer Treat. Rev. **133**, 69–127 (2007)
3. Gupta, R., Warren, T., Wald, A.: Genital herpes. Lancet **370**, 2127–2137 (2007)
4. Reddehase, M.J.: Special issue on cytomegalovirus. Med. Microbiol. Immunol. **197**, 65–256 (2008)
5. Schmidt-Chanasit J, Bialonski A, Heinemann P, Ulrich RG, Günther S, Rabenau HF, Doerr HW: A 12-year molecular survey of clinical herpes simplex virus type 2 isolates demonstrates the circulation of clade A and B strains in Germany. J Clin Virol. **48**, 208–211 (2010)

Genital Herpes

21

Adrian Mindel

Core Messages

- › Genital herpes simplex virus (HSV) infections are extremely common throughout the world and genital herpes is the leading cause of genital ulceration. In addition, genital HSV-2 infection is a major cofactor in HIV transmission and acquisition, especially in sub-Saharan Africa.
- › Most HSV infections are asymptomatic; however, viral shedding often occurs in the absence of symptoms and this is the most important factor in transmission.
- › Individuals with clinical infection often have recurrences. However, these are usually less severe than the first episode.
- › HSV infection may be transmitted from mother to baby at the time of delivery and the risk of transmission is highest when the mother acquires HSV infection for the first time close to delivery. Neonatal herpes is often severe and life-threatening.
- › Antiviral therapy with nucleoside analogs is very effective for the treatment of genital herpes.
- › Condoms offer some protection in reducing transmission and vaccines may offer benefit in the future.

A. Mindel
Sexually Transmitted Infections Research Centre (STIRC), University of Sydney, Westmead Hospital, Marian Villa, 170 Hawkesbury Road, Westmead, NSW 2145, Australia
e-mail: adrian.mindel@sydney.edu.au

21.1 Introduction

Genital herpes is a common sexually transmitted infection throughout the world. It is caused by either of the two herpes simplex viruses (HSV), HSV type 1 (HSV-1) or HSV type 2 (HSV-2), and is the most common cause of genital ulceration. HSV-2 infection has increased in some populations over recent years and the morbidity associated with the infection and the observations of a complex interaction between HSV and HIV have highlighted its public health importance.

21.2 Virology

There are two herpes simplex viruses (HSV), designated type 1 (HSV-1) and 2 (HSV-2), and they belong to the alpha-herpes virus subfamily [1]. The alpha-herpes viruses are rapidly replicating neurotropic viruses [2]. HSV-1 and HSV-2 have a diameter of 150 nm and have a similar structure, consisting of four components. The inner core contains the double-stranded, circular DNA genome; surrounding this is an icosahedral capsid consisting of 162 capsomers and seven proteins. The amorphous tegument surrounds the capsid, and this in turn is surrounded by the lipid membrane containing embedded glycoproteins [3]. The DNA genome codes more than 85 genes, some of which are essential for viral growth, others for viral replication and for encoding proteins that modify or prevent a variety of host immune responses, thus allowing for infection to occur.

Some of the surface glycoproteins (B, C, D, H, and L) are responsible for binding to cellular receptors, thus

G. Gross and S.K. Tyring (eds.), *Sexually Transmitted Infections and Sexually Transmitted Diseases*,
DOI: 10.1007/978-3-642-14663-3_21, © Springer-Verlag Berlin Heidelberg 2011

mediating viral entry into the cell, and others (C, E, and I) modulate host immune functions, including binding to the Fc portion of immunoglobulin and fixing complement.

HSV-1 and HSV-2 have sufficient differences in their DNA to differentiate them as separate species. However, most of the proteins and antigens are similar. A more detailed account of virology may be found in Chapter 20.

21.3 Latency and Reactivation

The virus gains access to the skin or mucous membranes following exposure to an infected individual, probably via microabrasions. After initial epidermal infection, the virus crosses into sensory nerve endings and is rapidly transported to the sacral nerve ganglia. Productive infection then occurs in some neurons, whereas other neurons restrict replication, resulting in the virus becoming latent and expressing only a small proportion of its genome called *latency-associated transcripts*. No viral proteins are expressed, so the neuron is not subject to the normal immune mechanisms. This is mainly because the infected neuron does not express major histocompatibility complex (MHC) class-I antigens.

Reactivation occurs extremely frequently. However, the mechanisms underlying latency and reactivation are still obscure. Following reactivation, the virus is actively transported via the microtubules to the nerve endings and crosses into the epidermis of the genital tract or adjacent skin, where it replicates. Virus replication may result in obvious lesions. However, more commonly, it will only cause small, often inapparent, lesions or viral replication in the absence of lesions.

A more detailed account of latency may be found in Chapter 20.

21.4 Epidemiology

The availability of type-specific HSV serology has facilitated our understanding of the epidemiology of HSV infections, by accurately differentiating between the two viruses and allowing detection of HSV-2 in the presence of HSV-1 and vice versa. A detailed description of these tests can be found below.

21.4.1 Seroprevalence and Seroincidence

A large number of seroepidemiological studies from around the world have shown that the majority of people infected with these viruses do not have any symptoms that can be attributable to herpes [4–11] (Table 21.1). In addition, the seroprevalence of HSV-1 and HSV-2 infections shows considerable geographic variation. Most of the seroepidemiological studies have been conducted in selected "high-risk populations" such as sexually transmitted infection (STI) clinic attendees, female commercial sex workers, and HIV positive individuals; or in convenience samples, such as women attending antenatal clinics or individuals attending other hospital departments, and only a handful of studies have looked at representative population-based samples. Despite these reservations, we now have a very extensive overview of HSV seroepidemiology worldwide.

Antibodies to HSV-2 are associated with a number of demographic, social, and sexual factors, including age, gender, ethnic origin, level of education, socioeconomic status, age at first sexual encounter, and lifetime number of sexual partners. Two of the most important demographic factors determining HSV-2 seropositivity are age and gender. Despite the fact that there are far fewer studies in men than in women, a consistent finding throughout the world is that HSV-2 infection is more common in women [5–7, 11, 12]. In some areas, including Australia, prevalence rates in women are twice those seen in men (16% versus 8%) [7], and in one study from South Africa, HSV-2 antibody rates in 24-year-olds were 80% in men and 40% in women [12].

Age is a very strong determinant of HSV-2 seropositivity. Antibodies are rarely detected before puberty [10]. In most populations, HSV-2 prevalence increases with increasing age [8–10]. In common with many STIs, women usually acquire HSV-2 at a younger age than men [10]. In many communities, HSV-2 is more common in individuals from lower socioeconomic backgrounds [8, 14–21]. However, the socioeconomic associations are complex and reflect the patterns of social mixing within different communities [13]. In some communities there are ethnic differences in HSV-2 seroprevalence. Such differences have been noted in the USA, where HSV-2 prevalence was higher in African-Americans than in White Americans [11],

Table 21.1 HSV seroprevalence in different communities

Population	HSV-2 Seroprevalence	HSV-1 Seroprevalence	References
Population based surveys			
USA population based 1976–1980	Men 13.4% Women 18.4%	Not reported	[8]
USA population based 1988–1994	Men 17% Women 25.2%	Men 59% Women 65%	[8, 11]
USA population based 1999–2004	Men 11.2% Women 22.8%	Men 55.9% Women 59.5%	[11]
Australia population based 1999–2000	Men 8.4% Women 15.6%	Men 71.3% Women 80.4%	[7]
Europe – using serum banks	Age standardized rates	Age standardized rates	[216, 217]
	Bulgaria 24%	Finland 52%	
	Germany 14%	Netherlands 57%	
	Finland 13%	Belgium 67%	
	Belgium 11%	Czech Republic 81%	
	Netherlands 9%	Bulgaria 84%	
	Czech Republic 6%	England and Wales	
	England and Wales 4.2%	46% in men and 49% in women	
High-risk populations			
Female commercial sex workers	74–98%	78–100%	[10, 27–35, 218, 219]
Men who have sex with men	24–87% Higher rates in those who are HIV co-infected	51–73%	[23, 26, 38, 220]
HIV infected	30–90%	73–84%	[26, 30, 34, 35, 220–224]
STI clinic attendees	13–75%	56–92%	[6, 24, 26, 30, 36, 37, 222, 225–228]
Low-risk populations			
Women attending antenatal clinics	0–54%	57–100%	[5, 25, 37, 229–242]
Adolescents	1–11%	40–72%	[218, 233, 243, 244]
Blood donors	5–26%	68–95%	[5, 6, 30]

and in Australia, where rates in Aboriginal Australians were 18% compared with 12% in the non-Aboriginal counterparts [7].

Numerous studies have shown that HSV-2 prevalence is directly related to the lifetime number of sexual partners, and individuals with previous or concurrent STIs and early age at first sex are also more likely to be HSV-2-positive [6, 22–26].

In high-risk populations, particularly in female sex workers, HSV-2 prevalence is extremely high, ranging from 74% to 98% [10, 27–35]. It is also high in STI clinic attendees (13–75%) [6, 24, 26, 36, 37] and in men who have sex with men (MSM) (24–87%), particularly in those who are HIV coinfected [6, 23, 26, 38].

21.4.2 Prevalence and Incidence of Clinical Disease

Many patients, who are infected with HSV-1 or HSV-2 at the genital site, never develop any symptoms. Some may have mild symptoms that are not recognized as genital herpes by the patients or their health-care providers. In addition, in many resource-poor settings, laboratory diagnosis is limited or unavailable. These factors will influence the reported incidence and prevalence of clinically apparent genital herpes in different communities. Despite these caveats, studies of patients who present with genital ulceration suggest that the majority of these ulcers worldwide are due to HSV infection. Over the recent years, a number of studies have been conducted around the world using molecular techniques to diagnose genital ulcers. In North America, Europe, Asia, and some parts of Africa, HSV accounts for between 13–84% of genital ulcers [39–48]. In some parts of Africa and in India, chancroid remains a leading cause of genital ulceration [43, 46–48]. However, in studies in a mining community in Carletonville, South Africa, where genital ulceration remains a major problem, the proportion of genital ulcers due to chancroid decreased from 69% to 51% between the years 1993/1994 and 1998, whereas the proportion due to HSV increased from 17% to 35% [43]; similar changes have been documented from Botswana and Uganda [49, 50].

In the UK, the number of cases of genital herpes diagnosed at genitourinary medicine (GUM) clinics between 1971 and 2006 increased fivefold in males and 22-fold in females. In 2006, over 21,000 cases were diagnosed, with the highest rates seen in the 20–24-year-old age group [51]. In the USA, the number of first-episode genital herpes diagnoses made by physicians increased from 16,986 in 1970 to over 370,000 in 2006, an increase of 15-fold [52, 53].

Over the recent years, a number of studies have shown that the proportion of cases of genital herpes due to HSV-1 has increased in the USA, Europe, Israel, and Australia, particularly in women under the age of 25, and in some populations, HSV-1 has become more common as a cause of genital herpes than HSV-2 [4, 54–62]. These studies do not have linked behavioral data, and consequently, one can only postulate the possible reasons for this change, which may include lower rates of prepubertal HSV-1 as a consequence of improved standards of living in most of the developed world, earlier age of first sexual intercourse, and changes in sexual behavior, in particular, the growing popularity of orogenital sex [55].

21.4.3 Transmission and Viral Shedding

Transmission occurs by close personal contact with an infected individual. Such contact, in the case of HSV-2, is usually genital-to-genital or mouth-to-genital, in the case of HSV-1. Transmission can occur during periods of symptomatic or, more commonly, asymptomatic shedding of the virus. Consequently, some individuals may become "silently" infected and then transmit the virus to their current or future sexual partner months or even years after infection. The overall transmission rate for HSV-2 infection to a seronegative partner is estimated to be 3–12% per year with higher rates noted in men [63–66]. Infected individuals are at an increased risk of transmission during the first year of the infection, when rates of asymptomatic viral shedding are at their highest. However, asymptomatic viral shedding can occur at any time and at a population level, the majority of infections are acquired as a consequence of asymptomatic viral shedding.

As mentioned above, viral shedding occurs from lesions from inapparent micro-abrasions, and from apparently intact skin and mucous membranes. While vesicles and ulcers are highly infectious, many infected individuals avoid sexual contact when they are present, first because they are often painful and second because they are aware of their infectivity and are anxious to avoid transmitting the infection to a sexual partner. Consequently, most transmission occurs when lesions are not present or from individuals who are unaware that they have the infection [67–69]. Studies in men and women, using polymerase chain reaction (PCR) and frequent self-swabbing, have shown that asymptomatic viral shedding is extremely common, occurring in up to 30% of days. Shedding lasts more than 1 day in 25% of cases, occurs in clusters, from multiple anatomical sites (in women from the cervix, vagina, vulva, and perianal area and in males from the penile skin, scrotal skin, and perianal area, and from the oral cavity in both sexes), often close to the time of clinical recurrences and intermittently in >90% of individuals who are asymptomatic but have detectable HSV-2 antibodies [70–73]. In addition, periods of shedding vary from just a few hours to several days and at times switching "on and off" very frequently. Quantitative PCR has shown that the number of viral copies in subclinical lesions is just as high as in clinical episodes, underpinning the observation that most transmissions occur as a result of asymptomatic viral shedding.

21.4.4 HSV and HIV Co-infection

Since the beginning of the HIV epidemic, numerous longitudinal studies have revealed that ulcerative STIs are associated with increased risk of HIV acquisition and transmission. Meta-analyses of these studies have suggested that ulcerative STIs increase the susceptibility to HIV by fourfold in males and threefold in women [74, 75].

Ulcerative STIs lead to disruption of the mucosal or skin surface – the portal of entry for HIV– and to an up-regulation of pro-inflammatory and immunoregulatory cytokines. In addition, ulcers may bleed, thus increasing the risk of HIV transmission. Finally, the treatment of genital ulcers results in a decrease in HIV detection.

In the "Explore Study" from the USA, among 4,295 high-risk, HIV-negative men, HIV risk was increased in those with recent incident (at the time of first visit) HSV-2, (HR = 3.6, 95% CI 1.7–7.8); in those with remote incident HSV-2 (within the previous 2 years of the first visit) (HR = 1.7, 95% CI 0.8–3.3); and, finally, in those with prevalent HSV-2 (adjusted HR = 1.5, 95% CI 1.1–2.1) [76].

A meta-analysis of transmission studies by Freeman et al. showed that relative risk (RR) of HIV acquisition in HSV-2-positive females in the general population was calculated at 3.1 (95% CI 1.7–5.6) and in high-risk females (commercial sex workers and bar workers), the risk was 1.0 (95% CI 0.53–2.0); in the general population of males, the RR was 2.7 (95% CI 1.9–3.9) and in men who had sex with men (MSM), the RR was 1.7 (95% CI 1.2–2.4) [77]. What this means is that in the general population, considering new HIV infections in women, 38–60% are attributable to HSV, and in men, 8–49% are attributable to HSV [76, 77].

There is also some epidemiological information that in MSM, HSV-1 may also be associated with an increased risk of HIV acquisition. In Sydney, Australia, 1,427 gay men were followed for 3 years: neither prevalent nor incident HSV-2 was associated with HIV; however, prevalent HSV-1 was associated with increased risk of HIV seroconversion in men under the age of 40 (HR = 8.21, 95% CI 1.11–60.93) [78]. With HSV-1 increasingly becoming the cause of anogenital herpes in MSM in some settings, it may be as important as HSV-2 in HIV acquisition [78, 79].

The biological plausibility of the link between HSV-2 infection and HIV transmission and the possible benefit of treatment for HSV-2 have been studied in MSM in Peru and in heterosexual women in Burkina Faso. Participants coinfected with HSV-2 and HIV and not receiving highly active antiretroviral therapy (HAART) were treated with valaciclovir 500 mg bd or placebo for between 8 and 12 weeks. In women and MSM, valaciclovir suppression resulted in a statistically significant reduction in HIV RNA levels in the cervix or rectum, as well as a decrease in plasma HIV RNA levels [80, 81]. Similar, though less consistent, findings have been noted from coinfected women in Burkina Faso, who were receiving HAART [82].

These observations suggested that treatment of HSV-2 infections may have a role in reducing HIV acquisition and transmission, and three large studies were conducted to evaluate these two hypotheses. The first was a study conducted in rural Tanzania. Eight hundred and twenty-one HIV-negative, HSV-2-positive women who were at high risk for the acquisition of HIV (commercial sex workers and bar workers) were randomized to receive acyclovir 400 mg bd or placebo for 30 months. The intention to treat analysis revealed no difference in HIV incidence between the two groups [83].

The second study was a large multinational, multicenter study to evaluate whether treatment of genital herpes in HIV-positive individuals would result in decreased sexual transmission to their noninfected partners. Over 3,000 (one partner HIV and HSV-2 coinfected, the other HIV-negative) were recruited. The coinfected individuals included 1,350 heterosexual women from South Africa, Zimbabwe, and Zambia; 1,355 MSM from Peru; and 459 MSM from the USA. The coinfected partners were randomized to receive either acyclovir 400 mg bd or matching placebo. Treatment continued for 18 months, and the primary endpoint was HIV infection in the uninfected partner. The final analysis revealed no difference in HIV acquisition in the two groups [84]. The final study was conducted in 14 African countries and included 3,408 serodiscordant couples (one partner HIV and HSV-2 coinfected, the other HIV-negative). As in the previous study, the coinfected partners were randomized to receive either acyclovir 400 mg bd or matching placebo, and the primary endpoint was HIV infection in the uninfected partner. The only difference was that treatment continued for 24 months. The final analysis revealed no difference in HIV acquisition in the two groups [85].

Several possible explanations have been put forward to explain these results. The first is that HSV-2 is not a risk factor for HIV acquisition or transmission; however, this seems unlikely due to the strength of the epidemiological evidence. The second suggestion is that HSV in Africa responds less well to acyclovir. However, this too seems unlikely as about half the participants in the transmission study were gay men from the USA and Peru. The third explanation is that these studies used either the wrong dose of acyclovir or, indeed, the wrong drug. Acyclovir has poor absorption and limited bioavailability, and the optimum dose for suppression is 200 mg four times daily [86]. However, this is not a convenient dose and the researchers chose a twice-daily dose. With compliance between 80% and 85% for these two studies, participants receiving acyclovir would have had long periods each day with no detectable acyclovir present in their systems. The prodrugs, namely valaciclovir and famciclovir, have far better absorption and bioavailability, but are more expensive and the researchers chose the cheaper option. Finally, it is possible that reactivation occurs far more frequently than previously believed and this, coupled with the poor bioavailability and suboptimal dose, may offer the best explanation.

21.4.5 Maternal HSV-2 and Perinatal HIV-1 Transmission

Perinatal transmission of HIV is a major public health problem, particularly in women in sub-Saharan Africa, and is associated with low CD4 counts and high viral loads. Two case-control studies looking at the association between HSV-2 and perinatal HIV-1 transmission have recently been published. The first was a relatively small study from the USA involving 26 HIV-positive women and 52 controls and this study showed no association between the HSV-2 prevalence and HIV transmission [87]. However, a much larger study from Zimbabwe involving 509 cases and 1,018 controls showed that 28.4% (95% confidence intervals 7.3–44.7%) of perinatal HIV-1 transmissions were potentially attributable to HSV-2 [88]. In both studies HSV-2 prevalence was extremely high in patients and controls (over 80%) and the reason for the different findings between these two studies may have been due to lack of power in the first study due to the small sample size. Further studies are underway to determine whether antiviral treatment of HSV-2 in late pregnancy will reduce HIV-1 transmission.

21.5 Clinical Features

21.5.1 First Episode Genital Herpes

Although the majority of people who are infected at the genital site with HSV-1 or HSV-2 are asymptomatic, when symptoms do occur, they can be severe and prolonged. The signs, symptoms, and duration of infection are indistinguishable when infections due to HSV-1 and HSV-2 are compared. In those patients who develop genital disease, the incubation period is 2–7 days. The severity of initial genital herpes depends upon whether there is prior cross-reactive immunity following infection with HSV-1, usually following orolabial herpes in infancy or childhood. In nonimmune individuals, systemic symptoms and signs are much more severe [89]. These symptoms include fever, malaise, myalgia, and headache and can last from 2 to 10 days.

In women, the genital symptoms include genital pain, dysuria, and a vaginal discharge, and on examination, lesions may be noticed on the vulva, suprapubic area, perineum, perianal area, buttocks, thighs, vagina, cervix, and the canal, depending upon the type of sexual activity that the person has had (Figs. 21.1 and 21.2). In males, lesions can occur anywhere on the penis, including the urinary meatus, scrotum, suprapubic area, perineum, perianal area, buttocks, thighs, and anal canal (Figs. 21.3 and 21.4). Lesions usually commence as erythema, and then painful vesicles or blisters occur. These then rupture to leave painful weeping ulcers, which eventually heal. On areas of dry skin, the healing occurs with scabs or crusts, but these do not occur on the mucous membranes. Lesions on the cervix, although not often visualized, may be atypical and the entire cervix may be erythematous or even appear to be necrotic [90]. Vesicles sometimes occur in crops over a period of 1–2 weeks and the entire episode can take anywhere between 2 and 4 weeks to heal. Lesions are mostly located at several anatomical sites and are often multiple and bilateral. During this time, the inguinal lymph nodes are usually enlarged and painful.

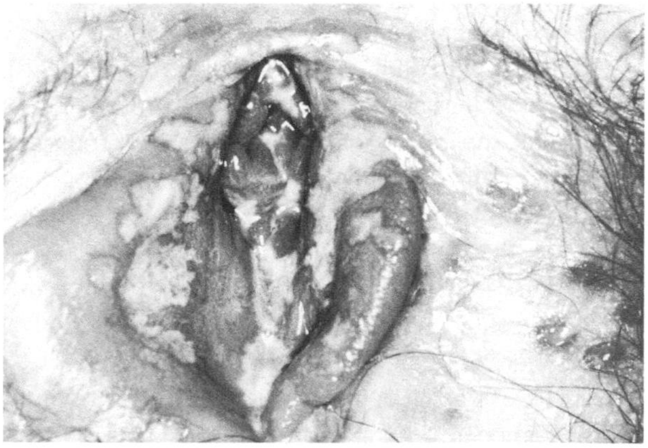

Fig. 21.1 Primary genital herpes, extensive vulval ulceration, and swelling

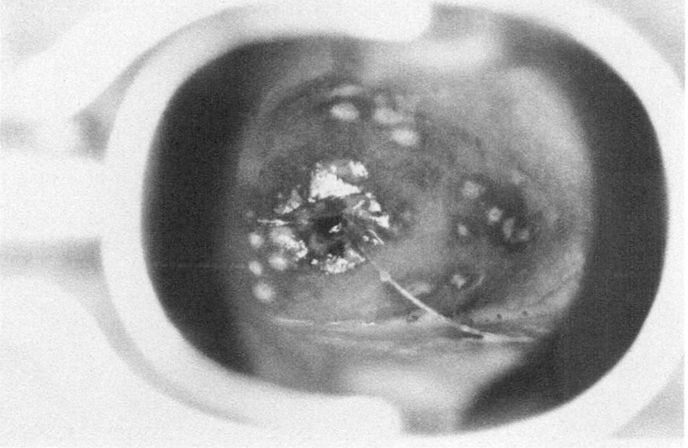

Fig. 21.2 Primary genital herpes, discrete ulcers on the ectocervix

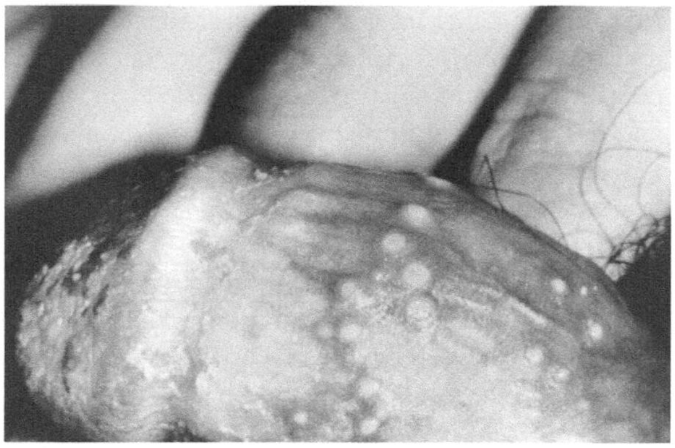

Fig. 21.3 Primary genital herpes, diffuse ulceration on the shaft of the penis

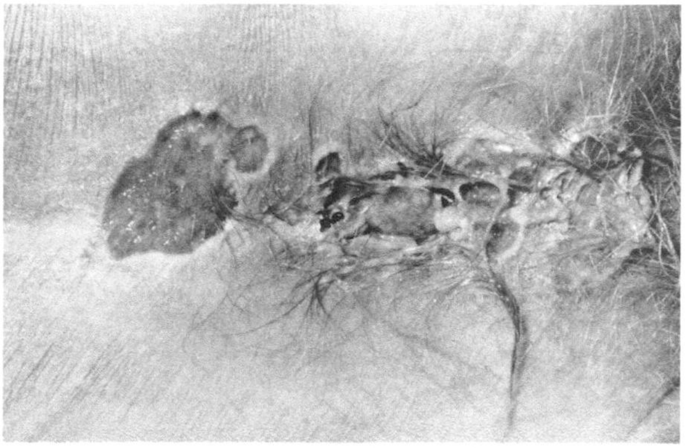

Fig. 21.4 Primary perianal herpes, extensive ulceration on the perianal skin

In males, urethritis may be the only manifestation of the infection, with men presenting with dysuria and a urethral discharge. The condition may be difficult to distinguish from other causes of urethritis, although the level of pain is sometimes more severe with genital herpes than with the other causes of urethritis.

In addition, tender inguinal lymphadenopathy may be noted. Patients with proctitis usually present with rectal pain, tenesmus, and rectal discharge [91]. In women and in patients with proctitis, prolonged local symptoms can occur. Symptoms are generally more severe in women than in men [89].

In patients who have had orogenital sex, pharyngeal infection is occasionally seen either in conjunction with genital herpes or, on occasion, when only orogenital contact has occurred, alone [92]. The condition appears similar to other infective causes of pharyngitis. Clinical signs can vary from mild erythema to very painful, ulcerative pharyngitis [93]. In severe infections systemic symptoms can occur and tender cervical lymphadenopathy is noted.

The most common complications of genital herpes are extragenital cutaneous lesions and aseptic meningitis (Mollaret's meningitis) presenting with neck stiffness, photophobia, and headache [94]. This condition runs a benign course with no long-term neurological sequelae, occurs in about 10% of patients, and is more common in women and in men who have had anal intercourse than in heterosexual men. Other complications include sacral radiculomyelitis [89], usually resulting in urinary retention (urinary retention is most often due to severe local pain rather than sacral radiculomyelitis) and, extremely rarely, a transverse myelitis [91, 95, 96], erythema multiforme [97], hepatitis [98, 99], pneumonitis [100], thrombocytopenia [101] and monoarticular arthritis [102].

Extragenital lesions, usually involving the buttocks, groin, or thighs or, less commonly, the fingers and eyes, occur in about 20% of patients [103–105] (Fig. 21.5). These lesions appear within 7–14 days, and are probably caused by direct inoculation at the time when the infection is first acquired.

Cutaneous dissemination from genital herpes may occur in patients with atopic eczema [106, 107]. Disseminated cutaneous and visceral infections occur rarely in severely immunocompromised [108, 109] or pregnant patients [110–112] and have a high mortality if not promptly treated.

21.5.2 Recurrent Genital Herpes

In recurrent disease, systemic symptoms are uncommon and the duration of episodes is shorter than the first episode, usually lasting for 4–7 days [89]. Many recurrences are preceded by prodromal or warning symptoms consisting of pain, burning, itching, paresthesia or sacral neuralgia in the genital area, thigh, buttocks, or legs [113]. These occur in up to 50% of recurrences and commence anywhere from 2 to 24 h before the lesions appear; they usually resolve once the lesions are apparent. For many patients, the prodromal symptoms can be the most troublesome aspect of infection [114, 115].

When the lesions eventually occur, they mostly consist of a single lesion or a small crop of lesions that occur particularly on the keratinized skin of the vulva, perianal area, thigh, buttock, or penis (Fig. 21.6). Internal lesions are uncommon. Tender inguinal lymphadenopathy may also occur. Recurrences may be more painful and prolonged in women than in men. Extra-genital cutaneous lesions can also recur, with or without genital lesions.

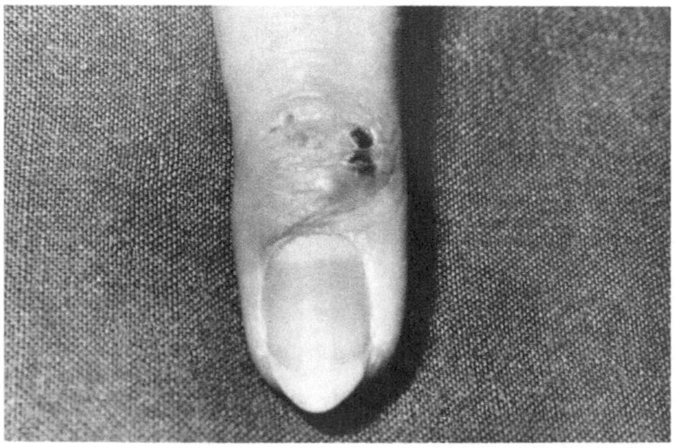

Fig. 21.5 Herpes infection on the finger

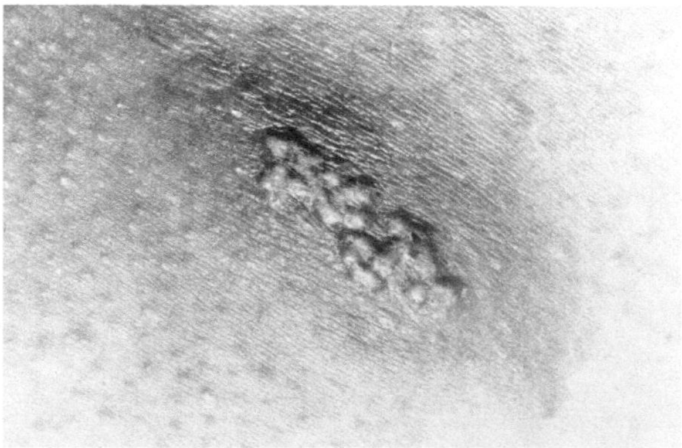

Fig. 21.6 Recurrent herpes, crop of vesicles on the buttocks

21.5.3 Atypical Clinical Features

Many recurrences are atypical, with erythema or small excoriations of the skin being the only visible manifestations of the infection. In women these are often misdiagnosed as genital dematoses, trauma, or thrush [116]. In an STI clinic setting, HSV can be isolated from up to 33% of "genital lesions." Consequently, in a high-risk setting such as STI clinics and among commercial sex workers, all genital lesions should routinely be swabbed for HSV detection.

21.5.4 HSV Infections HIV Coinfected Individuals

HSV infections are extremely common in individuals infected with HIV and may be the presenting symptom in some. In those who are profoundly immunosuppressed, chronic persistent ulcers are sometimes seen [117] (Fig. 21.7). Such lesions were common in the pre-HAART era, but are now seldom seen.

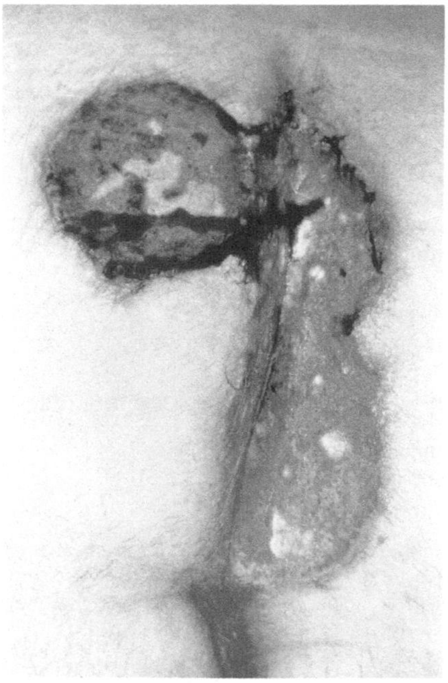

Fig. 21.7 Extensive chronic perianal ulceration in a profoundly immunosuppressed HIV-positive patient

Some coinfected individuals will have more frequent recurrences of their genital herpes [118]; however, most will respond to treatment with antiviral therapy [119–121] although resistance is occasionally seen in those with very low CD4 lymphocyte counts.

21.6 HSV Infections and Pregnancy

Neonatal herpes is a devastating infection with high mortality and considerable morbidity, and despite its rarity, the risk of transmission of HSV from mother to baby is a major cause of concern for many women with genital herpes.

The prevalence of neonatal herpes varies widely around the world. However, few countries collect accurate data. The highest reported incidence (2–50/100,000 live births) is from parts of the USA [122]; in Canada, it is 6/100,000 [123]; in Australia, 4/100,000 [124], and in the UK, 2/100,000 [125]. In the UK, national surveillance suggests that the incidence of neonatal herpes has increased over the past 20 years, but the infections still remains extremely rare [126]. There are no data available from the developing world, although anecdotal reports suggest that neonatal herpes is rare.

The neonate is at greatest risk (~50%) if the mother acquires the infection for the first time during pregnancy. However, many women (60–80%) who acquire genital herpes do not have any symptoms of the infection. With recurrent infection, the risk is much smaller (<1%) [127].

This has raised the question of whether there are ways of preventing neonatal transmission. One suggestion has been the use of antiviral suppression during the final weeks of pregnancy in women who have established recurrent genital herpes, or those who are HSV-2 antibody positive. This approach has been evaluated in a number of randomized controlled trials and has shown that the treatment is safe, that the number of recurrences was reduced, and that fewer Caesarean sections were performed to prevent HSV transmission [128–135]. However, none of these studies looked at the rates of neonatal herpes. Consequently, while this approach may be useful for individual patients, its usefulness as a public health initiative to prevent neonatal herpes remains unproven. Those women who prefer not to use antiviral suppression should be advised to present early at the onset of labor. If lesions are present, abdominal delivery should be recommended, but if not, a normal vaginal is appropriate [127, 136].

The second approach is to use type-specific serology as a method of establishing who is at risk of transmitting the infection to the neonate. This approach will allow identification of women who are seronegative, and if their sexual partner(s) are seropositive, they can be counseled about the risk and advised to avoid sexual contact, or to use condoms and/or antiviral suppression to reduce this risk. However, the efficacy of this approach is unproven.

21.7 Diagnosis

Genital herpes can often be diagnosed on the basis of the clinical features, particularly during the first episode. These include the presence of vesicles and/or painful ulcers which may be present at several anatomical sites and tender inguinal lymphadenopathy. Matted lymph nodes and rubbery, non-tender lymph nodes should always raise the suspicion of a non-herpes diagnosis. However, when ulceration is present in the absence of vesiculation, several other conditions need to be considered (see Table 21.2). This is particularly true in HIV-infected individuals. Also, simultaneous infections with two or more STIs also occur from time to time [137]. Consequently, basing the diagnosis on clinical features alone has very poor sensitivity and specificity. All genital ulcers, irrespective of their appearance, should be swabbed for HSV.

Herpes is a lifelong infection, with the potential for recurrences over many years, implications for current and future sexual partners and future pregnancies, and possible psychosexual implications. Consequently, where the test is available and resources exist, microbiological confirmation of the diagnosis is imperative.

21.7.1 Lesion Derived Specimens

Herpes simplex viruses can be identified from lesion-derived specimens using a variety of techniques. These include cell culture and polymerase chain

Table 21.2 Infective causes of genital ulceration

Condition and Causative Organism	Clinical Features	Laboratory Diagnosis
Genital herpes Herpes simplex type 1 (HSV-1) or type 2 (HSV-2)	Multiple, superficial, painful ulcers preceded by vesicles, with tender inguinal lymphadenopathy	Culture or PCR
Primary syphilis *Treponema pallidum*	Painless indurated ulcer – usually single, painless with painless, unilateral inguinal lymphadenopathy	Dark ground microscopy Serology
Chancroid *Haemophilus ducreyi*	Painful rapidly destructive ulcers, history of sexual contact with someone from an endemic area	PCR
Lymphogranuloma venereum *Chlamydia trachomatis serotypes L1–L3*	Ulcers are usually transient Inflammation and swelling of the inguinal lymph nodes (the bubo) occurs weeks or months after the ulcer	Culture or PCR Serology
Donovanosis *Klebsiella granulomatis*[a]	Exuberant fleshy painless ulcers that bleed easily and smell foul. Lesions are slowly destructive	Tissue smear stained with Giemsa PCR
Candidiasis (thrush) *Candida albicans*	Superficial erythema or excoriations especially in women	Gram stain Culture

[a]There is dispute about classification with some authorities still using the older name *Calymmatobacterium granulomatis*

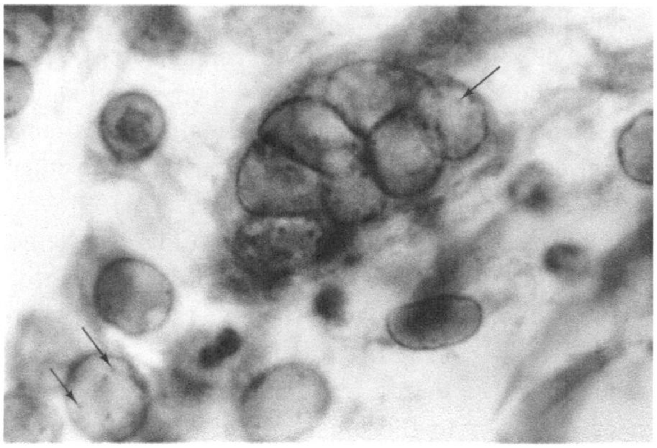

Fig. 21.8 HSV cytology (Tzanck test). Multinucleated giant cells with numerous intracellular inclusions

reaction (PCR), direct microscopy (Tzanck test), and antigen detection using immunofluorescence or ELISA [138, 139], with the majority of laboratories now relying on culture and PCR. The Tzanck test has the advantage of quick results. Direct swabs obtained from lesions are stained with Giemsa or Wrights stain and multinucleated giant cells visible on microscopy (Fig. 21.8). However, this test has a very low sensitivity [140].

HSV can be cultured in a variety of cell lines although human diploid fibroblasts such as the MRC-5 cell lines are usually selected [141]. The virus produces a typical cytopathic effect, evident as early as 12 h or as late as 7 days after inoculation [142].

PCR is more sensitive than culture and is now the method of choice for HSV detection in many laboratories [139, 143, 144]. A number of commercial PCR test kits are now available. PCR has the added advantage of speed and no requirement for viral transport media. Modifications such as real-time, nested, and multiplex PCR have the advantage of improved turnaround time, enhanced sensitivity, and the possible detection of other STIs [145] (see Chapter 56).

As viral titres are highest during the early phases of the infection, this is the ideal time to take a swab for culture or PCR. However, with improved sensitivity of PCR, microbiological confirmation is possible for longer during each episode. Suitable specimens for culture or PCR include vesicle fluid, material from the base of ulcers, and material from the base of scabs. Vesicle fluid is highly infectious and extreme caution should be taken when swabbing vesicles as fluid may spray into eyes or mucous membranes. A simple method of reducing the risk is to de-roof the vesicle using a sterile needle pointing away from the operator and held parallel to the skin surface.

For viral culture, specimens need to be transported to the laboratory in a timely fashion, using viral transport medium. However, for PCR, as HSV DNA is stable, transport time and storage conditions are less critical.

21.7.2 Serology

Non-type-specific HSV serology has limited usefulness in diagnosing HSV infection and has largely been replaced by the newer type-specific assays. Glycoprotein G from the viral envelope HSV-1 (glycoprotein G1) or HSV-2 (glycoprotein G2) has been used as an antigen in solid phase enzyme immunoassays [146]. Only glycoprotein G is sufficiently different to use as an antigen for type specific serology. Glycoprotein G2 is approximately 600 amino acids long, whereas glycoprotein G1 is 150 amino acids long and lacks the large central immunodominant region of glycoprotein G2. A number of these assays are now commercially available, however, the sensitivity and specificity of these assays shown considerable variation [147, 148]. Overall the specificity of the type-specific ELISA tests is high for HSV-2 but lower for HSV-1. Additional limitations of serology include the observation that antibodies may not develop for 6–8 weeks after exposure and that about 5% of exposed individuals never develop antibodies. The Western blot assay can also be used to test for type-specific antibodies, by detecting many individual HSV proteins, including glycoprotein G2 [149]. It can be useful to diagnose HSV-2 infection in those patients with prior HSV-1 infection and can also be used as a supplementary test to ELISA, enhancing the specificity of the HSV-2 antibody testing [150].

As mentioned above, type-specific serology has been widely used in epidemiological studies. However, there is still considerable debate about the clinical utility of type-specific serology. The test can be helpful when the clinical history is suggestive of herpes, but culture or PCR are repeatedly negative. In addition, the test can also be used in couples where one partner is infected and the other apparently not. However, in these circumstances the test should be done with caution and informed consent obtained, as many individuals who do not believe they have herpes may turn out to be positive, and determining where the infection came from and who may have given it to whom is impossible.

Whether serology should be widely used, particularly in high-risk populations, such as STI clinics, to diagnose asymptomatic infection, has been widely debated [151–153], with advocates suggesting that testing will enable health-care providers to counsel patients about risk-reduction strategies, and opponents suggesting that testing may result in undue anxiety and that evidence for benefit at a personal or public health level is lacking. To date, there is no consensus.

21.8 Psychological, Psychosexual, and Quality of Life Implication of Genital Herpes

Sexually transmitted infections (STIs) often cause psychological and psychosexual morbidity and anecdotal reports suggest that the psychosexual morbidity associated with genital herpes may be more profound and long-lasting than that associated with other STIs and that some of this morbidity may be responsible for "triggering" recurrences. There are difficulties in evaluating the scientific validity of these observations. First is the large number of psychological questionnaires that have been used, creating difficulties in the comparison of studies [154]. A second problem is that many of the studies have included mostly patients who have self-identified as having psychosexual problems and these patients may represent a minority view of herpes sufferers.

Nonetheless, patients with genital herpes have more psychosexual problems and have more concerns about their health and well-being than patients with other STIs [155]. The range of emotional responses that have been described relative to herpes include depression, anguish, distress, anger, diminution of self-esteem, and hostility to the one believed to be the source of infection [156–159]. However, the validity of these observations is difficult to ascertain, as mentioned above, as we cannot determine whether they would have had these psychological difficulties or coping problems prior to their herpes diagnosis, or whether, in fact, these difficulties would arise in the presence of any other illnesses [154]. A number of factors have been described as being important in terms of exacerbating the psychological morbidity associated with genital herpes. These include the site of the lesions and their sexual nature, the recurrent nature of the infection, social stigma, emotive and often inaccurate popular press coverage, and the perceived lack of adequate therapy [159].

One of the more intriguing questions is whether "stress" can precipitate recurrence. Most of the information comes from retrospective studies, where patients were asked after the development of a recurrence, whether there were any stressful events that occurred prior to the episode and not surprisingly, patients in these studies were often able to identity a stressful event [156–158, 160]. However, the results from prospective studies have been less consistent, suggesting that stress and recurrences may occur concurrently [161] and in some circumstances" persistent stress" particularly anxiety, may lead to a recurrence over the following week [162]. However, when patients with recurrent genital herpes are treated with suppressive antiviral treatment, measurable psychosexual morbidity is decreased suggesting that in some individuals it is the actual recurrences that cause stress rather than the other way round [163].

As mentioned above, a number of psychological measures have been used to evaluate the burden of disease from the patients' perspective. However, recently, quality of life measures have also been employed, including the SF-36 and a specific recurrent genital herpes quality of life questionnaire (RGHQoL). The SF-36 is a 36-question, multipurpose, short-form health survey, revealing a profile of functional health and well-being, as well as a psychometrically based physical and mental health summary [164]. The RGHQoL has been extensively evaluated in patients with recurrent genital herpes [165–168].

Studies, using the SF-36, on patients with established recurrent genital herpes and recruited from STD or dermatology clinics in Denmark, the Netherlands, the UK, Italy, and Australia showed that patients with genital herpes had scores for bodily pain, general health, vitality, social functioning, role emotion, and mental health that were all statistically lower when compared with documented population norms [167]. The frequency of pain, severity of recurrences, and previous suppressive antiviral therapy had no impact on scores. In contrast the RGHQoL score was significantly lower in patients experiencing more frequent and severe recurrence [167].

Both suppressive and episodic antiviral therapy of patients with recurrent genital herpes results in a sustained improvement in RGHQoL scores [169, 170].

21.8.1 Management of Psychosexual Problems

The backbone of management of psychosexual morbidity is the provision of accurate, up-to-date information to the patient about the clinical features, long-term implications, risks of transmission, and possible drug treatments. Some patients may require specialist counseling, and many will benefit from antiviral therapy.

21.9 Treatment

The treatment of herpes simplex virus infections is complicated by the fact that at present none of the available therapies will eliminate latent infection. The objectives of treatment depend on whether the patient is presenting with a first episode of genital herpes or whether they have recurrent infection. With the first episode, the objectives are to reduce the duration and severity of symptoms, to hasten healing, to prevent new lesion formation, and to prevent or reduce the likelihood of the development of complications, including viral meningitis and other neurological complications, and urinary retention.

With recurrent infections, the objectives of therapy are to reduce the duration and severity of symptoms, including the prodromal symptoms, the duration of lesions, and the likelihood of further recurrences.

21.9.1 Antiviral Drugs

The nucleoside analogues have been the backbone of therapy for genital herpes for 25 years. Acyclovir, a guanosine analogue, was the first of these drugs to be assessed. Acyclovir selectively inhibits HSV-1, HSV-2, and varicella zoster virus replication. The drug is activated by an enzyme called *thymidine kinase* that converts acyclovir to acyclovir monophosphate. Cellular enzymes then convert the monophosphate into acyclovir diphosphate and ultimately acyclovir triphosphate, which competes with guanosine triphosphate as a substrate, thereby inhibiting DNA polymerase. Acyclovir has poor oral bioavailability with only 10–20% of the drug being absorbed [171].

Valaciclovir is the prodrug of acyclovir and is converted into acyclovir by intestinal and liver enzymes [172], resulting in improved bioavailability of acyclovir [173] and levels of acyclovir equivalent to those achieved by intravenous dosing.

Famciclovir is converted in the bowel wall and liver to its active agent penciclovir and has a high bioavailability. Penciclovir, like acyclovir, requires triphosphorylation, the initial phosphorylation being dependant on viral thymidine kinase. Penciclovir triphosphate has an extremely long intracellular half-life of about 10 h compared with the 1 h for acyclovir triphosphate.

21.9.2 Treatment of First Episode Genital Herpes

All patients who present with a first episode of genital herpes, within 5 days of onset, or where vesicles or extensive ulceration are still present, should be treated with antiviral therapy (Table 21.3). In addition, if there are signs of meningitis, urinary problems, or sacral radiculomyelitis, antiviral therapy should also be given.

All three nucleoside analogues (acyclovir, valaciclovir, and famciclovir) have been evaluated in placebo-controlled, randomized controlled trials (RCTs) in patients with first episode genital herpes, including herpes proctitis. Topical, oral, and intravenous acyclovir are significantly better than placebo with regard to healing time, duration of viral shedding, and duration of symptoms, with systemic therapy being superior to topical [174–182]. Treatment with acyclovir has no measurable effect on the frequency or severity of subsequent recurrences [178, 183].

A RCT showed that valaciclovir 1,000 mg twice daily was equivalent to acyclovir 200 mg five times daily for the treatment of first episode genital herpes and both drugs were well tolerated [184]. A similar RCT that compared famciclovir with acyclovir also showed that the two drugs were comparable in relation to duration of symptoms, lesion healing times, and the duration of viral shedding [185].

Table 21.3 Treatment of first episode genital herpes

Drug	Dose and Route	Duration	Comments	References
Acyclovir	Intravenous 5–10 mg/kg three times a day	5 days, however it is often possible to switch to oral therapy after 1 or 2 days	Usually reserved for very severe infections	[175, 179]
Acyclovir	Oral 200 mg five times daily	5–10 days	Poor bioavailability and hence frequent dosing are inconvenient. However, lower cost is an advantage	[174, 178, 180, 181]
Valaciclovir	Oral 500 mg twice daily	5–10 days	Advantages include good bioavailability allowing for less frequent dosing	[184]
Famciclovir	Oral 250 mg three times daily	5–10 days	Advantages include good bioavailability allowing for less frequent dosing	[185]

Adverse events with all three drugs are rare and, in the placebo-controlled trials, occurred with similar frequency in the placebo and treated groups. The most commonly reported side effects are nausea and headache. All three drugs can be used for the treatment of first episode genital herpes and the recommended doses are shown in Table 21.3. In order to slow or stop progression and reduce the likelihood of the development of complications, treatment should be started as soon as the patient presents, irrespective of the severity of the episode and before viral confirmation is available. The use of suppressive antiviral therapy (see below) soon after diagnosis of an initial infection with HSV-2 has also been evaluated. Such treatment shows a reduction in the frequency of recurrences and viral shedding, and given the fact that viral shedding and clinical recurrences are more common at this time, such an approach may be considered in some patients [166, 186]. In addition to antiviral therapy, many patients will require analgesia and at times the pain will be so severe that narcotic analgesics may be required. Advice about keeping the lesions clean and dry is also helpful. Women with urinary difficulties may find that urination while in a bath of warm water is of assistance, and some women will need to be advised to try and separate the labia at the time of urination to stop the urine touching the lesions. On occasion, catheterization may be required. However, extreme caution should be exercised if there are lesions in or around the urethra, and in these circumstances, a suprapubic catheter is the preferred option.

Finally, it is always prudent to offer to screen all patients who present with a first episode of genital herpes for other sexually transmitted infections.

21.9.3 Treatment of Recurrent Genital Herpes

The antiviral treatment of recurrent genital herpes has adopted two different approaches. The first is to treat each episode when it occurs, sometimes called episodic treatment, and the second is to use daily treatment to prevent clinical recurrences, called suppressive therapy; both forms of treatment have been extensively evaluated in numerous RCTs with all three nucleoside analogues.

21.9.3.1 Episodic (Intermittent) Treatment

Episodic treatment, usually with 5 days of medication, reduces the duration of symptoms and viral shedding and hastens the time to healing, with oral therapy superior to topical and no apparent difference in efficacy between the three agents [176, 177, 180, 187–192] (Table 21.4). However, with less frequent daily dosing, patients usually prefer famciclovir and valaciclovir, and patient-initiated therapy means that treatment can be

Table 21.4 Traditional episodic (intermittent) treatment of recurrent genital herpes

Drug	Dose and Route	Duration	Comments	References
Acyclovir	Oral 200 mg five times daily	5–10 days	Poor bioavailability and hence frequent dosing are inconvenient. However, lower cost is an advantage	[180, 187, 189, 191]
Valaciclovir	Oral 500 mg twice daily	5–10 days	Advantages include good bioavailability allowing for less frequent dosing	[187, 192, 193]
Famciclovir	Oral 250 mg three times daily	5–10 days	Advantages include good bioavailability allowing for less frequent dosing	[190]

Table 21.5 Short-course episodic treatment of recurrent genital herpes

Drug	Dose and Route	Duration	Comments	References
Acyclovir	Oral 800 mg three times daily	2 days		[198]
Valaciclovir	Oral 500 mg twice daily	3 days	Early treatment may result in aborted lesions	[194, 197]
Famciclovir	Oral		Early treatment may result in aborted lesions	[194–196]
	1,000 mg twice daily or	1 day		
	500 mg statim, then 250 mg twice daily	2 days		

initiated very early in the episode, resulting in a greater proportion of aborted episodes [187, 192, 193].

A number of studies have recently been conducted with short courses of treatment (1–3 days versus 5 days) [194–198]. These studies suggest that a short-course therapy is equivalent to the standard 5-day course and this is now the preferred option for many patients (Table 21.5).

21.9.3.2 Suppressive Treatment

Suppressive antiviral therapy is highly successful in the management of recurrent genital herpes (Table 21.6). All three drugs are effective and the vast majority of people who are compliant with treatment will have no recurrences during treatment. Recurrences that do occur are mostly minor and short-lived [199–205]. Several studies have considered the question of the optimal dose for suppressive therapy and have shown that the likelihood of complete suppression is highly dose-dependent. With acyclovir, a dose-ranging study showed that the optimum dose for suppression was 200 mg qds, with 400 mg bd, 200 mg tds and 200 mg bd being slightly less effective, but virtually equivalent, and once daily dosing with 800, 400, or 200 mg being the least effective [86]. A study with valaciclovir showed that, in terms of time to first recurrence, 1 g od was superior to 500 mg od which, in turn, was superior to 250 mg od. The 250 mg bd dose was equivalent to 1 g od. Interestingly, a subgroup analysis of this study revealed that valaciclovir 1 g od and 250 mg bd, as well as acyclovir 400 mg bd, were more effective in patients with ≥10 recurrences/year [206]. Suggested doses for suppressive therapy are shown in Table 21.6.

Observational studies have shown that the efficacy of therapy is maintained for as long as the individual remains on treatment, and that both short- and long-term therapy is well tolerated and not associated with any significant side-effects [207, 208].

Table 21.6 Suppressive treatment of recurrent genital herpes

Drug	Dose and Route	Duration	Comments	References
Acyclovir	Oral Many doses been studied. However for convenience the following doses are recommended 200 mg twice or three times daily 400 mg twice daily	1 year and then reconsider	Long-term safety for over 10 years has been demonstrated Less frequent doses are more likely to result in breakthrough recurrences	[86, 200, 202, 204, 207, 208]
Valaciclovir	Oral 500 mg once daily 500 mg twice daily 1,000 mg once daily	1 year and then reconsider	Patients with more frequent recurrences may benefit from twice daily therapy	[203, 205, 206]
Famciclovir	Oral 125 or 250 mg three times daily or 250 mg twice daily. However, 250 mg twice daily is the most commonly used dose	1 year and then reconsider	Studies have been for 52 weeks, but repeated courses of are often prescribed	[199, 205]

21.9.3.3 Choosing the Best Treatment (Fig. 21.9)

Episodic and suppressive therapy with valaciclovir has been compared in two studies. The first was a crossover study where 225 patients with recurrent genital herpes were randomized to receive either 24 weeks of intermittent therapy, followed by 24 weeks of suppressive therapy or vice versa. Overall, patients on suppression had significantly fewer recurrences than those on episodic treatment and satisfaction with treatment and quality of life were significantly greater in those receiving suppressive therapy [209]. In the second smaller study, 80 participants were randomized to receive either episodic or suppressive treatment for 1 year. Patients who received suppression had fewer recurrences and fewer days with pain, lesions, and other genital symptoms. Patients in both the treatment groups had a statistically significant improvement in their quality of life scores while on treatment, with no significant differences between the two groups, although the scores in the suppression arm were lower throughout the study [169]. Consequently, when considering treatment for patients with recurrent genital herpes, a number of factors need to be taken into consideration and discussed with the patient, including the frequency and severity of recurrences, psychosexual concerns and quality of life issues, and details of sexual relationships. Perhaps most important is the frequency of recurrences. Clearly, patients with frequent recurrence will benefit most from suppression. However, there is no absolute minimum frequency, and the decision may also depend on the duration and severity of recurrences, whether the individual is in a sexual relationship, and on any associated psychosexual morbidity. The choice of the drug to use will depend on local availability and cost; however, patients with more than ten recurrences per year should probably commence treatment with a twice daily regimen. Suppression should probably continue for a year and then be stopped to consider whether a further period of suppression is desirable or whether episodic treatment is now the preferred option. Those with less-frequent episodes may well prefer episodic treatment and the short-course regimens offer the best option for patients. Again, the decision about which drug to use will depend on local availability and cost.

When patients present with a first episode of genital herpes, the usual approach has been to treat the first episode and then wait for the pattern and frequency of recurrence to be established, before considering patients for suppression. However, recent studies have suggested that starting suppressive therapy in patients recently diagnosed with first episode genital herpes results in a decreased frequency of recurrences and an improved quality of life [166, 210]. This approach may be particularly useful in adolescent females and in individuals who have profound psychosexual morbidity [154, 211].

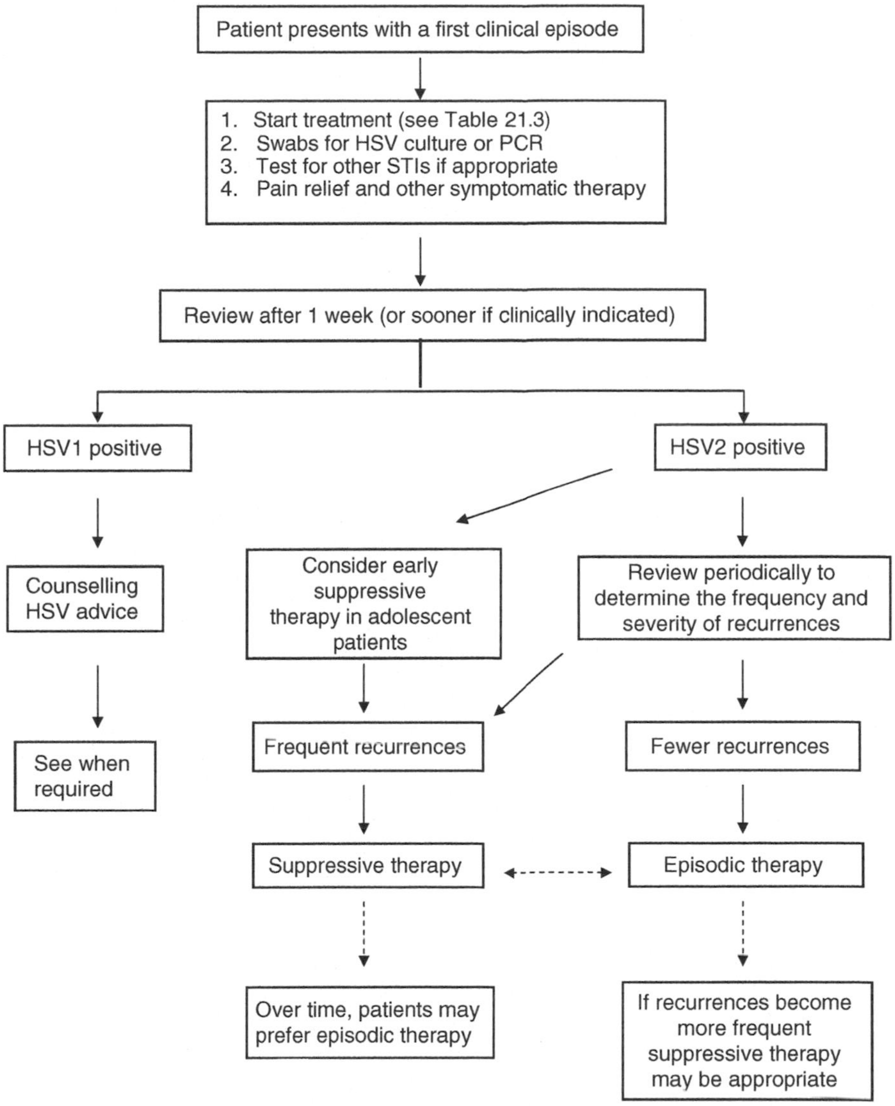

Fig. 21.9 Management of genital herpes

21.10 Prevention

The prevention of transmission is an important public health objective, as well as a major consideration for patients. A number of strategies need to be employed. First, it is vital that patients are informed about the infectious nature of genital herpes and that as a consequence of asymptomatic viral shedding, transmission to a susceptible partner is possible at any time. This may prompt some couples to seek serological testing to determine their "risk status." Other strategies include the use of condoms and suppressive antiviral therapy.

Most of the data in regard to condom efficacy for HSV reduction has been derived from secondary analysis of a failed, large, multinational HSV-2 candidate vaccine RCT. In this study, participants reporting more frequent use of condoms were at lower risk for acquiring HSV-2 than participants who used condoms less frequently (HR, 0.74 [95% CI, 0.59–0.95]). The effect of condom use on HSV-2 acquisition among men (HR, 0.69 [95% CI, 0.51–0.93]) and women (HR, 0.87 [95% CI, 0.58–1.30]) did not differ significantly ($P = 0.39$ for interaction) [212]. More recently, a pooled analysis of six prospective studies with individual condom-use data was published. These prospective studies involved 5,384 HSV-2 negative people who contributed over 2 million days of follow-up, and included three HSV-2 candidate vaccine trials, a treatment trial, an observational STI incidence study, and a behavioral STI intervention study. All six studies included laboratory confirmation of HSV-2 infection. Individuals who used condoms for 100% of sex acts had a 30% lower risk of HSV-2 acquisition compared with those who never used condoms (HR 0.70; 95% CI, 0.40–0.94; $P = 0.01$). In addition the risk of HSV-2 acquisition increased with each unprotected sex act (HR 1.16; 95% CI, 1.08–1.25 $P < 0.001$) [213]. Consistent condom use is associated with lower rates of HSV-2 acquisition in men and women and remains an important tool in prevention of transmission of genital herpes. However, despite patient awareness, condom use in serodiscordant couples is poor [212].

The second method that can used beneficially is suppressive therapy with valaciclovir, and this has been evaluated in a large, multicenter RCT. In this study, 1,484 heterosexual, monogamous couples, one partner having a symptomatic genital HSV-2 infection and the other susceptible to HSV-2, were recruited. Partners with HSV-2 infection were randomly allocated to receive either valaciclovir 500 mg or placebo for 8 months. Among those who received valaciclovir, symptomatic HSV-2 infection developed in 4 of 743 (0.5%) partners, compared with 16 of 741 (2.2%) whose partners were given placebo (HR, 0.25; 95% confidence interval, 0.08 to 0.75; $P = 0.008$) and overall, acquisition of HSV-2 was observed in 14 of the susceptible partners who received valaciclovir (1.9%), as compared with 27 (3.6%) who received placebo (HR, 0.52; 95% confidence interval, 0.27–0.99; $P = 0.04$) [214].

So at a personal level, advice on infection, condom use, and possible serological testing to determine susceptibility and suppressive antiviral therapy are all useful strategies.

At a population level, while all of these may be beneficial, the introduction of an effective vaccine will clearly be more useful. Details of vaccine development can be found in chapter 52. In brief, there have been several randomized placebo controlled trials (RCT) using subunit vaccines against genital herpes. However, the only RCTs that have shown efficacy so far are those of the HSV-2 glycoprotein-D–alum–MPL vaccine (Simplirix) developed by GlaxoSmithKline (GSK). These two studies, with a combined total of over 2,500 subjects aged 18–45, demonstrated that the vaccine was over 70% effective in preventing genital herpes disease, but only in women who were seronegative for both HSV-1 and -2 prior to receiving the vaccine [66]. The vaccine had no measurable effect in men. Further large phase III studies involving over 8,000 young women have just been completed and showed that the vaccine was ineffective [245].

A second method that may have some benefit is male circumcision. Observational studies have been inconsistent and, in addition, many studies are subject to confounding by sexual practices correlated with high risk of transmission or limited statistical power. However, secondary analysis of a recent randomized control trial evaluating adult circumcision to reduce HIV acquisition showed that the adjusted Hazard ratio for HSV-2 seroconversion was 0.72 (95% CI, 0.56–0.92; $P = 0.008$) [215]. In other words, at a population level, circumcision reduces the risk of HSV-2 acquisition by about 70%, and this should now be considered part of the public health armamentarium in reducing the prevalence of HSV-2 in the community.

Take-Home Pearls

- Genital HSV is one of the commonest sexually transmitted infections (STIs) worldwide.
- HSV infections are the leading cause of genital ulcers worldwide.
- HSV-2 is a major cofactor in HIV transmission.
- Most individuals with genital HSV infection are asymptomatic.
- Transmission commonly occurs from asymptomatic individuals.
- Genital herpes may recur frequently causing considerable physical and psychosexual distress.
- Transmission from mother to baby can occur, especially if the mother is infected for the first time close to the time of delivery.
- Antiviral drugs including acyclovir, valaciclovir, and famciclovir are highly effective for the treatment of first episode and recurrent genital herpes and also when used continuously to prevent clinical recurrences.
- Condoms reduce the risk of HSV transmission by about 30%.

References

1. Schneweis, K.E.: Serological studies on the type differentiation of Herpesvirus hominis. Z. Immun. Exp. Ther. **124**, 24–48 (1962)
2. Batterson, W., Roizman, B.: Characterization of the herpes simplex virion-associated factor responsible for the induction of alpha genes. J. Virol. **46**(2), 371–377 (1983)
3. Roizman, B.: The family Herpesvirdae. A brief introduction. In: Roizman, B., Whitley, R.J., Lopez, C. (eds.) The Human Herpesviruses, pp. 1–9. Raven Press, New York (1993)
4. Cowan, F.M., Copas, A., Johnson, A.M., et al.: Herpes simplex virus type 1 infection: a sexually transmitted infection of adolescence? Sex. Transm. Infect. **78**(5), 346–348 (2002)
5. Cowan, F.M., French, R.S., Mayaud, P., et al.: Seroepidemiological study of herpes simplex virus types 1 and 2 in Brazil, Estonia, India, Morocco, and Sri Lanka. Sex. Transm. Infect. **79**(4), 286–290 (2003)
6. Cowan, F.M., Johnson, A.M., Ashley, R., et al.: Antibody to herpes simplex virus type 2 as serological marker of sexual lifestyle in populations. BMJ **309**, 1325–1329 (1994)
7. Cunningham, A.L., Taylor, R., Taylor, J., et al.: Prevalence of infection with herpes simplex virus types 1 and 2 in Australia: a nationwide population based survey. Sex. Transm. Infect. **82**(2), 164–168 (2006)
8. Fleming, D.T., McQuillan, G.M., Johnson, R.E., et al.: Herpes simplex virus type 2 in the United States, 1976 to 1994. N. Engl. J. Med. **337**(16), 1105–1111 (1997)
9. Hashido, M., Kawana, T., Matsunaga, Y., et al.: Changes in prevalence of herpes simplex virus type 1 and 2 antibodies from 1973 to 1993 in the rural districts of Japan. Microbiol. Immunol. **43**(2), 177–180 (1999)
10. Smith, J.S., Robinson, N.J.: Age-specific prevalence of infection with herpes simplex virus types 2 and 1: a global review. J. Infect. Dis. **186**(suppl 1), S3–S28 (2002)
11. Xu, F., Sternberg, M.R., Kottiri, B.J., et al.: Trends in herpes simplex virus type 1 and type 2 seroprevalence in the United States. JAMA **296**(8), 964–973 (2006)
12. Auvert, B., Ballard, R., Campbell, C., et al.: HIV infection among youth in a South African mining town associated with herpes simplex virus-2 seropositivity and sexual behaviour. AIDS **15**(7), 931–934 (2001)
13. Page, A., Taylor, R., Richters, J., et al.: Upstairs and downstairs: socio-economic and gender interactions in herpes simplex virus type 2 seroprevalence in Australia. Sex. Transm. Dis. **36**(6), 344–349 (2009)
14. Buchacz, K., McFarland, W., Hernandez, M., et al.: Prevalence and correlates of herpes simplex virus type 2 infection in a population-based survey of young women in low-income neighborhoods of Northern California: The Young Women's Survey Team. Sex. Transm. Dis. **27**(7), 393–400 (2000)
15. Bunzli, D., Wietlisbach, V., Barazzoni, F., et al Seroepidemiology of Herpes Simplex virus type 1 and 2 in Western and Southern Switzerland in adults aged 25-74 in 1992–93: a population-based study. BMC Infect. Dis. **4**, 10 (2004)
16. Flom, P.L., Zenilman, J.M., Sandoval, M., et al.: Seroprevalence and correlates of herpes simplex virus type 2 infection among young adults in a low-income minority neighborhood. J. Infect. Dis. **191**(5), 818–820 (2005); author reply 820–821
17. Konda, K.A., Klausner, J.D., Lescano, A.G., et al.: The epidemiology of herpes simplex virus type 2 infection in low-income urban populations in coastal Peru. Sex. Transm. Dis. **32**(9), 534–541 (2005)
18. Malkin, J.E., Morand, P., Malvy, D., et al.: Seroprevalence of HSV-1 and HSV-2 infection in the general French population. Sex. Transm. Infect. **78**(3), 201–203 (2002)
19. McFarland, W., Gwanzura, L., Bassett, M.T., et al.: Prevalence and incidence of herpes simplex virus type 2 infection among male Zimbabwean factory workers. J. Infect. Dis. **180**(5), 1459–1465 (1999)
20. Mindel, A., Marks, C., Tideman, R., et al.: Sexual behaviour and social class in Australian women. Int. J. STD AIDS **14**(5), 344–349 (2003)
21. Uribe-Salas, F., Hernandez-Avila, M., Juarez-Figueroa, L., et al.: Risk factors for herpes simplex virus type 2 infection among female commercial sex workers in Mexico City. Int. J. STD AIDS **10**(2), 105–111 (1999)
22. Breinig, M.K., Kingsley, L.A., Armstrong, J.A., et al.: Epidemiology of genital herpes in Pittsburgh: serologic, sexual, and racial correlates of apparent and inapparent herpes simplex infections. J. Infect. Dis. **162**(2), 299–305 (1990)
23. Dukers, N.H., Bruisten, S.M., van den Hoek, J.A., et al.: Strong decline in herpes simplex virus antibodies over time among young homosexual men is associated with changing sexual behavior. Am. J. Epidemiol. **152**(7), 666–673 (2000)
24. Langeland, N., Haarr, L., Mhalu, F.: Prevalence of HSV-2 antibodies among STD clinic patients in Tanzania. Int. J. STD AIDS **9**(2), 104–107 (1998)
25. Tideman, R.L., Taylor, J., Marks, C., et al.: Sexual and demographic risk factors for herpes simplex type 1 and 2 in women attending an antenatal clinic. Sex. Transm. Infect. **77**(6), 413–415 (2001)
26. van de Laar, M.J., Termorshuizen, F., Slomka, M.J., et al.: Prevalence and correlates of herpes simplex virus type 2 infection: evaluation of behavioural risk factors. Int. J. Epidemiol. **27**(1), 127–134 (1998)
27. Chen, X.S., Yin, Y.P., Liang, G.J., et al.: Sexually transmitted infections among female sex workers in Yunnan, China. AIDS Patient Care STDs **19**(12), 853–860 (2005)
28. Dada, A.J., Ajayi, A.O., Diamondstone, L., et al.: A serosurvey of Haemophilus ducreyi, syphilis, and herpes simplex virus type 2 and their association with human immunodeficiency virus among female sex workers in Lagos, Nigeria. Sex. Transm. Dis. **25**(5), 237–242 (1998)
29. Davies, S.C., Taylor, J.A., Sedyaningsih-Mamahit, E.R., et al.: Prevalence and risk factors for herpes simplex virus type 2 antibodies among low- and high-risk populations in Indonesia. Sex. Transm. Dis. **34**(3), 132–138 (2007)
30. Kim, O., Kim, S.S., Park, M.S., et al.: Seroprevalence of sexually transmitted viruses in Korean populations including HIV-seropositive individuals. Int. J. STD AIDS **14**(1), 46–49 (2003)
31. Limpakarnjanarat, K., Mastro, T.D., Saisorn, S., et al.: HIV-1 and other sexually transmitted infections in a cohort of female sex workers in Chiang Rai, Thailand. Sex. Transm. Infect. **75**(1), 30–35 (1999)

32. Nzila, N., Laga, M., Thiam, M.A., et al.: HIV and other sexually transmitted diseases among female prostitutes in Kinshasa. AIDS **5**(6), 715–721 (1991)
33. Qutub, M., Akhter, J.: Epidemiology of genital herpes (HSV-2) among brothel based female sex workers in Bangladesh. Eur. J. Epidemiol. **18**(9), 903–905 (2003)
34. Rabenau, H.F., Buxbaum, S., Preiser, W., et al.: Seroprevalence of herpes simplex virus types 1 and type 2 in the Frankfurt am Main area, Germany. Med. Microbiol. Immunol. **190**(4), 153–160 (2002)
35. Suligoi, B., Dorrucci, M., Volpi, A., et al.: Prevalence and determinants of herpes simplex virus type 2 infection in a cohort of HIV-positive individuals in Italy. Sex. Transm. Dis. **29**(11), 665–667 (2002)
36. Cunningham, A.L., Lee, F.K., Ho, D.W., et al.: Herpes simplex virus type 2 antibody in patients attending antenatal or STD clinics. Med. J. Aust. **158**(8), 525–528 (1993)
37. Hashido, M., Lee, F.K., Nahmias, A.J., et al.: An epidemiologic study of herpes simplex virus type 1 and 2 infection in Japan based on type-specific serological assays. Epidemiol. Infect. **120**(2), 179–186 (1998)
38. Russell, D.B., Tabrizi, S.N., Russell, J.M., et al.: Seroprevalence of herpes simplex virus types 1 and 2 in HIV-infected and uninfected homosexual men in a primary care setting. J. Clin. Virol. **22**(3), 305–313 (2001)
39. Ahmed, H.J., Mbwana, J., Gunnarsson, E., et al.: Etiology of genital ulcer disease and association with human immunodeficiency virus infection in two Tanzanian cities. Sex. Transm. Dis. **30**(2), 114–119 (2003)
40. Beyrer, C., Jitwatcharanan, K., Natpratan, C., et al.: Molecular methods for the diagnosis of genital ulcer disease in a sexually transmitted disease clinic population in northern Thailand: predominance of herpes simplex virus infection. J. Infect. Dis. **178**(1), 243–246 (1998)
41. Bruisten, S.M., Cairo, I., Fennema, H., et al.: Diagnosing genital ulcer disease in a clinic for sexually transmitted diseases in Amsterdam, The Netherlands. J. Clin. Microbiol. **39**(2), 601–605 (2001)
42. Dillon, S.M., Cummings, M., Rajagopalan, S., et al.: Prospective analysis of genital ulcer disease in Brooklyn, New York. Clin. Infect. Dis. **24**(5), 945–950 (1997)
43. Lai, W., Chen, C.Y., Morse, S.A., et al.: Increasing relative prevalence of HSV-2 infection among men with genital ulcers from a mining community in South Africa. Sex. Transm. Infect. **79**(3), 202–207 (2003)
44. Mertz, K.J., Trees, D., Levine, W.C., et al.: Etiology of genital ulcers and prevalence of human immunodeficiency virus coinfection in 10 US cities. The Genital Ulcer Disease Surveillance Group. J. Infect. Dis. **178**(6), 1795–1798 (1998)
45. Moodley, P., Sturm, P.D., Vanmali, T., et al.: Association between HIV-1 infection, the etiology of genital ulcer disease, and response to syndromic management. Sex. Transm. Dis. **30**(3), 241–245 (2003)
46. Morse, S.A., Trees, D.L., Htun, Y., et al.: Comparison of clinical diagnosis and standard laboratory and molecular methods for the diagnosis of genital ulcer disease in Lesotho: association with human immunodeficiency virus infection. J. Infect. Dis. **175**(3), 583–589 (1997)
47. Risbud, A., Chan-Tack, K., Gadkari, D., et al.: The etiology of genital ulcer disease by multiplex polymerase chain reaction and relationship to HIV infection among patients attending sexually transmitted disease clinics in Pune, India. Sex. Transm. Dis. **26**(1), 55–62 (1999)
48. Totten, P.A., Kuypers, J.M., Chen, C.Y., et al.: Etiology of genital ulcer disease in Dakar, Senegal, and comparison of PCR and serologic assays for detection of Haemophilus ducreyi. J. Clin. Microbiol. **38**(1), 268–273 (2000)
49. Paz-Bailey, G., Rahman, M., Chen, C., et al.: Changes in the etiology of sexually transmitted diseases in Botswana between 1993 and 2002: implications for the clinical management of genital ulcer disease. Clin. Infect. Dis. **41**(9), 1304–1312 (2005)
50. Pickering, J.M., Whitworth, J.A., Hughes, P., et al.: Aetiology of sexually transmitted infections and response to syndromic treatment in southwest Uganda. Sex. Transm. Infect. **81**(6), 488–493 (2005)
51. Health Protection Agency. Genital herpes statistics (cited 4 Aug 2008). http://www.hpa.org.uk/webw/HPAweb& HPAwebStandard/HPAweb_C/1195733854250?p=1192454969657
52. Becker, T.M., Blount, J.H., Guinan, M.E.: Genital herpes infections in private practice in the United States, 1966 to 1981. JAMA **253**(11), 1601–1603 (1985)
53. Division of STD Prevention: Sexually Transmitted Disease Surveillance P.H.S. In: US Department of Health and Human Services (ed.) Centers for Disease Control and Prevention, Atlanta (2006)
54. Coyle, P.V., O'Neill, H.J., Wyatt, D.E., et al.: Emergence of herpes simplex type 1 as the main cause of recurrent genital ulcerative disease in women in Northern Ireland. J. Clin. Virol. **27**(1), 22–29 (2003)
55. Haddow, L.J., Dave, B., Mindel, A., et al.: Increase in rates of herpes simplex virus type 1 as a cause of anogenital herpes in western Sydney, Australia, between 1979 and 2003. Sex. Transm. Infect. **82**(2), 255–259 (2006)
56. Langenberg, A.G., Corey, L., Ashley, R.L., et al.: A prospective study of new infections with herpes simplex virus type 1 and type 2 Chiron HSV Vaccine Study Group. N. Engl. J. Med. **341**(19), 1432–1438 (1999)
57. Ribes, J.A., Steele, A.D., Seabolt, J.P., et al.: Six-year study of the incidence of herpes in genital and nongenital cultures in a central Kentucky medical center patient population. J. Clin. Microbiol. **39**(9), 3321–3325 (2001)
58. Roberts, C.M., Pfister, J.R., Spear, S.J.: Increasing proportion of herpes simplex virus type 1 as a cause of genital herpes infection in college students. Sex. Transm. Dis. **30**(10), 797–800 (2003)
59. Ross, J.D., Smith, I.W., Elton, R.A.: The epidemiology of herpes simplex types 1 and 2 infection of the genital tract in Edinburgh 1978–1991. Genitourin. Med. **69**(5), 381–383 (1993)
60. Samra, Z., Scherf, E., Dan, M.: Herpes simplex virus type 1 is the prevailing cause of genital herpes in the Tel Aviv area, Israel. Sex. Transm. Dis. **30**(10), 794–796 (2003)
61. Scoular, A., Norrie, J., Gillespie, G., et al.: Longitudinal study of genital infection by herpes simplex virus type 1 in Western Scotland over 15 years. BMJ **324**(7350), 1366–1367 (2002)
62. Tran, T., Druce, J.D., Catton, M.C., et al.: Changing epidemiology of genital herpes simplex virus infection in Melbourne, Australia, between 1980 and 2003. Sex. Transm. Infect. **80**(4), 277–279 (2004)

63. Bryson, Y., Dillon, M., Bernstein, D., et al.: Risk of acquisition of genital herpes simplex virus type 2 in sex partners of persons with genital herpes: a prospective couple study. J. Infect. Dis. **167**, 942–946 (1993)
64. Corey, L., Langenberg, A.G., Ashley, R., et al.: Recombinant glycoprotein vaccine for the prevention of genital HSV-2 infection: two randomized controlled trials Chiron HSV Vaccine Study Group. JAMA **282**(4), 331–340 (1999)
65. Mertz, G.J., Benedetti, J., Ashley, R., et al.: Risk factors for the sexual transmission of genital herpes. Ann. Intern. Med. **116**(3), 197–202 (1992)
66. Stanberry, L.R., Spruance, S.L., Cunningham, A.L., et al.: Glycoprotein-D-adjuvant vaccine to prevent genital herpes. N. Engl. J. Med. **347**(21), 1652–1661 (2002)
67. Corey, L.: The current trend in genital herpes Progress in prevention. Sex. Transm. Dis. **21**(2 Suppl), S38–S44 (1994)
68. Mertz, G.J., Coombs, R.W., Ashley, R., et al.: Transmission of genital herpes in couples with one symptomatic and one asymptomatic partner: a prospective study. J. Infect. Dis. **157**(6), 1169–1177 (1988)
69. Rooney, J.F., Felser, J.M., Ostrove, J.M., et al.: Acquisition of genital herpes from an asymptomatic sexual partner. N. Engl. J. Med. **314**(24), 1561–1564 (1986)
70. Gupta, R., Wald, A., Krantz, E., et al.: Valacyclovir and acyclovir for suppression of shedding of herpes simplex virus in the genital tract. J. Infect. Dis. **190**(8), 1374–1381 (2004)
71. Wald, A., Huang, M.L., Carrell, D., et al.: Polymerase chain reaction for detection of herpes simplex virus (HSV) DNA on mucosal surfaces: comparison with HSV isolation in cell culture. J. Infect. Dis. **188**(9), 1345–1351 (2003)
72. Wald, A., Zeh, J., Selke, S., et al.: Genital shedding of herpes simplex virus among men. J. Infect. Dis. **186**(suppl 1), S34–S39 (2002)
73. Wald, A., Zeh, J., Selke, S., et al.: Reactivation of genital herpes simplex virus type 2 infection in asymptomatic seropositive persons. N. Engl. J. Med. **342**(12), 844–850 (2000)
74. Rottingen, J.A., Cameron, D.W., Garnett, G.P.: A systematic review of the epidemiologic interactions between classic sexually transmitted diseases and HIV: how much really is known? Sex. Transm. Dis. **28**(10), 579–597 (2001)
75. Steen, R., Dallabetta, G.: Genital ulcer disease control and HIV prevention. J. Clin. Virol. **29**(3), 143–151 (2004)
76. Brown, E.L., Wald, A., Hughes, J.P., et al.: High risk of human immunodeficiency virus in men who have sex with men with herpes simplex virus type 2 in the EXPLORE study. Am. J. Epidemiol. **164**(8), 733–741 (2006)
77. Freeman, E.E., Weiss, H.A., Glynn, J.R., et al.: Herpes simplex virus 2 infection increases HIV acquisition in men and women: systematic review and meta-analysis of longitudinal studies. AIDS **20**(1), 73–83 (2006)
78. Jin, F., Prestage, G.P., Imrie, J., et al.: Anal sexually transmitted infections and risk of HIV infection in homosexual men. J. Acquir. Immune Defic. Syndr. [epub ahead of print; doi: 10.1097/QAI.0b013e3181b48f33].
79. Jin, F., Prestage, G.P., Mao, L., et al.: Transmission of herpes simplex virus types 1 and 2 in a prospective cohort of HIV-negative gay men: the health in men study. J. Infect. Dis. **194**(5), 561–570 (2006)
80. Nagot, N., Ouedraogo, A., Foulongne, V., et al.: Reduction of HIV-1 RNA levels with therapy to suppress herpes simplex virus. N. Engl. J. Med. **356**(8), 790–799 (2007)
81. Zuckerman, R.A., Lucchetti, A., Whittington, W.L., et al.: Herpes simplex virus (HSV) suppression with valacyclovir reduces rectal and blood plasma HIV-1 levels in HIV-1/HSV-2-seropositive men: a randomized, double-blind, placebo-controlled crossover trial. J. Infect. Dis. **196**(10), 1500–1508 (2007)
82. Ouedraogo, A., Nagot, N., Vergne, L., et al.: Impact of suppressive herpes therapy on genital HIV-1 RNA among women taking antiretroviral therapy: a randomized controlled trial. AIDS **20**(18), 2305–2313 (2006)
83. Watson-Jones, D., Weiss, H.A., Rusizoka, M., et al.: Effect of herpes simplex suppression on incidence of HIV among women in Tanzania. N. Engl. J. Med. **358**(15), 1560–1571 (2008)
84. Celum, C., Wald, A., Hughes, J., et al.: Effect of aciclovir on HIV-1 acquisition in herpes simplex virus 2 seropositive women and men who have sex with men: a randomised, double-blind, placebo-controlled trial. Lancet **371**, 2109–2119 (2008)
85. Celum, C., Wald, A., Lingappa, J., et al.: Twice-daily acyclovir to reduce HIV-1 transmission from HIV-1/HSV-2 co-infected persons with HIV-1 serodiscordant couples: a randomized, double-blind, placebo-controlled trial. In: 5th IAS Conference on HIV Pathogenesis Treatment and Prevention, Cape Town, South Africa, 19–22 July 2009
86. Mindel, A., Faherty, A., Carney, O., et al.: Dosage and safety of long-term suppressive acyclovir therapy for recurrent genital herpes. Lancet **1**(8591), 926–928 (1988)
87. Chen, K.T., Tuomala, R.E., Chu, C., et al.: No association between antepartum serologic and genital tract evidence of herpes simplex virus-2 coinfection and perinatal HIV-1 transmission. Am. J. Obstet. Gynecol. **198**(4), 399.e1–5 (2008)
88. Cowan, F.M., Humphrey, J.H., Ntozini, R., et al.: Maternal Herpes simplex virus type 2 infection, syphilis and risk of intra-partum transmission of HIV-1: results of a case control study. AIDS **22**(2), 193–201 (2008)
89. Corey, L., Adams, H.G., Brown, Z.A., et al.: Genital herpes simplex virus infections: clinical manifestations, course, and complications. Ann. Intern. Med. **98**(6), 958–972 (1983)
90. Barton, I.G., Kinghorn, G.R., Walker, M.J., et al.: Association of HSV-1 with cervical infection. Lancet **2**(8255), 1108 (1981)
91. Samarasinghe, P.L., Oates, J.K., MacLennan, I.P.B.: Herpetic proctitis and sacral radiomyelopathy: a hazard for homosexual men. BMJ **ii**, 365–366 (1979)
92. Embil, J.A., Manuel, F.R., McFarlane, E.S.: Concurrent oral and genital infection with an identical strain of herpes simplex virus type 1 Restriction endonuclease analysis. Sex. Transm. Dis. **8**(2), 70–72 (1981)
93. Evans, A.S., Dick, E.C.: Acute Pharyngitis and Tonsillitis in University of Wisconsin Students. JAMA **190**, 699–708 (1964)
94. Craig, C.P., Nahmias, A.J.: Different patterns of neurologic involvement with herpes simplex virus types 1 and 2: isolation of herpes simplex virus type 2 from the buffy coat of two adults with meningitis. J. Infect. Dis. **127**(4), 365–372 (1973)
95. Goldmeier, D., Bateman, J.R., Rodin, P.: Urinary retention and intestinal obstruction associated with ano-rectal Herpes simplex virus infection. Br. Med. J. **2**(5968), 425 (1975)

96. Shturman-Ellstein, R., Borkowsky, W., Fish, I., et al.: Myelitis associated with genital herpes in a child. J. Pediatr. **88**(3), 523 (1976)
97. Bastuji-Garin, S., Rzany, B., Stern, R.S., et al.: Clinical classification of cases of toxic epidermal necrolysis, Stevens-Johnson syndrome, and erythema multiforme. Arch. Dermatol. **129**(1), 92–96 (1993)
98. Flewett, T.H., Parker, R.G., Philip, W.M.: Acute hepatitis due to Herpes simplex virus in an adult. J. Clin. Pathol. **22**(1), 60–66 (1969)
99. Joseph, T.J., Vogt, P.J.: Disseminated herpes with hepatoadrenal necrosis in an adult. Am. J. Med. **56**(5), 735–739 (1974)
100. Corey, L., Spear, P.G.: Infections with herpes simplex viruses (2). N. Engl. J. Med. **314**(12), 749–757 (1986)
101. Whitaker 3rd, J.A., Hardison, J.E.: Severe thrombocytopenia after generalized herpes simplex virus-2 (HSV-2) infection. South Med. J. **71**(7), 864–865 (1978)
102. Friedman, H.M., Pincus, T., Gibilisco, P., et al.: Acute monoarticular arthritis caused by herpes simplex virus and cytomegalovirus. Am. J. Med. **69**(2), 241–247 (1980)
103. Benedetti, J.K., Zeh, J., Selke, S., et al.: Frequency and reactivation of nongenital lesions among patients with genital herpes simplex virus. Am. J. Med. **98**(3), 237–242 (1995)
104. Gill, M.J., Arlette, J., Buchan, K.: Herpes simplex virus infection of the hand. A profile of 79 cases. Am. J. Med. **84**(1), 89–93 (1988)
105. Mindel, A., Carney, O., Williams, P.: Cutaneous herpes simplex infections. Genitourin. Med. **66**(1), 14–15 (1990)
106. Mailman, C.J., Miranda, J.L., Spock, A.: Recurrent eczema herpeticum widespread cutaneous herpes simplex in atopic patient without active atopic dermatitis. Arch. Dermatol. **89**, 815–818 (1964)
107. Wheeler, C.E.J., Abele, D.C.: Eczema herpeticum, primary and recurrent. Arch. Dermatol. **93**, 162–173 (1966)
108. Linnemann, C.C.J., First, M.R., Alvira, M.M., et al.: Herpesvirus hominis type 2 meningoencephalitis following renal transplant. Am. J. Med. **61**, 703–708 (1976)
109. St Geme Jr., J.W., Prince, J.T., Burke, B.A., et al.: Studies of persistent herpes virus infection in children with the Aldrich syndrome. J. Pediatr. **61**, 302–303 (1962)
110. Goyette, R.E., Donowho Jr., E.M., Hieger, L.R., et al.: Fulminant herpesvirus hominis hepatitis during pregnancy. Obstet. Gynecol. **43**(2), 191–195 (1974)
111. Kobbermann, T., CL, L., Griffin, W.T.: Maternal death secondary to disseminated herpesvirus hominis. Am. J. Obstet. Gynecol. **137**(6), 742–743 (1980)
112. Young, E.J., Killam, A.P., Greene Jr., J.F.: Disseminated herpesvirus infection association with primary genital herpes in pregnancy. JAMA **235**(25), 2731–2733 (1976)
113. Guinan, M.E., MacCalman, J., Kern, E.R., et al.: The course of untreated recurrent genital herpes simplex infection in 27 women. N. Engl. J. Med. **304**(13), 759–763 (1981)
114. Parker, J.D., Banatvala, J.E.: Herpes genitalis; clinical and virological studies. Br. J. Vener. Dis. **43**(3), 212–216 (1967)
115. Sacks, S.L.: Frequency and duration of patient-observed recurrent genital herpes simplex virus infection: characterization of the nonlesional prodrome. J. Infect. Dis. **150**(6), 873–877 (1984)
116. Koutsky, L.A., Stevens, C.E., Holmes, K.K., et al.: Underdiagnosis of genital herpes by current clinical and viral-isolation procedures. N. Engl. J. Med. **326**(23), 1533–1539 (1992)
117. Siegal, F.P., Lopez, C., Hammer, G.S., et al.: Severe acquired immunodeficiency in male homosexuals, manifested by chronic perianal ulcerative herpes simplex lesions. N. Engl. J. Med. **305**(24), 1439–1444 (1981)
118. Schacker, T., Zeh, J., Hu, H.L., et al.: Frequency of symptomatic and asymptomatic herpes simplex virus type 2 reactivations among human immunodeficiency virus-infected men. J. Infect. Dis. **178**(6), 1616–1622 (1998)
119. Conant, M.A.: Prophylactic and suppressive treatment with acyclovir and the management of herpes in patients with acquired immunodeficiency syndrome. J. Am. Acad. Dermatol. **18**(1 Pt 2), 186–188 (1988)
120. DeJesus, E., Wald, A., Warren, T., et al.: Valacyclovir for the suppression of recurrent genital herpes in human immunodeficiency virus-infected subjects. J. Infect. Dis. **188**(7), 1009–1016 (2003)
121. Romanowski, B., Aoki, F.Y., Martel, A.Y., et al.: Efficacy and safety of famciclovir for treating mucocutaneous herpes simplex infection in HIV-infected individuals Collaborative Famciclovir HIV Study Group. AIDS **14**(9), 1211–1217 (2000)
122. Sullivan-Bolyai, J., Hull, H.F., Wilson, C., et al.: Neonatal herpes simplex virus infection in King County Washington Increasing incidence and epidemiologic correlates. JAMA **250**(22), 3059–3062 (1983)
123. Kropp, R.Y., Wong, T., Cormier, L., et al.: Neonatal herpes simplex virus infections in Canada: results of a 3-year national prospective study. Pediatrics **117**(6), 1955–1962 (2006)
124. Jones, C.A., Isaacs, D., McIntyre, P., et al.: Neonatal herpes simplex virus infection. In: Ninth Annual Report, Australian Paediatric Surveillance Unit, pp. 31–32 (2001)
125. Tookey, P., Peckham, C.S.: Neonatal herpes simplex virus infection in the British Isles. Paediatr. Perinat. Epidemiol. **10**(4), 432–442 (1996)
126. British Paediatric Surveillance Unit: British Paediatric Surveillance Unit 21st Anniversary Annual Report 2006/2007, London (2007)
127. Brown, Z.A., Wald, A., Morrow, R.A., et al.: Effect of serologic status and cesarean delivery on transmission rates of herpes simplex virus from mother to infant. JAMA **289**(2), 203–209 (2003)
128. Braig, S., Luton, D., Sibony, O., et al.: Acyclovir prophylaxis in late pregnancy prevents recurrent genital herpes and viral shedding. Eur. J. Obstet. Gynecol. Reprod. Biol. **96**(1), 55–58 (2001)
129. Brocklehurst, P., Kinghorn, G., Carney, O., et al.: A randomised placebo controlled trial of suppressive acyclovir in late pregnancy in women with recurrent genital herpes infection. Br. J. Obstet. Gynaecol. **105**(3), 275–280 (1998)
130. Scott, L.L., Hollier, L.M., McIntire, D., et al.: Acyclovir suppression to prevent clinical recurrences at delivery after first episode genital herpes in pregnancy: an open-label trial. Infect. Dis. Obstet. Gynecol. **9**(2), 75–80 (2001)
131. Scott, L.L., Hollier, L.M., McIntire, D., et al.: Acyclovir suppression to prevent recurrent genital herpes at delivery. Infect. Dis. Obstet. Gynecol. **10**(2), 71–77 (2002)

132. Scott, L.L., Sanchez, P.J., Jackson, G.L., et al.: Acyclovir suppression to prevent cesarean delivery after first-episode genital herpes. Obstet. Gynecol. **87**(1), 69–73 (1996)
133. Sheffield, J.S., Hill, J.B., Hollier, L.M., et al.: Valacyclovir prophylaxis to prevent recurrent herpes at delivery: a randomized clinical trial. Obstet. Gynecol. **108**(1), 141–147 (2006)
134. Sheffield, J.S., Hollier, L.M., Hill, J.B., et al.: Acyclovir prophylaxis to prevent herpes simplex virus recurrence at delivery: a systematic review. Obstet. Gynecol. **102**(6), 1396–1403 (2003)
135. Stray-Pedersen, B.: Acyclovir in late pregnancy to prevent neonatal herpes simplex. Lancet **ii**, 756 (1990)
136. Prober, C.G., Sullender, W.M., Yasukawa, L.L., et al.: Low risk of herpes simplex virus infections in neonates exposed to the virus at the time of vaginal delivery to mothers with recurrent genital herpes simplex virus infections. N. Engl. J. Med. **316**(5), 240–244 (1987)
137. Chapel, T.A., Jeffries, C.D., Brown, W.J.: Simultaneous infection with Treponema pallidum and herpes simplex virus. Cutis **24**(2), 191–192 (1979)
138. Reina, J., Saurina, J., Fernandez-Baca, V., et al.: Evaluation of a direct immunofluorescence cytospin assay for the detection of herpes simplex virus in clinical samples. Eur. J. Clin. Microbiol. Infect. Dis. **16**(11), 851–854 (1997)
139. Slomka, M.J., Emery, L., Munday, P.E., et al.: A comparison of PCR with virus isolation and direct antigen detection for diagnosis and typing of genital herpes. J. Med. Virol. **55**(2), 177–183 (1998)
140. Corey, L.: The diagnosis and treatment of genital herpes. JAMA **248**(9), 1041–1049 (1982)
141. Johnston, S.L.: Comparison of human rhabdomyosarcoma, HEp-2, and human foreskin fibroblast cells for the isolation of herpes simplex virus from clinical specimens. Diagn. Microbiol. Infect. Dis. **14**(5), 373–375 (1991)
142. Herrmann, K.L., Stewart, J.A.: Diagnosis of herpes simplex type 1 and 2 infections. In: Nahmias, A., Dowdle, W.R., Schinazi, R.F. (eds.) The Human Herpesviruses, pp. 343–350. Elsevier, New York (1981)
143. Jain, S., Wyatt, D., McCaughey, C., et al.: Nested multiplex polymerase chain reaction for the diagnosis of cutaneous herpes simplex and herpes zoster infections and a comparison with electronmicroscopy. J. Med. Virol. **63**(1), 52–56 (2001)
144. Markoulatos, P., Georgopoulou, A., Kotsovassilis, C., et al.: Detection and typing of HSV-1, HSV-2, and VZV by a multiplex polymerase chain reaction. J. Clin. Lab. Anal. **14**(5), 214–219 (2000)
145. O'Neill, H.J., Wyatt, D.E., Coyle, P.V., et al.: Real-time nested multiplex PCR for the detection of herpes simplex virus types 1 and 2 and varicella zoster virus. J. Med. Virol. **71**(4), 557–560 (2003)
146. Cherpes, T.L., Ashley, R.L., Meyn, L.A., et al.: Longitudinal reliability of focus glycoprotein G-based type-specific enzyme immunoassays for detection of herpes simplex virus types 1 and 2 in women. J. Clin. Microbiol. **41**(2), 671–674 (2003)
147. Ashley, R.L.: Sorting out the new HSV type specific antibody tests. Sex. Transm. Infect. **77**(4), 232–237 (2001)
148. van Dyck, E., Buve, A., Weiss, H.A., et al.: Performance of commercially available enzyme immunoassays for detection of antibodies against herpes simplex virus type 2 in African populations. J. Clin. Microbiol. **42**(7), 2961–2965 (2004)
149. Ho, D.W., Field, P.R., Irving, W.L., et al.: Detection of immunoglobulin M antibodies to glycoprotein G-2 by western blot (immunoblot) for diagnosis of initial herpes simplex virus type 2 genital infections. J. Clin. Microbiol. **31**(12), 3157–3164 (1993)
150. Golden, M.R., Ashley-Morrow, R., Swenson, P., et al.: Herpes simplex virus type 2 (HSV-2) Western blot confirmatory testing among men testing positive for HSV-2 using the focus enzyme-linked immunosorbent assay in a sexually transmitted disease clinic. Sex. Transm. Dis. **32**(12), 771–777 (2005)
151. Mindel, A., Taylor, J.: Debate: the argument against. Should every STD clinic patient be considered for type-specific serological screening for HSV? Herpes **9**(2), 35–37 (2002)
152. Patel, R., Rompalo, A.: Managing patients with genital herpes and their sexual partners. Infect. Dis. Clin. North Am. **19**(2), 427–438 (2005)
153. Patrick, D.M., Money, D.: Debate: the argument for. Should every STD clinic patient be considered for type-specific serological screening for HSV? Herpes **9**(2), 32–34 (2002)
154. Mindel, A., Marks, C.: Psychological symptoms associated with genital herpes virus infections: epidemiology and approaches to management. CNS Drugs **19**(4), 303–312 (2005)
155. Carney, O., Ross, E., Bunker, C., et al.: A prospective study of the psychological impact on patients with a first episode of genital herpes. Genitourin. Med. **70**(1), 40–45 (1994)
156. Bierman, S.M.: Recurrent genital herpes simplex infection: a trivial disorder. Arch. Dermatol. **121**(4), 513–517 (1985)
157. Luby, E.D., Klinge, V.: Genital herpes. A pervasive psychosocial disorder. Arch. Dermatol. **121**(4), 494–497 (1985)
158. Manne, S., Sandler, I.: Coping and adjustment to genital herpes. J. Behav. Med. **7**(4), 391–410 (1984)
159. Mindel, A.: Psychological and psychosexual implications of herpes simplex virus infections. Scand. J. Infect. Dis. Suppl. **100**, 27–32 (1996)
160. Goldmeier, D., Johnson, A.: Does psychiatric illness affect the recurrence rate of genital herpes? Br. J. Vener. Dis. **58**(1), 40–43 (1982)
161. Rand, K.H., Hoon, E.F., Massey, J.K., et al.: Daily stress and recurrence of genital herpes simplex. Arch. Intern. Med. **150**(9), 1889–1893 (1990)
162. Cohen, F., Kemeny, M.E., Kearney, K.A., et al.: Persistent stress as a predictor of genital herpes recurrence. Arch. Intern. Med. **159**(20), 2430–2436 (1999)
163. Carney, O., Ross, E., Ikkos, G., et al.: The effect of suppressive oral acyclovir on the psychological morbidity associated with recurrent genital herpes. Genitourin. Med. **69**(6), 457–459 (1993)
164. Ware Jr., J.E., Kosinski, M., Gandek, B., et al.: The factor structure of the SF-36 Health Survey in 10 countries: results from the IQOLA Project International Quality of Life Assessment. J. Clin. Epidemiol. **51**(11), 1159–1165 (1998)

165. Doward, L.C., McKenna, S.P., Kohlmann, T., et al.: The international development of the RGHQoL: a quality of life measure for recurrent genital herpes. Qual. Life Res. **7**(2), 143–153 (1998)
166. Handsfield, H.H., Warren, T., Werner, M., et al.: Suppressive therapy with valacyclovir in early genital herpes: a pilot study of clinical efficacy and herpes-related quality of life. Sex. Transm. Dis. **34**(6), 339–343 (2007)
167. Patel, R., Boselli, F., Cairo, I., et al.: Patients' perspectives on the burden of recurrent genital herpes. Int. J. STD AIDS **12**(10), 640–645 (2001)
168. Taboulet, F., Halioua, B., Malkin, J.E.: Quality of life and use of health care among people with genital herpes in France. Acta Derm. Venereol. **79**(5), 380–384 (1999)
169. Fife, K.H., Almekinder, J., Ofner, S.: A comparison of one year of episodic or suppressive treatment of recurrent genital herpes with valacyclovir. Sex. Transm. Dis. **34**(5), 297–301 (2007)
170. Patel, R., Tyring, S., Strand, A., et al.: Impact of suppressive antiviral therapy on the health related quality of life of patients with recurrent genital herpes infection. Sex. Transm. Infect. **75**(6), 398–402 (1999)
171. de Miranda, P., Blum, M.R.: Pharmacokinetics of acyclovir after intravenous and oral administration. J. Antimicrob. Chemother. **12**(Suppl B), 29–37 (1983)
172. Burnette, T.C., Harrington, J.A., Reardon, J.E., et al.: Purification and characterization of a rat liver enzyme that hydrolyzes valaciclovir, the L-valyl ester prodrug of acyclovir. J. Biol. Chem. **270**(26), 15827–15831 (1995)
173. Soul-Lawton, J., Seaber, E., On, N., et al.: Absolute bioavailability and metabolic disposition of valaciclovir, the L-valyl ester of acyclovir, following oral administration to humans. Antimicrob. Agents Chemother. **39**(12), 2759–2764 (1995)
174. Bryson, Y.J., Dillon, M., Lovett, M., et al.: Treatment of first episodes of genital herpes simplex virus infection with oral acyclovir A randomized double-blind controlled trial in normal subjects. N. Engl. J. Med. **308**(16), 916–921 (1983)
175. Corey, L., Fife, K.H., Benedetti, J.K., et al.: Intravenous acyclovir for the treatment of primary genital herpes. Ann. Intern. Med. **98**(6), 914–921 (1983)
176. Corey, L., Nahmias, A.J., Guinan, M.E., et al.: A trial of topical acyclovir in genital herpes simplex virus infections. N. Engl. J. Med. **306**(22), 1313–1319 (1982)
177. Fiddian, A.P., Kinghorn, G.R., Goldmeier, D., et al.: Topical acyclovir in the treatment of genital herpes: a comparison with systemic therapy. J. Antimicrob. Chemother. **12 suppl B**, 67–77 (1983)
178. Mertz, G.J., Critchlow, C.W., Benedetti, J., et al.: Double-blind placebo-controlled trial of oral acyclovir in first- episode genital herpes simplex virus infection. J. Am. Med. Assoc. **252**(9), 1147–1151 (1984)
179. Mindel, A., Adler, M.W., Sutherland, S., et al.: Intravenous acyclovir treatment for primary genital herpes. Lancet **1**(8274), 697–700 (1982)
180. Nilsen, A.E., Aasen, T., Halsos, A.M., et al.: Efficacy of oral acyclovir in the treatment of initial and recurrent genital herpes. Lancet **2**(8298), 571–573 (1982)
181. Rompalo, A.M., Mertz, G.J., Davis, L.G., et al.: Oral acyclovir for treatment of first-episode herpes simplex virus proctitis. JAMA **259**(19), 2879–2881 (1988)
182. Thin, R.N., Nabarro, J.M., Parker, J.D., et al.: Topical acyclovir in the treatment of initial genital herpes. Br. J. Vener. Dis. **59**(2), 116–119 (1983)
183. Corey, L., Mindel, A., Fife, K.H., et al.: Risk of recurrence after treatment of first-episode genital herpes with intravenous acyclovir. Sex. Transm. Dis. **12**(4), 215–218 (1985)
184. Fife, K.H., Barbarash, R.A., Rudolph, T., et al.: Valaciclovir versus acyclovir in the treatment of first-episode genital herpes infection. Results of an international, multicenter, double-blind, randomized clinical trial. The Valaciclovir International Herpes Simplex Virus Study Group. Sex. Transm. Dis. **24**(8), 481–486 (1997)
185. Loveless, M., Harris, W., Sacks, S.: Treatment of first episode genital herpes with famciclovir. In: 35th Interscience Conference on Antimicrobial Agents and Chemotherapy, San Francisco (1995)
186. Martens, M.G., Fife, K.H., Leone, P.A., et al.: Once daily valacyclovir for reducing viral shedding in subjects newly diagnosed with genital herpes. Infect. Dis. Obstet. Gynecol. **2009**, 105376 (2009)
187. Bodsworth, N.J., Crooks, R.J., Borelli, S., et al.: Valaciclovir versus aciclovir in patient initiated treatment of recurrent genital herpes: a randomised, double blind clinical trial International Valaciclovir HSV Study Group. Genitourin. Med. **73**(2), 110–116 (1997)
188. Kinghorn, G.R., Turner, E.B., Barton, I.G., et al.: Efficacy of topical acyclovir cream in first and recurrent episodes of genital herpes. Antiviral Res. **3**(5–6), 291–301 (1983)
189. Reichman, R.C., Badger, G.J., Mertz, G.J., et al.: Treatment of recurrent genital herpes simplex infections with oral acyclovir. A controlled trial. JAMA **251**(16), 2103–2107 (1984)
190. Sacks, S.L., Aoki, F.Y., Diaz-Mitoma, F., et al.: Patient-initiated, twice-daily oral famciclovir for early recurrent genital herpes. A randomized, double-blind multicenter trial. Canadian Famciclovir Study Group. JAMA **276**(1), 44–49 (1996)
191. Salo, O.P., Lassus, A., Hovi, T., et al.: Double-blind placebo-controlled, trial of oral acyclovir in recurrent genital herpes. Eur. J. Sex Transm. Dis. **1**, 95–98 (1983)
192. Spruance, S.L., Tyring, S.K., DeGregorio, B., et al.: A large-scale, placebo-controlled, dose-ranging trial of peroral valaciclovir for episodic treatment of recurrent herpes genitalis Valaciclovir HSV Study Group. Arch. Intern. Med. **156**(15), 1729–1735 (1996)
193. Saiag, P., Praindhui, D., Chastang, C.: A double-blind, randomized study assessing the equivalence of valacyclovir 1000 mg once daily versus 500 mg twice daily in the episodic treatment of recurrent genital herpes Genival Study Group. J. Antimicrob. Chemother. **44**(4), 525–531 (1999)
194. Abudalu, M., Tyring, S., Koltun, W., et al.: Single-day, patient-initiated famciclovir therapy versus 3-day valacyclovir regimen for recurrent genital herpes: a randomized, double-blind, comparative trial. Clin. Infect. Dis. **47**(5), 651–658 (2008)
195. Aoki, F.Y., Tyring, S., Diaz-Mitoma, F., et al.: Single-day, patient-initiated famciclovir therapy for recurrent genital herpes: a randomized, double-blind, placebo-controlled trial. Clin. Infect. Dis. **42**(1), 8–13 (2006)

196. Bodsworth, N., Bloch, M., McNulty, A., et al.: 2-day versus 5-day famciclovir as treatment of recurrences of genital herpes: results of the FaST study. Sex. Health **5**(3), 219–225 (2008)
197. Leone, P.A., Trottier, S., Miller, J.M.: Valacyclovir for episodic treatment of genital herpes: a shorter 3-day treatment course compared with 5-day treatment. Clin. Infect. Dis. **34**(7), 958–962 (2002)
198. Wald, A., Carrell, D., Remington, M., et al.: Two-day regimen of acyclovir for treatment of recurrent genital herpes simplex virus type 2 infection. Clin. Infect. Dis. **34**(7), 944–948 (2002)
199. Diaz-Mitoma, F., Sibbald, R.G., Shafran, S.D., et al.: Oral famciclovir for the suppression of recurrent genital herpes: a randomized controlled trial Collaborative Famciclovir Genital Herpes Research Group. JAMA **280**(10), 887–892 (1998)
200. Douglas, J.M., Critchlow, C., Benedetti, J., et al.: A double-blind study of oral acyclovir for suppression of recurrences of genital herpes simplex virus infection. N. Engl. J. Med. **310**(24), 1551–1556 (1984)
201. Halsos, A.M., Salo, O.P., Lassus, A., et al.: Oral acyclovir suppression of recurrent genital herpes: a double-blind, placebo-controlled, crossover study. Acta Derm. Venereol. **65**(1), 59–63 (1985)
202. Mindel, A., Weller, I.V., Faherty, A., et al.: Prophylactic oral acyclovir in recurrent genital herpes. Lancet **2**(8394), 57–59 (1984)
203. Patel, R., Bodsworth, N.J., Woolley, P., et al.: Valaciclovir for the suppression of recurrent genital HSV infection: a placebo controlled study of once daily therapy International Valaciclovir HSV Study Group. Genitourin. Med. **73**(2), 105–109 (1997)
204. Straus, S.E., Takiff, H.E., Seidlin, M., et al.: Suppression of frequently recurring genital herpes. A placebo-controlled double-blind trial of oral acyclovir. N. Engl. J. Med. **310**(24), 1545–1550 (1984)
205. Wald, A., Selke, S., Warren, T., et al.: Comparative efficacy of famciclovir and valacyclovir for suppression of recurrent genital herpes and viral shedding. Sex. Transm. Dis. **33**(9), 529–533 (2006)
206. Reitano, M., Tyring, S., Lang, W., et al.: Valaciclovir for the suppression of recurrent genital herpes simplex virus infection: a large-scale dose range-finding study International Valaciclovir HSV Study Group. J. Infect. Dis. **178**(3), 603–610 (1998)
207. Fife, K.H., Crumpacker, C.S., Mertz, G.J., et al.: Recurrence and resistance patterns of herpes simplex virus following cessation of > or = 6 years of chronic suppression with acyclovir Acyclovir Study Group. J. Infect. Dis. **169**(6), 1338–1341 (1994)
208. Goldberg, L.H., Kaufman, R., Kurtz, T.O., et al.: Long-term suppression of recurrent genital herpes with acyclovir. A 5-year benchmark. Acyclovir Study Group. Arch. Dermatol. **129**(5), 582–587 (1993)
209. Romanowski, B., Marina, R.B., Roberts, J.N.: Patients' preference of valacyclovir once-daily suppressive therapy versus twice-daily episodic therapy for recurrent genital herpes: a randomized study. Sex. Transm. Dis. **30**(3), 226–231 (2003)
210. Fife, K.H., Warren, T.J., Justus, S.E., et al.: An international, randomized, double-blind, placebo-controlled, study of valacyclovir for the suppression of herpes simplex virus type 2 genital herpes in newly diagnosed patients. Sex. Transm. Dis. **35**(7), 668–673 (2008)
211. Batalden, K., Bria, C., Biro, F.M.: Genital herpes and the teen female. J. Pediatr. Adolesc. Gynecol. **20**(6), 319–321 (2007)
212. Wald, A., Langenberg, A.G.M., Krantz, E., et al.: The relationship between condom use and herpes simplex virus acquisition. Ann. Intern. Med. **143**(10), 707–713 (2005)
213. Martin, E.T., Krantz, E., Gottlieb, S.L., et al.: A pooled analysis of the effect of condoms in preventing HSV-2 acquisition. Arch. Intern. Med. **169**(13), 1233–1240 (2009)
214. Corey, L., Wald, A., Patel, R., et al.: Once-daily valacyclovir to reduce the risk of transmission of genital herpes. N. Engl. J. Med. **350**(1), 11–20 (2004)
215. Tobian, A.A., Serwadda, D., Quinn, T.C., et al.: Male circumcision for the prevention of HSV-2 and HPV infections and syphilis. N. Engl. J. Med. **360**(13), 1298–1309 (2009)
216. Pebody, R.G., Andrews, N., Brown, D., et al.: The seroepidemiology of herpes simplex virus type 1 and 2 in Europe. Sex. Transm. Infect. **80**(3), 185–191 (2004)
217. Vyse, A.J., Gay, N.J., Slomka, M.J., et al.: The burden of infection with HSV-1 and HSV-2 in England and Wales: implications for the changing epidemiology of genital herpes. Sex. Transm. Infect. **76**(3), 183–187 (2000)
218. Suligoi, B., Tchamgmena, O., Sarmati, L., et al.: Prevalence and risk factors for herpes simplex virus type 2 infection among adolescents and adults in northern Cameroon. Sex. Transm. Dis. **28**(12), 690–693 (2001)
219. Theng, T.S., Sen, P.R., Tan, H.H., et al.: Seroprevalence of HSV-1 and 2 among sex workers attending a sexually transmitted infection clinic in Singapore. Int. J. STD AIDS **17**(6), 395–399 (2006)
220. Smit, C., Pfrommer, C., Mindel, A., et al.: Rise in seroprevalence of herpes simplex virus type 1 among highly sexual active homosexual men and an increasing association between herpes simplex virus type 2 and HIV over time (1984–2003). Eur. J. Epidemiol. **22**(12), 937–944 (2007)
221. Andreoletti, L., Piednoir, E., Legoff, J., et al.: High seroprevalence of herpes simplex virus type 2 infection in French human immunodeficiency virus type 1-infected outpatients. J. Clin. Microbiol. **43**(8), 4215–4217 (2005)
222. Da Rosa-Santos, O.L., Goncalves Da Silva, A., Pereira Jr., A.C.: Herpes simplex virus type 2 in Brazil: seroepidemiologic survey. Int. J. Dermatol. **35**(11), 794–796 (1996)
223. Mbopi-Keou, F.X., Gresenguet, G., Mayaud, P., et al.: Interactions between herpes simplex virus type 2 and human immunodeficiency virus type 1 infection in African women: opportunities for intervention. J. Infect. Dis. **182**(4), 1090–1096 (2000)
224. Ramaswamy, M., Sabin, C., McDonald, C., et al.: Herpes simplex virus type 2 (HSV-2) seroprevalence at the time of HIV-1 diagnosis and seroincidence after HIV-1 diagnosis in an ethnically diverse cohort of HIV-1-infected persons. Sex. Transm. Dis. **33**(2), 96–101 (2006)

225. Roest, R.W., van der Meijden, W.I., van Dijk, G., et al.: Prevalence and association between herpes simplex virus types 1 and 2-specific antibodies in attendees at a sexually transmitted disease clinic. Int. J. Epidemiol. **30**(3), 580–588 (2001)
226. Shivaswamy, K.N., Thappa, D.M., Jaisankar, T.J., et al.: High seroprevalence of HSV-1 and HSV-2 in STD clinic attendees and non-high risk controls: a case control study at a referral hospital in south India. Indian J. Dermatol. Venereol. Leprol. **71**(1), 26–30 (2005)
227. Singh, A.E., Romanowski, B., Wong, T., et al.: Herpes simplex virus seroprevalence and risk factors in 2 Canadian sexually transmitted disease clinics. Sex. Transm. Dis. **32**(2), 95–100 (2005)
228. Suligoi, B., Calistri, A., Cusini, M., et al.: Seroprevalence and determinants of herpes simplex type 2 infection in an STD clinic in Milan, Italy. J. Med. Virol. **67**(3), 345–348 (2002)
229. Alanen, A., Kahala, K., Vahlberg, T., et al.: Seroprevalence, incidence of prenatal infections and reliability of maternal history of varicella zoster virus, cytomegalovirus, herpes simplex virus and parvovirus B19 infection in South-Western Finland. BJOG **112**(1), 50–56 (2005)
230. Arseven, G., Tuncel, E., Tuncel, S., et al.: Distribution of HSV-1 and HSV-2 antibodies in pregnant women. Mikrobiyol. Bül. **26**(4), 359–366 (1992)
231. Bodeus, M., Laffineur, K., Kabamba-Mukadi, B., et al.: Seroepidemiology of herpes simplex type 2 in pregnant women in Belgium. Sex. Transm. Dis. **31**(5), 297–300 (2004)
232. Brown, Z.A., Selke, S., Zeh, J., et al.: The acquisition of herpes simplex virus during pregnancy. N Engl J. Med. **337**(8), 509–515 (1997)
233. Carvalho, M., de Carvalho, S., Pannuti, C.S., et al.: Prevalence of herpes simplex type 2 antibodies and a clinical history of herpes in three different populations in Campinas City, Brazil. Int. J. Infect. Dis. **3**(2), 94–98 (1998)
234. Dan, M., Sadan, O., Glezerman, M., et al.: Prevalence and risk factors for herpes simplex virus type 2 infection among pregnant women in Israel. Sex. Transm. Dis. **30**(11), 835–838 (2003)
235. Gaytant, M.A., Steegers, E.A., van Laere, M., et al.: Seroprevalences of herpes simplex virus type 1 and type 2 among pregnant women in the Netherlands. Sex. Transm. Dis. **29**(11), 710–714 (2002)
236. Ghebrekidan, H., Ruden, U., Cox, S., et al.: Prevalence of herpes simplex virus types 1 and 2, cytomegalovirus, and varicella-zoster virus infections in Eritrea. J. Clin. Virol. **12**(1), 53–64 (1999)
237. Haddow, L.J., Sullivan, E.A., Taylor, J., et al.: Herpes simplex virus type 2 (HSV-2) infection in women attending an antenatal clinic in the South Pacific island nation of Vanuatu. Sex. Transm. Dis. **34**(5), 258–261 (2007)
238. Levett, P.N.: Seroprevalence of HSV-1 and HSV-2 in Barbados. Med. Microbiol. Immunol. **194**(1–2), 105–107 (2005)
239. Lo, J.Y., Lim, W.W., Ho, D.W., et al.: Difference in seroprevalence of herpes simplex virus type 2 infection among antenatal women in Hong Kong and southern China. Sex. Transm. Infect. **75**(2), 123 (1999)
240. Nilsen, A., Mwakagile, D., Marsden, H., et al.: Prevalence of, and risk factors for, HSV-2 antibodies in sexually transmitted disease patients, healthy pregnant females, blood donors and medical students in Tanzania and Norway. Epidemiol. Infect. **133**(5), 915–925 (2005)
241. Patrick, D.M., Dawar, M., Cook, D.A., et al.: Antenatal seroprevalence of herpes simplex virus type 2 (HSV-2) in Canadian women: HSV-2 prevalence increases throughout the reproductive years. Sex. Transm. Dis. **28**(7), 424–428 (2001)
242. Uuskula, A., Nygard-Kibur, M., Cowan, F.M., et al.: The burden of infection with herpes simplex virus type 1 and type 2: seroprevalence study in Estonia. Scand. J. Infect. Dis. **36**(10), 727–732 (2004)
243. Enders, G., Risse, B., Zauke, M., et al.: Seroprevalence study of herpes simplex virus type 2 among pregnant women in Germany using a type-specific enzyme immunoassay. Eur. J. Clin. Microbiol. Infect. Dis. **17**(12), 870–872 (1998)
244. Garcia-Corbeira, P., Dal-Re, R., Aguilar, L., et al.: Is sexual transmission an important pattern for herpes simplex type 2 virus seroconversion in the Spanish general population? J. Med. Virol. **59**(2), 194–197 (1999)
245. National Institute of Allergy and Infectious Diseases. Study Finds Genital Herpes Vaccine Ineffective in Women. 2010; http://www.niaid.nih.gov/news/newsreleases/2010/Pages/Herpevac.aspx. Accessed 26 October 2010.

Clinical Aspects of HCMV Infections in Immunocompromised Patients

22

Miriam Wittek, Lutz Gürtler, and Hans Wilhelem Doerr

Core Messages

- Cytomegalovirus (CMV), a member of the herpesvirus family, induces permanent latent and recurrent infection in humans (HCMV). 50–100% of mankind are virus carriers.
- Beginning with the fetal period, the virus can be transmitted life-long, postnatally by intimate (saliva) and sexual or fresh blood contacts, and sometimes also by smear infection.
- The virus is transmitted by saliva, urine, and genital secretions.
- While immunocompetent hosts only rarely fall ill with an infectious mononucleosis (IM)-like disease, in immunocompromised patients a broad spectrum of diseases are caused by primary and by recurrent ("opportunistic") infections affecting nearly all organs.
- In non-treated AIDS patients, severe chorioretinitis (loss of vision) and colitis are most typical, while in immunosuppressed recipients of organs or bone marrow, pneumonia is most feared.
- Pre- and perinatal infections are rather frequent when the child-bearing woman is the virus carrier.
- In the newborn, severe organ damages, particularly of the CNS (due to prenatal infection), of the lung (due to perinatal infection) occur.
- HCMV infection induces some immune escape mechanisms (reduction of antigen presentation by MHC I).
- Cytomegalic inclusion histology (also falsely termed "disease", CID) is present in every HCMV carrier.
- Laboratory diagnosis is established by direct detection of virus, viral antigen, or nucleic acid using cell cultures, leukocyte smears, and preferentially PCR techniques (viral load determination in full blood or blood plasma) and indirectly by Ig class-differentiated antibody determination.
- Several drugs are licensed for effective usage in chemoprophylaxis and chemotherapy.
- Resistance is investigated by genotyping and by phenotypic cell culture experiments.
- Passive immunization is controversially discussed. An active vaccine is under development.

22.1 Introduction and General Aspects

Cytomegalovirus (CMV) is a virus that induces permanent and latent infection, cell fusion with giant cell formation, and partial cell death.

Cell cultures infected with CMV develop typical changes described as cytomegalic inclusion effect. Cells are enlarged or fusioned to syncytia and reveal typical intranuclear inclusion bodies ("owl eyes"). Such

H.W. Doerr (✉) and M. Wittek
Institut für Med Virologie,
Universitätsklinikum Frankfurt am Main,
Paul-Ehrlich-Straße 40, 60596 Frankfurt,
Germany
e-mail: h.w.doerr@em.uni-frankfurt.de

L.G. Gürtler
Max von Pettenkofer Institut,
Universität München, Pettenkofer Straße 9A,
80336 München, Germany

G. Gross and S.K. Tyring (eds.), *Sexually Transmitted Infections and Sexually Transmitted Diseases*,
DOI: 10.1007/978-3-642-14663-3_22, © Springer-Verlag Berlin Heidelberg 2011

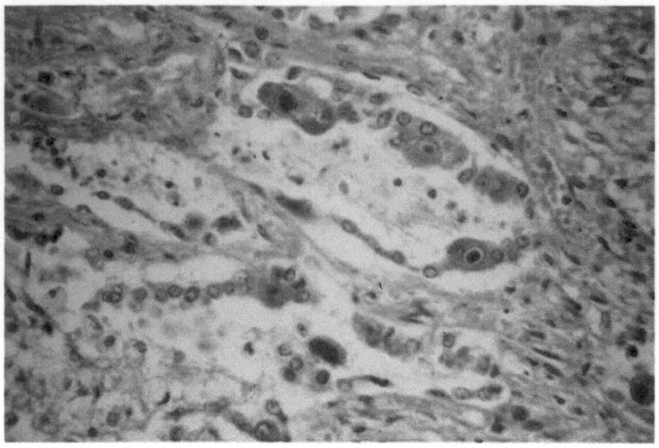

Fig. 22.1 Typical owl eye cells in tissue due to giant cell and parachromosomal episome formation induced by CMV replication (hemotoxylin–eosin stain)

histology was first detected by the German pathologist H. Ribbert in 1881 in salivary glands of newborns died from other reasons (Fig. 22.1). For many decades, pathologists called it the cytomegalic inclusion "disease" (CID), although no disease was apparent. Since 1950 it became clear that CID played a role in fetopathy and other diseases of the newborn, especially where premature infants were concerned. In 1956, CMV was isolated and identified as a herpesvirus by Rowe et al. (1956). Later on, similar viruses were isolated from monkeys and rodents. So, CMV of humans was termed HCMV. There are no cross infections indicating a strict species specificity of these herpesviruses. In 1967, transfusion-associated cases of infectious mononucleosis (IM) were described. Those patients produced antibodies to HCMV, but not to heterophilic antibodies against antigens on bovine erythrocytes in contrast to classical IM caused by Epstein-Barr virus (EBV), which was discovered at that time.

IM is a syndrome of fever (1–2 weeks), hepatitis, splenomegaly, tonsillitis, and cervical lymphadenopathy. The most characteristic feature is the formation of atypical, mononuclear cells in the blood ("mononucleosis"). Part of these cells are cytotoxic CD8 lymphocytes attacking other infected blood cells. After acquisition of HCMV via contact with saliva, breast milk, genital secretions, and urine, the virus is spread in the blood mainly by leukocytes, especially by mononuclear cells (monocytes). In these cells or their precursors, the virus replicates inducing cytotoxicity. In some cells, virus replication is not initiated, but HCMV-DNA remains as a parachromosomal episome. By this way the virus escapes humoral and cell-mediated immune reactions and establishes a life-long persistent infection. Latency is considered to be under the control of CD4 and CD8 cells, since recurrences reflect corresponding immunologic reactions as determined by the change in the number of such lymphocytes. HCMV infection is frequently reactivated hormonally, especially in women during the menstruation cycle. Most recurrences are like primary infections – silent, i.e., without clinical relevance. Compared to EBV infection of adolescents, HCMV is rarely an agent of IM. In this case, tonsillitis, which is typical of EBV IM, is absent, but a nonspecific sore throat occurs. Transfusion IM has been eradicated, since blood units are leukocyte depleted. Single CID cells may be found in nearly all organs of the body indicating a low-level productive infection besides (and supported by recurrency of) latent infection, especially in the salivary glands and kidney, which yields infectivity of saliva and urine, and also of genital secretions. HCMV triggers the infected cell to escape signal cascades of innate and specific immune reactions, in part by antigen presentation by the MHC class I pathway. Spread of HCMV throughout the organism is significantly promoted by the distinct tropism to endothelial cells of blood vessels. So, HCMV has been considered to contribute to atherosclerosis. In summary, each organ is affected by HCMV infection, but clinically evident pathogenesis is rare. Nevertheless, in single cases of immunocompetent hosts, deadly inflammation of many organs have been described, like hepatitis, myocarditis, encephalitis and neuritis, oesophagitis/gastritis, colitis, etc. However, an increasing number of therapeutically immunosuppressed or pathologically immunocompromised patients have revealed the entire spectrum of severe HCMV-associated diseases under therapy. Furthermore, the evidence of oncomodulation by HCMV has become stronger.

22.2 HCMV Infection in HIV Carriers and AIDS Patients

HCMV infection is sexually transmitted like HIV. Thus, most of HIV carriers were also found to be HCMV seropositive. While in immunocompetent hosts recurrences of HCMV infection is usually restricted by cell-mediated immune response before the onset of clinical signs of disease, in HIV carriers presenting less than 200 CD4 cells/mL blood, single cytomegalic "owl eye" cells (may) disseminate infection resulting in inflammatory symptoms. This is frequently observed in the gastrointestinal tract. Patients suffer from esophagitis and colitis with penetrating ulcers, which are easily confirmed by presence of HCMV bioptic histology. More rare are gastritis and hepatitis. Nearly pathognomonic for CID in AIDS patients is a necrotinizing chorioretinitis with the consequence of visual loss. Other, but more rare infections of CNS are encephalitis and peripheral neuropathy (polyradiculoneuritis). Single severe and life-threatening episodes of HCMV pneumonia have also been described during the course of AIDS. After the advent of HAART and its subsequent immune reconstitution, HCMV-associated diseases in HIV carriers have significantly reduced, but not eliminated.

22.3 HCMV Infection in Patients Under Immunosuppressive Therapy

Polytransfusion of blood units induces a light immunosuppression. As mentioned above, in recipients of fresh blood containing leukocytes HCMV-associated infectious mononucleosis was first discovered. In other cases, only hepatitis was recorded by elevated serum transaminase activities. This problem has been nearly eradicated, since blood units are depleted of the leukocyte fraction, but HCMV disease still occurs due to reactivation of the patient's CMV and undetected transmission. For special cases, HCMV seronegative donors are selected.

Solid organ transplantation (e.g., kidney, liver, lung) may also transmit considerable amounts of HCMV from seropositive donors. Latent virus may be reactivated by even slight immune reactions between graft and recipient via TNF-a, as mentioned in the Chap. 20. Since HCMV infects and damages mononuclear cells, therapeutic immunosuppression against potential organ rejection contributes to virus spread in the sense of a *circulus vitiosus*. Furthermore, because of the HCMV tropism to the endothelium of blood vessels, organ rejection might be initiated at this point of junction of blood vessels to the organism of the recipient. From human case studies and experiments in rats, some evidence has been collected for the hypothesis that HCMV is one of the etiologic factors of atherosclerosis. Most frequent symptoms of CID in immunosuppressed recipients of solid organs are febrile, sometimes sepsis-like illness ("CMV syndrome"), hepatitis, and hematopoietic disorders (thrombocytopenia, granulocytopenia). Life-threatening pneumonia is more common, and retinitis more rare than in AIDS patients. To avoid CID in transplantation recipients, organs are selected in terms of HCMV serologic results seen in the donor (D) and the recipient (R). The risk of CID is decreasing for these combinations: D+/R–, D+/R+, D–/R+. In the last case, an endogenous HCMV reactivation due to the immunosuppressive therapy might cause disease. Nearly no CID is to be expected, if both D and R are seronegative, i.e., virus free.

In *allogenic hematopoetic stem cell transplantation* (HSCT), HCMV disease was the most frequent and life-threatening infectious complication. Up to 25% of all recipients concerned, usually suffering from severe CID of lungs (pneumonitis), were associated with a very poor prognosis (85% mortality). By applying strict measures of prophylaxis before and after transplantation, today the risk has significantly decreased. Those measures include careful donor selection in terms of D/R carriership of HCMV (see above), prophylactic application of antiviral drugs, and "preemptive" antiviral therapy on the basis of consequent laboratory diagnostic monitoring, even before the onset of illness. Nevertheless, in 2–3% of HSCT patients, severe CID of the lungs and the gastrointestinal tract (from esophagitis to colitis) still occur depending on and correlating with major immunosuppressive therapy, which has to be individually applied or reduced. However, a graft versus host reaction may also activate CID in a sense of *circulus vitiosus*. So the different ways of immunosuppression like T cell depletion (by anti-CD52 or anti-thymocyte globulin), mycophenolate mofetil, cyclosporine A, or high-dose steroids should be carefully considered.

From a *dermatological point of view*, it should not be forgotten that HCMV reveals a distinct endothelium tropism and stimulates the generation of a broad range of autoimmune antibodies. The potential role for atherosclerosis has been already mentioned. Furthermore, systemic necrotizing vasculitis, polyarteritis nodosa, lupus erythematosus, and Sjögren's syndrome, etc., may be triggered by HCMV infection in terms of etiology or modulation.

22.4 HCMV Infection in Pregnancy, Fetal Development, and Infantal Life

During pregnancy, women undergo a physiological, minor immunosuppression. So, in HCMV-seropositive pregnant women, who are 50% of all females in this age of life in the developed world, may undergo a CID reactivation, while the other half of HCMV infection in pregnancy is caused by primary HCMV infection. It is assumed that 3–5% of all pregnancies face such HCMV infections.

Urine sample screening revealed that up to 5% of seropositive pregnant women excrete the virus at term of birth. Presumably 1/3 of women infected with or reactivating HCMV transmit the virus to the fetus; about 10% of them show CID-specific lesions. All visceral organs may be affected. Since the virus reveals a distinct neurotropism, brain damages are frequent leading to visual or auditive impairments or mental retardation.

Primary HCMV infection during pregnancy is considered more dangerous than reactivation or secondary reinfection. Figure 22.2 compiles the possible outcome of congenital infections in infants.

Besides prenatal infection, ten times more perinatally acquired infections or early postnatal infections occur. It is assumed that in developed countries up to 0.5% of all newborns prenatally and 5% perinatally are HCMV infected, and that 10% are symptomatic.

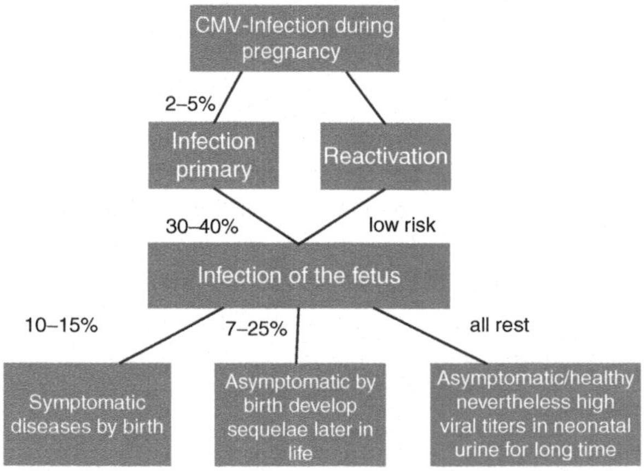

Fig. 22.2 Scheme of the course of CMV transmission during pregnancy and possibilities of the outcome of the fetal infection

A typical disease of perinatal infection is pneumonitis, frequently associated with pneumocystis infection. Since the immune defense of infants is still under development, especially premature infants suffer from HCMV life-threatening infections.

22.5 Diagnosis and Therapy

Clinical signs of HCMV infection are not usually as typical that diagnosis can be confirmed without laboratory tests. Today, the most important HCMV test is the determination of viral load by the use of PCR that has been developed in different modifications. HCMV DNA can be detected in whole-blood specimens and in plasma. To assess viral absence, whole blood should be used; to evaluate the clinical course of infection and therapy, plasma is the preferential sample. An alternate, and sometimes even more pathognomonic investigation, is testing for the HCMV pp65 antigen in smears of blood leukocytes. PCR may also be applied for the investigation of viral load in saliva and urine samples. However, virus isolation using the rapid "shell vial technology", i.e., detection of virus-specific antigen in cell culture inoculated with urine or saliva specimens, is nearly as efficient and cheaper, but still PCR is the method of choice for the detection of HCMV.

Antibody detection in blood samples yields information on HCMV carriership, not on immunity. Presence of virus-specific IgM may complement diagnosis of recent or recently reactivated HCMV infections in addition to the more rapid virus detection. In AIDS patients, quantitative virus-specific IgA determination has proven to be valuable and sometimes superior to other methods of laboratory CID diagnosis. As of now, five antiviral drugs have been licensed and are in reliable use for CID therapy. Ganciclovir, valganciclovir, and cidofovir are nucleoside analogs. Foscarnet is a phosphate bridge inhibitor of NA synthesis. Fomivirsen, which is only licensed for intraocular application against HCMV retinitis, is an anti-sense oligonucleotide. Other drugs are in clinical evaluation or under development. Application of HCMV hyperimmunoglobulins is now considered not to be efficient enough to justify the costs. A vaccine for active immunization against HCMV infection is under development, but as of now no breakthrough has been achieved.

Take-Home Pearls

- HCMV is transmitted by sexual intercourse and other intimate (saliva) contacts. It induces permanent infections, which cause "opportunistic" diseases of the lung, colon, brain, and other organs in humans who are immunocompromised from physiologic (newborns), pathologic (AIDS), or therapeutic reasons (immunosuppressive treatment).
- Main therapeutic tool of primary or course of infection-evaluating laboratory diagnosis is the determination of viral load in blood (plasma) specimens.
- Potent antiviral drugs are available.
- Drug resistance can be rapidly checked by virus genotyping.

Literature (Further Reading)

Michaelis, M., Doerr, H.W., Cinatl, J.: Oncomodulation by human cytomegalovirus: Evidence becomes stronger. Med. Microbiol. Immunol. **198**, 79–81 (2009)

Mocarsci Jr., E.S., Shenk, T., Pass, R.F.: Cytomegaloviruses. In: Knipe, M., Howley, P.M. (eds.) Fields Virology, 5th edn. Lippincott, Williams & Wilkins, Philadelphia. pp. 2701–2772 (2007)

Rowe, W.P., Hartley, J.W., Waterman, S., Turner, H.C., Huebner, R.J.: Cytopathogenic agent resembling human salivary gland virus recovered from tissue cultures of human adenoids. Proc. Soc. Exp. Biol. Med. **92**, 418–424 (1956)

Schleiss, M.R.: Cytomegalovirus vaccine development. Curr Top Microbiol Immunol. **325**, 361–382 (2008)

Weinberg, A., Lurain, N. (guest ed.): J. Clin. Virol. CMV. **41**, 173–241; Special Issue (2008)

Global Epidemiology of HIV

23

Osamah Hamouda

Core Messages

- The global percentage of adults living with HIV has leveled off since 2000.
- In 2007, there were 2.7 million new HIV infections and 2 million HIV-related deaths.
- The rate of new HIV infections has fallen in several countries, but globally these favorable trends are at least partially offset by increases in new infections in other countries.
- In 14 of 17 African countries with adequate survey data, the percentage of young pregnant women (ages 15–24) who are living with HIV has declined since 2000–2001. In seven countries, the drop in infections has equaled or exceeded the 25% target decline for 2010 set out in the Declaration of Commitment.
- As treatment access has increased over the last 10 years the annual number of AIDS deaths has fallen.
- Sub-Saharan Africa remains the region most heavily affected by HIV, accounting for 67% of all people living with HIV and for 75% of AIDS deaths in 2007. However, some of the most worrisome increases in new infections are now occurring in populous countries in other regions, such as Indonesia, the Russian Federation, and various high-income countries.
- Globally, the percentage of women among people living with HIV has remained stable (at 50%) for several years, although women's share of infections is increasing in several countries.
- In virtually all regions outside sub-Saharan Africa, HIV disproportionately affects injecting drug users, men who have sex with men, and sex workers.

23.1 Status of the Global HIV Epidemic (Summary)

On a global scale, the HIV epidemic has stabilized, although with unacceptably high levels of new HIV infections and AIDS deaths. Globally, there were an estimated 33 million (30.3 million–36.1 million) people living with HIV in 2007 (Fig. 23.1). The annual number of new HIV infections declined from 3.0 million (2.6 million–3.5 million) in 2001 to 2.7 million (2.2 million–3.2 million) in 2007. Overall, 2.0 million (1.8 million–2.3 million) people died due to AIDS in 2007, compared with an estimated 1.7 million (1.5 million– 2.3 million) in 2001 [1].

While the percentage of people (aged 15–49) living with HIV has stabilized since 2000, the overall number of people living with HIV has steadily increased as new infections occur each year, HIV treatments extend life, and as new infections still outnumber AIDS deaths (Fig. 23.2).

O. Hamouda
Abteilung für Infektionsepidemiologie, Robert Koch-Institut, Postfach, 65 02 61 D-13302, Berlin, Germany
e-mail: hamoudao@rki.de

G. Gross and S.K. Tyring (eds.), *Sexually Transmitted Infections and Sexually Transmitted Diseases*,
DOI: 10.1007/978-3-642-14663-3_23, © Springer-Verlag Berlin Heidelberg 2011

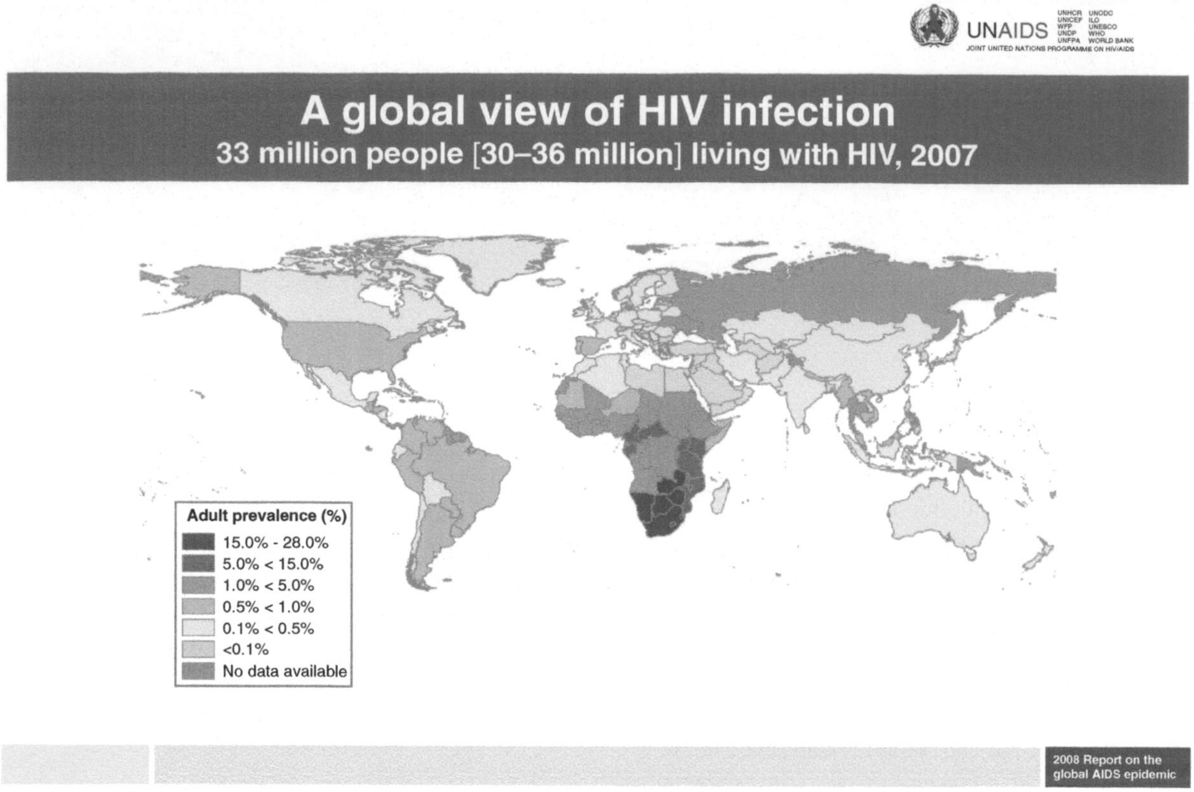

Fig. 23.1 A global view of HIV infection. 33 million people [30–36 million] living with HIV, 2007

Southern Africa continues to bear a disproportionate share of the global burden of HIV: 35% of HIV infections and 38% of AIDS deaths in 2007 occurred in that subregion. Altogether, sub-Saharan Africa is home to 67% of all people living with HIV.

Women account for half of all people living with HIV worldwide, and nearly 60% of HIV infections in sub-Saharan Africa. Over the last 10 years, the proportion of women among people living with HIV has remained stable globally, but has increased in many regions (Fig. 23.3).

Young people aged 15–24 account for an estimated 45% of new HIV infections worldwide. An estimated 370,000 (330,000–410,000) children younger than 15 years became infected with HIV in 2007.

Globally, the number of children younger than 15 years living with HIV increased from 1.6 million (1.4 million–2.1 million) in 2001 to 2.0 million (1.9 million–2.3 million) in 2007. Almost 90% live in sub-Saharan Africa.

23.2 Sub-Saharan Africa

An estimated 1.9 million (1.6 million–2.1 million) people were newly infected with HIV in sub-Saharan Africa in 2007, bringing to 22 million (20.5 million–23.6 million) the number of people living with HIV. Two thirds (67%) of the global total of 32.9 million (30.3 million–36.1 million) people with HIV live in this region, and three quarters (75%) of all AIDS deaths in 2007 occurred there.

Sub-Saharan Africa's epidemics vary significantly from country to country in both scale and scope (Fig. 23.4). Adult national HIV prevalence is below 2% in several countries of West and Central Africa, as well as in the horn of Africa, but in 2007 it exceeded 15% in seven southern African countries (Botswana, Lesotho, Namibia, South Africa, Swaziland, Zambia, and Zimbabwe), and was above 5% in seven other countries, mostly in Central and East Africa (Cameroon, the Central African Republic, Gabon,

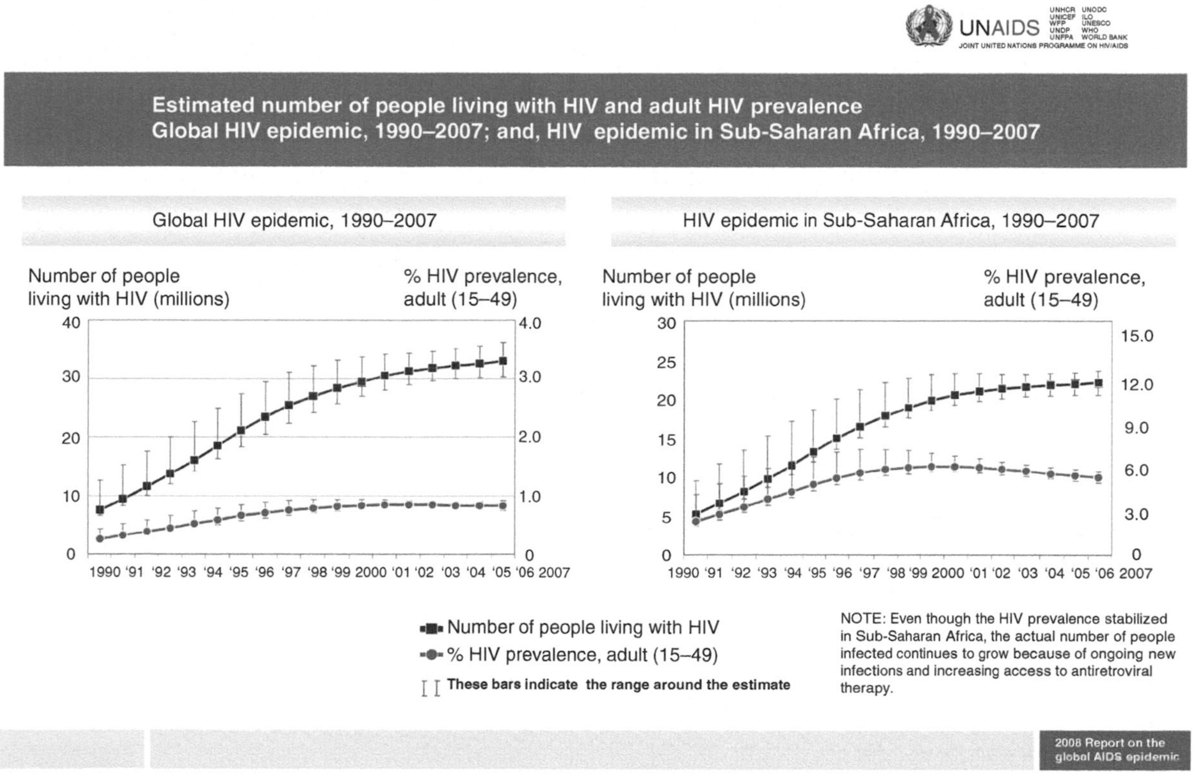

Fig. 23.2 Estimated number of people living with HIV and adult HIV prevalence. Global HIV epidemic, 1990–2007; and, HIV epidemic in Sub-Saharan Africa, 1990–2007

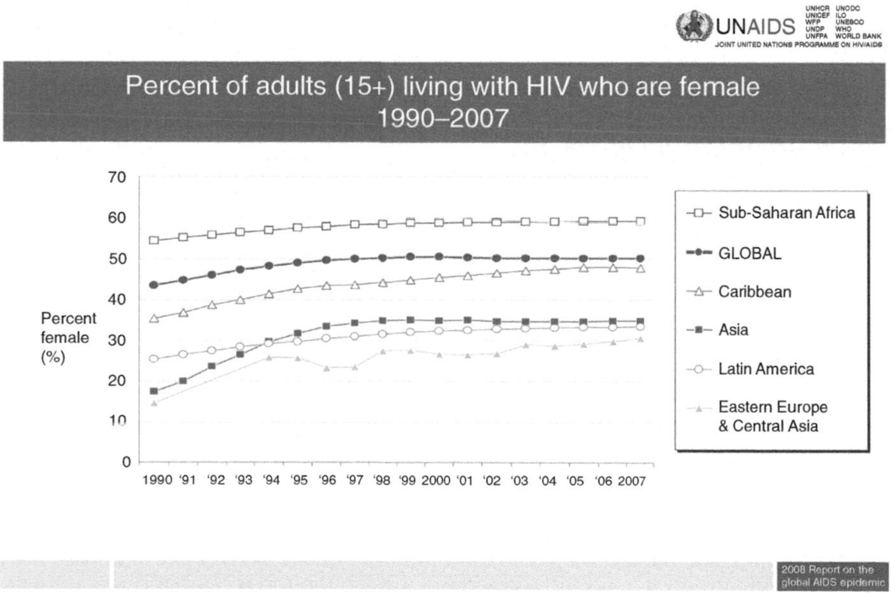

Fig. 23.3 Percent of adults (15+) living with HIV who are female 1990–2007

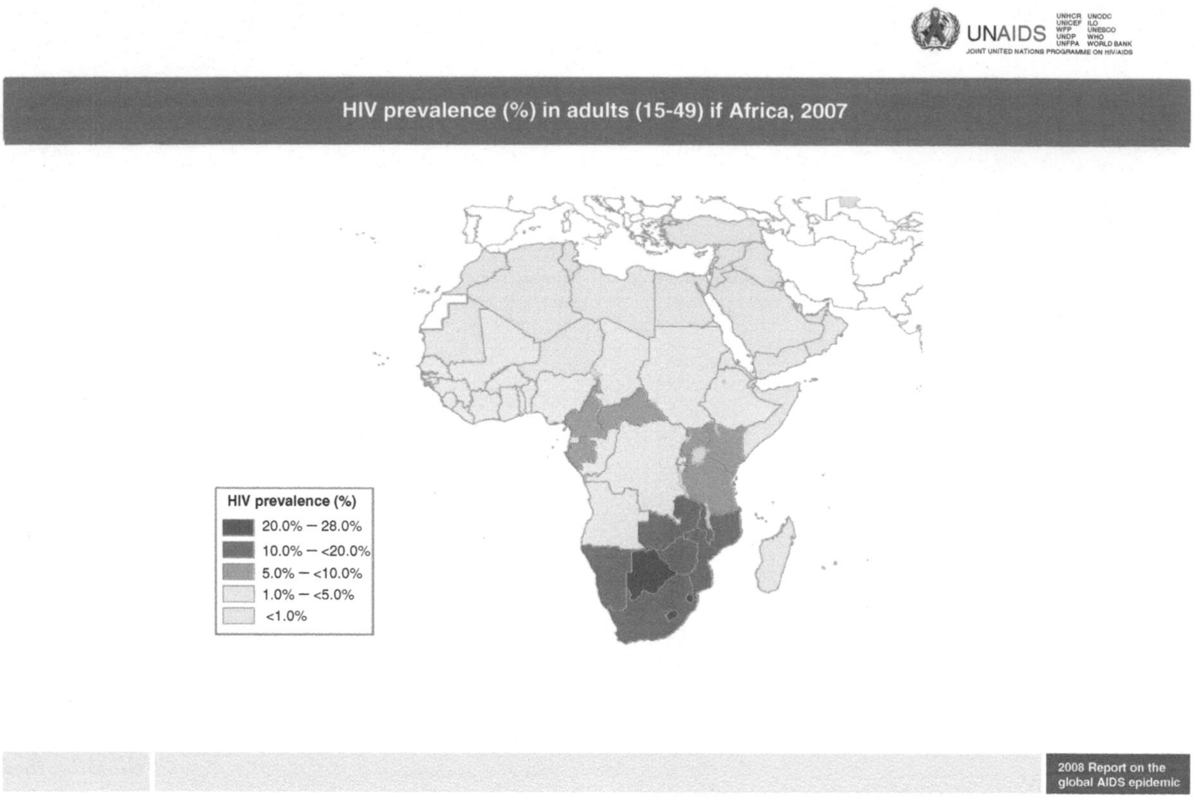

Fig. 23.4 HIV prevalence (%) in adults (15–49) in Africa, 2007

Malawi, Mozambique, Uganda, and the United Republic of Tanzania).

23.2.1 Recent Epidemiological Trends

Most epidemics in sub-Saharan Africa appear to have stabilized, although often at very high levels, particularly in southern Africa. Additionally, in a growing number of countries, adult HIV prevalence appears to be falling. For the region as a whole, women are disproportionately affected in comparison with men, with especially stark differences between the sexes in HIV prevalence among young people (Fig. 23.5).

In southern Africa, reductions in HIV prevalence are especially striking in Zimbabwe, where HIV prevalence in pregnant women attending antenatal clinics fell from 26% in 2002 to 18% in 2006 [2]. In Botswana, a drop in HIV prevalence among pregnant 15–19-year-olds (from 25% in 2001 to 18% in 2006) suggests that the rate of new infections could be slowing [3]. The epidemics in Malawi and Zambia also appear to have stabilized, amid some evidence of favorable behavior changes [4, 5] and signs of declining HIV prevalence among women using antenatal services in some urban areas [6–8].

HIV data from antenatal clinics in South Africa suggest that the country's epidemic might be stabilizing [9], but there is no evidence yet of major changes in HIV-related behavior. The estimated 5.7 million (4.9 million–6.6 million) South Africans living with HIV in 2007 make this the largest HIV epidemic in the world. Meanwhile, the 26% HIV prevalence found in adults in Swaziland in 2006 is the highest prevalence ever documented in a national population based survey anywhere in the world [10].

In Lesotho and parts of Mozambique, HIV prevalence among pregnant women is increasing. In some of the provinces in the central and southern zones of the country, adult HIV prevalence has reached or exceeded 20%, while infections continue to increase among young people (ages 15–24) [11].

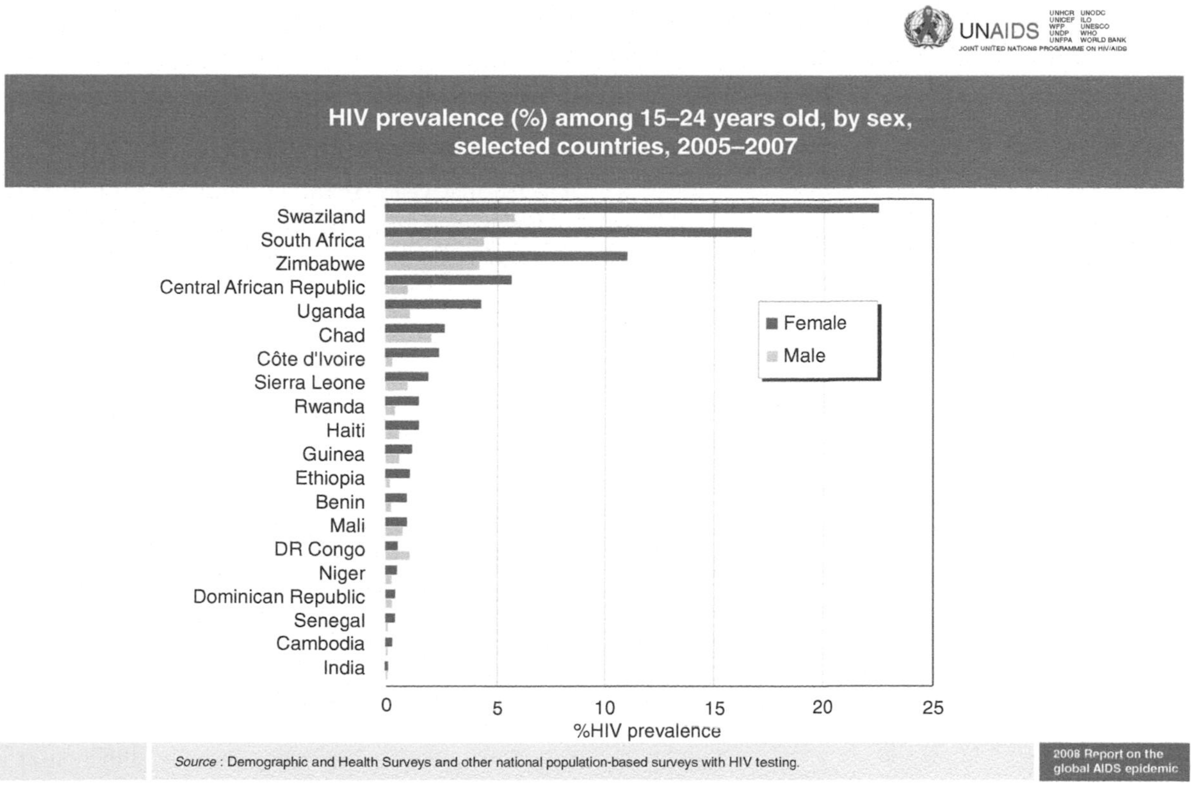

Fig. 23.5 HIV prevalence (%) among 15–24 years old, by sex, selected countries, 2005–2007

HIV prevalence in the comparatively smaller epidemics in East Africa has either reached a plateau or is receding. After dropping dramatically in the 1990s [12, 13], adult national HIV prevalence in Uganda has stabilized at 5.4% (5.0%–6.1%). However, there are signs of a possible resurgence in sexual risk-taking that could cause the epidemic to grow again. For example, the proportion of adult men and women who say they had sex with a person who was not a spouse and did not live with the respondent has grown since 1995 (from 12% to 16% for women and 29% to 36% for men) [13, 14].

Most of the comparatively smaller HIV epidemics in West Africa are stable or are declining – as is the case for Burkina Faso, Côte d'Ivoire, and Mali. In Côte d'Ivoire, HIV prevalence among pregnant women in urban areas fell from 10% in 2001 to 6.9% in 2005. The largest epidemic in West Africa – in Nigeria, the continent's most populous country – appears to have stabilized at 3.1% (2.3%–3.8%), according to HIV infection trends among women attending antenatal clinics [15].

23.2.2 Main Modes of HIV Transmission

Heterosexual intercourse remains the epidemic's driving force in sub-Saharan Africa. The high rate of sexual transmission has also given rise to the world's largest population of children living with HIV. However, recent epidemiological evidence has revealed the region's epidemic to be more diverse than previously thought.

23.2.2.1 Heterosexual Intercourse Related to Serodiscordant Couples

According to Demographic and Health Surveys in five African countries (Burkina Faso, Cameroon, Ghana, Kenya, and the United Republic of Tanzania), two thirds of HIV infected couples were serodiscordant, that is only one partner was infected. Condom use was found to be rare: in Burkina Faso, for example, almost 90% of the surveyed cohabiting couples said they did not use a condom the last time they had sex [16]. A separate, community-based study in Uganda has shown that, among serodiscordant heterosexual couples, the uninfected partner has an estimated 8% annual chance of contracting HIV [17]. Strikingly, in about 30–40% of the serodiscordant couples surveyed, the infected partner was female. Indeed, it appears that more than half of the surveyed HIV-infected women who were married or cohabiting had been infected by someone other than their current partner [16].

23.2.2.2 Sex Work

Sex work is an important factor in many of West Africa's HIV epidemics. More than one third (35%) of female sex workers surveyed in 2006 in Mali were living with HIV [18], and infection levels exceeding 20% have been documented among sex workers in Senegal [19] and Burkina Faso [20]. Sex work plays an important, but less central, role in HIV transmission in southern Africa, where exceptionally high background prevalence results in substantial HIV transmission during sexual intercourse unrelated to sex work.

23.2.2.3 Injecting Drug Use

Injecting drug use is a factor to some extent in several of the HIV epidemics in East and southern Africa, including Mauritius, where the use of contaminated injecting equipment is the main cause of HIV infection [21]. In various studies, about half of the injecting drug users tested in the Kenyan cities of Mombasa (50%) [22] and Nairobi (53%) were HIV-positive [23].

23.2.2.4 Sex Between Men

Several recent studies suggest that unprotected anal sex between men is probably a more important factor in the epidemics in sub-Saharan Africa than is commonly thought. In Zambia, one in three (33%) surveyed men who have sex with men tested HIV-positive [24]. In the Kenyan port city of Mombasa, 43% of men who said they had sex only with other men were found to be living with HIV [25]. HIV prevalence of 22% was found among the 463 men who have sex with men who participated in a study in Dakar, Senegal [26].

23.3 Asia

In Asia, an estimated 5.0 million (4.1 million–6.2 million) people were living with HIV in 2007, including the 380,000 (200,000–650,000) people who were newly infected that year. Approximately 380,000 (270,000–490,000) died from AIDS-related illnesses. National HIV infection levels are highest in Southeast Asia (Fig. 23.6), where there are disparate epidemic trends.

23.3.1 Recent Epidemiological Trends

The epidemics in Cambodia, Myanmar, and Thailand all show declines in HIV prevalence, with national HIV prevalence in Cambodia falling from 2% in 1998 to an estimated 0.9% in 2006 [27]. However, epidemics in Indonesia (especially in its Papua province), Pakistan, and Vietnam are growing rapidly. In Vietnam, the estimated number of people living with HIV more than doubled between 2000 and 2005 [28]. New HIV infections are also increasing steadily, although at a much slower pace, in populous countries such as Bangladesh and China.

23.3.2 Main Modes of HIV Transmission

The several modes of HIV transmission make Asia's epidemic one of the world's most diverse.

23.3.2.1 Injecting Drug Use

Injecting drug use is a major risk factor in the epidemics of several Asian countries. Slightly fewer than half the people living with HIV in China in 2006 are believed to have been infected through use of contaminated injecting equipment [29]. High infection levels have been detected among injecting drug users in the northeastern part of India and in several large cities outside the northeast, including in southern state Tamil Nadu, where 24% of drug users were believed to be infected in 2006 [30]. Use of contaminated injecting equipment (as well as unprotected sex between injecting drug users and their regular partners) is also the driving force

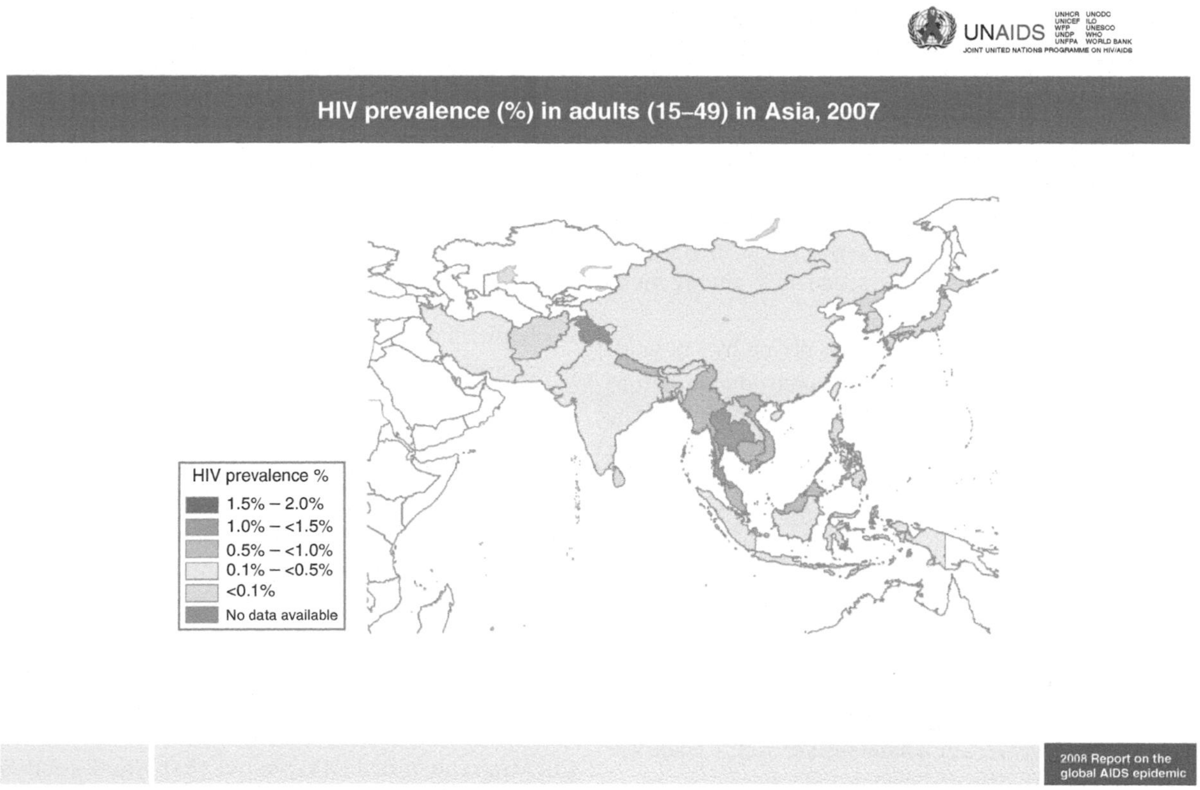

Fig. 23.6 HIV prevalence (%) in adults (15–49) in Asia, 2007

of the epidemic in Vietnam [31], and in Malaysia, where more than two thirds of HIV infections to date have been among injecting drug users [32].

23.3.2.2 Overlap of Sex Work and Injecting Drug Use

An increasing number of women are injecting drugs in China, and substantial proportions of them (about 56% in some cities) also sell sex [33] (Liu et al., 2006). Many male injecting drug users also buy sex, and often do not use condoms [34]. For example, in a 2005–2006 survey in Vietnam, between 20% and 40% of injecting drug users (depending on the area surveyed) said that they had bought sex in the previous 12 months, and up to 60% said that they regularly had sex with a steady partner. Between 16% and 36% said that they consistently used condoms with regular partners [35]. The overlap of injecting drug use and sex work is also a potentially worrisome phenomenon in India and Pakistan [36] (Ministry of Health [Pakistan], 2006).

Projections of the long-term effects of the intersection between injecting drug use and sex work in Jakarta, Indonesia – a metropolis in which an estimated 40,000 people inject drugs [37] show that although the epidemic was initially powered by HIV transmission among injecting drug users, about 15 years later, injecting drug users no longer comprise the majority of people infected with HIV. Indonesia's fast-growing epidemic is spreading quickly into sex-work networks [38, 39].

The most recent HIV outbreak has been in Afghanistan, where narcotics are now also being injected (opium traditionally was either inhaled or ingested orally) [40]. In Kabul, 3% of injecting drug users surveyed were HIV-positive, although this number may well rise because half of the survey participants said they had shared needles or syringes [41].

23.3.2.3 Sex Work

Unprotected sex (commercial and otherwise) is the most important risk factor for the spread of HIV in several parts of Asia. Sex-trafficked women and girls face especially high risks of HIV infection. HIV prevalence of 38% has been found among sex-trafficked females who have been repatriated to Nepal, while up to a half of the women and girls trafficked to Mumbai, India, who have been tested were HIV-positive [42, 43]. In Indian state Karnataka, HIV prevalence of 16% has been found among home-based sex workers, 26% among their street-based peers, and 47% among those working in brothels [44].

Some countries with epidemics driven by sex work have experienced declines in infections, due in part to an increase in the use of condoms during paid sex. For example, Cambodia's decline in HIV prevalence occurred at the same time that consistent condom use during commercial sex rose from 53% in 1997 to 96% in 2003 in Battambang, Kampong Cham, Phnom Penh, Siem Reap, and Sihanoukville [45]. HIV prevalence among sex workers dropped significantly – from 46% in 1998 to 21% in 2003 – among brothel-based sex workers, and from 44% to 8% over the same period among sex workers older than 20 [46]. Similar trends have been observed in Thailand and Tamil Nadu (in southern India), over the past decade.

The serious epidemic under way in Indonesia's Papua province is somewhat anomalous in Asia, in that HIV transmission appears to be occurring mainly due to both unprotected sex with a regular partner and paid sex. In a province-wide population-based survey in 2006, adult HIV prevalence was 2.4% (2.9% among men and 1.9% among women). Given that only 14% of men who buy sex say that they use condoms with sex workers [39], it is not surprising that high HIV infection levels (14–16%) have been found among sex workers in parts of the province [47].

23.3.2.4 Heterosexual Intercourse

Although paid sex has become safer in Cambodia, the spouses and regular partners of people infected due to indulging in commercial sex now account for a growing percentage of new infections [48]. Similarly, Thailand's epidemic has diminished but has also become more heterogeneous [49], and HIV is increasingly affecting people traditionally considered to be at lower risk of infection. About 43% of new infections in 2005 were among women, most of whom were infected by husbands or partners who had had unprotected sex or had used contaminated injecting equipment [50]. In India, a significant proportion of women with HIV have probably been infected by regular partners who paid for sex [51].

23.3.2.5 Sex Between Men

As in most other regions in the world, unprotected anal sex between men is a potentially significant but under-researched factor in the HIV epidemics in Asia. In Bangkok, HIV prevalence among men who have sex with men rose from 17% in 2003 to 28% in 2005 [52], and it is estimated that as many as one in five (21%) new HIV infections in Thailand in 2005 were attributable to unprotected sex between men [53]. In China's younger epidemic, it has been estimated that up to 7% of HIV infections might be attributable to unprotected sex between men [29].

Male sex workers face a particularly high risk of HIV infection. In Vietnam, one in three (33%) male sex workers recruited from more than 70 sites in Ho Chi Minh City tested HIV-positive [54]. Studies earlier this decade documented high HIV infection levels among transgender sex workers in Jakarta, Indonesia, and Phnom Penh, Cambodia, in 2003 [55, 56].

23.4 Eastern Europe and Central Asia

The estimated number of people living with HIV in Eastern Europe and Central Asia rose to 1.5 million (1.1 million–1.9 million) in 2007; almost 90% of those infected live in either the Russian Federation (69%) or Ukraine (29%). It is estimated that 110,000 (67,000–180,000) people in this region became infected with HIV in 2007, while some 58,000 (41,000–88,000) died of AIDS (Fig. 23.7).

23.4.1 Recent Epidemiological Trends

The HIV epidemic in the Russian Federation (already the largest in this region) continues to grow, although apparently at a slower pace than in Ukraine, where annual new HIV diagnoses have more than doubled

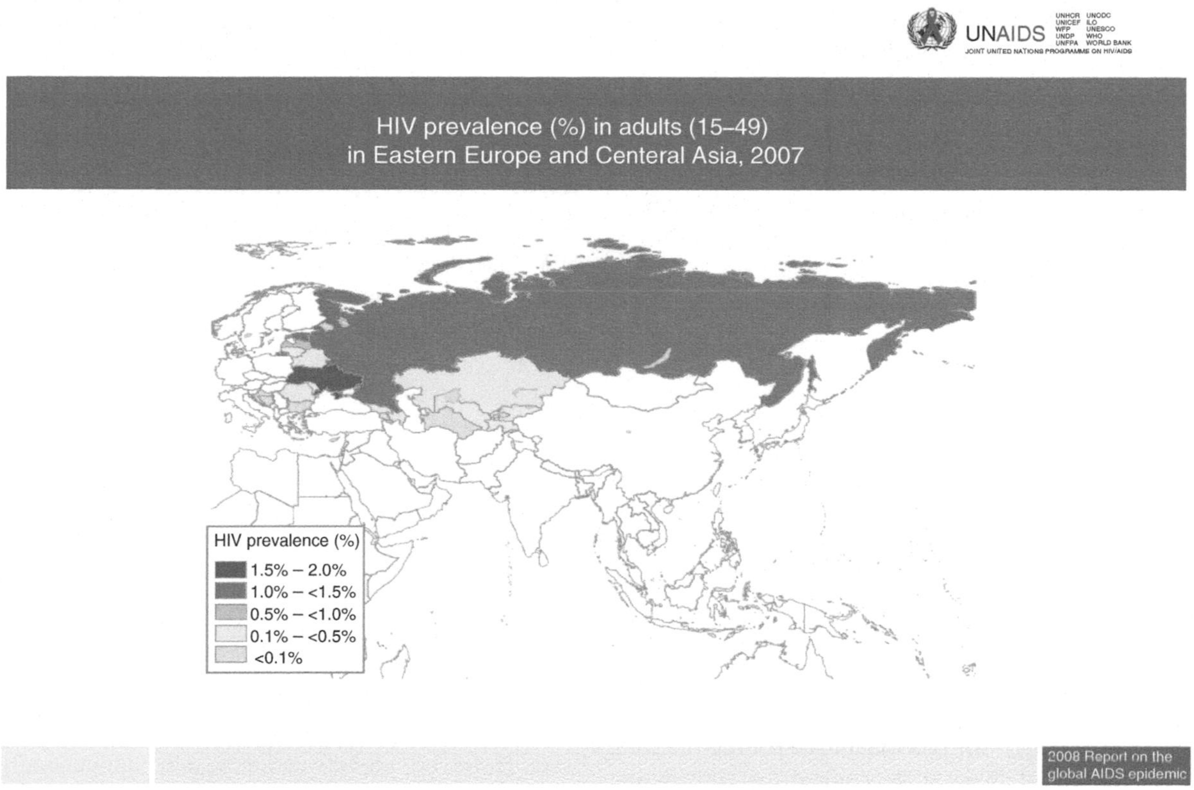

Fig. 23.7 HIV prevalence (%) in adults (15–49) in Eastern Europe and Central Asia, 2007

since 2001 [57, 58]. The annual numbers of newly reported HIV diagnoses are also rising in Azerbaijan, Georgia, Kazakhstan, Kyrgyzstan, the Republic of Moldova, Tajikistan, and Uzbekistan (which now has the largest epidemic in Central Asia).

23.4.2 Main Modes of HIV Transmission

Each of the HIV epidemics in this region is concentrated largely among injecting drug users, sex workers, and their various sexual partners.

23.4.2.1 Injecting Drug Use

Of the new HIV cases reported in this region in 2006 for which information is available on the mode of transmission, about 62% were attributed to injecting drug use. In the Russian Federation, HIV prevalence among injecting drug users ranges from 3% in Volgograd to more than 70% in Biysk [59]. Prevalence is also high among injecting drug users in Ukraine; among surveyed injecting drug users in national diagnostic studies prevalence increased from 11% in 2001 to 17% in 2006 [58]; also, local HIV prevalence as high as 63% has been found [60]. High infection levels have been detected among injecting drug users in Tashkent, Uzbekistan (30%, 2003–2004) [58, 61]; in Zlobin, Belarus (52%) [58]; and in Kazakhstan [62].

23.4.2.2 The Overlap of Sex Work and Injecting Drug Use

The overlap of sex work and injecting drug use features prominently in the region's epidemics. For example, 39% of female sex workers in the Samara oblast, Russian Federation (Population Services International, 2007), 37% in a St. Petersburg study [63], and up to 30% of sex workers participating in other studies [64] said that they had injected drugs.

Nowhere in this region have HIV epidemics reached a stage where they are likely to evolve independently of HIV transmission among injecting drug users and sex workers.

23.4.2.3 Heterosexual Intercourse

As the epidemics in this region evolve, the proportion of women infected with HIV is growing. About 40% of newly registered HIV cases in Eastern Europe and Central Asia in 2006 were among women [58]. Exceptionally high HIV prevalence was reported among pregnant women in several regions of central and eastern Ukraine. Three large, densely populated regions reported HIV prevalence among pregnant women exceeding 1% including Odessa oblast, Kiev oblast, and Mykolaev oblast [65]. Most of these women were probably infected during sex with a partner who had been infected through use of contaminated drug-injecting equipment [58, 66]. In the region overall, it is estimated that some 35% of HIV-positive women were infected through use of contaminated drug-injecting equipment, and about 50% acquired the virus during unprotected sex with drug-injecting partners [67].

23.4.2.4 Sex Between Men

In 2006, less than 1% of newly registered HIV cases (where the mode of transmission was known) were attributed to unprotected sex between men [58]; this is probably an underestimate of the role of this mode of HIV transmission. In the Russian Federation, HIV prevalence found in this population group has varied from 0.9% in Moscow [68, 69] to 9% in Nizhni Novgorod in 2006 [70]. Of men who have sex with men who participated in a study in Tashkent, Uzbekistan, 11% tested HIV-positive in 2005 [71], as did 5% of their peers in a study in Georgia [72].

23.5 Caribbean

An estimated 230,000 (210,000–270,000) people were living with HIV in the Caribbean in 2007 (about three quarters of them in the Dominican Republic and Haiti), while an estimated 20,000 (16,000–25,000) people were newly infected with HIV in this region, and some 14,000 (11,000–16,000) people died of AIDS (Fig. 23.8).

23.5.1 Recent Epidemiological Trends

HIV surveillance systems are still inadequate in several Caribbean countries, but available information indicates that most of the epidemics in the region appear to have stabilized, while a few have declined in urban areas. The latter trend is especially evident in the Dominican Republic and Haiti. In the Dominican Republic, for example, HIV prevalence declined from 1.0% in 2002 to an estimated 0.8% in 2007 [73].

23.5.2 Main Modes of HIV Transmission

The main mode of HIV transmission in the Caribbean is unprotected heterosexual intercourse, paid or otherwise. However, sex between men, although generally denied by society, is also a significant factor in several national epidemics.

23.5.2.1 Heterosexual Intercourse

In Haiti, which has the biggest epidemic in the Caribbean, HIV prevalence among pregnant women attending antenatal clinics declined from 5.9% in 1996 to 3.1% in 2004 [74], and has subsequently remained stable [75]. Although positive behavior changes appear to be at least partly responsible for the decline [74, 76, 77], significant levels of high-risk behavior have been documented in Haiti's rural areas and among young people [74, 76, 78].

23.5.2.2 Sex Work

As HIV prevalence has declined in the Dominican Republic, surveys have indicated that more sex workers are protecting themselves (and their clients) against HIV infection, especially in the main urban and tourist centers [79]. Among female sex workers, HIV prevalence of 9% has been documented in Jamaica and 31% in Guyana [80–83].

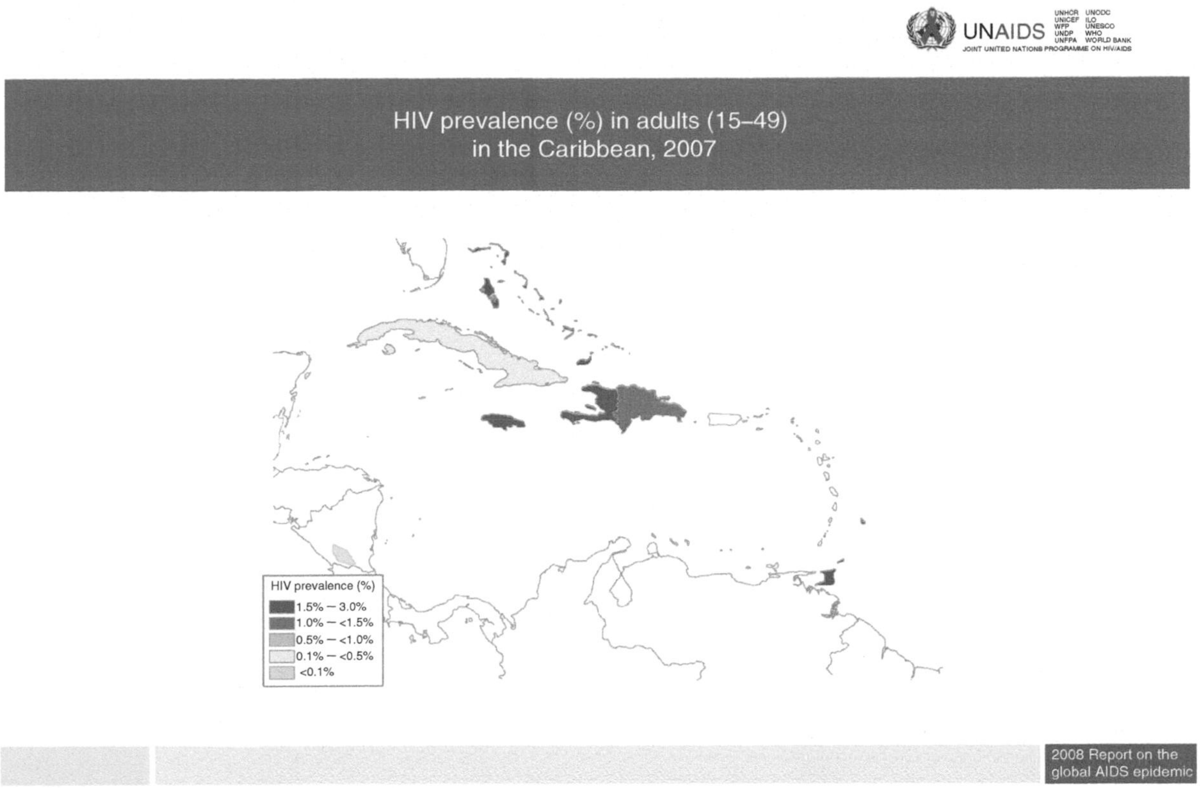

Fig. 23.8 HIV prevalence (%) in adults (15–49) in the Caribbean, 2007

23.5.2.3 Sex Between Men

As many as one in eight (12%) reported HIV infections in the region occurred through unprotected sex between men [84, 85]. Unprotected sex between men is the main mode of HIV transmission in Cuba, where men account for more than 80% of all reported HIV cases [86], and in Dominica, where almost three quarters (71% of the 319 HIV infections reported to date) have been in men [87]. Studies have found HIV prevalence of 20% among men who have sex with men in Trinidad and Tobago [88], 21% in Guyana's Region 4 [89], and 11% in the Dominican Republic [90].

23.6 Latin America

New HIV infections in 2007 totaled an estimated 140,000 (88,000–190,000), bringing to 1.7 million (1.5 million–2.1 million) the number of people living with HIV in this region. An estimated 63,000 (49,000–98,000) people died of AIDS last year (Fig. 23.9).

23.6.1 Recent Epidemiological Trends

The overall levels of HIV infections in Latin America have changed little in the past decade.

23.6.2 Main Modes of HIV Transmission

HIV transmission in this region is occurring primarily among men who have sex with men, sex workers, and (to a lesser extent) injecting drug users.

23.6.2.1 Sex Between Men

High HIV prevalence has been documented among men who have sex with men in several countries: 18–22% in Peru, in studies conducted between 1996 and 2002 [91, 92]; 14% in Buenos Aires, Argentina, in 2000–2001 [93]; 22% in Montevideo, Uruguay [94]; 15% in four Bolivian cities and in Quito,

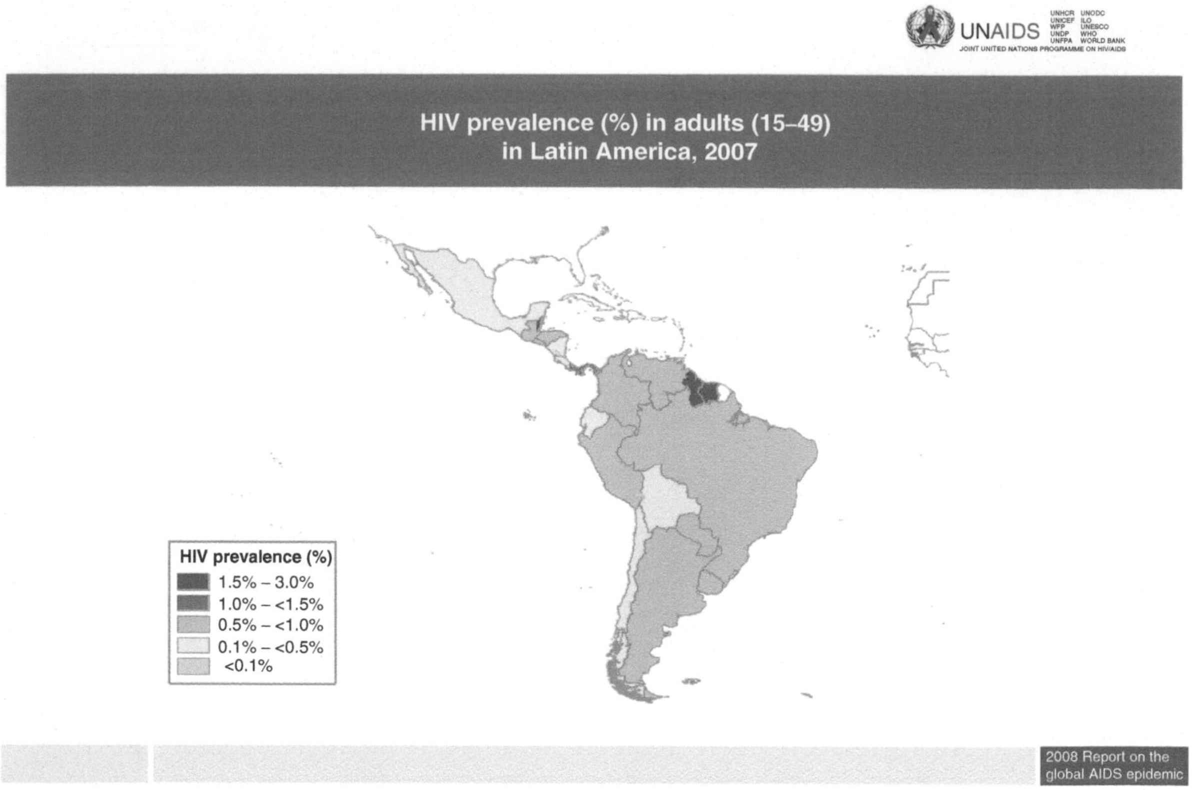

Fig. 23.9 HIV prevalence (%) in adults (15–49) in Latin America, 2007

Ecuador [94]; and 10–25% in some cities in Colombia [95, 96].

Research has uncovered hidden epidemics of HIV among men who have sex with men in several Central American countries, including Belize, Costa Rica, El Salvador, Guatemala, Mexico, Nicaragua, and Panama [97, 98]. More than half (57%) of the HIV diagnoses to date in Mexico have been attributed to unprotected sex between men [99]. Between one quarter and one third of men who have sex with men in those countries (except for Panama) also have sex with women – and between 30% and 40% of those men said that they had had unprotected sex with both men and women in the previous month [98].

23.6.2.2 Sex Work

Across South America, levels of HIV infection among female sex workers tend to be much lower than those among men who have sex with men [100]. HIV prevalence among female sex workers has been found to be 10% in Honduras, 4% in Guatemala, and 3% in El Salvador [98]. However, there is recent evidence of a steep decline in HIV prevalence among female sex workers in Honduras, where condom promotion efforts were stepped up in recent years. [101, 102].

23.6.2.3 Injecting Drug Use

HIV transmission as a result of injecting drug use still features in several of South America's epidemics. Regionally, this mode of transmission appears to be accounting for a smaller number of new infections than was the case previously. In Argentina, injecting drug use accounted for only about 5% of new HIV infections in Buenos Aires between 2003 and 2005 [103], and HIV infection levels in injecting drug users have declined in some Brazilian cities [104–106]. Notable HIV transmission has been occurring among injecting drug users in the capitals of Paraguay (12% HIV-positive in various surveys) and Uruguay (19% HIV-positive) [107, 108].

23.6.2.4 Heterosexual Intercourse

Increasing numbers of women are becoming infected in several countries in the region, including Argentina, Brazil, Peru, and Uruguay [91, 103, 109–111]. In Uruguay, for example, unprotected sex (mostly heterosexual) is believed to account for approximately two thirds of newly reported HIV cases [94]. Most of the women are being infected by male sexual partners who acquired HIV during unprotected sex with another man or through use of contaminated drug-injecting equipment [91, 103, 112].

23.7 North America and Western and Central Europe

The USA accounted for an estimated 1.2 million (690,000 – 1.9 million) of the 2.0 million (1.4 million–2.8 million) people living with HIV in North America, and in Western and Central Europe in 2007. Overall in those regions, 81,000 (30,000–170,000) people were newly infected with HIV in 2007. Comparatively few people – 31,000 in a range of 16,000–67,000 – died of AIDS last year (Fig. 23.10).

23.7.1 Recent Epidemiological Trends

In North America, annual numbers of new HIV diagnoses have remained relatively stable over recent years, but access to life-prolonging antiretroviral therapy has led to an increase in the estimated number of people living with HIV [113, 114]. In Western Europe, new HIV diagnoses are increasing, as is the total number of people living with HIV (the latter also because of wide access to antiretroviral treatment).

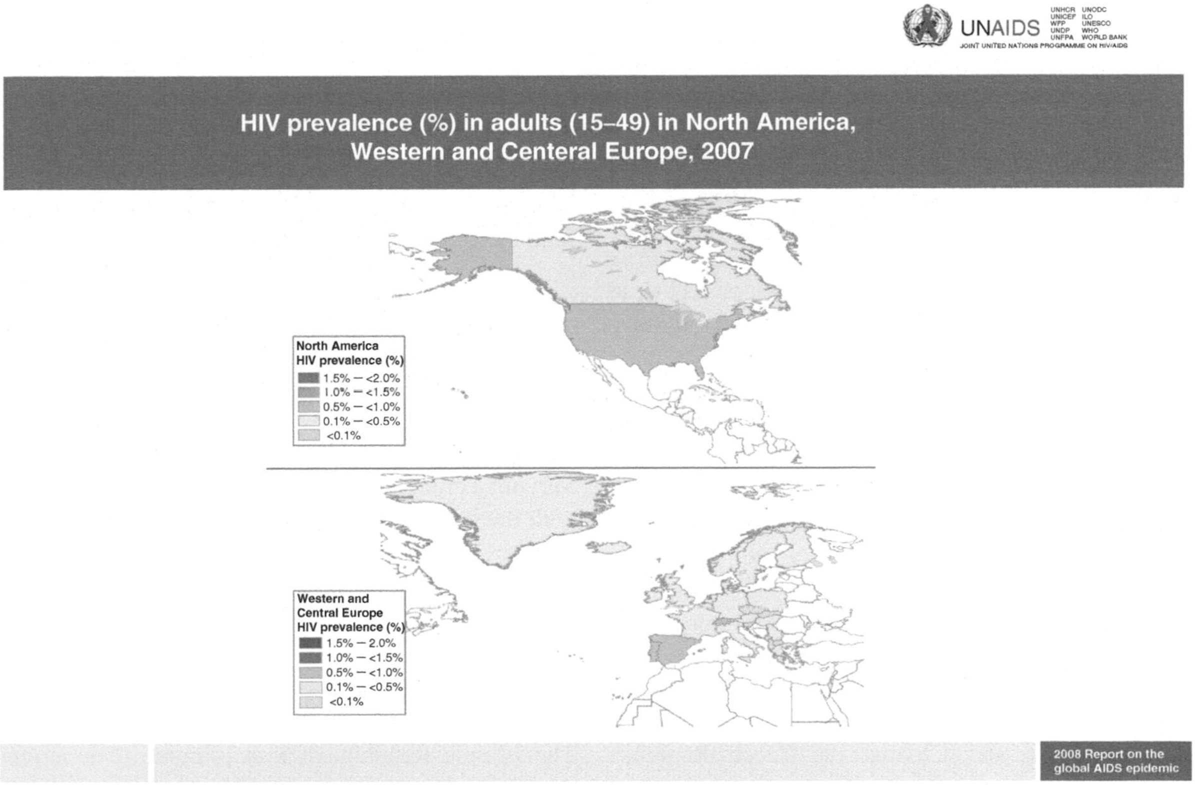

Fig. 23.10 HIV prevalence (%) in adults (15–49) in North America, Western and Central Europe, 2007

23.7.2 Main Modes of HIV Transmission

These high-income countries have diverse epidemics, although their epidemiological profiles have diverged as the epidemic has evolved. In general, injecting drug use is accounting for a smaller share of new HIV infections than before.

23.7.2.1 Sex Between Men

Unprotected sex between men is still the main mode of HIV transmission in both Canada and the USA – 40% of new HIV diagnoses in Canada in 2006 and 53% in the USA in 2005 [114, 115]. Men who have sex with men continue to be the population group most at risk of acquiring HIV within most Western European countries. Indeed, the number of new HIV diagnoses attributed to unprotected sex between men has increased sharply in recent years in Western Europe, and appears to be associated with reported increases in higher-risk unprotected sex between men in several countries [116–119]. In Germany, for example, the number of new HIV diagnoses among men who have sex with men rose by 96% (to 1,370) between 2002 and 2006 [120].

23.7.2.2 Heterosexual Intercourse

About one third (32%) of newly diagnosed HIV infections and AIDS cases in the USA in 2005 were attributable to high-risk heterosexual intercourse [114], as were 33% of new HIV infections in Canada in 2006. However, in Canada, a substantial proportion of those infections were in people born in countries with high HIV prevalence (mainly sub-Saharan Africa and the Caribbean) [115, 121]. A similar situation was seen in Western Europe, where unprotected heterosexual intercourse accounted for the largest share (42%) of new HIV diagnoses in Western Europe in 2006 (compared with the 29% that were attributed to unprotected sex between men). Unprotected heterosexual intercourse is the main reported mode of transmission in most countries of Central Europe, except for Estonia, Latvia, Lithuania, and Poland, where the main mode is injecting drug use, and Croatia, the Czech Republic, Hungary, and Slovenia, where it is unprotected sex between men [58, 122–124].

23.7.2.3 Injecting Drug Use

Transmission by multiple use of contaminated injecting equipment accounts for 18% of new HIV diagnoses in the USA (2005) and 19% in Canada (2006) [114, 115]. In Western Europe, a diminishing proportion of HIV diagnoses (6%) are related to the use of contaminated injecting equipment in 2006 [125]. In Denmark and the Netherlands, the number of new HIV diagnoses among injecting drug users fell by 72% and by 91%, respectively in 2002–2006 [125]. In Central Europe, too, newly reported HIV diagnoses in injecting drug users have decreased [125].

23.8 Middle East and North Africa

The limited HIV information available for the Middle East and North Africa indicates that approximately 380,000 [280,000–510,000] people were living with HIV in 2007, including the 40,000 [20,000–66,000] people who were newly infected with the virus in that year (2007) (Fig. 23.11).

23.8.1 Recent Epidemiological Trends

With the exception of the Sudan, the epidemics in this region are comparatively small.

23.8.2 Primary Sources of HIV Transmission

Varying combinations of risk factors are associated with the epidemic; chief among them are unprotected paid sex and the use of contaminated drug-injecting equipment [126].

23.8.2.1 Injecting Drug Use

The Islamic Republic of Iran is home to a serious drug-related epidemic, with HIV prevalence of between 15% and 23% documented among male injecting

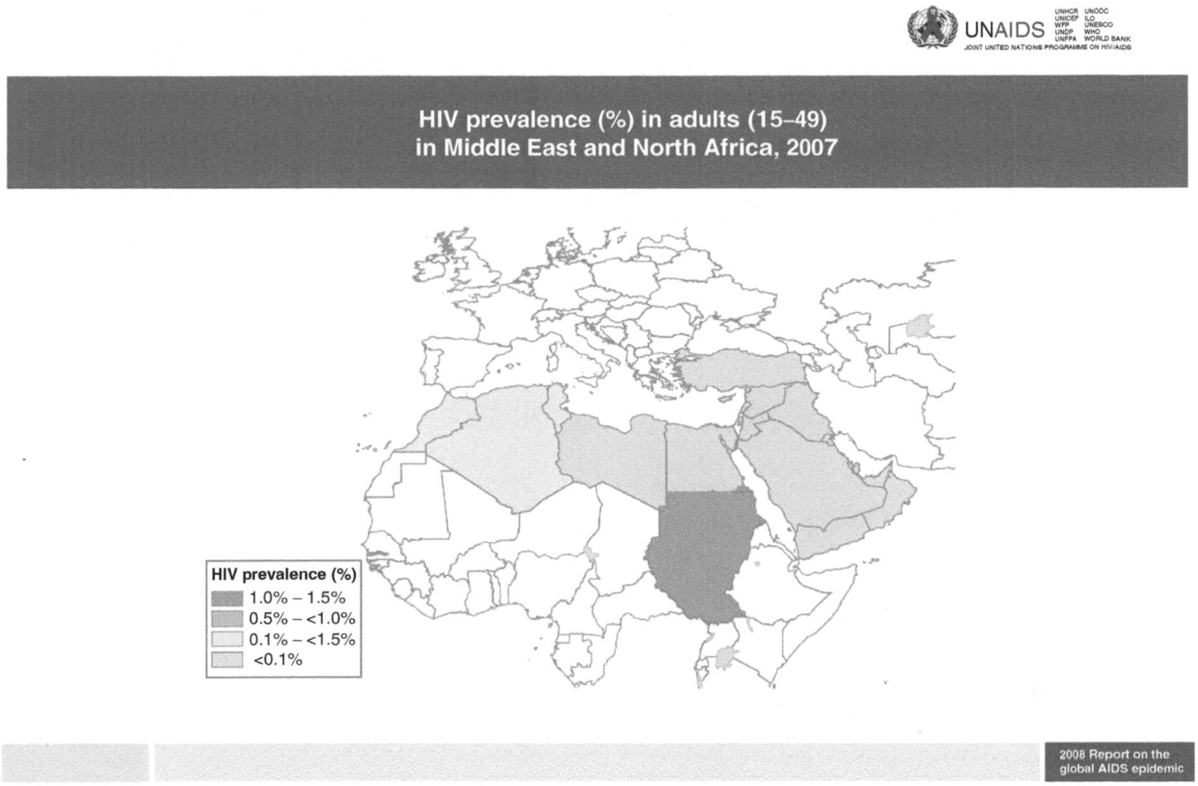

Fig. 23.11 HIV prevalence (%) in adults (15–49) in Middle East and North Africa, 2007

drug users who make use of drop-in or drug-treatment services in Tehran [127, 128]. Exposure to contaminated drug-injecting equipment is also the main route of HIV transmission in the Libyan Arab Jamahiriya and Tunisia, and it features in the epidemics of Algeria, Morocco, and the Syrian Arab Republic [126, 129, 130].

23.8.2.2 Overlap of Injecting Drug Use and Sex Work

A combination of injecting drug use and sex work may be facilitating the spread of HIV in Algeria, Egypt, Lebanon, and the Syrian Arab Republic, where one third or more of surveyed injecting drug users said that they recently either bought or sold sex. In the Syrian Arab Republic, more than half (53%) of the drug users interviewed in one study said they sold sex, and 40% of those users said they never used condoms [131].

23.8.2.3 Heterosexual Intercourse

Unprotected heterosexual intercourse is the main factor in Sudan's epidemic – the most extensive in the region – with national adult HIV prevalence estimated at 1.4% (1.0–2.0%) in 2007. In several other countries, increasing numbers of women are being diagnosed with HIV, most of them infected by husbands or boyfriends who had acquired HIV through injecting drug use or paid sex. In Morocco, for example, one third (33%) of women diagnosed with AIDS were married [132].

23.8.2.4 Sex Between Men

Although socially stigmatized and officially censured throughout the region, unprotected sex between men is probably a factor in several of the region's epidemics. A recent study in Egypt, for example, found that 6.2% of men who have sex with men were infected with HIV

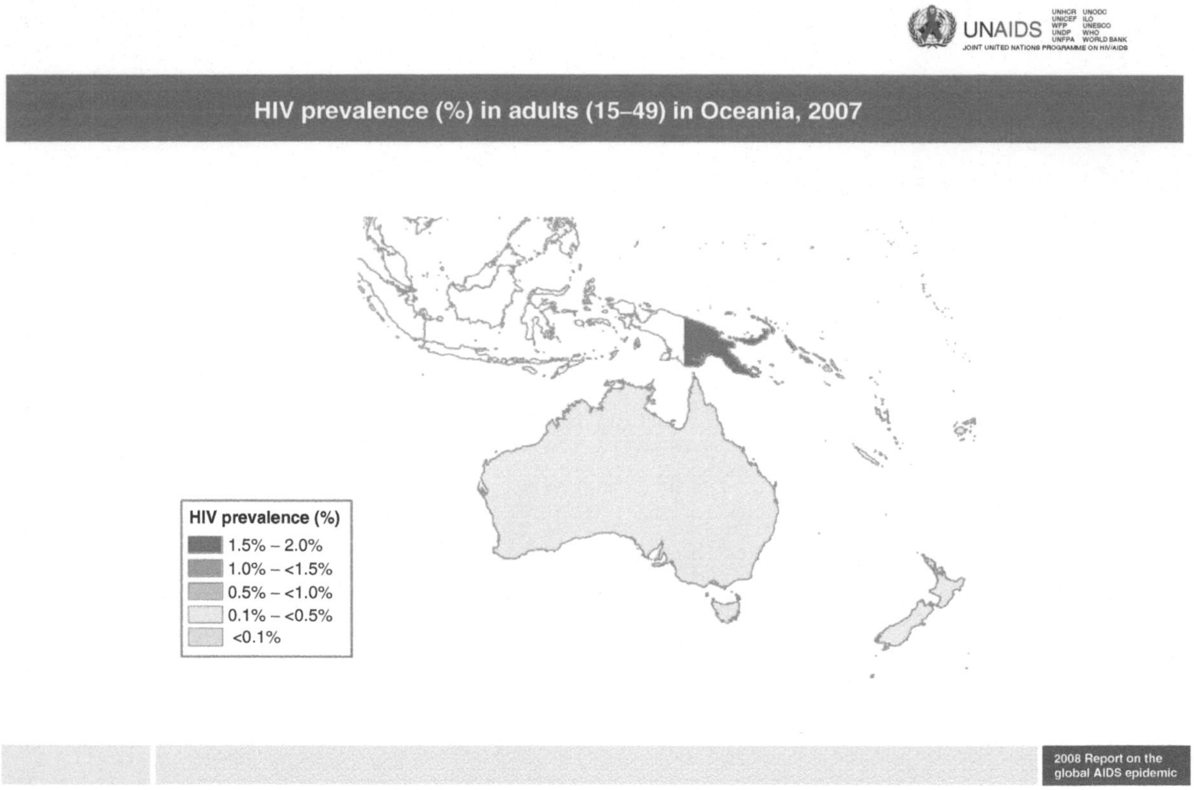

Fig. 23.12 HIV prevalence (%) in adults (15–49) in Oceania, 2007

[133], while 9% prevalence was found among their counterparts in state of Khartoum, Sudan [134].

23.9 Oceania

Overall, an estimated 74,000 (66,000–93,000) people were living with HIV in Oceania in 2007, about 13,000 (12,000–15,000) of whom were newly infected in the same year (Fig. 23.12).

23.9.1 Recent Epidemiological Trends

Most of the region's epidemics are small, except in Papua New Guinea, where the annual number of new HIV diagnoses more than doubled between 2002 and 2006, when 4,017 new HIV cases were reported [135].

23.9.2 Primary Sources of HIV Transmission

23.9.2.1 Heterosexual Intercourse

Unprotected heterosexual intercourse is the main mode of HIV transmission in Papua New Guinea [136], and unprotected paid sex in particular appears to be a central factor. In one recent survey, 60–70% of truck drivers and military personnel and 33% of port workers said they had bought sex in the previous year [136]. Community-based studies in ten provinces have shown that about 40% of participants were infected with at least one sexually transmitted infection [137].

23.9.2.2 Sex Between Men

Unprotected sex between men is the primary cause of HIV infection in Australia [138] and New Zealand

[139]. After declining sharply in the 1990s, new HIV diagnoses in Australia have increased, from the 763 reported in 2000 to 998 reported in 2006. There is evidence that the prevalence of unprotected sex between men has increased or remained at high levels in recent years in several cities including Adelaide, Brisbane, Canberra, Perth [140], and Sydney [141]. Unprotected sex between men also could be a factor in Papua New Guinea's epidemic. When surveyed, more than one in ten (12%) young men said they had had sex with men, and condom use was rare [142].

Take-Home Pearls

- Globally, there were an estimated 33 million [30 million–36 million] people living with HIV in 2007. The annual number of new HIV infections declined from 3.0 million [2.6 million–3.5 million] in 2001 to 2.7 million [2.2 million–3.2 million] in 2007.
- Overall, 2.0 million [1.8 million–2.3 million] people died due to AIDS in 2007, compared with an estimated 1.7 million [1.5 million–2.3 million] in 2001.
- While the percentage of people living with HIV has stabilized since 2000, the overall number of people living with HIV has steadily increased as new infections occur each year, HIV treatments extend life, and as new infections still outnumber AIDS deaths.
- Southern Africa continues to bear a disproportionate share of the global burden of HIV: 35% of HIV infections and 38% of AIDS deaths in 2007 occurred in that subregion. Altogether, sub-Saharan Africa is home to 67% of all people living with HIV.
- Women account for half of all people living with HIV worldwide, and nearly 60% of HIV infections in sub-Saharan Africa. Over the last 10 years, the proportion of women among people living with HIV has remained stable globally, but has increased in many regions.
- Young people aged 15–24 account for an estimated 45% of new HIV infections worldwide.
- An estimated 370 000 [330 000–410 000] children younger than 15 years became infected with HIV in 2007. Globally, the number of children younger than 15 years living with HIV increased from 1.6 million [1.4 million–2.1 million] in 2001 to 2.0 million [1.9 million–2.3 million] in 2007. Almost 90% live in sub-Saharan Africa.

References

1. UNAIDS/WHO. 2008 Report on the global AIDS epidemic. http://www.unaids.org/en/KnowledgeCentre/HIVData/GlobalReport/2008/
2. Ministry of Health and Child Welfare [Zimbabwe]. 2006 ANC preliminary report. Harare. Ministry of Health and Child Welfare [Zimbabwe] (2007).
3. Ministry of Health [Botswana]. 2006 Botswana Second-Generation HIV/AIDS Surveillance Technical Report. Gabarone (2006).
4. Heaton, L., Fowler, T., Palamuleni, M.: The HIV/AIDS epidemic in Malawi – putting the epidemic in context. XVI International AIDS Conference, Toronto, Ontario. 13–18 August (Abstract CDC0062) (2006).
5. Sandoy, I.F. et al.: Associations between sexual behaviour change in young people and decline in HIV prevalence in Zambia. BMC Public Health, 23 April. http://www.biomedcentral.com/content/pdf/1471-2458-7–60.pdf (2007). Accessed 8 May 2008.
6. Ministry of Health and Population [Malawi]: HIV and syphilis sero survey and national HIV prevalence estimates report. Ministry of Health and Population Malawi, Lilongwe (2005)
7. Ministry of Health [Zambia]: Zambia Antenatal Clinic Sentinel Surveillance Report, 1994–2004. November. Ministry of Health [Zambia]. Ministry of Health [Zambia], Lusaka (2005)
8. Michelo, C. et al.: Steep HIV prevalence declines among young people in selected Zambian communities: population-based observations (1995–2003). BMC Public Health, 10 November, http://www.biomedcentral.com/1471–2458/6/279 (2006). Accessed 8 May 2008.
9. Department of Health [South Africa]: National HIV and syphilis antenatal prevalence survey, South Africa 2006. Department of Health [South Africa], Pretoria (2007)
10. Central Statistical Office [Swaziland] and Macro International Inc (2007). Swaziland Demographic and Health Survey 2006–2007: preliminary report. Calverton (June).
11. Conselho Nacional de Combate ao HIV/SIDA: Relatório de actividades por 2005. Maputo, Ministério de Saúde (2006)

12. Asamoah-Odei, E., Garcia-Celleja, J.M., Boerma, T.: HIV prevalence and trends in sub-Saharan: no decline and large subregional differences. Lancet **364**, 35–40 (2004)
13. Kirungi, W.L., et al.: Trends in antenatal HIV prevalence in urban Uganda associated with uptake of preventive sexual behaviour. Sex. Transm. Infect. **82**(Suppl. 1), 136–141 (2006)
14. Uganda Bureau of Statistics, Macro International Inc: Uganda Demographic and Health Survey 2006. Uganda Bureau of Statistics, Macro International Inc., Calverton, MD (2007)
15. Federal Ministry of Health [Nigeria] (2006). The 2005 national HIV seroprevalence sentinel survey among pregnant women attending antenatal clinics in Nigeria: summary position paper. Abuja (April). Federal Ministry of Health [Nigeria].
16. de Walque, D.: Sero-discordant couples in five African countries: implications for prevention strategies. Popul. Dev. Rev. **33**(3), 501–523 (2007)
17. Wawer, M.J., et al.: Rates of HIV-1 transmission per coital act, by stage of HIV-1 infection, in Rakai, Uganda. J. Infect. Dis. **191**, 1403–1409 (2005)
18. Ministère de la Santé du Mali (2006). Résumé des résultats de l'enquête ISBS 2006. Bamakó. Ministère de la Santé et de l'Hygiène Publique de la Côte d'Ivoire, CDC/RETRO–CI/MEASURE Evaluation (2007). Enquête de surveillance sentinelle du VIH de 2005. Abidjan.
19. Gomes do Espirito Santo, M.E., Etheredge, G.D.: Male clients of brothel prostitutes as a bridge for HIV infection between high risk and low risk groups of women in Senegal. Sex. Transm. Infect. **81**, 342–344 (2005)
20. Kintin, F.D. et al.: Enquete de prevalence des IST/VIH et des comportements sexuels chez les travailleuses due sexe et leurs partenaires masculins a Ouagadougou, Burkina Faso. Ouagadougou, Conseil national de lutte contre le sida et les IST, CIDA, CCSID (November) (2004).
21. Sulliman, F.T., Ameerberg, S.A.G., Dhannoo, M.I.: Report of the Rapid Situation Assessment and Responses on Drug Use in Mauritius and Rodrigues. Ministry of Health, Mauritius (2004)
22. Ndetei, D.: Study on the Assessment of the Linkages Between Drug Abuse, Injecting Drug Abuse and HIV/AIDS in Kenya: A Rapid Situation Assessment 2004. United Nations Office on Drugs and Crime, Nairobi (2004)
23. Odek-Ogunde, M.: World Health Organization Phase II Drug Injecting Study: Behavioural and Seroprevalence (HIV, HBV, HCV) Survey Among Injecting Drug Users in Nairobi. Nairobi, WHO (2004)
24. Zulu, K.P., Bulawo, N.D., Zulu, W.: Understanding HIV risk behaviour among men who have sex with men in Zambia. XVI International AIDS Conference, Toronto, Ontario. 13–18 August. (Abstract WEPE0719) (2006).
25. Sanders, E.J., et al.: HIV-1 infection in high risk men who have sex with men in Mombassa, Kenya. AIDS **21**, 2513–2520 (2007)
26. Wade, A.S., et al.: HIV infection and sexually transmitted infections among men who have sex with men in Senegal. AIDS **19**(18), 2133–2140 (2005)
27. National Centre for HIV/AIDS, Dermatology and STIs (2007). HIV sentinel surveillance (HSS) 2006/2007: results, trends and estimates. Phnom Penh. National Centre for HIV/AIDS, Dermatology and STIs.
28. Ministry of Health [Vietnam]. HIV/AIDS estimates and projections 2005–2010. Hanoi, General Department of Preventive Medicine and HIV/AIDS Control, Ministry of Health (2005).
29. Lu, F. et al.: HIV/AIDS epidemic in China: Increasing or decreasing? XVI International AIDS Conference, Toronto, Ontario. 13 – 18 August. (Abstract MOPE0462) (2006).
30. National Institute of Health and Family Welfare, National AIDS Control Organisation (2007). Annual HIV Sentinel Surveillance Country Report 2006. New Delhi. National Institute of Health and Family Welfare, National AIDS Control Organisation.
31. Tuang, N.A., et al.: Human immunodeficiency virus (HIV) infection patterns and risk behaviours in different population groups and provinces in Vietnam. Bull. World Health Organ. **85**(1), 35–41 (2007)
32. Reid, G., Kamarulzaman, A., Sran, S.K.: Malaysia and harm reduction: the challenges and responses. Int. J. Drug Policy **18**(2), 136–140 (2007)
33. Choi, S.Y.P., Cheung, Y.W., Chen, K.: Gender and HIV risk behaviour among intravenous drug users in Sichuan province, China. Soc. Sci. Med. **62**(7), 1672–1684 (2006)
34. Hesketh, T. et al.: Risk behaviours in injecting drug users in Yunnan province, China: lessons for policy. XVI International AIDS Conference, Toronto, Ontario. 13–18 August. (Abstract CDD0591) (2006).
35. Ministry of Health [Vietnam]: Results from the HIV/STI integrated biological and behavioural surveillance (IBBS) in Vietnam, 2005–2006. Ministry of Health [Vietnam], Hanoi (2006)
36. Chandrasekaran, P., et al.: Containing HIV/AIDS in India: the unfinished agenda. Lancet Infect. Dis. **6**(8), 508–521 (2006)
37. Commission on AIDS in Asia: Redefining AIDS in Asia: Crafting An Effective Response. Oxford University Press, New Delhi (2008)
38. Statistics Indonesia and Ministry of Health [Indonesia]: Situation of Risk Behaviour for HIV in Indonesia. Results of BSS 2004–2005. Statistics Indonesia and Ministry of Health, Jakarta (2006)
39. Ministry of Health [Indonesia] and Statistics Indonesia: Risk Behavior and HIV Prevalence in Tanah Papua, 2006. Ministry of Health [Indonesia] and Statistics Indonesia, Jakarta (2007)
40. UNODC: Afghanistan Drug Use Survey 2005. Kabul, UNODC (2005)
41. Todd, C.S., et al.: HIV, Hepatitis C, and Hepatitis B infections and associated risk behavior in injection drug users in Kabul, Afghanistan. Emerg. Infect. Dis. **13**(9), 1327–1331 (2007)
42. Silverman, J.G., et al.: HIV prevalence and predictors among rescued sex-trafficked women and girls in Mumbai, India. J. Acquir. Immune Defic. Syndr. **43**(5), 588–593 (2006)
43. Silverman, J.G., et al.: HIV prevalence and predictors of infection in sex-trafficked Nepalese girls and women. JAMA **298**(5), 536–542 (2007)
44. Ramesh, B. et al.: Sex work typology and risk for HIV in female sex workers: findings from an integrated biological and behavioural assessment in the southern Indian state of Karnataka. XVI International AIDS Conference, Toronto, Ontario. 13 – 18 August. (Abstract WEAC0305) (2006).

45. Gorbach, P.M., et al.: Changing behaviors and patterns among Cambodian sex workers: 1997–2003. J. Acquir. Immune Defic. Syndr. **42**(2), 242–247 (2006)
46. Ministry of Health [Cambodia]. Report on HIV sentinel surveillance in Cambodia, 2003. Phnom Penh (July). Ministry of Health [Cambodia] (2006).
47. National AIDS Commission [Indonesia]: Country Report on the Follow Up to the Declaration of Commitment on HIV/AIDS (UNGASS) 2004–2005. National AIDS Commission [Indonesia], Jakarta (2006)
48. National Centre for HIV/AIDS, Dermatology and STIs: HIV Sentinel Surveillance (HSS) 2003: Trends Results, and Estimates. National Centre for HIV/AIDS, Dermatology and STIs, Phnom Penh (2004)
49. Over, M., et al.: The economics of effective AIDS treatment in Thailand. AIDS **21**(Suppl. 4), S105–S116 (2007)
50. WHO: HIV/AIDS in the South-East Asia region. New Delhi, WHO Regional Office for South-East Asia (March). http://www.searo.who.int/hiv-aids (2007). Accessed 8 May 2008.
51. Anonymous: India in the spotlight (editorial). Lancet **367**:1876 (2006).
52. Van Griensven, F., et al.: HIV prevalence among populations of men who have sex with men – Thailand, 2003 and 2005. Morb. Mortal. Wkly Rep. **55**(31), 844–848 (2006)
53. Gouws, E. et al.: Short-term estimates of adult HIV incidence by mode of transmission: Kenya and Thailand as examples. Sex. Transm. Infec. **82**(Suppl. 3):iii51–iii5 (2006); WHO: HIV/AIDS in the South-East Asia region. New Delhi, WHO Regional Office for South-East Asia (March), http://www.searo.who.int/hiv-aids (2007). Accessed 8 May 2008.
54. Nguyen, T.A., et al.: Prevalence and risk factors associated with HIV infection among men having sex with men in Ho Chi Minh City, Vietnam. AIDS Behav. **12**(3), 476–482 (2008)
55. Girault, P., et al.: HIV, STIs and sexual behaviors among men who have sex with men in Phnom Penh, Cambodia. AIDS Educ. Prev. **6**(1), 31–44 (2004)
56. Pisani, E., et al.: HIV, syphilis infection, and sexual practices among transgenders, male sex workers, and other men who have sex with men in Jakarta, Indonesia. Sex. Transm. Infect. **80**(6), 536–540 (2004)
57. UNAIDS Reference Group on Estimates, Modelling and Projections: Improving parameter estimation, projection methods, uncertainty estimation, and epidemic classification, http://www.epidem.org/Publications/Prague2006report.pdf (2006). Accessed 24 April 2008.
58. EuroHIV: HIV/AIDS surveillance in Europe: mid-year report 2007, No 76. Institut de Veille Sanitaire. Saint-Maurice (No 76), http://www.eurohiv.org (2007). Accessed 8 May 2008.
59. Pasteur Scientific and Research Institute of Epidemiology: Epidemiological Surveillance and Monitoring of HIV in Risk Behaviour Groups in Volgogradskaya Oblast. Pasteur Scientific and Research Institute of Epidemiology, St. Petersburg (2005)
60. Ministry of Health [Ukraine] (2007). HIV infection in Ukraine: Information bulletin no. 27. Kyiv, Ukraine. Ministry of Health [Ukraine].
61. Sanchez, J.L., et al.: High HIV prevalence and risk factors among injection drug users in Tashkent, Uzbekistan, 2003–2004. Drug Alcohol Depend. **82**(Suppl. 1), S15–S22 (2006)
62. Ministry of Health [Kazakhstan] et al.: Results of investigation of the real situation with drug abuse in Kazakhstan. Almaty (in Russian) (2005).
63. Benotsch, E.G., et al.: Drug use and sexual risk behaviors among female Russian IDUs who exchange sex for money or drugs. Int. J. STD AIDS **15**(5), 343–347 (2004)
64. Rhodes, T., et al.: HIV transmission and HIV prevention associated with injecting drug use in the Russian Federation. Int. J. Drug Policy **15**(1), 1–16 (2004)
65. Ministry of Health [Ukraine]: Ukraine: National Report on Monitoring Progress Towards the UNGASS Declaration of Commitment on HIV/AIDS (Reporting Period: January 2006–December 2007). Kyiv, Ukraine. Ministry of Health [Ukraine] (2008).
66. Scherbinska, A.: HIV infection in Ukraine: a review of epidemiological data. XVI International AIDS Conference, Toronto, Ontario. 13–18 August. (Abstract CDC0398), (2006).
67. EuroHIV: HIV/AIDS surveillance in Europe: end-year report 2005. Saint-Maurice, Institut de Veille Sanitaire (No 73) (2006).
68. Smolskaya, T.T. et al.: Sentinel HIV surveillance among risk groups in Azerbaijan, Moldova and Russian Federation. WHO Regional office for Europe. Ministry of Health [Ukraine] (2008).
69. Smolskaya, T.T.: Studying HIV prevalence and risks among men having sex with men in Moscow and Saint Petersburg. Saint Petersburg Scientific and Research Institute of Epidemiology and Microbiology named after Pasteur, World Health Organization (2006).
70. Ladnaya, N.N.: The national HIV and AIDS epidemic and HIV surveillance in the Russian Federation. Presentation to Mapping the AIDS Pandemic meeting. June 30, Moscow (2007).
71. Ministry of Health [Uzbekistan]: Strategic Programme of Response to HIV in the Republic of Uzbekistan for 2007–2011. Ministry of Health [Uzbekistan], Tashkent (2007)
72. EuroHIV: HIV/AIDS Surveillance in Europe: Mid-Year Report 2005. Saint-Maurice, Institut de Veille Sanitaire (No 72) (2006).
73. Centro de Estudios Sociales y Demograficos et al.: Republica Dominicana Encuesta Demografica y de Salud 2007 Informe Preliminar. Noviembre. Santo Domingo and Calverton (2007).
74. Gaillard, E.M., et al.: Understanding the reasons for decline of HIV prevalence in Haiti. Sex. Transm. Infect. **82**(Suppl. 1), 14–20 (2006)
75. Ministère de la Santé Publique et de la Population: Etude de serosurveillance par methode sentinelle de la prevalence du VIH, de la syphilis, de l'hépatite B et de l'hépatite C chez les femmes enceintes en Haiti, 2006/2007. Juillet, Port au Prince (2007)
76. Cayemittes, M. et al.: Enquête mortalité, morbidité et utilisation des services EMMUS-IV: Haïti 2005–2006. Juillet. Pétion ville et Calverton, Institut Haïtien de l'Enfance et ORC Macro (2006).
77. Hallett, T.B., et al.: Declines in HIV prevalence can be associated with changing sexual behaviour in Uganda,

urban Kenya, Zimbabwe and urban Haiti. Sex. Transm. Infect. **82**(Suppl. 1), i1–i8 (2006)
78. Centre d'Evaluation et de Recherche Appliquée (CERA) et Family Health International: Résultats préliminaires. Enquêtes de Surveillance des Comportements. Haiti 2006, FHI BSS III (2006).
79. Kerrigan, D., et al.: Environmental-structural interventions to reduce HIV/STI risk among female sex workers in the Dominican Republic. Am. J. Public Health **96**(1), 120–125 (2006)
80. Secretaría de Estado de Salud Pública y Asistencia Social de Republica Dominica: Encuestas de vigilancia del comportamiento sobre VIH/ SIDA/ ITS en RSX y HSH del Área V de Salud. Enero. Santo Domingo (2005).
81. Allen, C.F., et al.: Sexually transmitted infection use and risk factors for HIV infection among female sex workers in Georgetown, Guyana. J. Acquir. Immune Defic. Syndr. **43**(1), 96–101 (2006)
82. Gebre, Y. et al.: Tracking the course of the HIV epidemic through second generation surveillance in Jamaica: Survey of female sex workers. XVI International AIDS Conference, Toronto, Ontario. 13 – 18 August. (Abstract CDC0313) (2006).
83. Pan American Health Organization: AIDS in the Americas: The Evolving Epidemic, Response and Challenges Ahead. Pan American Health Organization, Washington, DC (2007)
84. Caribbean Commission on Health and Development: Report of the Caribbean Commission on Health and Development for the 26th Meeting of the CARICOM Heads of Government: Overview. 3 – 6 July, Saint Lucia (2005)
85. Inciardi, J.A., Syvertsen, J.L., Surratt, H.L.: HIV/AIDS in the Caribbean Basin. AIDS Care **17**(Suppl. 1), S9–S25 (2005)
86. Programa Nacional de Prevención y control de las ITS/ VIH/Sida. Actualización de la situación Nacional hasta el 31 de Dic 2006. Diciembre. Dirección Nacional de Epidemiología, MINSAP. La Habana (2006).
87. Ministry of Health and Social Security [Dominica]: HIV/ AIDS Epidemiology and Information in Dominica. Ministry of Health and Social Security [Dominica], Roseau (2007)
88. Lee, R.K. et al.: Risk behaviours for HIV among men who have sex with men in Trinidad and Tobago. XVI International AIDS Conference, Toronto, Ontario. 13 – 18 August. (Abstract CDD0366) (2006).
89. Ministry of Health [Guyana]: Behavioural surveillance survey, Round I: 2003/2004 – Executive Summary. Ministry of Health [Guyana], Georgetown (2005)
90. Toro-Alfonso, J., Varas-Díaz, N.: Identificación y descripción de conocimiento, actitudes, creencias y comportamientos de riesgo para la transmisión del VIH en población de homosexuales y hombres que tienen sexo con hombres en la República Dominicana. USAID and Projecto Conecta, Santo Domingo (2008)
91. Ministerio de Salud de Peru (2005). Sentinel surveillance report. Lima, Ministerio de Salud de Peru, Directorate of Epidemiology. Ministerio de Salud de Peru (2006). Análisis de la situación epidemiológica del VIH/SIDA en el Perú – Bases Epidemiológicas para la Prevención y el Control. Lima (Noviembre).
92. Sanchez, J., et al.: HIV-1, sexually transmitted infections, and sexual behavior trends among men who have sex with men in Lima, Peru. J. Acquir. Immune Defic. Syndr. **44**(5), 578–585 (2007)
93. Pando, M.A., et al.: Epidemiology of human immunodeficiency virus, viral hepatitis (B and C), Treponema pallidum, and human T-cell lymphotropic I/II virus among men who have sex with men in Buenos Aires, Argentina. Sex. Transm. Dis. **33**(5), 307–313 (2006)
94. Montano, S.M., et al.: Prevalences, genotypes and risk factors for HIV transmission in South America. J. Acquir. Immune Defic. Syndr. **40**(1), 57–64 (2005)
95. Mejía, A. et al.: HIV seroprevalence and associated risk factors in men who have sex with men in the Villavicencio city, Colombia, 2005. XVI International AIDS Conference, Toronto, Ontario. (Abstract CDC0734) (2006).
96. Ministerio de la Protecciòn Social de Colombia y ONUSIDA Grupo Tematico: Infeccion por VIH y SIDA en Colombia, Estado del arte. 2000–2005. Mayo. Bogota, Ministerio de la Proteccion Social de Colombia y ONUSIDA Gruupo Tematico (2006).
97. Magis, C. et al.: HIV prevalence and factors associated with the possession of condoms among male sex workers in two cities: Guadalajara and Mexico City, Mexico. XVI International AIDS Conference, Toronto, Ontario. 13–18 August. (Abstract CDC0336) (2006).
98. Soto, R.J., et al.: Sentinel surveillance of sexually transmitted infection/HIV and risk behaviours in vulnerable populations in 5 Central American countries. J. Acquir. Immune Defic. Syndr. **46**(1), 101–111 (2007)
99. Bravo-Garcia, E., Magis-Rodriquez, C., Saavedra, J.: New estimates in Mexico: more than 180,000 people living with HIV. XVI International AIDS Conference, Toronto, Ontario. 13 – 18 August. (Abstract CDC0411) (2006).
100. Bautista, C.T., et al.: Seroprevalence of and risk factors for HIV-1 infection among female commercial sex workers in South America. Sex. Transm. Infect. **82**(4), 311–316 (2006)
101. Secretaría de Salud de Honduras et al: Estudio Centroamericano de vigilancia de comportamiento sexual y prevalencia de VIH/ITS en poblaciones vulnerables: Trabajadoras Sexuales. Agosto, Tegucigalpa (2007)
102. Secretaría de Salud de Honduras et al: Estudio Centroamericano de vigilancia de comportamiento sexual y prevalencia de VIH/ITS en poblaciones vulnerables: Hombres que tienen sexo con hombres (HSH). Julio, Tegucigalpa (2007)
103. Cohen, J.: Up in smoke: epidemic changes course. Science **313**, 487–488 (2006)
104. Fonseca, M.E., et al.: Os programas de reducao de danos ao uso de drogas no Brasil: caacterizacao preliminar de 45 programas. Caderna de Saude Publica **2**(4), 761–770 (2006)
105. Okie, S.: Fighting HIV – lessons from Brazil. N. Eng. J. Med. **354**(19), 1977–1981 (2006)
106. Rossi, D., et al.: The HIV/AIDS epidemic and changes in injecting drug use in Buenos Aires, Argentina. Cad. Saúde Pública **22**(4), 741–750 (2006)
107. IDES, et al.: HIV, HBV, HCV prevalence related to sexual behavior and drug use in 200 injecting drug users in Montevideo. Montevideo, Ministry of Health, Uruguay (2005)

108. National AIDS Program [Paraguay]: HIV/STI sentinel prevalence and behavioral study on clients of female sex workers and injecting drug users. National AIDS Program Paraguay, PRONASIDA. Asunción (2006).
109. National AIDS Program [Argentina]: Epidemiological surveillance report. Buenos Aires (December). National AIDS Program [Argentina] (2005).
110. Martínez, G.P., Elea, N.A., Chiu, A.M.: Epidemiology of HIV infection and acquired immune deficiency disease syndrome in Chile. Revista Chilena Infectología **23**(4), 321–329 (2006)
111. Dourado, I., et al.: HIV-1 seroprevalence in the general population of Salvador, Bahia State, Northeast Brazil. Cad. Saúde Pública **23**(1), 25–32 (2007)
112. Silva, A.C.M., Barone, A.A.: Risk factors for HIV infection among patients infected with hepatitis C virus. Rev. Saúde Pública **40**(3), 482–488 (2006)
113. Public Health Agency of Canada: HIV and AIDS in Canada: surveillance report to June 30, 2006, Ottawa, http://www.phac-aspc.gc.ca/aids-sida/publication/index.html#surveillance (2006). Accessed 8 May 2008.
114. US Centers for Disease Control and Prevention: HIV/AIDS surveillance report: Cases of HIV infection and AIDS in the United States and Dependent Areas, 2005. Atlanta, Georgia, Centers for Disease Control and Prevention (Revised June 2007, Vol 17) (2007).
115. Public Health Agency of Canada: HIV and AIDS in Canada. Selected surveillance tables to June 30, 2007. Ottawa, Surveillance and Risk Assessment Division, Centre for Infectious Disease Prevention and Control, Public Health Agency of Canada, http://www.phac-aspc.gc.ca/aids-sida/publication/index.html#surveillance (2007). Accessed 8 May 2008.
116. Dodds, J.P., et al.: Increasing risk behaviour and high levels of undiagnosed HIV infection in a community sample of homosexual men. Sex. Transm. Infect. **80**, 236–240 (2004)
117. Balthasar, H., Jeannin, A., Dubois-Arber, F.: VIH/SIDA: augmentation des expositions au risque d'infection par le VIH chez les homes ayant des rapports sexuels avec des hommes: premiers résultats de Gay Survey 04 (2005).
118. Moreau-Gruet, F., Dubois-Arber, F., Jeannin, A.: Long-term HIV/AIDS-related prevention behaviours among men having sex with men: Switzerland 1992–2000. AIDS Care **18**, 35–43 (2006)
119. Hamouda, O., et al.: Epidemiology of HIV infections in Germany. Bundesgesundheitsblatt **50**(4), 399–411 (2007)
120. Robert Koch Institut: Epidemiologisches Bulletin. Berlin (5 October) (2007).
121. Boulos, D., et al.: Estimates of HIV prevalence and incidence in Canada, 2005. Can. Commun. Dis. Rep. **32**, 165–174 (2006)
122. Hamers FF, Devaux I, Alix J, Nardone A. HIV/AIDS in Europe: trends and EU-wide priorities. Euro Surveill. 2006;11(47):pii=3083. Available online: http://www.eurosurveillance.org/ViewArticle.aspx?ArticleId=3083
123. Rosinska, M.: Current trends in HIV/AIDS epidemiology in Poland, 1999–2004. Eurosurveillance **11**(4–6), 94–97 (2006)
124. Brucková M, Maly M, Vandasova J, Maresova M. HIV/AIDS in the Czech Republic, 2006. Euro Surveill. 2007; **12**(14):pii=3170. Available online: http://www.eurosurveillance.org/ViewArticle.aspx?ArticleId=3170
125. EuroHIV: HIV/AIDS surveillance in Europe: end-year report 2006, No 75. Institut de Veille Sanitaire. Saint-Maurice (No 75), http://www.eurohiv.org (2007). Accessed 8 May 2008.
126. Obermeyer, C.M.: HIV in the Middle East. Br. Med. J. **333**, 851–854 (2006)
127. Zamani, S., et al.: Prevalence of and factors associated with HIV-1 infection among drug users visiting treatment centers in Tehran, Iran. AIDS **19**, 709–716 (2005)
128. Zamani, S., et al.: High prevalence of HIV infection associated with incarceration among community-based drug users in Tehran, Iran. J. Acquir. Immune Defic. Syndr. **42**(3), 342–346 (2006)
129. Kilani, B. et al.: Sero-epidemiology of HCV-HIV co-infection in Tunisia. IAS Conference on HIV Pathogenesis and Treatment. 13–16 July. Antivir. Ther. **8**(Suppl. 1):S452–S453 (Abstract No. 952) http://www.aegis.org/conferences/IASHIVPT/2003/952.html (2003). Accessed 8 May 2008.
130. Mimouni, B., Remaoun, N.: Etude du Lien Potentiel entre l'Usage Problématique de Drogues et le VIH/SIDA en Algérie 2004–2005. Alger, Ministerie de education (2006)
131. Ministry of Health [Syria], UNODC, UNAIDS: Assessment on Drug Use and HIV in Syria. Damascus (Draft Report, July). Ministry of Health [Syria], UNODC, UNAIDS (2007).
132. Ministère de la Santé [Maroc]: Surveillance sentinelle du VIH: Resultats 2006 et tendances de la séroprévalence du VIH. Janvier, Rabat (2007)
133. Ministry of Health [Egypt], USAID, Impact and FHI: HIV/AIDS Biological and Behavioral Surveillance Survey; Summary Report; Egypt 2006. National AIDS Programme, Cairo (2006)
134. Elrashied, S.: Prevalence, knowledge and related risky sexual behaviours of HIV/AIDS among receptive men who have sex with men (MSM) in Khartoum State, Sudan, 2005. XVI International AIDS Conference, Toronto, Ontario. 13–18 August. (Abstract TUPE0509) (2006).
135. National AIDS Council Secretariat [Papua New Guinea]: The 2007 consensus report on the HIV epidemic in Papua New Guinea. National AIDS Council Secretariat [Papua New Guinea], Port Moresby (2007)
136. National AIDS Council Secretariat [Papua New Guinea] and National HIV/AIDS Support Project. HIV/AIDS Behavioural Surveillance Survey Within High Risk Settings Papua New Guinea: BSS Round 1, 2006.Port Moresby. National AIDS Council Secretariat [Papua New Guinea] and National HIV/AIDS Support Project (2007).
137. Institute of Medical Research. "It's in Every Corner Now": A nationwide study of HIV, AIDS and STIs. Gorokoa, Papua New Guinea Institute of Medical Research, Operational Research Unit (2007).
138. National Centre in HIV Epidemiology and Clinical Research: Australian HIV Surveillance Report **23**(1) January: (2007).
139. Ministry of Health [New Zealand]: AIDS – New Zealand. February. Auckland (Issue 59) http://www.moh.govt.nz/moh.nsf/indexmh/aids-nz-issue59 (2007). Accessed 8 May 2008.
140. National Centre in HIV Epidemiology and Clinical Research. HIV/AIDS, viral hepatitis and sexually transmissible infec-

tions in Australia Annual Surveillance Report 2007. Sydney, NSW , National Centre in HIV Epidemiology and Clinical Research, The University of New South Wales. Canberra, ACT, Australian Institute of Health and Welfare (2007)
141. Prestage, G., et al.: Trends in unprotected anal intercourse among Sydney gay men. XVI International AIDS Conference, Toronto, Ontario. 13–18 August. (Abstract WEPE0721) (2006).
142. Maibani-Michie, G., Yeka, W.: A Baseline Research for Poro Sapot Project: A Program for Prevention of HIV/AIDS among MSM in Port Moresby and FSW in Goroka and Port Moresby Papua New Guinea. Papua New Guinea (IMR/FHI Research Report to USAID) (2005)
143. Liu H et al. (2006). Drug users: Potentially important bridge population in the transmission of sexually transmitted diseases, including AIDS, in China. Sexually Transmitted Diseases, **33**(2):111–117

Immunology of HIV

24

Heribert Stoiber and Doris Wilflingseder

Core Messages

- Human immunodeficiency virus (HIV) escapes both the innate and the adaptive immune responses. Only few infected but treatment-naive individuals control viral replication.
- The viral escape from the innate immune response is mediated by the neutralization of complement attacks and the impairment of the cellular arm of the innate immune system such as macrophages, dendritic cells (DCs), natural killer (NK) cells, and natural killer T (NKT) cells. The identification of a putative cellular antiviral factor secreted by CD8 cells remains elusive. However, individuals with a deletion in the CCR5 gene exhibit a decreased risk for infection.
- HIV efficiently impairs T cell responses and depletes T helper cells by direct (infection) or indirect mechanisms (induction of apoptosis).
- The induction of long-lasting neutralizing antibodies is a rare event in vivo. Approaches to induce broadly neutralizing antibodies in HIV-infected individuals have failed so far.

H. Stoiber (✉) and D. Wilflingseder
Department of Hygiene and Medical Microbiology, Innsbruck Medical University, Fritz-Pregl Strasse 3, A-6020 Innsbruck, Austria
e-mail: heribert.stoiber@i-med.ac.at; doris.wilflingseder@i-med.ac.at

24.1 Introduction

In 1983, the human immunodeficiency virus (HIV) was identified as the causative agent of the acquired immunodeficiency syndrome (AIDS) [13, 40, 112]. This immunodeficiency is characterized by opportunistic infections and the loss of $CD4^+$ T cells in the peripheral blood and the gastrointestinal (GI) tract (Fig. 24.1). HIV affects all arms of the immune response in infected individuals and undermines the immunity of the host [40, 112]. This includes escape mechanisms against both the innate and the adaptive immune responses. However, the clinical course of infection varies among individuals. The median time from infection to the development of AIDS is approximately 10 years (Fig. 24.1) [38]. Around 10% of the patients can control HIV despite prolonged periods of infection and are therefore referred to as long-term non-progressors (LTNPs). They remain asymptomatic, suffer no loss in $CD4^+$ T-cell counts, and keep the viral load close to the detection limit without any therapy. In contrast, about 10% of infected individuals are rapid progressors, who develop AIDS within 5 years [79]. In addition, groups were identified that remain uninfected in spite of living at high risk for HIV infection. These "exposed but uninfected" individuals include commercial sex workers, discordant couples having unprotected sex, or infants of seropositive mothers, to name only a few [40, 112]. Responsible for these differences in the pathogenesis of the infection is a complex interaction of host immune and viral factors. Thus, understanding the interplay of the immune system with HIV will provide the basis to identify the mechanisms that protect from infection by this virus.

G. Gross and S.K. Tyring (eds.), *Sexually Transmitted Infections and Sexually Transmitted Diseases*,
DOI: 10.1007/978-3-642-14663-3_24, © Springer-Verlag Berlin Heidelberg 2011

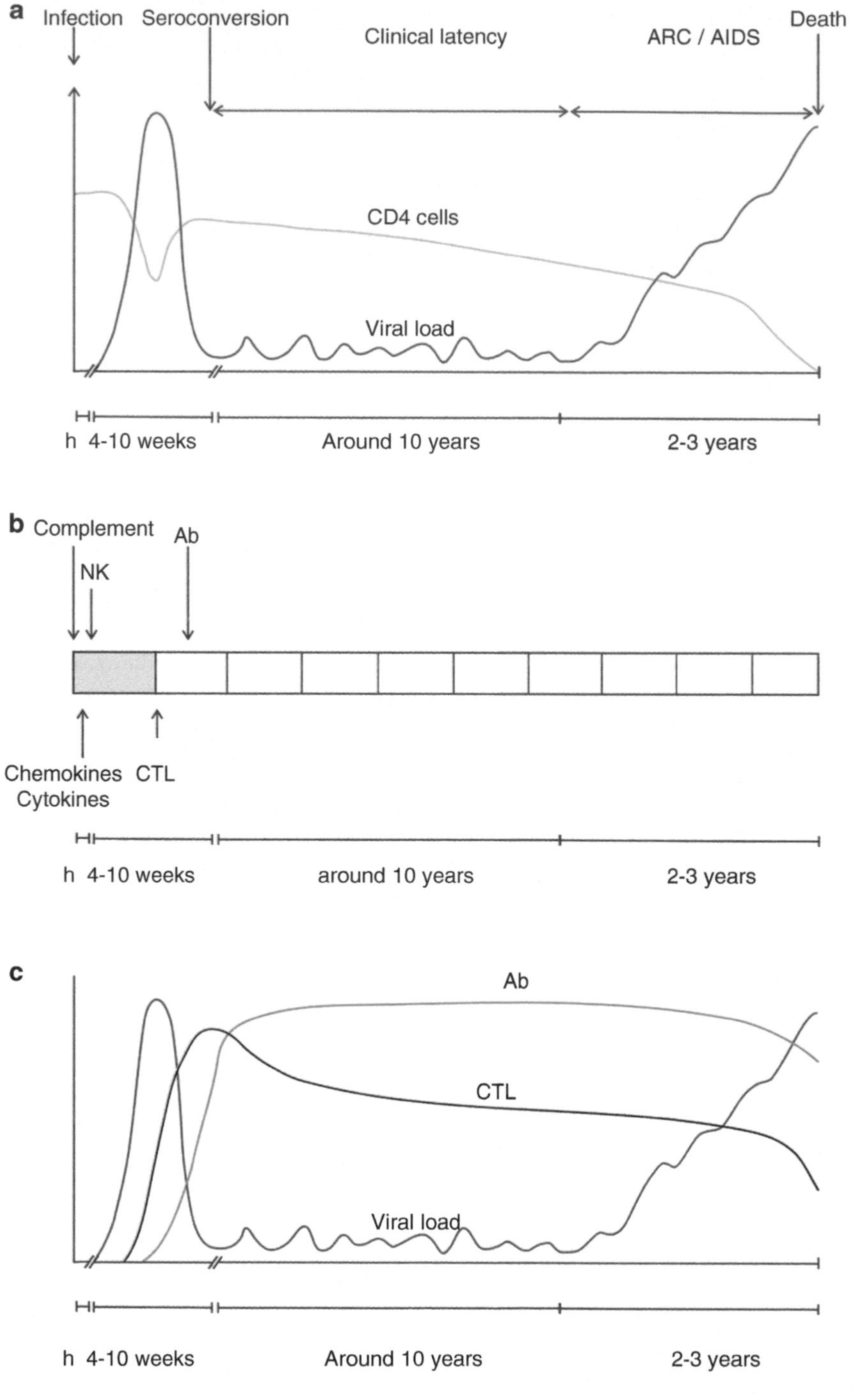

Fig. 24.1 Typical course of untreated HIV-1 infected individuals. (**a**) A burst in viral replication with an associated loss of $CD4^+$ T-cell counts during the first weeks upon infection with HIV-1 followed by partial control of the virus. After 4 to 10 weeks, HIV-specific antibodies arise in the serum of the patients. When the $CD4^+$ T-cell counts decrease below 200 cells/mm^3, the viral titer rises again. At this stage of the disease – usually 10 years postinfection – opportunistic infections occur. The patients suffer from AIDS-related complexes (ARC) and AIDS leading finally to the death of infected individuals. (**b**) Already during the first minutes after the exposure of HIV on the mucosal surface and upon entrance of the virus, complement is activated. Within a few hours, further effector functions of the innate immune response are triggered such as chemokine/cytokine responses, interferon release, or activation of NK-cells. The adaptive immunity is responding not before the second week after viral challenge. (**c**) During peak viremia, the induced CTL response starts to partially control viral replication. HIV-specific antibodies which arise several weeks later are thought to further contribute to determine the individual viral set-point over the next 10 years. Despite a continuous CTL and antibody response, the virus is not cleared and rises again parallel to the decline of the $CD4^+$ T cells below 200 cells/mm^3

24.2 The Innate Immune Response

The innate immune response gains increasing attention in its contribution to the control of HIV infection. The concerted action of a wide range of humoral and cellular components induces a rapid first-line immune defense and provides the basis for a robust adaptive immune response [100]. The complement system is among the first components activated during the innate immune response (Fig. 24.1). Together with interferons, cytokines, and chemokines, complement fragments activate innate immune cells, such as natural killer (NK) cells and natural killer T (NKT) cells, monocytes, macrophages, and dendritic cells (DCs), steering the antiviral defense and helping to bridge the time until adaptive immune effectors are available. To trigger a robust adaptive immunity, the components of the cellular arm of innate immunity are essential. Natural killer (NK) cells and macrophages provide essential chemokines and cytokines for B- and T-cell responses. Dendritic cells are the main antigen-presenting cells in the periphery. Thus, the coordinated action of the innate immune system is essential to control the viral burden at initial phases of infection and to trigger a robust adaptive immune response (Fig. 24.1).

24.2.1 Complement

Among the components of the innate immunity, the complement system is the first barrier to control HIV propagation. More than 35 proteins comprise the family of complement proteins. It provides the first-line defense against invading pathogens and bridges the innate with the adaptive immunity [97].With the classical, the mannose-binding lectin (MBL), and the alternative pathway, three different routes of activation are identified, all of which converge at the cleavage of C3. Upon C3 activation, the terminal complement pathway is triggered. Activated C5 (C5b) associates with C6, C7, C8, and C9. This complex is referred to as the terminal membrane attack complex (MAC). The formation of the MAC disrupts the membrane resulting in lysis of infected cells or pathogens [97]. Regulators of complement activation (RCAs) are crucial to avoid potential self-damage of host cells and tissue by complement-mediated lysis (CoML). Although HIV has acquired membrane-anchored and fluid-phase RCAs, which provide intrinsic resistance against human complement [101], the protection is not complete. Mainly at early stages of infection, CoML might contribute to the control of the virus before factors of the adaptive immunity appear [43]. At later stages of infection, CoML seems to play a minor role in reducing the viral burden in infected individuals [43]. HIV-1 that survives complement attacks remains covered with C3 fragments. Thus, opsonized HIV accumulates in all complement-enriched compartments of the host, such as blood, lymphatic tissue (LT), brain, mother's milk, or seminal fluid and interacts with complement receptor (CR) positive cells, such as macrophages, DCs, NK cells, B cells, or follicular dendritic cells (FDCs). The possible complement-mediated enhancement of infection in "cis" and/or in "trans" may counteract the contribution of the complement system in viral clearance via CoML and phagocytosis [101–103]. Trapping of complement-coated virions to CR2-positive cells has been shown in ex vivo studies for FDCs [11, 45]. This is of importance as up to 90% of viral particles are extracellularly bound to FDCs, representing by far the largest viral reservoir in HIV-infected individuals (Fig. 24.2) [36, 77]. Trapped virions remain infectious for T cells migrating through GC even in the presence of neutralizing antibodies [11]. Besides CRs, additional molecules such as Fcγ receptors or adhesion molecules such as ICAM-1 and LFA-1 have been suggested to contribute to FDC-mediated trapping of HIV, yet the complement-dependent interaction of opsonized HIV with CRs expressed on FDCs is mainly responsible for the generation of this huge viral reservoir in infected individuals (Fig. 24.2).

24.2.2 Chemokines and Cytokines

First indications that soluble host factors of the innate immune response interfere with HIV infection were provided in the early 1990s by the group of J. Levy reporting on a cellular antiviral factor (CAF) exclusively produced and secreted by $CD8^+$ T cells [59]. Although the identification of CAF remains still elusive, several members of the CC-chemokine family were identified, which inhibit viral replication in vitro. Chemokines are chemotactic cytokines, which bind to seven transmembrane G-protein-coupled receptors (GPCRs) and are involved in immune homeostasis and cell trafficking. The first three factors of the chemokine family, which were identified as suppressors of HIV infection, were RANTES (CCL5), MIP-1a (CCL3),

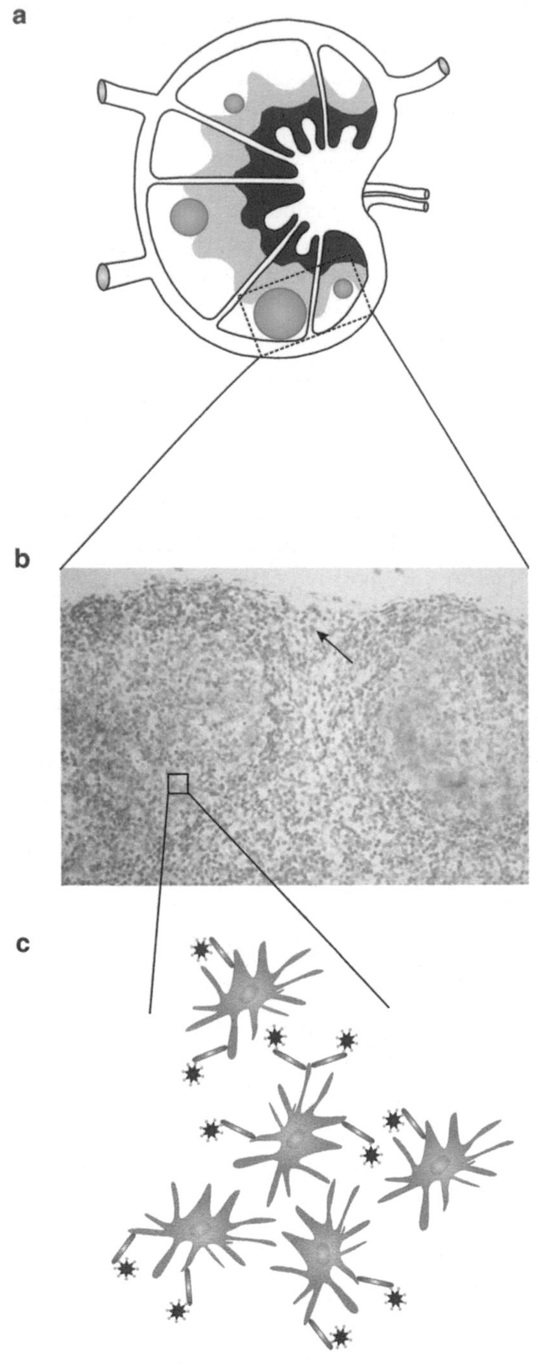

Fig. 24.2 Trapping of opsonized HIV in the germinal center (GC) of the lymphatic tissue. (**a**) The simplified model of a lymph node (LN) shows germinal centers in blue, which mainly constitute B cells and follicular dendritic cells (FDCs). (**b**) HIV-RNA is detected in a LN of an individual chronically infected with the virus by in situ hybridization (stained in turquoise). Although some viral RNA can be detected outside the germinal center (see arrow for an example) this lymphatic compartment sustains by far the largest viral reservoir within an infected patient. (**c**) Trapping of HIV in the germinal centers is driven by complement and complement receptors, as complement-opsonized virus is binding to CR2 (shown in gray) expressed by FDCs

and MIP-1b (CCL4) [20]. All these chemokines bind to the GPCR CCR5. This receptor was identified a year later as a co-receptor for so-called macrophage-tropic HIV-1 strains, now termed R5-tropic viruses. Similarly, the CXC chemokine SDF-1 (CXCL12), which naturally binds to CXCR4, suppresses the infection with T-cell tropic strains [14, 74]. These viral isolates use CXCR4 as a second receptor and are referred to as X4-tropic. The discovery of the chemokine receptors as co-factors for viral entry led to the discovery that polymorphisms in the CCR5, especially a 32 base-pair gene deletion (CCR5Δ32) leads to an impairment of this receptor, resulting in a decreased susceptibility to infection with R5-tropic virus strains [56]. Individuals, who are heterocygotous for the CCR5Δ32 are susceptible to infection with CCR5-tropic HIV strains, but exhibit a significantly lower disease progression. Carriers of the homocygotic CCR5Δ32 genes are resistant to infection with R5-tropic isolates, but can be infected with X4-tropic viruses.

24.2.3 HIV and NK Cells

About 2% of the lymphocytes circulating in the blood are natural killer (NK) cells. NK cells derive from bone marrow precursors and circulate as mature populations in blood and spleen. Besides their direct cytotoxic activity, which is regulated by a balance of activating and inhibitory NK cell receptors [55], NK cells additionally suppress viral replication by secretion of several chemo- and cytokines, such as MIP-1α (CCL3), MIP-1β (CCL4), RANTES (CCL5), IFN-γ, TNF, or GM-CSF [22] (Fig. 24.3). NK cells interact with dendritic cells, too. At low NK cell/DC ratios, NK cells are able to activate dendritic cells (DCs, see Sect. 24.2.6) and induce their maturation. Activation and maturation of DCs occur by either cell–cell contact or secretion of TNF-α [81, 119]. Vice versa, many groups described the key role of DC-derived cytokines and membrane-bound molecules in the activation process of NK cells e.g., [7, 69, 71].

NK cells play an important role in prevention and control of HIV infection, since they can kill HIV-infected target cells by direct lysis, or by antibody-dependent cell-mediated cytotoxicity (ADCC) [15]. Additionally, they initiate priming of the adaptive immunity by their cross-talk with DCs. Their killer inhibitory receptors (KIRs), which transmit an inhibitory signal upon encounter with MHC class I molecules on a cell surface, are pivotal in killing virus-infected cells, since many viruses, including HIV, down-regulate MHC class I on infected cells. Killing is performed by exocytosis of granules containing perforin and granzymes. Two subsets of NK cells are characterized by their expression of CD16 (FcγRIII) and CD56. The $CD16^{high}CD56^{low}$ subset (>95%) is responsible for direct lysis of cells and ADCC [22] and this subset was very recently reported to decline during HIV infection [42]. By contrast, the $CD16^{low/-}CD56^{high}$ subset (<5% of NK cells in blood) produces high amounts of IFN-γ and TNF-α, but exhibits poor cytotoxic properties. As shown, in HIV-infected individuals, NK cell responses are impaired [3]. The dysfunction comprises both cytotoxic activity of NK cells in terms of virus-infected cells and the capacity of NK cells to secrete CCR5-ligands (MIP-1α, MIP-1β, RANTES) [63]. The cytotoxic activity of NK cells is suggested to be inefficient due to HIV-mediated down-regulation of activating receptors on the cell surface [63]. By suppressing the secretion of CCR5-ligands, infected cells are not effectively eliminated and virus replication is not limited. Though it is known that HIV modulates NK phenotype and function in vitro and in vivo, the exact mechanisms of the interactions between virus and killer cell is presently not clear and needs further investigations.

24.2.4 HIV and NKT Cells

Natural killer T cells (NKT) cells are a unique subgroup of T lymphocytes that are involved in the innate immune response against auto-antigens and pathogens, but also appear to be susceptible to HIV infection [70]. NKT cells secrete high amounts of IFN-γ (double-negative NKT cells), a major T_H1 cytokine, or IL-4 and IL-13 ($CD4^+$ NKT cells), the main T_H2-type cytokines. This may accelerate the help for a cell- (IFN-γ) or antibody-mediated (IL-4) response compared to conventional T cells. They express a semi-invariant TCR (NKT TCR) that comprises an invariant α-chain, and a restricted TCR-β-chain repertoire [reviewed in 29]. The TCR expressed on NKT cells recognizes self or foreign glycolipids presented by the non-polymorphic MHC class I-like molecule CD1d. Full activation of NKT cells requires secretion of type-I interferons (IFN-α, IFN-β) or pro-inflammatory cytokines (IL-15, IL-12, IL-18). Therefore, NKT cells rely on a cross-talk with other cells, in particular, with different DC subtypes to show a fully activated phenotype (plasmacytoid DCs: type-I IFNs, myeloid DCs: IL-12).

Despite the potential of NKT cells to control HIV, several studies have shown that NKT cells are dramatically reduced in HIV-infected individuals compared to healthy donors [70, 91]. In vivo studies [70, 91] have also demonstrated that the decline in $CD4^+$ NKT cell counts significantly correlate with higher viremia in infected individuals. This subset of $CD4^+$ NKT cells is highly susceptible to infection with R5-tropic viruses, which are shown to cause rapid destruction of the cells in vitro [70]. Therefore, $CD4^+$ NKT cells were assumed as gateways for R5-tropic HIV during the primary stage of infection due to their high CCR5 expression. Furthermore, NKT cells are supposed to activate resting bystander $CD4^+$ T cells, thereby contributing to the spread of the virus [108]. Due to the loss of their regulatory functions, the decline of NKT cells during HIV pathogenesis may have severe consequences for the development of autoimmune-like symptoms observed in HIV-infected individuals and account for the loss of antitumor responses, in particular for the increased incidence of tumors, such as Kaposi's sarcoma or non-Hodgkin's lymphoma in AIDS patients.

24.2.5 HIV and Macrophages

Like DCs and NK cells, macrophages are key players in the innate and adaptive immunity. These cells are also infected and modulated by HIV. Macrophages and latently infected resting $CD4^+$ T cells comprise the two major intracellular reservoirs during HIV pathogenesis (Fig. 24.3). Productively infected macrophages have been detected in both untreated patients and those receiving HAART [95]. By its accessory genes, HIV converts macrophage immune responses, affects the cell cycle, and enhances the viral replication in these cells [25, 35, 50]. Microarray studies revealed that HIV induced a pro-inflammatory gene expression pattern in macrophages, which is associated with an enhanced virus replication and the persistence of chronically activated macrophages in vivo. Additionally, IFN-/NFκB-responsive chemo- and cytokines that are supposed to promote recruitment of CD4+ T cells and macrophages to sites of infection were shown to be up-regulated [116]. Macrophages express only low levels of CD4, but high levels of heparan sulfate proteoglycans (such as syndecan), macrophage mannose receptor (MR), and

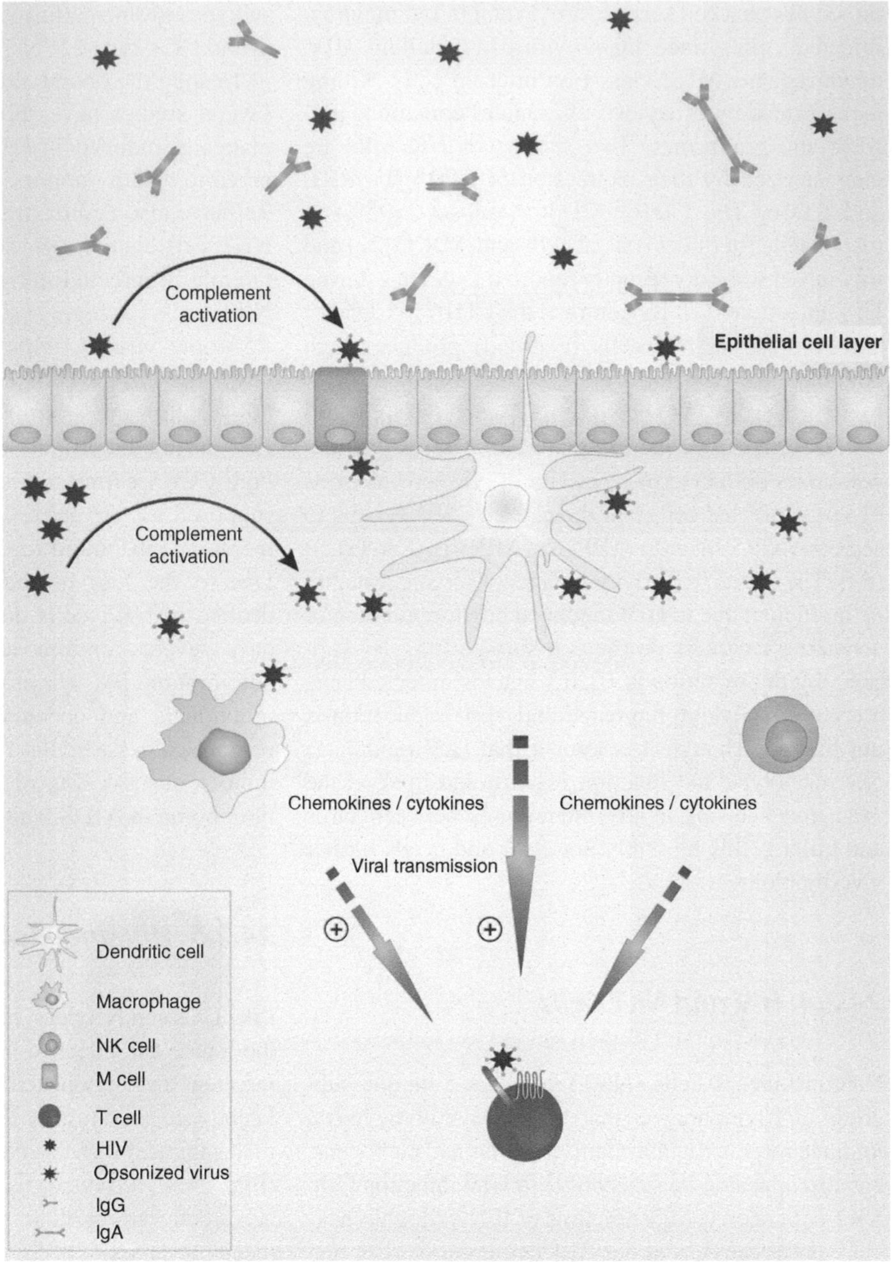

Fig. 24.3 Mucosal transmission of HIV and infection of T cells. Complement-opsonized virus is crossing the epithelial layer by yet undefined mechanisms. Once across the border, HIV interacts with different cells of the innate immune system, such as macrophages, DCs, or NK cells. Macrophages and DCs can transmit the virus in "cis" or in "trans" to T cells indicated by "+" in the figure. Additionally, the interaction of HIV with cells of the innate immune system induces a whole array of cytokines and chemokines, which directly act upon T cells. These humoral factors can promote or inhibit infection and/or viral replication in T cells

elastase [72]. Therefore, even in a host cell expressing low levels of CD4, HIV interacts alternatively with abundant receptors on the cell for attachment, and internalization. Primary human macrophages express CCR5 as well as CXCR4, and infection with both R5- and X4-tropic virus isolates has been reported in vitro and in vivo [18]. Once taken up by macrophages, HIV accumulates in endocytic compartments similar to multivesicular bodies, which facilitate HIV assembly and escape immune surveillance [54]. This accumulation of HIV in the cytoplasmic vesicles of macrophages results in prolonged storage of infectious virions, which can rapidly infect $CD4^+$ T cells even after months [96]. Upon formation of a virological synapse between macrophage and T cell, the virus is efficiently transmitted. Therefore, tissue macrophages were claimed to act as a "Trojan horse", hiding the virus from the immune system.

24.2.6 HIV and Monocytes

Monocytes express CD4 and the chemokine receptors that allow the viral interaction, in particular with macrophage-tropic HIV strains. Besides macrophages, also monocytes are resistant to the cytopathic effects following HIV infection, and persist throughout the course of the disease. They act as important viral reservoirs and may disseminate the infection to different tissues [49]. Infectious HIV was shown to be recovered from patients obtaining HAART. Both macrophages and monocytes were demonstrated to play a crucial role in the neuropathogenesis of HIV-infection and to contribute to HIV-mediated dementia due to production of pro-inflammatory cytokines and neurotoxins [49]. HIV-1 Tat induces activation of microglial and perivascular cells to produce pro-inflammatory proteins, thereby leading to monocyte infiltration into the brain. Other features promoted by Tat following infection with HIV are chemotaxis of monocytes, their adhesion to the endothelium, and their recruitment into extravascular tissues. This modulation of the chemotactic activity seemed to be mediated by the Tat cysteine-rich domain [4]. HIV thus affects multiple immune functions of monocytes/macrophages (chemotaxis, phagocytosis, intracellular killing, APC function, cytokine production) and thereof allows establishment as well as reactivation of opportunistic infections [49].

24.2.7 DCs and HIV

Among the first cells that interact with HIV upon entry via mucosal surfaces are dendritic cells that play a key role against invading pathogens. DCs initiate, shape, and control the immune response. They act as linker between innate and adaptive immunity [10]. DCs produce high amounts of cytokines, such as IL-12 or interferons, which belong to the first line of the host defense against invading organisms (Fig. 24.3). They are also able to activate natural killer (NK) cells and produce cytokines to attract other cells of the immune system [66]. In addition to their contribution to innate responses, DCs play an essential role in initiating and shaping the adaptive immunity [9]. They can be functionally divided into immature dendritic cells (iDCs) and mature dendritic cells (mDCs) based on their capacity to stimulate T cells [9]. iDCs sample antigens at the mucosal epithelia via their endocytic and phagocytic receptors. Following uptake of the antigen, iDCs undergo major changes and mature. This functional maturation correlates with the down-regulation of the antigen-capturing machinery and with an increased antigen-presenting capacity due to up-regulation of specific cell surface molecules such as MHC class I and class II, adhesion or co-stimulatory molecules [57, 92, 110]. The maturation is closely linked to migration of DCs from peripheral tissues to secondary lymphoid organs due to up-regulation of CCR7 [90, 113]. Following CCR7-dependent migration along an MIP-3β/SLC-gradient to lymphoid organs, DCs present the processed antigen to naive T cells, thus initiating T_H1 or T_H2 immune responses. DCs are furthermore involved in the generation of regulatory T cells (T reg) [99] and are thus pivotal to inducing both immunity and tolerance. At least three subsets of human DCs are known: myeloid "conventional" DCs, Langerhans cells (LCs), and plasmacytoid DC (pDCs) [86]. The subsets exhibit differences in their abilities to regulate T-cell responses (T_H1, T_H2, T_{reg}), to produce type-I interferon – a property of pDCs – and to cross-present exogenous antigens to $CD8^+$ T cells.

Upon entry of HIV into the host, the virus has to be transported from mucosal surfaces to LT, where it is transmitted to its primary targets, $CD4^+$ T lymphocytes (Fig. 24.3). As mentioned above, this process is thought to be contrived by DCs. By clustering and activating T cells, DCs may both activate antiviral immunity as well as facilitate the spread of the virus. In vitro experiments indicate that DCs efficiently capture and transmit HIV to T cells and initiate a vigorous infection [64, 85, 114]. This implies that HIV exploits DCs at mucosal sites as shuttles to $CD4^+$ T cells in the lymph nodes in vivo (Fig. 24.3). Independent of the route of transmission, the majority of HIV strains isolated at the beginning are R5-tropic isolates [109]. The reason for the pronounced negative selection of X4- or dual (R5X4)-tropic HIV at the beginning of infection is suggested but not elucidated in detail yet. The preference for R5-tropic viruses is not explainable by a single "gatekeeping" mechanism at the site of exposure, but it is mediated by multiple simultaneous or sequential mechanisms [reviewed in 62]. First levels of X4-restriction at the site of infection are the preferential expression of CCR5 on LCs and DCs. Kawamura et al. [48] demonstrated very recently that epithelial Langerhans cells accounted for >95% of HIV dissemination from skin explants. Furthermore, ex vivo analyses revealed that R5-tropic viruses replicate much more efficient in DCs and LCs compared to X4-tropic HIV [31, 48]. Although HIV infects LCs and other types of myeloid DCs both in vivo and in vitro [98, 106], productive infection of DCs and LCs with HIV is relatively inefficient compared to HIV-infection of $CD4^+$ T cells and it is difficult to detect HIV- or SIV-infected DCs in vivo [reviewed in 83]. A low productive virus replication of IFN-α-producing pDCs has been shown in vivo and in vitro by both, R5- and X4-tropic HIV variants [94]. Constant exposure of pDCs to HIV results in their chronic hyperactivation along with production of type-I interferon and indoleamine 2,3-dioxygenase (IDO), which in turn may exert cytotoxic and suppressive effects on T cells [39]. Despite this low-level infection of DCs, the virus is very efficiently transferred to T cells either via de novo ("cis"-transfer) or without ("trans"-) infection [107]. C-type lectin receptors (CLRs), in particular DC-SIGN (DC-specific intercellular adhesion molecule 3 (ICAM-3) grabbing nonintegrin), Langerin on LCs, or CD206 (mannose receptor) were implicated in the process of "trans"-infection [28, 105, 107]. Besides C-type lectins, other molecules, such as cholesterol [33] or adhesion molecules, e.g., ICAM-1 [85] are described to further contribute to DC-HIV interaction. Additionally, complement receptors (CRs) or Fc receptors (FcR) may contribute to the attachment of the virus, as HIV is opsonized in vivo with C3 fragments and, after seroconversion, with virus-specific IgG. In this constellation, the DC-SIGN- or ICAM-dependent interactions seem to play a minor role for attachment and infection of DCs and the transfer of HIV to T cells [85]. Vigorous trans-infection of $CD4^+$ T cells by DCs is promoted via formation of an infectious synapse independent of the attachment mechanism (CLRs, adhesion molecules, CRs; Fig. 24.3) [82 and own unpublished observations]. The receptors involved have to be rearranged and recruited to the dendritic cell–T-cell junctions [64]. The exact mechanism of translocation of the molecules to the infectious synapse is presently not clear, but microscopic analyses of DC-$CD4^+$ T-cell conjugates showed recruitment of CD4, and the chemokine co-receptor (CXCR4, CCR5) on the T cell, and of HIV on the DC to the junction [64]. Therefore, besides inducing specific immune responses, DCs efficiently assist in transmission to, and infection of, T cells with HIV (Fig. 24.3).

24.3 Adaptive Immunity

Although HIV infection affects the cellular arm of the innate immune response, the pathogenesis of HIV comprises mainly $CD4^+$ T cells. Replication within $CD4^+$ T cells and their subsequent destruction causes the profound immune suppression and progression to AIDS observed in HIV infected individuals, which goes in parallel with a rapid and dramatic loss of $CD4^+$ T cells in lymphoid tissues (LT) of the GI tract during acute infection with HIV [65, 112]. The induction of neutralizing antibodies (nAbs) is thought to further contribute to the control of the viral burden. At the beginning of infection a massive expansion of oligoclonal $CD8^+$ T cells [76], and appearance of HIV-specific $CD8^+$ T cells [16, 53] can be observed that are associated with decline of extremely high viral burdens. Not only direct killing by CTLs, but also secretion of cytokines, chemokines, or other soluble factors is associated with decreasing viremia. Although HIV is inducing a vast array of specific and nonspecific immune responses, most of the infected individuals cannot control or eradicate the virus completely. The ongoing viral replication during the chronic phase of the disease is accompanied by a continuous gradual loss of $CD4^+$ T cells, which is further accelerated during AIDS [58]. Increased levels of T-cell activation markers and lymphoid hyperplasia suggest that chronic T-cell activation persists in immune-compromised hosts, and contributes to the exhaustion of immune functions.

24.3.1 HIV and T Lymphocytes

Naive T cells, which are trafficking through lymphoid organs, interact with DCs upon recognition of specific antigens in an MHC context. Subsequent to the DC–T-cell cross-talk, primed T cells undergo major changes and proliferate extensively. The activated T cells migrate to tissues to combat the pathogen directly. Subsequent to the clearance of the antigen, approximately 90–95% of the activated effector T cells are deleted. Only a pool of antigen-experienced memory T cells survives, which is quickly reactivated upon re-encounters with the same antigen. In most of the infected individuals, the pathogenesis of HIV infection is characterized by a progressive loss of $CD4^+$ T cells, by enormous immune activation and poor control of the virus. The immune response exerts selective pressure on the virus that leads to rapid accumulation of virus variants, so-called escape mutants. This phenomenon has been observed for $CD8^+$ T cells [24, 80] as well as $CD4^+$ T cells [34]. However, the severe qualitative modifications in both $CD4^+$ and $CD8^+$ T cells that are observed in individuals during HIV-infection are still not well understood [reviewed in 60].

24.3.1.1 HIV and Cytotoxic T Cell (CTL) Response

CTLs recognize and kill target cells that present virus-specific peptides in an HLA class I context. Several studies showed that HIV-specific CTLs are crucial for the control of the virus and that many long-term non-progressors (LTNPs) maintain a vigorous HIV-specific T-cell response [67, 77]. Not only the quantity but also the quality of the CTL response may play a role as LTNPs show a broad specificity toward various HIV-1 proteins, while rapid progressors were found to express a narrow, static CTL response [37]. As recently shown [5], $CD8^+$ T cells from HIV-1-infected patients with slow disease progression exhibited potent polyfunctionality and HIV-suppressive activity. Elimination of HIV-infected cells occurs due to direct cell–cell contact between infected cells and HLA class I-restricted cytotoxic T cells [117] or non-cytolytic mechanisms [118]. $CD8^+$ T cells from HIV-infected individuals exhibit a strong soluble anti-HIV activity that inhibits HIV-replication in autologous and allogeneic cultures. Despite this potent initial CTL response, the virus continues to replicate during the course of infection. This viral escape is probably due to multiple factors such as CTL escape mutants, down-modulation of MHC class I on target cells by nef, lack of perforin and immature phenotype, PD1 expression on $CD8^+$ T cells [41, 78], T-cell dysfunction with reduced proliferative capacity and cytokine production. During primary infection, activated CTLs are capable of controlling the viremia [16, 53], which is associated with slower decrease in $CD4^+$ T-cell count (Fig. 24.1). Macaques infected with simian immunodeficiency virus (SIV) that were depleted of $CD8^+$ T cells using an anti-CD8 mAb showed a significantly increased viral load during acute and chronic SIV infection [44]. Therefore, low viral loads, sustained HIV-specific CTL activity, and slow disease progression are associated with a protective function of CTLs. Studies of individuals exposed to, but not infected with, HIV indicate that these persons elicited effective HIV-specific CTL responses. These findings further underline the important role of CTLs for the prevention of infection [84, 88]. Continued antigenic exposure might be necessary for maintaining the resistance against HIV infection, since a follow-up study in a cohort of commercial sex workers in Kenya demonstrated that seroconversion in several former exposed but not infected women occurred [47].

$CD8^+$ T cells may also become infected with HIV [89] in particular at late stages of the disease. De novo expression of CD4 upon co-stimulation of $CD8^+$ lymphocytes might explain the observed infection of $CD8^+$ T cells [52]. However, the frequency of infected memory $CD8^+$ T cells was described as only marginal [17]. Among the T-cell subsets harboring HIV, ~95% were $CD4^+$ memory T cells, ~3% naive $CD4^+$ T cells, 1.7% memory $CD8^+$ T cells (0% HIV-specific $CD8^+$ T cells) and 0% naïve $CD8^+$ T cells [17].

24.3.1.2 HIV and T Helper (T_H1/T_H2) Immune Response

$CD4^+$ T helper cells are antigen-specific and they are activated upon recognition of a viral epitope presented by MHC class II. T_H1 cells primarily produce IL-2 and IFN-γ, thereby supporting effector functions of the immune system (CTLs, NK cells, macrophages), while T_H2 cells mainly secrete IL-4, IL-5, IL-10, and IL-6, thus inducing a humoral immune response. Depletion of $CD4^+$ T cells occurs early during pathogenesis, since HIV preferentially infects activated $CD4^+$ cells. This loss in $CD4^+$ T-cell count and a functional loss with respect to an impaired cytokine production may contribute to the immune dysfunction during ongoing pathogenesis. Less attention has been paid to the protective role of $CD4^+$ T cells against HIV compared to $CD8^+$ T cells although studies reveal that both HIV-specific CTLs as well as helper T cells are essential for the control of viremia [46, 87]. Additionally, exposed but uninfected individuals show an increased anti-HIV-specific $CD4^+$ T-cell activity, and this argues for a protective role of HIV-specific helper T-cell responses [19, 84]. T helper cells of exposed but noninfected individuals secreted IL-2 following in vitro stimulation with HIV env antigens and peptides in contrast to control cells. Also, treatment during acute infection was shown to help in preserving the HIV-specific T-helper function [87], while treatment during the chronic phase was not able to reestablish an effective T helper cell response [8, 21].

24.3.1.3 HIV and T_{regs}

$CD4^+$ $CD25^+$ forkhead box transcription factor $(Foxp)^{3+}$ regulatory T cells (T_{regs}) that are crucial for maintaining T-cell tolerance to self-antigens and for avoiding autoimmune disorders were recently described as responsible for the suppression of T-cell responses to foreign antigens, including HIV. There is a substantial debate about beneficial versus detrimental effects of T_{regs} for the pathogenesis of HIV infection. On the one hand, T_{regs} are hypothesized to correlate with low immune activation and lower viral loads [75], and on the other, T_{reg} cells are said to hinder the control of HIV/SIV infection or facilitate the infection [1, 23, 51]. As recently published [73], numbers of T_{reg} cells in gut-associated lymphatic tissues (GALT) are increased in HIV-infected individuals, which might reflect the general depletion of $CD4^+$ T-cell counts in GALT [32]. The increased T_{reg} cell number may be induced by direct interaction of the cells with gp120 on HIV. The gp120-T_{reg} interaction was shown to induce proliferation of T_{regs} in vitro [73], resulting in an effective suppression of the immune response against HIV.

Human T_{reg} cells isolated from healthy donors were shown to express the HIV-co-receptor CCR5, to be highly susceptible to HIV infection dependent on the HIV-1 strain used [68] and to be killed by viral replication [75]. Further work is necessary to elucidate the timing and full implications of the expansion of this subset in tissues.

24.3.2 B cell Response

Several weeks after the initial phase of infection, HIV-1-specific antibodies (Abs) are detectable in the plasma of infected individuals (Fig. 24.1). Unfortunately, most of the putative neutralizing epitopes on the viral glycoproteins gp120 and gp41, which are involved in receptor binding and/or fusion events are shielded by carbohydrates and are thus not exposed and limited accessible. The ongoing mutations and recombination of the viral genome further contributes to the escape of HIV-1 to antibody-mediated immune responses. Therefore, only a limited fraction of HIV-specific antibodies in infected individuals exhibit a direct antiviral activity. These Abs are referred to as neutralizing Abs (nAbs). Although very few of the induced Abs can reduce the viral load, Abs are thought to contribute to the reduction of the viremia already during early stages of infection [2, 61, 111]. Their mode of action is still not completely defined. Some of the nAbs may inhibit viral entry by interfering either with structures of the gp120/gp41 complex or with epitopes that bind to chemokine receptors. Alternatively, they may cross-link virus particles and induce clearance of immune-complexed viruses by phagocytosis. Additionally, antibody-dependent cellular cytotoxicity (ADCC) is thought to appear early during acute infection [93] and can be detected at later stages of disease progression, too. ADCC has been studied in the SIV monkey model, was associated with the control of HIV in infected humans [12, 27, 30] and may contribute to a slower disease progression in long-term non-progressors [6]. In concert with Abs, complement activation and the subsequent CoML may further reduce the viral titer [102].

Presently only few monoclonal Abs (mAbs) have been established that have broad antiviral potency against HIV-1 [43, 115]. Among the best characterized mAbs are b12, 2G12, 2F5, and 4E10. The first two Abs are directed against gp120. While b12 is recognizing the CD4-binding site of gp120, 2G12 is directed against clusters of carbohydrate residues of oligomannose-type sugars on gp120. Thus, both Abs seem to interfere with viral binding to target cells. The mAbs 2F5 and 4E10 recognize adjacent but distinct epitopes on the ectodomain of gp41 and are thought to inhibit the fusion process. The broad antiviral effect of these mAbs has been shown in vitro for different strains and clades of HIV-1. A combination of the Abs was successfully tested in animal models too [26]. Vaccine approaches, which aim to induce Abs with 2G12 or 2F5 and 4G12 specificity did not elicit potent neutralizing Ab responses and the proof of viral control upon passive transfer of the Abs in phase I clinical trials remains circumstantial. However, passive transfer approaches to control viral replication in chronically infected individuals revealed a delay of HIV-1 rebound after the cessation of drug therapy [104]. The successful intervention of the antibodies in HIV-1 infected individuals may be limited due to the rapid selection of escape variants within the HIV-1 pool. Additionally host factors such as the complement system may counteract the nAb response by enhancing the infection [101–103, 115].

24.4 Concluding Remarks

The study of HIV and AIDS over the past decade has provided insights into the multifactorial interactions of HIV with the immune system. Specifically, cohort studies including investigations with LTNPs or rapid progressors helped to elucidate mechanisms contributing to the control of the viral replication in infected individuals. Although our understanding of the complex orchestration of the immune response is steadily growing, further intensive and extensive investigations are needed. Only the complete understanding of the multifaceted interplay of the immune system with HIV will provide the basis for the development of therapeutic and preventive vaccines.

Take-Home Pearls

- The innate immune response gains increasing attention in its contribution to control HIV infection.
- The complement system is among the first components activated.
- Together with interferons, cytokines, and chemokines, complement fragments activate innate immune cells, such as NK and NKT cells, monocytes, macrophages, and dendritic cells (DCs).
- Among the first identified HIV-suppressing chemokines (not identical with CAV) were RANTES, MIP-1α, MIP-1β, and SDF-1, which are also secreted by NK cells.
- NK cells also directly kill HIV-infected target cells by lysis or antibody-dependent cell-mediated cytotoxicity (ADCC).
- Despite NKT cells being involved in the innate immune response against auto-antigens and pathogens, they also appear to be susceptible to HIV infection.
- Both macrophages and monocytes are resistant to the cytopathic effects of HIV, and persist throughout the course of the disease, thereby acting as important viral reservoirs.
- Among the first cells interacting with HIV upon entry via mucosal surfaces are dendritic cells (DCs).
- DCs initiate, shape, and control the immune response, but they also efficiently assist in transmission to and infection of T cells with HIV.
- Although HIV infection affects the cellular arm of the innate immune response, the pathogenesis of HIV comprises mainly $CD4^+$ T cells.
- Ongoing viral replication during the chronic phase of the disease is accompanied by a continuous gradual loss of $CD4^+$ T cells.
- HIV interacts at multiple levels with the immune system and affects innate and adaptive immune responses.
- Only the complete understanding of the multifaceted interplay of the immune system with HIV will provide the basis for the development of therapeutic and preventive vaccines.

References

1. Aandahl, E.M., Michaelsson, J., Moretto, W.J., Hecht, F.M., Nixon, D.F.: Human CD4+ CD25+ regulatory T cells control T-cell responses to human immunodeficiency virus and cytomegalovirus antigens. J. Virol. **78**, 2454–2459 (2004)
2. Aasa-Chapman, M.M., Hayman, A., Newton, P., Cornforth, D., Williams, I., Borrow, P., et al.: Development of the

antibody response in acute HIV-1 infection. AIDS **18**, 371–381 (2004)

3. Ahmad, A., Menezes, J.: Antibody-dependent cellular cytotoxicity in HIV infections. FASEB J. **10**, 258–266 (1996)
4. Albini, A., et al.: Identification of a novel domain of HIV tat involved in monocyte chemotaxis. J. Biol. Chem. **273**, 15895–15900 (1998)
5. Almeida, J.R., Sauce, D., Price, D.A., Papagno, L., Shin, S.Y., Moris, A., Larsen, M., Pancino, G., Douek, D.C., Autran, B., Sáez-Cirión, A., Appay, V.: Antigen sensitivity is a major determinant of CD8+ T-cell polyfunctionality and HIV-suppressive activity. Blood **113**(25), 6351–6360 (2009)
6. Alsmadi, O., Herz, R., Murphy, E., Pinter, A., Tilley, S.A.: A novel antibody-dependent cellular cytotoxicity epitope in gp120 is identified by two monoclonal antibodies isolated from a long-term survivor of human immunodeficiency virus type 1 infection. J. Virol. **71**, 925–933 (1997)
7. Andrews, D.M., Scalzo, A.A., Yokoyama, W.M., Smyth, M.J., Degli-Esposti, M.A.: Functional interactions between dendritic cells and NK cells during viral infection. Nat. Immunol. **4**, 175–181 (2003)
8. Autran, B., et al.: Thymocyte and thymic microenvironment alterations during a systemic HIV infection in a severe combined immunodeficient mouse model. AIDS **10**, 717–727 (1996)
9. Banchereau, J., Steinman, R.M.: Dendritic cells and the control of immunity. Nature **392**, 245–252 (1998)
10. Banki, Z., et al.: Cross-linking of CD32 induces maturation of human monocyte-derived dendritic cells via NF-kappa B signaling pathway. J. Immunol. **170**, 3963–3970 (2003)
11. Bánki, Z., Kacani, L., Rusert, P., Pruenster, M., Wilflingseder, D., Falkensammer, B., Stellbrink, H.J., van Lunzen, J., Trkola, A., Dierich, M.P., Stoiber, H.: Complement dependent trapping of infectious HIV in human lymphoid tissues. AIDS **19**, 481–486 (2005)
12. Banks, N.D., Kinsey, N., Clements, J., Hildreth, J.E.: Sustained antibody-dependent cell-mediated cytotoxicity (ADCC) in SIV-infected macaques correlates with delayed progression to AIDS. AIDS Res. Hum. Retroviruses **18**, 1197–1205 (2002)
13. Barré-Sinoussi, F., Chermann, J.C., Rey, F., Nugeyre, M.T., Chamaret, S., Gruest, J., Dauguet, C., Axler-Blin, C., Vézinet-Brun, F., Rouzioux, C., Rozenbaum, W., Montagnier, L.: Isolation of a T-lymphotropic retrovirus from a patient at risk for acquired immune deficiency syndrome (AIDS). Science **220**, 868–871 (1983)
14. Bleul, C.C., Farzan, M., Choe, H., Parolin, C., Clark-Lewis, I., Sodroski, J., Springer, T.A.: The lymphocyte chemoattractant SDF-1 is a ligand for LESTR/fusin and blocks HIV-1 entry. Nature **382**, 829–833 (1996)
15. Bonaparte, M.I., Barker, E.: Killing of human immunodeficiency virus-infected primary T-cell blasts by autologous natural killer cells is dependent on the ability of the virus to alter the expression of major histocompatibility complex class I molecules. Blood **104**, 2087–2094 (2004)
16. Borrow, P., Lewicki, H., Hahn, B.H., Shaw, G.M., Oldstone, M.B.: Virus-specific CD8+ cytotoxic T-lymphocyte activity associated with control of viremia in primary human immunodeficiency virus type 1 infection. J. Virol. **68**, 6103–6110 (1994)
17. Brenchley, J.M., et al.: CD4+ T cell depletion during all stages of HIV disease occurs predominantly in the gastrointestinal tract. J. Exp. Med. **200**, 749–759 (2004)
18. Clapham, P.R., McKnight, A.: Cell surface receptors, virus entry and tropism of primate lentiviruses. J. Gen. Virol. **83**, 1809–1829 (2002)
19. Clerici, M., et al.: HIV-specific T-helper activity in seronegative health care workers exposed to contaminated blood. JAMA **271**, 42–46 (1994)
20. Cocchi, F., DeVico, A.L., Garzino-Demo, A., Arya, S.K., Gallo, R.C., Lusso, P.: Identification of RANTES, MIP-1 alpha, and MIP-1 beta as the major HIV-suppressive factors produced by CD8+ T cells. Science **270**, 1811–1815 (1995)
21. Connors, M., et al.: HIV infection induces changes in CD4+ T-cell phenotype and depletions within the CD4+ T-cell repertoire that are not immediately restored by antiviral or immune-based therapies. Nat. Med. **3**, 533–540 (1997)
22. Cooper, M.A., Fehniger, T.A., Fuchs, A., Colonna, M., Caligiuri, M.A.: NK cell and DC interactions. Trends Immunol. **25**, 47–52 (2004)
23. Estes, J.D., et al.: Premature induction of an immunosuppressive regulatory T cell response during acute simian immunodeficiency virus infection. J. Infect. Dis. **193**, 703–712 (2006)
24. Evans, D.T., et al.: Virus-specific cytotoxic T-lymphocyte responses select for amino-acid variation in simian immunodeficiency virus Env and Nef. Nat. Med. **5**, 1270–1276 (1999)
25. Federico, M., et al.: HIV-1 Nef activates STAT1 in human monocytes/macrophages through the release of soluble factors. Blood **98**, 2752–2761 (2001)
26. Ferrantelli, F., Rasmussen, R.A., Buckley, K.A., Li, P.L., Wang, T., Montefiori, D.C., Katinger, H., Stiegler, G., Anderson, D.C., McClure, H.M., Ruprecht, R.M.: Complete protection of neonatal rhesus macaques against oral exposure to pathogenic simian-human immunodeficiency virus by human anti-HIV monoclonal antibodies. J. Infect. Dis. **189**, 2167–2173 (2004)
27. Forthal, D.N., Landucci, G., Keenan, B.: Relationship between antibody-dependent cellular cytotoxicity, plasma HIV type 1 RNA, and CD4+ lymphocyte count. AIDS Res. Hum. Retroviruses **17**, 553–561 (2001)
28. Geijtenbeek, T.B., van Kooyk, Y.: DC-SIGN: a novel HIV receptor on DCs that mediates HIV-1 transmission. Curr. Top. Microbiol. Immunol. **276**, 31–54 (2003)
29. Godfrey, D.I., MacDonald, H.R., Kronenberg, M., Smyth, M.J., Van Kaer, L.: NKT cells: what's in a name? Nat. Rev. Immunol. **4**, 231–237 (2004)
30. Gómez-Román, V.R., Patterson, L.J., Venzon, D., Liewehr, D., Aldrich, K., Florese, R., et al.: Vaccine-elicited antibodies mediate antibody-dependent cellular cytotoxicity correlated with significantly reduced acute viremia in rhesus macaques challenged with SIVmac251. J. Immunol. **174**, 2185–2189 (2005)
31. Granelli-Piperno, A., Delgado, E., Finkel, V., Paxton, W., Steinman, R.M.: Immature dendritic cells selectively replicate macrophagetropic (M-tropic) human immunodeficiency virus type 1, while mature cells efficiently transmit both M- and T-tropic virus to T cells. J. Virol. **72**, 2733–2737 (1998)
32. Guadalupe, M., et al.: Viral suppression and immune restoration in the gastrointestinal mucosa of human

immunodeficiency virus type 1-infected patients initiating therapy during primary or chronic infection. J. Virol. **80**, 8236–8247 (2006)
33. Gummuluru, S., Rogel, M., Stamatatos, L., Emerman, M.: Binding of human immunodeficiency virus type 1 to immature dendritic cells can occur independently of DC-SIGN and mannose binding C-type lectin receptors via a cholesterol-dependent pathway. J. Virol. **77**, 12865–12874 (2003)
34. Harcourt, G.C., Garrard, S., Davenport, M.P., Edwards, A., Phillips, R.E.: HIV-1 variation diminishes CD4 T lymphocyte recognition. J. Exp. Med. **188**, 1785–1793 (1998)
35. Hassaine, G., et al.: The tyrosine kinase Hck is an inhibitor of HIV-1 replication counteracted by the viral vif protein. J. Biol. Chem. **276**, 16885–16893 (2001)
36. Haase, A.T.: Population biology of HIV-1 infection: viral and CD4+ T cell demographics and dynamics in lymphatic tissues. Annu. Rev. Immunol. **17**, 625–656 (1999)
37. Hay, C.M., et al.: Lack of viral escape and defective in vivo activation of human immunodeficiency virus type 1-specific cytotoxic T lymphocytes in rapidly progressive infection. J. Virol. **73**, 5509–5519 (1999)
38. Haynes, B.F., Pantaleo, G., Fauci, A.S.: Toward an understanding of the correlates of protective immunity to HIV infection. Science **271**, 324–328 (1996)
39. Herbeuval, J.P., Shearer, G.M.: HIV-1 immunopathogenesis: how good interferon turns bad. Clin. Immunol. **123**, 121–128 (2007)
40. Hogan, C.M., Hammer, S.M.: Host determinants in HIV infection and disease. Part 1: cellular and humoral immune responses. Ann. Intern. Med. **134**, 761–776 (2001)
41. Holm, M., Pettersen, F.O., Kvale, D.: PD-1 predicts CD4 loss rate in chronic HIV-1 infection better than HIV RNA and CD38 but not in cryopreserved samples. Curr. HIV Res. **6**, 49–58 (2008)
42. Hong, H.S., Eberhard, J.M., Keudel, P., Bollmann, B.A., Ballmaier, M., Bhatnagar, N., Zielinska-Skowronek, M., Schmidt, R.E., Meyer-Olson, D.J.: HIV infection is associated with a preferential decline in less differentiated CD56dim CD16+ NK cells. J. Virol. **84**(2), 1183–1188 (2009)
43. Huber, M., Olson, W.C., Trkola, A.: Antibodies for HIV treatment and prevention: window of opportunity? Curr. Top. Microbiol. Immunol. **317**, 39–66 (2008)
44. Jin, X., et al.: Dramatic rise in plasma viremia after CD8(+) T cell depletion in simian immunodeficiency virus-infected macaques. J. Exp. Med. **189**, 991–998 (1999)
45. Kacani, L., Prodinger, W.M., Sprinzl, G.M., Schwendinger, M.G., Spruth, M., Stoiber, H., Döpper, S., Steinhuber, S., Steindl, F., Dierich, M.P.: Detachment of human immunodeficiency virus type 1 from germinal centers by blocking complement receptor type 2. J. Virol. **74**, 7997–8002 (2000)
46. Kalams, S.A., et al.: Association between virus-specific cytotoxic T-lymphocyte and helper responses in human immunodeficiency virus type 1 infection. J. Virol. **73**, 6715–6720 (1999)
47. Kaul, R., et al.: Late seroconversion in HIV-resistant Nairobi prostitutes despite pre-existing HIV-specific CD8+ responses. J. Clin. Invest. **107**, 341–349 (2001)
48. Kawamura, T., et al.: Significant virus replication in Langerhans cells following application of HIV to abraded skin: relevance to occupational transmission of HIV. J. Immunol. **180**, 3297–3304 (2008)
49. Kedzierska, K., Crowe, S.M.: The role of monocytes and macrophages in the pathogenesis of HIV-1 infection. Curr. Med. Chem. **9**, 1893–1903 (2002)
50. Kino, T., Gragerov, A., Kopp, J.B., Stauber, R.H., Pavlakis, G.N., Chrousos, G.P.: The HIV-1 virion-associated protein vpr is a coactivator of the human glucocorticoid receptor. J. Exp. Med. **189**, 51–62 (1999)
51. Kinter, A., McNally, J., Riggin, L., Jackson, R., Roby, G., Fauci, A.S.: Suppression of HIV-specific T cell activity by lymph node CD25+ regulatory T cells from HIV-infected individuals. Proc. Natl. Acad. Sci. USA **104**, 3390–3395 (2007)
52. Kitchen, S.G., Korin, Y.D., Roth, M.D., Landay, A., Zack, J.A.: Costimulation of naive CD8(+) lymphocytes induces CD4 expression and allows human immunodeficiency virus type 1 infection. J. Virol. **72**, 9054–9060 (1998)
53. Koup, R.A., et al.: Temporal association of cellular immune responses with the initial control of viremia in primary human immunodeficiency virus type 1 syndrome. J. Virol. **68**, 4650–4655 (1994)
54. Kramer, B., Pelchen-Matthews, A., Deneka, M., Garcia, E., Piguet, V., Marsh, M.: HIV interaction with endosomes in macrophages and dendritic cells. Blood Cells Mol. Dis. **35**, 136–142 (2005)
55. Lanier, L.L.: NK cell recognition. Annu. Rev. Immunol. **23**, 225–274 (2005)
56. Liu, R., Paxton, W.A., Choe, S., Ceradini, D., Martin, S.R., Horuk, R., MacDonald, M.E., Stuhlmann, H., Koup, R.A., Landau, N.R.: Homozygous defect in HIV-1 coreceptor accounts for resistance of some multiply-exposed individuals to HIV-1 infection. Cell **86**, 367–377 (1996)
57. Lechmann, M., Berchtold, S., Hauber, J., Steinkasserer, A.: CD83 on dendritic cells: more than just a marker for maturation. Trends Immunol. **23**, 273–275 (2002)
58. Levy, J.A.: Pathogenesis of human immunodeficiency virus infection. Microbiol. Rev. **57**, 183–289 (1993)
59. Levy, J.A.: The search for the CD8+ cell anti-HIV factor (CAF). Trends Immunol. **24**, 628–632 (2003)
60. Lieberman, J., Shankar, P., Manjunath, N., Andersson, J.: Dressed to kill? A review of why antiviral CD8 T lymphocytes fail to prevent progressive immunodeficiency in HIV-1 infection. Blood **98**, 1667–1677 (2001)
61. Lindbäck, S., Thorstensson, R., Karlsson, A.C., von Sydow, M., Flamholc, L., Blaxhult, A., et al.: Diagnosis of primary HIV-1 infection and duration of follow-up after HIV exposure. Karolinska Institute Primary HIV Infection Study Group. AIDS **14**, 2333–2339 (2000)
62. Margolis, L., Shattock, R.: Selective transmission of CCR5-utilizing HIV-1: the 'gatekeeper' problem resolved? Nat. Rev. Microbiol. **4**, 312–317 (2006)
63. Mavilio, D., et al.: Natural killer cells in HIV-1 infection: dichotomous effects of viremia on inhibitory and activating receptors and their functional correlates. Proc. Natl. Acad. Sci. USA **100**, 15011–15016 (2003)
64. McDonald, D., Wu, L., Bohks, S.M., KewalRamani, V.N., Unutmaz, D., Hope, T.J.: Recruitment of HIV and its receptors to dendritic cell-T cell junctions. Science **300**, 1295–1297 (2003)
65. Mehandru, S., Poles, M.A., Tenner-Racz, K., Horowitz, A., Hurley, A., Hogan, C., Boden, D., Racz, P., Markowitz, M.:

Primary HIV-1 infection is associated with preferential depletion of CD4+ T lymphocytes from effector sites in the gastrointestinal tract. J. Exp. Med. **200**, 761–770 (2006)
66. Mellman, I., Steinman, R.M.: Dendritic cells: specialized and regulated antigen processing machines. Cell **106**, 255–258 (2001)
67. Miedema, F., Klein, M.R.: AIDS pathogenesis: a finite immune response to blame? Science **272**, 505–506 (1996)
68. Moreno-Fernandez, M.E., Zapata, W., Blackard, J.T., Franchini, G., Chougnet, C.A.: Human regulatory T cells are targets for HIV infection and their susceptibility differs depending on the HIV-1 strain. J. Virol. **83**(24), 12925–12933 (2009)
69. Moretta, L., et al.: Effector and regulatory events during natural killer-dendritic cell interactions. Immunol. Rev. **214**, 219–228 (2006)
70. Motsinger, A., Haas, D.W., Stanic, A.K., Van Kaer, L., Joyce, S., Unutmaz, D.: CD1d-restricted human natural killer T cells are highly susceptible to human immunodeficiency virus 1 infection. J. Exp. Med. **195**, 869–879 (2002)
71. Newman, K.C., Korbel, D.S., Hafalla, J.C., Riley, E.M.: Cross-talk with myeloid accessory cells regulates human natural killer cell interferon-gamma responses to malaria. PLoS Pathog. **2**, e118 (2006)
72. Nguyen, D.G., Hildreth, J.E.: Involvement of macrophage mannose receptor in the binding and transmission of HIV by macrophages. Eur. J. Immunol. **33**, 483–493 (2003)
73. Nilsson, J., et al.: HIV-1-driven regulatory T-cell accumulation in lymphoid tissues is associated with disease progression in HIV/AIDS. Blood **108**, 3808–3817 (2006)
74. Oberlin, E., Amara, A., Bachelerie, F., Bessia, C., Virelizier, J.L., Arenzana-Seisdedos, F., Schwartz, O., Heard, J.M., Clark-Lewis, I., Legler, D.F., Loetscher, M., Baggiolini, M., Moser, B.: The CXC chemokine SDF-1 is the ligand for LESTR/fusin and prevents infection by T-cell-line-adapted HIV-1. Nature **382**, 833–835 (1996)
75. Oswald-Richter, K., et al.: HIV infection of naturally occurring and genetically reprogrammed human regulatory T-cells. PLoS Biol. **2**, E198 (2004)
76. Pantaleo, G., et al.: Major expansion of CD8+ T cells with a predominant V beta usage during the primary immune response to HIV. Nature **370**, 463–467 (1994)
77. Pantaleo, G., et al.: Studies in subjects with long-term non-progressive human immunodeficiency virus infection. N. Engl. J. Med. **332**, 209–216 (1995)
78. Petrovas, C., et al.: PD-1 is a regulator of virus-specific CD8+ T cell survival in HIV infection. J. Exp. Med. **203**, 2281–2292 (2006)
79. Phair, J., Jacobson, L., Detels, R., Rinaldo, C., Saah, A., Schrager, L., Muñoz, A.: Acquired immune deficiency syndrome occurring within 5 years of infection with human immunodeficiency virus type-1: the Multicenter AIDS Cohort Study. J. Acquir. Immune. Defic. Syndr. **5**, 490–496 (1992)
80. Phillips, R.E., et al.: Human immunodeficiency virus genetic variation that can escape cytotoxic T cell recognition. Nature **354**, 453–459 (1991)
81. Piccioli, D., Sbrana, S., Melandri, E., Valiante, N.M.: Contact-dependent stimulation and inhibition of dendritic cells by natural killer cells. J. Exp. Med. **195**, 335–341 (2002)
82. Piguet, V., Sattentau, Q.: Dangerous liaisons at the virological synapse. J. Clin. Invest. **114**, 605–610 (2004)
83. Piguet, V., Steinman, R.M.: The interaction of HIV with dendritic cells: outcomes and pathways. Trends Immunol. **28**, 503–510 (2007)
84. Plummer, F.A., Ball, T.B., Kimani, J., Fowke, K.R.: Resistance to HIV-1 infection among highly exposed sex workers in Nairobi: what mediates protection and why does it develop? Immunol. Lett. **66**, 27–34 (1999)
85. Pruenster, M., et al.: C-type lectin-independent interaction of complement opsonized HIV with monocyte-derived dendritic cells. Eur. J. Immunol. **35**, 2691–2698 (2005)
86. Pulendran, B.: Variegation of the immune response with dendritic cells and pathogen recognition receptors. J. Immunol. **174**, 2457–2465 (2005)
87. Rosenberg, E.S., et al.: Immune control of HIV-1 after early treatment of acute infection. Nature **407**, 523–526 (2000)
88. Rowland-Jones, S., et al.: HIV-specific cytotoxic T-cells in HIV-exposed but uninfected Gambian women. Nat. Med. **1**, 59–64 (1995)
89. Saha, K., Zhang, J., Zerhouni, B.: Evidence of productively infected CD8+ T cells in patients with AIDS: implications for HIV-1 pathogenesis. J. Acquir. Immune. Defic. Syndr. **26**, 199–207 (2001)
90. Sallusto, F., et al.: Rapid and coordinated switch in chemokine receptor expression during dendritic cell maturation. Eur. J. Immunol. **28**, 2760–2769 (1998)
91. Sandberg, J.K., et al.: Selective loss of innate CD4(+) V alpha 24 natural killer T cells in human immunodeficiency virus infection. J. Virol. **76**, 7528–7534 (2002)
92. Santin, A.D., et al.: Expression of surface antigens during the differentiation of human dendritic cells vs macrophages from blood monocytes in vitro. Immunobiology **200**, 187–204 (1999)
93. Sawyer, L.A., Katzenstein, D.A., Hendry, R.M., Boone, E.J., Vujcic, L.K., Williams, C.C., et al.: Possible beneficial effects of neutralizing antibodies and antibody-dependent, cell-mediated cytotoxicity in human immunodeficiency virus infection. AIDS Res. Hum. Retroviruses **6**, 341–356 (1990)
94. Schmidt, B., et al.: Low-level HIV infection of plasmacytoid dendritic cells: onset of cytopathic effects and cell death after PDC maturation. Virology **329**, 280–288 (2004)
95. Sharkey, M.E., et al.: Persistence of episomal HIV-1 infection intermediates in patients on highly active anti-retroviral therapy. Nat. Med. **6**, 76–81 (2000)
96. Sharova, N., Swingler, C., Sharkey, M., Stevenson, M.: Macrophages archive HIV-1 virions for dissemination *in trans*. EMBO J. **24**, 2481–2489 (2005)
97. Speth, C., Prodinger, W.M., Würzner, R., Stoiber, H., Dierich, M.P.: Complement. In: Fundamental Immunology, 6th edn, pp. 1047–1078. Lippincott-Raven, Philadelphia, New York (2008)
98. Stahl-Hennig, C., et al.: Rapid infection of oral mucosal-associated lymphoid tissue with simian immunodeficiency virus. Science **285**, 1261–1265 (1999)
99. Steinman, R.M.: The dendritic cell advantage: New focus for immune-based therapies. Drug News Perspect. **13**, 581–586 (2000)
100. Stoiber, H., Speth, C., Dierich, M.P.: Editorial. Mol. Immunol. **42**, 143–144 (2005)

101. Stoiber, H., Banki, Z., Wilflingseder, D., Dierich, M.P.: Complement-HIV interactions during all steps of viral pathogenesis. Vaccine **26**(24), 3046–3054 (2008)
102. Stoiber, H., Soederholm, A., Wilflingseder, D., Gusenbauer, S., Hildgartner, A., Dierich, M.P.: Complement and antibodies: a dangerous liaison in HIV infection? Vaccine **26**(Suppl 8), I79–I85 (2008)
103. Stoiber, H.: Complement, Fc receptors and antibodies: a Trojan horse in HIV infection? Curr. Opin. HIV AIDS **4**, 394–399 (2009)
104. Trkola, A., Kuster, H., Rusert, P., Joos, B., Fischer, M., Leemann, C., Manrique, A., Huber, M., Rehr, M., Oxenius, A., Weber, R., Stiegler, G., Vcelar, B., Katinger, H., Aceto, L., Günthard, H.F.: Delay of HIV-1 rebound after cessation of antiretroviral therapy through passive transfer of human neutralizing antibodies. Nat. Med. **11**, 615–622 (2005)
105. Trumpfheller, C., Park, C.G., Finke, J., Steinman, R.M., Granelli-Piperno, A.: Cell type-dependent retention and transmission of HIV-1 by DC-SIGN. Int. Immunol. **15**, 289–298 (2003)
106. Tschachler, E., et al.: Epidermal Langerhans cells: a target for HTLV-III/LAV infection. J. Invest. Dermatol. **88**, 233–237 (1987)
107. Turville, S., Wilkinson, J., Cameron, P., Dable, J., Cunningham, A.L.: The role of dendritic cell C-type lectin receptors in HIV pathogenesis. J. Leukoc. Biol. **74**, 710–718 (2003)
108. Unutmaz, D., KewalRamani, V.N., Marmon, S., Littman, D.R.: Cytokine signals are sufficient for HIV-1 infection of resting human T lymphocytes. J. Exp. Med. **189**, 1735–1746 (1999)
109. van't Wout, A.B., et al.: Macrophage-tropic variants initiate human immunodeficiency virus type 1 infection after sexual, parenteral, and vertical transmission. J. Clin. Invest. **94**, 2060–2067 (1994)
110. Weissman, D., Li, Y., Orenstein, J.M., Fauci, A.S.: Both a precursor and a mature population of dendritic cells can bind HIV. However, only the mature population that expresses CD80 can pass infection to unstimulated CD4+ T cells. J. Immunol. **155**, 4111–4117 (1995)
111. Wei, X., Decker, J.M., Wang, S., Hui, H., Kappes, J.C., Wu, X., et al.: Antibody neutralization and escape by HIV-1. Nature **422**, 307–312 (2003)
112. Weiss, R.A.: Special anniversary review: twenty-five years of human immunodeficiency virus research: successes and challenges. Clin. Exp. Immunol. **152**, 201–210 (2008)
113. Wilflingseder, D., et al.: HIV-1-induced migration of monocyte-derived dendritic cells is associated with differential activation of MAPK pathways. J. Immunol. **173**, 7497–7505 (2004)
114. Wilflingseder, D., et al.: IgG opsonization of HIV impedes provirus formation in and infection of dendritic cells and subsequent long-term transfer to T cells. J. Immunol. **178**, 7840–7848 (2007)
115. Willey, S., Aasa-Chapman, M.M.I.: Humoral immunity to HIV-1: neutralisation and antibody effector functions. Trends in Microbiol. **16**(12), 596–604 (2008)
116. Woelk, C.H., et al.: Interferon gene expression following HIV type 1 infection of monocyte-derived macrophages. AIDS Res. Hum. Retroviruses **20**, 1210–1222 (2004)
117. Yang, O.O., et al.: Suppression of human immunodeficiency virus type 1 replication by CD8+ cells: evidence for HLA class I-restricted triggering of cytolytic and noncytolytic mechanisms. J. Virol. **71**, 3120–3128 (1997)
118. Yewdell, J.W., Norbury, C.C., Bennink, J.R.: Mechanisms of exogenous antigen presentation by MHC class I molecules in vitro and in vivo: implications for generating CD8+ T cell responses to infectious agents, tumors, transplants, and vaccines. Adv. Immunol. **73**, 1–77 (1999)
119. Zitvogel, L.: Dendritic and natural killer cells cooperate in the control/switch of innate immunity. J. Exp. Med. **195**, F9–F14 (2002)

HIV in Children

25

Sasan Mohammadsaeed, James R. Murphy, and Gloria P. Heresi

Core Messages

- A basic difference between pediatric and adult HIV infection is the main route of transmission which is mother to child, Vertical transmission, to infants and children.
- VT makes serological tests of limited use for diagnosis of HIV infected infants. PCR is the main and primary diagnostic test for them.
- Immaturity of fetus and newborn immune system leads to rapid disease progression in some HIV infected infants.
- HIV has important adverse effects on the developing central nervous system (CNS) and normal linear growth and weight gain; hence encephalopathy and growth retardation are early and common problems in HIV infected children.
- Because disease progression is unpredictable in HIV infected infants, all *HIV exposed* infants have to get PJP prophylaxis and all *HIV infected* infants have to be treated with cART.
- VT of HIV is an important impediment to disease control in developing countries. The keys of successful prevention are: 1) Universal screening of pregnant women. 2) Antiretroviral therapy for all HIV infected mothers and exposed neonates. 3) Withholding of breast feeding when safe.

S. Mohammadsaeed, J.R. Murphy, and G.P. Heresi (✉)
Department of Pediatrics, University of Texas Health Science Center at Houston, Pediatric Infectious Diseases,
6431 Fannin, MSB 6.132a, Houston, TX, USA
e-mail: gloria.p.heresi@uth.tmc.edu

25.1 Introduction

Important features distinguish HIV infection in infants and children from the infection in adults. A supermajority of infections is acquired by maternal-to-child transmission (MTCT). There is clear evidence from resource-rich countries that existing interventions can prevent most MTCT [26, 73]. However, these interventions are not deployed against the majority of about 1,500 MTCT that occur daily, mostly in sub-Saharan Africa [71] and postnatally a very small fraction of these children even receive antiretroviral treatment [6]. Possibly because HIV infection in newborns [43] is less well immunologically controlled than that of adults, infection progresses more rapid following MTCT. Half of these infected children may die before the age of 2 years [17, 54]. Thus, for most HIV-infected children the natural history of HIV disease is that of an infection progressing without antiretroviral therapy. This pattern results in significant excess morbidity in addition to mortality.

Pediatric HIV is the area in which the major advance in reducing HIV morbidity and mortality has occurred, i.e., the capacity to stop nearly all MTCT. Dissemination of this known effective intervention to populations in need stands second only to finding a cure for infection as an important goal in HIV control.

25.2 Epidemiology of Pediatric AIDS

25.2.1 Global Vision

As of November 2007, 33.2 million people worldwide were living with HIV [72] and 2.5 million of these were children under 15 years old [71, 72]. Children

G. Gross and S.K. Tyring (eds.), *Sexually Transmitted Infections and Sexually Transmitted Diseases*,
DOI: 10.1007/978-3-642-14663-3_25,

(<15 years) account for 16.5% of all new HIV infections, 7.5% of total HIV infections, and 15.7% of deaths from HIV/AIDS [71]. The number of children living with HIV increased from 1.5 million in 2001 to 2.5 million in 2007 with nearly 90% of cases occurring in sub-Saharan Africa. In this century, global deaths due to HIV/AIDS in children range from 330,000 to 360,000 per year [71, 72]. Worldwide approximately 4% of all child deaths (<5 years) is attributable to HIV/AIDS [40].

25.2.1.1 Two Pediatric HIV Epidemics

Worldwide pediatric HIV resolves into two distinct epidemiological patterns. One is occurring in resource-rich regions and is characterized by low rates of HIV infection, prolonged survival, complications of long-term combination antiretroviral therapy (cART), problems with adherence to ART, ART resistance, chronic and acute mental health morbidity, and issues of transitions of children to adolescents and then to adults. These characteristics are directly related to the wide availability of effective ART in an environment where diagnosis, education, and counseling services are generally available and where formula feeding is practical [34, 71].

The opposite is true for the 95% of HIV-infected children who reside in the developing world where lack of early infant diagnosis, breast feeding, late or no access to care and treatment, and limited treatment options lead to increased early mortality [50].

25.2.2 Male–Female Ratio in Pediatric HIV

In Africa, a strong association of infant HIV infection and female gender was observed in Malawi [67], with 12.6% of girls, compared with 6.3% of boys, infected at birth (m/f = 1/2). Results from studies in Europe [68, 75] and Cote d'Ivoire [4] had similar findings. In the Malawian study [67], female infants continued to acquire infections postnatally more frequently than boys through to 6–8 weeks of age, but the difference was not statistically significant. Other studies, however, including major clinical trials in the USA [14] and Africa [33], did not show a significantly increased risk of HIV among newborn girls. And, in the USA from 1992 up to 2004, there were no notable gender differences in number of MTCT [47]. There is no apparent explanation for these discrepant results and the possibility that HIV-infected males in certain circumstances may have higher in utero death rates has not been excluded.

25.2.3 Migration

In countries of low HIV incidence, migration-related infection in children may be an emerging epidemic. In 2002, Canada introduced routine, mandatory HIV-antibody screening for residency applicants, including selected children. From January 2002 to February 2005, 36 pediatric HIV cases were detected (14/100,000 applicants) with 32 (89%) originating in Africa and the major mode of acquisition being MTCT; 94% of infected children were eligible for entry into Canada [44]. For children less than 15 years old immigrating to the USA no laboratory testing is required [63]. A study of 119 HIV-infected children born before or after immigration to Belgium documented seven infections attributed to blood product transfusion and 112 MTCT [21, 36]. Migration can be a significant source of pediatric HIV, including MTCT in countries of low incidence, especially under circumstances where migrants avoid prenatal care [18, 19].

25.2.4 International Adoption

Significant numbers of children from resource-poor high-HIV-risk environments are adopted by residents in resource-rich settings; from 1986 to 2003 nearly 220,000 children were adopted from other countries by US residents [49]. Despite widespread public concern about HIV infection in international adoptees, the risk is low. In seven studies that present a total of 1,089 children adopted by persons resident in the USA, Australia, and France, no child with HIV infection was identified [49].

25.2.5 Pediatric HIV/AIDS in Africa

Although globally more than 68% of HIV infected adults live in Africa, nearly 90% of children infected with HIV live in this region. There are an estimated 2 million HIV-infected children and 11.4 million orphans due to HIV/AIDS in southern Africa [71]. HIV/AIDS is the single largest cause of mortality in sub-Saharan Africa. Major modes of acquisition of pediatric HIV in Africa include in rank MTCT, breast feeding, and transfusion of blood products. Because seroprevalence in the general population is high, even in African regions where HIV screening of blood donors is available, the risk of HIV infection from donors who are in the seroconversion window is significant.

25.2.6 Pediatric AIDS in the USA

Although the USA had an estimated 1.1 million HIV-infected persons at the end of 2007 [31] of which 9,590 were less than 13 years old [12] and had >35,000 new HIV/AIDS cases diagnosed in 2007 [12], there is now very little MTCT. MTCT cases in the USA decreased from a peak of 945 in 1992 to 48 in 2008. The prevalence of HIV infection among children was 7.4 per 100,000 at the end of 2005 [11]. As in adults there is a large race/ethnicity discrepancy in the prevalence of pediatric HIV cases with black children constituting 67% of the total US cases [46], where blacks comprise 13.4% of the US population [70]. Of the estimated 9,590 children living with HIV/AIDS (in 2007), 92% had been exposed perinatally, 6% from a transfusion of blood or blood products (2% from transfusion because of hemophilia) [12]. However, for children with hemophilia and coagulation disorders there have been no new HIV/AIDS cases in children <13 years in the USA since 2001 [71]. The annual death rate for HIV-infected children in the USA declined from 13% in 1995 to 1% in 2004–2005 [40]. A notable problem in some large metropolitan regions in the USA is that up to 50% of MTCT cases of HIV are in recent migrants, most of whom do not receive prenatal care [18, 19].

25.2.7 Pediatric AIDS in Europe

In the WHO European region (up to December 31, 2005) most (80%) MTCT HIV infections have been reported from the western Europe region (38.2% of total cases from the UK). Reported cases of MTCT in western Europe increased through to 2002, and have since decreased to 200 cases in 2005. In eastern Europe, reported MTCT cases increased from 12 in 2001 to 83 cases in 2005 [25]. Because the European region comprises numerous countries with differing reporting requirements and a number of larger countries that have not reported, incidence rates and regional distributions of cases can be misleading. The overall picture of pediatric HIV in Europe is consistent with that seen in North America with indications that migration may be more of a factor in the western, and IV drug abuse in the eastern regions. Clusters of special circumstances exist. Romania, for example, had a reported 4,611 pediatric AIDS cases through December 1997, which, at that time, represented more than one-half of all European pediatric AIDS cases [39, 46]. Children represented 90% of all Romanian AIDS cases and were born mostly to uninfected mothers (4% MTCT). An iatrogenic procedure was found responsible for most of this transmission and its discontinuance resulted in termination of this epidemic [41]. In Kazakhstan, a blood transfusion-associated outbreak infecting more than 130 children was reported [71].

25.2.8 Pediatric AIDS in Asia

The number of HIV-positive children in Asia and the Pacific continues to grow. In 2005, more than 138,000 children and adolescents were living with HIV in the region. By 2006, that number increased 38%, to more than 190,000 – a figure that will continue to climb given the relative absence of mother-to-child transmission-prevention programs and improvements in reporting. Many HIV-positive women are understandably reluctant to seek antiretroviral therapy or to bottle-feed their infants for fear of arousing suspicion regarding their HIV status and confronting the stigma surrounding HIV/AIDS in some locations [2].

25.3 Pathogenesis

The pathogenesis of untreated HIV infection in children shares major characteristics with disease in untreated adults. Shortly after infection, high-level viremia occurs, and then drops to a lower-level set point that is maintained for a varying, but usually extended, interval until viral load again increases in late-stage disease. In parallel, the number and percentage of CD4+ lymphocytes progressively declines. Notable differences as compared to adults for MTCT infection include that high-level initial viremia, which usually persists for weeks in adults, may persist for years following MTCT. Viral-specific cytotoxic T-cells (CTL) that are associated with control of infection appear in weeks following infection of adults and rapidly rise to high levels in parallel with decline in viral load. These do not appear until months after MTCT and thereafter may not reach substantial levels through a year of more after infection [43]. Reasons proposed for infection being less well controlled following MTCT include that infection occurs before the immune system is fully developed, the newborn shares HLA alleles with the mother and to which the transmitted virus is adapted, and that passive transfer of maternal antibodies may inhibit generation of virus-specific immunity by the newborn [57].

25.4 Transmission

Transmission of HIV-l occurs via sexual contact, other exposures to live-virus-containing fluids and tissues including vertical transmission (VT) from mother to child. VT can occur before (intrauterine), during (intrapartum), or after delivery (mostly through breast-feeding) and is the cause of 90% of pediatric HIV globally and is predominantly a disease of resource-poor regions.

In resource-rich regions, VT is well controlled. The combination of maternal cART, neonatal ART, and cesarean section results in very limited VT, with the notable exceptions of mothers in whom HIV infection is not controllable because of ineffectiveness of cART (usually because of multi-ART-resistant viruses), noncompliance with ART, or failure to receive prenatal care. Although fewer neonates are acquiring HIV by VT in these regions, those that become infected are likely to live through sexual debut and potentially become sources for further spread by means usually associated with the epidemiology of infection in adults. Acquisition of HIV through sexual abuse of children is increasingly recognized.

In resource-poor regions, ART, prenatal care, and cesarean section are not readily available and VT rates are between 25% and 40%. These rates show that VT is a significantly more efficient mode of transfer of HIV than sexual contact and second only to implantation of HIV-infected blood or tissues where a 90% transmission rate can be seen. About 15–20% of HIV infection at birth is attributable to intrauterine acquisition of the virus and 60–80% intrapartum infection. Intrauterine transmission is identifiable by a positive HIV DNA PCR test on a newborn by age 48 h [22]. Intrapartum transfer is evidenced by infants that do not show viremia before 1 week of age [33], that cesarean section results in decreased transmission, and that first-born twins are three times more likely to be infected than the paired sibling. Longer exposure to the birth canal associates with enhanced transmission.

A comparison of rates of VT before and after the introduction of cART and between resource-rich and -poor regions reveals conditions that enhance transmission of HIV. Before the use of ART, MTCT rates ranged between 13% and 40% [29, 61] with the highest rates reported from Africa [61]. This regional disparity most likely reflects differences in the severity of maternal disease, nutritional status, rates of breast feeding, and concomitant STD. And, it has been clearly established that mothers at both extremes of the clinical evolution of HIV infection with either acute primary infection [23, 42, 55, 66] or advanced, symptomatic disease [61] are more likely to transmit HIV to their infants than asymptomatic seropositive women. For women whose HIV-positive status is known during pregnancy, the most important risk factor for VT is the maternal HIV viral load [37, 51]. However, globally, the main risk factor for VT is lack of awareness of HIV status. Use of illicit drugs during pregnancy and low-antenatal CD4 count are also associated with increased risk for MTCT as are obstetric factors that disrupt the maternal–fetal barrier (chorioamnionitis, preterm delivery, or prolonged rupture of membranes).

Breast feeding is an efficient mode of transmission of HIV and can be responsible for up to 50% of cases of VT in some regions; between 320,000 and 800,000 infections per year globally [28]. Although transmission can occur at any point during breast feeding, the first 6 weeks of life entail the greatest risk comprising about 67% of transmissions [28, 52, 75]. The greater cellular composition of colostrum and early milk has been suggested as a mechanism. However, the risk of transmission by breast milk, although remaining significant, is less for exclusive breast feeding; combinations of breast feeding with solid foods or formula result in higher transmission rates. The frequency of breast-milk transmission is also increased if the mother's $CD4^+$ count is less than 200 cells/μL.

The World Health Organization (WHO) recommends that women be counseled about the risk of HIV transmission through breast feeding. When replacement feeding is affordable, feasible, acceptable, sustainable, and safe, avoidance of all breast feeding by HIV-infected mothers is recommended. When replacement feeding is not possible, exclusive breast feeding is recommended and breast feeding should be discontinued as soon as possible [15, 79].

In some regions and cultures, premastication of solid foods by an adult prior to feeding of an infant occurs. If the adult is HIV-infected, this practice can result in infection of the child [30].

In regions where exclusive formula feeding is readily available and socially acceptable, breast-feeding transmission of HIV has been essentially eliminated.

25.5 Clinical Manifestations

Important differences exist between clinical manifestations of HIV in adults and children: The immune system is immature in infants and young children and perhaps because of this they can develop severe immune deficiency while maintaining high CD4 counts. Lymphocytic interstitial pneumonitis (LIP) and multiple or recurrent serious bacterial infections are AIDS-defining conditions only for children. Certain types of cytomegalovirus (CMV) and herpes simplex virus (HSV) infections and toxoplasmosis of the brain are AIDS-defining only for adults and for children older than 1 month of age [8]. Overall, HIV disease progression in children is more rapid and *Pneumocystis jiroveci* pneumonia (PJP) and encephalopathy occur early in the course of HIV infection (especially in infants). Cerebral toxoplasmosis, cryptococcal meningitis and pneumonia, progressive multifocal leukoencephalopathy (PML), all forms of Kaposi's sarcoma, bacillary angiomatosis, cytomegalovirus retinitis, and hypersensitivity to trimethoprim and sulfamethoxazole [20] are rare in children.

Clinical presentation of HIV infection in children varies by age. Infants with vertically acquired HIV infection usually are clinically normal during the neonatal period. Infrequently, they may present similar to other congenital infections with growth retardation, skin rash, lymphadenopathy, hepatosplenomegaly, and cytopenias. In infants, common presentations of HIV infection are PJP, generalized adenopathy, hepatomegaly, splenomegaly, failure to thrive (FTT), and, recurrent invasive bacterial infections. Progression to moderate or severe immune suppression is also frequent in infected infants. By 12 months of age, approximately 50% of children develop moderate immune suppression and 20% severe immune suppression [32]. The 1-year risk of AIDS or death is substantially higher in younger than older children at any CD4 percentage, particularly for infants age <12 months [9].

School-aged children may present with progressive cognitive delay, recurrent otitis media, pneumonia, sinusitis, and lymphoid interstitial pneumonitis.

Older children present with opportunistic infections suggestive of very low $CD4^+$ T-cell counts, such as oral candidiasis, recurrent diarrhea, cardiomyopathy, HIV encephalopathy, and malignancies [33]. In recent years with earlier diagnosis and with expanded use of cART, these manifestations are less common.

Growth abnormalities were among the first recognized manifestations of HIV infection in children [13, 48]. Growth retardation is often apparent within 3–4 months after birth, and the magnitude of height and weight impairment increases with age [20]. Wasting syndrome (as defined in Ped HIV Classification [Box 25.1]), is not as common as FTT in pediatric patients. Before the cART era, at least one-third of HIV-infected children experienced severe growth delay (Table 25.1) [48].

Recurrent bacterial infections (Box 1) are second only to PJP as an AIDS-defining infection. HIV-infected patients have a rate of invasive pneumococcal disease that is approximately 40 times that of the general population. The most common serious infections are bacteremia, sepsis, and bacterial pneumonia.

Lymphocytic interstitial pneumonitis LIP is the most common chronic lower respiratory tract abnormality (historically occurring in 20–40%) [3] and the second most common AIDS-defining illness (about 20% of cases) in children with HIV infection. It is the only AIDS-defining condition that does not belong to CDC class 3 status, because the prognosis of children with LIP is better than that of children with other AIDS-defining illnesses [8, 69]. The cause of LIP is unclear, although it is speculated that an exaggerated

Box 25.1: 1994 Revised Human Immunodeficiency Virus Pediatric Classification System: Clinical Categories

Category N: Not symptomatic
No signs or symptoms considered to be the result of HIV infection or only one of the conditions listed in Category A.

Category A: Mildly symptomatic
Two or more of the following without any of the conditions listed in Categories B and C: lymphadenopathy (0.5 cm at more than two sites; bilateral – one site); hepatomegaly; splenomegaly; dermatitis; parotitis; recurrent or persistent upper respiratory infection, sinusitis, or otitis media.

Category B: Moderately symptomatic
Symptomatic conditions attributed to HIV infection other than those listed for Category A or C including but not limited to anemia (<8 g/dL), neutropenia (<1,000/μL), or thrombocytopenia (<100,000/μL) persisting 30 days; bacterial meningitis, pneumonia, or sepsis (single episode); oropharyngeal candidiasis persisting for >2 months; cardiomyopathy; cytomegalovirus (CMV) infection with onset before age 1 month; recurrent or chronic diarrhea; hepatitis; recurrent herpes simplex virus (HSV) stomatitis (more than two episodes within 1 year); HSV bronchitis, pneumonitis, or esophagitis with onset before age 1 month; herpes zoster involving at least two distinct episodes or more than one dermatone; leiomyosarcoma; lymphoid interstitial pneumonia (LIP) or pulmonary lymphoid hyperplasia (PLH) complex; nephropathy; nocardiosis; fever lasting >1 month; toxoplasmosis with onset before age 1 month; disseminated varicella.

Category C: Severely symptomatic
Any condition listed in the 1987 surveillance case definition for AIDS, with the exception of LIP (which is a category B condition): Serious bacterial infections, multiple or recurrent (i.e., any combination of at least two culture confirmed infections within a 2-year period) of the following types: septicemia, pneumonia, meningitis, bone or joint infection, or abscess of an internal organ or body cavity; candidiasis esophageal or pulmonary; coccidioidomycosis, disseminated; cryptococcosis, extrapulmonary; cryptosporidiosis or isosporiasis with diarrhea persisting >1 month; cytomegalovirus disease with onset of symptoms at age >1 month (at a site other than liver, spleen, or lymph nodes); encephalopathy (at least one of the following progressive findings present for at least 2 months in the absence of a concurrent illness other than HIV infection that could explain the findings): (a) failure to attain or loss of developmental milestones or loss of intellectual ability; (b) impaired brain growth or acquired microcephaly or brain atrophy demonstrated by CT scan or MRI; (c) acquired symmetric motor deficit manifested by two or more of the following: paresis, pathologic reflexes, ataxia, or gait disturbance; herpes simplex virus infection causing a mucocutaneous ulcer that persists for >1 month; or bronchitis, pneumonitis, or esophagitis for any duration affecting a child >1 month of age; histoplasmosis, disseminated (at a site other than or in addition to lungs or cervical or hilar lymph nodes); Kaposi's sarcoma; lymphoma, primary, in brain; lymphoma, small, noncleaved cell (Burkitt's), or immunoblastic or large cell lymphoma of B-cell or unknown immunologic phenotype; Mycobacterium tuberculosis, disseminated or extrapulmonary; Mycobacterium, other species or unidentified species, disseminated; Mycobacterium avium complex or *Mycobacterium kansasii*, disseminated; *Pneumocystis jiroveci* pneumonia; progressive multifocal leukoencephalopathy; *Salmonella* (nontyphoid) septicemia, recurrent; toxoplasmosis of the brain with onset at >1 month of age; wasting syndrome in the absence of a concurrent illness other than HIV infection that could explain the following findings: (a) persistent weight loss >10% of baseline; OR (b) downward crossing of at least two of the following percentile lines on the weight-for-age chart (e.g., 95th, 75th, 50th, 25th, 5th) in a child ≥1 year of age; OR (c) <5th percentile on weight-for-height chart on two consecutive measurements, ≥30 days apart PLUS: (1) chronic diarrhea (i.e., ≥2 loose stools per day for >30 days),OR (2) documented fever (for ≥30 days, intermittent or constant).

Table 25.1 Revised HIV pediatric classification system (immunologic categories)

Immune category	<12 months		1–5 years		6–12 years	
	CD4 number	CD4 (%)	CD4 number	CD4 (%)	CD4 number	CD4 (%)
Category 1 – no suppression	>1,500	25	1,000	25	500	25
Category 2 – moderate suppression	750–1,499	15–24	500–999	15–24	200–499	15–24
Category 3 – severe suppression	<750	<15	<500	<15	<200	<15

CDC 1994, MMWR [9]

local response to Epstein–Barr virus or HIV, or both may be causative [3].

CNS involvement is frequent in pediatric HIV infection, and encephalopathy is an AIDS-defining condition. At the beginning of the epidemic, 50–60% of children with advanced HIV infection developed progressive encephalopathy; but in recent estimates the frequency of this complication ranged from 20% to 40% [24]. HIV encephalopathy usually presents as peripheral spasticity, followed or accompanied by developmental delay or loss of developmental milestones and cognitive decline, with or without microcephaly [1]. The course may be progressive or it may plateau and become static. It may resemble, and may be difficult to differentiate from, cerebral palsy. Neuroradiographic findings include cerebral atrophy, white matter lesions, and basal ganglia calcifications. Of these, atrophy is most closely related to the clinical findings of HIV encephalopathy [56].

Opportunistic infections (OI) are generally seen in children with severe depression of the CD4 count. PJP is the most common serious OI in children with HIV infection and is associated with a high mortality [65]. PJP occurs most frequently in infants between 3 and 6 months of age, but it can occur in younger infants, beginning as early as 4–6 weeks of age [77]. Infants and children characteristically develop a subacute, diffuse pneumonitis with dyspnea at rest, tachypnea, oxygen desaturation, nonproductive cough, and fever [77]. Other common opportunistic infections that occur as a presentation in children with AIDS include *Candida* esophagitis, disseminated cytomegalovirus infection, chronic or disseminated herpes simplex virus, and varicella–zoster virus infections. The rate of *M. avium* complex infection and *Cryptococcus* infection in HIV-infected children is less than 14% and 1%, compared with 18–36% and 5–15%, respectively, in adults.

Hepatitis C virus and HIV coinfection in children is much less common than in adults (2% versus 33%) [62]. Malignant disorders are more common in HIV-infected children (representing 2% of pediatric AIDS-defining illnesses). As in adults, the most common malignancy is B-cell lymphoma [74]. Kaposi's sarcoma is rare in children.

25.6 Diagnosis

Diagnosis of HIV infection in children older than 18 months, as in adults, is routinely based on serologic tests and except for a window of the first few weeks after infection; these tests are highly sensitive and specific. During the first weeks following infection, HIV viral load by RNA assay is the preferred method for diagnosis.

A different approach is required for children younger than 18 months because serological tests may yield false-positive results due to the presence of maternal antibodies to HIV and tests for the presence of HIV RNA in plasma may yield false-negative results because of influences of maternal cART. Because of this confounding, the most commonly used definitive test for diagnosis of HIV infection before 18 months of age is HIV DNA PCR [7].

25.6.1 HIV DNA PCR

HIV DNA PCR detects specific HIV sequences in integrated proviral DNA in patient's peripheral blood mononuclear cells. The sensitivity of a single HIV DNA PCR test performed at <48 h of age is less than 40%, but increases to over 90% by 2–4 weeks of age [53].

25.6.2 *HIV RNA Assays*

HIV RNA assays detect extracellular viral RNA in plasma. It has been speculated that false-negative results can be obtained with the HIV RNA test if the mother of a newborn received cART [16, 59]. Positive results from either RNA or DNA tests have similar specificities. Some prefer to use an HIV RNA test as a confirmatory test for infants who have an initial positive HIV DNA PCR test. This strategy has benefits beyond confirming the diagnosis: it saves money because of the relative costs of the tests and defines plasma viral load, which is a benchmark for evaluating ART. HIV RNA assays may be more sensitive than HIV DNA PCR for detecting HIV non-subtype B [76].

25.6.2.1 Approach to Diagnosis

For infants born to an HIV-positive mother and who are not breast fed, virologic tests (DNA PCR, RNA assays, p24 Ag, culture) are the only acceptable methods of diagnosis of HIV infection in the first months of life. For reasons of cost and availability, DNA PCR and RNA PCR are preferred over cultures and preferred over p24 Ag tests because of the relative poor sensitivity of the p24 Ag test in the first months of life [76]. Tests for antibodies to HIV become increasingly reliable after 6 months of age and can be used alone for definitive diagnosis of HIV infection after 18 months of age.

Based on characteristics of HIV-infected young children and test performance it has become common practice to perform virologic tests on exposed infants at 14–21 days of life, 1–2 and 4–6 months of life, and HIV antibody tests at 6 months or more of life. HIV infection is considered presumptively excluded by two negative virologic tests (at ≥14 and ≥30 days of life) or one negative virologic test at ≥2 and one negative HIV antibody test at ≥6 months of life. Definitive exclusion of HIV infection is based on two blood samples negative by virologic tests or HIV antibody tests (at ≥1 and ≥4 months or ≥6 months, respectively) [60, 76]. Additionally, the child should be free of clinical evidence of HIV infection.

For infants born to an HIV-positive mother and who are breast fed, definitive testing for HIV infection status should be started not sooner than 6 weeks after termination of breast feeding. The tests selected should be a function of infant age at termination of breast feeding using the guidelines in the preceding paragraph.

HIV infection is diagnosed by two positive HIV virologic tests performed on separate blood samples (regardless of age, cord blood sample is not acceptable) or for children ≥18 months old a positive HIV antibody test with confirmatory Western blot (or IFA) [10].

25.7 Antiretroviral Treatment

The use of potent combination ARV therapy has dramatically improved the quality of life and survival of HIV-infected children. However, cure of HIV infection is not achieved. Recommendations on when to start ART have evolved with time. There are currently guidelines on when to start treatment issued by European [64] and US [76] sources and by the World Health Organization for children in resource-limited regions [77]. The ability to differentiate children at risk of rapid versus slower disease progression by clinical and laboratory parameters is also very limited. No specific "at-risk" viral or immunologic threshold can be easily identified, and progression of HIV disease and opportunistic infections can occur in young infants with normal CD4 counts [35]. A randomized clinical trial conducted in South Africa found that initiation of therapy at <12 weeks of age in asymptomatic infants with normal immune status resulted in lower mortality (75% reduction in early death) than waiting to initiate therapy in such children until they reached standard criteria for initiation of therapy [5]. Most of the deaths in the children in the delayed treatment arm occurred in the first 6 months after study entry. In a French study there were no opportunistic infections or development of encephalopathy during the first 2 years of life among 40 infants who started cART before age 6 months, whereas 6 of 43 infants who started cART after age 6 months had seven AIDS-defining events, three of which were encephalopathy [27]. A current recommendation for initiation of therapy in HIV-infected infants is to start cART for all infants before 12 months of age, regardless of clinical status, CD4 percentage,

Table 25.2 Indications for initiation of antiretroviral therapy in children infected with HIV (Updated August 16, 2010)

Age	Criteria	Recommendation
<12 months	Regardless of clinical symptoms, immune status, or viral load	Treat (AI)
1 to <5 years	AIDS or significant HIV-related symptoms[a]	Treat (AI)
	CD4 < 25%, regardless of symptoms or HIV RNA level	Treat (AI)
	Asymptomatic or mild symptoms[b] and CD4 ≥ 25% and HIV RNA ≥ 100,000 copies/mL	Treat (BII)
	Asymptomatic or mild symptoms[b] and CD4 ≥ 25% and HIV RNA <100,000 copies/mL	Consider (CIII)
≥5 years	AIDS or significant HIV-related symptoms[a]	Treat (AI)
	CD4 < 350 cells/mm	Treat (AI)
	Asymptomatic or mild symptoms[b] and CD4 ≥ 350 cells/mm[b] and HIV RNA ≥ 100,000 copies/mL	Treat (BII)
	Asymptomatic or mild symptoms[b] and CD4 ≥ 350 cells/mm[b] and HIV RNA < 100,000 copies/mL[c]	Consider (CIII)

[a]CDC Clinical Category C and B (except for the following Category B conditions: single episode of serious bacterial infection or lymphoid interstitial pneumonitis)

[b]CDC Clinical Category A or N or the following Category B conditions: single episode of serious bacterial infection or lymphoid interstitial pneumonitis

[c]Clinical and laboratory data should be reevaluated every 3–4 months

The table is from the Guidelines for the Use of Antiretroviral Agents in Pediatric HIV Infection; August 16, 2010

or viral load [76]. Table 25.2 presents indications for starting cART after the first year of life.

A combination antiretroviral regimen in treatment-naive children generally contains one non-nucleoside analogue reverse transcriptase inhibitor (NNRTI) plus a nucleoside/nucleotide analogue reverse transcriptase inhibitors (2-NRTI) backbone or one PI (protease inhibitor) plus a 2-NRTI backbone. A 3-NRTI regimen consisting of zidovudine, abacavir, and lamivudine is recommended only if a PI (protease inhibitor) or NNRTI-regimen cannot be used [8].

Recommendation on current optimal antiretroviral regiments frequently change as new drugs and knowledge become. Current recommendation can be found at sites that are continuously updated [76, 77].

25.8 Prevention of Opportunistic Infections

Children with AIDS need prophylaxis against opportunistic infections (mainly PJP and MAC), the major differences specific to children are PJP prophylaxis with co-trimoxazole (C-TX) is started for all HIV-exposed infants at 4–6 weeks of age until HIV is ruled out. All HIV-positive infants should receive C-TX prophylaxis regardless of symptoms or CD4 percentage in the first year of life; after 1 year of age, initiation of C-TX prophylaxis is recommended for symptomatic children (WHO clinical stages 2, 3, or 4) or children with CD4 < 25%. Adult clinical staging and CD4 count thresholds for C-TX initiation or discontinuation apply to children older than 5 years of age [78]. $CD4^+$ T lymphocyte thresholds for starting prophylaxis (azithromycin or clarithromycin) against disseminated MAC infections in children <13 years are age >6 years, <50 cells/μL; 2–6 years, <75 cells/μL; 1–2 years, <500 cells/μL, and <12 months, <750 cells/μL [38].

25.9 Prevention of HIV Transmission

The near elimination of new cases of HIV infection and AIDS among children in resource-rich countries (due to the success of efforts to prevent MTCT) is one of few major public health success stories in the nearly 25 year history of the epidemic. Effective interventions to reduce VT in developed countries include cesarean delivery, avoiding breast feeding, and use of antiretroviral drugs. Benefits of cART are well documented. The first successful trial in preventing MTCT to non-breast-fed newborns, ACTG 076 was published in 1994 [14]. The study included five doses of zidovudine to pregnant women (ZDV) intrapartum, and ZDV to the newborn for 6 weeks. The trial showed a 67% decrease in transmission. Presently, in the developed world, transmission rates have dropped to <2%.

A major risk factor in transmission of HIV and a barrier to prevention of VT is lack of awareness of HIV status among pregnant women. Approximately 25% of HIV-infected people in the USA (and 90% of them globally) do not know their HIV status [10]. In the USA, 45% of people with new sexually acquired HIV infections do not know their HIV status [45]. Thanks to widespread prenatal HIV screening, 95% of HIV-exposed neonates who were reported to the CDC in 2005 were born to women who were tested before or at the time of birth and thus received appropriate HIV prophylaxis. On the other hand, only 48% of perinatally HIV infected infants had a mother who was tested before or at the time of birth [11].

ART for prevention of HIV transmission during pregnancy should be recommended to all HIV-infected mothers regardless of plasma HIV RNA copy number or CD4 cell count. For women with severe HIV disease, treatment should be initiated as soon as possible, including in the first trimester. For HIV-infected pregnant women who do not require immediate treatment, initiation of cART prophylaxis (with three antiretrovirals) can be delayed until after the first trimester. Use of ZDV prophylaxis alone during pregnancy may be considered for those women initiating prophylaxis with plasma HIV RNA levels <1,000 copies. Intrapartum intravenous ZDV is recommended for all HIV-infected pregnant women, regardless of their antepartum regimen. The addition of intrapartum/newborn single-dose NVP is not recommended [58].

HIV RNA levels should also be assessed at approximately 34–36 weeks of gestation to guide decisions on the mode of delivery. For women who have received antepartum antiretroviral drugs but have suboptimal viral suppression near delivery (i.e., >1,000 copies/mL), scheduled cesarean delivery is recommended [8].

Prophylaxis of HIV-exposed neonates is based primarily on ZDV monotherapy for the first 6 weeks of life. ZDV should be initiated as close to the time of birth as possible, preferably within 6–12 h of delivery. Some experts consider the use of ZDV in combination with other antiretroviral drugs in certain situations, although the optimal prophylactic regimen for infants born to women in these circumstances is unknown. These include infants born to mothers who received antepartum and intrapartum ART but have suboptimal viral suppression at delivery, infants born to mothers who have received only intrapartum ART, infants born to mothers who have received no antepartum or intrapartum ART; and infants born to mothers with known antiretroviral drug-resistant virus [58].

25.10 Summary/Conclusion

An increasing fraction of the global HIV infection burden is HIV infections of children, a group in which infection is most often acquired by peripartum mother-to-child transmission. Children generally have higher rates of mortality from HIV and more rapid progression to sever disease than adults. The majority of HIV infections of children are preventable by proven interventions. However, these have been difficult to deploy to resource-limited regions; the areas of the majority of HIV infections. In most cases, application of antiretroviral therapy to infected children can result in persistent infection where most children can remain in good health through at least early adulthood – antiretroviral therapies have not been available long enough to document longer survival. Again, availability of proven effective antiretroviral therapies are limited in resource-limited regions.

Take-Home Pearls

- Vertical transmission (VT) is the cause of 90% of pediatric HIV globally.
- Breast-feeding is responsible for 30-50% of VT in developing countries.
- The rate of VT of HIV varies from 40% (in Africa before cART) to less than 2% (in US in recent years).
- The main risk factor for VT which is also the main barrier to the prevention of perinatal HIV

transmission is lack of awareness of HIV status among pregnant women.

- Disease progression in children (especially infants) is more rapid.
- *Pneumocystis jiroveci* pneumonia (PjP) and encephalopathy occur early in the course of HIV infection (especially in infants).
- LIP and multiple serious bacterial infections are AIDS-defining only for children.
- The standard test for diagnosis of HIV infection before 18 months of age is HIV DNA PCR.
- HIV antibody tests are used for exclusion of HIV infection only after 6 month of age.
- HAART should be started for all HIV infected infants (<12 months) regardless of clinical status, CD4 percentage or viral load.
- PJP prophylaxis with (TMP-SMX) is started for all HIV exposed infants at 4-6 weeks of age until HIV is ruled out.
- All HIV positive infants should receive TMP-SMX prophylaxis regardless of symptoms or CD4 percentage.

References

1. Features of children perinatally infected with HIV-I surviving longer than 5 years. Italian Register for HIV Infection in Children. Lancet, **343**(8891):191–5 (1994)
2. American Foundation for AIDS Research (AmFAR) 2007 Annual Report AIDS in Asia and the Pacific Overview of the epidemic in Asia. (2007)
3. Andiman, W.A., Shearer, W.T.: Lymphoid interstitial pneumonitis. In: Pizzo, P.A., Wilfert, C.M. (eds.) Pediatric AIDS: The Challenge of HIV Infection in Infants, Children and Adolescents, pp. 323–334. Lippincott Williams & Wilkins, Baltimore (1998)
4. Beau, J.P., Imboua-Coulibaly, L.: HIV-related gender biases among malnourished children in Abidjan, Cote D'Ivoire. J. Trop. Pediatr. **45**(3), 169–171 (1999)
5. Becquet, R., Mofenson, L.M.: Early antiretroviral therapy of HIV-infected infants in resource limited countries: possible, feasible, effective and challenging. AIDS **22**(11), 1365–1368 (2008)
6. Boerma, J.T., Stanecki, K.A., Newell, M.L., et al.: Monitoring the scale-up of antiretroviral therapy programmes: methods to estimate coverage. Bull. World Health Organ. **84**(2), 145–150 (2006)
7. Bremer, J.W., Lew, J.F., Cooper, E., et al.: Diagnosis of infection with human immunodeficiency virus type 1 by a DNA polymerase chain reaction assay among infants enrolled in the Women and Infants' Transmission Study. J. Pediatr. **129**(2), 198–207 (1996)
8. Centers for Disease Control: Revised classification system for human immunodeficiency virus infection in children less than 13 years of age. MMWR **43**(RR-12), 1–10 (1994)
9. Centers for Disease Control and Prevention: 1994 revised guidelines for the performance of CD4+ T-cell determinations in persons with human immunodeficiency virus (HIV) infections. MMWR **43**(RR-3), 1–21 (1994)
10. Centers for Disease Control and Prevention US: Revised guidelines for HIV counseling, testing, and referral. MMWR Recomm. Rep. **50**(RR-19), 1–57 (2001). quiz CE1-19a1-CE6-a1
11. Centers for Disease Control and Prevention US: Cases of HIV Infection and AIDS in the United States and Dependent Areas. US Department of Health and Human Services, Atlanta (2005)
12. Center for Disease Control and Prevention US (2008), Pediatric HIV/AIDS surveillance (through 2007) http://cdc.gov/HIV/topics/surveillance/resources/slides/pediatric/index.htm
13. Chantry, C.J., Byrd, R.S., Englund, J.A., Baker, C.J., McKinney Jr., R.E.: Growth, survival and viral load in symptomatic childhood human immunodeficiency virus infection. Pediatr. Infect. Dis. J. **22**(12), 1033–1039 (2003)
14. Connor, E.M., Sperling, R.S., Gelber, R., et al.: Reduction of maternal-infant transmission of human immunodeficiency virus type 1 with zidovudine treatment. Pediatric AIDS Clinical Trials Group Protocol 076 Study Group [see comments]. N. Engl. J. Med. **331**(18), 1173–1180 (1994)
15. Coutsoudis, A., Coovadia, H.M., Wilfert, C.M.: HIV, infant feeding and more perils for poor people: new WHO guidelines encourage review of formula milk policies. Bull. World Health Organ. **86**(3), 210–214 (2008)
16. Cunningham, C.K., Charbonneau, T.T., Song, K., et al.: Comparison of human immunodeficiency virus 1 DNA polymerase chain reaction and qualitative and quantitative RNA polymerase chain reaction in human immunodeficiency virus 1-exposed infants. Pediatr. Infect. Dis. J. **18**(1), 30–35 (1999)
17. Dabis, F., Elenga, N., Meda, N., Leroy, V., Viho, I., et al.: 18-month mortality and perinatal exposure to zidovudine in West Africa. AIDS **15**(6), 771–779 (2001)
18. Del Bianco, G., Perez, N., Hilliard, M., Murphy, J.R., Heresi, G.P.: Current patterns of perinatal transmission of HIV in the HAART era in Houston, TX. In: Infectious Diseases Society of America, p. Poster 902, Toronto (2006).
19. Del Bianco, G., Perez, N., Wall, V., Oliver, G., Hilliard, M., Murphy, J.R., Heresi, G.P.: Risk factors associated with maternal child transmission of HIV in Houston, Texas 2000–2005. In: European Society for Paediatric Infectious Diseases, p. Poster 353, Porto, Portugal (2007).
20. Domachowske, J.B.: Pediatric human immunodeficiency virus infection. Clin. Microbiol. Rev. **9**(4), 448–468 (1996)
21. Doyle, M.: HIV infection in children born before and after immigration to Belgium. J. Travel Med. **2**(3), 151–152 (1995)
22. Dunn, D.T., Brandt, C.D., Krivine, A., et al.: The sensitivity of HIV-1 DNA polymerase chain reaction in the neonatal period and the relative contributions of intra-uterine and intra-partum transmission. AIDS **9**(9), F7–F11 (1995)

23. Ehrnst, A., Lindgren, S., Dictor, M., et al.: HIV in pregnant women and their offspring: evidence for late transmission. Lancet **338**(8761), 203–207 (1991)
24. Epstein, L.G., Sharer, L.R., Oleske, J.M., et al.: Neurologic manifestations of human immunodeficiency virus infection in children. Pediatrics **78**(4), 678–687 (1986)
25. EuroHIV: HIV/AIDS Surveillance in Europe: Mid-year report 2006 (2006).
26. European Collaborative Study: Mother-to-child transmission of HIV infection in the era of highly active antiretroviral therapy. Clin. Infect. Dis. **40**(3), 458–465 (2005)
27. Faye, A., Le Chenadec, J., Dollfus, C., et al.: Early versus deferred antiretroviral multidrug therapy in infants infected with HIV type 1. Clin. Infect. Dis. **39**(11), 1692–1698 (2004)
28. Fowler, M.G., Newell, M.L.: Breast-feeding and HIV-1 transmission in resource-limited settings. J. Acquir. Immune Defic. Syndr. **30**(2), 230–239 (2002)
29. Gabiano, C., Tovo, P.A., de Martino, M., et al.: Mother-to-child transmission of human immunodeficiency virus type 1: risk of infection and correlates of transmission. Pediatrics **90**(3), 369–374 (1992)
30. Gaur, A.H., Dominguez, K.L., Kalish, M.L., et al.: Practice of feeding premasticated food to infants: a potential risk factor for HIV transmission. Pediatrics. **124**(2), 658–66 (2009)
31. Centers for Disease Control and Prevention. Diagnosis of HIV infection and AIDS in the United States and defendant area. **20** (2008)
32. Gray, L., Newell, M.L., Thorne, C., Peckham, C., Levy, J.: Fluctuations in symptoms in human immunodeficiency virus-infected children: the first 10 years of life. Pediatrics **108**(1), 116–122 (2001)
33. Guay, L.A., Musoke, P., Fleming, T., et al.: Intrapartum and neonatal single-dose nevirapine compared with zidovudine for prevention of mother-to-child transmission of HIV-1 in Kampala, Uganda: HIVNET 012 randomised trial. Lancet **354**(9181), 795–802 (1999)
34. Ferris, M., Kline, M. Pediatric AIDS: Worlds apart. Semin Pediatr Infect Dis. **11**(2), 148–154 (2000)
35. HIV Paediatric Prognostic Markers Collaborative Study: Predictive value of absolute CD4 cell count for disease progression in untreated HIV-1-infected children. AIDS **20**(9), 1289–1294 (2006)
36. Irova, T.I., Burtonboy, G., Ninane, J.: HIV infection in children born before and after immigration to Belgium. J. Travel Med. **2**(3), 169–173 (1995)
37. Jamieson, D.J., Sibailly, T.S., Sadek, R., et al.: HIV-1 viral load and other risk factors for mother-to-child transmission of HIV-1 in a breast-feeding population in Cote d'Ivoire. J. Acquir. Immune Defic. Syndr. **34**(4), 430–436 (2003)
38. Kaplan, J.E., Masur, H., Holmes, K.K.: Guidelines for preventing opportunistic infections among HIV-infected persons–2002. Recommendations of the U.S. Public Health Service and the Infectious Diseases Society of America. MMWR Recomm. Rep. **51**, 1–52 (2002)
39. Kline, M.W.: No greater gift than hope. Semin. Pediatr. Infect. Dis. **14**(4), 309–313 (2003)
40. Kline, M.W.: Perspectives on the pediatric HIV/AIDS pandemic: catalyzing access of children to care and treatment. Pediatrics **117**(4), 1388–1393 (2006)
41. Kozinetz, C.A., Matusa, R., Cazacu, A.: The burden of pediatric HIV/AIDS in Constanta, Romania: a cross-sectional study. BMC Infect. Dis. **1**, 7 (2001)
42. Kuhn, L., Steketee, R.W., Weedon, J., et al.: Distinct risk factors for intrauterine and intrapartum human immunodeficiency virus transmission and consequences for disease progression in infected children. Perinatal AIDS Collaborative Transmission Study. J. Infect. Dis. **179**(1), 52–58 (1999)
43. Luzuriaga, K., McManus, M., Catalina, M., et al.: Early therapy of vertical human immunodeficiency virus type 1 (HIV-1) infection: control of viral replication and absence of persistent HIV-1-specific immune responses. J. Virol. **74**(15), 6984–6991 (2000)
44. MacPherson, D.W., Zencovich, M., Gushulak, B.D.: Emerging pediatric HIV epidemic related to migration. Emerg. Infect. Dis. **12**(4), 612–617 (2006)
45. Marks, G., Crepaz, N., Janssen, R.S.: Estimating sexual transmission of HIV from persons aware and unaware that they are infected with the virus in the USA. AIDS **20**(10), 1447–1450 (2006)
46. McKenna, M.T., Hu, X.: Recent trends in the incidence and morbidity that are associated with perinatal human immunodeficiency virus infection in the United States. Am. J. Obstet. Gynecol. **197**(3 Suppl), S10–S16 (2007)
47. McKinney Jr., R.E., Maha, M.A., Connor, E.M., et al.: A multicenter trial of oral zidovudine in children with advanced human immunodeficiency virus disease. The Protocol 043 Study Group. N. Engl. J. Med. **324**(15), 1018–1025 (1991)
48. McKinney Jr., R.E., Wilfert, C.: Growth as a prognostic indicator in children with human immunodeficiency virus infection treated with zidovudine. AIDS Clinical Trials Group Protocol 043 Study Group. J. Pediatr. **125**(5 Pt 1), 728–733 (1994)
49. Miller, L.C.: International adoption: infectious diseases issues. Clin. Infect. Dis. **40**(2), 286–293 (2005)
50. Mofenson, L.: Challenges in pediatric and adolescent HIV care. In: 15th Conference on Retroviruses and Opportunistic Infections, Boston (2008)
51. Mofenson, L.M., Lambert, J.S., Stiehm, E.R., et al.: Risk factors for perinatal transmission of human immunodeficiency virus type 1 in women treated with zidovudine. Pediatric AIDS Clinical Trials Group Study 185 Team. N. Engl. J. Med. **341**(6), 385–393 (1999)
52. Nduati, R., John, G., Mbori-Ngacha, D., Richardson, B., et al.: Effect of breastfeeding and formula feeding on transmission of HIV-1: a randomized clinical trial. JAMA **283**(9), 1167–1174 (2000)
53. New York State Department of Health: HIV Testing and Diagnosis in Infants and Children. Health NYSDo, New York (2005)
54. Obimbo, E.M., Mbori-Ngacha, D.A., Ochieng, J.O., et al.: Predictors of early mortality in a cohort of human immunodeficiency virus type 1-infected african children. Pediatr. Infect. Dis. J. **23**(6), 536–543 (2004)
55. Patterson, K.B., Leone, P.A., Fiscus, S.A., et al.: Frequent detection of acute HIV infection in pregnant women. AIDS **21**(17), 2303–2308 (2007)
56. Pearson, D.A., McGrath, N.M., Nozyce, M., et al.: Predicting HIV disease progression in children using measures of neuropsychological and neurological functioning. Pediatric

AIDS clinical trials 152 study team. Pediatrics **106**(6), E76 (2000)
57. Prendergast, A., Tudor-Williams, G., Jeena, P., Burchett, S., Goulder, P.: International perspectives, progress, and future challenges of paediatric HIV infection. Lancet **370**(9581), 68–80 (2007)
58. Panel on Treatments of HIV infected Pregnant Women and Prevention of Perinatal Transmission. Recommendations for use of antiretroviral drugs in pregnant HIV-1 infected women for maternal health and intervention to reduce perinatal HIV transmission in the United States. May 24, 2010, pp1–117. http://aidsinfo.nih.gov
59. Pugatch, D.: Testing infants for human immunodeficiency virus infection. Pediatr. Infect. Dis. J. **21**(7), 711–712 (2002)
60. Read, J.S.: Diagnosis of HIV-1 infection in children younger than 18 months in the United States. Pediatrics **120**(6), e1547–e1562 (2007)
61. Ryder, R.W., Nsa, W., Hassig, S.E., et al.: Perinatal transmission of the human immunodeficiency virus type 1 to infants of seropositive women in Zaire. N. Engl. J. Med. **320**(25), 1637–1642 (1989)
62. Schuval, S., Dyke, R.V., Lindsey, J., et al., AIDS Clinical Trials Group: Hepatitis C Prevalence in Perinatally-Infected HIV-Positive Children, p. 144. American Society for Microbiology, San Diego (2003)
63. Schwarzwald, H.: Illnesses among recently immigrated children. Semin. Pediatr. Infect. Dis. **16**(2), 78–83 (2005)
64. Sharland, M., Blanche, S., Castelli, G., Ramos, J., Gibb, D.M.: PENTA guidelines for the use of antiretroviral therapy, 2004. HIV Med. **5**(Suppl 2), 61–86 (2004)
65. Simonds, R.J., Oxtoby, M.J., Caldwell, M.B., Gwinn, M.L., Rogers, M.F.: Pneumocystis carinii pneumonia among US children with perinatally acquired HIV infection. JAMA **270**(4), 470–473 (1993)
66. Taha, T.E., Gray, R.H.: Genital tract infections and perinatal transmission of HIV. Ann. NY Acad. Sci. **918**, 84–98 (2000)
67. Taha, T.E., Nour, S., Kumwenda, N.I., et al.: Gender differences in perinatal HIV acquisition among African infants. Pediatrics **115**(2), e167–e172 (2005)
68. Thorne, C., Newell, M.L.: Are girls more at risk of intrauterine-acquired HIV infection than boys? AIDS **18**(2), 344–347 (2004)
69. Tovo, P.A., de Martino, M., Gabiano, C., et al.: Prognostic factors and survival in children with perinatal HIV-1 infection. The Italian Register for HIV Infections in Children. Lancet **339**(8804), 1249–1253 (1992)
70. U.S. Census Bureau: B02001. RACE – Universe:TOTAL POPULATION. U.S. Census Bureau (2006).
71. UNAIDS/World Health Organization: AIDS Epidemic Update, December, 2006
72. UNAIDS/World Health Organization: 2007 AIDS epidemic update
73. US Public Health Service Task Force: Recommendations of the U.S. Public Health Service Task Force on the use of zidovudine to reduce perinatal transmission of human immunodeficiency virus. MMWR Recomm. Rep. **43**(RR-11), 1–20 (1994)
74. Verneris, M.R., Tuel, L., Seibel, N.L.: Pediatric HIV infection and chronic myelogenous leukemia. Pediatr. AIDS HIV Infect. **6**(5), 292–294 (1995)
75. Weinberg, G.A.: The dilemma of postnatal mother-to-child transmission of HIV: to breastfeed or not? Birth **27**(3), 199–205 (2000)
76. Panel on antiretroviral Therapy and Medical Management of HIV-Infected Children. Guidelines for the use of antiretroviral agents in pediatric HIV infection. Available at http://aidsinfo.nih.gov/contentfiles/pediatricguidelines.pdf (2010)
77. World Health Organization: Antiretroviral Therapy of HIV Infection in Infants and Children in Resource-Limited Settings: Towards Universal Access. WHO, Geneva (2006)
78. World Health Organization: Guidelines on Co-trimoxazole Prophylaxis for HIV-Related Infection Among Children, Adolescents and Adults. WHO, Geneva (2006)
79. World Health Organization: HIV and Infant Feeding Technical Consultation Held on Behalf of the Inter-agency Task Team on Prevention of HIV Infections in Pregnant Women, Mothers and Their Infants. WHO, Geneva (2006)

Clinical Manifestations of HIV Infections

26

Norbert H. Brockmeyer and Anja V. Potthoff

Core Messages

- The incidence of opportunistic infections decreased dramatically with the introduction of highly active antiretroviral therapy.
- While Kaposi's sarcoma, TBC, lymphoma and pneumonia occur at any CD4 cell count, CMV retinitis and atypical mycobacteriosis are almost exclusively seen in highly immunosuppressed patients.
- Opportunistic infection can still be life-threatening but long-term prognosis of AIDS-patients has greatly improved.
- HIV patients should be treated in specialized centers.
- New antiretroviral drugs have reduced side effects and opened new treatment opportunities.

26.1 Diagnosis

HIV infection is a chronic infectious disease with different phases. A great problem is the diagnostic window period when the HIV test can be false-negative. It takes 6–12 weeks until HIV antibodies are detectable. For screening HIV ELISA is used. A positive result has to be confirmed by a western blot test or HIV-PCR. Rapid tests can be useful in certain setting, e.g., emergency rooms. For early diagnosis HIV-PCR can be helpful [26].

In the first weeks of an acute HIV infection, flu-like symptoms, fever, lymphadenopathy, and rash occur in 40–90% of all patients. They normally resolve after a maximum of 4 weeks and do not result in further diagnostic steps in most cases. After this most patients have no health problems for several years or mild symptoms like lymphadenopathy. Later HIV-related symptoms show a deterioration of the immune competence. The skin is a reflection of the immune system. HIV-positive patients often present with skin or mucosal problems (e.g., herpes zoster, thrush) as the first sign of the infection. AIDS is the last stage of the HIV infection. AIDS-defining illnesses (opportunistic infections and tumors) are listed in the CDC classification of HIV (Table 26.1, [14]). Before the era of antiretroviral therapy most patients died within 2 years of the first manifestation of AIDS-defining complications. Without antiretroviral therapy up to 90% of all HIV-infected patients die from AIDS [48].

26.2 Opportunistic Infections (OI)

The incidence of opportunistic infections decreased dramatically with the introduction of highly active antiretroviral therapy. Most patients presenting with severe opportunistic infections are not aware of their HIV infection. Earlier HIV testing would not only improve the prognosis of these patients, but would also help to avoid new infections. While opportunistic infection can still be life-threatening long-term prognosis of AIDS patients has greatly improved. The CD4 cell count can help for differential diagnosis of some HIV-associated conditions. While Kaposi's sarcoma,

N.H. Brockmeyer (✉) and A.V. Potthoff
St. Josef Hospital Bochum, Gudrunstr. 56, 44791
Bochum, Germany
e-mail: n.brockmeyer@derma.de;
a.potthoff@klinikum-bochum.de

G. Gross and S.K. Tyring (eds.), *Sexually Transmitted Infections and Sexually Transmitted Diseases*,
DOI: 10.1007/978-3-642-14663-3_26, © Springer-Verlag Berlin Heidelberg 2011

Table 26.1 Clinical categories of the CDC classification system in HIV-infected persons [14]

Category A	*Category C* – AIDS-defining illnesses
Asymptomatic HIV infection	Candidiasis of bronchi, trachea, or lungs
Acute (primary) HIV infection with accompanying illness or history of acute HIV infection	Candidiasis, esophageal Cervical cancer, invasive
Persistent generalized lymphadenopathy	Coccidioidomycosis, disseminated or extrapulmonary Cryptococcosis, extrapulmonary
Category B	Cryptosporidiosis, chronic intestinal (greater than 1 month's duration)
Symptomatic conditions that are not included among conditions listed in clinical Category C. Examples include, but are not limited to:	Cytomegalovirus disease (other than liver, spleen, or nodes) Cytomegalovirus retinitis (with loss of vision)
Bacillary angiomatosis	Encephalopathy, HIV-related
Candidiasis, oropharyngeal (thrush)	Herpes simplex: chronic ulcer(s) (greater than 1 month's duration); or bronchitis, pneumonitis, or esophagitis
Candidiasis, vulvovaginal; persistent, frequent, or poorly responsive to therapy	Histoplasmosis, disseminated or extrapulmonary
Cervical dysplasia (moderate or severe)/cervical carcinoma in situ	Isosporiasis, chronic intestinal (greater than 1 month's duration) Kaposi's sarcoma
Constitutional symptoms, such as fever (38.5° C) or diarrhea lasting longer than 1 month	Lymphoma, Burkitt's (or equivalent term) Lymphoma, immunoblastic (or equivalent)
Hairy leukoplakia, oral	Lymphoma, primary, of brain
Herpes zoster (shingles), involving at least two distinct episodes or more than one dermatome	Mycobacterium avium complex or *M. kansasii*, disseminated or extrapulmonary
Idiopathic thrombocytopenic purpura	Mycobacterium tuberculosis, any site (pulmonary or extrapulmonary)
Listeriosis	Mycobacterium, other species or unidentified species, disseminated or extrapulmonary
Pelvic inflammatory disease, particularly if complicated by tubo-ovarian abscess	Pneumocystis pneumonia Pneumonia, recurrent
Peripheral neuropathy	Progressive multifocal leukoencephalopathy Salmonella septicemia, recurrent Toxoplasmosis of brain Wasting syndrome due to HIV

TBC, lymphoma, and pneumonia occur at any CD4 cell count, CMV retinitis and atypical mycobacteriosis are seen almost exclusively in highly immunosuppressed patients (<50 CD4/μL) (Table 26.2).

26.2.1 *Pneumocystis jiroveci (carinii)* Pneumonia (PCP)

PCP is still the most common opportunistic infection. In the early years of the HIV epidemic most patients died from PCP. With antiretroviral therapy and sufficient prophylaxis PCP is mainly seen in patients without sufficient antiretroviral therapy. Mortality rates of PCP are still high. Patients should be treated in specialized centers. Artificial respiration is often necessary. Classical symptoms are unproductive cough, elevated body temperature, and dyspnea especially after exercise. Many patients also present with other opportunistic infections like oral candidosis and weight loss. Respiratory decompensation can be fast. All patients with dyspnea and suspected PCP should be hospitalized immediately. Ambulatory treatment can be feasible only in cases of mild PCP (BGA: PO_2 > 70–80 mmHg). Clinical examination and chest X-ray can be without pathological findings in the beginning. In this case, high-resolution computer

Table 26.2 Differential diagnosis for different CD4 values (important: this is only for orientation, there can be exceptions)

No limits (but rising incidence with lower CD4 cell count)	Kaposi's sarcoma, lung TBC, shingles, bacterial pneumonia, lymphoma
<250/μL	PCP, candida esophagitis, PML, HSV
<100/μL	Cerebral toxoplasmosis, HIV-encephalopathy, cryptococcosis, miliary TBC
<50/μL	CMV retinitis, MAC

tomography is indicated. For final diagnosis a bronchoalveolar lavage is needed. Treatment should be started immediately without waiting for the final diagnostic results. LDH is a good progression parameter. Pneumothorax and superinfections are common complications. For treatment cotrimoxazole 3 × 2,400 mg is given for 21 days. Additionally prednisone 2 × 20–40 mg for 5–10 days reduces mortality. With high-dose cotrimoxazole treatment, total blood count, transaminases, electrolytes, and retention parameter have to be controlled regularly. Exanthema and drug fever are common. In this case, after stopping antibiotic treatment for 24–48 h treatment reinitiation can be tried with half of the dose and addition of steroids. After 10–14 days and clinical improvement daily pentamidine inhalation (300 mg) is an option for the last days. Alternative treatment with intravenous pentamidine, atovaquone 2 × 750–1,500 mg or clindamycin 3–4 × 600 mg i.v. and primaquine 30 mg is less efficient.

Patients with <200/μL $CD4^+$ cells should take cotrimoxazole 480 mg daily or 960 mg 3×/week for PCP and toxoplasmosis prophylaxis. Monthly inhalation with 300 mg pentamidine can be an alternative for patients with cotrimoxazole intolerance.

Bacterial pneumonia can occur with good immunological status. Diagnosis and treatment are the same as in non HIV infected patients. Auscultation almost always allows distinction from PCP. If something can be heard, PCP is unlikely [20]. Bacterial pneumonia mostly appears in HIV-infected drug users. More than one episode in the last year is considered AIDS-defining.

For prophylaxis, all HIV-infected patients with more than 200 CD4/μL should have pneumococcal conjugate vaccine.

26.2.2 Candidosis

Candida species are facultative pathogens. Oral thrush often occurs with helper cells between 300 and 400/μL. Taste disorders and a burning sensation together with a white to yellow film on the tongue are characteristic symptoms. It can be treated with oral amphotericin B suspension 4 × 1 mL (100 mg) or nystatin 4 × 1 mL (100.000 I.E.) at least for 48 h after symptoms have stopped. Additional chlorhexidine has shown good effectiveness. If symptoms cannot be controlled fluconazole 50 mg–100 1×/day or itraconazole solution 200 mg/day can be initiated for 7–14 days [3, 61]. For *Candida glabrata* and *Candida krusei* there is a known resistance to fluconazole and itraconazole [66]. Miconazole buccal tablets 50 mg/day are a new option even for fluconazole-resistant species and showed good effectiveness for treatment of oropharyngeal candidiasis, but are not available in all countries [7]. Posaconazole 200 mg on the first day, then 100 mg for 13 days has proven efficacy in HIV-positive patients with oral thrush. Higher doses (2 × 400 mg for 3 days and then 1 × 400 mg for 125 days) can be used for recalcitrant candidosis [76, 82]. Voriconazole and caspofungin are only approved for invasive mycosis. Dysphagia, retrosternal pain especially in patients with oral candidosis should be suspicious of esophagitis, which is AIDS-defining. Gastroscopy is indicated if treatment with fluconazole 200 mg for 1 week is not successful. Dose escalation to 800 mg, itraconazole 200–400 mg, amphotericin (0.1–0.5 mg/kg bw i.v.), voriconazole (initial dose 2 × 400 mg, then 2 × 200 mg) and caspofungin (initial dose 70 mg, then 50 mg; i.v. application) are therapeutic options for recalcitrant disease [32, 40].

In women, vulvovaginal candidosis is a common problem with discharge and pruritus. Local treatment includes nystatin, amphotericin B, imidazole, and ciclopiroxolamine treatment of the recalcitrant disease. Treatment of recalcitrant disease should be initiated with fluconazole 150–300 mg orally and maintenance therapy with the same dose every 1–4 weeks should be continued for several months [78].

Oral hairy leukoplakia is an important differential diagnosis for oral lesions in HIV-infected patients. This EBV-associated tongue alteration does not need treatment, but is an important marker disease for progressive immunodeficiency. White films at the side of

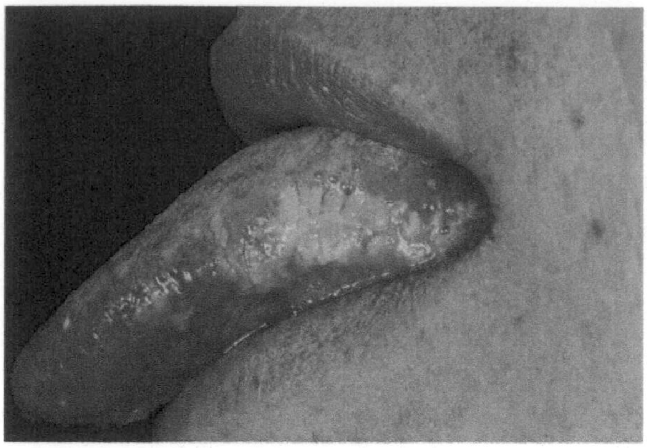

Fig. 26.1 Oral hairy leukoplakia: white films at the side of the tongue cannot be removed

the tongue cannot be removed (Fig. 26.1). With immune reconstitution after initiation of antiretroviral therapy, they resolve without further treatment. Acyclovir or other antiherpes drugs are able to cure the lesions, but after treatment discontinuation a rapid recurrence is often noticed [55].

26.2.3 Herpes Simplex

Recurrent herpes simplex infections are a common problem in HIV patients. First episodes are often more severe and should be treated with acyclovir 3 × 400 mg or valacyclovir 2 × 1,000 mg or famciclovir 3 × 250 mg for 7–10 days. Recurrent episodes can be treated with 3 × 400–800 mg or 2 × 1,000 mg valacyclovir or 2 × 500 mg famciclovir for 5 days. Suppressive treatment with 800 mg acyclovir or 500–1,000 mg valacyclovir or 1,000 mg famciclovir reduces recurrence rates. Dissemination with esophagitis, encephalitis, keratoconjunctivitis, or pneumonitis is AIDS-defining and has to be treated with high-dose intravenous acyclovir 3 × 5–10 mg/kg bw i.v. for 7–14 days [34].

26.2.4 Shingles

Herpes zoster is known to be associated with immunosuppression and is considered an HIV-related illness when localized in more than one dermatome. Patients with HIV infection have a 300-fold higher risk to suffer from herpes zoster than HIV-negative persons [37]. They also suffer more frequently from disseminated disease and complications like post-zoster neuralgia. It often occurs in patients with mild immunodeficiency around 300 CD4/μL. When starting antiretroviral therapy, herpes zoster can be part of an immune reconstitution syndrome [38, 65, 81]. After prodrome with headache, reduced general condition, and hypoesthesia, small blisters occur in one or more dermatome. Systemic treatment with acyclovir should be initiated as soon as possible. Oral treatment with 5 × 800 mg acyclovir or 3 × 1,000 mg valacyclovir or 125 mg brivudine may be sufficient in a very initial stage. Severe cases should be treated with acyclovir 3 × 10 mg/kg bw i.v. Analgesia is very important. Gabapentin (start with 300 mg, increase by 300 mg every day, up to 1,200–2,400 mg/day) can be added for neuropathic pain, but drug interactions with antiretroviral therapy have to be considered [83].

26.2.5 Progressive Multifocal Leukoencephalopathy (PML)

PML may present with any combination of weakness, speech disturbances, limb incoordination, cognitive deficits, and visual impairment. Diagnosis is obtained by MRI with high sensitivity but low specificity, revealing T2-hyperintense lesions in the white matter, sparing the subcortical U-fibers. JC viral DNA amplification from cerebrospinal fluid has a sensitivity of 80% and a specificity approximating 100%. JC are the initials of the first patient from whom this polyomavirus was isolated. There is no association with Creutzfeldt–Jakob disease. In the pre-HAART era most patients died within 3–6 months. The only therapy is successful restoration of the immune system with effective antiretroviral treatment. Though up to two-thirds of all patients still live after 2 years, full recovery is seen only in few cases. Cidofovir 5 mg/kg bw every 7–14 days has been used experimentally with minimum success [84].

26.2.6 Toxoplasmosis

Cerebral toxoplasmosis is still the most important neurological opportunistic infection. In Europe up to 90%

of all adults have had contact with this parasite and symptomatic disease is almost always due to reactivation in severely immunocompromised patients with <100/μL CD4 cells.

Clinical symptoms develop within days with pareses, speech disorder, or paresthesia. Seizures together with headache and fever without meningism are also common. In the MRT or CT, often multiple foci with circular contrast medium enhancement can be found. Differential diagnosis includes abscesses or lymphoma. Before taking a biopsy probationary treatment can be tried. Cerebral fluid shows pleocytosis and protein elevation but PCR is often negative.

The 5-year survival rate of cerebral toxoplasmosis has risen to 78% in 2007 [35]. Primary treatment is initiated with sulfadiazine 4 × 1,000–1,500 mg plus pyrimethamine 2 × 50 mg plus calcium foliate 15 mg 3×/week orally for 4–6 weeks. Patients with cerebral edema can profit from short-term treatment with fortecortin up to 4 × 8 mg. Dose reduction (half of acute therapy) is recommended after 75% remission. Treatment can be stopped 6 months after first MRT without contrast medium enhancement and 6 months after CD4 cell count >200/μL. Primary prophylaxis with cotrimoxazole 480 mg/day is recommended in patients with <200/μL CD4 cells. Alternative treatment options are clindamycin 4 × 600 mg in combination with pyrimethamine or atovaquone 2 × 1,500 mg with pyrimethamine [21].

26.2.7 CMV

About 50–70% of adults have experienced CMV infection. In patients with <50/μL CD4 reactivation can cause retinitis that leads to blindness in up 30% of the patients. Impaired vision is an alarm symptom. Treatment can only stop progress, but full recovery is often not achievable. Other manifestations are pneumonia, esophagitis, colitis, or encephalitis. The most important differential diagnosis is chorioretinitis due to *Toxoplasma gondii*. In patients with >100/μL CD4 cells herpes virus infection or syphilis are more likely. For diagnosis pp65 or CMV-PCR are helpful. All patients should initiate or optimize antiretroviral therapy. Oral application of valganciclovir 2 × 900 mg for 3 weeks has displaced intravenous ganciclovir therapy. Total blood count should be checked regularly because of myelotoxicity. Intravenous foscarnet or cidofovir are therapeutic options but very nephrotoxic. Secondary prophylaxis with 2 × 450 mg valganciclovir should be maintained for 6 months (and CD4 > 100–150/μL).

Patients with <200/μL CD4 should have fundoscopy every 3–6 months. Before initiation of antiretroviral therapy especially in patients with low helper cells fundoscopy is mandatory to avoid acute manifestations during immune reconstitution [47].

26.2.8 Cryptococcosis

Cryptococcus neoformans infections are rare in Europe, but quite common in the USA and southeastern Asia. Mortality rates are between 6% and 25%. In most HIV patients, lung infection is the beginning of a disseminated disease with manifestation in the central nervous system. Patients present with headache, fever, and disorientation. A high-resolution computer tomography can help to detect pulmonary manifestation. Ink preparation of cerebrospinal fluid is the best way of diagnosis. Other localizations are the skin, lymph nodes, and the urogenital and gastrointestinal system. The introduction of new antifungal agents and the adoption of strategies for controlling elevated intracranial pressure in cryptococcal meningitis have added to our therapeutic options. A combination of liposomal amphotericin B 3 mg/kg bw, fluconazole 2 × 200 mg and 4 × 2.5 g flucytosin for 6 weeks still is the first treatment of choice. Total blood count, transaminases, electrolytes, and retention parameter have to be controlled regularly. Fluconazole 200–400 mg should be given for secondary prophylaxis for at least 6 months (and >200/μL CD4). In patients with high cryptococcus-antigen lifelong treatment can be necessary [63].

26.2.9 Tuberculosis TBC

Nearly 10% of all tuberculosis infections worldwide occur in HIV positive patients. One third of all HIV patients are coinfected with tuberculosis. Symptoms are the same as in HIV-negative patients, e.g., fever, weight loss, night sweat, cough, and hemoptysis.

Chest X-ray can show characteristic hiliary infiltrates or caverns. Sputum or bronchial lavage fluid should be preserved for diagnostic analysis. Lymph node or transbronchial lung biopsy can secure diagnosis. If cultures are positive, resistance testing is mandatory. Lymph node tuberculosis is the most common extrapulmonary manifestation. Tuberculin skin testing is not reliable in HIV patients [74]. Standard tuberculostatic treatment should be initiated for 6 months. Adverse drug reactions are common. After drug interruption reinitiation can be tried with reduced initiation dose. Simultaneous beginning of antiretroviral and tuberculostatic therapy is problematic because of drug interactions and toxicity. In addition, immune reconstitution (see below) can worsen the clinical condition of the patient. Rifampicin should not be used with protease inhibitors. Alternatively rifabutin can be used as a weaker inducer of the cytochrome p450 system. In patients with <100/μL CD4 cell count antiretroviral therapy should be started after 2 weeks. In patients with 100–200/μL CD4 cell count antiretroviral therapy can be initiated after 2 months when tuberculostatic treatment is deescalated [50].

26.2.10 Atypical Mycobacteriosis (MAC)

Symptoms of disseminated MAC infection are anemia, fever, weight loss, elevated alkaline phosphatase, and diarrhea in patients with <100/μL CD4 cells. Localized forms, mostly lymph node abscesses, are seen in patients with better CD4 cells or immune reconstitution syndrome. Diagnosis in blood cultures and biopsies is difficult. First-line therapy is a combination of clarithromycin 2 × 500 mg, ethambutol 1,200 mg, and rifabutin 300 mg. Azithromycin 600 mg can be tried instead of clarithromycin. Rifabutin can be stopped a few weeks after clinical improvement. Treatment should be maintained for 6 months (and CD4 > 100/μL) [17].

26.2.11 Cryptosporidiosis

Cryptosporidiosis is usually self-limiting but may cause persistent and prolonged diarrhea in immunocompromised patients. There have been case reports of the successful use of nitazoxanide 2 × 500 mg daily. Symptomatic treatment and optimizing antiretroviral therapy are the most important procedures [1].

26.2.12 Wasting Syndrome

Wasting syndrome is defined as a weight loss of more than 10% and persistent diarrhea, fatigue, or fever for more than 30 days. Underlying infections and testosterone deficiency have to be excluded. Parenteral nutrition is only indicated in patients with malabsorption.

With the occurrence of opportunistic infections antiretroviral therapy should be initiated. OI treatment can be toxic, and there are many drug–drug interactions. In some cases, it can be beneficial for the patient to first start OI therapy (Table 26.3) and to postpone HAART for a few days or weeks. For PML or cryptosporidiosis there is no specific treatment and HAART should be optimized immediately [46].

26.2.13 Lipodystrophy Syndrome

Lipodystrophy syndrome describes clinical and metabolic changes associated with antiretroviral therapy and HIV. The mechanism is not fully understood. Mitochondrial toxicity seems to play an important role. Stavudine and zidovudine are the most common associated drugs. Change to tenofovir or abacavir should be considered. Abdominal lipoaccumulation, gynecomasty, fat accumulation in the neck and lipoatrophy in the face, (Fig. 26.2) or limbs can be disfiguring features. Insulin resistance, pathological glucose tolerance, hyperlipidemia, and low HDL are metabolic changes associated with lipodystrophy syndrome. For lipoatrophy injections with fillers (e.g., hyaluronic acid) can be considered. Diet and exercise have some positive effects on lipoaccumulation. Localized fat accumulation can be treated with excision or liposuction but results are often not satisfying [6]. Hyperlipidemia should be treated with statins or fibrates but drug interactions have to be considered.

26.3 HIV and Tumors

A survey in French clinics specialized in HIV showed that 28% of all HIV-positive patients' deaths were tumor-related; 45% of those were non-AIDS-defining tumors [9]. In the beginning of the HIV epidemic,

Table 26.3 First-line therapy of opportunistic infections

Opportunistic infection	First-line therapy	Length of therapy
PCP	Cotrimoxazole 3 × 2,400 mg i.v.+	21 days
	Prednisone 2 × 20–40 mg	5–10 days
Bacterial pneumonia	Community-acquired: Clarithromycin 2 × 500 mg or Roxithromycin 1 × 300 mg or Cefpodoxim 2 × 200 mg Hospital-acquired: Piperacillin 3 × 4.5 g i.v. or Ceftriaxon 2 g i.v. or Cefuroxim 3 × 1.5 g i.v. + Roxithromycin 300 mg or Clarithromycin 2 × 500 mg	7–10 days
Oral candidosis	Amphotericin B suspension 4 × 1 mL or nystatin 4 × 1 mL	For 48 h after symptoms have stopped
Candida esophagitis	Fluconazole 2 × 100 mg or Itraconazole 2 × 100–200 mg	Minimum10 days
Oral hairy leukoplakia	Initiation of antiretroviral therapy, in special cases acyclovir 2 × 800 mg	7 days
Herpes simplex	Acyclovir 3 × 400 mg or valacyclovir 2 × 1,000 mg or 2 × 500 mg famciclovir	5 days 7–14 days
	Severe infections:	
	Acyclovir 3 × 5–10 mg/kg i.v.	
Herpes zoster	Acyclovir 3 × 5–10 mg/kg i.v. analgesia	7–10 days
PML	Initiation of antiretroviral therapy Consider cidofovir 5 mg/kg	Every 7–14 days
Toxoplasmosis	Sulfadiazine 4 × 1,000–15,000 mg + pyrimethamine 1 × 50 mg + calcium foliate 15 mg 3 × 7 weeks	4–6 weeks then reduced dose for at least 6 months
CMV	Valganciclovir 2 × 900 mg	3 weeks then reduced dose for at least 6 months
Cryptococcosis	Amphotericin B 3 mg/kg + Fluconazole 2 × 200 mg + Flucytosine 4 × 2.5 g	6 weeks, then only fluconazole 200–400 mg for at least 6 months
TBC	Standard tuberculostatic treatment Avoid rifampicin in patients treated with PIs	6 months
MAC	Clarithromycin 2 × 500 mg + Ethambutol 1,200 mg + Rifabutin 300 mg	6 months Rifabutin can be stopped a few weeks after clinical improvement
Cryptosporidiosis	Initiation of antiretroviral therapy	

Kaposi's sarcoma was a common stigma in AIDS patients and one of the leading causes of death (Chapter 31). While Kaposi's sarcoma is seen less frequently after the introduction of antiretroviral therapy, lymphoma and other malignancies are increasingly challenging [8].

HIV-positive patients have an eight times higher risk of developing lung cancer. They are younger and the tumor (predominantly adenocarcinoma) grows rapidly. Smoking is an important additional risk factor. The risk of developing hepatocellular carcinoma is determined by hepatitis B and C coinfection. Chronic hepatitis is more common in HIV-positive patients and leads faster to cirrhosis. Early hepatitis treatment and prevention of hepatitis B by vaccination are important to reduce liver-associated deaths [9].

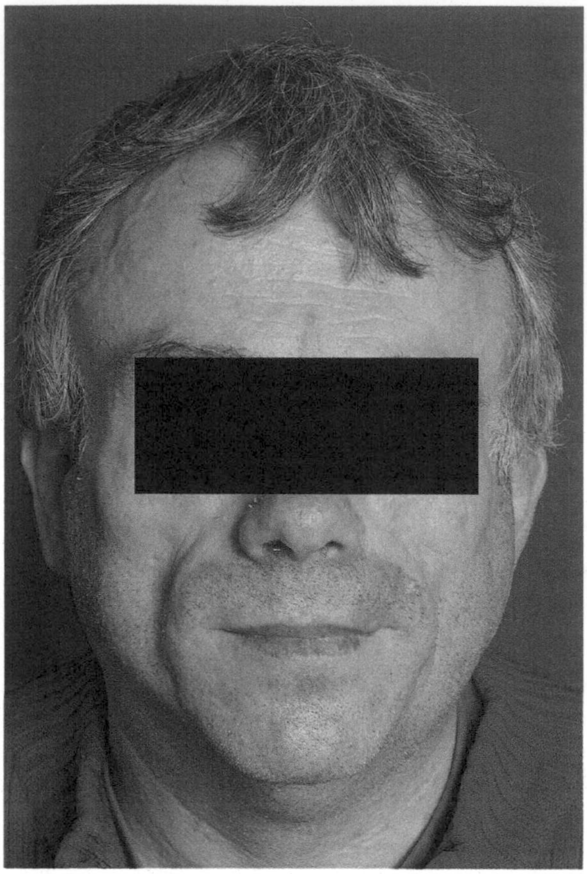

Fig. 26.2 Lipodystrophy syndrome: lipoatrophy in the face

26.3.1 Lymphoma

26.3.1.1 Non-Hodgkin Lymphoma

HIV-associated lymphomas are the second most-common AIDS-defining neoplasias. On first diagnosis disseminated disease is seen in 90% of patients with non-Hodgkin lymphoma (NHL). Involvement of the gastrointestinal tract, the bone marrow, and the liver are common. Up to 30% affect the central nervous system, primarily and secondarily. Body-cavity lymphomas (primary effusion lymphoma) clinically appear as pleura effusion or ascites. This aggressive tumor is almost exclusively seen in HIV-positive patients. An association with Epstein–Barr virus (EBV) has been described [68]. Most HIV-related NHL are highly malignant blastic B-cell lymphoma. HIV is associated with a TH2 cytokine profile that is associated with B-cell proliferation. These cytokines also enhance HIV proliferation, immune evasion, angiogenesis, and transcription of oncogenes [18]. Long-term persistence of HIV-1 structural protein and glycoproteins in the germinal centers of lymph nodes play a potential role in chronic antigenic stimulation and subsequent lymphoma formation. They could be found in the absence of detectable virus replication in patients under highly active antiretroviral therapy [62]. It can be difficult to distinguish between HIV-related lymph adenopathy and lymphoma. A lymph node biopsy is mandatory. Most NHL occur in patients with about 100/μL CD4 cells, but helper cells can be much higher. Staging should include chest X-ray, abdominal ultrasound, bone marrow biopsy, and CTs. ECG and echocardiography are needed before initiation of chemotherapy that may have cardiotoxic effects. Most patients are treated with CHOP (day 1 cyclophosphamide 750 mg/m^2, doxorubicin 50 mg/m^2, vincristine 1.4 mg/m^2, day 1–5 prednisone 100 mg) regimen (four to six cycles). Treatment with rituximab has been discussed controversially, but recently published studies showed equal outcomes in HIV negative and positive lymphoma patients in combination with CHOP [69].

Burkitt's lymphoma is an especially aggressive tumor entity. Intensified chemotherapy regimens (e.g., B-ALL) showed better survival rates than CHOP [10].

Primary effusion lymphoma has been a poor prognosis. There is no standard treatment. High-dose MTX and initiation of antiretroviral therapy are the most successful regimes [72].

Primary CNS lymphomas are a late complication of HIV infection. In the pre-HAART era most patients died within 3 months. Seizures, personality changes, headaches, and pareses are clinical symptoms. Differential diagnosis includes toxoplasmosis and other opportunistic infections, glioblastomas, and metastases of other tumors. Radiation or high-dose MTX are therapeutic options. Optimization of antiretroviral therapy is very important [31].

26.4 CD30$^+$ Large-Cell Lymphoma

Patients with CD 30$^+$ large-cell lymphoma typically present with a rapidly growing deep skin nodule or plaque. Histologically, there is a predominance of the

T-cell lineage in HIV-associated cutaneous CD30$^+$ large-cell lymphoma in contrast with B-cell types that occur at other sites [42]. In NHL, early therapeutic intervention is necessary because of the fast progression of the tumor. Diagnosis and treatment does not differ from HIV-negative patients. Prior to antiretroviral therapy, patients with CD30$^+$ large-cell lymphoma had a very poor prognosis. Improved survival has been reported with the addition of rituximab to CHOP in patients with HIV-associated diffuse large B-cell lymphoma [27]. A previous study had seen a higher rate of treatment-related infectious deaths [39].

26.5 Hodgkin's Lymphoma

Hodgkin's lymphoma is often seen in patients with antiretroviral therapy. Staging should be performed analogous to non-Hodgkin's lymphoma (see above). Radiochemotherapy (ABVD or BEACOPP) is frequently used, but prospective studies should be performed [80].

Diagnosis of *multicentric Castleman's disease* is difficult. Association with HHV 8 is obligatory. Half of the patients also suffer from Kaposi's sarcoma. Lymph node swelling, fever, night sweat, and weight loss are typical. Diagnostic features are hepatosplenomegaly, respiratory symptoms, edema, with hypoalbuminemia and hypergammaglobulinemia. Lymph nodes show a lymphoproliferative disease with malignant aspects and have to be sent to specialized centers. Experimental treatment includes virostatics, chemotherapy, and rituximab. There are no established therapy regimens [54].

26.6 Cutaneous T-Cell Lymphoma (CTCL)

Lymphomas in HIV-positive patients rarely affect the skin. Mycosis fungoides and Sézary syndrome are rare conditions in HIV-infected persons. In most cases the immune system is still relatively intact. Standard and antiretroviral therapies should be applied. Immunosuppressive substances such as methotrexate should be avoided if possible because of their potential to worsen the immune status. Interferon alfa-2a has been used safely for other indications in HIV-infected persons [85].

26.6.1 Human Papilloma Virus (HPV)-Related Tumors

Human papilloma virus is known to induce not only warts but also tumors and its precursor lesions. Association with high-risk HPV types (e.g., 16, 18) has first been described in cervical cancer [53]. All HIV-positive women should be screened carefully for cervical intraepithelial neoplasia (CIN) and AIDS-defining cervical cancer. The relative risk for developing cervical cancer in HIV-positive women compared with HIV-negatives varies widely across the globe [12] (Fig. 26.3). The incidence of HPV-related anal carcinoma and its precursor lesions

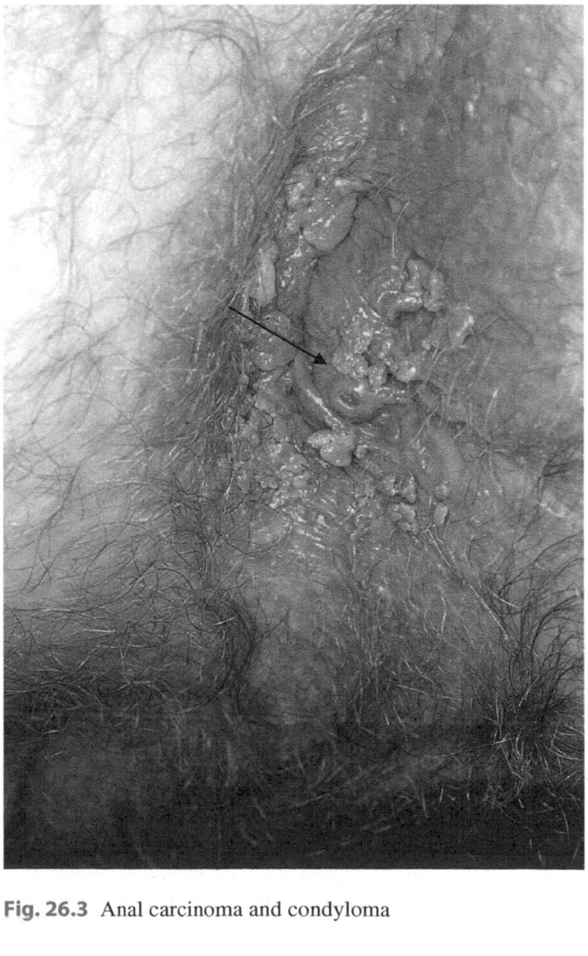

Fig. 26.3 Anal carcinoma and condyloma

are rising dramatically. Diamond et al. saw 2.8/1,000 AIDS cases in 1992 and 24.7/1,000 AIDS cases in 2000; 32% of the patients died of anal cancer (median survival 37 months). Compared with the general population, concomitant HIV infection drastically increases the relative risk for anal intraepithelial neoplasia (AIN, 60×) and anal cancer (37×). In HIV-positive patients under the age of 30 there is a 130–162 times higher risk of developing AIN than in the general population [23]. Perianal human papillomavirus (HPV) infections have been detected in up to 93% of men who are HIV-positive and a high incidence of high-grade AIN has been reported. Kreuter et al. found AIN in 19.4% of his patients. With high-resolution anoscopy this number rises up to 40–50% [15, 44, 58]. Screening programs with high-resolution anoscopy and cytology as they are already established for cervical carcinoma should be implemented. HIV-positive men also carry a 36-fold higher risk of developing penile cancer. Regular clinical screening is suggested.

Imiquimod has shown good clearance rates and safety when applied in the form of anal tampons and creams for anal intraepithelial neoplasia [41, 45]. There is a tendency to higher incidence of anal, penile, or cervical cancer in patients with lower CD4 levels, but antiretroviral therapy does not lead to a reduction of intraepithelial dysplasia [58]. So far, there are no studies with the new HPV vaccines in HIV-infected patients. Vaccination has to be considered on an individual basis.

26.6.2 Non-melanoma Skin Cancer (NMSC)

An increase of basal cell carcinomas, squamous cell carcinoma, and Merkel cell carcinoma in persons with HIV-infections has been observed. For basal cell carcinoma, the age-adjusted rate in Caucasian males was 795 per 100,000 person years compared to 475 per 100,000 in HIV-negative persons. The rate for squamous cell skin carcinoma was 159 per 100,000, which is also higher than the general Caucasian US population [9]. HIV-positive patients with NMSC tend to be younger than HIV-negative patients.

26.6.2.1 Basal and Squamous Cell Carcinoma

Basal cell carcinoma in immunosuppressed patients appears to show a more aggressive behavior [57]. The risk factors including sun exposure, blond hair, blue eyes, and a family history of skin cancer are the same as in HIV-negative persons. Higher exposure to recreational UV radiation in homosexual men has been reported [28, 49]. Patients with HIV-infection more commonly experience treatment-associated complication such as infection and recurrence.

26.6.2.2 Squamous Cell Carcinoma

The ratio of squamous cell carcinoma to basal cell carcinoma in HIV-infected patients is approximately 1:7 unlike in organ transplant recipients were it is 1.8:1. An uncontrolled retrospective case series reports a strikingly aggressive nature of squamous cell carcinomas in HIV-infected patients. The authors suggest adjunctive modalities, such as sentinel lymph node biopsy for high-risk tumors. Primary prevention with avoidance of UV radiation and aggressive management of precancerous lesions should be recommended. Infection with unusual HPV-types is more common in HIV-related squamous cell carcinoma of the anogenital region, the nail unit, and in epidermodysplasia verruciformis [85].

26.6.2.3 Merkel Cell Carcinoma

Several cases of Merkel cell carcinoma (MCC) in persons with HIV infection have been described [4]. The patients' mean age was 48 years, while 85% of MCC patients uninfected by HIV-1 are over 60 years old. The relative risk of Merkel cell carcinoma compared with the general population was 13.4 (95% confidence interval 4.9–29.1). It can develop before AIDS diagnosis. The role of sun exposure in addition to the immune deficiency is discussed. The tumor is particularly aggressive in HIV-positive patients resulting in a poor prognosis (medium survival time 18 months) [24]. A standard therapy has not been established. Surgical removal in combination with radiation with or without chemotherapy is indicated in localized tumors. A safety margin of at least 3 cm including the fascia should be chosen where possible. When distant metastases are diagnosed only palliative care is possible. The cKIT inhibitor imatinib showed lack of efficacy in some case reports [86].

26.6.3 Melanoma

It is not clear whether melanoma is more common in HIV-infected patients [9, 59]. However they tend to have an atypical appearance. A number of case reports have been published [11]. Metastatic disease with poor prognosis is common. In a case-control study, 17 HIV-positive patients were matched with HIV-negative patients. HIV-positive patients had a significantly shorter disease-free survival ($p=0.03$) and overall survival ($p = 0.045$). Low CD4 cell counts led to earlier melanoma recurrence [73]. Standard guidelines for melanoma treatment including surgical margins for excision procedures have been proposed. Adjuvant treatments with chemotherapy or interferon-alpha should be considered on a case-by-case basis [11]. Collaboration with an oncologist who has experience with melanoma and HIV patients is highly recommended. The safety of adjuvant interferon-alpha has been documented in the treatment of HIV-related Kaposi's sarcoma [64].

Therapeutic options should be chosen according to the stage of the disease. Antiretroviral therapy should be continued if possible. Interaction between HAART und chemotherapy has to be considered. Treatment should be confined to specialized centers.

26.7 Other Dermatological Signs

Mollusca contagiosa in adults are a sign of severe immunodeficiency (<200/μL CD4). Papules can be treated with curettage or cryotherapy [77].

Ulcerating papules are characteristic for bacillary angiomatosis (BA). BA is caused by two species: *Bartonella heneslae* and *Bartonella quintana*. *Bartonella* have to be treated with macrolides for several months [70].

Seborrheic dermatitis is seen in 20–60% of all HIV-infected patients. Scaling and erythema in the seborrheic areas are characteristic. Antimycotic treatment or metronidazole have shown clinical efficacy. It is sometimes discussed if seborrheic dermatitis is a minimal form of psoriasis. Although psoriasis is not seen more often than in the general population worsening of the disease and first manifestation have been seen in association with HIV infection or deterioration of the immunocompetence. The dermatoproliferative effect of HIV and cytokine induction is discussed as pathogenetic effects. After initiation of antiretroviral therapy, skin lesions often resolve. Case reports have described the successful use of antipsoriatic agents including biological ones [2, 5, 43].

Oral aphthosis is often seen in acute and advanced stages of HIV infection. Differential diagnosis are HSV or CMV ulcers. Symptomatic treatment is carried out with disinfecting solutions, local steroids, and local anesthesia [67].

Pruritus is a common problem in patients with and without antiretroviral therapy. Pathogenesis is not known. If patients also suffer from Xerosis cutis moisturizing creams with addition of polidocanol can reduce itch.

26.8 HIV and STDs

About 80% of HIV-infected patients have also experienced syphilis infection. Severe clinical courses of syphilis infection are more common with neurosyphilis occurring within months after infection. Cerebrospinal liquor puncture should be considered in all patients. Some physicians recommend more intensive treatment because treatment failure is common. Benzathine penicillin 2.4 Mio i.E. i.m. (if duration is not known repeat in week 2 and 3) is the first line treatment in early syphilis. Neurosyphilis is treated with penicillin G 5 × 6 Mio, i.e., or 3 × 10 Mio i.E. i.v. All sexually transmitted diseases increase the risk of HIV transmission and should be treated consequently. Atypical manifestations and locations (e.g., anal, pharyngeal) (Fig. 26.4) should be considered. This is also true for gonorrhea and chlamydia infection.

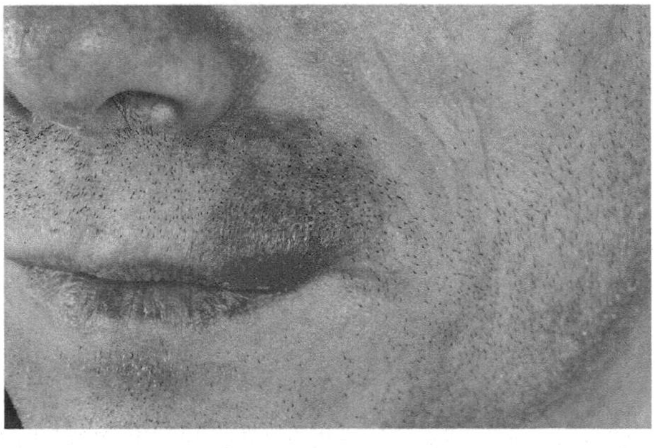

Fig. 26.4 Early syphilis with atypical chancre at the lip

Since 1993, single-dose fluoroquinolones (e.g., ciprofloxacin 500 mg) have been first-line treatment for gonorrhea. Considering rising resistance rates of up to 29% in men, who have sex with men in the USA, ceftriaxone 250 mg i.m. or cefixime 400 mg p.o. are the best single-dose treatment options now. Chlamydia coinfection should always be excluded [13]. Clinical course and treatment do not differ from HIV-negative patients, but the incidence is much higher. Screening should be considered in all HIV-positive patients.

26.9 Antiretroviral Therapy

There is hardly any other medical field that has experienced changes and developments as dramatic as in the treatment of HIV infection in the last years. Twenty-three antiretroviral substances are approved worldwide (Table 26.4). A turning point was the introduction of the *protease inhibitors* (PI) saquinavir and indinavir in 1995 and nevirapine and the class of *NNRTIs* in 1996. This was the beginning of the HAART (highly active antiretroviral therapy) era. The combination of a "backbone" of two NRTI and a NNRTI or protease inhibitor still form the basis of antiretroviral therapy [26]. Addition of low-dose ritonavir to protease inhibitors ("booster") results in a high plasma concentration of coadministrated PI and decreases pill burden, number of doses, and food restrictions [52].

Enfuvirtide so far is the only substance of the class of *fusion inhibitors*. By binding to gp41, it inhibits the fusion of the HIV with the cellular membrane of CD4 cells. Parenteral administration and local side reactions are the disadvantage of this promising substance [16]. The *CCR5 receptor antagonist* Maraviroc (approved 10/2007) can only be used after tropism testing. Patients with CXCR4 tropic viruses do not profit from the treatment. In addition the dose has to be adjusted to background therapy. Hopes for less side effects and better efficacy have risen for the class of *integrase inhibitors*. Raltegravir (MK0518) is the first substance of this class and was approved in 10/2007 [36].

Shortly after the first antiretroviral substances were available, the problem of resistance could be seen [19]. Primary resistance has been seen in up to 14% of therapy-naive patients [22]. Although genotypic resistance testing and the combination of at least two active substances have improved the outcome even of heavily pretreated patients, further research is needed.

26.10 Side Effects

The use of antiretroviral therapy is also limited by side effects. The mitochondrial toxicity of the old NRTIs is associated with lipodystrophy, hepatotoxicity, and other metabolic disorders [25]. Some side effects are substance-specific, e.g., zidovudine is known to cause macrocytic anemia [51] and abacavir associated with the hypersensitivity syndrome in HLA B5701-positive patients [79]. Pancreatitis can be seen after treatment with didanosine [33] and tenofovir can cause nephrotoxicity [75]. Nevirapine can cause severe allergic skin reactions and liver toxicity, especially in women with high CD4 cell count [70]. The effects on the central nervous system of efavirenz can lead to dizziness, depression, and nightmares [71]. Gastrointestinal problems are often seen when protease inhibitors are given. Hyperglycemia, lipodystrophy, and hyperlipidemia are also attributed to them [56]. Substance specific side effects are nephrolithiasis and paronychia after indinavir treatment [30] and hyperbilirubinemia during atazanavir treatment [29]. A good relationship and communication between the patient and the therapist can help to minimize compliance problems due to side effects, but new substances with fewer side effects would permanently solve the problem. In addition, in order to succeed, a potent impact of pharmacogenomics and individualized therapy should be taken into account.

26.11 Immune Reconstitution Syndrome

The immune reconstitution syndrome is still a challenge to the therapist. Especially in patients with <200/μL $CD4^+$ T-cells who start antiretroviral therapy, subclinical infections can demask after immune reconstitution. Before the beginning of therapy a screening for opportunistic infections with chest X-ray, ultrasound of the abdomen, and a fundoscopy should be standard procedures. Patients have to be watched carefully during the first weeks of antiretroviral therapy.

Table 26.4 Antiretroviral drugs

Trade name (abbreviation)	Drug	Dose
Nucleoside and nucleotide reverse transcriptase inhibitors (NRTIs)		
Combivir (CBV)	Zidovudine + Lamivudine	2 × 300 mg/150 mg
Emtriva (FTC)	Emtricitabine	1 × 200 mg
Epivir (3TC)	Lamivudine	2 × 150 mg or 1 × 300 mg
Hivid (ddC)	Zalcitabine	Distribution ceased
Kivexa/Epzicom (KVX)	Abacavir + Lamivudine	1 × 600 mg/300 mg
Retrovir (AZT)	Zidovudine	2 × 250 mg
Trizivir (TZV)	Zidovudine + Abacavir + Lamivudine	2 × 300 mg/300 mg/150 mg
Videx (ddI)	Didanosine	<60 kg 1 × 250 mg
		≥60 kg 1 × 400 mg
Viread (TDF)	Tenofovir	1 × 300 mg
Truvada (TDF/FTC)	Tenofovir/Emtricitabine	300 mg/200 mg
Zerit (d4T)	Stavudine	<60 kg 2 × 30 mg
		≥60 kg 2 × 40 mg
Ziagen (ABC)	Abacavir	2 × 300 mg
Non-nucleoside reverse transcriptase inhibitors (NNRTIs)		
Intelence (TMC 125)	Etravirine	2 × 100 mg
Rescriptor (DLV)	Delavirdine	3 × 400 mg
Sustiva/Stocrin (EFV)	Efavirenz	1 × 600 mg or 3 × 200 mg
Viramune (NVP)	Nevirapine	2 × 200 mg
NRTI/NNRTI combination		
Atripla (ATR)	Tenofovir + Emtricitabine + Efavirenz	1 × 300 mg/200 mg/600 mg
Protease-inhibitors (PIs)		
Aptivus (TPV)	Tipranavir	2 × 250 mg + 2 × 200 mg RTV
Agenerase (APV)	Amprenavir	2 × 20 mg/kg
Crixivan (IDV)	Indinavir	2 × 800 mg + 2 × 100 mg RTV
Invirase 500 (SQV)	Saquinavir	2 × 1,000 mg + 2 × 100 mg RTV
Kaletra (LPV)	Lopinavir/Ritonavir	2 × 400 mg/100 mg
Norvir (RTV)	Ritonavir	Only as booster
Prezista (DRV)	Darunavir	2 × 300 mg + 1 × 100 mg RTV
Reyataz (ATV)	Atazanavir	1 × 300 mg + 1 × 100 mg RTV or 1 × 400 mg
Telzir/Lexiva (FPV)	Fosamprenavir	2 × 700 mg + 1 × 200 mg RTV
Viracept (NFV)	Nelfinavir	2 × 1,250 mg
Fusion inhibitors		
Fuzeon (T20)	Enfuvirtide	2 × 1 mL at 90 mg s.c.

(continued)

Table 26.4 (continued)

Trade name (abbreviation)	Drug	Dose
Entry inhibitors		
Celsentri (MCV)	Maraviroc	2 × 300 mg
Integrase inhibitors		
Isentress (RAL)	Raltegravir	2 × 400 mg

26.12 Summary

HIV-positive patients often present with skin or mucosal problems as first sign of the infection. Highly immunosuppressed patients with opportunistic infections or tumors are often not aware of their HIV infection. Earlier HIV testing would not only improve the prognosis of these patients, but would also help to avoid new infections. HIV patients should be treated in specialized centers. Differential diagnosis can be highly complex and drug interactions have to be considered when treating opportunistic infections and concomitant diseases. Lifespan has increased immensely but side effects of lifelong antiretroviral therapy and non-AIDS-defining tumors in aging patients have to be managed.

Take-Home Pearls

- HIV positive patients often present with skin or mucosal problems as first sign of the infection.
- Earlier HIV testing would not only improve the prognosis of these patients, but would also help to avoid new infections.
- Most patients presenting with severe opportunistic infections are not aware of their HIV-infection.
- Management of comorbidities is the new challenge in aging HIV patients.
- 28% of all HIV positive patients´ deaths were tumor-related. 45% of those were non AIDS-defining tumors.
- STD-Screening (including HPV) should be considered in all HIV-positive patients.

References

1. Abubakar, I., Aliyu, S.H., Arumugam, C.: Treatment of cryptosporidosis in immunocompromised individuals: systematic review and meta-analysis. Br. J. Clin. Pharmacol. **63**, 387–393 (2007)
2. Akaraphanth, R., Lim, H.W.: HIV, UV and immunosuppression. Photodermatol. Photoimmunol. Photomed. **15**, 28–31 (1999)
3. Albougy, H.A., Naidoo, S.: A systematic review of management of oral candidiasis associated with HIV/AIDS. SADJ **57**, 457–466 (2002)
4. An, K.P., Ratner, D.: Merkel cell carcinoma in the setting of HIV infection. J. Am. Acad. Dermatol. **45**, 309–312 (2001)
5. Bartke, U., Venten, I., Kreuter, A., et al.: Human immunodeficiency virus-associated Psoriasis and psoriatic arthritis treated with infliximab. Br. J. Dermatol. **150**, 784–786 (2004)
6. Bechara, F.G., Sand, M., Potthoff, A., et al.: HIV-associated facial lipoatrophy-review of current therapy option. Eur. J. Med. Res. **13**, 93–99 (2008)
7. Bensadoun, R., Daoud, J., Gueddari, B., et al.: Comparison of the efficacy and safety of miconazole 50 mg mucoadhesive buccal tablets with miconazole 500 mg gel in the treatment of oropharyngeal candidiasis: a prospective randomized, single-blind, multicenter, comparative, phase III treal in patients treated with radiotherapy for head and neck cancer. Cancer **112**, 204–211 (2008)
8. Bonnet, F., Lewden, C., May, T., et al.: Malignancy-related causes of death in human immunodeficiency virus-infected patients in the era of highly active antiretroviral therapy. Cancer **101**, 317–324 (2004)
9. Burgi, A., Brodine, S., Wegner, S., et al.: Incidence and risk factors for the occurrence of non-AIDS-defining cancers among human immunodeficiency virus-infected individuals. Cancer **104**, 1505–1511 (2005)
10. Blinder, V.S., Chadburn, A., Furman, R.R., et al.: Improving outcomes for patients with Burkitt lymphoma and HIV. AIDS Patients Care STDS **22**, 175–187 (2008)
11. Calista, D.: Five cases of melanoma in HIV positive patients. Eur. J. Dermatol. **11**, 446–449 (2001)
12. Castellsague, X., Diaz, M., de Sanjose, S., et al.: International Agency for Research on Cancer Multicenter Cervical Cancer Study Group. Worldwide human papillomavirus etiology of cervical adenocarcinoma and its cofactors: implications for screening and prevention. J. Natl Cancer Inst. **98**, 303–315 (2006)
13. CDC: Update to CDC's sexually transmitted diseases treatment guidelines, 2006: fluoroquinolones no longer recommended

for treatment of gonococcal infections. MMWR Morb. Mortal. Wkly. Rep. **56**, 332–336 (2007)
14. Centers for Disease Control: 1993 revised classification system for HIV infection and expanded surveillance case definition for aids among adolescents and adults. MMWR **41**, RR-17 (1993)
15. Chin-Hong, P.V., Vittinghoff, E., Cranston, R.D.: Age-related prevalence of anal cancer precursors in homosexual men: the EXPLORE study. J. Natl Cancer Inst. **97**, 896–905 (2005)
16. Clotet, B., Raffi, F., Cooper, D., et al.: Clinical management of treatment-experienced, HIV infected patients with the fusion inhibitor enfuvirtide: consensus recommendations. AIDS **18**, 1137–1146 (2004)
17. Corti, M., Palmero, D.: Mycobacterium avium complex infection in HIV/AIDS patients. Expert Rev. Anti-infect. Ther. **6**, 351–363 (2008)
18. Dalgleish, A.G., O´ Byrne, K.J.: Chronic immune activation and inflammation in the pathogenesis of AIDS and cancer. Adv. Cancer Res. **84**, 231–276 (2002)
19. D'Aquila, R.T., Johnson, V.A., Welles, S.L., et al.: Zidovudine resistance and HIV-1 disease progression during antiretroviral therapy. Ann. Intern. Med. **122**, 401–408 (1995)
20. Davis, J.L., Fei, M., Huang, L.: Respiratory infection complicating HIV infection. Curr. Opin. Infect. Dis. **21**, 184–190 (2008)
21. Dedicoat, M., Livesley, N.: Management of toxoplasmic encephalitis in HIV-infected adults – a review. S. Afr. Med. J. **98**, 31–32 (2008)
22. DeGruttola, V., Dix, L., A'Aquila, R., et al.: The relationship between baseline HIV drug resistance and response to antiretroviral therapy: re-analysis of retrospective and prospective studies using a standardized data analysis plan. Antivir. Ther. **5**, 43–50 (2000)
23. Diamond, C., Taylor, T.H., Aboumrad, T., et al.: Increased incidence of squamous cell anal cancer among men with AIDS in the era of highly active antiretroviral therapy. Sex. Transm. Dis. **32**, 314–320 (2005)
24. Engels, E.A., Frisch, M., Goerdert, J.J., et al.: Merkel cell carcinoma and HIV infection. Lancet **359**, 497–498 (2002)
25. Esser, S., Helbig, D., Hillen, U., et al.: Side effects of HIV therapy. J. Dtsch Dermatol. Ges. **5**(9), 745–754 (2008)
26. European AIDS Clinical Society (EACS), European Guidelines for the Clinical Management and Treatment of HIV Infected Adults in Europe 2008. http://www.eacs.eu/guide/index.htm.
27. Ezzat, H., Filipenko, D., Vickars, L., et al.: Improved survival in HIV-associated diffuse large B-cell lympoma with the addition of rituximab to chemotherapy in patients receiving highly active antiretroviral therapy. HIV Clin. Trials **8**, 132–144 (2007)
28. Flegg, P.J.: Potential risks of ultraviolet radiation in HIV infection. Int. J. STD AIDS **1**, 46–48 (1990)
29. Fuster, D., Clotet, B.: Review of atazanavir: a novel HIV protease inhibitor. Expert Opin. Pharmacother. **6**, 1565–1572 (2005)
30. Garcia-Silva, J., Almagro, M., et al.: Indinavir-induced retinoid-like effects: incidence, clinical features and management. Drug Saf. **25**, 993–1003 (2002)
31. Gerstner, E., Batchelor, T.: Primary CNS lymphoma. Expert Rev. Anticancer Ther. **7**, 689–700 (2007)
32. Ghannoum, M.A., Kuhn, D.M.: Voriconazole-better chances for patients with invasive mycoses. Eur. J. Med. Res. **7**, 242–256 (2002)
33. Guo, J.J., Jang, R., Louder, A., Cluxton, R.J.: Acute pancreatitis associated with different combination therapies in patients infected with human immunodeficiency virus. Pharmacotherapy **25**, 1044–1054 (2005)
34. Gupta, R., Warren, T., Wald, A.: Genital herpes. Lancet **370**, 2127–2137 (2007)
35. Hoffmann, C., Ernst, M., Meyer, P., et al.: Evolving characteristics of toxoplasmosis in patients infected with human immunodeficiency virus-1: clinical course and Toxoplasma gondii-specific immune responses. Clin. Microbiol. Infect. **13**, 510–515 (2007)
36. Hughes, A., Barber, T., Nelson, M.: New treatment options for HIV salvage patients: an overview of second generation PIs, NNRTIs, integrase inhibitors and CCR5 antagonists. J. Infect. **57**(1), 1–10 (2008)
37. Hung, C.C., Hsiao, C.F., Wang, J.L., et al.: Herpes zoster in HIV-1-infected patients in the era of highly active antiretroviral therapy: a prospective observational study. Int. J. STD AIDS **16**(10), 673 (2005)
38. Jevtovic, D.J., Salemovic, D., Ranin, J., et al.: The prevalence and risk of immune restoration disease in HIV-infected patients treated with highly active antiretroviral therapy. HIV Med. **6**(2), 140–143 (2005)
39. Kaplan, L.D., Lee, J.Y., Ambinder, R.F., et al.: Rituximab does not improve clinical outcome in a randomized phase 3 trial of CHOP with or without rituximab in patients with HIV-associated non-Hodgkin lymphoma: AIDS-Malignancies Consortium Trial 010. Blood **106**, 15–43 (2005)
40. Karsonis, N., Di Nubile, M.J., Bartizal, K., et al.: Efficacy of caspofungin in the treatment of esophageal candidiasis resistant to fluconazole. J. Acquir. Immune Defic. Syndr. **31**, 183–187 (2002)
41. Kaspari, M., Gutzmer, R., Kaspari, T., et al.: Application of imiquimod by suppositories (anal tampons) efficiently prevents recurrences after ablation of anal canal condyloma. Br. J. Dermatol. **147**, 757–759 (2002)
42. Kerschmann, R.L., Berger, T.G., Weiss, L.M., et al.: Cutaneous presentations of lymphoma in human immunodeficiency virus disease. Predominance of T cell lineage. Arch. Dermatol. **131**, 1281–1288 (1995)
43. Kreuter, A., Schugt, I., Rasokat, H., et al.: Dermatological diseases and signs of HIV-infection. Eur. J. Med. Res. **7**, 57–62 (2002)
44. Kreuter, A., Brockmeyer, N.H., Hochdorfer, B., et al.: Clinical spectrum and virologic characteristics of anal intraepithelial neoplasia in HIV infection. J. Am. Acad. Dermatol. **52**, 603–608 (2005)
45. Kreuter, A., Potthoff, A., Brockmeyer, N.H.: Imiquimod leads to a decrease of human papillomavirus DNA and to a sustained clearance of anal intraepithelial neoplasia in HIV-infected men. J. Invest. Dermatol. **128**, 2078–2083 (2008)
46. Kulstad, R., Schöller, D.A.: The energetics of wasting disease. Curr. Opin. Clin. Nutr. Metab. Care **10**, 488–493 (2007)

47. Lalonde, R.G., Voivin, G., Deschênes, J., et al.: Canadian consensus guidelines for the management of cytomegalovirus disease in HIV/AIDS. Can. J. Infect. Dis. Med. Microbiol. **15**, 327–335 (2004)
48. Lewden, C., May, T., Rosenthal, E., et al.: Changes in causes of death among adults infected by HIV between 2000 and 2005: The "Motalité 2000 and 2005" Surveys (ANRS EN 19 and Mortavic). J. Acquir. Immune Defic. Syndr. **48**, 590–598 (2008)
49. Lobo, D.V., Chu, P., Grekin, R.C., Berger, T.G.: Nonmelanoma skin cancers and infection with the human immunodeficiency virus. Arch. Dermatol. **128**, 623–627 (1992)
50. Mc Illeron, H., Meintjes, G., Burman, W.J., Maartens, G.: Complications of antiretroviral therapy in patients with tuberculosis: drug interactions, toxicity, and immune reconstitution inflammatory syndrome. J. Infect. Dis. **196**(Suppl 1), 63–75 (2007)
51. Mildvan, D., Greagh, T., Leitz, G., The Anemia Prevalence Study Group: Prevalence of anemia and correlation with biomarkers and specific antiretroviral regimens in 9690 human-immunodeficiency-virus-infected patients: findings of the Anemia Prevalence Study. Curr. Med. Res. Opin. **23**, 343–355 (2007)
52. Motwani, B., Khayr, W.: Pharmacoenhancement of protease inhibitors. Am. J. Ther. **13**, 57–63 (2006)
53. Munoz, N., Bosch, F.X., de Sanjose, S., et al.: International Agency for Research on Cancer Multicenter Cervical Cancer Study Group: Epidemiologic classification of human papillomavirus types associated with cervical cancer. N Engl J. Med. **348**, 518–527 (2003)
54. Mylona, E.E., Barabutis, I.G., Lekakis, L.J.: Multicentric castleman's disease in HIV infection: a systematic review of the literature. AIDS Rev. **10**, 25–35 (2008)
55. Nokta, M.: Oral manifestations associated with HIV infection. Curr. HIV/AIDS Rep. **5**, 5–12 (2008)
56. Nolan, D., Mallal, S.: Antiretroviral-therapy-associated lipoatrophy: current status and future directions. Sex. Health **2**, 153–163 (2005)
57. Oram, Y., Orengo, I., Griego, R.D., et al.: Histologic patterns of basal cell carcinoma based upon patient imunostatus. Dermatol. Surg. **21**, 611–614 (1995)
58. Palefsky, J.M., Holly, E.A., Efirdc, J.T., et al.: Anal intraepithelial neoplasia in the highly active antiretroviral therapy era among HIV-positive men who have sex with men. AIDS **19**, 1407–1414 (2005)
59. Pantanowitz, L., Schlecht, H.P., Dezube, B.J.: The growing problem of non-AIDS-defining malignancies in HIV. Curr. Opin. Oncol. **18**, 469–478 (2006)
60. Peytavin, G., Gautran, C., Otoul, C., et al.: Evaluation of pharmacokinetic interaction between cetirizine and ritonavir, an HIV-1 protease inhibitor, in healthy male volunteers. Eur. J. Clin. Pharmacol. **61**, 267–273 (2005)
61. Phillips, P., De Beule, K., Frechette, G., Tchamouroff, S., Vandercam, B., Weitner, L., Hoepeman, A., Stingl, G., Clotet, B.: A double-blind comparison of itraconazole oral solution and fluconazole capsules for the treatment of oropharyngeal candidiasis in patients with AIDS. Clin. Infect. Dis. **26**, 1368–1373 (1998)
62. Popovic, M., Tenner-Racz, K., Pelser, C., et al.: Persistence of HIV-1 structural proteins and glycoproteins in lymph nodes of patients under highly active antiretroviral therapy. Proc. Natl. Sci. USA **102**, 14807–14812 (2005)
63. Pukkila-Worley, R., Mylonakis, E.: Epidemiology and mangement of crytococcal meningitis: developments and challenges. Expert Opin. Pharmacother. **9**, 551–560 (2008)
64. Rasokat, H., Haussermann, L., Minnemann, M.: Response of AIDS-related Kaposi's sarcoma to treatment with recombinant interferon alpha depends on the stage of underlying immunodeficiency. J. Invest. Dermatol. **89**, 444–445 (1989)
65. Ratnam, I., Chiu, C., Kandala, N.B., et al.: Incidence and risk factors for immune reconstitution inflammatory syndrome in an ethnically diverse HIV type 1-infected cohort. Clin. Infect. Dis. **42**(3), 418–427 (2006)
66. Revankar, S.G., Kirkpatrick, W.R., McAtee, R.K., Dib, O.P., Fothergill, A.W., Redding, S.W., Rinaldi, M.G., Hilsenbeck, S.G., Patterson, T.F.: A randomized trial of continuous or intermittent therapy with fluconazole for oropharyngeal candidiasis in HIV-infected patients: clinical outcomes and development of fluconazole resistance. Am. J. Med. **105**, 7–11 (1998)
67. Reichart, P.A.: Oral ulcerations in HIV infection. Oral Dis **3**(Suppl 1), 180–182 (1997)
68. Resk, S.A., Weiss, L.M.: Epstein-Barr virus-associated lymphoproliferative disorders. Hum. Pathol. **38**, 1293–1304 (2007)
69. Ribera, J.M., Oriol, A., Morgades, M., et al.: Safety and efficacy of cyclophosphamide, adriamycin, vincristine, prednisone and rituximab in patients with human immunodeficiency virus-associated diffuse large B-cell lymphoma:results of a phase II trial. Br. J. Haematol. **140**, 411–419 (2008)
70. Rigopoulos, D., Paparizos, V., Katsambas, A.: Cutaneous markers of HIV infection. Clin. Dermatol. **22**, 487–498 (2004)
71. Rihs, T.A., Begley, K., Smith, D.E., et al.: Efavirenz and chronic neuropsychiatric symptoms: a cross-sectional case control study. HIV Med. **7**, 544–548 (2006)
72. Ripamonti, D., Marini, B., Rambaldi, A., Suter, F.: Treatment of primary effusion lymphoma with highly active antiviral therapy in the setting of HIV infection. AIDS **22**, 1236–1237 (2008)
73. Rodrigues, L.K., Klencke, B.J., Vin-Christian, K., et al.: Altered clinical course of malignant melanoma in HIV-positive patients. Arch. Dermatol. **138**, 765–770 (2002)
74. Roehr, B.: WHO says more HIV patients should be screened for tuberculosis. BMJ **337**, a1181 (2008)
75. Sax, P.E., Gallant, J.E., Klotman, P.E.: Renal safety of tenofovir disoproxil fumarate. AIDS Read. **17**, 90–92 (2007). 99-104, C3
76. Skiest, D.J., Vazquez, J.A., Anstead, G.M., Graybill, J.R., Reynes, J., Ward, D., Hare, R., Boparai, N., Isaacs, R.: Posaconazole for the treatment of azole-refractory oropharyngeal and esophageal candidiasis in subjects with HIV infection. Clin. Infect. Dis. **44**, 607–614 (2007)
77. Smith, K.J., Skelton, H.: Molluscum contagiosum: recent advances in pathogenic mechanisms and new therapies. Am. J. Clin. Dermatol. **3**, 535–545 (2002)
78. Sobel, J.D.: Treatment of vaginal Candidia infections. Expert Opin. Pharmacother. **3**, 1059–1065 (2002)
79. Stekler, J., Maenza, J., Stevens, C., et al.: Abacavir hypersensitivity reaction in primary HIV infection. AIDS **20**, 1269–1274 (2006)

80. Tanaka, P.Y., Pessoa Jr., V.P., Pracchia, L.F., et al.: Hodgkin lymphoma among patients infected with HIV in post-HAART era. Clin. Lmyphoma Myeloma **7**, 364–368 (2007)
81. Vanhems, P., Voisin, L., Gayet-Ageron, A., et al.: The incidence of herpes zoster is less likely than other opportunistic infections to be reduced by highly active antiretroviral therapy. J. Acquir. Immune Defic. Syndr. **38**, 111–113 (2005)
82. Vazquez, J.A., Skiest, D.J., Nieto, L., Northland, R., Sanne, I., Gogate, J., Greaves, W., Isaacs, R.: A multicenter randomized trial evaluating posaconazole versus fluconazole for the treatment of oropharyngeal candidiasis in subjects with HIV/AIDS. Clin. Infect. Dis. **42**, 1179–1186 (2006)
83. Volpi, A., Stanberry, L.: Herpes zoster in immunocompromized patients. Herpes **14**, 31 (2007)
84. Weber, T.: Progressive multifocal leukoencephalopathy. Neurol. Clin. **26**, 833–854 (2008)
85. Wilkens, K., Turner, R., Dolev, J.C., et al.: Cutaneous malignancy and human immunodeficiency virus disease. J. Am. Acad. Dermatol. **54**, 189–206 (2006)
86. Yang, Q., Hornick, JL., Granter, SR., Wang, L.C.: Merkel cell carcinoma: lack of KIT positivity and implications for the use of imatinib mcsylate. Appl Immunohistochem Mol Morphol. **17**, 276–281 (2009).

HIV in Eastern Europe

27

Nikolai Mashkilleyson and Jeffrey V. Lazarus

Core Messages

- Between 2001 and 2008, the number of people living with HIV in the countries of the former Soviet Union rose from an estimated 0.9 million to 1.5 million.
- HIV outbreaks in the region have been characterized by the rapid spread of infections among people who inject drugs, who are often criminalized or denied access to prevention interventions and treatment for their drug use and/or HIV.
- The HIV epidemic among MSM is well established in many Eastern European countries, but is often under-reported due to high levels of discrimination and violence toward men who have sex with men.
- The HIV epidemic in Eastern Europe has been exacerbated by frequent coinfection with sexually transmitted infections, tuberculosis, hepatitis B, hepatitis C, and other infections. In countries where the HIV epidemic is driven by injecting drug use, coinfection with hepatitis C ranges from 10% to 80%.
- Starting in 2006, antiretroviral therapy coverage has expanded significantly in the region, which should improve the quality of life and long-term survival for many people living with HIV, as well as decrease HIV transmission rates.
- One of the major challenges facing Eastern Europe is ensuring equitable access to HIV treatment and making key prevention interventions available, including needle and syringe exchange programs and opioid substitution therapy.

27.1 Introduction

By the end of 2008, more than 33 million people in the world were estimated to be living with HIV [117]. Although Eastern European countries[1] were not seriously affected by the epidemic until the late 1990s, the increase in their HIV rates at that time was unprecedented in the history of the HIV epidemic. This is especially true with regards to Estonia, the Russian Federation, and Ukraine. For example, there was a 100-fold increase in HIV seroprevalence among

[1]In the context of this chapter the term Eastern Europe refers to the countries of the former Soviet Union situated in Europe, namely the Baltic states (Estonia, Latvia, and Lithuania), Transcaucasia (Armenia, Azerbaijan, and Georgia) and other former Soviet states (Belarus, the Republic of Moldova, the Russian Federation, and Ukraine). The term Central Asia refers to the five former Soviet republics of Kazakhstan, Kyrgyzstan, Tajikistan, Turkmenistan, and Uzbekistan. All of these countries have shown similarities in how the HIV epidemic developed. Most of these countries inherited the Soviet surveillance system.

N. Mashkilleyson (✉)
Independent Consultant,
Bulevardi 13, 00120 Helsinki, Finland
e-mail: nikolai.mashkilleyson@gmail.com

J.V. Lazarus
Copenhagen School of Global Health,
University of Copenhagen, Øster Farimagsgade 5,
Bd. 9, DK-1353 Copenhagen K, Denmark
e-mail: jefflaz@pubhealth.ku.dk

G. Gross and S.K. Tyring (eds.), *Sexually Transmitted Infections and Sexually Transmitted Diseases*,
DOI: 10.1007/978-3-642-14663-3_27, © Springer-Verlag Berlin Heidelberg 2011

women giving birth in St. Petersburg, the Russian Federation, between 1998 and 2002 [48]. The estimated number of people living with HIV (PLHIV) in Eastern Europe and Central Asia shows more than a 20-fold increase in the past decade. The purpose of this chapter is to describe the HIV epidemic in Eastern Europe from a historical prospective, to illustrate the current status of the epidemic and its trends, to examine the groups in the region that are at risk for HIV, and to summarize recent national prevention and treatment efforts.

27.2 A Short History of the HIV Epidemic in Eastern Europe

The first documented AIDS case of a Soviet citizen was recorded in 1987, when someone who had become infected with HIV while working in Africa was registered in Leningrad (now St. Petersburg, the Russian Federation). After that, for almost a decade, the virus spread slowly, mainly via homosexual transmission. In 1987–1988, several persons became infected through blood transfusions. The number of cases reported among men and women was roughly equal. At the end of 1988, the official number of HIV-positive individuals totaled 71 [85].

In 1989, outbreaks of HIV among children were recorded at children's hospitals in the cities of Elista, Volgograd, and Rostov-on-Don in what is now the southern part of the Russian Federation. They were caused by the regular use of contaminated syringes. Ultimately, more than 250 children became infected in this manner [69, 87].

After 1987, Soviet health authorities undertook a massive program of HIV screening. They believed that compulsory screening would identify the carriers of HIV and allow them to take appropriate action to prevent the spread of the virus [101]. However, in the early years, tests of 19,000 Russian homosexuals revealed just 2 who were HIV-positive. And out of more than 120,000 drug users in the Soviet Union who were tested, none were found to be positive [18]. At that time, the Soviet mass media introduced the slogan "AIDS – the plague of the 20th century." The infection was regarded as imported and limited to certain risk groups: homosexuals, sex workers (SWs), and injecting drug users (IDUs). A full-scale epidemic was considered impossible.

Out of more than 18 million HIV tests performed in the Soviet Union in 1990, 557 were found to be HIV-positive. Such extensive screening was continued in the region after the collapse of the Soviet Union. In the Russian Federation, for instance, 20–24 million tests were performed annually in 1991–1995. However, the detection rate remained very low, rising from 81 cases in 1991 to 198 in 1995. Half of the PLHIV detected were men who have sex with men (MSM), while the other half were heterosexuals of both sexes [94].

HIV prevalence in the region remained very low until 1995–1996. The situation changed dramatically when the virus started spreading among IDUs in the principal cities of Ukraine, the Russian Federation, Belarus, and the Republic of Moldova. The first outbreaks were reported in the southern Ukrainian cities of Odessa and Nikolayev in 1995 [22, 23, 39, 51]. In 1995–1996, 6,750 new HIV infections were diagnosed among IDUs tested in Ukraine [41]. By 1997, the number of diagnosed HIV infections in Ukraine had jumped from virtually zero before 1995 to around 20,000 [118].

The HIV outbreaks in Ukraine were followed by other explosively expanding, drug-related outbreaks in other countries of the former Soviet Union. In 1996, a rapidly emerging outbreak of HIV was registered in the region (oblast) of Kaliningrad, an exclave of the Russian Federation situated on the Baltic Sea between Poland and Lithuania [62, 63, 67]. Soon thereafter, outbreaks of HIV were registered in the Russian regions of Krasnodar, Nizhny Novgorod, Rostov-on-Don, Saratov, Tver, and Tyumen [22, 90]. In 1996, the number of people diagnosed with HIV in the Russian Federation totaled over 2,500 [97].

In 1996–1997, outbreaks of HIV among IDUs were recorded in Belarus and in the Republic of Moldova [23]. Belarus had a sharp increase in registered cases of HIV among IDUs, starting in June 1996, particularly in the city of Svetlogorsk. There, according to the local police, most adolescents younger than 17 had experimented with drug injecting. It was estimated that 4,000–7,000 IDUs lived in Svetlogorsk. Before June 1996, nearly all HIV test results from Svetlogorsk had been negative. In June, 6 of 33 IDUs (18%) tested positive for HIV. In July, 173 of 333 (50%) tested positive.

By October, 482 cases of HIV were registered, mostly among IDUs [75].

In 1997–1998, the first cases of HIV among IDUs began to be detected in the Baltic States and the countries of the Caucasus, leading to a rapid increase in the total number of cases reported there [22]. From 1987 until the end of 1997, the number of newly reported cases of HIV in Latvia remained low and all transmission was reported to be sexual, mostly among MSM. By the end of this period, there were 88 Latvians known to be living with HIV. The country experienced an outbreak of HIV at the end of 1997, and by the end of 1998, IDUs constituted approximately 50% of its known HIV cases (122 of 251 cases) [35]. The rate of newly reported cases peaked in 2001, when 807 new HIV cases were registered. Since 2004, the reported number of newly diagnosed cases has been relatively stable [119, 120, 130].

The first HIV case in Lithuania was documented in 1989. Up to 1997, HIV in Lithuania was reported as being transmitted through sexual contacts, mostly among MSM and among sailors who had contracted the virus heterosexually in countries with generalized epidemics. Since 1997, there has been a rapid spread of HIV infections among IDUs, especially in prisons. The reported number of newly diagnosed cases peaked in 2002, when 397 new infections were registered, including 263 among prisoners at the Alytus prison. Before the tests at the prison, Lithuania had reported just 300 cases of HIV in the whole country. Since 2002, the number of new HIV cases has remained relatively stable, with an average of 116 new cases reported annually [131].

Overall, the number of new HIV diagnoses in Eastern European countries increased dramatically, from 234 cases in 1994 to 99,499 in 2001, mostly as a result of an increase in cases diagnosed among IDUs. The number of cases attributed to heterosexual contact also rose, but to a lesser extent, from less than 100 annually through 1994, to 4,621 in 2001 [40]. By mid-2001, of the total number of PLHIV in the Russian Federation, homosexual transmission was reported in 0.5% of all cases, heterosexual transmission in 2.8%, mother-to-child transmission in 0.7%, and nosocomial transmission in 0.2%. Less than 0.1% of the cases were attributed to blood transfusion, whereas injecting drugs comprised 57.8% of the total. A transmission route was not identified in 37.9% of cases. However, it is assumed that these infections were also usually contracted via injecting drugs [94]. At least three in every four new HIV infections in the Eastern Europe so far this decade have been in people under the age of 30, with unsafe drug-injecting practices the main cause of infection [29].

The spread of HIV in the countries of the former Soviet Union is closely linked to the trafficking of heroin from Afghanistan and its surrounding countries to Europe through Central Asia and Eastern Europe, and to a substantial rise in drug consumption [8, 77, 90]. HIV outbreaks in the region have been characterized by the rapid spread of infections in the IDU community, a high proportion of young adults among the infected and a high prevalence of risk factors.

27.3 Current Epidemic Status and Trends

The unprecedented expansion of HIV in Eastern Europe in the beginning of the twenty-first century brought the region to the world's attention as an HIV crisis area for the first time. Between 2001 and 2008, the number of PLHIV in the countries of the former Soviet Union rose from 0.9 million to 1.5 million (see Fig. 27.1), a 67% increase [117]. HIV prevalence in adults (15–49 years) in the region rose correspondingly from 0.5% in 2001 [43] to 0.7% in 2008 [44]. In contrast, over the same period, HIV prevalence in sub-Saharan Africa was

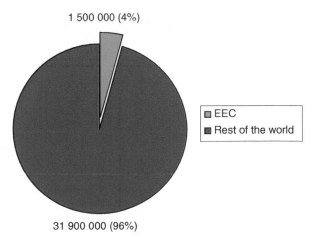

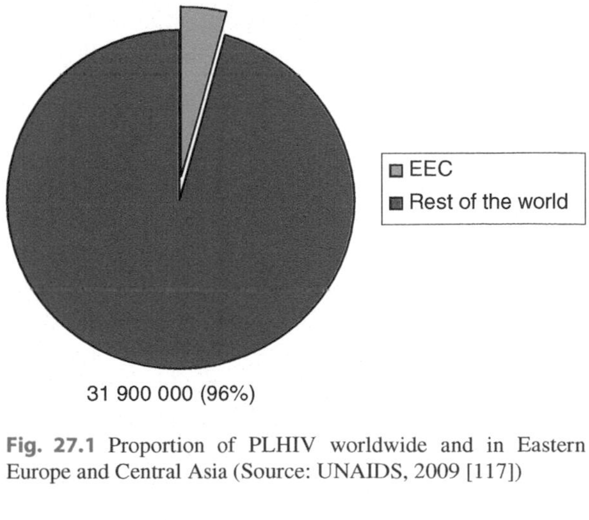

Fig. 27.1 Proportion of PLHIV worldwide and in Eastern Europe and Central Asia (Source: UNAIDS, 2009 [117])

estimated to have fallen from 5.8% to 5.2%, and to have stabilized in South and Southeast Asia at 0.3% [117].

27.3.1 Socioeconomic Factors Contributing to the Development of the Epidemic

The collapse of the Soviet Union in the 1990s and the consequent break in linkages among its 15 republics, coupled with the major political changes, economic chaos, and social stratification of the subsequent transition period, led to widespread social destabilization, unemployment, and the marginalization of large population groups. In the Russian Federation, the country with by far the largest number of reported HIV cases in Europe, it is estimated that the gross domestic product fell by roughly 12% in real terms in 1991 and continued to contract until 1995, while inflation rose to triple digits. This economic decline had a major impact on living standards, dramatically heightening income inequalities and increasing the percentage of Russians living in poverty [108].

Vulnerable populations experienced the worst effects of the transition years, which were eventually reflected in overall increases in the incidence rates for suicide, substance abuse, sex work, HIV, and sexually transmitted infections (STIs). For instance, since the early 1990s, most countries of the former Soviet Union have experienced a dramatic growth in the number of reported syphilis cases. The extent of this increase has varied significantly, with 1997 rates exceeding 250 reported cases per 100,000 population in the Russian Federation and 200/100,000 in Belarus and the Republic of Moldova. The next highest syphilis rates were reported in Ukraine, which had around 150/100,000, and the Baltic States, where they ranged from 72/100,000 (Estonia) to 125/100,000 (Latvia) [23].

The HIV epidemic highlighted the emerging inequity of a society that had once been more uniform and the inability of health systems to respond to a public health crisis adequately. The transition processes made failures in health-care systems more evident and more acute. These failures were related not only to a lack of resources and to changing priorities, but also to the ways in which health-care systems were organized and to the "systemic obstacles" that communicable diseases can reveal [19]. Outdated, unresponsive centralized systems were slow to cope with the emergent HIV epidemic, as well as with recrudescent epidemics such as tuberculosis (TB) [21, 101]. Despite evidence to the contrary from the World Health Organization and countries that had successfully reduced the spread of HIV among injecting drug users, the former Soviet republics continued to favor population-based approaches, for example, mass screening, over interventions targeting the groups most at risk, such as IDUs and SWs. Even in 2002, more than 24 million tests were carried out in the Russian Federation, yet only around a third of those estimated to be living with HIV were detected. Old attitudes and views, including a rigid demarcation of responsibilities, thus continued to prevail in medical services [25] – with serious public health consequences that continue to date.

27.3.2 General Characteristics of the Epidemic

The existing HIV/AIDS surveillance system in Eastern Europe is insufficient and incomplete. Most of the national data are based on national case reporting, which includes newly diagnosed HIV cases and AIDS-related deaths. Several factors make this reporting less accurate and thus less useful than other methods. Prevalence data are mostly based on diagnostic testing and are subject to participation bias and the availability of tests. For example, the sharp decrease in reported HIV cases in the Russian Federation in 2002 can be explained by the significant decrease in HIV testing among IDUs and prisoners in comparison to the previous year [95]. In addition, statistics from some countries and cities apply only to the citizens of their respective jurisdictions, and not foreigners or unregistered residents/migrants, whose infection rates are often much higher. Another important reason for the systematic underreporting of HIV cases in Eastern Europe is the large number of patients who do not return for confirmation testing and who are thus often excluded from the statistics. And, finally, although schools of public health have begun to open in Eastern Europe, there is still a lack of trained epidemiologists in the region who are familiar with modern epidemiological methods and statistics.

Due to all these factors, there are numerous gaps in what is known about the HIV situation in many Eastern European countries. Official HIV prevalence rates in the region are estimated to be about one third of the actual figures [120]. The lack of adequate surveillance hampers the implementation of effective HIV prevention strategies [21]. As public health authorities have begun to recognize the weaknesses inherent in national case reporting, they have slowly begun to shift to sentinel surveillance, which collects data from major risk groups.

The HIV epidemic has a different pattern in Eastern Europe than in other parts of the world. For instance, in the USA and many Western European countries, the HIV epidemic started and remains heavily concentrated among MSM, while in sub-Saharan Africa, the heaviest burden of HIV is borne by heterosexuals, though with homosexuality illegal in most countries is there, the exact percentages stratified by mode of transmission are unknown. In contrast, as described in the previous section, injecting drug use has been the main driving force in Eastern Europe's HIV epidemic. The fastest growing national HIV epidemics in the region have been the result of a combination of factors that include disintegrating health systems, widespread unemployment, economic crises, and drug-use epidemics [21, 36, 40, 45, 47]. To some extent, these factors have played a role in the spread of HIV in all the countries of the former Soviet Union.

27.3.3 Molecular Epidemiology of HIV in Eastern Europe

There is epidemiological evidence of close links among the outbreaks of HIV in the region. Molecular studies of outbreaks among IDUs in different countries of the former Soviet Union in the late 1990s have shown that these outbreaks were caused by HIV-1 subtypes A, B and recombinant A/B, with little genetic diversity, and that at least some of these events were closely interrelated [12, 13, 35, 63, 64, 79, 103, 109, 145]. A recent study demonstrated that three HIV-1 subtype A viruses collected in St. Petersburg from heterosexually transmitted cases in 1992–1994 derived from a strain that earlier propagated heterosexually in Ukraine and originated in Central Africa [106]. In some studies, HIV-1 subtype A1 has spread more quickly than subtype B, which has been attributed to non-drug users and shown somewhat less virulence [10, 34].

27.3.4 Geographic Differences

Estonia, the Russian Federation, and Ukraine are the three countries in the region that have estimated HIV prevalence rates greater than 1% in their adult populations [117]. Reported HIV cases are on the rise in Azerbaijan, Georgia, Kazakhstan, Kyrgyzstan, the Republic of Moldova, Tajikistan, and Uzbekistan, which has the largest HIV epidemic in Central Asia [116]. In 2008, Eastern Europe and Central Asia had 110,000 new HIV cases and 87,000 AIDS-related deaths [117].

That same year, the vast majority of the region's newly reported HIV cases were concentrated in two countries: the Russian Federation (69%) and Ukraine (29%) [116]. HIV prevalence in the Russian Federation and Ukraine had become as high by then as in many countries of sub-Saharan Africa (see Fig. 27.2).

In absolute terms, the *Russian Federation* now has the largest HIV epidemic in Europe, in part due to its large population, and it continues to grow, although not as rapidly as in the late 1990s. In 2008, the country conducted almost 24 million HIV tests and reported 54,046 new HIV cases [96], indicating a considerable increase in positive results compared to previous years [97]. According to official data from the Russian Federal AIDS Center, the total number of the HIV cases registered in the country from the beginning of the epidemic reached 504,537 by the end of 2008, including 3,837 children and 5,282 people who died of AIDS [97]. The administrative divisions of the Russian Federation most affected by the HIV epidemic are, in descending order, Samara region, Irkutsk region, Leningrad region,[2] Orenburg region, St. Petersburg, Sverdlovsk region, Khanty-Mansi autonomous territory, Ulyanovsk region, and Chelyabinsk region. Overall, HIV prevalence grew 14% from 2007 to 2008 [97]. The annual number of HIV tests performed in the

[2]Leningrad region – a territory around St. Petersburg – is a separate administrative entity of the Russian Federation.

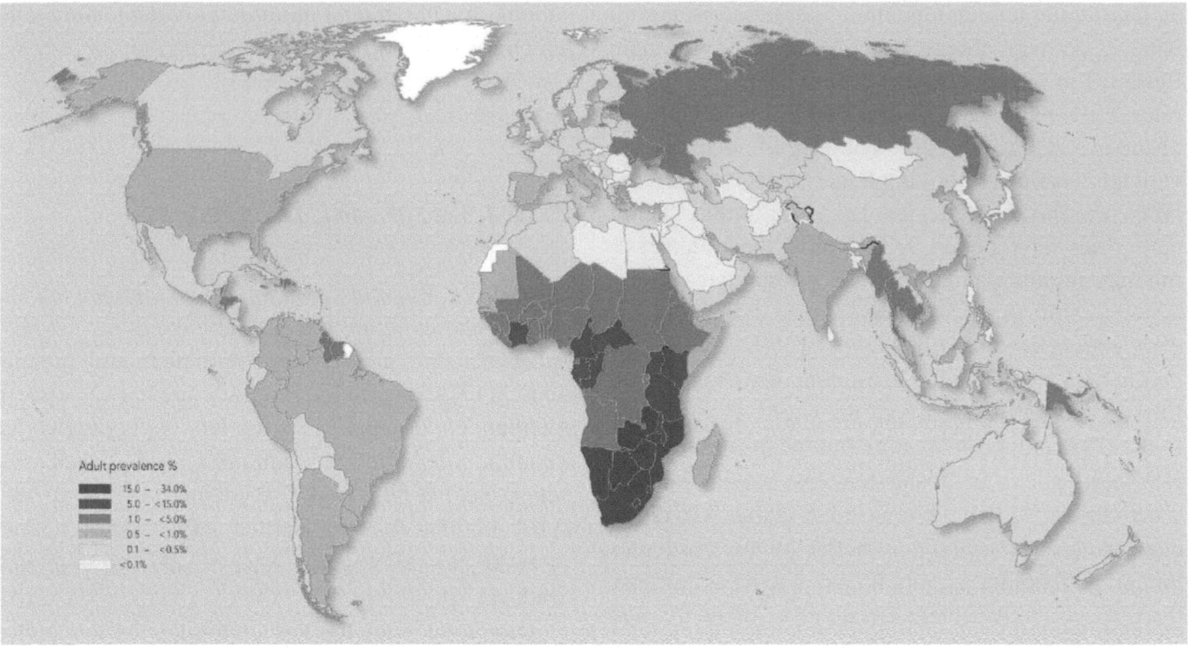

Fig. 27.2 Adult HIV prevalence by country (Source: UNAIDS, 2008 [116])

Russian Federation has remained fairly stable in recent years. About two thirds of all HIV cases are still attributed to injecting drug use [117].

With adult HIV prevalence around 1.5%, *Ukraine* has the highest reported infection level of the 53 countries in the WHO European Region [55], and is experiencing Eastern Europe's fastest-growing epidemic [116]. By the end of 2006, Ukrainian authorities reported a cumulative total of 91,057 adult HIV cases [133]. Ukraine has also reported the highest number of annual AIDS-related deaths in the European Region [31]. Southeastern Ukraine and the capital city Kiev together represent more than 70% of all registered cases of HIV in Ukraine [72]. The HIV epidemic there is still heavily concentrated among high-risk groups (IDUs, SWs, and MSM). In HIV sentinel surveys undertaken in six cities in 2007, prevalence rates among IDUs ranged from 10% in Lugansk and 13% in Kiev to 89% in Krivoi Rog [111]. Among SWs, prevalence ranged from 4% in Kiev to 24% in Donetsk and 27% in Nikolayev [15].

Belarus had reported a cumulative total of 7,747 HIV cases and 603 AIDS cases by the end of 2006 [31]. Most new HIV infections were reported in and around the capital, Minsk, and in the provinces of Brest and Vitebsk [70]. As in other Eastern European countries, the epidemic in Belarus is largely concentrated among IDUs, with prevalence in this population varying from 17% in Gomel to 34% in Zhlobin [117].

In the *Republic of Moldova*, there were 3,464 registered HIV cases by the end of 2006 [132]. Although the country has been experiencing an HIV epidemic that is similar to other Eastern European countries in most respects, the proportion of its cases attributed to heterosexual transmission was over 50% [31].

In the Baltic countries, following the sudden increase of HIV at the end of 1990s, HIV prevalence began increasing at a slower pace. By the end of 2006, the cumulative number of HIV cases in *Estonia, Latvia,* and *Lithuania* was 5,731, 3,631, and 1,200, respectively [31, 113]. Estonia has the second-highest estimated prevalence rate in the European region (after Ukraine), comprising 1.3% of the adult population. However, as mentioned above, the reported incidence rate has been steadily decreasing in the Baltic countries.

In contrast, the number of new HIV cases in the Caucasian countries of *Georgia, Armenia,* and *Azerbaijan* has been rising. Most of the HIV cases in these countries have been reported during the last 5 years. The main route of transmission reported among men is injecting drug use, whereas for women it is heterosexual contact [117]. By the end of 2006, Georgia reported a cumulative total of 1,156 HIV cases, of which 516 had developed AIDS, including 213 who had died. Most Georgian PLHIV (89%) were age 25 or older at the time of HIV diagnosis, and most (78%) were also male. Among the cumulative HIV cases with a known route of transmission, 63% were infected through injecting drug use, 32% through heterosexual contact, 3% through male-to-male sex, and 1.6% through perinatal transmission. In 2006, Georgian authorities registered 276 new HIV cases and 134 new AIDS cases, the highest figures ever reported for the country [129].

In *Armenia*, a cumulative total of 429 HIV cases were reported by the end of 2006. Of these, 151 were reported as having developed AIDS, including 42 people who had died. Men constituted 76% of all HIV cases registered in Armenia, while 83% of all cases were older than 25 [125].

By the end of 2006, *Azerbaijan* reported 1,010 cumulative HIV cases. Among them, 193 had been diagnosed with AIDS, including 140 who died. Of the cases that were registered with a known transmission mode (86%), 56% had been infected through injecting drug use and 22% reported infection through heterosexual contact [126].

27.3.5 HIV Trends

Injecting drug use remains the predominant mode of HIV transmission in Eastern Europe, with approximately two thirds of all cases attributed to the sharing of infected needles [117]. In 2001, men accounted for 110,584, or 79%, of the HIV cases reported among the region's IDUs, and for 174,433, or 75%, of all reported cases. At the same time, more than half (7,753, or 52%) of the heterosexually transmitted cases were women. One of the trends observed in the evolution of the HIV epidemic in Eastern Europe has been the increasing proportions of women among the infected, and of HIV cases attributed to unprotected heterosexual intercourse, especially in areas with comparatively mature epidemics. This trend is evident in all countries of the region [30]. According to the Russian Federal AIDS Center, since 2004 the proportion of new diagnoses among women has exceeded 42% annually, peaking at 44% in 2006 – a larger share than ever before [96]. In Ukraine, the number of heterosexual cases is increasing year-by-year and reached 44% in 2006 [133]. In Belarus, the proportion of cases attributed to heterosexual transmission was 64% in 2006 [127]. Because about 90% of the infected women are of childbearing age, Eastern Europe may well see an increase in mother-to-child transmission in the next few years unless preventive measures are taken.

27.3.6 HIV and Coinfections

The HIV epidemic in Eastern Europe has been exacerbated by frequent coinfection with STIs, TB, hepatitis B, hepatitis C, and other infections. In countries where the HIV epidemic is driven by injecting drug use, coinfection with hepatitis C ranges from 10% to 80% [59]. More than a third of PLHIV, including more than half of those who are also IDUs, are estimated to be coinfected with hepatitis C [3, 88].

Eastern Europe has the highest incidence of TB and multidrug-resistant (MDR) TB in the European Region – and TB is by far most common indicative disease for AIDS [59]. Among people living with AIDS, TB coinfection is associated with a higher morbidity and mortality; and among people living with TB, HIV coinfection is associated with increased TB transmission to the general population [20]. A recent study on HIV/TB coinfections found that only 45% of the patients from Eastern Europe diagnosed with HIV/TB had begun first-line TB treatment, while 31% had begun antiretroviral therapy, in contrast compared to 87% and 77%, respectively, in Western Europe [105].

TB patients in some countries of the region, such as the Baltic States and the Russian Federation, are ten times more likely to have MDR strains than TB patients in the rest of the world [135]. National data indicate a rapid growth in the cumulative number of TB/HIV coinfection cases in the Russian Federation, from 515 in 1991 to 2,354 in 2002. In Moscow, the number of such patients doubled between 2004 and 2005. Most of TB/HIV patients from Moscow are young males aged 30–39 who are drug and alcohol addicts with other diseases. A large proportion of the TB cases from Moscow are also multidrug-resistant, which complicates treatment and results in high mortality [76]. Another study from the Russian Federation indicates a high prevalence of generalized TB in HIV-infected patients, and very low treatment efficiency and high mortality rates among those who were thus coinfected [80]. The deadly combination of HIV and TB is also a serious concern in Ukraine, where 10–15% of TB cases are estimated to be multidrug-resistant, and where TB has become the leading cause of death among PLHIV [112]. TB, especially its MDR strains, is a serious threat in other Eastern European countries too [31, 60]. Fifteen countries from the region feature among the 27 countries that have the highest burdens of MDR TB in the world [117].

27.3.7 HIV Risk Groups and Transmission Routes

The HIV epidemic in Eastern European region is still heavily concentrated among "traditional" risk groups, which overlap a good deal: IDUs, SWs, prisoners, and MSM [117], although HIV in the last group is greatly underreported [16]. Understanding the behavior and characteristics of the major risk groups is a crucial part of the fight against HIV. However, according to a recent assessment of HIV serosurveillance in low- and middle-income countries, only one country in Eastern Europe and Central Asia – Ukraine – has a fully functioning serosurveillance system [66]. The key weaknesses identified were countries' overreliance on HIV and AIDS case reporting in long-term surveillance and not enough studies of risk groups other than IDUs [16, 66]. Public health systems, rooted in Soviet traditions, are struggling to respond effectively to the challenges of resurgent infectious diseases, such as tuberculosis and HIV. Among Eastern European policy specialists, there is widespread concern about the poor quality of population health data in the region, and of the quality of TB and HIV data in particular, and their limited usefulness for informing policy decisions, especially in conjunction with the weak infrastructure for communicable disease control found in Eastern European countries [19].

27.3.8 Injecting Drug Users (IDUs)

Injecting drug use is the predominant mode of HIV transmission in Eastern Europe and Central Asia. In 2008, 45% of the region's newly reported cases for which transmission data were available were caused by injecting drug use [32]. However, the percentage may be higher, since the countries there greatly underestimate the total number of HIV cases [32] and there is a continuing stigmatization and discrimination that IDUs experience in the region, which discourage IDUs from being tested and, when they are, from admitting to drug use. HIV prevalence among IDUs is accordingly high. It is estimated that between 38.5% and 50.3% of Ukraine's 375,000 IDUs are HIV-positive, as are 37% of the Russian Federation's 2 million IDUs and 72% of Belarus's 49,896 IDUs [68, 117]. Likewise, in 2005–2007, HIV prevalence among IDUs was as high as 30% and 52%, respectively, in parts of Uzbekistan and of Belarus [116].

The collapse of the Soviet Union, with its draconian antidrug policies and strict enforcement, was followed by a striking rise in injecting drug use in many Eastern European countries [22, 36]. Other reasons that have been attributed for the region's drug-injecting epidemic, which continues today, include the severe socioeconomic crisis that followed the collapse, as well as significant increases in opiate demand and supply. The number of youth in the region who have turned to drugs is unprecedented. As reported by the Russian Federation's minister of the interior in 2005, 4 million Russian teenagers were drug users (of a total of 144 million) and 1 million of those were hardened addicts. According to the minister, "the average age of drug users has fallen from 17 to 11 in recent years, and addiction rates in the young are now 2.5 times higher than those in the adult population" [78].

The main mode of HIV transmission among IDUs is the sharing of contaminated needles and syringes; however, sexual transmission is not uncommon. IDUs in Eastern European countries have had a tendency to be very young and as a result quite active sexually, facilitating the transmission of HIV to their sexual partners and to the general population [45, 47]. Adolescents, who are neither in school nor living with a family and spend most of their time on the street, are especially vulnerable to many negative health outcomes, including HIV infection [7]. A recent study in St. Petersburg found extraordinarily high HIV seroprevalence among 313 street youth aged 15–19 (37.4%) [49]. Subgroups with the highest seroprevalences included those currently sharing needles (86.4%) and those currently using injection drugs (78.6%). Most HIV-infected street youth were sexually active (96.6%), had multiple partners (65.0%), and used condoms inconsistently (80.3%) [49]. As might have been expected, the rise in injecting drug use after the collapse of the Soviet Union was soon followed by the rapid spread of HIV infection. HIV outbreaks among IDUs were reported in many Russian, Ukrainian, and Belarusian cities, including, respectively, Irkutsk, Kaliningrad, Moscow, Orel, Rostov-on-Don, and St. Petersburg; Nikolayev and Odessa; and Svetlogorsk [6, 12, 24, 51, 52, 54, 100, 144].

Evidence shows that IDUs tend to have little concern for their own health. Up to two thirds of IDUs tested positive for HIV in different regions of the Russian Federation were not aware of HIV and shared injecting equipment [53, 91, 92].

Injecting drug use also overlaps with sex work, further fuelling spread of the virus. The overlap is reflected in the high prevalence of STIs among IDUs [1, 92]. Studies suggest that one third of SWs in the Russian Federation also inject drugs [117]. As mentioned above, HIV infection transmitted heterosexually between infected IDUs and their partners is becoming an increasing problem in Eastern Europe [117], contributing to the rise in HIV cases among women, who accounted for 40% of all new cases in 2006 [116]. In the same year, it was estimated that 35% of HIV-positive women in Eastern Europe and Central Asia were infected through the use of contaminated injecting equipment and 50% through unprotected sexual intercourse with partners who were IDUs [116].

Despite very high HIV seroprevalence among IDUs, the provision of any kind of services to this population is extremely difficult in Eastern Europe due to stigma and discrimination associated with drug injecting, reflected in an absence of effective drug rehabilitation programs there and the very limited availability of harm-reduction programs for IDUs [14]. For example, neither of the two programs that are considered most effective in reducing HIV transmission among IDUs – needle exchange and methadone maintenance programs [38, 141] – has received adequate governmental support in the region [14, 37].

27.3.9 Sex Workers (SWs)

The emergence of sex work on a large and organized scale in Eastern Europe is associated with the cultural, social, and economic changes that occurred there during the last decade of the twentieth century [47]. Due to a variety of factors, SWs are disproportionately affected by the HIV epidemic. To begin with, one characteristic of commercial sex work in Eastern Europe is the substantial overlap with injecting drug use [104], which facilitates heterosexual HIV transmission and the epidemic's spread to the general population [1]. It is estimated that between 15% and 50% of female IDUs in the Russian Federation are involved in commercial sex work, many of them as a means of obtaining drugs. One study documented that every third female IDU in St. Petersburg had been exchanging sex for money or drugs [53]. Surveys carried out in several Russian cities indicate that most SWs there were aged 17–23 years [7, 83, 84, 99], and that condom use in Russian sex work is an exception rather than the rule [11, 56].

Nonetheless, SWs commonly become infected with HIV through injecting drug use, rather than sex. In the city of St. Petersburg in 2003, 48% of SWs were found to be HIV-infected, a high prevalence attributed to the fact that most of the SWs also injected drugs [102]. By contrast, in the capital city Moscow, where the sex industry is better organized and actively discourages drug use, only 3% of SWs in 2005 were estimated to be infected with HIV [120]. In 2004, in Odessa, 67% of drug-injecting SWs were HIV-positive, as were 35–50% of those in the Ukrainian cities of Donetsk, Lutsk, Poltava, and Simferopol [110].

Many studies have noted that Eastern European SWs have a high prevalence of risky sexual and drug use behavior. They use condoms inconsistently and are more likely to share needles; they also have higher levels of STIs, which are indicative of unsafe sexual behaviors [11, 83, 99, 110].

Due to all these factors, commercial sex is playing an increasingly prominent role in the HIV epidemics of many countries in the region [114]. HIV transmission from SWs to their male clients is common, and these clients may serve as a "bridge" population, infecting subsequent sex partners and thus spreading HIV to the general population [65].

27.3.10 Men Who Have Sex with Men (MSM)

MSM have long been considered one of the population groups most at risk for HIV. However, throughout the course of the epidemic in Eastern Europe, the number of new HIV diagnoses reported among homosexual and bisexual men has remained low and stable, averaging a total for all countries of about 100 cases per year in 1996–2001. In comparison to other risk groups, the data on HIV epidemiology among MSM are less available, which has been partly attributed to stigmatization of homosexuality in these transitional, post-Communist societies [89, 143]. In some countries of the former Soviet Union, homosexual relationships were punishable by law until the mid-1990s or later; even today, Turkmenistan and Uzbekistan still explicitly criminalize homosexuality [58]. Available data from surveillance surveys and special studies show high levels of discrimination and violence toward gay people [16]. The lack of evidence for the homosexual spread of HIV in Eastern Europe may thus reflect the social vulnerability of homosexual and bisexual men in the region rather than an accurate epidemiological portrait of this population [40], since the considerable stigmatization that MSM still face in the Russian Federation and other countries of the region leads to underreporting of cases [5]. Less than 1% of newly registered HIV cases in the Russian Federation were attributed to unsafe sex between men in 2006 [31]. According to the European Centre for the Epidemiological Monitoring of AIDS (EuroHIV), the cumulative number of newly reported infections among MSM from the start of reporting through the end of 2006 was 3,101 for Central Europe and 1,828 for Eastern Europe and Central Asia, out of 18,253 and 343,047 total new infections, respectively, among all men for the same period [16]. By contrast, the 23 countries of Western Europe reported a cumulative total of 84,561 new cases among MSM through 2006, out of a cumulative total of 179,135 new cases among all men [31].

The HIV epidemic among MSM is well established in Estonia, Latvia, the Republic of Moldova, Ukraine, Uzbekistan, and some Russian cities [16]. In addition, small-sample surveys show an increase in HIV prevalence among MSM in Armenia [73]. A study conducted in four Ukrainian cities found HIV prevalence among MSM ranged from 4% in the capital Kiev to 23% in Odessa. Of the HIV-positive men identified in the study, only 34% reported using a condom the last time they had sex with a male partner [111].

A 2006 survey of MSM in Moscow and St. Petersburg showed an HIV prevalence of 0.93% and 3.8%, respectively [136]. Another study of St. Petersburg MSM revealed that most of them were bisexual, 79% had had female partners during their lifetime, 23% exchanged sex for money, 38% had had unprotected anal sex in the last 3 months, and 70% used condoms inconsistently or not at all [4]. More generally, HIV-risk behaviors among Eastern European MSM are associated with frequent commercial sex activity and sexual partnerships with women [16].

27.3.11 Prisoners

Prison systems have been disproportionately affected by HIV, with prevalence in the world's prison population estimated to be at least four times that of the general population [115]. A large proportion of prisoners are IDUs, which when coupled with the high turnover and severe overcrowding typical behind bars, leads to a high potential for HIV transmission.

Prisons in Eastern Europe (and elsewhere) pose a high risk for many adverse health outcomes due to poor nutrition, inadequate medical care, and HIV risk behaviors. In many countries of Eastern Europe and Central Asia, HIV prevalence in prisons has been found to be above 10% [117], partly due to injecting drug use. In Latvia, it has been estimated that prisoners may account for up to one third of the total PLHIV population [117].

The Russian Federation has the third highest incarceration rate in the world, behind the USA and China, and very high turnover [112, 142]. A study among juvenile detainees and women at a temporary detention centre in Moscow found HIV prevalence to be 30–120 times higher than in the general population [99]. In addition to widespread injecting drug use and needle-sharing, sex between men (both voluntary and forced) was reported as a risk factor for HIV and other STIs. Condoms and sterile injection equipment are typically unavailable in Russian prisons. In 2003, according to the Federal Correctional Service of the Russian Federation, 74,000 of the total population of 847,000 inmates in Russian penal institutions had TB, and 26,000 had syphilis (S. Selivanov, personal communication, 2003).

Due to factors such as these, prisons in the Eastern Europe often serve as incubators for HIV and other infectious diseases [121].

27.3.12 HIV-Exposed Infants

Because recent HIV trends show increasing rates of heterosexual transmission and increasing prevalence among women in Eastern Europe, preventing perinatal transmission has become a public health priority for the region.

In the Russian Federation, general HIV prevalence among pregnant women was 0.4% in 2005 and 2006 [57], but seroprevalences of at least 1% have been recorded in some areas, including Orenburg and St. Petersburg [61, 122]. In Ukraine, 95% of all pregnant women were tested for HIV in 2006. The high take-up is due to a combination of factors: the integration of various government programs for preventing HIV infection in infants, a universal opt-out strategy for voluntary counseling and testing during pregnancy, and access to antiretroviral prophylaxis. In all, 91% of the 2,575 HIV-positive Ukrainian women who gave birth in 2006 received antiretroviral prophylaxis to prevent vertical transmission during pregnancy and delivery. As a result, of the 2,822 infants born to PLHIV, just 168 (5.6%) were infected with HIV. By way of contrast, the cumulative number of children reported born to HIV-positive mothers through the end of 2006 was 13,647, while the cumulative number of verified mother-to-child HIV transmission cases was 1,367 (10.0%), with another 4,611 (33.8%) still pending diagnostic confirmation [72].

The overall rate of mother-to-child transmission in Eastern Europe ranges from 7% to 10% [33, 46, 97], a figure that is substantially higher than the rate in Western Europe and North America, which is below 2% [33]. There are several explanations for why Eastern Europe lags behind these other regions, despite the efforts of its governmental and nongovernmental organizations to reduce the risk of mother-to-child transmission. First, the region's HIV-positive women often do not have access to effective contraception and therefore have high rates of unintended pregnancies [42]. Secondly, up to 25% of pregnant PLHIV do not receive adequate prenatal care and only show up at maternity hospital once labor begins [33, 50]. The absence of prenatal care not only limits knowledge of a mother's HIV status, but also her prophylactic choices. Although many maternity hospitals now have rapid HIV testing programs, the single-dose nevirapine prophylaxis indicated for a positive result in such a situation is not the most effective way to prevent mother-to-child transmission, as it only decreases the transmission rate to about 10% [9, 17, 50], which is not acceptable in the present era of highly active antiretroviral therapy (HAART). Even among women who start receiving prenatal care in early pregnancy, the most effective prophylaxis regimen is not always provided – because in most parts of Eastern Europe, monotherapy remains the method of choice, while combination therapy (which is recommended for prophylaxis among all pregnant women [81]) is only used for women with advanced disease [71].

HIV-exposed infants are often abandoned in maternity hospitals. In St. Petersburg in 2004, half of the HIV-infected women who delivered without the benefit of prenatal care relinquished their infants to the state [42]. The most common reason that they reported for abandonment was that their pregnancy was unintended and resulted from a lack of effective contraception [82].

27.4 Prevention Programs and Antiretroviral Treatment

Around the world, there have been efforts in recent years to integrate HIV prevention and treatment efforts with existing reproductive health services, such as antenatal care or STI clinics. However, since injecting drug use is so widespread in many countries of Eastern Europe, and because it plays such a prominent role in HIV transmission there, effective HIV control in the region requires measures well beyond those aimed at reducing sexual transmission [58]. The most successful initiatives seek to reduce the harm that drug users subject themselves to from drugs and injecting equipment. Proven harm-reduction interventions include most significantly opioid substitution therapy and needle and syringe exchange, both of which have been shown to be an essential part of successful HIV prevention and care programs for IDUs [123, 124]. However, substitution therapy is still not accepted in many countries of Eastern Europe, especially where it is most needed: the Russian Federation. Moreover, needle- and syringe-exchange programs have not been implemented widely enough to affect the course of the epidemic [2, 101].

Meanwhile, the groups that are at highest risk for HIV, including IDUs, SWs, and inmates, still have poor access to prevention and treatment [98]. In 2004, HIV prevention programs covered just 10% of SWs, less than 8% of IDUs, and only 4% of MSM in Eastern Europe and Central Asia [119]. According to several different sources, needle- and syringe-exchange programs do not cover >3–20% of the IDU population.

In signing the Dublin Declaration [27] in February 2004, the 53 countries in the WHO European Region, including all those that comprise the former Soviet Union, committed themselves to providing universal access to effective, affordable, and equitable HIV prevention, treatment, and care. Since then, progress in expanding treatment coverage has been quite substantial, and the number of patients receiving HAART has increased dramatically [139]. However, IDUs access to HAART in Eastern Europe is still inequitable [26], and treatment gaps in many countries of the region remain immense – and widening [137]. Among the major obstacles to timely, uninterrupted access to HAART are a lack of clear policies and regulations for providing treatment to IDUs, a lack of infrastructure, a shortage of trained staff for providing treatment, and, in some countries, the absence of interventions such as methadone treatment programs to support IDUs receiving HAART [14].

A recent survey carried out among multiple stakeholders in Volgograd Oblast in the Russian Federation [107] showed a diversity of opinion on harm reduction and suggested that harm-reduction supporters and opponents have reached a state of parity in the country. The main factors that the study identified as obstacles to scaling up harm-reduction efforts included insufficient financial resources, a lack of information on the effectiveness of harm reduction, a perception of harm reduction as culturally unacceptable, the reluctance of IDUs to use harm-reduction services, opposition from law enforcement agencies and the Russian Orthodox Church, and vague regulations and laws.

For MSM in Eastern Europe, key barriers to the implementation of targeted HIV prevention services are the stigmatization of MSM, weak HIV surveillance systems, a lack of intervention evaluation studies, and insufficient funding for prevention efforts [16].

In 2004, only about 11% of the Eastern Europeans who needed HAART received it, and for those who were IDUs in the worst-hit countries it was rare or nonexistent [119]. By mid-2006, this figure had only risen slightly, to 13% of the estimated 190,000 people in need, or less than 24,000 [113]. In the Russian Federation, HAART was administered in 2005 to a mere 5,000 of the estimated 100,000 people in need [140]. Two major hurdles were the high costs of antiretrovirals and poor protocols for HIV treatment and care. The latter obstacle was remedied with the 2004 launch of the WHO Regional Office for Europe protocols on HIV/AIDS treatment and care [134], which initially appeared in English and Russian and targeted the Commonwealth of Independent States. This was followed by a comprehensive volume covering all aspects of the disease, including coinfection with TB and hepatitis, and Chap. 5 specifically addressed the needs of IDUs in 2007 [138].

More recently, vastly improved access to HAART has dramatically changed the prognosis for Eastern European PLHIV [137]. This development has reversed the pessimistic forecasts in previously elaborated models of HIV-related disability, life expectancy, and the consequent economic burden for the countries of the former Soviet Union [28, 74, 86, 93].

In the *Russian Federation*, a total of 135,340 HIV patients were seen for medical care in 2006, and HAART was initiated for 14,681 of them, although 1,430 of these PLHIV dropped out of treatment within a year. Another 16,403 patients in the country began HAART in 2007 [96].

Ukraine had 50 HAART facilities in 2003, but they were providing HAART to only 37 people [140]. In 2006, Ukrainian providers offered some type of medical services to approximately 72,000 PLHIV. As of May 2007, the number of PLHIV on HAART had increased to 5,572, including 1,776 infected through drug injecting and 46 prisoners [72]. By January 1, 2008, the number of Ukrainian HAART recipients had increased to 7,657 [133].

In *Belarus*, 6,406 people were seen for HIV-related care in 2006, of whom 9% were prisoners and 4% IDUs. As of December 2007, 884 Belarusians were receiving HAART, an increase of 879 since the end of 2002 [127]. Of those on HAART as of April 2006, 54% were male, 42% were IDUs and 25% were younger than 15 [140].

In the *Republic of Moldova*, 1,380 PLHIV were treated for HIV in 2006. As of December 2007, 464 people were receiving HAART at three treatment facilities. Of those on HAART, 55% were male, 41% were IDUs, and 9% were prisoners [132].

Estonia provided 2,500 people with regular medical care for HIV 2006; 75% of them had been infected through injecting drug use. The number of Estonians receiving HAART increased from 47 in 2003 to 772 at five treatment facilities by December 31, 2007, including 67% who were IDUs and 15% prisoners [128].

In 2006, *Latvia* provided 2,442 PLHIV with medical care for their condition [130]. As of May 2007, the country had 323 PLHIV on HAART, of whom 57% were IDUs and 33% prisoners; 11% of the IDUs on HAART were also receiving opioid substitution therapy. Of the Latvians who had been on HAART in 2006, 37% stopped treatment, mostly due to low adherence; IDUs accounted for 99% of those who stopped.

In 2006, 433 *Lithuanians* were treated for HIV-related medical problems. They included 75 people who were on HAART at the end of 2006. Of the 19 IDUs on HAART, 6 were also receiving opioid substitution therapy. By December 2007, 98 Lithuanians were receiving HAART [131].

Since December 2004, all registered HIV patients in *Georgia* have had access to HAART. As of December 2006, a reported 738 PLHIV were covered by medical care, including 65% who had been infected through injecting drug use. The number covered also included 275 who were receiving HAART, of whom 147 were IDUs and 33 prisoners. By November 2007, a total of 334 Georgians were on HAART. Twelve per cent of the IDUs receiving HAART were also receiving opioid substitution therapy. Among PLHIV who were tested for major co-infections, 13% had hepatitis B, 35% hepatitis C and 17% active TB [129].

Armenia has a single treatment facility providing PLHIV with medical care. In 2006, it treated 170 people for HIV. By the end of the next year, 78 were receiving HAART, including 35 current or former IDUs. More than 30% of the Armenian PLHIV who were tested for coinfections were found to have active TB and/or hepatitis C [125].

Finally, *Azerbaijan* provided 628 PLHIV with HIV medical care in 2006. At the end of 2006, there were 8 Azerbaijanis on HAART, and in January 2008 there were 81 [126].

One of the biggest achievements in the AIDS response in the region has been the high coverage of services to prevent mother-to-child HIV transmission. In December 2008, the coverage of services to prevent mother-to-child transmission exceeded 90% in Eastern Europe and Central Asia [117].

27.5 Conclusion

For many countries in Eastern European, the continued high numbers of reported HIV cases, coupled with the fact that more than half of those living with HIV are unaware of their serostatus, pose a serious public health challenge. The region's HIV epidemic continues to be concentrated in risk groups, particularly IDUs. Unfortunately, the members of these risk groups remain sorely underserved in terms of their prevention, treatment, and care needs. However, starting in 2006, HAART coverage has expanded significantly in the region, which should improve the quality of life and long-term survival for many PLHIV, as well as decreasing HIV transmission rates. It is also hoped that broader coverage will encourage Eastern Europeans at risk to be tested for HIV, so that all PLHIV will receive the treatment and care they require.

Take-Home Pearls

- Injecting drug use has been the main HIV transmission factor in the countries of the Eastern Europe.
- HIV epidemic in the region is still concentrated in risk groups.
- More than half of those living with HIV in the region are unaware of their serostatus.
- The rates of heterosexual transmission of HIV in Eastern Europe are increasing along with HIV prevalence among women.
- Preventing perinatal transmission is a public health priority for the region.

Acknowledgments The authors would like to express their deep gratitude to Dmitry Kissin, M.D., M.P.H., Senior Service Fellow at the United States Centers for Disease Control and Prevention for his expert advice. We also would like to thank Misha Hoekstra for his many constructive comments and edits.

References

1. Abdala, N., Krasnoselskikh, T.V., Durante, A.J., et al.: Sexually transmitted infections, sexual risk behaviors and the risk of heterosexual spread of HIV among and beyond IDUs in St. Petersburg, Russia. Eur. Addict. Res. **14**, 19–25 (2008)
2. Aceijas, C., Hickman, M., Donoghoe, M.C., et al.: Access and coverage of needle and syringe programmes (NSP) in Central and Eastern Europe and Central Asia. Addiction **102**, 1244–1250 (2007)
3. Aceijas, C., Rhodes, T.: Global estimates of prevalence of HCV infection among injecting drug users. Int. J. Drug Policy **18**, 352–358 (2007)
4. Amirkhanian, Y.A., Kelly, J.A., Kukharsky, A.A., et al.: Predictors of HIV risk behavior among Russian men who have sex with men: an emerging epidemic. AIDS **15**, 407–412 (2001)
5. Amirkhanian, Y.A., Kelly, J.A., Kirsanova, A.V., et al.: HIV risk behaviour patterns, predictors, and sexually transmitted disease prevalence in the social networks of young men who have sex with men in St Petersburg, Russia. Int. J. STD AIDS **17**, 50–56 (2006)
6. Anonymous: Rapid increase in HIV rates – Orel Oblast, Russian Federation, 1999–2001. Morb. Mortal. Wkly. Rep. **52**, 657–660 (2003)
7. Aral, S.O., St Lawrence, J.S., Dyatlov, R., et al.: Commercial sex work, drug use, and sexually transmitted infections in St. Petersburg, Russia. Soc. Sci. Med. **60**, 2181–2190 (2005)
8. Atlani, L., Caraël, M., Brunet, J.B., et al.: Social change and HIV in the former USSR: the making of a new epidemic. Soc. Sci. Med. **50**, 1547–1556 (2000)
9. Ayouba, A., Tene, G., Cunin, P., et al.: Low rate of mother-to-child transmission of HIV-1 after nevirapine intervention in a pilot public health program in Yaounde, Cameroon. J. Acquir. Immune Defic. Syndr. **34**, 274–280 (2003)
10. Balode, D., Ferdats, A., Dievberna, I., et al.: Rapid epidemic spread of HIV type 1 subtype A1 among intravenous drug users in Latvia and slower spread of subtype B among other risk groups. AIDS Res. Hum. Retroviruses **20**, 245–249 (2004)
11. Benotsch, E.G., Somlai, A.M., Pinkerton, S.D., et al.: Drug use and sexual risk behaviours among female Russian IDUs who exchange sex for money or drugs. Int. J. STD AIDS **15**, 343–347 (2004)
12. Bobkov, A., Kazennova, E., Khanina, T., et al.: An HIV type 1 subtype A strain of low genetic diversity continues to spread among injecting drug users in Russia: study of the new local outbreaks in Moscow and Irkutsk. AIDS Res. Hum. Retroviruses **17**, 257–261 (2001)
13. Bobkov, A.F., Kazennova, E.V., Selimova, L.M., et al.: Temporal trends in the HIV-1 epidemic in Russia: predominance of subtype A. J. Med. Virol. **74**, 191–196 (2004)
14. Bobrova, N., Sarang, A., Stuikyte, R., et al.: Obstacles in provision of anti-retroviral treatment to drug users in Central and Eastern Europe and Central Asia: a regional overview. Int. J. Drug Policy **18**, 313–318 (2007)
15. Booth, R.E., Kwiatkowski, C.F., Brewster, J.T., et al.: Predictors of HIV sero-status among drug injectors at three Ukraine sites. AIDS **20**, 2217–2223 (2006)
16. Bozicevic, I., Voncina, L., Zigrovic, L., et al.: HIV epidemics among men who have sex with men in central and eastern Europe. Sex. Transm. Infect. **85**, 336–342 (2009)
17. Bulterys, M., Jamieson, D.J., O'Sullivan, M.J., et al.: Rapid HIV-1 testing during labor: a multicenter study. JAMA **292**, 219–223 (2004)
18. Burrows, D., Holmes, D., Schwalbe, N. HIV/AIDS in the Former Soviet Union. Global AIDS Link (Global Health Council) 72:12–13. Available at: http://globalhealth.org/publications/article.php3?id=700 (2002)
19. Coker, R.J., Atun, R.A., McKee, M.: Health-care system frailties and public health control of communicable disease on the European Union's new eastern border. Lancet **363**, 1389–1392 (2004)
20. Corbett, E.L., Watt, C.J., Walker, N., et al.: The growing burden of tuberculosis: global trends and interactions with HIV epidemic. Arch. Intern. Med. **163**, 1009–1021 (2003)
21. DeBell, D., Carter, R.: Impact of transition on public health in Ukraine: case study of the HIV/AIDS epidemic. BMJ **331**, 216–219 (2005)
22. Dehne, K.L., Grund, J.P.C., Khodakevich, L., et al.: The HIV/AIDS epidemic among drug injectors in Eastern Europe: patterns, trends and determinants. J. Drug Issues **29**, 729–776 (1999)
23. Dehne, K.L., Khodakevich, L., Hamers, F.F., et al.: The HIV/AIDS epidemic in Eastern Europe: recent patterns and trends and their implications for policy-making. AIDS **13**, 741–749 (1999)
24. Dehne, K.L., Pokrovskiy, V., Kobyshcha, Y., et al.: Update on the epidemics of HIV and other sexually transmitted infections in the newly independent states of the former Soviet Union. AIDS **14**(Suppl 3), S75–S84 (2000)
25. Donoghoe, M.C., Lazarus, J.V., Matic, S.: HIV/AIDS in the transitional countries of Eastern Europe and Central Asia. Clin. Med. **5**, 487–490 (2005)
26. Donoghoe, M.C., Bollerup, A.R., Lazarus, J.V., et al.: Access to highly active antiretroviral therapy (HAART) for injecting drug users in the WHO European Region 2002–2004. Int. J. Drug Policy **18**, 271–280 (2007)
27. Dublin Declaration on Partnership to Fight HIV/AIDS in Europe and Central Asia, Dublin, Ireland, 24 February 2004 http://www.eu2004.ie/templates/document_file.asp?id=7000, (2004). Accessed 2 December 2007.
28. Eberstadt, N.: The future of AIDS. Foreign Affairs November/December **81**(6) (2002).
29. EuroHIV: HIV/AIDS Surveillance in Europe: End-Year Report 2004. Institut de Veille Sanitaire, Saint-Maurice (2005). No. 71
30. EuroHIV: HIV/AIDS Surveillance in Europe. End-Year Report 2005. Institut de Veille Sanitaire, Saint-Maurice (2006). No. 73
31. EuroHIV: HIV/AIDS Surveillance in Europe. End-Year Report 2006. Institut de Veille Sanitaire, Saint-Maurice (2007). No. 75
32. European Centre for Disease Prevention and Control/WHO Regional Office for Europe: HIV/AIDS surveillance in Europe 2008. Stockholm: European Centre for Disease Prevention and Control. http://www.ecdc.europa.eu/en/publications/Publications/0912_SUR_HIV_AIDS_surveillance_in_Europe.pdf, (2009)

33. European Collaborative Study: The mother-to-child HIV transmission epidemic in Europe: evolving in the East and established in the West. AIDS **20**, 1419–1427 (2006)
34. Fel'dblium, I.V., Zverev, S.I., Ostapovich, A.V., et al.: The molecular epidemiological aspects of HIV-infection spreading in Perm region. Zh. Mikrobiol. Epidemiol. Immunobiol. **2**, 18–24 (2007)
35. Ferdats, A., Konicheva, V., Dievberna, I., et al.: An HIV type 1 subtype A outbreak among injecting drug users in Latvia. AIDS Res. Hum. Retroviruses **15**, 1487–1490 (1999)
36. Field, M.G.: HIV and AIDS in the former Soviet bloc. N. Engl. J. Med. **351**, 117–120 (2004)
37. Finnerty, E.: Opiate substitution treatment in the former Soviet Union. Lancet **368**, 1066 (2006)
38. Gowing, L., Farrell, M., Bornemann, R. et al.: Substitution treatment of injecting opioid users for prevention of HIV infection. Cochrane Database Syst. Rev. CD004145 (2008).
39. Hamers, F.F.: HIV infection in Ukraine (1987–1996). Rev. Épidémiol. Santé Publique **48**(Suppl 1), 3–15 (2000)
40. Hamers, F.F., Downs, A.M.: HIV in Central and Eastern Europe. Lancet **361**, 1035–1044 (2003)
41. Hamers, F.F., Batter, V., Downs, A.M., et al.: The HIV epidemic associated with injecting drug use in Europe: geographic and time trends. AIDS **11**, 1365–1374 (1997)
42. Hillis, S.D., Rakhmanova, A., Vinogradova, E., et al.: Rapid HIV testing, pregnancy, antiretroviral prophylaxis and infant abandonment in St Petersburg. Int. J. STD AIDS **18**, 120–122 (2007)
43. HIV/AIDS Policy Fact Sheet: US Global Health Policy. The Henry J. Kaiser Family Foundation. Publication 3030-02, July 2002. http:// www.kff.org/hivaids/upload/The-Global-HIV-AIDS-Epidemic-Fact-Sheet-Fact-Sheet.pdf, (2002).
44. HIV/AIDS Policy Fact Sheet: US Global Health Policy. The Henry J. Kaiser Family Foundation. Publication 3030-14, November2009.http://www.kff.org/hivaids/upload/3030-14.pdf, (2009).
45. Kalichman, S.C., Kelly, J.A., Sikkema, K.J., et al.: The emerging AIDS crisis in Russia: review of enabling factors and prevention needs. Int. J. STD AIDS **11**, 71–75 (2000)
46. Kallings, L.O.: Can we halt the epidemic in Eastern Europe and Central Asia? Facing the prevention challenges. In: Proceedings of the 1st EECAAC. Moscow, Russia, May 14–17 (2006).
47. Kelly, J.A., Amirkhanian, Y.A.: The newest epidemic: a review of HIV/AIDS in Central and Eastern Europe. Int. J. STD AIDS **14**, 361–371 (2003)
48. Khaldeeva, N., Hillis, S.D., Vinogradova, E., et al.: HIV-1 seroprevalence rates in women and relinquishment of infants to the state in St Petersburg, Russia, 2002. Lancet **362**, 1981–1982 (2003)
49. Kissin, D.M., Zapata, L., Yorick, R., et al.: HIV seroprevalence in street youth, St. Petersburg, Russia. AIDS **21**, 2333–2340 (2007)
50. Kissin, D.M., Akatova, N., Rakhmanova, A.G., et al.: Rapid HIV testing and prevention of perinatal HIV transmission in high-risk maternity hospitals in St. Petersburg, Russia. Am. J. Obstet. Gynecol. **198**, 183–187 (2008)
51. Kobyshcha, Y., Shcherbinskaya, A., Khodakevich, L. et al.: HIV infection among drug users in Ukraine: beginning of the epidemic. In: Proceedings of XI International Conference on AIDS. Vancouver, Canada, Abstract TuC204, (1996).
52. Kostikova, L.I., Firsova, N.P., Vasilevskaya, A.E., et al.: An analysis of an outbreak of HIV infection in the city of Svetlogorsk, the Republic of Byelarus, among persons using injected narcotics. Zh. Mikrobiol. Epidemiol. Immunobiol. **1**, 18–19 (1999)
53. Kozlov, A.P., Shaboltas, A.V., Toussova, O.V., et al.: HIV incidence and factors associated with HIV acquisition among injection drug users in St Petersburg, Russia. AIDS **20**, 901–906 (2006)
54. Kravchenko, V.F., Dunaev, A.G., Golubenko, I.A.: The results of conducting a rapid assessment of the situation in relation to intravenous narcotic abuse in the city of Rostov-on-Don. Zh. Mikrobiol. Epidemiol. Immunobiol. **1**, 93–96 (1999)
55. Kruglov, Y.V., Kobyshcha, Y.V., Salyuk, T., et al.: The most severe HIV epidemic in Europe: Ukraine's national HIV prevalence estimates for 2007. Sex. Transm. Infect. **84**(Suppl 1), i37–i41 (2008)
56. Ladnaya, N.N.: Epidemiologic situation with HIV/AIDS in Russia. In: Proceedings of the workshop on provision of access to HIV prevention, treatment, care and support for the population of the Russian Federation, 15–16 December 2005. Moscow, Russia (2005).
57. Ladnaya, N.N.: The national HIV and AIDS epidemic and HIV surveillance in the Russian Federation. Presentation at the workshop "Mapping the AIDS Pandemic", June 30, Moscow, Russia, (2007).
58. Lazarus, J.V.: The spread of HIV in Europe. Hidden epidemics and other barriers to universal access to prevention, treatment and care. Lund University, Faculty of Medicine Doctoral Dissertation Series, 19 (2008).
59. Lazarus, J.V., Shete, P.B., Eramova, I., et al.: HIV/hepatitis coinfection in eastern Europe and new pan-Europe an approaches to hepatitis prevention and management. Int. J. Drug Policy **18**, 426–432 (2007)
60. Lazarus, J.V., Olsen, M., Ditiu, L., et al.: TB/HIV coinfection: Policy and epidemiology in 25 countries in the European region. HIV Med. **9**, 406–414 (2008)
61. Lazutkina, I.: Vertical transmission and medical-social support to women and children born to HIV-positive mothers in Orenburg oblast. Presentation at the regional monitoring and evaluation workshop. Regional AIDS Center, Orenburg, Russia, June 5–7 (2007).
62. Leinikki, P.: AIDS epidemic in Kaliningrad. Lancet **349**, 1914–1915 (1997)
63. Liitsola, K., Tashkinova, I., Laukkanen, T., et al.: HIV-1 genetic subtype A/B recombinant strain causing an explosive epidemic in injecting drug users in Kaliningrad. AIDS **12**, 1907–1919 (1998)
64. Liitsola, K., Holm, K., Bobkov, A., et al.: An AB recombinant and its parental HIV type 1 strains in the area of the former Soviet Union: low requirements for sequence identity in recombination UNAIDS Virus Isolation Network. AIDS Res. Hum. Retroviruses **16**, 1047–1053 (2000)
65. Lowndes, C.M., Alary, M., Platt, L.: Injection drug use, commercial sex work, and the HIV/STI epidemic in the Russian Federation. Sex. Transm. Dis. **30**, 46–48 (2003)
66. Lyerla, R., Gouws, E., Garcia-Calleja, J.M.: The quality of sero-surveillance in low- and middle-income countries: status and trends through 2007. Sex. Transm. Infect. **84**(Suppl.1), i85–i91 (2008)

67. Mashkilleyson, N., Leinikki, P.: Evolution of the HIV epidemic in Kaliningrad, Russia. J. Clin. Virol. **12**, 37–42 (1999)
68. Mathers, B., Degenhardt, L., Phillips, B., et al.: Global epidemiology of injecting drug use and HIV among people who inject drugs: a systematic review. Lancet **372**, 1733–1745 (2008)
69. Medvedev, Z.A.: Evolution of AIDS policy in the Soviet Union: II – the AIDS epidemic and emergency measures. BMJ **7**, 932–934 (1990)
70. Ministry of Health of Belarus: HIV epidemic situation in the Republic of Belarus in 2006. Information bulletin No. 24. Minsk, Belarus (2007).
71. Ministry of Health of the Russian Federation: Instructions on prevention of mother-to-child transmission of HIV and the form of informed consent for initiation of HIV chemoprophylaxis (Executive order No. 606) [in Russian]. Moscow, Russia (2003).
72. Ministry of Health of Ukraine: HIV-infection in Ukraine. Information bulletin No. 27. Kiev, Ukraine (2007).
73. National Center for AIDS Prevention: Behavioural and biological HIV surveillance in the Republic of Armenia 2007. Yerevan, Armenia (2007)
74. National Intelligence Council: The next wave of HIV/AIDS: Nigeria, Ethiopia, Russia, India, and China. ICA 2002-04D. September 11–12 (2002).
75. Netherlands Institute of Mental Health and Addiction: HIV and injecting drug use in Belarus. Proceedings of the workshop organized in Svetlogorsk, 6–8 October 1996 by the Netherlands Institute of Mental Health and Addiction, Minsk (1996).
76. Nikitina, L.V., Sel'tsovskii, P.P., Kochetkova, E.I., et al.: Tuberculosis and HIV infection: detection, follow-up, treatment: Moscow data. Probl. Tuberk. Bolezn. Legk. **10**, 31–36 (2007)
77. ODCCP: World drug report. United Nations Office for Drug Control and Crime Prevention, Oxford (2000)
78. Osborn, A.: Russia's youth faces worst crisis of homelessness and substance misuse since second world war. BMJ **330**, 1348 (2005)
79. Pandrea, I., Descamps, D., Collin, G., et al.: HIV type 1 genetic diversity and genotypic drug susceptibility in the Republic of Moldova. AIDS Res. Hum. Retroviruses **17**, 1297–1304 (2001)
80. Panteleev, A.M., Savina, T.A., Suprun, T.I.: Extrapulmonary tuberculosis in HIV-infected patients. Probl. Tuberk. Bolezn. Legk. **7**, 16–19 (2007)
81. Perinatal HIV Guidelines Working Group/Public Health Service Task Force: Recommendations for use of antiretroviral drugs in pregnant HIV-infected women for maternal health and interventions to reduce perinatal HIV transmission in the United States. http://aidsinfo.nih.gov/ContentFiles/PerinatalGL.pdf, (2007), pp. 1–96.
82. Pervysheva, N., Zabina, H., Kissin, D. et al.: Child abandonment among HIV-infected mothers in Russian cities with a high seroprevalence of HIV. In: Proceedings of the 2nd EECAAC. Moscow, Russia, May 3–5 (2008).
83. Platt, L., Rhodes, T., Lowndes, C.M., et al.: Impact of gender and sex work on sexual and injecting risk behaviors and their association with HIV positivity among injecting drug users in an HIV epidemic in Togliatti City, Russian Federation. Sex. Transm. Dis. **32**, 605–612 (2005)
84. Platt, L., Rhodes, T., Judd, A., et al.: Effects of sex work on the prevalence of syphilis among injection drug users in 3 Russian cities. Am. J. Public Health **97**, 478–485 (2007)
85. Pokrovsky, V.V.: HIV epidemiology and control. Medicine, Moscow (1996)
86. Pokrovsky, V.V.: HIV infection in Russia: forecast. Issues Virol. **3**, 31–34 (2004)
87. Pokrovsky, V.V., Eramova, I.I., Deulina, M., et al.: An intrahospital outbreak of HIV infection in Elista. Zh. Mikrobiol. Epidemiol. Immunobiol. **4**, 17–23 (1990)
88. Results of mapping of situation with hepatitis C among drug users in countries of central and eastern Europe: Central and Eastern European Harm Reduction Network (2007). Vilnus, 2007.
89. Rhodes, T., Simic, M.: Transition and the HIV risk environment. BMJ **331**, 220–223 (2004)
90. Rhodes, T., Ball, A., Stimson, G.V., et al.: HIV infection associated with drug injecting in the Newly Independent States, Eastern Europe: the social and economic context of epidemics. Addiction **94**, 1323–1336 (1999)
91. Rhodes, T., Sarang, A., Bobrik, A., et al.: HIV transmission and HIV prevention associated with injecting drug use in the Russian Federation. Int. J. Drug Policy **15**, 1–16 (2004)
92. Rhodes, T., Platt, L., Maksimova, S., et al.: Prevalence of HIV, hepatitis C and syphilis among injecting drug users in Russia: a multi-city study. Addiction **101**, 252–266 (2006)
93. Rühl, C., Vinogradov, V., Pokrovsky, V., et al.: The economic consequences of HIV in Russia. World Bank, Moscow, Russia (2003)
94. Russian Federal AIDS Center: HIV-infection. Information bulletin No. 21. Moscow, Russia (2001).
95. Russian Federal AIDS Center: HIV infection. Information bulletin No. 27, Moscow, Russia (2005).
96. Russian Federal AIDS Center: HIV-infection in the Russian Federation. Information bulletin No. 33. Moscow, Russia (2009).
97. Russian Federal AIDS Center. Moscow, Russia. http://www.hivrussia.ru/stat.
98. Sarang, A., Stuikyte, R., Bykov, R.: Implementation of harm reduction in Central and Eastern Europe and Central Asia. Int. J. Drug Policy **18**, 129–135 (2007)
99. Shakarishvili, A., Dubovskaya, L.K., Zohrabyan, L.S., et al.: Sex work, drug use, HIV infection, and spread of sexually transmitted infections in Moscow, Russian Federation. Lancet **366**, 57–60 (2005)
100. Shchelkanov, M.I., Iaroslavtseva, N.G., Nabatov, A.A., et al.: Serotypical stratification of HIV-1 in populations of intravenous drug users in the South/Southwestern Ukraine. Vopr. Virusol. **43**, 176–182 (1998)
101. Schwalbe, N., Lazarus, J.V., Adeyi, O.: HIV/AIDS and tuberculosis control in post-soviet countries. In: Coker, R., Atun, R., McKee, M. (eds.) Health Systems and the Challenges of Communicable Diseases: Experiences from Europe and Latin America, pp. 154–170. Open University Press, McGraw-Hill, New York (2008)
102. Smolskaya, T., Rusakova, M., Tsekhanovich, A. et al.: Sentinel seroepidemiological and behavioural surveillance among female commercial sex workers in Saint Petersburg (Russian Federation) in 2003. In: Proceedings of XV International AIDS Conference. Bangkok, Thailand, [Abstract ThOrC1371] (2004).

103. Smolskaya, T., Liitsola, K., Zetterberg, V., et al.: HIV epidemiology in the Northwestern Federal District of Russia: dominance of HIV type 1 subtype A. AIDS Res. Hum. Retroviruses **22**, 1074–1080 (2006)
104. Somlai, A.M., Kelly, J.A., Benotsch, E., et al.: Characteristics and predictors of HIV risk behaviors among injection-drug-using men and women in St. Petersburg, Russia. AIDS Educ. Prev. **14**, 295–305 (2002)
105. The HIV/TB Study Writing Group: Mortality from HIV and TB coinfections is higher in Eastern Europe than in Western Europe and Argentina. AIDS **23**, 2485–2495 (2009)
106. Thomson, M.M., de Parga, E.V., Vinogradova, A., et al.: New insights into the origin of the HIV type 1 subtype A epidemic in former Soviet Union's countries derived from sequence analyses of preepidemically transmitted viruses. AIDS Res. Hum. Retroviruses **23**, 1599–1604 (2007)
107. Tkatchenko-Schmidt, E., Renton, A., Gevorgyan, R., et al.: Prevention of HIV/AIDS among injecting drug users in Russia: opportunities and barriers to scaling-up of harm reduction programmes. Health Policy **85**, 162–171 (2008)
108. Tragakes, E., Lessof, S.: Health care systems in transition: Russian Federation. WHO Regional Office for Europe, Copenhagen, Denmark (2003)
109. Turbina, G.I., Kirillova, L.D., Garaev, M.M.: Molecular epidemiologic characteristics of HIV-1 variants isolated in the Lipetsk region. Zh. Mikrobiol. Epidemiol. Immunobiol. **3**, 77–81 (2007)
110. Ukrainian AIDS Centre: Epidemiological surveillance of HIV-infection and sexually transmitted infections as a component of the system of second generation epidemiological surveillance of HIV infection in Ukraine. Kiev, Ukraine (2005).
111. Ukrainian Institute for Social Research, Ukrainian AIDS Centre, International HIV/AIDS Alliance in Ukraine: Linked surveillance among IDU and MSM. In: Materials of the Third National Conference on Monitoring and Evaluation in Ukraine. Kiev, Ukraine (2007).
112. UNAIDS: Report on the global AIDS epidemic. Geneva, Switzerland (2004).
113. UNAIDS: AIDS epidemic update: Special report on HIV/AIDS: December 2006. Geneva, Switzerland (2006).
114. UNAIDS: HIV and sexually transmitted infection prevention among sex workers in Eastern Europe and Central Asia. Geneva, Switzerland (2006).
115. UNAIDS: Report on the global AIDS epidemic. Geneva, Switzerland (2006).
116. UNAIDS: Report on the global AIDS epidemic. Geneva, Switzerland (2008).
117. UNAIDS: AIDS epidemic update. Geneva, Switzerland (2009).
118. UNAIDS/WHO: Workshop on HIV/AIDS and adult mortality in developing countries. New York, 8–13 September 2003. Geneva, Switzerland (2003).
119. UNAIDS/WHO: Fact sheet: AIDS in Eastern Europe and Central Asia. In: AIDS epidemic update 2004. Geneva, Switzerland (2004).
120. UNAIDS/WHO: AIDS epidemic update. Geneva, Switzerland (2006).
121. UNDP: HIV/AIDS in Eastern Europe and the Commonwealth of Independent States. Reversing the epidemic: facts and policy options. Bratislava, Slovakia (2004).
122. Volkova, G.V.: Trends of the HIV epidemic in St. Petersburg. In: Presentation at the regional monitoring and evaluation workshop. 18–20 April. City AIDS Center, St Petersburg, Russia (2007).
123. WHO: Effectiveness of drug dependence treatment in prevention of HIV among injecting drug users. Geneva, Switzerland (2004).
124. WHO: Effectiveness of sterile needle and syringe programming in reducing HIV among injecting drug users. Geneva, Switzerland (2004).
125. WHO: Armenia – HIV/AIDS country profile. http://www.euro.who.int/aids/ctryinfo/overview/20060118_2, (2008). Updated June 18 2008.
126. WHO: Azerbaijan – HIV/AIDS country profile. http://www.euro.who.int/aids/ctryinfo/overview/20060118_4, (2008). Updated June 18 2008.
127. WHO: Belarus – HIV/AIDS country profile. http://www.euro.who.int/aids/ctryinfo/overview/20060118_5, (2008). Updated June 18 2008.
128. WHO: Estonia – HIV/AIDS country profile. http://www.euro.who.int/aids/ctryinfo/overview/20060118_13, (2008). Updated June 2008.
129. WHO: Georgia – HIV/AIDS country profile. http://www.euro.who.int/aids/ctryinfo/overview/20060118_16, (2008). Updated June 18 2008.
130. WHO: Latvia – HIV/AIDS country profile. http://www.euro.who.int/aids/ctryinfo/overview/20060118_26, (2008). Updated June 19 2008.
131. WHO: Lithuania – HIV/AIDS country profile. http://www.euro.who.int/aids/ctryinfo/overview/20060118_27, (2008). Updated June 19 2008.
132. WHO: Moldova – HIV/AIDS country profile. http://www.euro.who.int/aids/ctryinfo/overview/20060118_34, (2008). Updated June 19 2008.
133. WHO: Ukraine – HIV/AIDS country profile. http://www.euro.who.int/aids/ctryinfo/overview/20060118_48, (2008). Updated June 19 2008.
134. WHO/Europe: HIV/AIDS treatment and care. WHO protocols for CIS countries. Version 1. Copenhagen, Denmark. http://euro.who.int/document/e83863.pdf, (2004).
135. WHO/Europe: The tuberculosis challenge in the European region. Copenhagen, Denmark, (2004).
136. WHO/Europe: HIV prevalence and risks among men having sex with men in Moscow and Saint Petersburg. Copenhagen, Denmark, (2006).
137. WHO/Europe: Sexually transmitted infections/HIV/AIDS programme. Survey on HIV/AIDS and antiretroviral therapy: 31 December 2006. Copenhagen, Denmark, (2007).
138. WHO/Europe: HIV/AIDS treatment and care. Clinical protocols for the WHO European region. Copenhagen, Denmark. http://www.euro.who.int/document/e90840.pdf, (2007)
139. WHO/Europe: Progress on implementing the Dublin Declaration on Partmership to Fight HIV/AIDS in Europe and Central Asia. Copenhagen, Denmark. http://www.euro.who.int/aids, (2008).
140. WHO/UNAIDS: Progress on global access to HIV antiretroviral therapy: a report on "3 by 5" and beyond. Geneva, Switzerland (2006).
141. Wodak, A., Cooney, A.: Do needle syringe programs reduce HIV infection among injecting drug users: a comprehensive

review of the international evidence. Subst. Use Misuse **41**, 777–813 (2006)
142. World Prison Population List: International Centre for Prison Studies. King's College, London, United Kingdom. http://www.kcl.ac.uk/depsta/law/research/icps/news.php?id=203, (2009).
143. Wright, M.T.: Homosexuality and HIV/AIDS prevention: the challenge of transferring lessons learned from Western Europe to Central and Eastern European Countries. Health Promot. Int. **20**, 91–98 (2005)
144. Zaznobova, N.A., Ivanova, N.V.: The HIV infection epidemic in the city of Irkutsk under the conditions of drug abuse prevalence. Zh. Mikrobiol. Epidemiol. Immunobiol. **4**, 38–39 (2000)
145. Zetterberg, V., Ustina, V., Liitsola, K., et al.: Two viral strains and a possible novel recombinant are responsible for the explosive injecting drug use-associated HIV type 1 epidemic in Estonia. AIDS Res. Hum. Retroviruses **20**, 1148–1156 (2004)

HIV/AIDS in India

28

Janak Maniar, Amar Uttamrao Surjushe,
Ratnakar Kamath, and Alok Maniar

Core Messages

- HIV infection is very prevalent in India
- The clinical presentations of AIDS in India are somewhat distinctive
- Although some states of India have had success in slowing the rate of increase of cases of HIV, other states are experiencing a steady increase in cases
- New cases of HIV in India are being reported most frequently from intravenous drug users and from MSMs (men having sex with men)
- The rate of HIV is also increasing rapidly in women and in young girls
- Although education is a key resource in controlling the spread of HIV, there are many cultural taboos against discussing sex in India
- Although most cases of AIDS in India are caused by HIV-1, there is a growing number of AIDS cases caused by HIV-2

J. Maniar (✉)
Dermatovenereology and HIV Medicine, Grant Medical College, Bombay, India and
Dermatovenereology and HIV Medicine, K.J. Somaiya Medical College, Bombay, India and
Jaslok Hospital and Research Centre, Bombay, India
e-mail: jkmaniar@vsnl.com

A.U. Surjushe
Shri Vasantrao Naik Government Medical College, Yavatmal, India

R. Kamath
Grant Medical College, Bombay, India

A. Maniar
HIV Trials Unit - Thomas Jefferson University,
834 Walnut St, suite 650, Philadelphia, PA, USA

28.1 Introduction

Acquired immunodeficiency syndrome or AIDS caused by human immunodeficiency virus (HIV) is a major public health problem in India, already contributing to a significant disease burden. The pandemic of HIV/AIDS is proving to be a modern scourge. Apart from known diseases and opportunistic infections occurring worldwide in HIV/AIDS, India like other countries in the tropics has a distinctive pattern of disease profile, both systemic and cutaneous, which health-care workers need to be familiar with for an early diagnosis and effective management. Because of this, diagnosis and management of HIV/AIDS and associated opportunistic infections and disease-specific conditions vary significantly.

28.2 Epidemiology

28.2.1 Estimate of HIV/AIDS in India

According to estimates released by the National AIDS Control Organization (NACO), UNAIDS and WHO, the prevalence of HIV in the adult population is 0.36%, which corresponds to about 2–3.1 million people living with HIV/AIDS (PLWHA) in India. The estimates were released at the time of launching the third phase of National AIDS Control Policy on July 6, 2007, after integration of data obtained by the National Family Health Survey (NFHS) and upgraded sentinel sites across the country [1]. These estimates are more accurate than those of previous years, as they are based on an expanded surveillance system and a revised and enhanced methodology. The estimates, although

G. Gross and S.K. Tyring (eds.), *Sexually Transmitted Infections and Sexually Transmitted Diseases*,
DOI: 10.1007/978-3-642-14663-3_28,

showing a decline from the previous figure of 5.7 million by UNAIDS in 2005 (including pediatric HIV cases), are alarming and the HIV epidemic still exists, albeit with few changing trends [2]. While overall, the HIV epidemic shows a stable trend in the recent years, there is variation between states and population groups. The good news is that in Tamil Nadu and other southern states (provinces) with high HIV burden, where effective interventions have been in place for several years, HIV prevalence has begun to decline or stabilize. HIV continues to emerge in new areas. The 2006 surveillance data has identified selected pockets of high prevalence in the northern states. There are 29 districts with high prevalence, particularly in the states of West Bengal, Orissa, Rajasthan, and Bihar. The 2006 surveillance figures show an increase in HIV infection among several groups at higher risk of HIV infection such as people who inject drugs and men who have sex with men (MSM). The HIV seropositivity among injecting drug users (IDUs) has been found to be significantly high in metro cities of Chennai, Delhi, Mumbai, and Chandigarh. Besides, the states of Orissa, Punjab, West Bengal, North East India, Uttar Pradesh and Kerala also show high prevalence among IDUs (Fig. 28.1).

Unlike developed countries, India lacks the scientific laboratories, research facilities, equipment, and medical personnel to deal with an AIDS epidemic. In addition, factors such as cultural taboos against discussion of sexual practices, poor coordination between local health authorities and their communities, widespread poverty and malnutrition, and a lack of capacity to test and store blood would severely hinder the ability of the government to control AIDS if the disease did become widespread.

Peter Piot, Executive Director of UNAIDS, stresses: “The statement that India has the AIDS problem under control is not true. There is a decline in prevalence in some of the Southern states. … In the rest of the county there are no arguments to demonstrate that AIDS is under control.”

28.2.2 HIV/AIDS Epidemic in India and High-Risk Groups

India has managed to keep its epidemic pattern similar to that in the developed world, where HIV circulates mostly within high-risk groups (sex workers and their clients, especially truckers; MSM; and IDUs; Fig. 28.2). However, the HIV/AIDS epidemic is increasingly affecting women and young girls, with heterosexual exposure remaining the main mode of transmission. Women are a vulnerable population in India. Male dominance, illiteracy, financial dependence on men, failure to make decisions on the use of condoms during sexual activity, and lack of power to negotiate with male partners make them susceptible for acquiring HIV infection.

The majority of HIV disease in India is caused by *HIV-1 virus subtype C*. Although HIV-2 infection is found primarily in West Africa (8–10% in Guinea-Bissau), significant numbers of cases are seen in southwest India, Angola, Mozambique, and Brazil [3, 4]. HIV-2 infection in India is quite often underdiagnosed because of the following reasons: (1) Not many physicians clinically suspect HIV-2 infection, (2) the Western blot test for HIV-2 infection is not readily available, and (3) the HIV-2 PCR test is not commercially marketed.

The natural history of HIV-2 infection, although not adequately studied, differs from commonly occurring HIV-1 infection in several ways. The HIV-2 infection does not spread as effectively as that of HIV-1, therefore people living with HIV-2 infection are estimated to be low, nearly 4%. It is difficult to have laboratory monitoring of HIV-2 infection under treatment. Currently available NNRTIs are not effective in the management of HIV-2 infection. The possibility of dual infection is estimated as low as 1–2%, but it is again poorly recognized.

28.2.3 Awareness of HIV/AIDS in India

Ironically, about 86% of people living with HIV/AIDS are still unaware of their HIV status. This is intricately related to their poor educational status and poor access to health infrastructure. Awareness of preventive methods is present in about 57% of the general population and 80% of commercial sex workers.

28.2.4 Modes of Transmission of HIV

HIV infection is transmitted in the following ways [5] (Fig. 28.3):

1. By sexual contact, both heterosexual and homosexual.
2. By transfusion of blood or blood products.

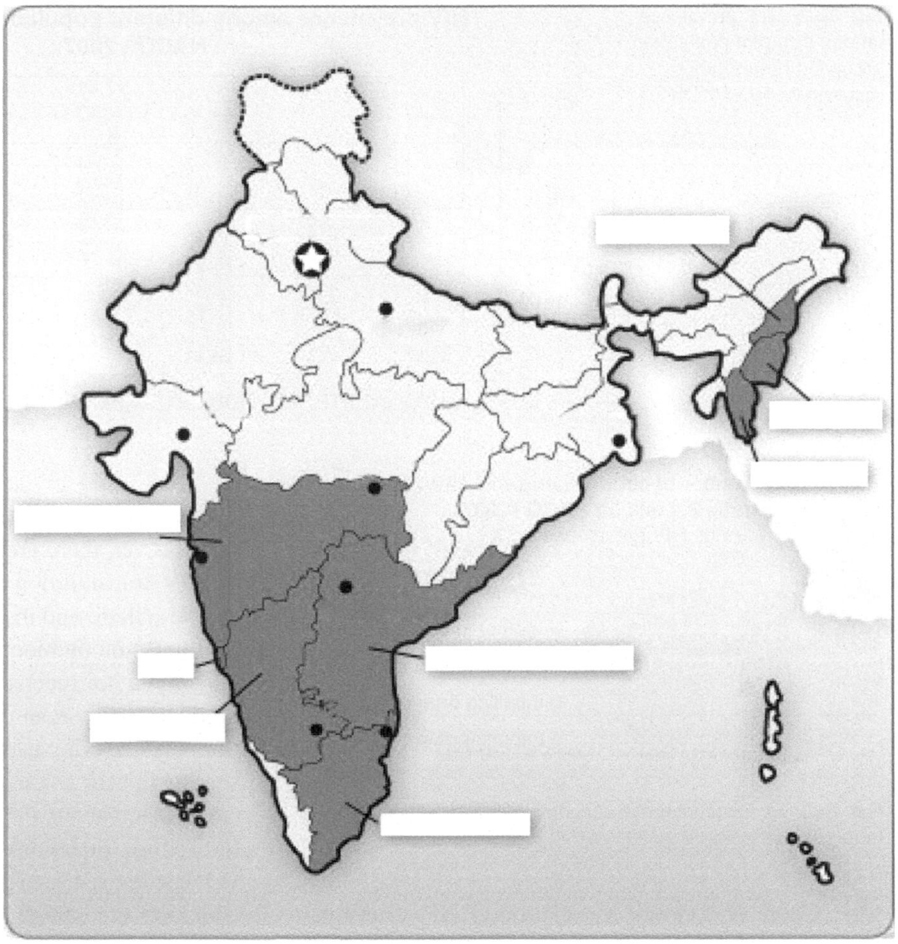

Fig. 28.1 (**a**) (Map) and (**b**) (Distribution of PLHA): Indian scenario on HIV/AIDS

3. From infected mother to infants, either antepartum, perinatally, or via breast milk.

As yet, there is no evidence to prove that HIV is transmitted by casual contact or insect bite.

1. Sexual transmission:
   Unprotected sexual intercourse is the major cause of HIV transmission worldwide. In the tropics including India or the African subcontinent, heterosexual transmission is the commonest mode of infection [6].
   - HIV has been demonstrated in semen, both within infected mononuclear cells and in the cell-free state. [7] The virus appears to concentrate in semen in inflammatory conditions such as urethritis and epididymitis, due to an increase in the number of mononuclear cells present. HIV has also been demonstrated in cervical and vaginal fluid.

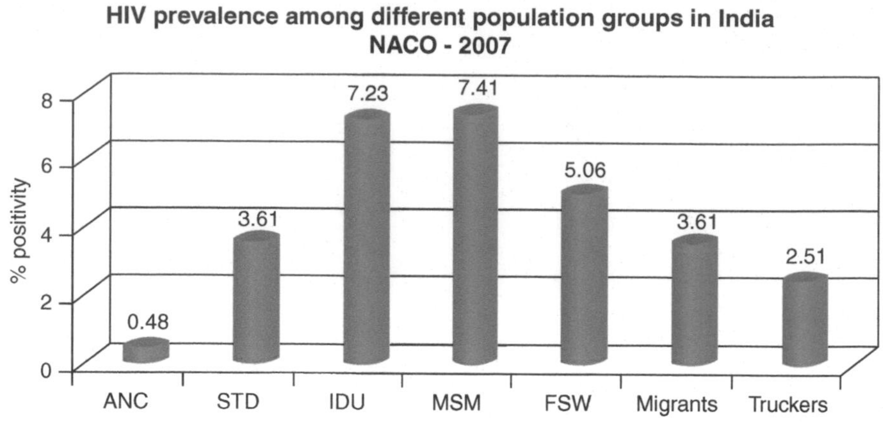

Fig. 28.2 HIV prevalence among different population groups in India; Indian scenario on HIV/AIDS

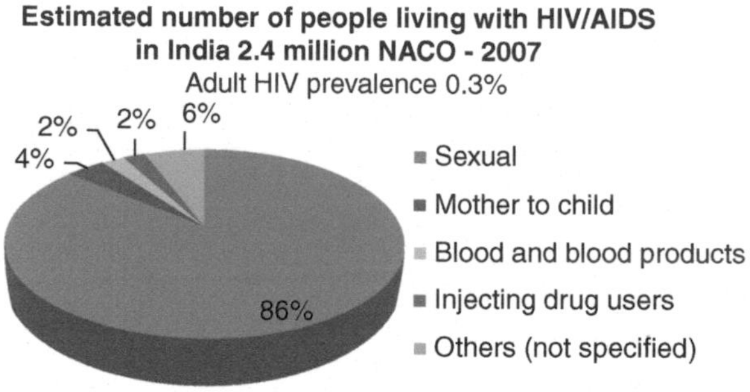

Fig. 28.3 Estimated number of people living with HIV/AIDS in India; Indian scenario on HIV/AIDS

- There is a strong association of HIV transmission with receptive anal sex [8]. The virus can also be transmitted to either partner through vaginal intercourse. A linear prospective study in the USA has shown that male-to-female transmission was approximately eight times more efficient than female-to-male transmission [5, 9].
- Sexually transmitted diseases (STDs), especially genital ulcer diseases (GUD), are also a major risk factor, with regards to infectivity and susceptibility to infection [5, 10]. Coinfection with syphilis, chancroid, and genital herpes infection, as well as non-ulcerative inflammation such as gonorrhea, non-gonococcal urethritis, trichomoniasis, bacterial vaginosis, and reproductive tract inflammation such as vaginitis, cervicitis, and salpingitis have been linked to an increased risk of transmission [11].
- Lack of male circumcision is also strongly associated with a higher risk. This may be due to an increased susceptibility to ulcerative STDs and increased trauma [12].
- Oral sex is much less efficient in this regard. However, there are several documented cases of HIV transmission resulting solely from receptive fellatio and insertive cunnilingus [5].

2. Transmission by blood and blood products:

Persons who receive contaminated blood/blood products and organ transplants are also at risk. Intravenous drug users (IVDUs) are affected by sharing injection material such as needles, syringes, etc. Subcutaneous (skin popping) or intramuscular (muscling) injections also can transmit HIV. In IVDUs, the risk increases with the duration of the addiction and a large number of sharing partners.

- Transfusions of whole blood, packed red blood cells, platelets, leukocytes, and plasma are also capable of transmitting HIV infection. In contrast, hyperimmune gamma-globulin, hepatitis immune globulin, plasma-derived hepatitis B vaccine, and RhO immune globulin have not been associated with transmission of HIV infection. The procedures involved in their production either inactivate or remove the virus. Due to these risks, the screening of donated blood/blood products as well as of organ donors has been made mandatory worldwide.
- There is also a small but definite occupational risk of HIV transmission in health-care workers (HCWs), laboratory employees, and in individuals working with HIV-infected specimens, especially sharp objects. The risk is increased with exposure involving a relatively large quantity of blood, a procedure that involves venesection or deep injury. The risk also increases with high concentration of the virus in the blood and also

with the presence of more virulent strains. The very occurrence of transmission of HIV as well as hepatitis B and C, to and from HCWs in the workplace underscores the importance of the use of universal precautions when caring for all patients [13].

3. Mother-to-child transmission (MTCT):
This is an important form of transmission of HIV infection in developing countries. HIV can be transmitted from mother to fetus as early as the first or second trimester of pregnancy. However, maternal transmission to the fetus occurs mainly in the perinatal period.
   - Maternal factors indicative of a high risk of transmission include high levels of plasma viremia, low $CD4^+$ T-cell counts, and anti-p24 antibody levels, vitamin A deficiency, prolonged labor, chorioamnionitis at delivery, or STDs during pregnancy, cigarette smoking and hard drug use during pregnancy, preterm labor and obstetric procedures such as amniocentesis and amnioscopy [14, 15].
   - Although MTCT occurs chiefly during pregnancy and at birth, breast-feeding may account for 5–15% of infants being infected after delivery. High levels of HIV in breast milk, presence of mastitis, low maternal $CD4^+$ T-cell counts and maternal vitamin A deficiency all increase the risk [16].

28.3 Natural Course of HIV-1 Infection

Within 2–3 weeks of viral transmission, the acute retroviral syndrome develops that lasts for about 2–3 weeks. It is followed by chronic HIV infection and after an average period of 8 years, the patient develops symptomatic infection/AIDS defining complex. The course of the disease from the time of initial infection to the development of full-blown AIDS is divided into the following stages (Fig. 28.4).

- *Primary HIV infection*: Acute retroviral syndrome is the symptom complex that follows infection, and is experienced by 80–90% of HIV infected patients, but this diagnosis is infrequently recognized [5, 17]. The time from the initial exposure to onset of symptoms is usually 2–4 weeks, but may be as long as 10 months in rare cases. The clinical symptoms include fever, lymphadenopathy, pharyngitis, erythematous maculopapular rash, arthralgia, myalgia, diarrhea, nausea, vomiting, headache, mucocutaneous ulceration involving the mouth, esophagus, or genitals, hepatosplenomegaly, and thrush. The neurological features include meningoencephalitis, peripheral neuropathy, facial palsy, Guillain–Barré syndrome, brachial neuritis, radiculopathy, cognitive impairment, and psychosis. The laboratory findings include lymphopenia followed by lymphocytosis with depletion of CD4

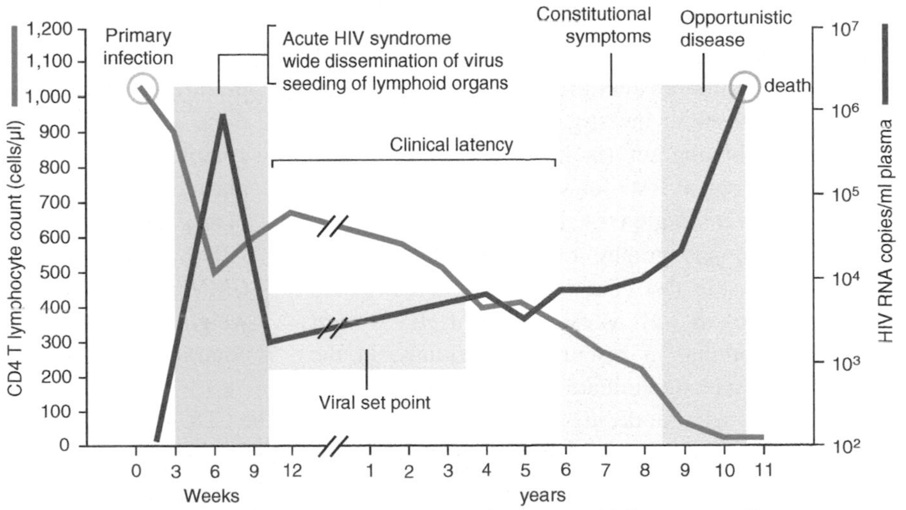

Fig. 28.4 Natural history of HIV-1 infection

From immunity: The immune response in infectious and inflammatory disease; DeFranco, Locksley and Robertson 1999–2007 New Science Press

cells, CD8 lymphocytosis, and often, atypical lymphocytes. The transaminase levels may be elevated. The diagnosis is established by demonstrating quantitative plasma HIV RNA or qualitative HIV DNA; and negative or indeterminate HIV serology. Complete clinical recovery with a reduction in plasma levels of HIV RNA follows. The preliminary studies indicate that aggressive antiretroviral therapy protects active HIV-specific CD4 cells from HIV infection to preserve a response analogous to the response seen in the non-progressor. The observation emphasizes the importance of early recognition and aggressive antiretroviral therapy. The seroconversion with positive HIV serology generally takes place at an average of 3 weeks after transmission, detectable with the standard third-generation enzyme immunoassay (EIA). By using standard serological tests, it now appears that more than 95% seroconvert within 5.8 months following transmission.

- *Asymptomatic chronic infection, with or without PGL*: During this period, the patient is clinically asymptomatic and generally has no findings on physical examination, except in some cases for persistent generalized lymphadenopathy (PGL) [5, 18]. PGL is defined as enlarged lymph nodes involving at least two noncontiguous sites, other than inguinal nodes, persisting for more than 3 months. Detailed history-taking followed by thorough clinical examination is necessary. Incidental findings could be scars from previous genital ulcer disease or herpes zoster, lymphadenopathy, oral hairy leukoplakia (OHL), and even asymptomatic dermatological manifestations. HIV screening of conjugal partners or relevant children after informed consent is essential. The baseline investigations should include a complete hemogram (including platelets count), ESR, serological tests for syphilis (STS), hepatitis B and C, liver function test, urine examination, chest radiograph, sonography of abdomen/pelvis, and tuberculin skin test. The evaluation of CD4/CD8 lymphocytes as well as estimation of HIV 1 viral load is optional in resource-poor setups, in the absence of a plan to initiate antiretroviral therapy. It may only help to decide regarding initiation of chemoprophylaxis against opportunistic infections. It is important to offer counseling emphasizing maintenance of food and water hygiene, lifestyle modification such as practicing safer sex and refraining from organ donation (blood, semen, kidney, etc.). The periodical follow-up visits (every 3–6 months) consisting of history-taking, clinical examination, baseline investigations, and counseling are of equal importance.
- *Symptomatic HIV infection*, previously known as AIDS-related complex (CD4 counts between 200 and 499 cells/mm^3, category B symptoms, CDC clinical classification): During the symptomatic HIV infection, the skin and mucous membranes are predominantly involved. Widespread seborrheic dermatitis is the most common presentation. Other features include multidermatomal herpes zoster, molluscum contagiosum, oral hairy leukoplakia (OHL), pruritic dermatitis, folliculitis, dermatophyte infection, recurrent vulvovaginal candidiasis, and oral candidiasis [18]. Upper and lower respiratory tract infections caused by *Streptococcus pneumoniae*, *Haemophilus influenzae*, and *Mycoplasma pneumonia* may also occur. Other features during this stage include Kaposi's sarcoma, pulmonary tuberculosis, cervical dysplasia, and idiopathic thrombocytopenic purpura (ITP).
- *AIDS* (CD4 counts between 50 and 200 cells/mm^3, category C symptoms, CDC clinical classification): This stage is characterized by opportunistic infection and malignancy. Other features are persistent and progressive constitutional symptoms, wasting disease, and neurological abnormalities [18].
- *Advanced HIV disease*, characterized by CD4 cell count of ≤50/mm^3: As in the previous stage, it is also characterized by AIDS-defining opportunistic infections and malignancy. Some of the infections are more frequently seen like *M. avium* complex, CMV, cryptococcal meningitis, histoplasmosis, slow virus disease, and cervical dysplasia. CNS involvement also is very prominent: AIDS dementia complex, CNS lymphoma, and CMV infection. AIDS wasting syndrome with a weight loss of > 10% of ideal body weight is common.

The CDC has proposed the following clinical classification for HIV infection in adults and adolescents. It is based on three ranges of CD4 cell counts and three clinical categories, as given in Table 28.1.

Table 28.1 1993 Revised classification for HIV infection and the expanded AIDS surveillance definition for adolescents and adults

CD4 Count (/mm^3)	A	B	C
>500	A1	B1	**C1**
200–500	A2	B2	**C2**
<200	**A3**	**B3**	**C3**

The bold areas indicate the expanded AIDS surveillance case definition

28.3.1 Clinical Categories of HIV Infection

A. *Acute retroviral syndrome*
   Persistent generalized lymphadenopathy
   Asymptomatic disease

B. *Symptoms of AIDS-related complex*
   Bacillary angiomatosis
   Candidiasis, mucosal (thrush, vulvovaginal: persistent, frequent or poorly responsive to therapy)
   Cervical dysplasia (moderate or severe)/cervical Ca in situ
   Constitutional symptoms, such as fever (38.5°C) or diarrhea lasting > 1 month
   Herpes zoster, recurrent and multidermatomal
   Idiopathic thrombocytopenic purpura (ITP)
   Listeriosis
   Oral hairy leukoplakia (OHL)
   Pelvic inflammatory disease, particularly tubo-ovarian abscess
   Peripheral neuropathy

C. *AIDS-defining conditions (CD4 count < 200)*
   Candidiasis, esophageal or pulmonary
   Cervical cancer, invasive
   Coccidioidomycosis, disseminated or extrapulmonary
   Cryptococcosis, extrapulmonary
   Cryptosporidiosis, chronic intestinal (>1 month)
   Cytomegalovirus infection (excluding liver, spleen, and lymph nodes) and retinitis (with loss of vision)
   Herpes esophagitis, bronchitis, pneumonia, or chronic cutaneous and/or oral ulcers (>1 month)
   HIV encephalopathy
   Toxoplasmosis, disseminated or extrapulmonary
   Isosporiasis, chronic intestinal (>1 month)
   Kaposi's sarcoma
   Lymphoma, primary CNS or Burkitt's
   Mycobacterial disease
   Pneumocystis jirovecii infection, commonly pneumonia (PCP)
   Pneumonia, recurrent bacterial
   Progressive multifocal leukoencephalopathy (PML)
   Salmonellosis
   Wasting syndrome

28.4 Clinical Manifestations

28.4.1 Dermatological Manifestations of HIV Infection

The skin is usually the first organ system that provides a clue to the presence of HIV infection [19–22]. There is a wide range of dermatological manifestations that should prompt the clinician to screen the individual for the presence of the virus. Each of these dermatological markers has a different positive predictive value for HIV/AIDS. A discussion of the entire spectrum of skin disease in HIV infection is beyond the scope of this chapter. The common conditions associated with HIV infection, and those that have high positive predictive value for diagnosis are enumerated and elucidated in Table 28.2. Almost all dermatological manifestations of HIV/AIDS respond to currently recommended combination antiretroviral therapy (cART).

28.4.2 Sexually Transmitted Infections (STI) and HIV/AIDS

There is a well-known synergistic relationship between STDs and HIV infection. It is a known fact that the presence of sexually transmitted infections (STI), namely, genital ulcer disease, urethritis, vaginitis, or cervicitis favors transmission of HIV during unprotected sexual intercourse. Therefore prompt diagnosis and treatment of the STI reduces HIV transmission. Besides, HIV-infected individuals may present with atypical or severe manifestations of common STIs. Depending upon the severity of immunosuppression, the clinical features of various STI show varying degrees of aggressiveness. The recommended therapy

Table 28.2 Dermatological manifestations of HIV/AIDS

Cutaneous Manifestations	Clinical Features
Herpes zoster (Fig. 28.5)	Painful rash of small fluid-filled blisters in distribution of a nerve supply on a hemorrhagic or erythematous background, and not crossing the midline, occurring currently or in the last 2 years. Ophthalmic division is commonly involved, eye complication common, multisegmental or bilateral, necrotic, hemorrhagic, sometimes generalized. Severe or frequently recurrent herpes zoster is usually associated with more advanced HIV disease
Herpes simplex infection (Fig. 28.6)	It is usually a reactivation of latent HSV, and disease may be recurrent, aggressive, and extensive. Bilateral, lumbar, or perianal lesions are common. Response to acyclovir is variable, with a high degree of resistance. Severe and progressive painful orolabial, genital, or anorectal lesions caused by recurrent HSV infection reported for more than 1 month. History of previous episodes may be present and scarring may be evident. Presence of active disease increases likelihood of transmission, unless safe sex is practiced
Seborrheic dermatitis (Fig. 28.7)	Chronic, itchy, scaly skin condition, particularly affecting scalp, face, upper trunk, and perineum. It may progress to erythroderma. It is, quite often, the presenting feature of HIV. Its severity correlates inversely with CD4 counts
Psoriasis (Fig. 28.8)	There seems to be a strong correlation between the initial onset of psoriasis and HIV infection, such as eruptive disease or sudden exacerbation of preexisting disease in a person at risk. Severe disease with widespread lesions, erythroderma, palmoplantar keratoderma, psoriatic arthritis, and pustular psoriasis are more common in HIV infected individuals. Phototherapy, retinoids, and antiretroviral therapy (ART) containing zidovudine (AZT) are effective
Reiter's syndrome (Fig. 28.9)	Presents with migratory arthritis, erythematous papules, and plaques with "limpet"-like scales. Circinate balanitis and plantar fasciitis are common, but urethritis and uveitis may or may not be present. Higher prevalence in HIV infection, hence considered almost as an AIDS-defining illness. Disease is persistent, of varied severity. Oral retinoids are the drug of choice
Pruritic papular eruptions (Fig. 28.10)	Pruritic papulovesicular lesions present on the face, exposed surfaces of the extremities, and the trunk are common, more than in uninfected adults. Note: scabies and obvious insect bites should be excluded. The disease is chronic, recurrent, or persistent; intensely pruritic; and difficult to treat
Molluscum contagiosum (Fig. 28.11)	In HIV infection, disease severity varies, with widespread and atypical lesions, as well as extragenital location. Giant, multiple, and inflamed lesions are common. Treatment is difficult
Norwegian (crusted) scabies (Fig. 28.12)	In advanced disease, crusted and hyperkeratotic lesions involving unusual sites such as palms, soles, face, scalp, and trunk may be seen and house millions of mites. Erythroderma may occur. The condition is chronic, and itching may be almost absent. Treatment is similar to HIV-uninfected individuals, but is to be continued for a longer duration
Cutaneous cryptococcosis	Usually associated with systemic disease such as meningitis or pneumonitis (Fig. 28.13). The skin lesions mimic molluscum contagiosum, and diagnosis requires histopathologic evidence. Treatment consists of systemic antifungals, such as amphotericin B, 5-fluorocytosine, and fluconazole
Pyomyositis (Fig. 28.14)	It is an AIDS-defining illness, and may be localized or extensive. It is associated with severe constitutional symptoms. Various bacteria have been implicated, and culture/sensitivity testing is essential to decide appropriate antibiotics. Surgical intervention may be required.
Candidiasis/angular cheilitis (Fig. 28.15)	Recurrent, oral, or esophageal, candidiasis is common, with a varied morphological appearance (erosive, membranous, vegetative, angular cheilitis). Systemic fluconazole is required for treatment and resistance is increasingly observed. Newer molecules such as voriconazole may be required in resistant cases
Oral hairy leukoplakia (Fig. 28.16)	Fine small linear patches on lateral borders of the tongue, generally bilaterally, which do not scrape off. It is a marker of HIV infection, and is sometimes difficult to distinguish from oral candidiasis. It is caused by Epstein–Barr virus (EBV) infection and is asymptomatic
Aphthae	Recurrent, occurring twice or more in 6 months, and difficult to treat
Stevens–Johnson syndrome (Fig. 28.17]	Adverse drug reactions (ADR) are more common in HIV infection than in uninfected adults. Commonly implicated drugs are sulphonamides (cotrimoxazole), nevirapine, abacavir, dilantin, pyrazinamide, rifampicin, and carbamazepine. Complications including toxic epidermal necrolysis, sepsis, electrolyte imbalance, renal failure, etc. are common and death may result

Table 28.2 (continued)

Cutaneous Manifestations	Clinical Features
Addisonian pigmentation (Fig. 28.18)	It may occur without adrenal dysfunction or as a consequence of adrenalitis due to TB or CMV infection. Diffuse melanotic pigmentation of skin on the face, photoexposed areas, skin creases and buccal mucosa, with longitudinal melanonychia is common, and progressive. The condition is cosmetically stigmatizing. Reversible pigmentation may occur with HAART as well
Erythroderma	It can be the presenting feature of the disease. Mostly it is primary HIV-related erythroderma, but it may also occur due to exacerbation of pre-existing dermatoses described above. It responds to HAART
Tuberculids (Fig. 28.19)	Papulonecrotic tuberculids or lichen scrofulosorum lesions are common, and most often associated with detectable tuberculous focus. It is a hypersensitivity state to the mycobacterial antigen and responds to antituberculous therapy (ATT)
ITP	It is chronic, of varied severity, and is difficult to correct
Ichthyosis/xerosis	It is acquired, quite often marked, and extensive. Disease severity correlates with CD4 counts. It is pruritic, and responsive to ART
Acne conglobata	Disease is severe and extensive, and responds to oral retinoids or HAART
Hair changes	Lusterless and thin hair, various types of alopecia, discoloration of hair, premature graying, and long eyelashes have been described
Nail changes	Leukonychia, pigmentation, half and half nail, clubbing, onychomycosis, paronychia, and yellow nail syndrome have been described. Fungal paronychia (painful red and swollen nail bed) or onycholysis (separation of the nail from the nail bed) of the fingernails is common. Proximal white/subungual onychomycosis is a marker of HIV infection

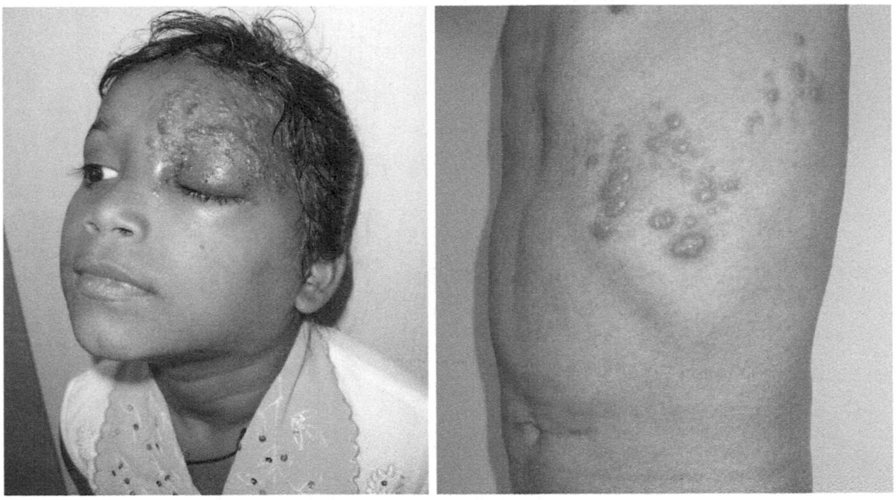

Fig. 28.5 (**a** and **b**) Herpes zoster

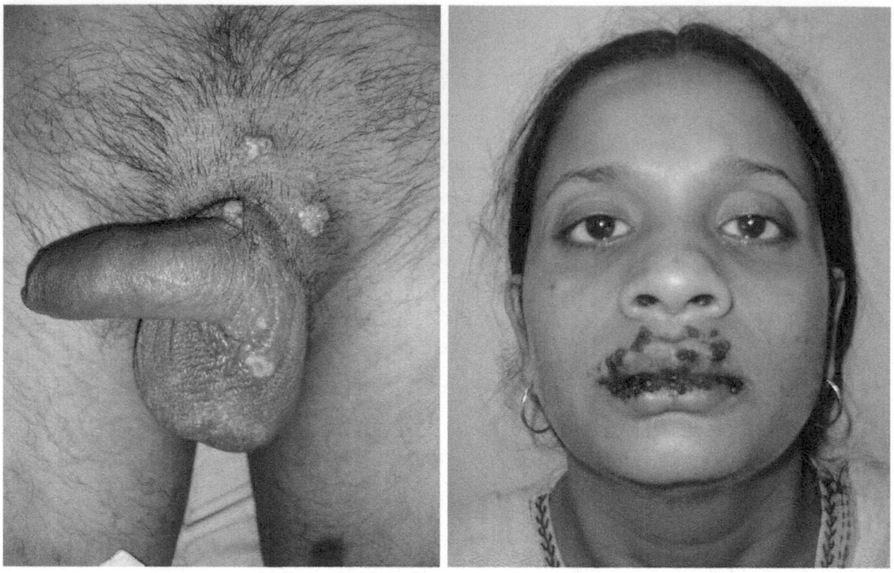

Fig. 28.6 (**a** and **b**) Herpes simplex

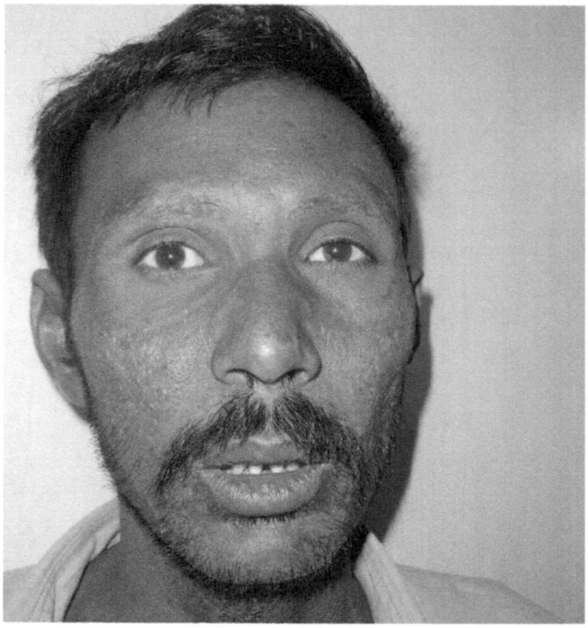

Fig. 28.7 Seborrheic dermatitis

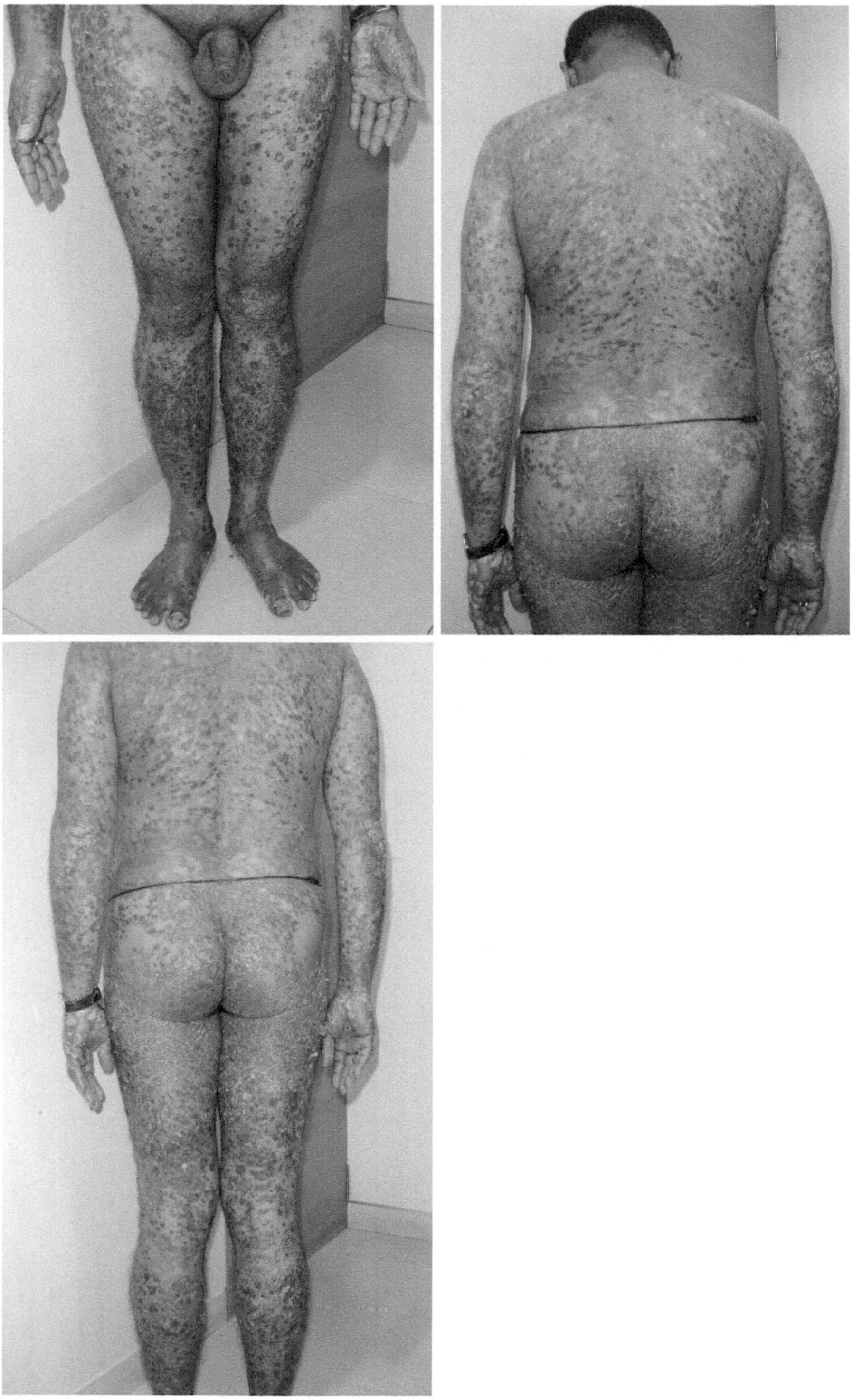

Fig. 28.8 (**a**, **b**, and **c**) Psoriasis

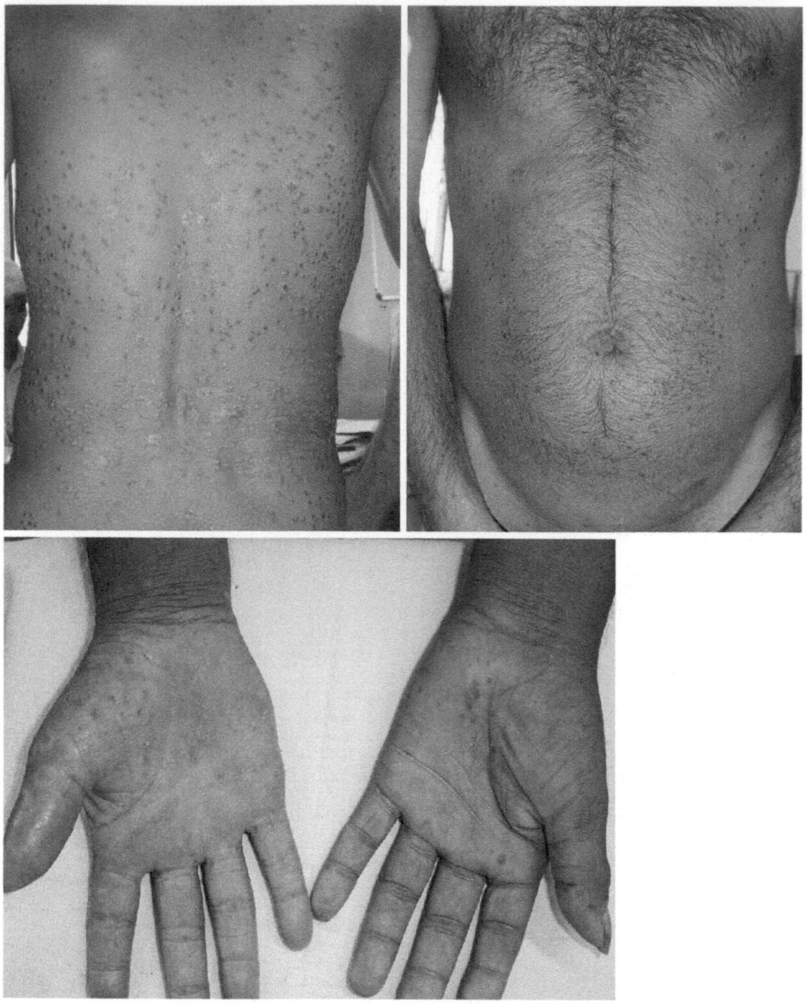

Fig. 28.9 (**a**, **b**, and **c**) Reiter's disease

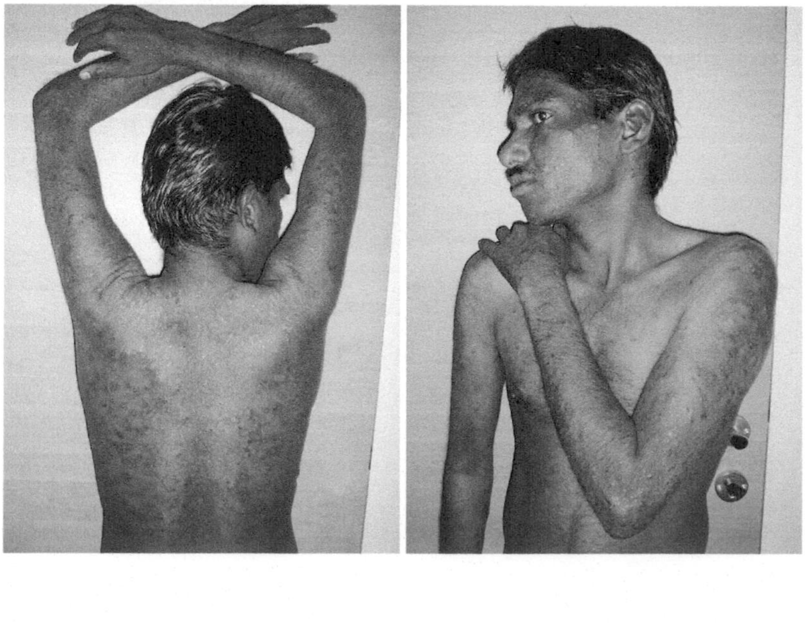

Fig. 28.10 (**a** and **b**) Papular eruption of HIV

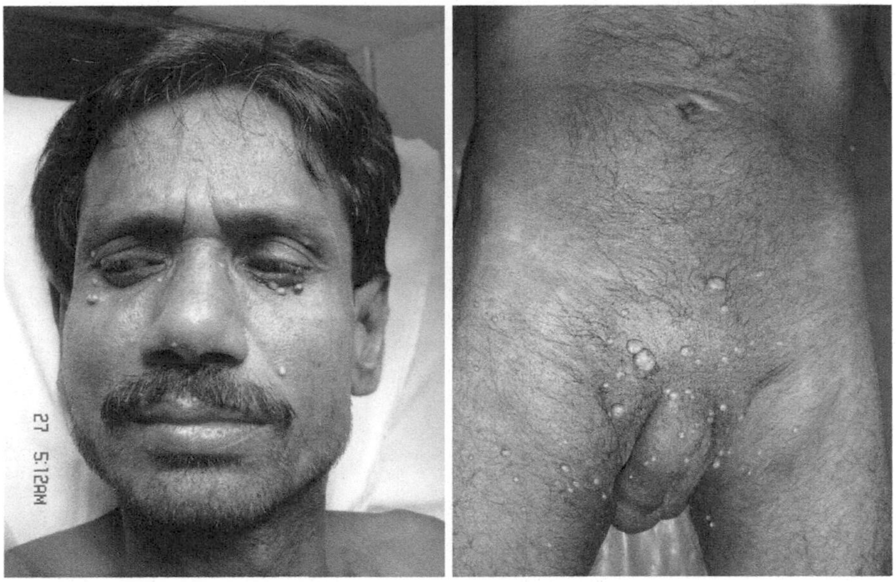

Fig. 28.11 (**a** and **b**) Molluscum contagiosum

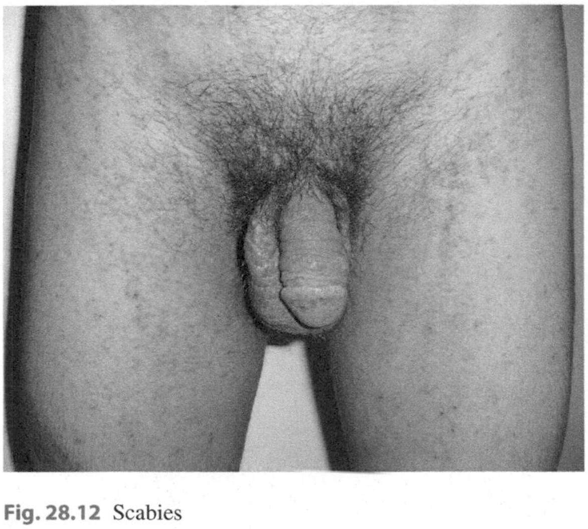

Fig. 28.12 Scabies

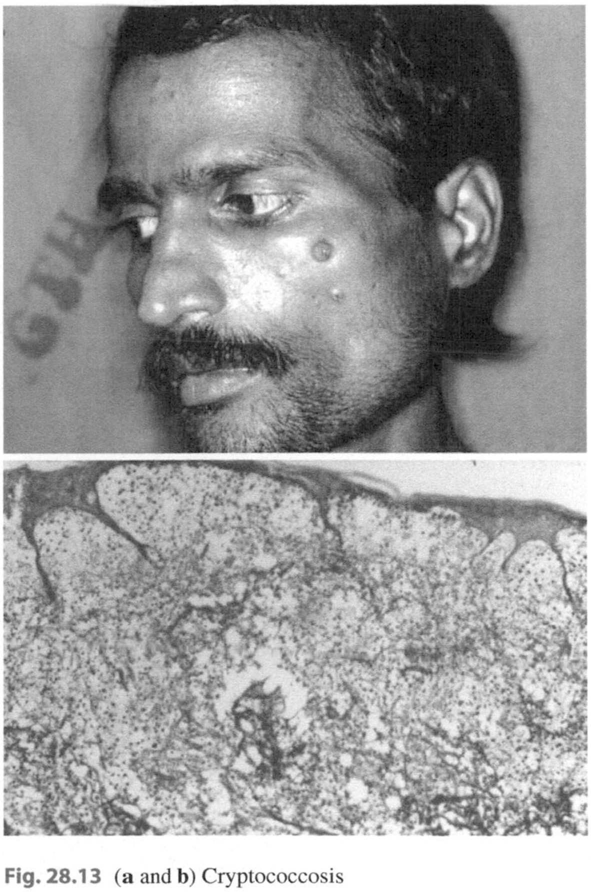

Fig. 28.13 (**a** and **b**) Cryptococcosis

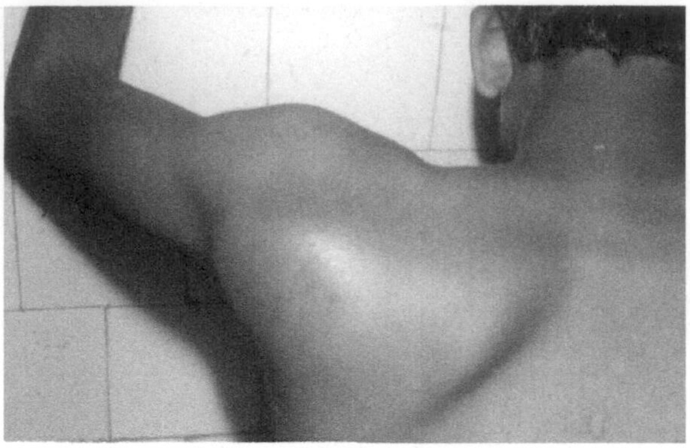

Fig. 28.14 Pyomyositis

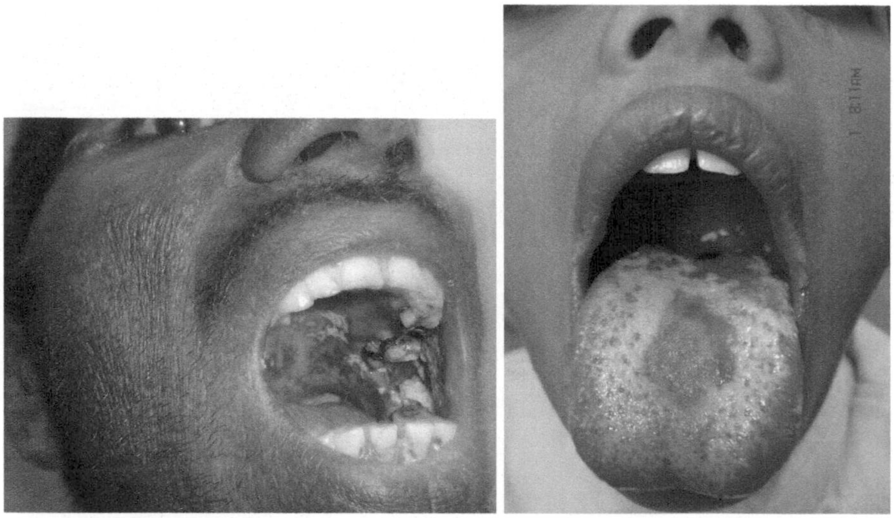

Fig. 28.15 (**a** and **b**) Oral candidiasis

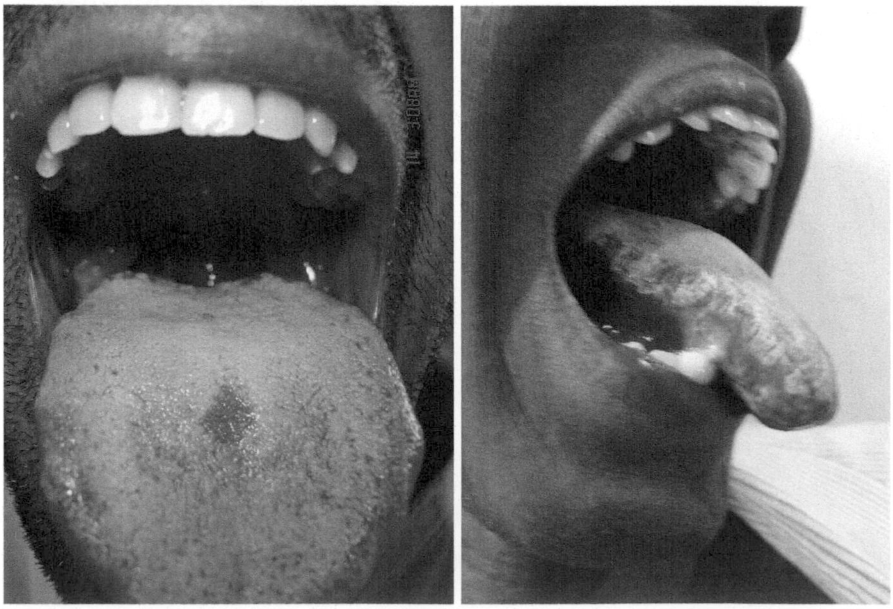

Fig. 28.16 (**a** and **b**) Oral hairy leukoplakia

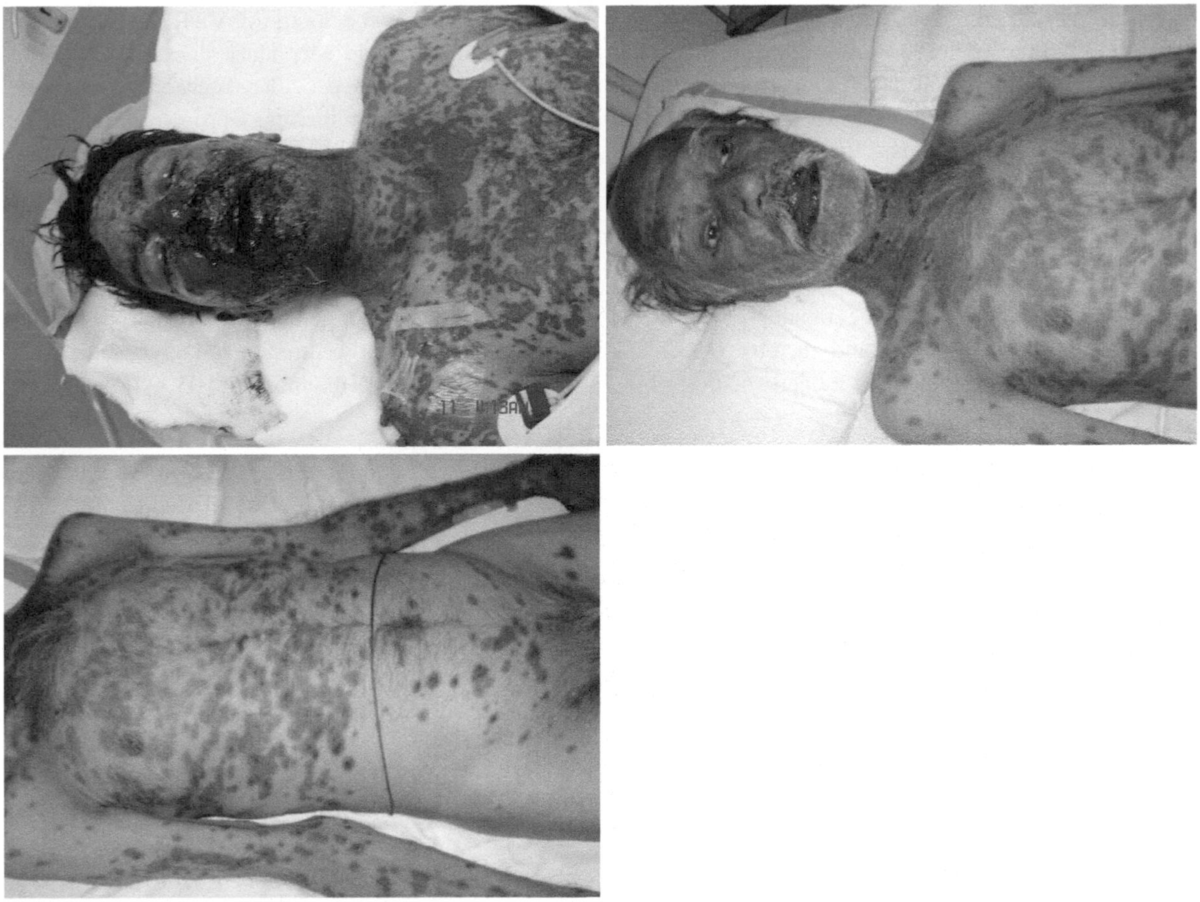

Fig. 28.17 (**a**, **b**, and **c**) Stevens–Johnson syndrome

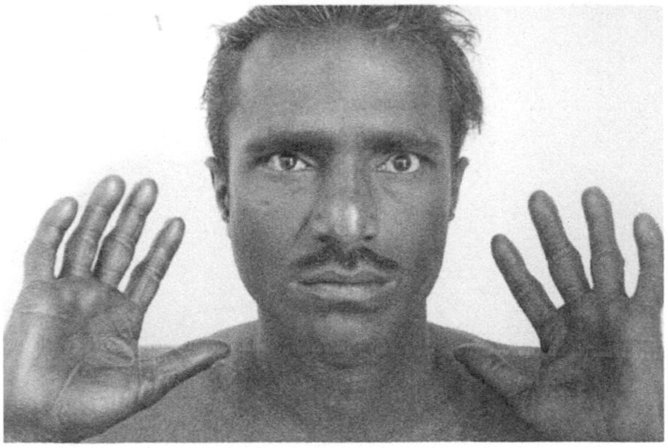

Fig. 28.18 Addisonian pigmentation

for a particular STI may need modification depending upon the individual case, i.e., severity of disease and extent of immunosuppression. Besides, the occurrence of more than one STI at a given time carries higher positive predictive value for HIV/AIDS.

Syphilis: Serological tests for syphilis (STS) may either be reactive in higher dilutions or may be false negative or false positive (Figs. 28.20 and 28.21). In such circumstances, specific tests for syphilis may be necessary to confirm the diagnosis, in addition to clinical suspicion. There could be rapid progression in natural history of syphilis, and thereby precocious occurrence of tertiary syphilis, namely, neurosyphilis or cardiovascular syphilis. HIV coinfection has been associated with higher titers of VDRL, multiple primary chancres, florid secondary disease, faster progression to tertiary and ocular disease, lues maligna, slower resolution after therapy, a propensity to develop the Jarisch–Herxheimer reaction and higher rates of relapse. Coinfection may increase the frequency or accelerate the development of neurologic sequelae, such as aseptic meningitis or CNS gummata.

Herpes simplex virus infection: As described earlier, the reactivation of genital/perianal herpes simplex virus infection is fairly common and its presence helps in algorithmic clinical diagnosis of HIV/AIDS. Chronic

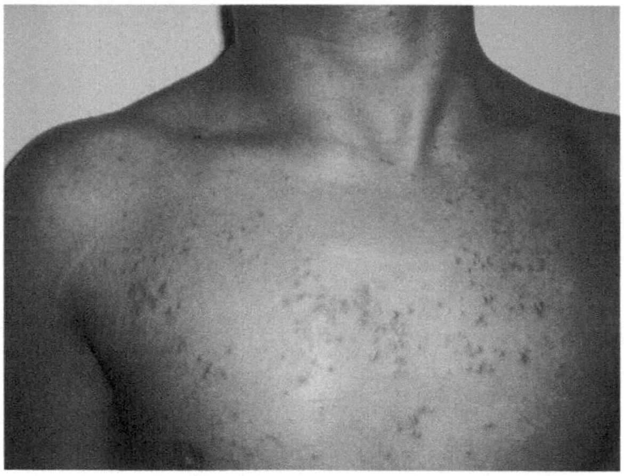

Fig. 28.19 Papular tuberculids

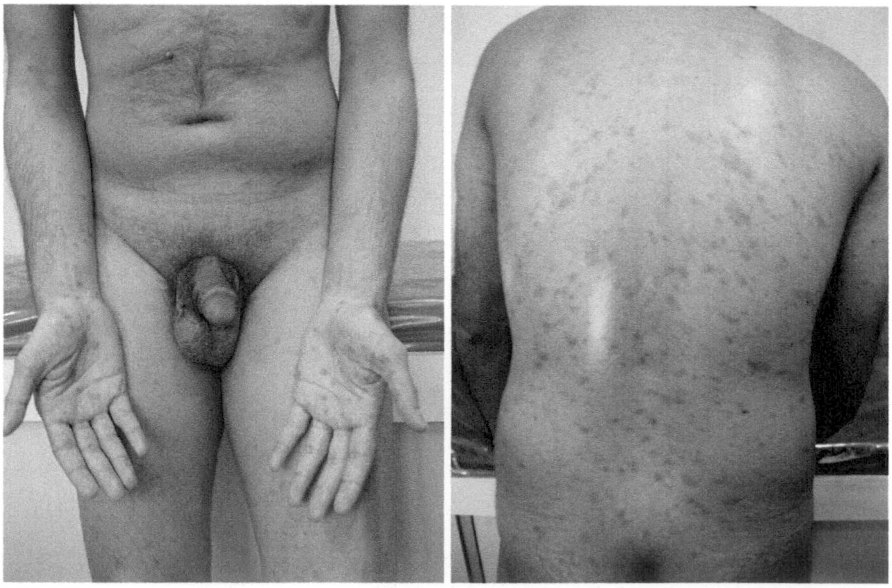

Fig. 28.20 (**a** and **b**) Secondary syphilis

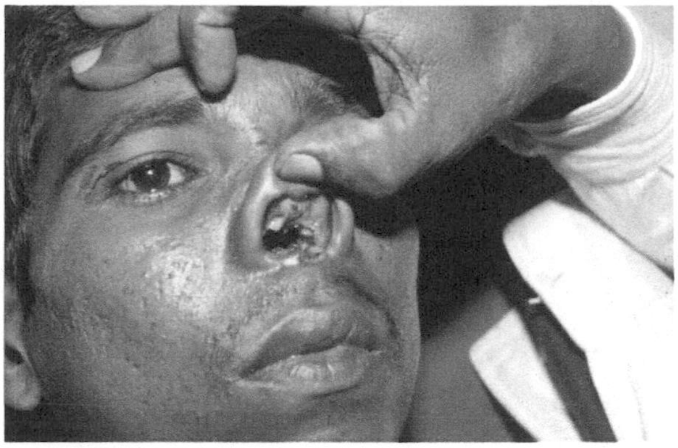

Fig. 28.21 Tertiary syphilis

erosive genital/perineal herpes (lasting > 6 weeks) recurrent and refractory disease, atypical lesions (follicular, necrotic, and nodular), and acyclovir-resistant herpes are more common.

Human papillomavirus (HPV) infection: Extensive and florid disease is more common in HIV disease. There is a tendency to dysplastic change and the incidence of malignant transformation in HPV infection, namely, cervical intraepithelial neoplasia (CIN), cancer of penis, vulva, or perianal area is higher in HIV-infected individuals (Figs. 28.22 and 28.23).

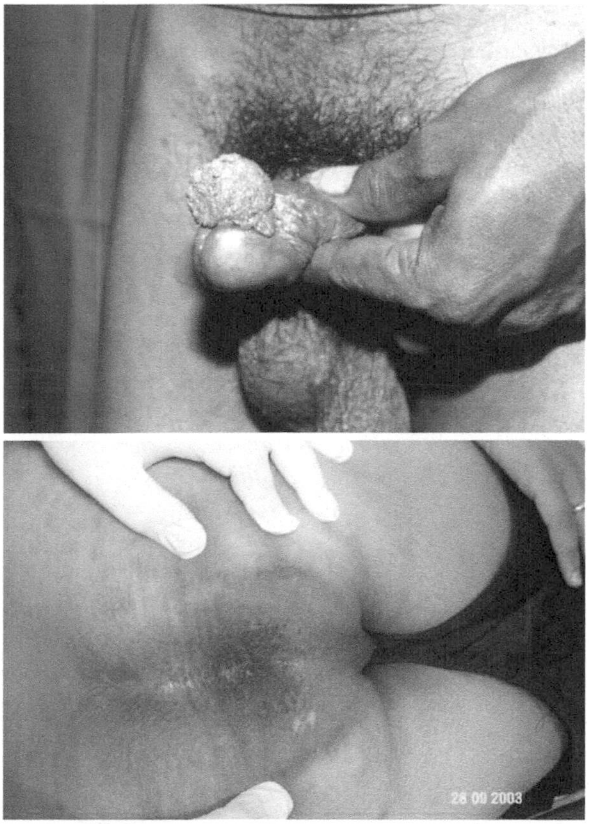

Fig. 28.22 (**a** and **b**) Human papillomavirus infection; condyloma acuminatum

28.4.3 Systemic Involvement in HIV Infection

28.4.3.1 Diseases of the Respiratory System

The lung is the most frequent site of opportunistic infection in AIDS, because, along with the gastrointestinal tract, it serves as an interface with all the potential pathogens in the environment. The clinical profile depends on the stage of the disease and CD4 counts [5]. At higher counts (>250 cells/mm^3), recurrent bacterial URTI, sinusitis, bronchitis, and otitis media are more common. As disease progresses, other manifestations appear. In the Western world, *Pneumocystis jirovecii* pneumonia (PCP) is the commonest respiratory complaint. In the developing world, however, tuberculosis remains the most common infection. Pulmonary involvement in HIV infection may have infective, neoplastic, or inflammatory causes. Infective agents implicated in pneumonitis/pneumonia in HIV infection include bacteria

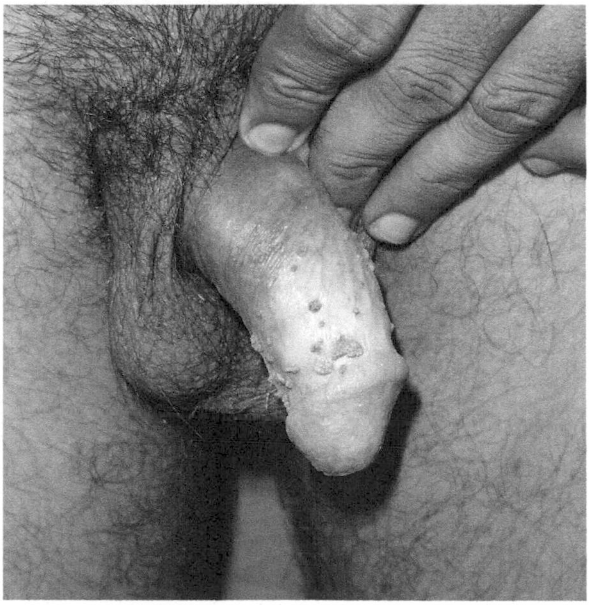

Fig. 28.23 Human papillomavirus infection; bowenoid papulosis

including of mycobacteria, viruses, fungi, and protozoa. The various pathogens described are:

- Bacteria: *Streptococcus pneumoniae*, *Haemophilus influenzae*, *Pseudomonas aeruginosa*, *Staphylococcus aureus*, *Moraxella catarrhalis*, *Rhodococcus equi*, *Nocardia asteroides*, *Mycobacterium tuberculosis*, *Mycobacterium avium* complex.
- Viruses: *Cytomegalovirus*, *Adenovirus*, *Herpes simplex*.
- Fungi: *Cryptococcus neoformans*, *Histoplasma capsulatum*, *Aspergillus fumigatus*, *Coccidioides immitis*, *Blastomyces dermatitidis*, *Pneumocystis jirovecii*, *Penicillium marneffei*.
- Protozoa: *Toxoplasma gondii*.
- Metazoa: *Strongyloides stercoralis*.

Tuberculosis: In the tropics, the almost ubiquitous presence of *Mycobacterium tuberculosis* leads to the flaring of hitherto quiescent lesions into active foci of infection, as a result of immunosuppression (Figs. 28.24 and 28.25). Tuberculosis may occur at any stage of the disease and is therefore the commonest presentation of HIV disease in the tropics. Over 15% of tuberculosis patients in India are likely to be HIV-positive. Approximately one-third of all AIDS-related deaths are due to tuberculosis. TB also hastens the onset and progression of other opportunistic infections, thus increasing the morbidity and mortality. At higher CD4 counts, the disease resembles that in immunocompetent individuals, while atypical presentation is common at lower counts. Extrapulmonary infections occur more commonly in advanced HIV disease. Pulmonary TB tends to be more occult and patients with advanced AIDS form poor granulomas and have large number of AFB in their sputum. They may be clinically and radiologically normal. However, radiologic evidence of diffuse, bilateral lower lobe infiltrates is commoner than the upper lobe lesions seen in immunocompetent patients. Patients with HIV are also highly prone to the development of active TB on exposure to bacilli in the community. Thus, TB in HIV patients may be as a result of new infections, rather than just reactivation of previous lesions. Treatment of TB in HIV does not differ from that in normal individuals, although multidrug-resistant and extensive drug-resistant diseases (MDR-TB/XDR-TB) are more common in HIV-infected individuals.

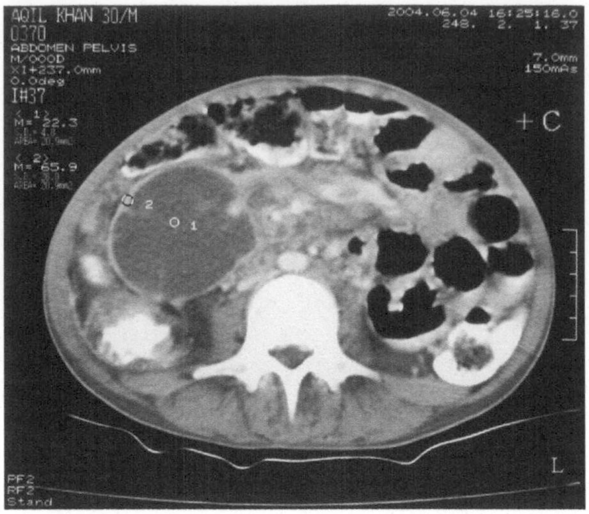

Fig. 28.25 Abdominal tuberculosis

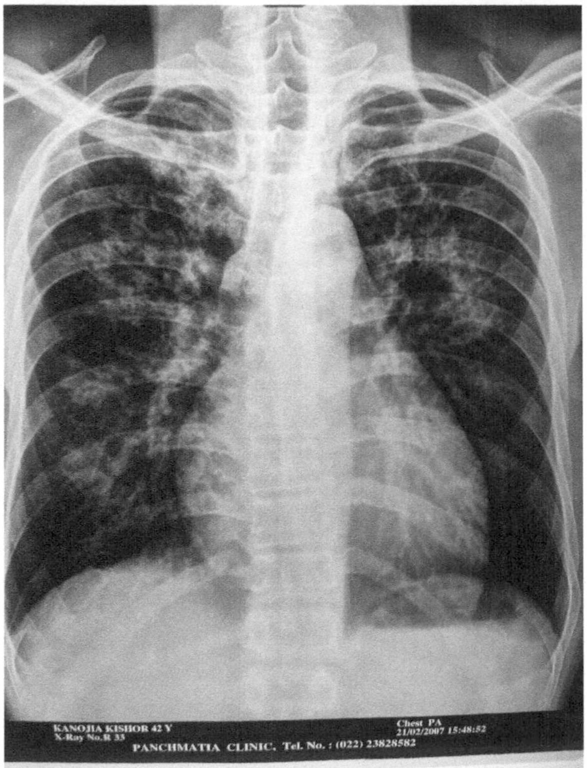

Fig. 28.24 Pulmonary tuberculosis

Other respiratory tract infections: Acute bronchitis and maxillary sinusitis are quite common, and recurrent respiratory tract infections (sinusitis, pneumonitis, otitis media, etc.) are markers of HIV infection. The most common manifestation of pulmonary disease is pneumonia. Both bacterial (pyogenic) and *P. jirovecii* pneumonia (PCP) occur in AIDS.

Pneumocystis jirovecii pneumonia (PCP): *Pneumocystis jirovecii* (formerly called *P. carinii*) is the organism causing the most common life-threatening opportunistic infection in most developed countries. The usual presentation is subacute (over 2–4 weeks), with malaise, fatigue, weight loss, characteristic retrosternal chest pain (that is typically worse on inspiration), and nonproductive cough. The patient may be breathless, but auscultation reveals no adventitious sounds. The chest radiograph may be normal or may show the classical finding of dense perihilar infiltrate. The arterial oxygen tension is usually low, and serum LDH (fraction LDH-3) is elevated. An LDH > 450 IU/L is strongly predictive of PCP, and higher levels are associated with poorer prognosis. The diagnosis is usually confirmed by direct demonstration of the trophozoite or the cyst in sputum induced with hypertonic saline or in bronchial lavage (BAL) obtained by fiber-optic bronchoscopy. A gallium scan may be contributory. Cotrimoxazole is the drug of choice. Pentamidine isethionate, trimetrexate with leucovorin, dapsone with trimethoprim, clindamycin, primaquine, and atovaquone are second-line drugs. Adjunctive corticosteroids are indicated in patients with moderate and severe disease (Fig. 28.26).

Atypical mycobacterial infections: These infections are also seen in AIDS patients, especially with *M. avium complex* (MAC). MAC infection is usually a late occurrence when the $CD4^+$ T-cell count is < 50 cell/mm^3. The most common presentation is disseminated disease with fever, weight loss, and night sweats. Other findings are abdominal pain, diarrhea, lower lobe infiltrates suggestive of miliary spread, and sometimes alveolar, nodular, hilar, or mediastinal adenopathy may occur.

Fungal infections: Pulmonary fungal infections, such as histoplasmosis, coccidioidomycosis, penicilliosis, and aspergillosis have been described, mostly in endemic areas. These infections are rare, and present with pneumonia with severe constitutional and respiratory symptoms. Demonstration of the fungus may be necessary to achieve a diagnosis. Amphotericin B remains the drug of choice.

Miscellaneous: Two forms of idiopathic interstitial pneumonia have been described – lymphoid interstitial pneumonitis (LIP) and nonspecific interstitial pneumonitis (NSIP). LIP is common in perinatally infected children < 13 years of age. The exact pathogenesis is

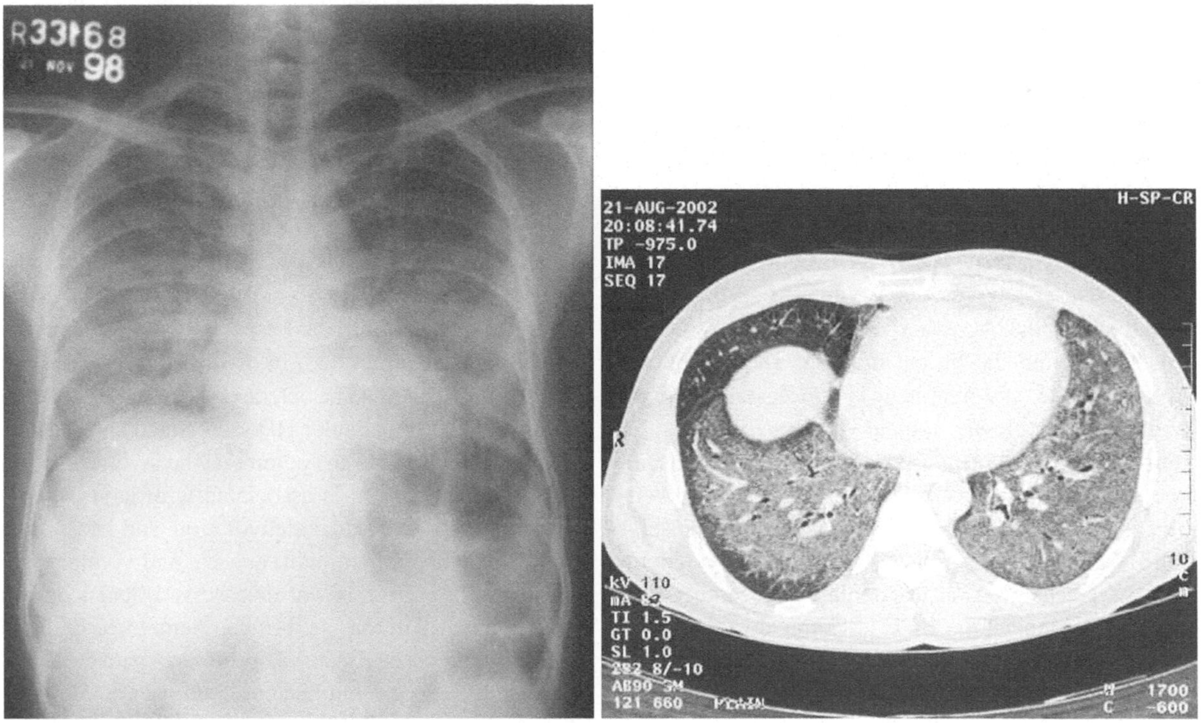

Fig. 28.26 (**a** and **b**) *Pneumocystis jirovecii* infection

unclear, although simultaneous infection by EBV and HIV may play a role. The most common radiographic features are bilateral reticulonodular infiltrates in the entire lung field or in the lower lobes. BAL shows CD8 lymphocytosis in the aspirate. No effective treatment is known. NSIP is similar to LIP, but more common in adults. It is a diagnosis of exclusion.

Primary pulmonary hypertension, emphysema, and bronchiectasis have also been reported.

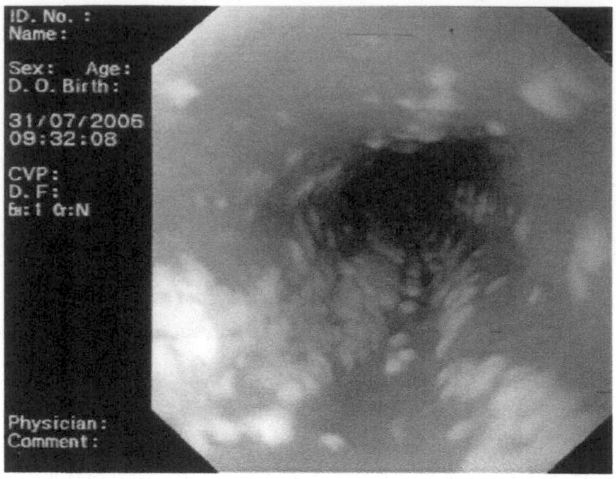

Fig. 28.27 Esophageal candidiasis

28.4.3.2 Disease of the Oropharynx and Gastrointestinal System

Most of the oropharyngeal and gastrointestinal diseases are due to opportunistic infection. The oral lesions are thrush, OHL, periodontal disease and aphthous ulcers [5].

Thrush (oral candidiasis): It is caused by *Candida albicans* and rarely by *C. krusei*. It is the most common HIV-associated condition and is reported in up to 70% of patients. The hyperplastic variant is more common, and appears as white, cheesy exudates often on an erythematous mucosa in the posterior oropharynx. The buccal mucosa and soft palate are the commonest sites but early lesions are seen along the gingival border. Other clinical variants include the acute erythematous/atrophic variant, angular cheilitis (perleche) and median rhomboid glossitis. Thrush is suggestive of advanced immunosuppression and is an indicator for introducing cotrimoxazole prophylaxis in affected individuals. Fluconazole is the drug of choice, although resistance has been reported.

Oral hairy leukoplakia (OHL): Caused by Epstein–Barr virus (EBV), presents as white frond-like lesions usually along the lateral borders of the tongue but sometimes involving the buccal mucosa. The condition is asymptomatic, and treatment is unnecessary, although high-dose acyclovir, topical podophyllotoxin, and retinoic acid have been tried. Thrush and OHL usually occur in patients with $CD4^+$ T-cell counts of $<250/cm^3$.

Periodontal disease: Three characteristic presentations have been described – necrotizing periodontal disease, linear gingival erythema (LGE), and exacerbated attachment loss. LGE is characterized by rapid process of bone and soft tissue destruction in patients with good oral hygiene, without any plaque or calculus. It has high predictive value for immunosuppression.

Aphthous stomatitis: Recurrent oral ulcers, with a characteristic erythematous halo, occurring at least twice over 6 months are a marker of HIV infection. Their cause is obscure, although a vasculitic process has been suggested, as is herpes simplex virus infection. The disease is refractory to therapy, and thalidomide may be prescribed in severe cases.

Gastrointestinal tract GIT involvement in HIV usually consists of esophagitis and diarrheal diseases.

Esophagitis: It presents with dysphagia and odynophagia and can be caused by candida, cytomegalovirus (CMV), or herpes simplex virus (HSV) (Fig. 28.27). CMV infection is associated with a single large ulcer, whereas herpetic infection presents with multiple small ulcers. Esophagitis is a sign of worsening immunosuppression.

Diarrhea: Diarrhea is the most common GI complaint in HIV infection. Infections of the small and large intestine with various bacteria, protozoa, and viruses can cause diarrhea and abdominal pain. Also, drug-associated diarrhea, especially with protease inhibitors is also reported. In one-fifth of all cases, no pathogen or cause can be detected. These cases are considered to be idiopathic or HIV-associated enteropathy. The small intestine or the colon may be involved. Small intestine involvement is associated with large-volume diarrhea, and associated dehydration and electrolyte anomalies. Abdominal pain, nausea, and vomiting are present, while large bowel disease is associated with low-volume diarrhea, tenesmus, hematochezia, and fecal leukocytosis. Bacteria, protozoa, parasites, and viruses have been implicated. *Salmonella*, *Shigella*, *Campylobacter*, and *Clostridium difficile* diarrhea have been described. Disease is more severe in HIV-infected individuals. MAC and *M. tuberculosis* are also implicated. *Cryptosporidia* spp., *Microsporidia*, and *Isospora belli* are the most common opportunistic protozoa that infect the GIT and cause noninflammatory diarrhea. *Giardia intestinalis* and *E. histolytica* infections are common in homosexual men. CMV colitis presents as non-bloody diarrhea, abdominal pain, weight loss, and anorexia. Endoscopic examination reveals multiple mucosal ulcerations and the biopsy shows characteristic intranuclear inclusion bodies. In advanced disease, various systemic fungal infections like histoplasmosis, coccidioidomycosis, etc. may also cause diarrhea. Nelfinavir causes diarrhea in up to 20% individuals, and disease may be severe enough to withhold therapy. Besides these secondary infections, HIV infection per se can cause AIDS enteropathy. The exact pathogenetic mechanism by which HIV causes diarrhea is unknown. Analysis of stool samples, with relevant special stains, is required for diagnosis. Sigmoidoscopy, colonoscopy, or upper GI endoscopy with biopsy may be indicated if stool analysis is inconclusive. Management of the diarrhea involves treatment of the cause, with relevant anti-infective agents. Maintenance of fluid–electrolyte balance is essential. Oral rehydration is mandatory, and total parenteral nutrition may be required in unresponsive cases. Luminal agents such as dietary fiber supplements may be helpful, but may bind medication as well. Antimotility agents may be used judiciously, and octreotide may be required in intractable AIDS-associated secretory diarrhea.

28.4.4 HIV and Nervous System (Neuro–AIDS)

Cerebral toxoplasmosis is the most frequent opportunistic infection of the central nervous system [5]. It usually results from reactivation of toxoplasma cysts in the brain, causing abscess formation. The abscess can be unifocal or multifocal. Clinically, it presents with features of a space-occupying lesion (SOL). CT scan shows ring-enhancing lesions with surrounding edema (Fig. 28.28).

Cryptococcal meningitis accounts for 5–10% of opportunistic infections in patients with HIV infection. The clinical presentation is subacute with headache, fever, and cranial nerve palsies. Neck stiffness is relatively rare. CSF analysis will demonstrate the yeast in 70% of the cases and antigen detection is positive in 100% of the patients.

Progressive multifocal leukoencephalopathy (PML) is a demyelinating disease (slow virus disease) caused by JC virus. Clinically there may be focal neurological deficits, ataxia, and personality changes (Fig. 28.29).

HIV Encephalopathy – Patients with this disorder have a form of dementia known as AIDS-related cognitive–motor complex. In the early stages, there is impairment of memory and concentration. Later, motor signs appear such as hyperreflexia, extensor plantar responses, lack of coordination, and ataxia.

Other neurological features in HIV infection are progressive vacuolar myelopathy (with spastic paraplegia, ataxia, and loss of sphincter control), transverse myelitis (due to VZV, HSV, and CMV infections), peripheral neuropathy, and psychiatric manifestations (acute psychosis, depression).

28.4.5 Disease of the Liver, Gall Bladder, and Pancreas

Liver involvement is usually in the form of coinfection with HBV/HCV [5]. Direct HIV infection of the liver may lead to functional defects, which may present as porphyria cutanea tarda (PCT). The liver is also affected as a result of drug administration, both HAART and therapy for opportunistic infections, especially antituberculous treatment.

Sclerosing cholangitis and papillary stenosis are reported in cryptosporidiosis, CMV infection, and Kaposi's sarcoma. Pancreatitis usually occurs secondary to drug toxicity, mainly with didanosine.

The HIV/AIDS and hepatitis coinfection is the current topic of interest globally. There is paucity of epidemiological data on HBV or HCV infection in India, namely, incidence, genotyping study, natural history of infection, and incidence of HIV and HBV/HCV co-infection [21]. It is believed that the effective mode of transmission for HBV or HCV in descending order would be transfusion > intravenous drug user > sexual > needle stick injury > unknown. According to Fauci, over 95% of HIV-infected individuals have evidence of infection with HBV; 5–40% are coinfected with HCV and coinfection with hepatitis D, E, and/or G viruses is common. There is approximately a threefold increase in the development of persistent hepatitis B surface antigenemia. Patients coinfected with HIV and HBV have a low incidence of inflammatory disease, presumably because of the

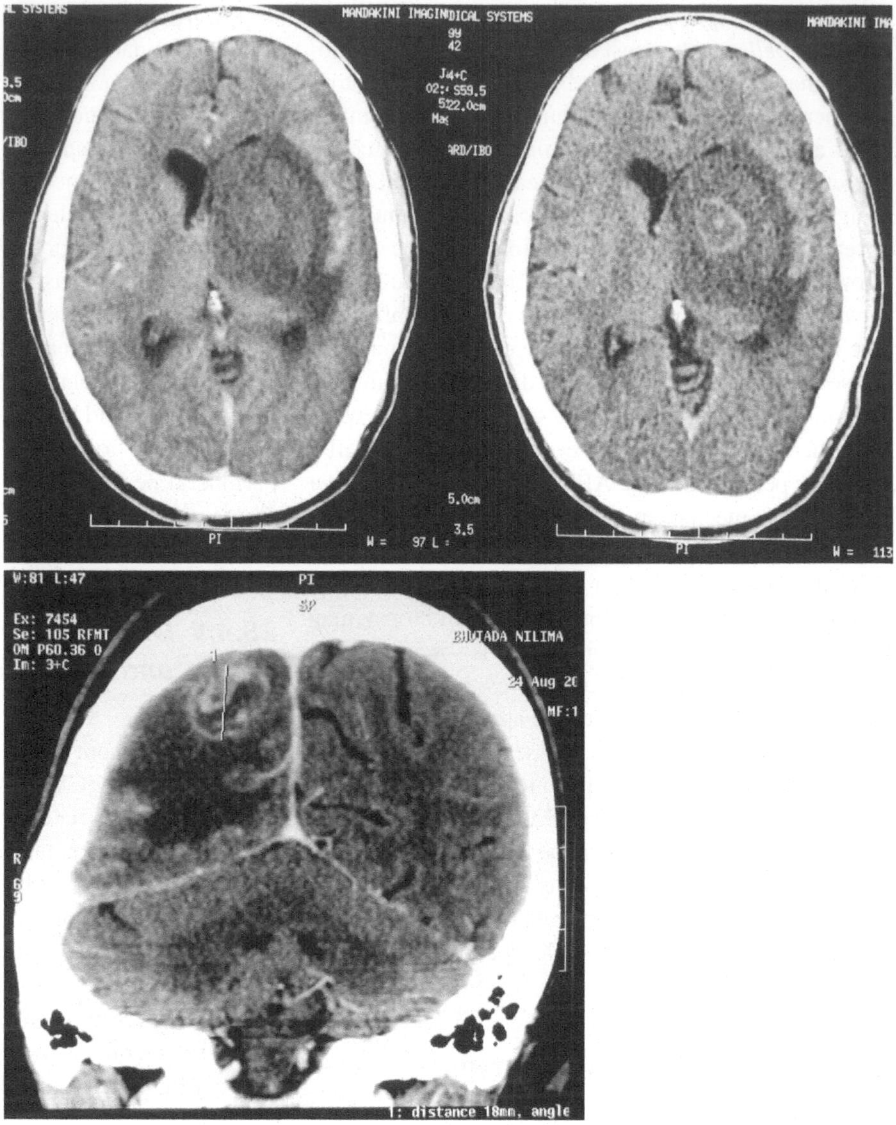

Fig. 28.28 (**a** and **b**) Toxoplasmosis

antecedent immunosuppression. Severe hepatitis may develop due to immune-reconstitution as a result of antiretroviral therapy. IFN-alpha is less successful as a treatment of HBV and lamivudine is the drug of choice. Since it is also a potent antiretroviral drug, it should never be used as a single agent in the treatment of HBV in HIV patients to prevent the development of resistant quasi-species.

In contrast, HCV infection is more severe in patients with HIV and levels of HCV are tenfold higher than in the HIV-negative patient, as also is the incidence of liver failure. It is recommended that all HIV-positive individuals who have not experienced natural infection be immunized with hepatitis A and/or hepatitis B vaccines. End-stage liver disease (ESLD) is the commonest cause of mortality amongst such individuals, especially if not treated with HAART.

28.4.6 Diseases of the Kidney

HIV-associated nephropathy (HIVAN): The kidneys can be involved in HIV infection and the most common presentation is with nephrotic syndrome and renal failure [5]. Focal segmental glomerulosclerosis and mesangial proliferative glomerulonephritis account for most of the cases of HIV-associated nephropathy. Renal disease can also occur as a side effect of therapy in HIV disease.

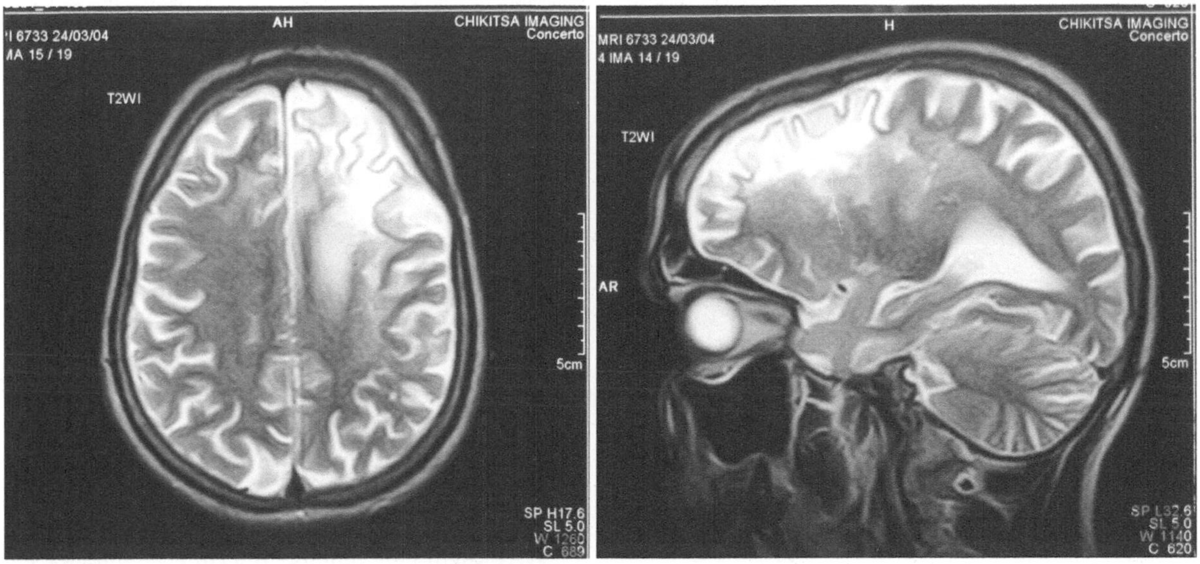

Fig. 28.29 (**a** and **b**) Progressive multifocal leukoencephalopathy

28.4.7 Diseases of the Eye

The most common ophthalmic opportunistic infection in India is CMV retinitis, which almost always occurs in patients with CD4 counts < 50 cells/mm^3 [23] (Fig. 28.30). The second most common manifestation is HIV retinopathy. This is a noninfectious condition seen in 13–15% patients, presenting with cotton wool spots on thc fundus.

Other conditions described are extensive blepharitis, spontaneous lid ulcerations, molluscum contagiosum, herpes simplex keratitis, frosted branch angiitis due to CMV retinitis, subretinal cysticercosis, acute retinal necrosis syndrome, squamous cell carcinoma,

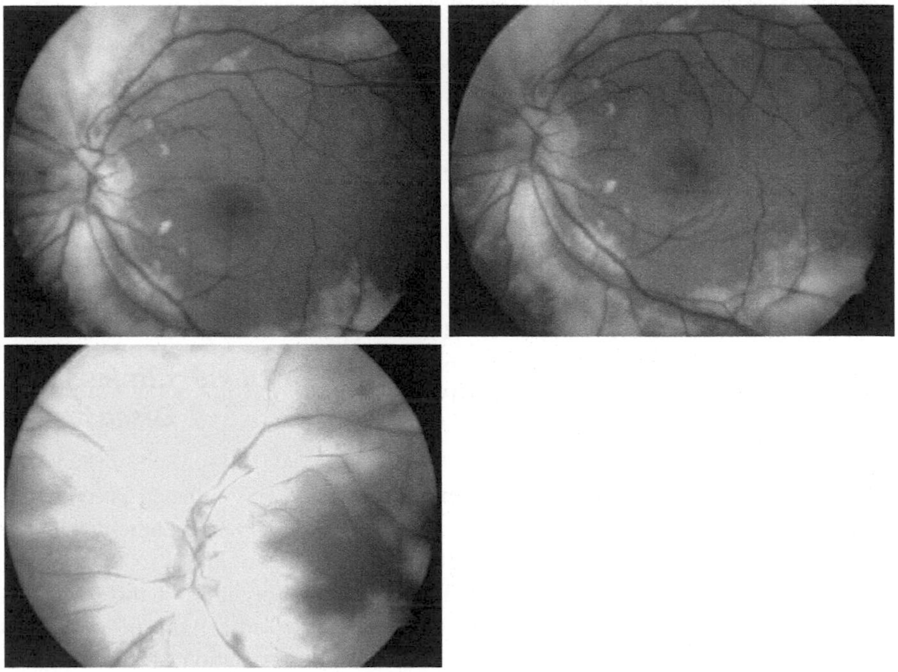

Fig. 28.30 (**a**, **b**, and **c**) Cytomegalovirus retinitis

and immune recovery vitritis following treatment with protease inhibitors.

28.4.8 HIV and Cancer

28.4.8.1 Kaposi's Sarcoma (KS)

KS was the first neoplasm reported in HIV disease. It is usually seen in gay and bisexual men, and in women in Africa. The worldwide incidence of KS in patients with AIDS may approach 34%. KS occurs at all stages of HIV disease, and its severity is not strictly correlated with the degree of immunosuppression. KS is believed to be a proliferation of endothelial cells induced by human herpes virus-type 8 (HHV-8), acquired through sexual transmission.

About one third of HIV-infected cases have a preponderance of tumors on the legs and feet. However, lesions may develop elsewhere on the skin, including the scalp, lips, hard palate, and gums. Lesions may occur singly or in groups. KS begins as pink, red, brown, or purple macules that disseminate and progress to violaceous plaques or nodules. They may easily be mistaken for bruises, purpura, or nevi. Lesions may be symmetrical with smooth borders or asymmetrical with jagged edges. They darken and become scaly as they age. Involvement of internal organs and mucosa is common. As a rule, a patient has approximately one internal lesion for every five skin lesions. Gastrointestinal involvement is common and may result in hemorrhage or obstruction. The course of KS in HIV-infected patients is more aggressive than the other clinical types of KS.

Incidentally, incidence of KS is extremely low in India for reasons not yet clear; however, there is low seroprevalence of HHV-8 in HIV-positive individuals in India. KS is seen among heterosexual HIV-positive individuals including females. There are not enough numbers of HIV-related KS patients who had an opportunity to receive HAART and see its impact including emergence of IRIS KS. Apparently HIV-2 infection has no impact on KS incidence as also observed in HIV-2 high-prevalence countries.

For limited disease, local therapy with liquid nitrogen, alitretinoin, or intralesional vincristine may be effective. Surgery, radiotherapy, and systemic single-agent chemotherapy, usually with vinblastine, vincristine, bleomycin, doxorubicin, or etoposide may be useful. However, systemic chemotherapy has not been shown to improve the long-term survival rates. Immune reconstitution after HAART may lead to remission of KS. Interferon (IFN)-alpha and IFN-beta, photodynamic therapy and systemic hyperthermia have also been used. Cryotherapy, laser irradiation, and electrodessication can be useful for localized solitary lesions of KS [5]. (For further reading, see chapter 31).

28.4.8.2 Non-Hodgkin's Lymphoma (NHL)

At least 6% of all AIDS patients develop lymphomas at some point during their illness (Fig. 28.31). The initiation of cART has no effect on the incidence. Most tumors are extralymphatic and histologically, they are high-grade, large-cell immunoblastic, or non-cleaved small-cell tumors. Burkitt's lymphoma has also been reported. Their pathogenesis may be related to EBV and also to HHV-8. The CNS is the most common site. Clinically, it presents with signs and symptoms of a space-occupying lesion (SOL). Systemic lymphoma is seen at an earlier stage of infection. In addition to lymph node involvement, the bone marrow (leading to pancytopenia), liver, lung, and gastrointestinal tract (~25% patients) may be involved. Any site in the GIT may be involved. Patients may present with dysphagia and pain. Pulmonary disease may present as a mass lesion, multiple nodules, or an interstitial infiltrate. A variant called primary effusion lymphoma or body cavity lymphoma has also been described. Lymphomatous pleural, pericardial, and/or peritoneal effusions, in the absence of discreet nodal or extranodal masses, are seen.

Other tumors that can occur in AIDS are Hodgkin's lymphoma, squamous cell carcinoma (Ca) of the anus especially in homosexual men, cervical cancer, adenocarcinoma, renal cell Ca, teratoma, and seminoma.

28.4.9 Clinical Manifestation of HIV Disease in India

HIV-infected individuals in India are exposed to various environmental factors like malnutrition and poverty and also to a host of tropical infections that are peculiar to this region [23–25]. Striking similarities and certain differences exist between the clinical presentation of AIDS in the Indian population and other

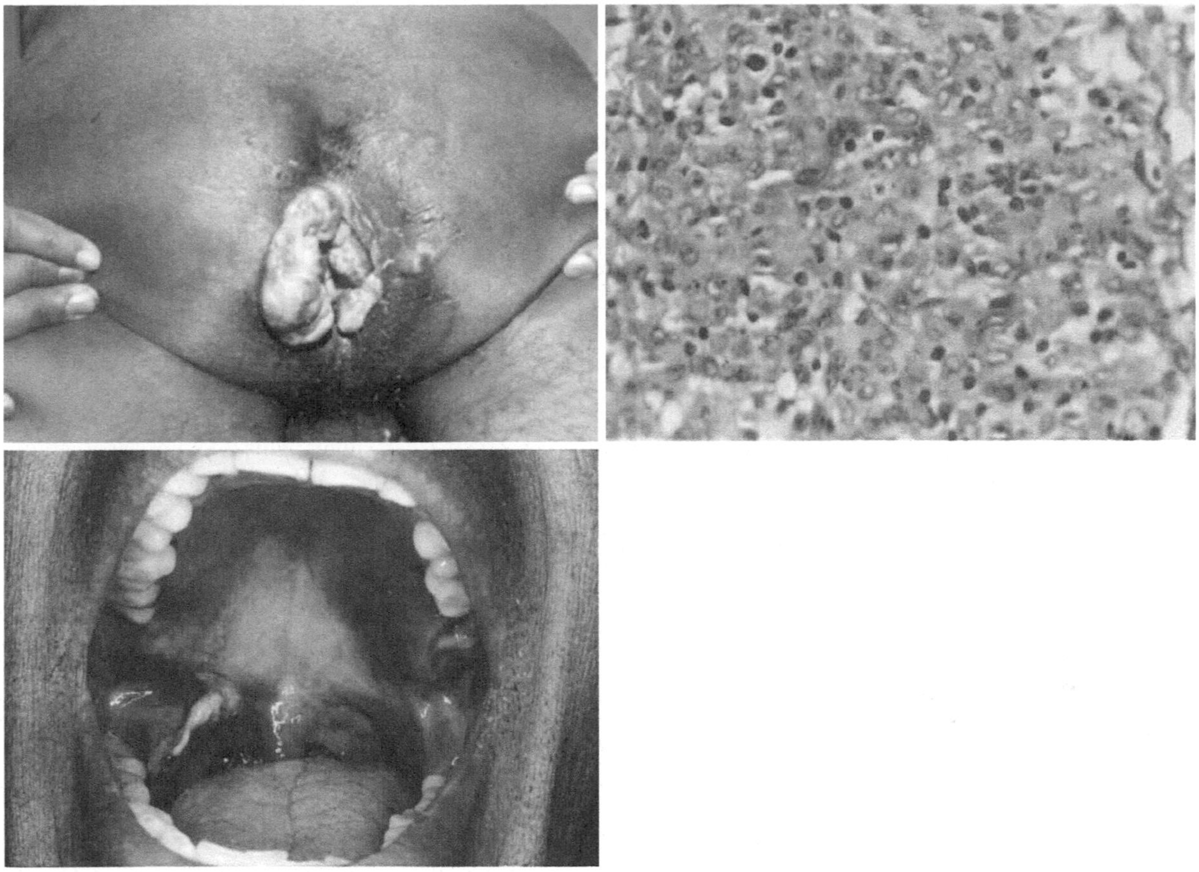

Fig. 28.31 (**a**, **b**, and **c**) Non-Hodgkin's lymphoma

countries. Slim disease or the wasting syndrome is the most common mode of presentation in Africa. A similar presentation was seen in 62% patients in a series from south India. *Pneumocystis jirovecii* pneumonia is the most common opportunistic infection in most of the developed countries. By contrast PCP is unusual in the Indian population and the most common opportunistic infection is tuberculosis. The rarity of PCP among the Indian patients may be due to the fact they have many other tropical infectious diseases prior to reaching the severe immunosuppressed state and consequent relatively early mortality due to these infections.

Mycobacterium avium intracellular is the most common of the mycobacterium isolated from patients in the USA, whereas *M. tuberculosis* is more frequently isolated in patients from India.

Candidiasis (oropharyngeal and esophageal) is the second most common opportunistic infection in India. Toxoplasmosis, histoplasmosis, Kaposi's sarcoma, and CNS lymphomas are uncommon in the Indian population compared to Western countries.

28.4.10 Diagnosis of AIDS

Clinical: For the purpose of AIDS surveillance, an adult or adolescent (>12 years of age) is considered to have AIDS if at least two of the following major signs are present in combination with at least one of the minor signs listed in Table 28.3, and if these signs are

Table 28.3 Major and Minor Signs of AIDS

Major signs
• Weight loss > 10% of body weight
• Chronic diarrhea for more than 1 month
• Prolonged fever for more than 1 month (intermittent or constant)
Minor signs
• Persistent cough for more than 1 month
• Generalized pruritic dermatitis
• History of herpes zoster
• Oropharyngeal candidiasis
• Chronic progressive or disseminated herpes simplex infection
• Generalized lymphadenopathy

not known to be due to a condition unrelated to HIV infection [5].

The presence of either generalized Kaposi's sarcoma or cryptococcal meningitis is sufficient for the diagnosis of AIDS for surveillance purposes.

Laboratory tests: The diagnosis of HIV infection is based on the demonstration of antibodies to HIV/AIDS antigens or the direct detection of viral antigens [5]. These tests may be classified as:

(1) Tests for HIV-specific antibodies in serum and plasma:
   (a) Screening tests
      (i) ELISA: The ELISA is the standard screening test used. It is a solid-phase assay in which the antibody is detected using the sandwich technique. It has a sensitivity of>99.5%, but the specificity is not optimal in low-risk cases. Also, a number of conditions may interfere with the test result and cause false-positive reactions.
      (ii) Rapid tests: These are visual tests in which a positive test appears as a dot on a tile or a comb; or as agglutination on a slide.
   (b) Supplemental tests
      (i) Western Blot assay: Viral antigens are separated on the basis of their molecular weights and antibodies to each are detected as distinct bands. The test is considered positive if antibodies to at least 2 out of p24, gp41 or gp120/160 are detected.
      (ii) Immunofluorescence tests.
(2) Tests on saliva: Although these kits are efficacious, there is some concern about how early following infection the antibody is detectable in saliva as compared to serum/plasma, as well as the minimum concentration of IgG at which each kit gives a correct result.
(3) Confirmatory tests:
   (a) Virus isolation: This assay is 100% specific, but its sensitivity varies with the stage of HIV infection. Both in adults and in children, the virus cannot be cultured from peripheral blood mononuclear cells (PBMCs) for approximately 6 weeks following the time of transmission. However, this procedure is labor-intensive and dangerous and hence undertaken in specialized laboratories only.
   (b) Detection of the p24 antigen: This test detects the unbound HIV p24 antigen in the serum. The test may be useful (a) during the window period, (b) during late disease when the patient is symptomatic, (c) to detect HIV infection in the newborn because diagnosis is difficult due to presence of maternal antibodies, (d) when neurologic involvement is suspected, the test is performed with CSF.
   (c) Detection of HIV RNA: Three different techniques, namely RT-PCR, nucleic acid sequence-based amplification (NASBA) and branched DNA (bDNA) assay have been employed to develop commercial kits.
(4) Monitoring tests:
   (a) $CD4^+$ T-cell counts: This is expressed as a product of the CD4 cell percentage, derived by flow cytometry, and the total lymphocyte count determined by the WBC counts. It is performed at diagnosis and every 3–6 months thereafter. Two determinations are usually performed before any decision to start or change ART is taken.
   (b) Viral load: This is the same as detection of HIV RNA copies.
(5) Surrogate tests: These include estimation of the following
   (a) Circulating levels of neopterin, beta-2-microglobulin, and soluble IL-2 receptors.
   (b) HIV IgA levels.
   (c) Levels of acid-labile endogenous interferon or TNF-alpha.

28.5 Antiretroviral Treatment

In September 2003, WHO declared a "global health emergency" due to the lack of access to antiretroviral (ARV) treatment. An emergency plan was announced by WHO/ UNAIDS in order to cover at least 3 million people by the end of 2005, which was popularly known as the "3-by-5" initiative [26]. The WHO guidelines for "Antiretroviral Use in Resource-Constrained Settings" have since been revised in December 2003 and in August 2006.

The Government of India launched the free ART program on April 1, 2004, starting with eight tertiary-level government hospitals in the six high-prevalence states, namely, Andhra Pradesh, Karnataka, Maharashtra, Tamil Nadu, Manipur, and Nagaland, as well as in Delhi.

Since then the ART centers are being scaled up in a phased manner and it is planned that free ART will be provided to 200,000 patients by the end of 2010 and 200,000 patients by 2011 in 250 centers across the country. The introduction of highly effective antiretroviral drugs at affordable costs has greatly transformed the AIDS epidemic in the resource-poor developing world. The World Health Organization and UNAIDS are aiming for "Universal Access to ART for all by 2010." [27]

28.5.1 Key Goals of the National ART Program Include [26, 28]

- To provide long-term ART to eligible patients.
- To monitor and report treatment outcomes on a quarterly basis.
- To attain individual drug adherence rates of 95% or more.
- To increase life span so that 50% of patients on ART are alive 3 years after starting the treatment.
- To ensure that 50% of patients on ART are engaged in, or can return to, their previous employment.

28.5.2 Protocol for ART Regimen [26, 28]

- Confirmation of HIV diagnosis.
- Counseling for ART.
- Baseline investigations.
- Indications of therapy.
- Selection of regimens.
- Monitoring of ART.
- Switching of regimens.

After confirming the diagnosis of HIV, patients should be counseled regarding the ART (cost, adverse effect, adherence, and long-term treatment). Investigations to rule out any opportunistic infections along with viral load and CD4 count should be done. Under the national program (due to cost factors) only CD4 is done. The following investigations should be considered before starting ART: Complete blood count with differential, ESR, serum electrolytes, liver and renal function tests, CD4 count and HIV viral load, chest radiograph, Mantoux (tuberculin) test, sputum stain and culture, and ultrasonography of the abdomen. For women annual Papanicolaou (PAP) smear screening or acetic acid cervical screening at district health-care facilities are recommended as are HBsAg and HCV screening for IDUs and those with transfusion-associated infections or elevated liver enzyme levels [27].

28.5.3 Antiretrovirals Available in India Are

Nucleoside reverse transcriptase inhibitors (NRTI): Zidovudine (AZT/ZDV)*, Stavudine (d4T)*, Lamivudine (3TC)*, Didanosine (ddl), Zalcitabine (ddC), Abacavir (ABC), Emtricitabine (FTC), Tenofovir (TDF).

Non-nucleoside reverse transcriptase inhibitors (NNRTI): Nevirapine* (NVP), Efavirenz*(EFV).

Protease inhibitors: Saquinavir (SQV), Ritonavir (RTV), Nelfinavir (NFV), Indinavir (INV), Lopinavir/Ritonavir (LPV), Atazanavir (ATV).

* Drugs available under the national program

28.5.4 Indication of ART [27, 28]

Initiation of ART based on CD4 count and WHO clinical staging

Classification of HIV-associated clinical disease	WHO clinical stage	CD4 test not available (or result pending)	CD4 test available
Asymptomatic	1	Do not treat	Treat if CD4 <200
Mild symptoms	2	Do not treat	
Advanced symptoms	3	Treat	Consider treatment if CD4 <350 and initiate ART before CD4 Drops below 200
Severe/advanced symptoms	4	Treat	Treat irrespective of CD4 count

28.5.5 Regimens [27, 28]

In resource-limited settings like in India, nucleoside analogs reverse transcriptase inhibitors (NRTI)/non-nucleoside analogs reverse transcriptase inhibitors (NNRTI) triple combinations form the backbone of ART. [29] Currently, the national program provides the following combinations for first-line regimens:

1. Stavudine (30 mg)+Lamivudine (150 mg).
2. Zidovudine (300 mg)+Lamivudine (150 mg).
3. Stavudine (30 mg)+Lamivudine (150 mg)+Nevirapine (200 mg).
4. Zidovudine (300 mg)+Lamivudine (150 mg)+Nevirapine (200 mg).
5. Efavirenz (600 mg).
6. Nevirapine (200 mg).

Fixed-dose combinations (FDCs) are preferred because they are easy to use, have distribution advantages (procurement and stock management), improve adherence to treatment, and thus reduce the chances of development of drug resistance.

28.5.6 Principles for Selecting the First-Line Regimen [26]

1. Choose 3TC (lamivudine) in all regimens
2. Choose one NRTI to combine with 3TC (AZT or d4T)
3. Choose one NNRTI (NVP or EFV)

First choice: AZT+3TC+NVP (for patients with Hb>8 g/dl).

Second choice: d4T+3TC+NVP.

Substitute NVP with EFV, for patients with TB or toxicity due to NVP.

28.5.7 Monitoring [29]

	1 month	3 months	6 months	Every 6 months thereafter
Clinical* (monthly)	Yes	Yes	Yes	Yes
CD4 counts	No	No	Yes	Yes
LFTs	Yes	No	Yes	Yes
CBC	Yes (AZT)	No	Yes	Yes
Other chemistry	As clinically indicated			

28.5.8 ARV Toxicities

The major class toxicities of NRTIs (Fig. 28.32) are bone marrow suppression and mitochondrial toxicity (lactic acidosis, steatohepatitis, peripheral neuropathy, insulin resistance, and lipodystrophy). While NNRTIs are associated with skin rash and hepatitis, PIs cause gastrointestinal intolerance and lipid metabolism anomalies. The major individual toxicities include bone marrow suppression (ZDV), pancreatitis (ddI), hypersensitivity (ABC), hepatic necrosis (NVP), neuropsychiatric complaints (EFV), and nephrolithiasis (IDV). Hyperlipidemias have emerged as an important concern with HAART, due to the potential for premature atherosclerosis and coronary artery disease.

28.5.9 Treatment Failure

Treatment failure is defined using the same variables that define the goals of antiretroviral therapy. Virologic failure is viral load (VL)>200/mL or a sustained VL>50/mL, after 24 weeks of therapy. Immunologic failure is arbitrarily defined as failure of the CD4 count to rise by 25–50 cells/mm^3 in the first year after HAART. Clinical failure is defined as the occurrence of an AIDS-defining opportunistic complication after 3 months of HAART, when immune reconstitution inflammatory syndrome (IRIS) has been excluded.

IRIS is defined as occurrence or worsening of clinical and/or laboratory parameters despite a favorable outcome in human immunodeficiency virus (HIV) surrogate markers (CD4 counts) and plasma viral load [30]. Both infective (clinical or subclinical) and noninfective conditions can act as triggering factors for precipitating IRIS [31]. The predisposing factors for IRIS include a very low CD4 count (below 50 cells/mm^3) and very high plasma viral load prior to initiation of therapy, undetected presence of antigens of nonviable microorganisms (e.g., cryptococci and CMV) and active or subclinical infection (*M. tuberculosis, M. leprae*, etc.). This forms the perfect milieu in India for the development of IRIS, which is reflected in an upsurge of number of cases of IRIS in the ART era. As about 40% of the Indian population harbors primary infection with *M. tuberculosis*, it is not surprising that large cases of tuberculous lymphadenopathy are seen as IRIS after initiation of ART (personal experience). In a cohort study of 144 HIV/TB co-infected patients, the incidence of IRIS was 15.2 cases/100 patient-years

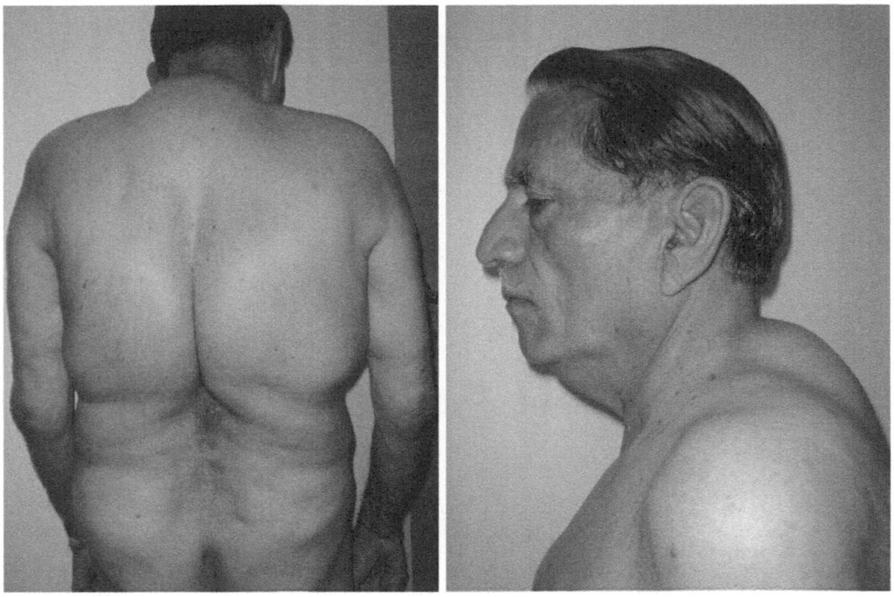

Fig. 28.32 (**a** and **b**) Lipodystrophy

and the median time for IRIS development was 42 days. Recently, cases of type-I lepra reaction and cryptococcal lymphadenitis have been described in India [32, 33]. As of now, there are no standard guidelines for the treatment of IRIS. Treatment includes continuation of primary therapy against the offending pathogen in order to decrease the antigenic load, continuation of effective cART (unless the IRIS is life-threatening) and judicious use of anti-inflammatory agents [31]. Causes of treatment failure include non-adherence or partial adherence, subtherapeutic drug levels, wrong choice of ART, and selection of mutant strains leading to drug resistance (Figs. 28.33 and 28.34).

28.5.10 ART Regimens for Failure [29]

First line regimens	Second-line regimens for treatment failure	Second-line regimens for treatment failure
	NRTI component	PI component
AZT+3TC+NVP	Choices:	First LPV/r
AZT+3TC+EFV	First TDF/ABC	Second ATV/r
D4T+3TC+NVP	Second ddI/ABC	Third SQV/r
D4T+3TC+EFV		Fourth IND/r
TDF+3TC+NVP	Choices:	
TDF+3TC+EFV	First ddI/ AZT/3TC*	
	Second ddI/ ABC	

In a nutshell, judicious use of HAART is essential for durable viral suppression and to ensure delayed development of resistance [34]. Prior to starting ARV in the HIV infected, it is essential to define treatment goals and to select the most appropriate tools to achieve these goals. Therefore, rational sequencing use of HAART is important so as to achieve virological, immunological, and clinical goals while maintaining treatment options, limit drug toxicities, and facilitate adherence. In resource-poor settings, ART drug regimens have often not been chosen with long-term treatment as the first priority. It is now time to take a different view, especially in settings where, in the foreseeable future, drug options will still be limited. It is mandatory to make the right choices from the very beginning of treatment [34].

28.5.11 Generic Antiretrovirals

Generic antiretrovirals have been marketed in India for more than 10 years. Most of the antiretrovirals are readily available (December 2008) except the latest molecules, namely, darunavir, tipranavir, raltegravir, or fosamprenavir. The prices of these antiretrovirals are fairly low as compared to those of internationally marketed ones. The quality control as well as bioequivalence study is periodically varied. Despite reasonably low prices, not many people living with HIV/AIDS can afford these antiretrovirals. Nearly 60% of antiretroviral requirement globally (especially in developing

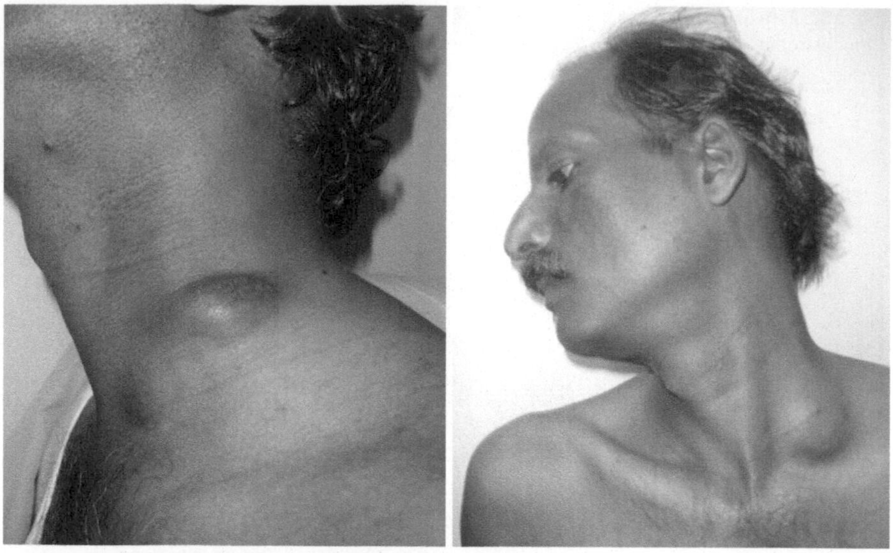

Fig. 28.33 (**a** and **b**) IRIS; tuberculosis nodes

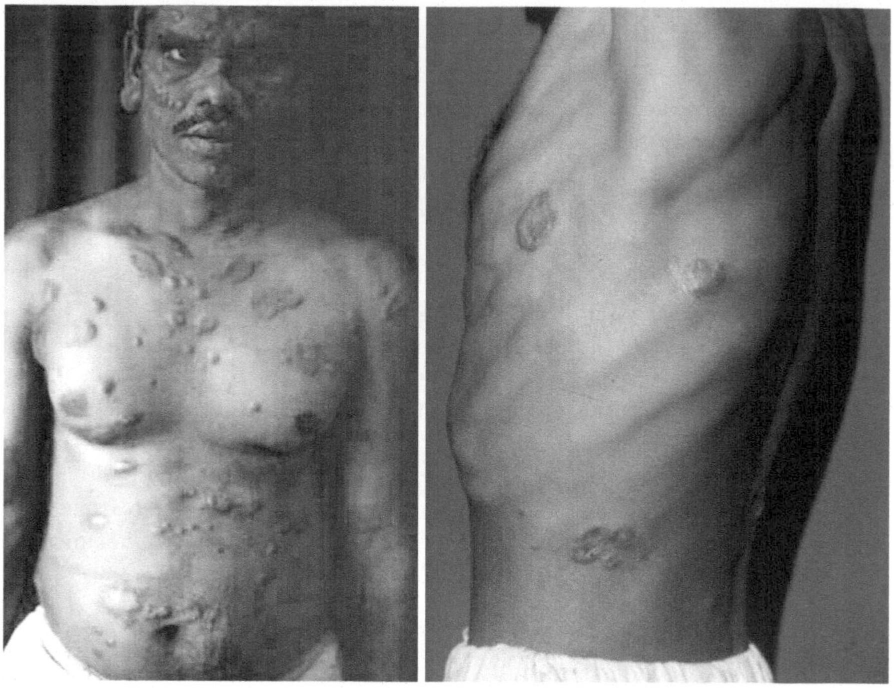

Fig. 28.34 (**a** and **b**) IRIS; Hansen's disease

countries) is supplied by Indian pharmaceutical companies. The National AIDS Control Organisation – NACO, Government of India-initiated antiretrovirals roll-out program is being scaled up, but has met with significant difficulties as regards cost-effectiveness. The perinatal HIV intervention has the highest beneficial impact because of generic preparations. Currently the health insurance scheme does not cover treatment of HIV/AIDS (even life insurance does not cover HIV/AIDS risk). Salient features that need to be addressed include the following: the shortage of skilled physicians, undiagnosed opportunistic infections (especially tuberculosis), poor counseling support, antiretroviral toxicities, poor adherence, irrational ART prescription, lack of family support, need for lifelong treatment, undiagnosed HIV-2 infection, hepatitis coinfection, poor health awareness, and advertisements misleading the public regarding cures for HIV/AIDS by alternate medicine experts.

28.6 Parent-to-Child Transmission (PTCT) of HIV

HIV can be transmitted during pregnancy especially in the last trimester, during childbirth, or breastfeeding [35]. The rate of perinatal transmission is 15–25% in developed countries, and 25–45% in developing countries. This difference is largely attributed to infant feeding practices especially breastfeeding, universality of its practice, and longer duration of breastfeeding in developing countries than in the developed world. Realizing the potential of nevirapine-based combination antiretroviral approaches, a feasibility study of offering nevirapine to HIV-infected mothers to reduce MTCT is in progress in India. In the developing countries like India, it is believed that husbands are mostly responsible for transmission of HIV to mothers through the sexual route, and therefore they are considered to be equally responsible for the transmission of HIV to their children. In India, therefore MTCT is termed as "parent-to-child transmission" so that mothers alone should not be blamed.

The feasibility study of AZT intervention and primary prevention was conducted among pregnant women at 11 institutions located in five states of India, namely, Maharashtra, Tamil Nadu, Andhra Pradesh, Karnataka, and Manipur, which are categorized as states with high prevalence of HIV infection. The feasibility study was conducted by the National AIDS Control Organization (NACO), Government of India (GOI), between April 2000 and September 2001 [1].

Although currently, India has an overall low prevalence of HIV among pregnant women in many parts of the country, with the progression of the epidemic in the general population, it is bound to rise in women in the reproductive age group and thereby increase the chances of MTCT of HIV infection. Therefore, the challenge for the future is how to keep the prevalence of HIV infection among women low and reduce parent-to-child transmission.

Antiretroviral prophylaxis, preferably in combination therapy or single agent, is recommended for all pregnant women with HIV-1 infection with careful and regular monitoring of the pregnancy and potential toxicities. Still the challenge remaining for the future is to find the most cost-effective and feasible intervention to achieve 0% transmission of HIV from an infected mother to her child.

Postexposure (occupational) prophylaxis in the form of combination antiretrovirals (TDF+FTC+LPV/r) is being increasingly used in India. The role of male circumcision to prevent HIV transmission from female to male is not being given due importance so far, and needs multicentric study in India. However there are a significant number of HIV-infected patients who have already been circumcised during infancy on religious grounds creating a cost-effective role of a mass campaign for male circumcision.

28.7 Pediatric AIDS

Pediatric HIV infection and AIDS is not adequately studied in India [36]. This is possibly due to emphasis on adult HIV disease in the initial stages of the HIV epidemic and lack of awareness, proper diagnostic facilities, and care rendered to the pediatric population in India. However, with the increased incidence of HIV cases due to parent-to-child transmission, parenteral transmission by contaminated blood, and intravenous drug abuse in adolescents, there is urgent need to study epidemiology, clinical profile, and natural course of HIV disease in the Indian pediatric population. Nevertheless, a few isolated case reports, smaller studies and personal experiences are invaluable to form an opinion about pediatric HIV disease in India.

Perinatal transmission remains the most common mode of acquiring HIV infection (82%) with an estimated risk of vertical transmission of 30–40% in HIV-infected mothers. As with pediatric HIV worldwide, perinatal transmission is affected by the mother's disease status, the route of delivery, maternal hemorrhage and infection, duration of rupture of membranes, and postnatal feeding practices.

After acquiring the disease perinatally, up to 25% develop symptoms in the first year of life in the form of opportunistic infections and neurodevelopmental disease indicating rapid progression. This is manifested clinically in the form of lymphadenopathy, hepatosplenomegaly, lymphocytic parotitis, and lymphoid interstitial pneumonia in early pediatric HIV disease.

In a 2-year Indian study of the clinical profile of HIV infection in children, symptomatic cases had protein-energy malnutrition (90%), fever>1 month (50%), weight loss>1 month (50%), persistent generalized lymphadenopathy (24%), and skin manifestations (79%). The gastrointestinal (62%) and respiratory (52%) were the most commonly involved organ systems.

Relatively immature immune systems and high viral load acquired perinatally exposes infants and children to a variety of bacterial, fungal, viral, and parasitic opportunistic infections. Among opportunistic infections, pulmonary tuberculosis is especially common in India. Recurrent bacterial infections of the skin of staphylococcal and streptococcal origin like impetigo, furunculosis, ecthyma, cellulitis, etc. usually occur early at 3–4 years. Candidiasis of the mucosa (oral, vulvovaginal, perianal) and intertriginous areas is more common in HIV-infected children in the intermediate stage of HIV disease especially when antibacterial usage is rampant. After a review of the literature, none of the studies from different parts of India have reported dermatophytosis or deep fungal infections in children. Viral infections usually develop during the intermediate stage of HIV infection commonly at 5 years. Recurrent herpetic gingivostomatitis (more than two episodes in a year), varicella infections, extensive and confluent molluscum contagiosum, as well as multiple viral warts are commonly seen viral infections of the skin. Up to 20% of children with chickenpox can develop complications like pneumonia, meningoencephalitis, severe skin lesions, and recurrence. Multidermatomal, ophthalmic, or recurrent herpes zoster in older children should raise a suspicion of HIV disease. HSV bronchitis or esophagitis is more common in neonates born to mothers with genital herpes infection.

Among systemic opportunistic infections, disseminated tuberculosis affecting the central nervous system and gastrointestinal system, recurrent lower respiratory tract infections, diarrhea due to *Salmonella, Shigella, Campylobacter* spp., *Giardia lamblia, and Entamoeba histolytica* are common. Although tuberculosis is less prevalent in children as compared to the adult HIV population, it is more common as compared to the non-HIV pediatric population in India. A common age for the presentation for tuberculosis is 2–5 years, and tuberculous pneumonitis is common as compared to cavitary disease. For the similar reason, diagnosis by routine sputum examination for AFB becomes difficult in HIV children, and chest radiography is an easier, cost-effective, and reliable option. Cutaneous TB like scrofuloderma is more common in Indian children infected with HIV but other forms like lupus vulgaris, TB chancre, tuberculids, etc. are definitely uncommon. The Mantoux test, a test of limited value in an endemic country like India, is nevertheless useful for diagnosis of progressive primary infection. Induration of more than 5 mm is considered as a positive Mantoux test in HIV-infected children. In children with protein energy malnutrition and those with advanced disease, the test may be false negative.

Diagnostic facilities provided under the voluntary counseling and testing centre (VCTC) and prevention of parent–child transmission (PPTCT) are now remodeled as Integrated Counselling and Testing Centers (ICTC). Currently, 4,000 ICTCs are spread across India and NACP III intends to expand testing sites to 5,000 and establish another 10,000 in the coming years. Currently, enzyme-linked immunosorbent assay (ELISA) is the standard screening test employed for the diagnosis of HIV infection. Unlike in the past, the test done with at least three different kits (third-generation ELISA) is required to make the diagnosis. The "Duo test," a combination of P24 antigen assay and ELISA test, is available in India and is popular among some physicians. However, in institutional settings, P24 antigen assay and Western blot test have become uncommon practices. During the window period and in neonates borne to seropositive mothers, qualitative HIV-DNA PCR has become the gold standard. However, the test is expensive, requires expertise, and has a risk of false positivity due to contamination. Other tests like indirect immunofluorescence, radioimmuno-precipitation tests, and latex agglutination tests are only of historical importance.

28.8 Summary

Acquired immunodeficiency syndrome or AIDS caused by human immunodeficiency virus (HIV) is a major public health problem in India, contributing to a significant negative impact on socioeconomic indicators. According to estimates released by the National AIDS Control Organization (NACO), UNAIDS, and WHO, the prevalence of HIV in the adult population is 2–3.1 million people. This high prevalence provides a large dormant group of patients that keeps the disease smoldering in the community. Also, the low socioeconomic and educational status of the at-risk groups makes them completely ignorant of the risk and propagates poor health-seeking behavior. Consequently, clinical assistance is sought only at a later stage in the disease evolution or when the patient is symptomatic. This lack of awareness forms the most formidable challenge to public health professionals and to the government. Promotion of health-seeking behavior, safe sex, and removal of stigma associated with the disease are the first steps that are required to improve the disease burden.

The clinical profile of HIV infection in India is also different as compared to the Western world. As in other countries of the developing world, opportunistic infections form the major cause of symptoms. Tuberculosis in its protean manifestations, especially extrapulmonary disease is the commonest OI in adults. It forms a significant cause of mortality and morbidity in pediatric disease as well. Management of HIV–TB coinfection requires intricate knowledge of drug interactions. This is important since nevirapine is one of the first line drugs provided by the government and has extensive interaction with antituberculous agents. Thorough clinical, microbiologic, and radiographic examination is a must to rule out TB, before initiating ART. Also, counseling of the patient and close relatives is extremely essential to ensure adherence with the drug regimen. The patient has to be given a fair idea of the adverse effect profile and drug–food interactions to ensure optimal drug delivery and viricidal effect. Emotional and psychological support of the patient goes a long way in ensuring complete compliance. At every opportunity, the clinician has to emphasize the importance of safe sex (especially in discordant couples), drug adherence, and health-seeking behavior.

Finally, the main focus of public health intervention should be directed at the vulnerable population groups, i.e., women and children. Due to gender discrimination and patriarchal societal attitudes, these most vulnerable groups are also the most overlooked, due to ignorance and poverty. Any health program created without factoring in the very special and specific needs of this group is bound to be a waste of time, money, and good intentions, besides being a colossal mistake on HIV disease control. Any clinician attending to a HIV-infected patient should give due importance to the status of the spouse, and any affected offspring.

The continuing research on antiretroviral drugs and the development of new agents such as the integrase inhibitors and chemokine antagonists provide hope for the future. Ensuring affordable medication in the form of generic molecules, and discovery of reliable and effective vaccines are the specific challenges facing researchers and clinicians in the developing world. Until that time, increasing awareness and promoting health-seeking behavior form the bedrock of HIV control in India.

Take-Home Pearls

- The public needs more education regarding protection against HIV as well as education regarding the signs and symptoms of AIDS
- Patients need to practice safer sex, including use of condoms
- Intravenous drug users should seek therapy for their addiction and not reuse needles
- All pregnant women should be tested for HIV and should be offered antiretroviral therapy if positive, in order to decrease transmission to their infants
- Persons at any risk for HIV should be tested regularly
- Persons with AIDS should be encouraged to seek therapy, not only for HIV, but also for opportunistic infections
- Because tuberculosis (TB) is a leading cause of death in patients with HIV in India, better control of TB would greatly improve morbidity and mortality
- Some opportunistic infections and cancers, e.g. Kaposi's sarcoma, are less common in Indian AIDS patients than in other parts of the world, but cutaneous manifestations of TB may be more common and need to be recognized as a possible sign of AIDS
- In order to decrease the spread of HIV, other sexually transmitted diseases need to be diagnosed and treated;
- All blood products need to be tested before they are used;
- Malnutrition and poverty in India significantly worsen the morbidity and mortality of AIDS and need to be addressed as part of the problem
- Many generic antiretroviral drugs are available in India, which decreases their price, thus increasing their availability, but more potential patients need testing, counseling and therapy

References

1. Marfatia, Y.S., Sharma, A., Modi, M.: Overview of HIV/AIDS in India. Indian J. Sex Transm. Dis. **28**, 1–5 (2007)
2. Health minister launches third phase of NACP, Friday 6 July 2007. Ministry of Health and Family Welfare. http://pib.nic.in/release/release.asp?relid=29036 (Cited 10 July 2007)
3. Rubsamen-Waigmann, H., Briesen, H.V., Maniar, J.K., Rao, P.K., Scholz, C., Pfutzner: Spread of HIV-2 in India. Lancet **337**, 550–551 (1991)
4. Andersson, S., Norrgren, H., da Silva, Z., Biague, A., Bamba, S., Kwok, S., Christopherson, C., Biberfeld, G., Albert, J.: Plasma viral load in HIV-1 and HIV-2 singly and dually infected individuals in Guinea-Bissau, West Africa: significantly lower plasma virus set point in HIV-2 infection than in HIV-1 infection. Arch. Intern. Med. **160**(21), 3286–3293 (27 Nov 2000)
5. Fauci, A.S., Lane, H.C.: Human Immunodeficiency Virus (HIV) disease. In: Braunwald, E., Fauci, A.S., Kasper, D.L. (eds.) Harrison's Principles of Internal Medicine, 15th edn, pp. 1852–1913. McGraw-Hill, New York (2001)
6. Joint United Nations Programme on HIV/AIDS (UNAIDS): Report on the Global HIV/AIDS Epidemic, Geneva (Dec 2002)
7. Fauci, A.S.: Host factors and the pathogenesis of HIV-induced disease. Nature **384**, 529 (1996)
8. Vittinghoff, E., et al.: Per-contact risk of human immunodeficiency virus transmission between male sexual partners. Am. J. Epidemiol. **150**, 306 (1999)
9. Padian, N.S., et al.: Heterosexual transmission of human immunodeficiency virus (HIV) in Northern California: Results from a ten-year study. Am. J. Epidemiol. **146**, 350 (1997)
10. Centers for Disease Control and Prevention: HIV/AIDS Surveillance Rep. 1999 **11**(2), 1 (2000)
11. Sewankambo, N., et al.: HIV-1 infection associated with abnormal vaginal flora morphology and bacterial vaginosis. Lancet **350**, 546 (1997)
12. Halperin, D.T., Bailey, R.C.: Male circumcision and HIV infection: 10 years and counting. Lancet **354**, 1813 (1999)
13. Centers for Disease Control and Prevention: Public Health Service guidelines for the management of health-care worker exposures to HIV and recommendations for postexposure prophylaxis. MMWR **47**(RR-7), 1 (1998)
14. Landesman, S.H., et al.: Obstetrical factors and the transmission of human immunodeficiency virus type 1 from mother to child. N. Engl. J. Med. **334**, 1617 (1997)
15. Garcia, P., et al.: Maternal level of plasma human immunodeficiency virus type 1 RNA and the risk of perinatal transmission. N. Engl. J. Med. **341**, 394 (1999)
16. Miotti, P., et al.: HIV transmission through breast-feeding: a study in Malawi. JAMA **212**, 744 (1999)
17. Severson, J.L., Tyring, S.K.: Relation between herpes simplex viruses and human immunodeficiency virus infections. Arch. Dermatol. **135**(11), 1393–1397 (1999)
18. Gulick, R.M., Heath-Chiozzi, M., Crumpacker, C.S.: Varicella-zoster virus disease in patients with human immunodeficiency virus infection. Arch. Dermatol. **126**(8), 1086–1088 (1990)
19. Resnick, L., Herbst, J.S., Raab-Traub, N.: Oral hairy leukoplakia. J. Am. Acad. Dermatol. **22**(6 Pt 2), 1278–1282 (1990)
20. Rajagopalan, B., Jacob, M., George, S.: Skin lesions in HIV-positive and HIV –negative in South India. Int. J. Dermatol. **35**, 489–492 (1996)
21. Kumarasamy, N., Solomon, S., Madhivanan, P., Ravikumar, B., Thyagarajan, S.P., Yesudian, P.: Dermatological manifestations among human immunodeficiency virus patients in South India. Int. J. Dermatol. **39**, 192–195 (2000)
22. Singh, A., Thappa, D.M., Hamide, A.: The spectrum of mucocutaneous manifestations during the evolutionary phases of HIV disease: an emerging Indian scenario. J. Dermatol. **26**, 294–304 (1999)
23. Kumarasamy, N., Vallabhaneni, S., Flanigan, T.P., Mayer, K.H., Solomon, S.: Clinical profile of HIV in India. Indian J. Med. Res. **121**, 377–394 (2005)
24. Chacko, S., John, T.J., Jacob, M., Kaur, A., Mathai, D.: Clinical profile of AIDS in India: a review of 61 cases. JAPI **43**, 535–538 (1995)
25. Maniar, J.K.: The HIV/AIDS epidemic in India - real challenge for Dermatovenereologists in the new millennium. 29th National Conference of IADVL, Agra, 1–4 Feb 2001
26. National AIDS Control Organization (NACO): Antiretroviral Therapy Guidelines for HIV-Infected Adults and Adolescents Including Post-exposure Prophylaxis, May 2007.
27. WHO and HIV/AIDS. http://www.who.int/hiv/en/. Last accessed: 29 Sept 2006
28. Antiretroviral therapy. In: Bartlett, J.G., Gallant, J.E. (eds.) Medical Management of HIV Infection. Johns Hopkins Medicine Health Publishing Business Group, Baltimore (2005–2006)
29. Scaling up antiretroviral therapy in resource limited settings: treatment guidelines for a public health approach, 2003 revision. World Health Organization, Geneva. http://www.who.int/hiv/pub/prev_care/en/arvrevision2003en.pdf (2004)
30. French, M.A., Price, P., Stone, S.F.: Immune restoration disease after antiretroviral therapy. AIDS **18**, 1615–1627 (2004)
31. Surjushe, A.U., Jindal, S.R., Kamath, R.R., Saple, D.G.: Immune reconstitution inflammatory syndrome. Indian J. Dermatol. Venereol. Leprol. **72**, 410–414 (2006)
32. Kharkar, V., Bhor, U.H., Mahajan, S., Khopkar, U.: Type I lepra reaction presenting as immune reconstitution inflammatory syndrome. Indian J. Dermatol. Venereol. Leprol. **73**, 253–256 (2007)
33. Tahir, M., Sharma, S.K., Sinha, S., Das, C.J.: Immune reconstitution inflammatory syndrome in a patient with cryptococcal lymphadenitis as the first presentation of acquired immunodeficiency syndrome. J. Postgrad. Med. **53**, 250–252 (2007)
34. Maniar, J.K.: Antiretroviral therapy: Need for a long-term view. Indian J. Dermatol. Venereol. Leprol. **72**, 401–404 (2006)
35. Guidelines for the prevention of mother to child transmission of HIV. National AIDS Control Organisation. http://www.nacoonline.org/guidelines/guideline_9.pdf
36. Shah, S.R., Tullu, M.S., Kamat, J.R.: Clinical profile of pediatric HIV infection from India. Arch. Med. Res. **36**, 24–31 (2005)

HIV in Africa

29

Lutz G. Gürtler

Core Messages

- AIDS is a zoonotic disease, caused by HIV-1, which originates from chimpanzees (*Pan troglodytes troglodytes*), and by HIV-2 from sooty mangabey monkeys (*Cercopithecus atys*).
- At least 12 separate events of transmission of these viruses to humans, most probably by blood, during the last 2 decades before its description in 1981–1983, can be estimated.
- Now AIDS is a human disease, mainly transmitted by sexual intercourse and contaminated blood, and until a vaccine is found, HIV will persist in the human population.

29.1 History

Three aspects dominate, with respect to HIV in Africa:

First: The heterogeneity of the population in the continent that may be roughly divided in HIV epidemiological terms into a population of northern Africa with a predominantly Arabic, Semitic, Berber, and Nilotic population. In this region, HIV is transmitted by heterosexual and homosexual intercourse, by drug consumption, and occasionally by blood transfusion and blood-contaminated medical equipment. Prevalence of HIV is low compared to sub-Saharan Africa. Availability of epidemiological data is partially restricted. This chapter deals mainly with the second aspect.

Second: Sub-Saharan Africa has a mixed population of mainly Bantu, Pygmies (rare), Khoisan, and others, such as Bushmen, Masai, etc. in which HIV is transmitted mainly by heterosexual contact, rarely by blood transfusion and contaminated medical equipment, and exceptionally by drug consumption.

Third: The evolution of humans started in Africa, as known from anthropologic studies and conserved human skulls and bones in East Africa and southern Africa, which suggest that most probably humans settled quickly in the whole central and southern continent. Evolution of primates started some 35 million years ago, that of humans by diverging from the common lineage with chimpanzees some 5–7 million years ago; humans kept company with the evolution of apes and monkeys, living in the neighborhood of these animals, also eating them. Humans in tropical Africa suffered from various zoonotic infectious diseases, such as malaria and yellow fever, leukemia induced by human T cell lymphotropic virus (HTLV) and a number of other infectious diseases, which killed part of the population. Yellow fever virus is an excellent example to show that man was, and still is, susceptible to infectious agents that evolved in, and adapted to, monkeys. The example of yellow fever virus demonstrates that the similar genetic background of man and monkey facilitates the transfer of other viruses, such as the immunodeficiency virus, from chimpanzees (SIVcpz) to man and gorilla (SIVgor), the topic that is discussed in this chapter. [1].

Survival of the various tribes in sub-Saharan Africa was governed by the number of members and their offspring, and thus the European Christian rules that

L.G. Gürtler
Max von Pettenkofer Institute of the University München, Pettenkofer Str 9A, D-80336, Munich, Germany and Spitzlberger Str 10, D-82166, Graefelfing, Germany
e-mail: lutzg.guertler@vodafone.de

G. Gross and S.K. Tyring (eds.), *Sexually Transmitted Infections and Sexually Transmitted Diseases*,
DOI: 10.1007/978-3-642-14663-3_29, © Springer-Verlag Berlin Heidelberg 2011

equated morality with monogamy was not a priority of people under pressure to survive. This liberty might be one of the reasons why sexually transmitted diseases (STD) still spread quickly in certain areas of Africa.

Human immunodeficiency virus (HIV) was recognized as an epidemiologically relevant, new infectious disease in 1981 [2]. At that time, HIV had already been spreading in central Africa for at least 2 decades, perhaps longer [3, 4]. Old descriptions from missionary colonial medical doctors' accounts describe the clinical symptoms of malaria, yellow fever, sleeping sickness, leprosy, and other diseases very well, so today the underlying infectious agent can easily be linked. Descriptions of the typical symptoms of AIDS with aggressive Kaposi sarcoma and wasting (slim disease being the African expression) from that time are lacking [5]. In conclusion, HIV is a further example of how a new human infectious agent, which is mainly transmitted by sexual contact, can be distributed worldwide.

29.2 HIV Groups and Subtypes

The animal reservoir of HIV-1 is the lentivirus simian immunodeficiency virus (SIV) from chimpanzees (SIVcpz), with several transfers within the different chimpanzee populations, *Pan troglodytes troglodytes* and also from this species to *Pan troglodytes schweinfurthii* [6]. The animal reservoir for HIV-2 is the sooty mangabey monkey and its subspecies that live in West Africa. The four chimpanzee species, *Pan troglodytes troglodytes*, *Pan troglodytes schweinfurthii*, and *Pan troglodytes verus*, which is found mainly in West Africa, had been separated by the big rivers in Central Africa, allowing the diversification of SIVcpz in *Pan troglodytes troglodytes* and finally in *Pan troglodytes schweinfurthii* in Central Africa. Only in the last few decades has the transmission of these adapted viruses to humans happened. There have been at least four transmissions of HIV-1 – group M to P – and probably eight for HIV-2,– group A to H. From the heterogeneity of group M subtypes, it can be estimated that at least 50 independent transmission events might have occurred.

The route of this transmission has been discussed: eating monkey meat is a less probable route as humans have been eating monkeys for more than a thousand years, and transmission could not have taken till only 2 decades ago to happen. Sexual intercourse with monkeys is only theoretical and it is hard to link it with human sexual behavior, especially in sub-Saharan Africa. More probable is the transfer by blood, be it by biting, or fighting with a pet animal or as a paramedical application to increase libido [7].

After transmission from chimpanzees, the divergence of HIV in man has continued, due to the high mutation rate of HIV during transcription (1 in 10.000) and by the selection pressure of the host immune system.

HIV is divided in two types, HIV-1 and HIV-2. HIV-1 is the most prevalent type; especially, HIV-1 group M is transmitted more efficiently by sexual contact compared to the other HIVs.

29.2.1 *HIV-1*

HIV-1 is divided in four groups: M, N, O and P [9, 10]. Group M is subdivided into subtypes and recombinants – circulating recombinant form (CRF). Recombination is a frequent event in HIV replication. It occurs when one cell is infected with two HIVs. Recombination takes place between all groups of HIV-1; the SIVcpz from *Pan troglodytes schweinfurthii* has evolved by recombination as well [6]. Recombinants like CRF A/E have spread very efficiently after transfer from Central Africa for example to Thailand. Until now recombinants between HIV-1 and HIV-2 have not been found; theoretically this mode of recombination is possible.

Group M: Among the four groups, group M viruses are the most pathogenic. Till date, only HIV-1 group M (HIV-1 M) is subdivided into subtypes A to K, among which E and I are missing as these are recombinants. In group M, subtype C is most efficiently transmitted by heterosexual contact in southern Africa [11]. Some modes of behavior seem to influence subtype transmission as well [12]. Since most of the presently available antiretroviral drugs are designed and checked for efficacy for HIV-1 M subtype B infected, failure of antiretroviral treatment might occur in patients carrying non-B subtypes.

Group N: This rare virus is to date prevalent only in Cameroon. According to recent knowledge, some 20 patients infected with group N virus have been identified. Group N virus is more close to group M than to group O.

Group O: Most of the group O-infected patients have been found in Cameroon, where the prevalence is declining in contrast to the rise of group M viruses.

Nucleic acid sequencing studies of various group O strains show a similar heterogeneity as in group M virus, but classification of subtypes is pending. Non-nucleoside reverse transcriptase inhibitors (NNRTI) are inefficient in inhibiting group O virus replication. The oldest-reported human HIV infection in Europe (Norway) in 1966 was caused by group O virus [13].

Group P: This virus was identified only in 2009. Origin is Cameroon and there has only one female patient been reported from the capital Yaounde with symptoms of AIDS, carrying this virus [10]. Thus prevalence seems to be very low. Group P virus is more close to O than to M, and evolutionary linked to SIVgor (see Sect. 29.1).

Modern diagnostic screening tests, that are used in Europe, detect all HIV-1 and HIV-2 by serology and all HIV-1 by nucleic acid testing.

29.2.2 HIV-2

HIV-2 has its origin in sooty mangabey monkeys (*Cercopithecus atys*) in West Africa. In humans, eight groups, formerly named subtypes, have been identified; among these, group A and B are the most common, while the others are rare. HIV-2 is primarily prevalent in West Africa, with higher prevalences in Mozambique and former Goa (Velha Goa) in India. In Guinea Bissau, where the HIV-2 prevalence was high at the beginning of the AIDS epidemic in 1985, HIV-1 group M has a higher prevalence today [14], indicating that HIV-2 was dominated by HIV-1 group M. HIV-2 is seldom transmitted from mother to child during pregnancy and delivery. HIV-2 causes AIDS, but usually only after 15 years, a period that is compared to the 10 years of HIV-1 prolonged. The reason for the lower pathogenicity of HIV-2 is still unknown.

Most of the drugs developed for the inhibition of HIV-1 replication are ineffective for growth inhibition of HIV-2.

29.3 Sexual HIV Transmission

Transmission of HIV is facilitated in the presence of other infectious diseases, especially when they are associated with ulcerative lesions of the genital mucosa [15] – there is no specialty of sexual transmission in Africa. The higher the viral load in the genital tract, the more easily HIV is transmitted [16].

29.4 Coinfections

Typical genital coinfections in African countries are chlamydia, gonorrhea, *Treponema pallidum*, and *Herpes simplex virus* type 2 some less frequent agents as *Haemophilus ducreyi*, *Klebsiella granulomatosis*, and HTLV-1. HTLV-1 is a well-known retrovirus that is transmitted commonly in Africa [17], and which can accelerate the deterioration of the immune function in the HIV-infected.

29.4.1 Tuberculosis

The most common severe coinfection in HIV-infected African patients is still tuberculosis. Mycobacteria are transmitted by the respiratory route and not by sexual intercourse, but since there is close contact, mycobacteria are transmitted as well. In the-HIV infected with minor immunodeficiency, open tuberculosis can be caused by reactivation of mycobacteria acquired during early childhood or by a newly acquired infection. Rates might be as high as 20% [18], and sub-Saharan Africa is the worst affected region in the world [8]. Treatment of mycobacteria is partially complicated by spread of multidrug-resistant strains that occur in all African countries [19] and are highly underreported [20].

29.5 Epidemiology of HIV in Africa

The oldest HIV containing blood samples originate from 1959 and 1960 from two stored specimens in Congo-Kinshasa. Both viruses are typically structured as SIVcpz [4] and so divergent that they most probably were introduced at that time from two different chimpanzees. The conclusion is that the HIV epidemic had started before 1960 in sub-Saharan Africa. Without a diagnostic assay and without knowledge of the symptoms of the disease and its identification there was no way of preventing the HIV transmission.

Prevalence of HIV and AIDS rose continuously from 1980 to 1990 in various African countries, with the highest prevalences of HIV-1 in Central Africa and of HIV-2 in West Africa. At the end of 2008, around 22.4 million people living with HIV/AIDS were reported to WHO (UNAIDS, report 2009), of whom 1.9 million had been infected and 1.4 million had died in 2008. The estimated general prevalence of HIV in sub-Saharan Africa was calculated to be approximately 5%. In countries like South Africa, Lesotho, and Botswana, prevalence in the sexually active urban population is estimated to be between 25% and 35% (www.who.int/whosis; http://data.unaids.org/2007 update and 2009 update), see Fig. 29.1, with a recent tendency to decline.

Since the beginning of reports of the AIDS epidemic, sub-Saharan Africa has had the highest burden of the AIDS disease worldwide, and this trend will not change in the coming years. In conclusion, people who enjoy having sexual contacts in Africa have a greater possibility of acquiring HIV and should be tested when there is any suspicion of transmission.

29.6 Outcome

There have been and there are a number of efforts being made to reduce HIV transmission in African countries, and in several other countries, for example, in Uganda, HIV prevalence has decreased. In the southern African countries, the HIV epidemic started later than in Central Africa; in these countries, the prevalence is very high (Fig. 29.2), and efforts to reduce HIV transmission has partially been hampered by political rulers.

Mankind has never lost an infectious agent transmitted by sexual contact including bacteria that might very easily be eradicated by appropriate antibiotic treatment. In conclusion HIV, both HIV-1 and HIV-2,

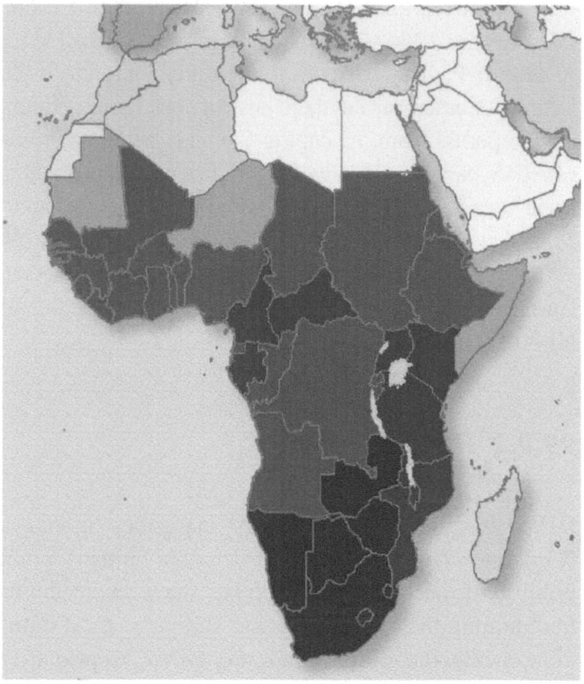

Fig. 29.2 Prevalence of HIV in Africa. The darker the colour, the higher the prevalence – it can easily be seen that southern African countries are the most severely affected. The dark colour corresponds to prevalence in adults: of 15–28% (The figure is taken from AIDS epidemic update 2009 [http://data.unaids.org/2009update])

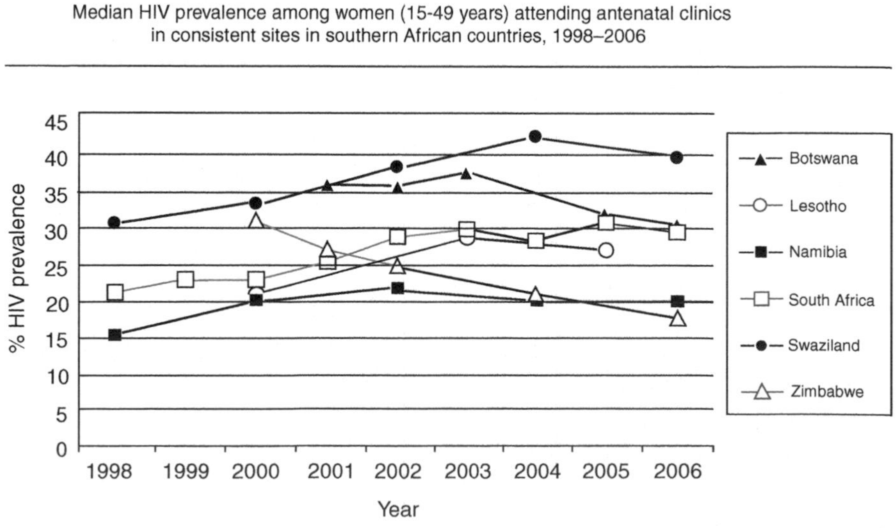

Fig. 29.1 Kinetic of the HIV prevalence in six southern African countries affected severely by the AIDS epidemic from 1999 to 2006 (The figure is taken from UNAIDS report 2007 [http://data.unaids.org/2007update])

will persist in humans despite the antiretroviral treatment, which is now available in most urban centers in sub-Saharan Africa. Diagnostic tests to measure CD4 cell count and viral load have been implemented by the Gates Foundation in recent years. This treatment however is limited by selection of resistant strains and by persistence of HIV in sanctuary sites in the organism.

From a long-term perspective, possibly some 1,000 years later, humans will adapt to the pathogenic action of HIV as has been the case in chimpanzees and in the other monkeys infected with similar lentiviruses.

Take-Home Pearls

› Risky sexual behavior will transmit HIV, especially in countries with a high prevalence. African subtypes of HIV-1 group M and the other groups might cause diagnostic and antiretroviral treatment problems. HIV will continue to be transmitted to human beings regardless of sex, age, ethnicity, and education.

Abbreviations

Cpz	Chimpanzee
CRF	Circulating recombinant form
Gor	Gorilla
HIV	Human immunodeficiency virus
HTLV-1	Human T cell lymphotropic virus type 1
NNRTI	Non-nucleoside reverse transcriptase inhibitors
SIV	Simian immunodeficiency virus

References

1. Takehisa, J., Kraus, M.H., Ayouba, A., Bailes, E., Van Heuverswyn, F., Decker, J.M., Li, Y., Rudicell, R.S., Learn, G.H., Neel, C., Mpoudi Ngole, E., Shaw, G.M., Peeters, M., Sharp, P.M., Hahn, B.H.: Origin and biology of simian immunodeficiency virus in wild-living western gorillas. J. Virol. **83**, 1635–1648 (2009)
2. Gottlieb, M.D., Schroff, R., Schanker, H.M., Weissman, J.D., Fan, P.T., Wolf, R.A., Saxon, A.: Pneumocystis carinii pneumonia and mucosal candidiasis in previously healthy homosexual men. N. Engl. J. Med. **305**, 1425–1431 (1981)
3. Woodman, Z., Williamson, C.: HIV molecular epidemiology: transmission and adaptation to human populations. Curr. Opin. HIVAIDS **4**, 247–252 (2009)
4. Worobey, M., Gemmel, M., Teuwen, D.E., Haselkorn, T., Kunstman, K., Bunce, M., Myembe, J.J., Kabongo, J.M., Kalengayi, R.M., van Marck, E., Gilbert, M.T., Wolinsky, S.M.: Direct evidence of extensive diversity of HIV-1 in Kinshasa by 1960. Nature **455**, 661–664 (2008)
5. Colven, R.: 25 years of HV/AIDS: a dermatologist epidemic watcher's perspective. Dermatol. Clin. **24**, 407–412 (2006)
6. Leitner, T., Dazza, M.C., Ekwalanga, M., Apetrei, C., Saragosti, S.: Sequence diversity among chimpanzee simian immunodeficiency virus (SIVcpz) suggests that SIVcpzPts was derived from SIVcpzPtt through additional recombination events. AIDS Res. Human Retroviruses **23**, 1114–1118 (2007)
7. Kashamura, A.: Famille, sexualité et culture. Payot, Paris
8. Lawn SD, Churchyard G. Epidemiology of HIV-associated tuberculosis (2009). Curr. Opin. HIV AIDS **4**, 325–333 (1973)
9. Neel, C., Etienne, L., Li, Y., Takehisa, J., Rudicell, R.S., Bass, I.N., Moudindo, J., Mebenga, A., Esteban, A., Van Heuverswyn, F., Liegois, F., Kranzusch, P.J., Walsh, P.D., Sanz, C.M., Morgan, D.B., Ndjango, J.B.N., Plantier, J.C., Locatelli, S., Gonder, M.K., Leendertz, F.H., Boesch, C., Todd, A., Delaporte, E., Mpoudi-Ngole, E., Hahn, B.H., Peeters, M.: Molecular epidemiology of simian immunodeficiency virus infection in wild-living gorillas. J. Virol. **84**, 1464–1476 (2010)
10. Plantier, J.C., Leoz, M., Dickerson, J.E., De Oliviera, F., Cordonnier, F., Lemée, V., Damond, F., Robertson, D.L., Simon, F.: A new human immunodeficiency virus derived from gorillas. Nat. Med. **15**, 871–872 (2009)
11. Tebit, D.M., Nankya, I., Arts, E.J., Goa, Y.: HIV diversity, recombination and disease progression: how does fitness "fit" into the puzzle? AIDS Rev. **9**, 75–87 (2007)
12. Morison, L., Buvé, A., Zekeng, L., Hendrickx, L., Anagonou, S., Musonda, R., Kahindo, M., Weiss, H.A., Hayes, R.L., Laga, M., Janssens, W., von der Groen, G.: HIV-1 subtypes and the HIV epidemics in four cities in sub-Saharan Africa. AIDS **15**(suppl 4), S109–S116 (2001)
13. Frøland, S.S., Jenum, P., Lindboe, C.F., Wefring, K.W., Linnestad, P.J., Böhmer, T.: HIV infection in Norwegian family before 1970. Lancet **i**, 144–1345 (1988)
14. Da Silva, Z.J., Oliviera, I., Andersen, A., Dias, F., Rodrigues, A., Holmgren, B., Andersson, S., Aaby, P.: Changes in prevalence and incidence of HIV-1, HIV-2 and dual infections in urban areas of Bissau, Guinea Bissau: is HIV-2 disappearing ? AIDS **19**, 1195–1202 (2008)
15. Johnson, L.F., Lewis, D.A.: The effect of genital tract infections on HIV-1 shedding in the genital tract: a systematic review and meta-analysis. Sex. Transm. Dis. **35**, 946–959 (2008)
16. Attia, S., Egger, M., Müller, M., Zwahlen, M., Low, N.: Sexual transmission of HIV according to viral load and antiretroviral therapy: systematic review and meta-analysis. AIDS **23**, 397–404 (2009)
17. Verdonck, K., Gonzalez, E., Van Dooren, S., Vandamme, A.M., Vanham, G., Goluzzo, E.: Human T-lymphotropic virus 1: recent knowledge about an ancient infection. Lancet Infect. Dis. **7**, 266–281 (2007)
18. Glynn, J.R., Murray, J., Bester, A., Nelson, G., Shearer, S., Sonnenberg, P.: High rates of recurrence in HIV-infected and HIV-uninfected patients with tuberculosis. J. Infect. Dis. **201**, 704–711 (2010)

19. Miotti, P., Saleri, N., Dembelé, M., Ouedraogo, M., Badoum, G., Pinsi, G., Migliori, G.B., Matteelli, A., Cirillo, D.M.: Molecular detection of rifampicin and isonizid resistance to guide chronic TB patient management in Burkina Faso. BMC Infect. Dis. **9**, 142 (2009)
20. Ben Amor, Y., Nemser, B., Singh, A., Sankin, A., Schluger, N.: Underreported threat of multidrug-resistant tuberculosis in Africa. Emerg. Infect. Dis. **14**, 1345–1352 (2008)

Cutaneous Conditions and HIV in Africa

30

Anisa Mosam and P.N. Naidu

Core Messages

- Sub-Saharan Africa has the highest incidence of HIV/AIDS in the world – approximately 70%.
- Skin disease occurs in 90% of individuals with HIV/AIDS.
- It is the first manifestation of HIV in at least a third of patients.
- Infections are the commonest conditions seen; however, they are more severe and frequently relapse.
- Dermatoses correlate with stage of HIV infection; from seroconversion illness through full-blown AIDS.
- As the CD4 count declines, the number of dermatoses increases and they become more severe.
- Several infectious, inflammatory, and neoplastic conditions are pathognomonic of HIV/AIDS.
- The advent of HAART has decreased the incidence of HIV-related dermatoses.
- Drug reactions and immune reconstitution-related dermatoses are still common in the era of HAART.
- Identification of dermatoses is important in monitoring HIV progression and the success of HAART.

A. Mosam (✉)
Department of Dermatology, Nelson R Mandela School of Medicine, University of KwaZulu-Natal, Rm 327 3rd Floor Medical School, Congella, Private Bag X 7, 4013 Durban, South Africa
e-mail: mosama@ukzn.ac.za

P.N. Naidu
Department of Dermatology, Nelson R Mandela School of Medicine, University of KwaZulu-Natal, Durban, South Africa

30.1 Introduction

Diseases of the skin and oral mucosa are one of the first barriers to be disrupted in Human Immunodeficiency Virus (HIV) infection and are the sentinel diagnosis for HIV infection in at least 37% [1] of individuals. Skin conditions are notoriously common in HIV infection, affecting 90% of individuals during the course of their illness. As the CD4 count declines and patients progress from HIV infection to AIDS, a number of skin conditions coexist, rashes are more severe and may respond less and relapse more frequently requiring multiple courses of therapy [2–4]. Most conditions are those that occur in the general population, but may be more severe and skin conditions can be used as a surrogate marker of severity of HIV infection. The prevalence of skin conditions increases with a declining CD4 count less than 200 cells/mm^3 [5]. In Africa, the following dermatoses, i.e., Kaposi's sarcoma, palmo-plantar rash, and herpes zoster had positive predictive values for the presence of HIV infection of more than 80% [1].

Cutaneous disorders can be divided into three categories: the infections, which comprise the largest category; inflammatory disorders; and tumors which are present on the skin.

Some of the commonest cutaneous conditions that have been noted to occur in the outpatient setting in Africa are: herpes simplex and zoster, seborrhoeic dermatitis, and papular eruptions [6]. However, the majority of dermatology admissions in order of frequency are: seborrhoeic dermatitis, psoriasis, drug eruptions, and erythroderma [7]. An exhaustive description of the skin conditions that occur in HIV is beyond the scope of this chapter hence our objective is to familiarize the reader with the common, important conditions that will improve the diagnosis and treatment of those with skin disease.

G. Gross and S.K. Tyring (eds.), *Sexually Transmitted Infections and Sexually Transmitted Diseases*,
DOI: 10.1007/978-3-642-14663-3_30,

30.2 Inflammatory Conditions in HIV

A discussion of all the inflammatory conditions that may be due to or exacerbated by HIV infection is beyond the scope of this chapter. We will therefore focus on the commonly seen and important conditions which the reader should have a thorough working knowledge of. These are:

- Seborrhoeic dermatitis
- Papular eruptions
- Pruritus/xerosis
- Photodermatitis
- Psoriasis
- Drug eruptions
- Immune reconstitution inflammatory syndrome

30.2.1 Seborrhoeic Dermatitis (Figs. 30.1–30.3)

This is an eczematous dermatitis and the one inflammatory condition that is the most frequently diagnosed in HIV infection, affecting 24% in the initial stages and 30% with AIDS [8]. It is one of the early skin conditions associated with HIV/AIDS, occurring while CD4 counts are between 200 and 500 cells/mm^3 [9]. It worsens as the CD4 count declines and the disease progresses from HIV infection to AIDS. It tends to be more severe and the onset more abrupt in HIV/AIDS as compared to the condition in healthy individuals[1]. The dermatitis may be subtle initially presenting as it does in nonimmunocompromised individuals, i.e., scaling, erythema, and pruritus involving the greasy areas of the scalp, eyebrows, perinasal areas, and flexures (Fig. 30.1). With more advanced HIV infection, there is more extensive involvement (Fig. 30.2) and may progress to erythroderma (>90% of the body is red and scaly). The flexures and scalp are most severely affected. The scalp is affected with dandruff initially and later is replaced by yellowish greasy crusted scales. In African children, the lesions often heal with postinflammatory hypopigmentation (Fig. 30.3). The flexures (retroauricular, axillae, inframammary folds, and groin) may be erythematous and later weeping and secondary bacterial infection occur and are associated with pain and are malodorous. Secondary herpes virus

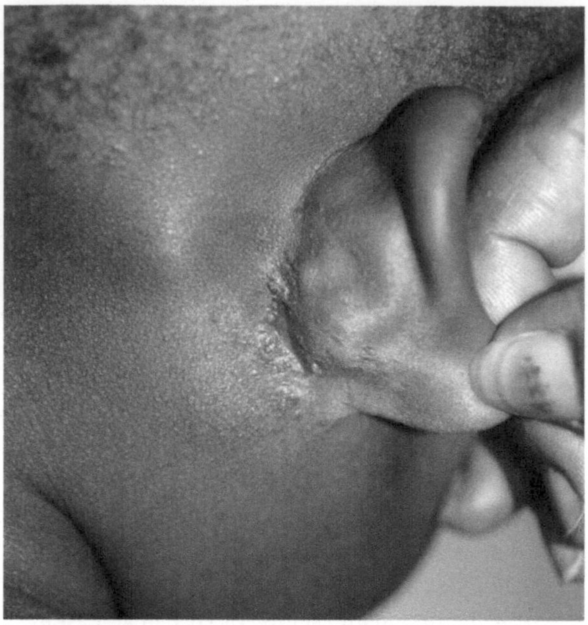

Fig. 30.1 Retroauricular erythema and scaling seen in early seborrhoeic dermatitis

infection may complicate extensive seborrhoeic dermatitis where the skin has been denuded. The dermatitis responds to topical steroid creams, while the scalp can be treated in addition with antidandruff and antifungal shampoos. Preparations containing sulfur and salicylic acid are effective in treating infection and debriding the crusts. *Malassezia* yeasts have been implicated in the pathogenesis of seborrhoeic dermatitis. In cases of extensive and resistant seborrhoeic dermatitis, oral antifungals, such as ketoconazole, itraconazole, and terbinafine, may be beneficial. Essentially, antifungal therapy reduces the number of yeasts on the skin, leading to an improvement in seborrhoeic dermatitis [10]. Symptomatic therapy with antihistamines is sometimes required for severe pruritus. Resistant cases may respond to ultraviolet light therapy, but highly active antiretroviral therapy (HAART) is essential to control the HIV infection and lead to immune restoration.

30.2.2 Papular Eruptions (Figs. 30.4 and 30.5)

Papular eruptions are an umbrella term for the itchy disorders eosinophilic folliculitis (EF) and papular

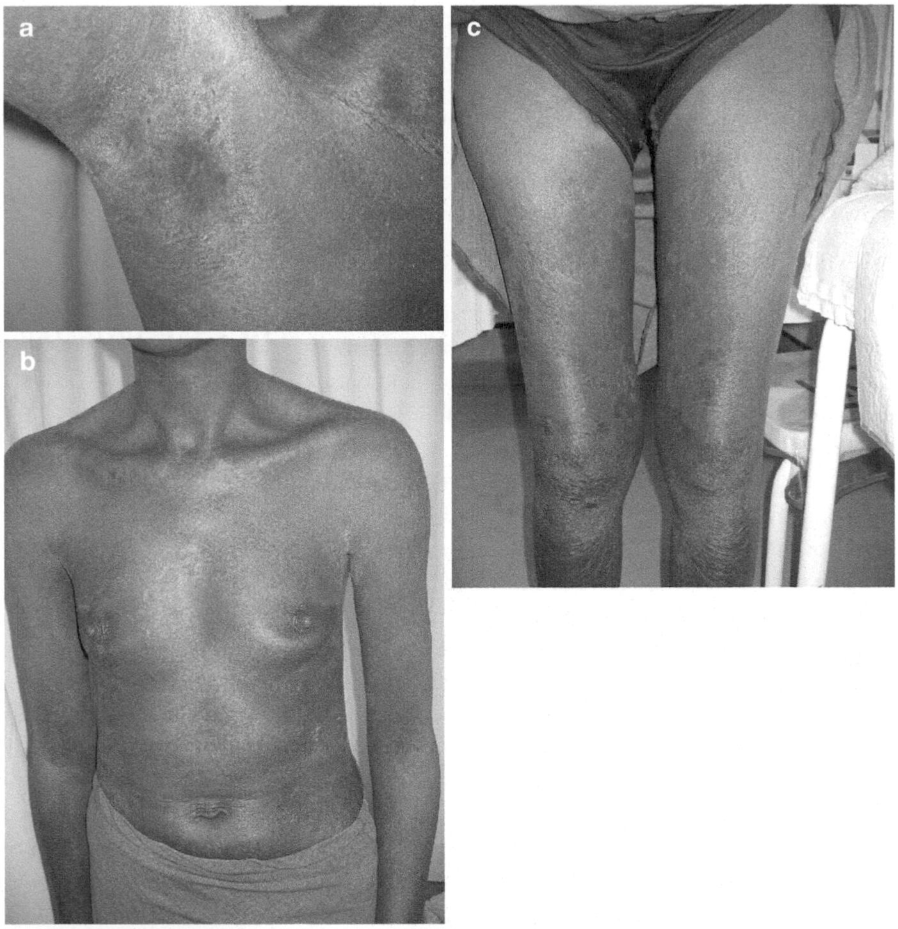

Fig. 30.2 Extensive seborrhoeic dermatitis with erythema and scaling and lichenification involving the flexures (**a**), the trunk and upper limbs (**b**), and the lower limbs (**c**)

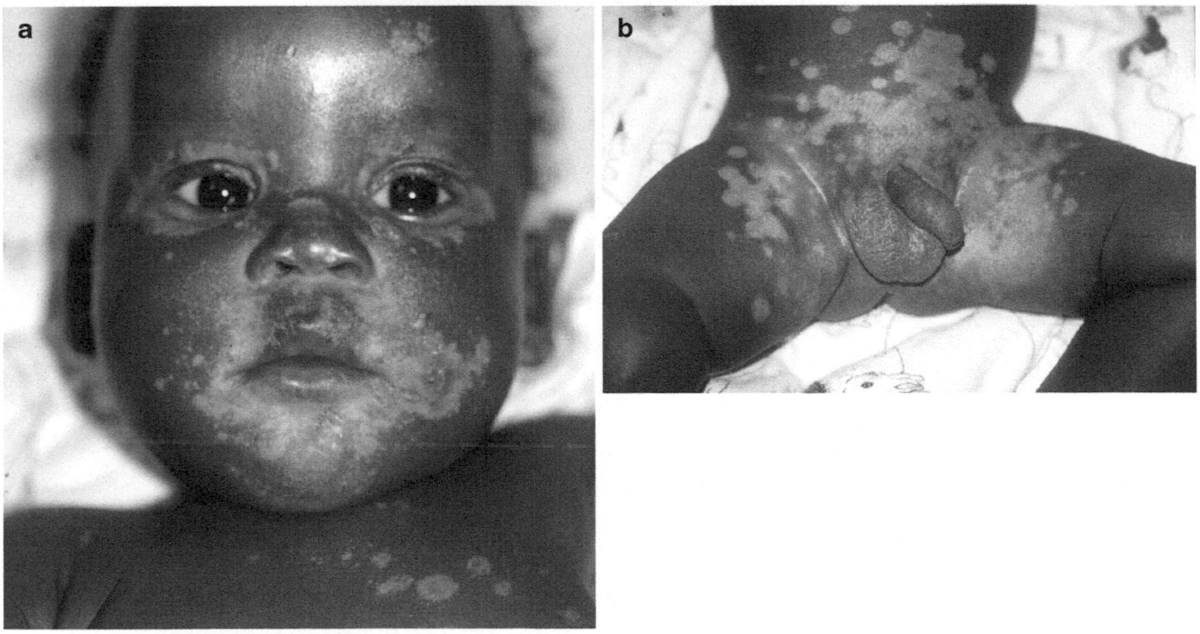

Fig. 30.3 Seborrhoeic dermatitis of the face (**a**) and groin (**b**) healing with hypopigmented macules in children

eruption of retroviral disease (PPE). Various organisms have been implicated in the pathogenesis: *Demodex folliculorum*, *Pityrosporum ovale*, and mites, but none have been conclusively proven. They are a presenting sign of HIV in at least 50% of individuals [11]. Papular eruptions have been associated with more advanced HIV infection, specifically with CD4 counts below 200 cells/mm^3 [9, 12]. The lesions are intensely itchy, folliculocentric, papules usually affecting the face, "V" of the neck, and extensors of upper arms. It can extend to involve the trunk, and upper and lower limbs. However, the web spaces, mucosae, and palms and soles are spared, helping to differentiate it from scabies [13]. The lesions are itchy, erythematous, urticarial papules in the early stage (Fig. 30.4) and subject to constant excoriation heal with postinflammatory hyperpigmentation (Fig. 30.5).

The condition causes great distress to individuals and therapy is symptomatic with oral antihistamines, topical steroids, and emollients. In cases that are not responsive to first-line therapy, oral tetracyclines, metronidazole, and dapsone [14] have been found to be effective on the basis of their anti-inflammatory and antimicrobial properties. Severe cases have warranted short courses of systemic steroids and phototherapy [15, 16].

Papular eruptions occur so frequently in African patients (12–46%) that they have been used as a clinical marker of successful HAART. In a Ugandan study, PPE was scored and correlated with HIV viral loads [17]. Lower PPE scores were associated with HIV viral load clearance and higher scores with failure of first-line HAART. At least 86% had disappearance of PPE within 6 months of initiation of HAART. However, EF has been known to recur as a manifestation of the immune reconstitution syndrome as a result of successful HAART [18].

30.2.3 Pruritus/Xerosis (Fig. 30.6)

Pruritus is a distressing and important symptom of HIV infection, often signifying advanced disease with CD4 counts below 50 cells/mm^3 [19–21]. It can be a manifestation of systemic disease, i.e., nutritional disorders, liver and renal impairment, and lymphoma. Most commonly, it is a manifestation of concurrent cutaneous disease, either infections like scabies, insect bites, or tinea or inflammatory conditions like papular eruptions, eczemas, or drug reactions. Hence, one should be vigilant for underlying systemic and concurrent skin conditions in the management of pruritus associated with HIV and a test for HIV should be included in the workup of any patient with pruritus.

However, idiopathic or HIV-associated pruritus has been recognized as an entity and is the development of intractable pruritus due to immune dysregulation and overgrowth of *Staphylococcus aureus* and *Demodex*

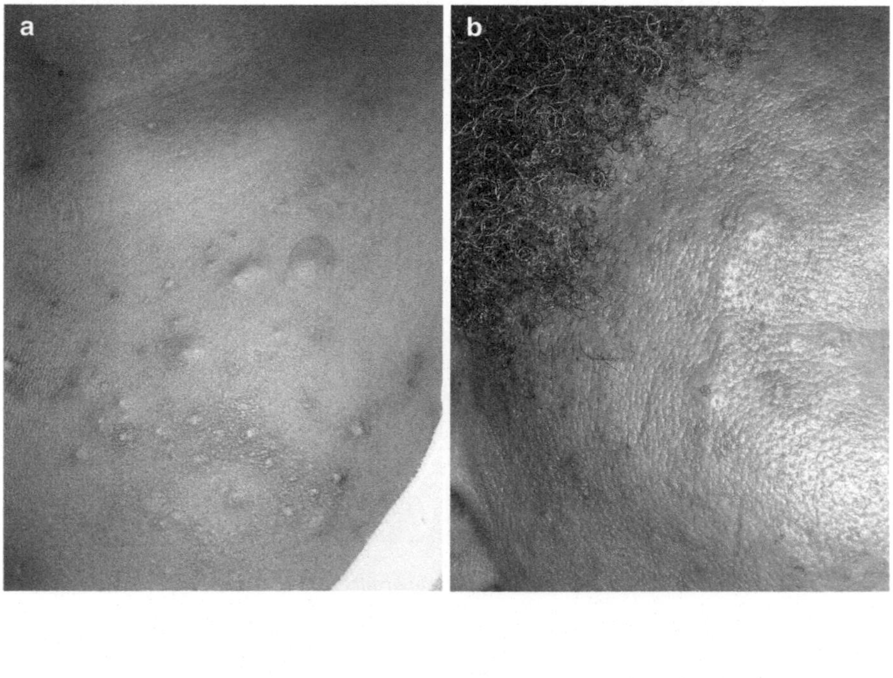

Fig. 30.4 The early lesions are erythematous, urticarial wheals involving the face (**a**) and "V" of the neck (**b**)

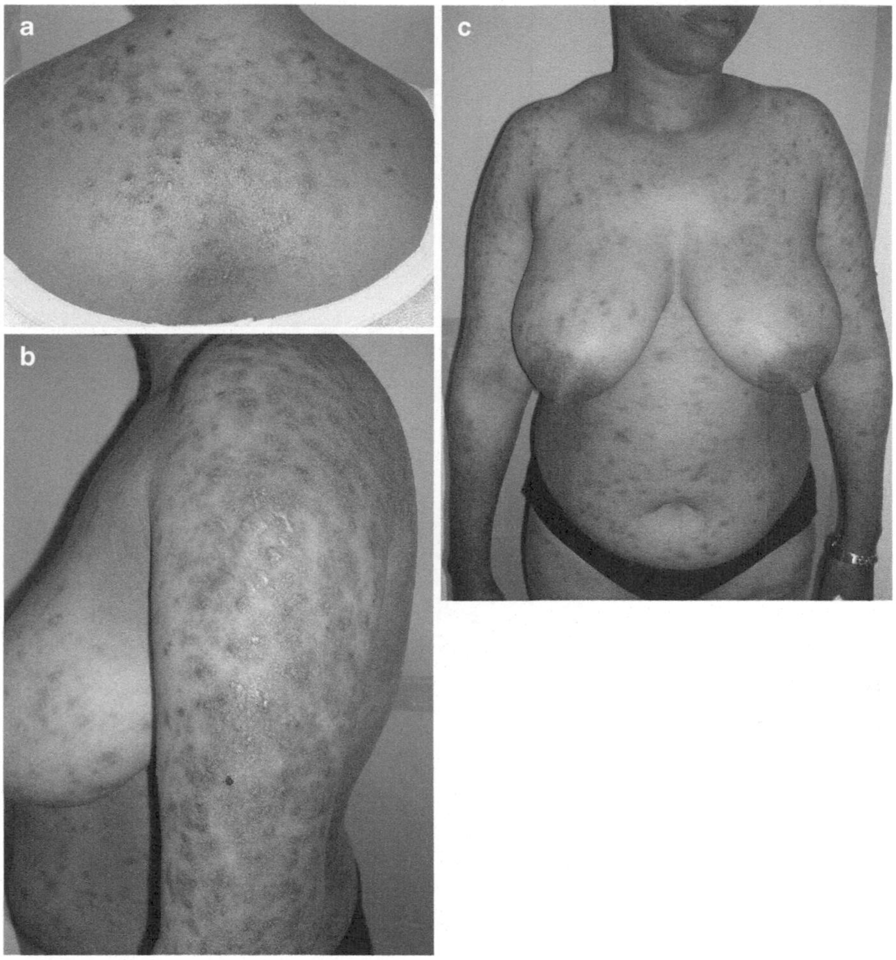

Fig. 30.5 Lesions healing with postinflammatory hyperpigmentation involving the upper back (**a**), extensors of the arms (**b**), and the trunk (**c**)

folliculorum [19]. It is notoriously difficult to treat and significantly hampers the quality of life of patients. First-line therapy is with emollients, topical steroids, and antihistamines. However, many patients will require second-line therapies which include: doxepin, indomethacin, amitriptyline, pentoxyfilline, and ultraviolet light [22, 23].

Xerosis, or dryness of the skin, occurs in approximately 30% of HIV patients. It is characterized by diffuse dryness, scaling, hyperpigmentation, and sometimes crusting. Eczema craquele may complicate xerosis with fissuring and secondary infection. Xerosis usually accompanies other dermatoses, for example, papular eruptions, as demonstrated in Fig. 30.6. The xerosis is thought to be due to malnutrition, chronic illness, and immunosuppression [24, 25]. Therapy is purely symptomatic with urea, lactate or salicylic acid containing emollients, and antihistamines.

30.2.4 Photodermatitis *(Figs. 30.7 and 30.8)*

Photosensitivity is one of the markers of HIV infection with a prevalence of 5.4% [26]. This has been based on the immune dysregulation or may be secondary to phototoxic or photoallergic drug ingestion. In the early stages, patients may complain of sun sensitivity or pruritus and rash involving the face. As the photosensitivity progresses, there is xerosis, scaling, and eventually frank eczema with lichenification over time involving the photo areas: face, "V" and nape of neck, extensors of forearms and lower legs (Fig. 30.7). If untreated, the rash may progress to involve the entire body with scaling and hyperpigmentation and results in erythroderma (Fig. 30.8). Therapy consists of identification and avoidance of any photosensitizing agents, avoidance of ultraviolet light, and symptomatic therapy in the form

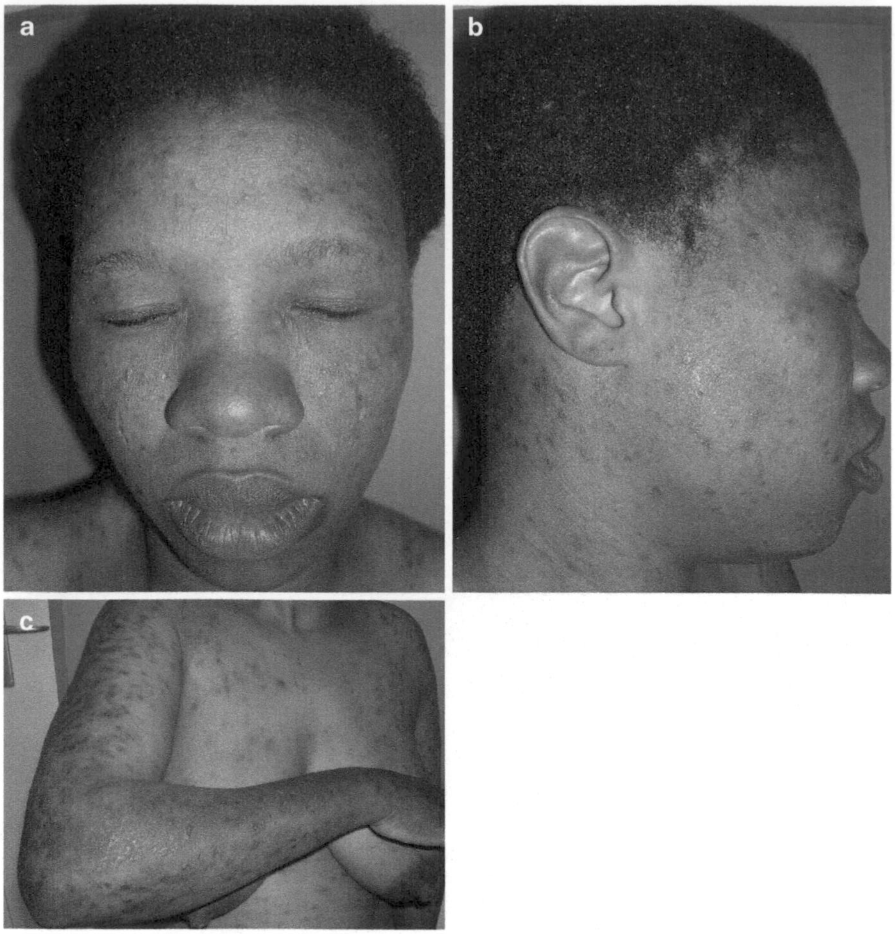

Fig. 30.6 Xerosis of the skin with hyperpigmentation and scaling associated with papular eruptions seen demonstrated on the face (**a**, **b**) and extensors of the arm (**c**)

of topical steroids, broad spectrum sunscreens, and antihistamines. If this fails, hydroxychloroquine may be beneficial as second-line therapy [27].

30.2.5 Psoriasis *(Figs. 30.9–30.11)*

The prevalence of psoriasis, psoriatic arthritis, and Reiter's disease is higher and occurs with increased severity in patients with HIV. The prevalence of psoriasis is 2–5% in patients with HIV and arthritis associated with it occurs in 10% of HIV-positive individuals [24, 28]. Many factors have been implicated in the pathogenesis and flares of HIV psoriasis: HIV-associated T helper 2 immune dysregulation, genetic predisposition, and underlying infection with *candida* and *staph* [28, 29]. The development of sudden and severe psoriasis should prompt a search for underlying HIV infection. Psoriasis may present as the characteristic well-defined salmon-colored plaques with silvery scaling (Fig. 30.9) similar to that in the nonimmunocompromised individual. It usually begins in the classic sites: scalp, retroauricular area, extensors of the upper and lower limbs, and nails. However, with advancing HIV/AIDS, it tends to be more extensive with hyperkeratotic scaling (Fig. 30.10) and erythroderma (Fig. 30.11). Psoriasis has been significantly associated with CD4 counts of less than 200 cells/mm^3 [12].

Localized plaques of psoriasis can be treated with topical preparations: Tar and salicylic acid, calcipotriol, vitamin A, anthranol, and topical steroids. However, more extensive disease requires systemic therapy with retinoids, for example, acitretin. Immunosuppressive therapy with methotrexate and the biologics are contraindicated in HIV psoriasis. However, phototherapy may be beneficial in those who do not respond or have side effects to retinoid therapy [30].

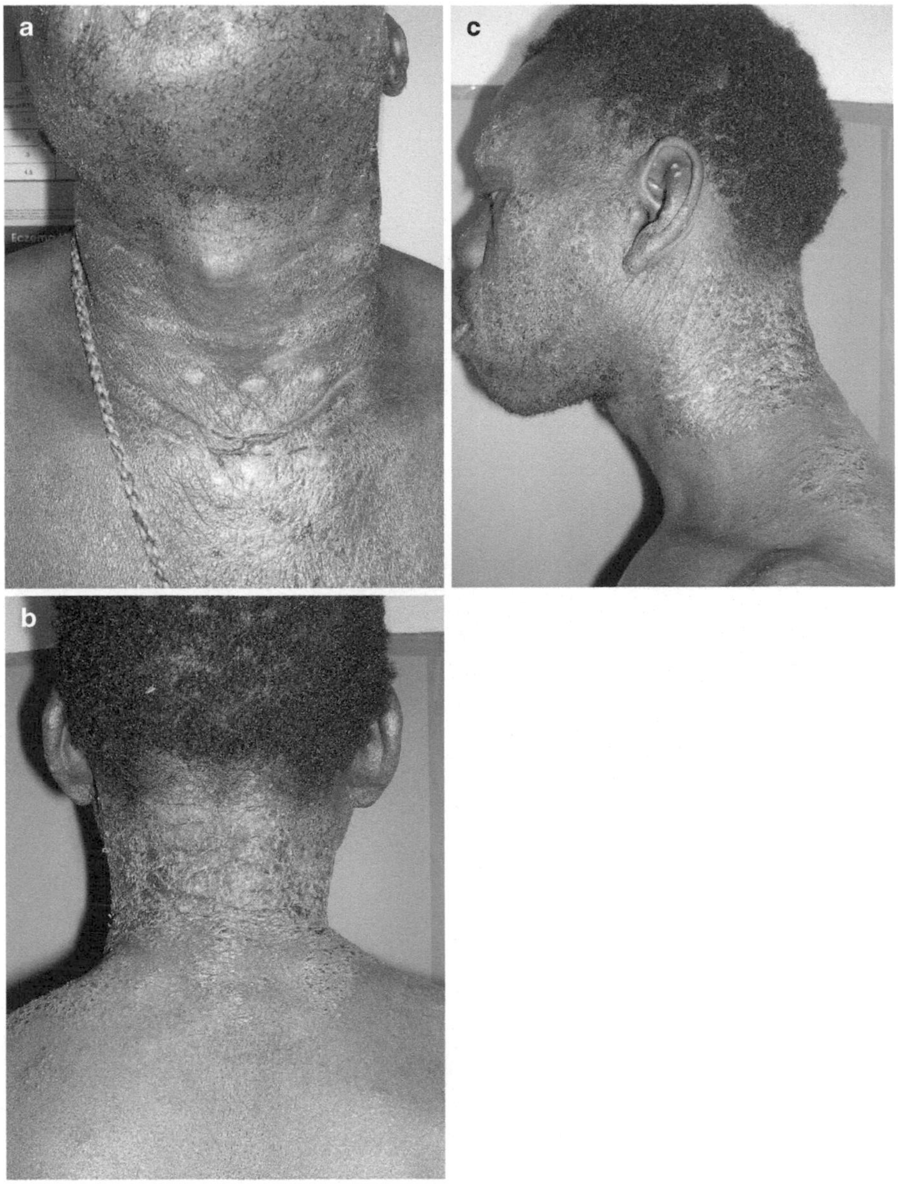

Fig. 30.7 Chronic eczema with lichenification involving the photodistributed areas of the "V" of the neck (**a**), the nape of the neck (**b**), and the face (**c**)

30.2.6 Drug eruptions *(Figs. 30.12–30.15)*

Drug eruptions are a 100 times commoner in those infected with HIV compared to the general population and their prevalence increases as immunodeficiency increases in severity [31, 32]. A number of factors are responsible for the pathogenesis of drug reactions in HIV/AIDS: polypharmacy, the type of drugs used for the therapy of opportunistic infections, genetic predisposition, CD4 counts <200 cells/mm^3 and >25 cells/mm^3, viral infections with EBV, altered renal and liver function which reduces the capacity to detoxify drugs, relative glutathione deficiency, and slow acetylator status [33–35]. Certain HLA types have been implicated, for example, HLAB *5701 in Abacavir hypersensitivity [36].

The drugs most likely to initiate hypersensitivity reactions are the group of antibiotics, responsible for at least 75% of reactions. Of these, it is trimethoprim-sulfamethoxazole which is the most notorious followed by the penicillin-containing antibiotics [32, 37, 38]. Others often implicated are: anticonvulsants, anti-tuberculous drugs, and antiretrovirals especially nevirapine. The pattern of drug eruption most commonly seen is the morbilliform (also called exanthematous or maculopapular)

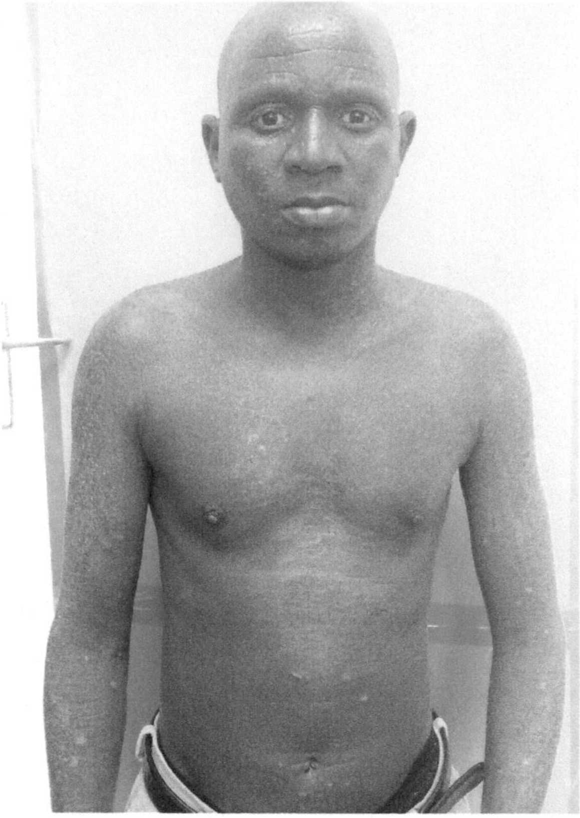

Fig. 30.8 Photodermatitis spilling over to the rest of the body seen as erythroderma

eruption (Fig. 30.12). Urticarial patterns are another manifestation, particularly with nevirapine (Fig. 30.13), and erythema multiforme or targetoid lesions (Fig. 30.14a, b) with central blisters and surrounding erythema should alert one to an underlying drug reaction. When these lesions extend to involve the mucosal surfaces the condition is termed Stevens–Johnson syndrome (SJS) (Fig. 30.15). The severe drug reaction occurs when there is stripping of at least 30% of the skin surface, i.e. toxic epidermal necrolysis (TEN). The diagnosis of a drug eruption depends on the timing of the reaction in relation to the introduction of the drug. It occurs at least 1–3 weeks after the initial exposure to a drug and 24–48 h after re-exposure.

Early reactions can be treated conservatively with antihistamines and topical steroids. However, SJS and TEN which are life threatening require immediate discontinuation of the most likely implicated drug and referral for dermatological opinion and admission.

30.2.7 Immune Reconstitution Inflammatory Syndrome

Immune Reconstitution Inflammatory Syndrome (IRIS) refers to the paradoxical worsening of a

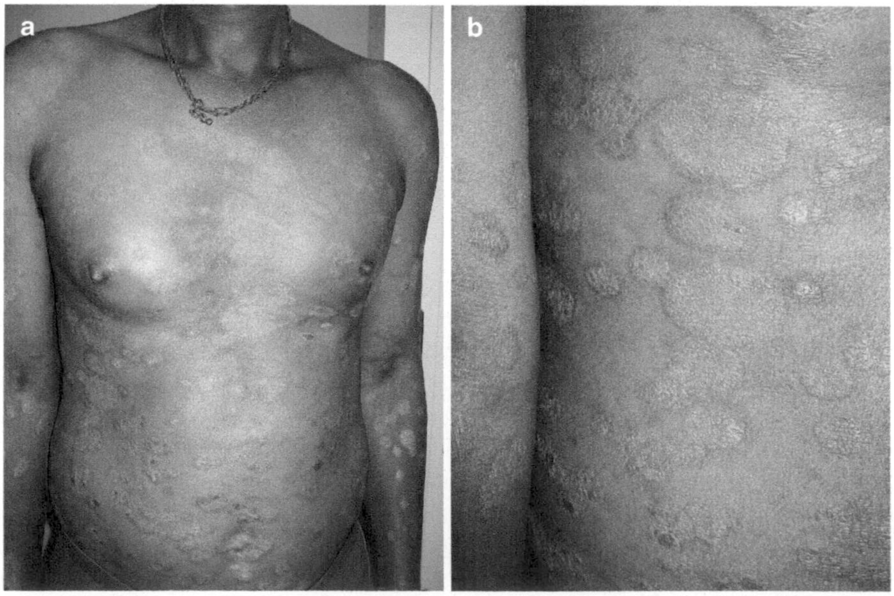

Fig. 30.9 (**a**, **b**) Plaques of psoriasis which are well defined and distributed on the trunk

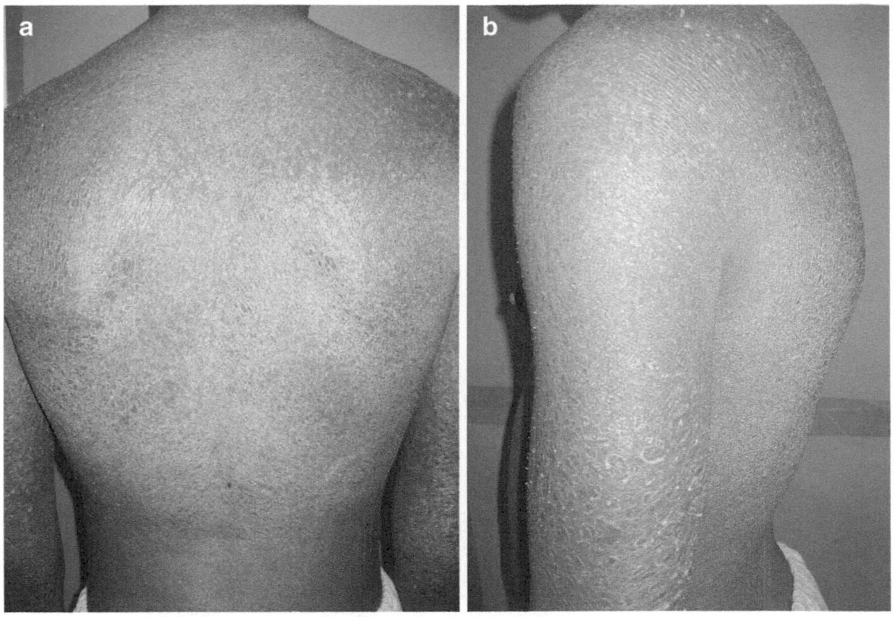

Fig. 30.10 (**a**, **b**) Erythrodermic, unstable psoriasis where there are no well-defined plaques but the body is red and scaly

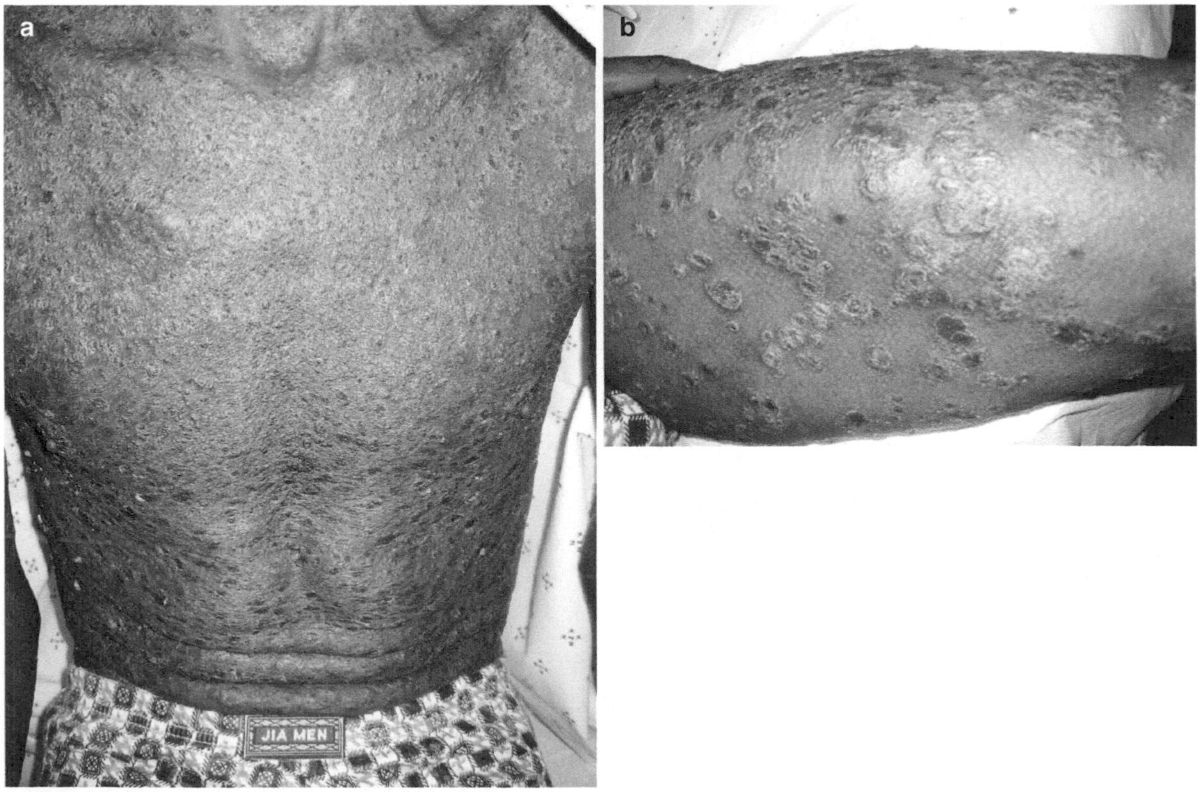

Fig. 30.11 Hyperkeratotic plaques of psoriasis seen on the trunk (**a**) and limbs (**b**)

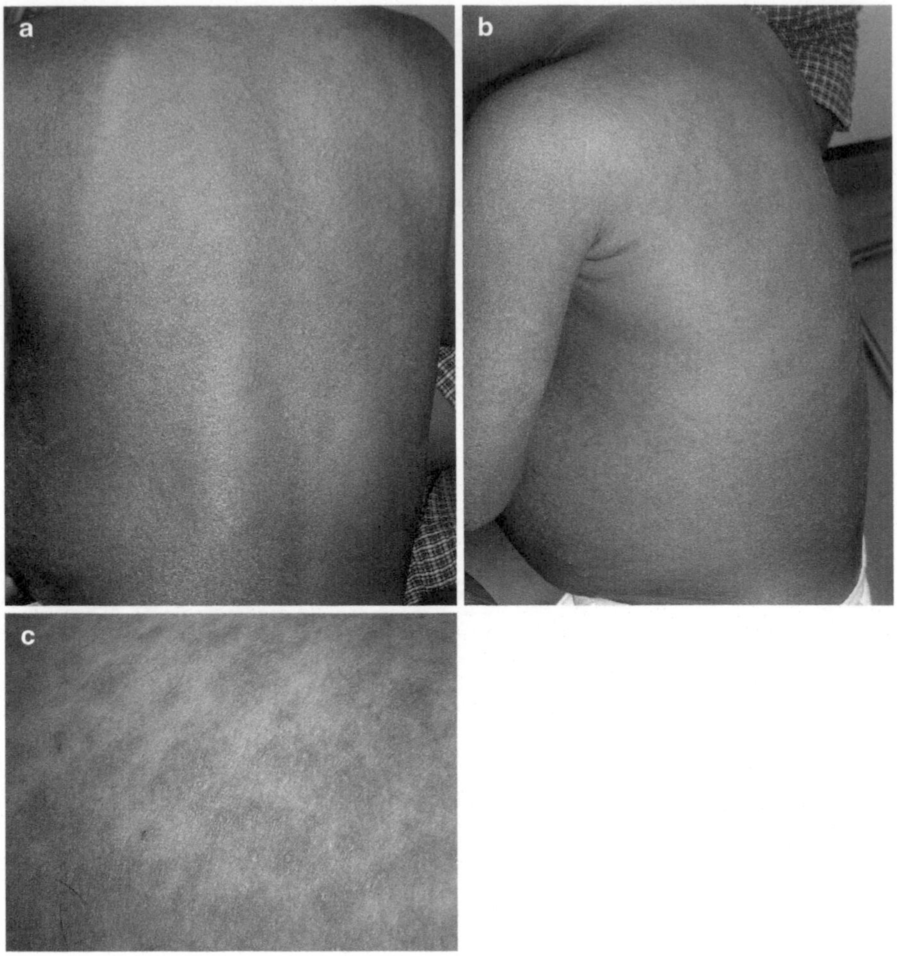

Fig. 30.12 (**a–c**) Morbilliform or exanthematous eruption seen on the trunk of an infant due to Trimethoprim-sulfamethoxazole. A close-up of the erythematous macules and papules is shown in (**c**)

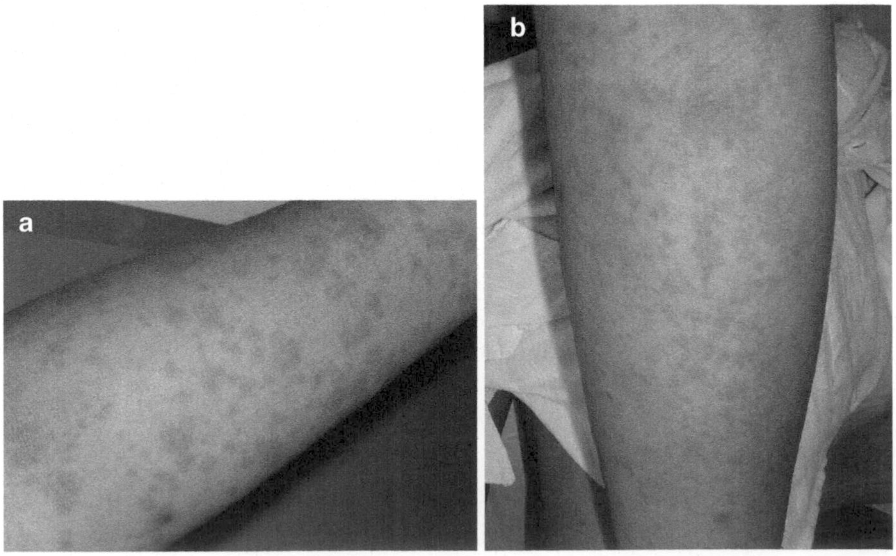

Fig. 30.13 (**a**, **b**) Urticarial papules seen on the arms due to nevirapine hypersensitivity

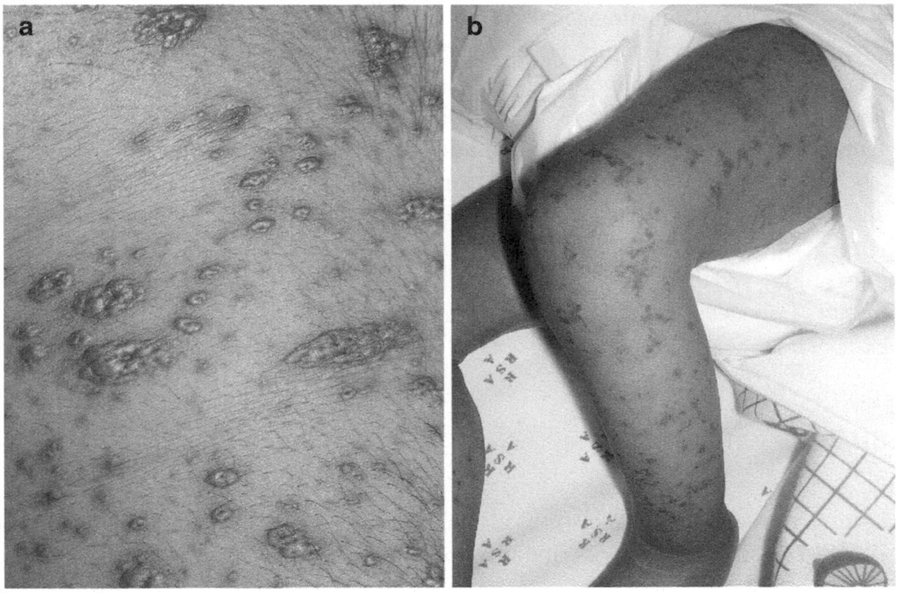

Fig. 30.14 **a, b** Erythema multiforme type lesions with blisters centrally and surrounding erythema in (**a**) and resolving lesions in (**b**)

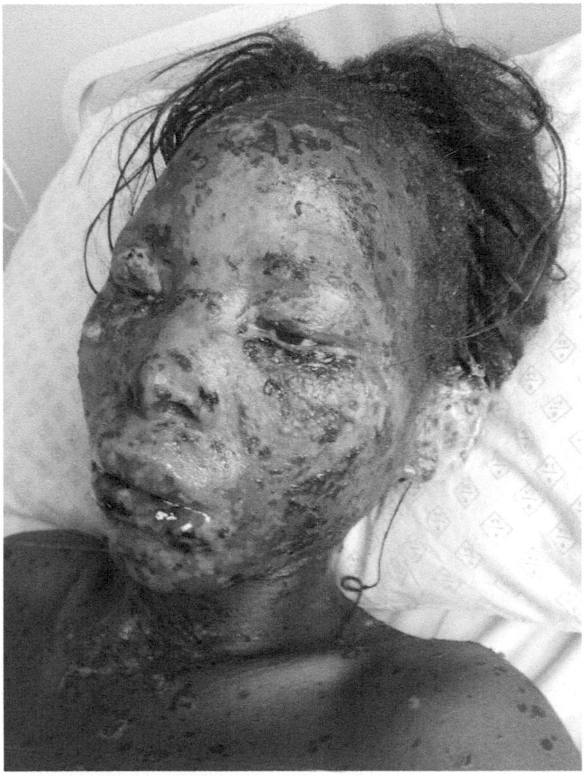

Fig. 30.15 Stevens–Johnson syndrome with involvement of mucosal surfaces

condition, either inflammatory or infectious, in the face of a successful response to antiretroviral therapy. Hence, within the first 12 weeks of initiation of HAART, there is CD4 cell recovery and good viral clearance [38–41]. The pathogenesis is thought to be related to the restoration of the T helper 1 response and some skin problems, paradoxically, make their appearance then [18]. Herpes zoster, mucocutaneous herpes, EF, molluscum contagiosum, and mycobacterial infections have been documented. This may be because immune restoration of a host's immunity causes recognition of silent or latent infection and results in development of the condition [18]. It is important for clinicians to be aware of these phenomena which require specific therapy for the IRIS dermatological event while continuing HAART.

30.3 Cancers and HIV/AIDS

30.3.1 *Kaposi's sarcoma* (Fig. 30.16)

This is the commonest cancer occurring in HIV/AIDS. It is associated with marked immune suppression and is thus AIDS defining. It is intimately linked with Human herpesvirus type 8 infection which is endemic in Africa. The skin is most commonly affected with violaceous macules, plaques, and tumors which are asymptomatic (Fig. 30.16a). Involvement of the lymphatics causes lymphedema (Fig. 30.16b, solid nonpitting) and pain. The gastrointestinal (Fig. 30.16c) and respiratory tracts and lymph nodes are commonly involved. Diagnosis requires biopsy for confirmation and referral for specific staging and therapy. Tuberculosis is the most commonly associated coinfection; hence it should be excluded in the workup of patients [42].

30.3.2 Lymphomas

Lymphomas are associated with advanced immunosuppression and present with nodules, some ulcerated on the skin. They are associated with generalized lymphadenopathy and patients should have a biopsy for diagnosis and staging purposes. They should then be referred for specific chemotherapy.

30.4 Infections and HIV/AIDS

Infections and infestations form the largest group of cutaneous manifestations in HIV and are mainly due to immunosuppression. Most infections occur with low CD4 counts, usually below 200 cells/mm^3. Infections are usually exaggerated, widespread, and more severe, unlike immunocompetent individuals. Infections can also occur as part of the IRIS.

The common infections are as follows.

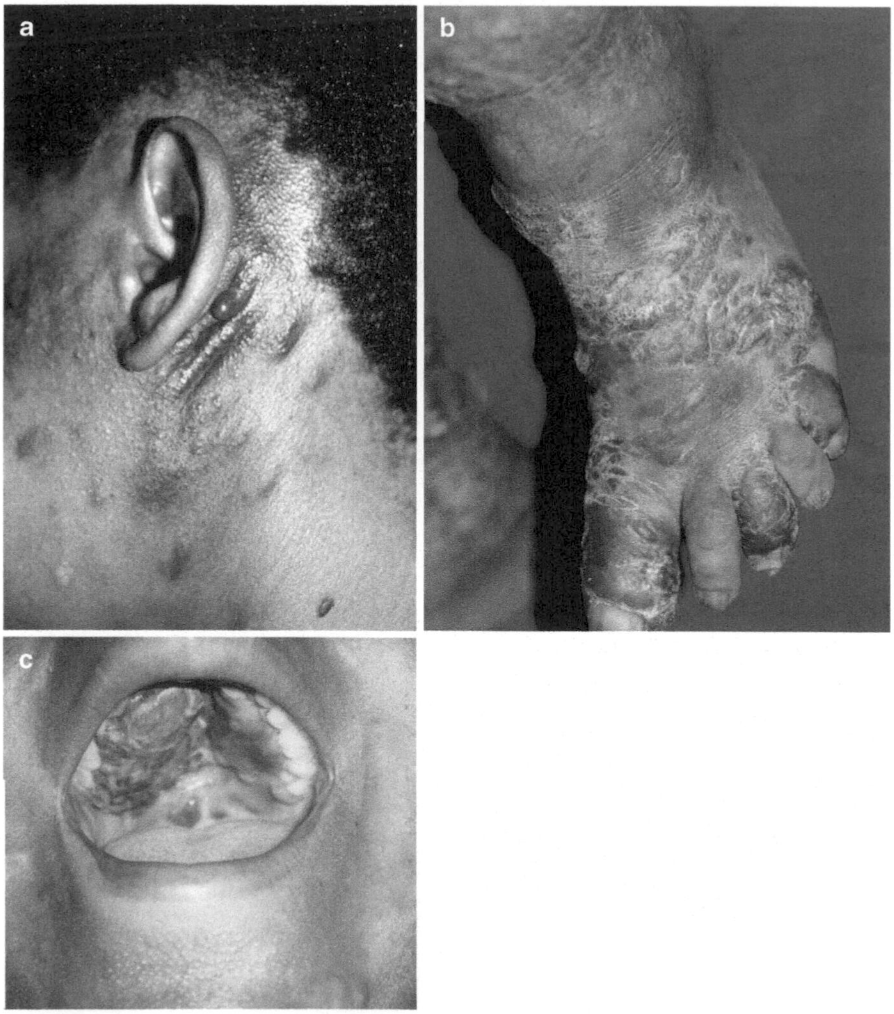

Fig. 30.16 (**a**) Violaceous plaques and nodules of Kaposi's sarcoma in skin crease lines in a retroauricular location. (**b**) Plaques on the lower limbs associated with lymphedema. (**c**) Nodular plaques involving the hard palate

30.4.1 Viral Infections

30.4.1.1 Herpes Simplex (Figs. 30.17 and 30.18)

The underlying cause is *Herpes simplex virus, type 1 and 2* (*HSV 1and 2*). Type 1 usually affects the face, oral and perioral areas, while type 2 affects the ano-genital areas. The initial lesions are painful, grouped vesicles on an erythematous base. Common sites are the oral cavity, lips, perioral areas, glans penis, vulva, and vagina. HSV 2 infection is one of the commonest sexually transmitted diseases in HIV, with 75% being coinfected in the developing world [43]. In HIV-infected individuals, multiple sites may be affected; by lesions that present atypically and are more common as the CD4 declines. Severe gingivostomatitis and pharyngitis with severe genital ulceration are often seen. In females vulvovaginitis, vaginal and cervical erosions may occur. Important clues to the diagnosis are pain and recurrence. The infection usually heals with residual scarring. Herpes

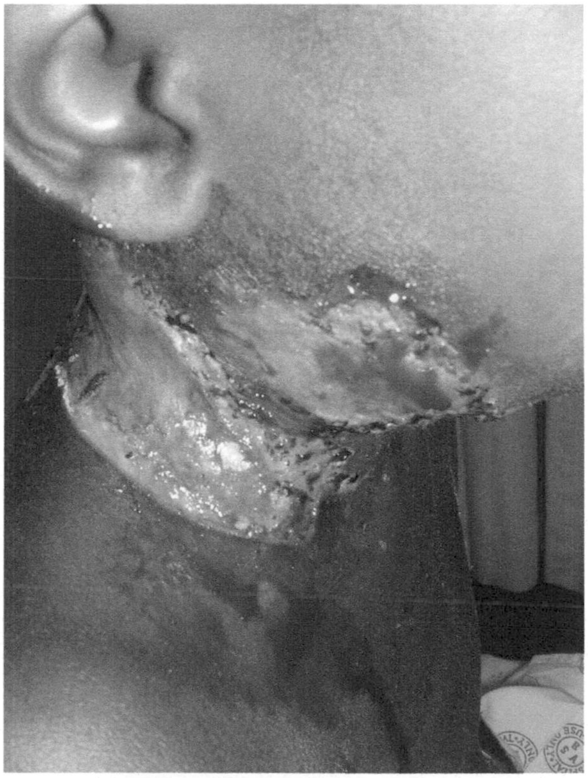

Fig. 30.17 Chronic painful ulcers manifesting as herpes as immunity declines

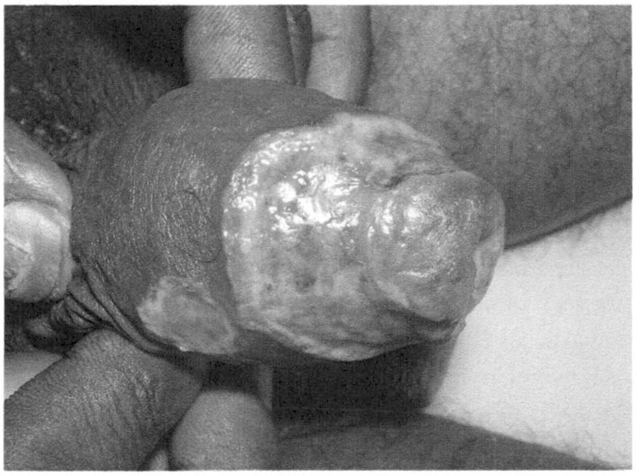

Fig. 30.18 Painful denuded ulcers of herpes genitalis

simplex if present for more than 1 month is AIDS defining. The natural course is healing in 10–14 days, but in AIDS the course is prolonged. HSV infection may worsen as immune restoration occurs on HAART. In fact, HSV 2 reactivation is responsible for more than half of IRIS events [44].

Diagnosis

Diagnosis is usually clinical, but in atypical cases, Tzanck smear, culture, or direct fluorescent test is necessary to differentiate from the following mimickers: cutaneous TB, syphilis, chancroid, and lymphogranuloma venereum.

Treatment

Prevention of spread is to be emphasized. Therapy with oral antivirals is effective: Valacyclovir 1 g twice a day for 7–10 days, Famciclovir 125–250 mg twice a day for 5–7 days, or Acyclovir 200 mg 5 times daily for 7 days. Ulcerated lesions can be treated with topical antibacterial creams (mupirocin or fucidic acid). If patients experience more than 8 attacks per year and has associated erythema multiforme, chronic suppressive antiviral treatment is indicated. In HIV/AIDS, resistance to acyclovir is becoming increasingly common and second-line agents like foscarnet and imiquimod are effective [45].

30.4.1.2 Chicken Pox

It is a childhood viral exanthem caused by the *varicella zoster virus*. The rash presents as erythematous vesicles with umbilication, which become pustules and crusted. The lesions begin on the head and face, spreading to the trunk and extremities. A disease predominantly of children, but when it occurs in adults, an underlying immunodeficiency like HIV must be excluded. Patients with AIDS usually have extensive, hyperkeratotic and hemorrhagic generalized lesions that heal with scarring. Other complications are bacterial superinfection, pneumonia, encephalitis, and hepatitis. Ataxia due to cerebellar inflammation may occur. In addition, in patients with HIV, the interval between chickenpox and herpes zoster is shortened. Although chickenpox is more severe in immunocompromised children, it is not associated with progression to AIDS. It is therefore considered safe to immunize HIV-infected children with the live attenuated virus [46, 47]. Immunization is beneficial in decreasing the risk of later development of herpes zoster. HAART at the time of primary varicella infection has also been found to reduce the incidence of herpes zoster and increase zoster-free survival [48].

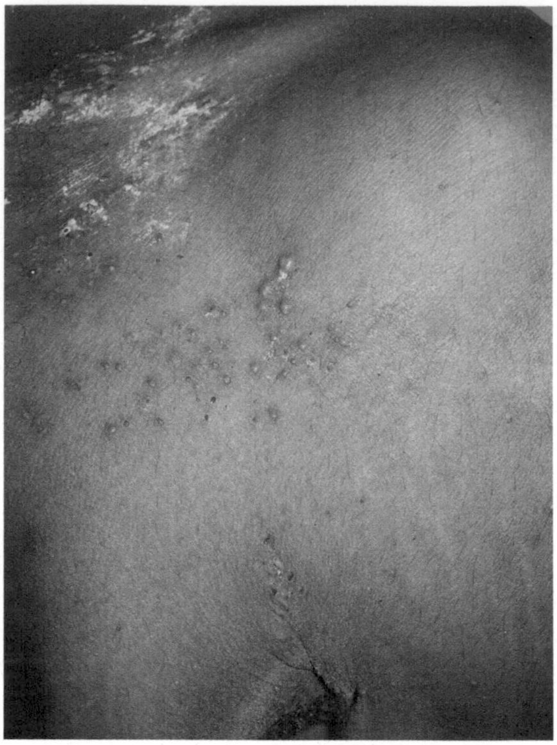

Fig. 30.19 Painful vesicles on an erythematous base in a dermatomal distribution indicative of herpes zoster

Diagnosis

Diagnosis is usually clinical; however, since lesions present atypically, a Tzanck smear and culture help to confirm the diagnosis. Adults with severe generalized infections should be tested for HIV.

Treatment

Oral treatment in immunocompromised patients is routinely recommended: Valacyclovir 1 gram thrice a day for 7 days, or famciclovir 250 mg three times a day for 7 days, or acyclovir 800 mg 5 times daily for 7 days. If patient is gravely ill or has complications, intravenous acyclovir may be required. The pediatric dose of acyclovir is 10 mg/kg 8 hourly. Patients with chicken pox should be isolated till all scabs fall off. Varicella zoster immune globulin is recommended for postexposure prophylaxis. Symptomatic treatment consists of bland calamine lotion, antibacterial creams, and antipyretics and/or antihistamines.

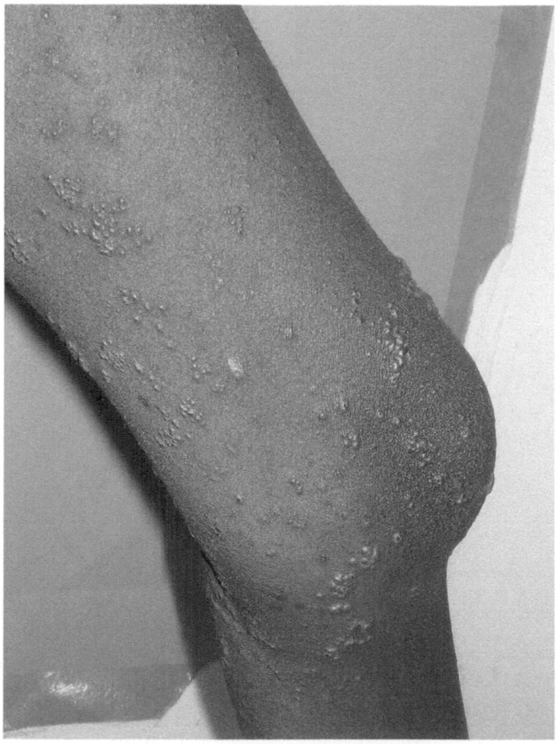

Fig. 30.20 Multidermatomal herpes zoster

30.4.1.3 **Herpes Zoster (Shingles)** (Figs. 30.19 and 30.20)

This very painful infection is almost pathognomonic of HIV especially in a young person. It is caused by the *varicella zoster* virus affecting either single or multiple dermatomes. Severe pain, itching, or burning may precede eruption by 4–5 days. Vesicles with umbilication usually present in a linear distribution over the dermatome. These later become pustular and ulcerate. Complications are postherpetic neuralgia, encephalitis, myelitis, and scarring. Ophthalmic nerve involvement can lead to severe complications (keratopathy, episcleritis, iritis, and blindness). Although HAART has reduced the incidence rates of herpes zoster in children, it still remains a frequent complication [49].

Diagnosis

Diagnosis is clinical. Tzanck smear and culture can be done.

Treatment

Oral antivirals should be started within 48–72 h of lesions appearing, but if lesions have not crusted or there are new vesicles occurring, oral therapy should be started immediately: Acyclovir 800 mg 5 times daily for 7 days, famciclovir 250 mg three times a day for 7 days, or valacyclovir 1 g 3 times a day for 7 days. Topical treatment consists of Castellani's paint, calamine lotion, or antibacterial creams. Analgesics are always indicated, for example, paracetamol, aspirin, and ibuprofen can be used. Amitriptyline 25 mg 3 times a day, carbamazepine 200–400 mg daily, and pregabalin 75–150 mg daily can be used for postherpetic neuralgia.

30.4.1.4 **Molluscum Contagiosum** (Figs. 30.21a, b)

It is a *molluscipox* virus infection characterized by discrete pearly, skin-colored, umblicated papules or nodules. They tend to be extensive and widespread in HIV.

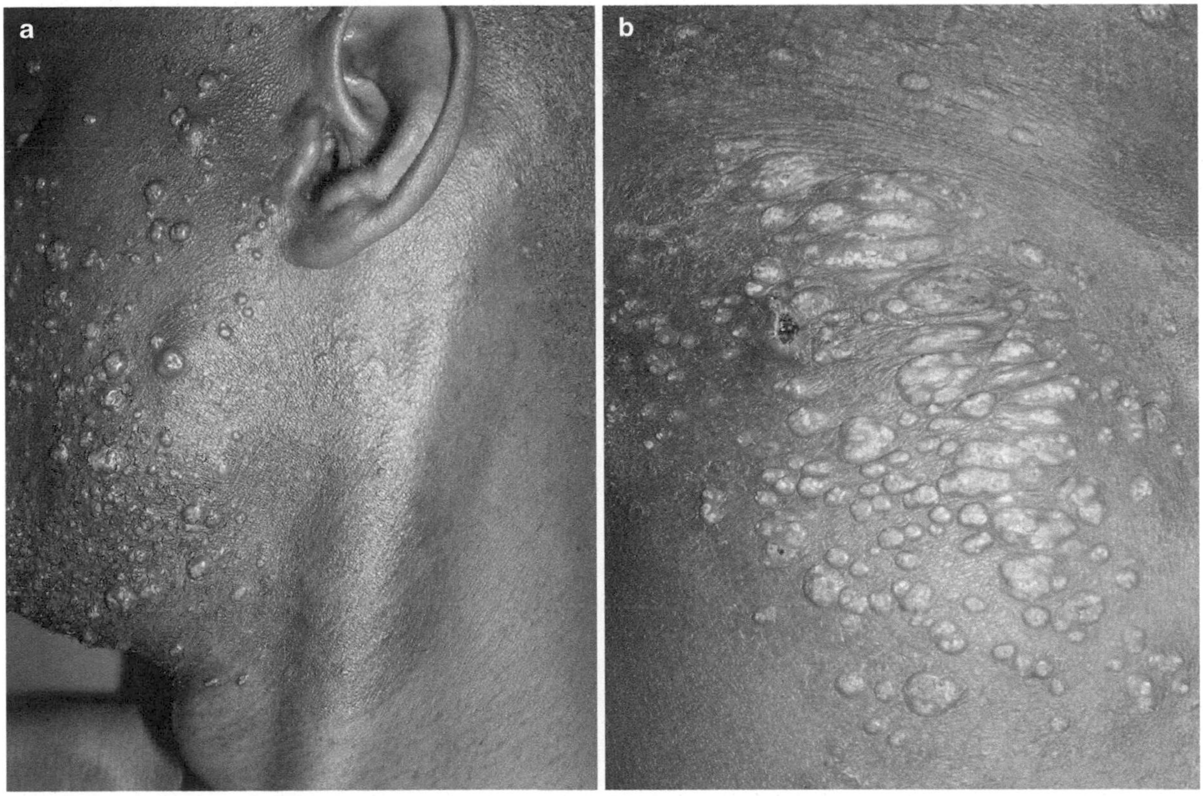

Fig. 30.21 (**a, b**) Extensive umbilicated papules and nodules with central white keratinous cores indicative of molluscum contagiosum in advanced HIV infection

Lesions in the genital areas are sexually transmitted. Lesions may be extremely large ("giant" mollusca) and disfiguring in HIV [49].

Patients presenting with generalized lesions and adults with extragenital mollusca should be investigated for HIV [50]. Lesions may recur as a manifestation of the immune reconstitution syndrome.

Diagnosis

Although diagnosis is usually clinical, biopsy of a lesion or the contents of a papule can be stained with toluidine blue or giemsa stain. In ill patients, molluscum-like lesions require differentiation from cryptococcosis and histoplasmosis.

Treatment

A recent Cochrane review reported that no therapies were found to be convincingly effective [50]. However, a variety of therapies can be attempted, for example, curettage and cautery and cryotherapy with application of iodized phenol applied to the lesions. For multiple large lesions, removal under general anesthesia may be required. A recent study documented the superiority of 100% trichloracetic acid to cryosurgery in multiple facial mollusca in HIV-infected individuals [51]. For recalcitrant lesions in HIV, a combination approach may be required, for example, CO_2 laser, trichloracetic acid, and pulsed dye laser [52]. Less effective therapies are retinoic creams, imiquimod cream, and salicylic and lactic acid preparations. Children and adults with mollusca should be educated not to scratch lesions in order to prevent transmission and autoinoculation [50].

30.4.1.5 Verrucae (Figs. 30.22–30.24)

These are benign epidermal hypertrophic lesions caused by the *human papilloma virus* subtypes 3 and 10. Usually, lesions are multiple over the face and extremities and have a verrucous or filiform appearance. Common variety seen in HIV is common warts, flat warts, epidermodysplasia-like lesions, and non-melanoma skin cancers [53, 54]. These usually occur as flat-topped slightly elevated papules on the face but may be generalized. Koebnerization usually occurs.

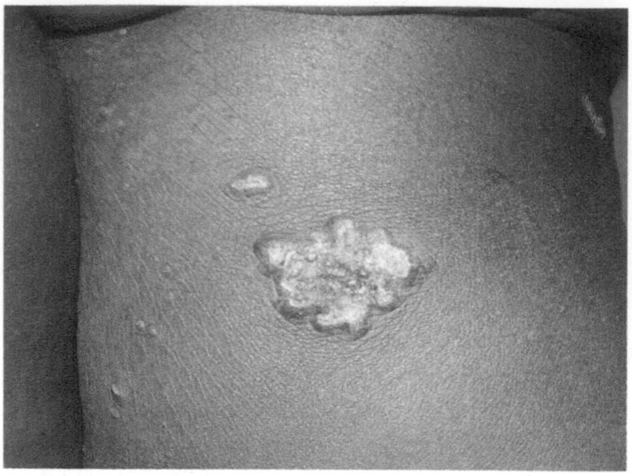

Fig. 30.22 Warty plaque of a giant verruca

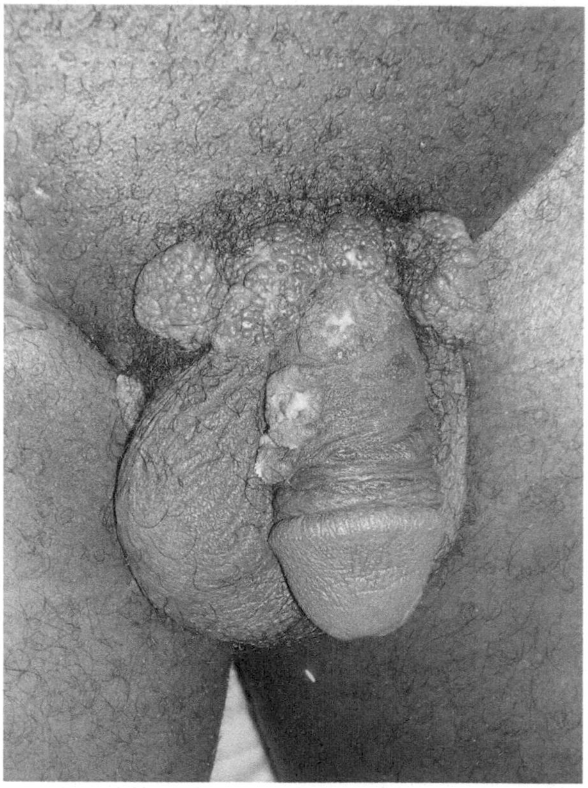

Fig. 30.23 Condylomata accuminata

Condylomata accuminata usually occur on genital areas and can present as small hypertrophic lesions or giant "cauliflower" growths. HIV-infected individuals are commonly coinfected with multiple types of HPV which are persistent [55]. Hence, the development of HPV-related tumors remains high, even in the era of

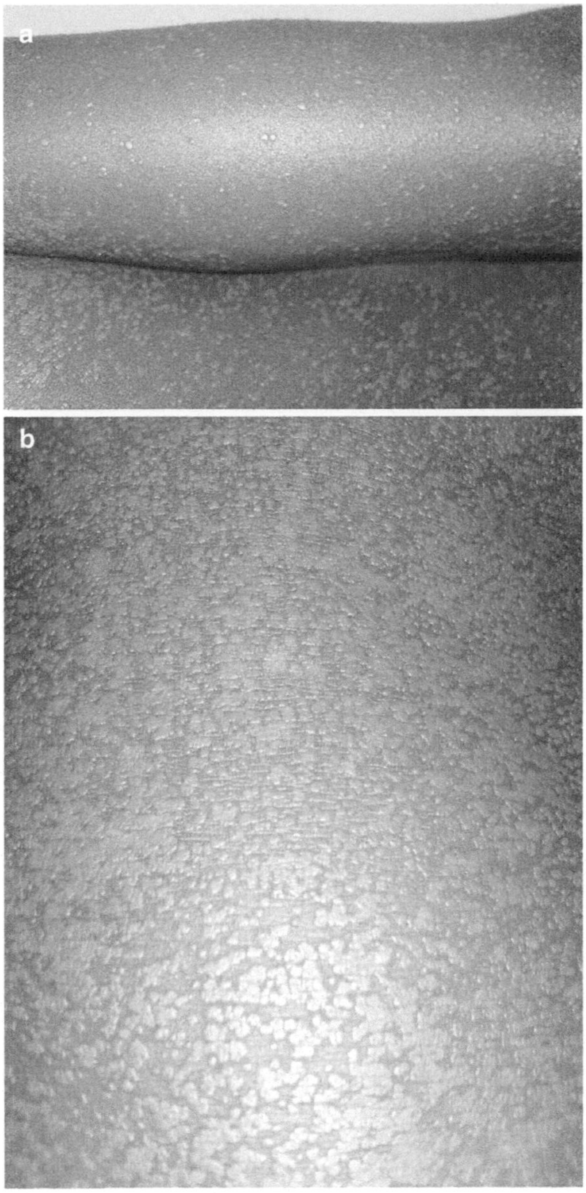

Fig. 30.24 (**a**, **b**) Flat topped, asymptomatic gray to skin-colored papules of verruca plana involving the limbs and trunk

HAART [56]. Genotyping of HPV types remains important for the development of vaccines in order to prevent malignancies [57].

Diagnosis

Diagnosis is clinical but if in doubt biopsy will confirm the diagnosis. Condylomata acuminata can be confused with condylomata lata (secondary syphilitic infection) where the lesions are usually moist and malodorous. If in doubt, serological tests for syphilis should be done.

Treatment

Cryotherapy or curetting and cauterization for small numbers of lesions may also be used. Large condylomata can be excised and cauterized. Other modalities of treatment are salicylic preparations, imiquimod, retinoic acid, cantharidin, and candida antigen. Imiquimod has been reported to be effective in facial warts, and genital and extragenital warts [57]. Warts may be quite persistent despite HAART and in fact, may become more profuse as a manifestation of immune reconstitution [58, 59, 60].

30.4.2 Bacterial

30.4.2.1 Acute bacterial infections (Fig. 30.25)

Impetigo

This is a common bacterial infection usually caused by *Staphylococcus aureus* and *Streptococcus pyogenes.* Initial lesions are thin-walled bullae, containing cloudy or yellowish fluid that easily rupture leading to honey colored crusted lesions. In HIV patients, lesions may be widespread with thick crusts. Satellite lesions may appear beyond the periphery and they may recur after therapy.

Diagnosis

Diagnosis is made by clinical presentation. Pus swab for microscopy, culture, and sensitivity can aid in the diagnosis, identification of the causative organism, and antibiotic resistance.

Treatment

Treatment of impetigo in HIV patients requires oral antibiotics, for example, penicillin, erythromycin, amoxicillin, and clavulanic acid. Topical antibiotics like mupirocin, fucidic acid, and neomycin may be useful. Recurrent episodes are common in HIV patients and require longer courses of therapy and cephalosporins.

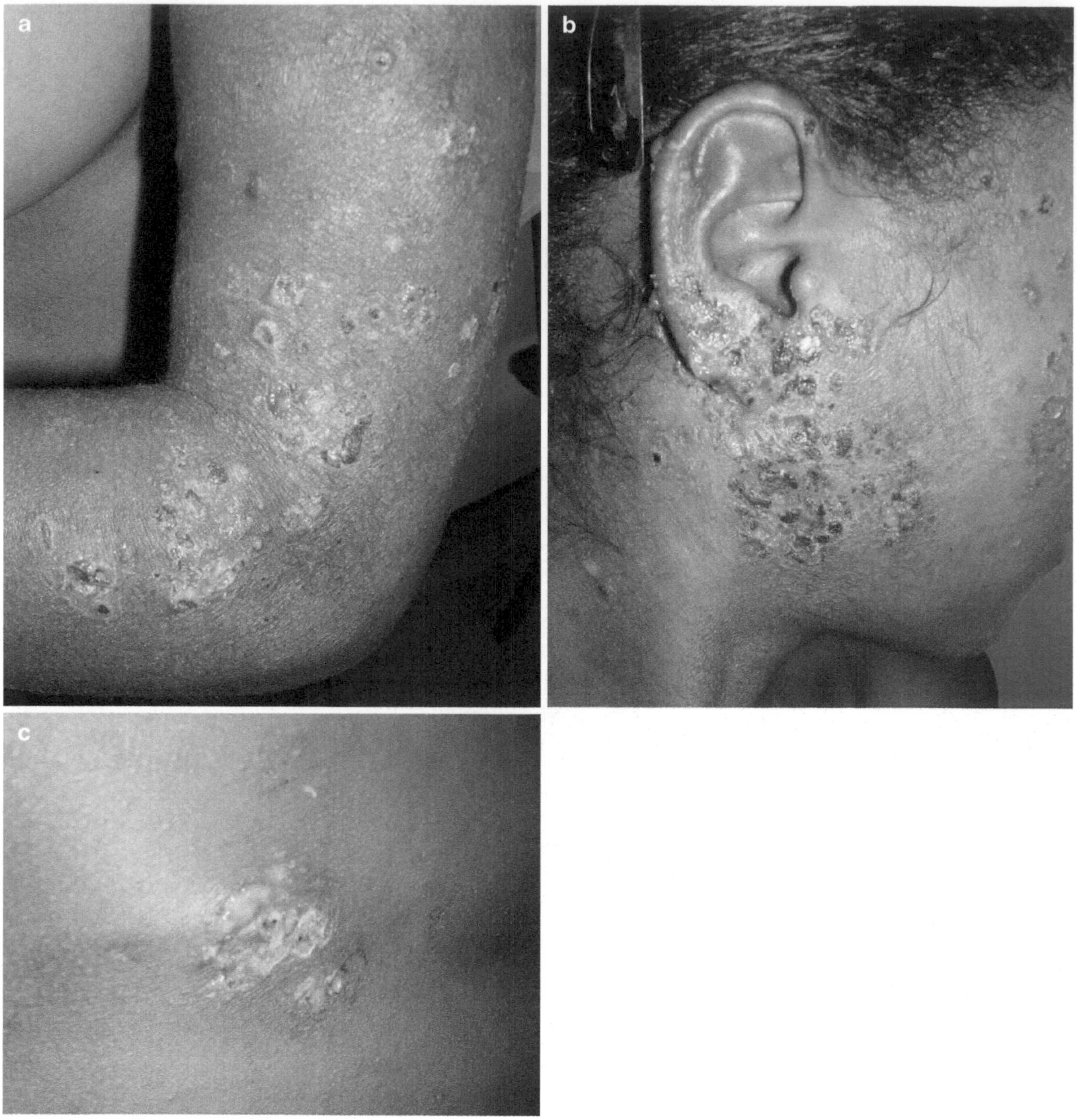

Fig. 30.25 (**a**–**c**) Erythematous nodules and plaques, purulent discharge and crusting involving the trunk, face, and limbs

Folliculitis

This is *Staphylococcus aureus* infection affecting the hair follicles of the scalp, arms, legs, axillae, and trunk. It presents as small dome shaped pustules with an erythematous halo with a hair shaft centrally. Patients with HIV have a higher staphylococcus carriage and are prone to recurrent folliculitis.

Diagnosis

Diagnosis can be confirmed by pus swab and biopsy.

Treatment

Minimize heat, friction, and occlusion. If widespread oral antibiotics are required. Topical antibiotics are effective in localized lesions. Nasal and perineal carriage of both **Staphylococci** and **Streptococci** should be treated with topical antibiotics.

Furuncles and Carbuncles

Furuncles are walled off, deep painful, firm or fluctuant masses enclosing a collection of pus, often evolving from superficial folliculitis. **Staphylococcus** *aureus* is the most common cause, but other organisms like *E. coli*, *Pseudomonas aeruginosa, and* **Streptococcus**. *faecalis* may also be the cause. Carbuncles or "boils" are deep interconnected aggregates of furuncles and are extremely painful.

Diagnosis

Painful throbbing, tender erythematous fluctuant swelling.

Treatment

Incision and drainage are required and a pus swab for culture and sensitivity should be done.

Appropriate antibiotics (amoxicillin and clavunate, erythromycin, flucloxacillin, or clindamycin) should be prescribed for 5–7 days. Wound cleansing and topical antibiotics are also required. Since HIV-infected patients have greater incidence of nasal **staphylococci**, topical antibiotics should be prescribed. If there is no response, biopsy should be done to exclude other infections, for example, atypical mycobacterial infection.

The bacterial infections are known to recur as a manifestation of immune reconstitution syndrome; hence, systemic antibiotic therapy should be continued while maintaining HAART.

Bacillary Angiomatosis (Fig. 30.26)

This uncommon condition is caused by a spirochaete, *Bartonella henselae and B. quintana*. It usually occurs in severely immunocompromised patients with CD4 counts <50 cells/mm^3. They present with a pyrexial illness and sudden eruption of angiomatous papules and nodules leading to abscesses. This condition may be confused clinically with Kaposi's sarcoma, but unlike Kaposi's sarcoma, there is no oral involvement or lymphedema. Patients may also have systemic involvement with hepatic, cardiac, pulmonary, and bone involvement.

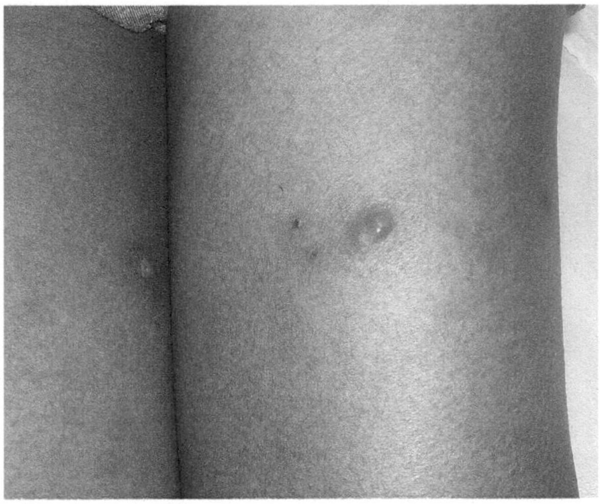

Fig. 30.26 Violaceous dermal and subcutaneous nodule of bacillary angiomatosis on the limb

Diagnosis

Histology and culture will confirm the diagnosis.

Treatment

Erythromycin 600 mg 6 hourly or doxycycline 100 mg 12 hourly until all lesions resolve.

30.4.2.2 Chronic Bacterial Infections

Tuberculosis (Figs. 30.27–30.29)

Pulmonary tuberculosis is one of the commonest coinfections associated with HIV/AIDS in Africa. Hence, cutaneous tuberculosis is on the increase and presents both with primary and secondary hypersensitivity lesions. The hypersensitivity manifestations of tuberculosis have become more common and usually occur in those with higher CD4 counts. The common primary lesion is lupus vulgaris. The characteristic lesions are plaques consisting of nodules ("apple jelly"), extending irregularly with tissue destruction and scarring. In severe cases, there may be deep ulcerations

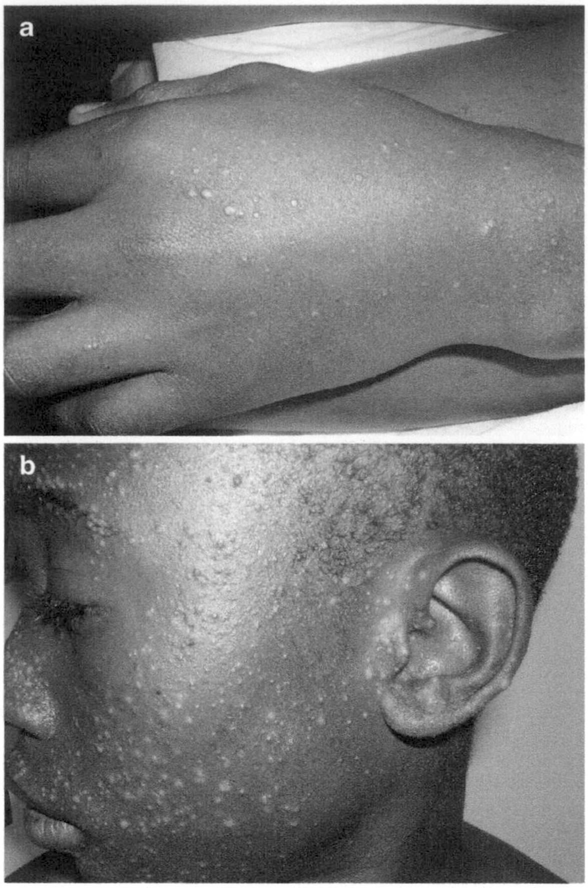

Fig. 30.27 (**a**, **b**) Asymptomatic follicular papules of lichen scrofulosorum on the limbs and face in a child

with vegetating lesions and tumors. Although any site of the body may be involved, the tip of the nose is common. The differential diagnosis includes sarcoidosis, leprosy, syphilis, and deep fungal infections. Cutaneous tuberculosis can present more aggressively than it does in the healthy individual. Scrofuloderma, draining sinuses overlying affected lymph nodes occur at lower CD4 counts.

The hypersensitivity types are:

1. Papulonecrotic tuberculid consisting of papules and pustules which ulcerate and involve acral sites: ear lobes, elbows, knees, and the buttocks.
2. Lichen scrofulosorum: grouped papules on the trunk occurring with underlying lymphadenopathy and bone TB.
3. Erythema induratum: nodules on the calves which ulcerate and have a distinct bluish edge.

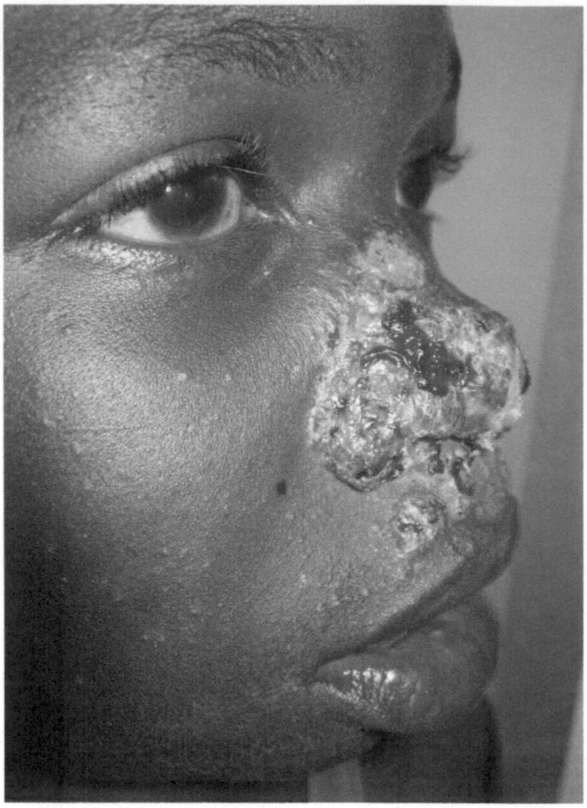

Fig. 30.28 Chronic, destructive crusted plaque of lupus vulgaris

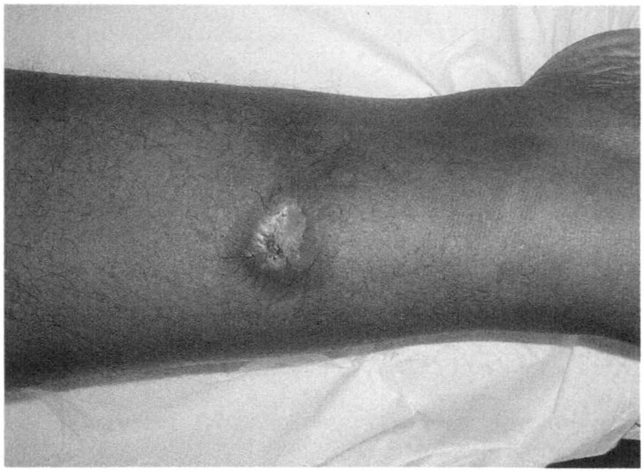

Fig. 30.29 Ulcer with bluish edges indicating erythema induratum on the lower leg

Diagnosis

The diagnosis is strongly supported by a blistering mantoux test, histology, and a search for underlying TB (sputum examination and chest X-rays). Recently, a serological test, the Quantiferon Gold test has been used as an adjunct.

Treatment

Full anti-TB treatment consisting of rifampicin, isoniazid, ethambutol, and pyrazinamide for 6 months is required. It is also important to screen contacts. If clinical response after 6 months is suboptimal, therapy should be continued for 9 months. If response is still suboptimal, lesions should be biopsied and cultured to identify resistant strains.

Syphilis (Fig. 30.30)

Syphilis is a sexually transmitted disease caused by the spirochaete *Treponema pallidum* and often coexists with HIV. Untreated syphilis passes through stages; primary, secondary, latent, and tertiary. The primary lesion is classically a painless ulcer on the genitalia. If untreated, this heals in 10–14 days and passes through the secondary stage. This presents approximately 6 weeks after the initial infection. Because of immunosuppression, acceleration from secondary to tertiary infection occurs. Secondary lesions present as a papular squamous eruption of the trunk, annular plaques over the "muzzle" area of the face, split papules at the corners of the mouth, snail track ulcers of the tongue and hyperpigmentation of the palms and soles and lymphadenopathy. There may also be annular syphilide lesions and patchy alopecia (moth eaten) of the scalp. In immunocompromised HIV patients, the course may be more aggressive and profuse with severe ulceration (lues maligna). These patients convert quicker to the tertiary stage.

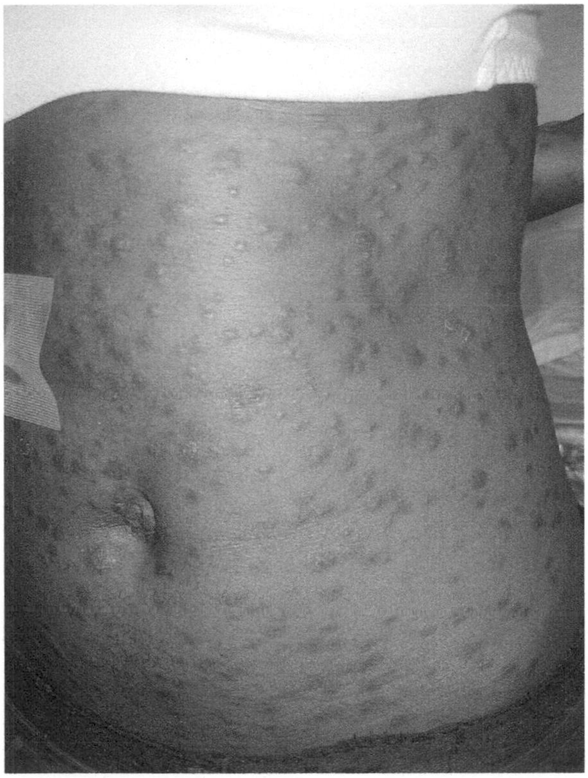

Fig. 30.30 Erythematous papules and nodules involving the trunk in secondary syphilis

Condyloma lata occurs in the genital areas and present as moist, malodorous warty lesions.

Diagnosis

In the latent phase, serological tests are positive with absence of active disease.

Diagnosis can be made serologically (WR, RPR, VDRL, TPHA, and FTA). Titres that are greater than 1:8 should be regarded as positive. However, HIV patients may have false negative serology; hence one should treat based on clinical suspicion.

Treatment

Drug of choice is benzathine penicillin 2.4 million units intramuscularly weekly for 3 weeks. Other antibiotics used are erythromycin 500 mgm 4 times daily for 28 days or doxycycline 100 mgm twice daily for 3 weeks. Successful therapy is indicated by a falling RPR titre. Partners must be treated as well. However, in HIV infection, there may be a poor serological response. HAART and macrolide therapy for opportunistic infections in HIV ensures a better serological response to therapy for syphilis [60].

30.4.3 Fungal Infections

30.4.3.1 Pityriasis (Tinea) versicolor

This common infection is caused by the lipophilic yeast *Pityrosporum orbiculare* (*Malassezia furfur*) usually affecting the seborrhoeic areas of the body (trunk, neck, and face). It presents as scaly hypopigmented or hyperpigmented macules. In HIV, lesions may be widespread with frequent relapses. Generally patients are asymptomatic.

Diagnosis can be confirmed by microscopic examination of skin scrapings treated with 20% potassium hydroxide ("spaghetti and meatball" pattern of mycelia and spores).

Treatment

Selenium or ketoconazole shampooing of the body alternate nights combined with 20% sodium hyposulfite solution is the treatment of choice. Facial lesions can be treated with imidazole creams. For extensive and resistant cases, short courses of oral ketoconazole (200 mg for 10 days) or itraconazole (100 mg twice daily for 7 days) or fluconazole (150 mg weekly for 1–2 weeks) may be used.

30.4.3.2 **Candidiasis** (Fig. 30.31)

This yeast infection is caused by *Candida albicans* and is the most common mucocutaneous infection in HIV-infected patients. It presents as pseudomembranous (thrush), erythematous macules, hyperplastic (thick whitish-yellow plaques on the buccal mucosa) and angular cheilitis.

Symptoms of pain and burning may be present. Oral candida defines the patient as WHO stage 3 illnesses and is a reliable marker of HIV progression. Other areas affected are the genital areas (glans penis and vagina), groin, submammary areas, and the interdigital clefts. In the intertriginous areas, candida presents as red moist glistening plaques extending to the opposing skin folds. Satellite lesions may be present along the periphery.

Diagnosis

Skin scrapings treated with KOH and microscopic examination can confirm diagnosis.

Treatment

Topical treatments consist of fluoride mouthwashes and antifungal suspensions and creams.

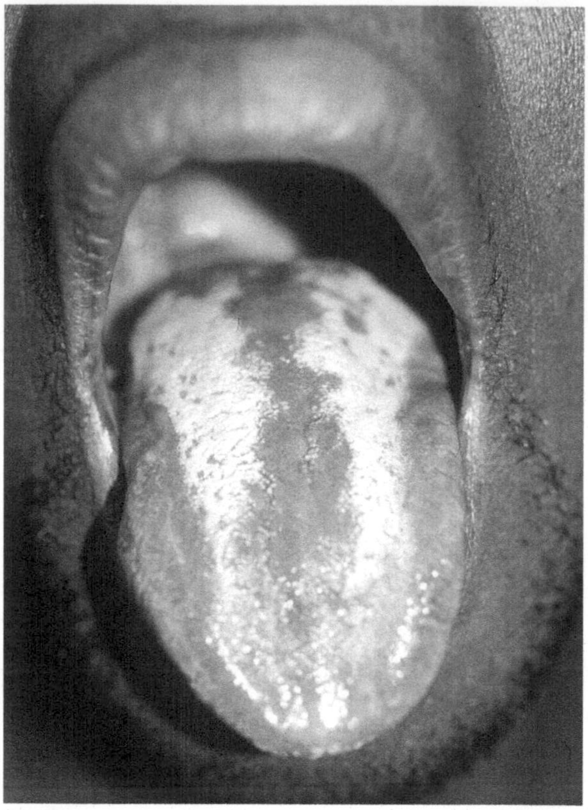

Fig. 30.31 Pseudomembranous candidiasis of the tongue

Oral fluconazole 200 mg daily for 7 days can be effective. Other azoles used are ketoconazole 200 mg daily for 7 days or itraconazole 200 mg daily for 7 days. In patients with candida balanitis or vaginitis, partners should be treated as well.

30.4.3.3 **Dermatophytosis (Tinea)** (Figs. 30.32–30.34)

This superficial fungal infection is caused by three dermatophytes commonly affecting man – *trichophyton*, *epidermophyton*, and *microsporum* species. It usually presents as a scaly erythematous patch with a well-defined active border consisting of papules and vesicles.

In HIV, lesions may be well widespread, atypical, and severe with a higher incidence of nail involvement [61]. Sites affected are the face, palms, axillae, groin, buttock, feet, and nails. Tinea capitis is rare in adults, but in HIV patients, the lesions may be extensive, with patches of broken-off hairs, scaling, pustulation, crusting, and abscesses (kerion). Patients treated with steroid creams have ill-defined inflammatory lesions (tinea incognito).

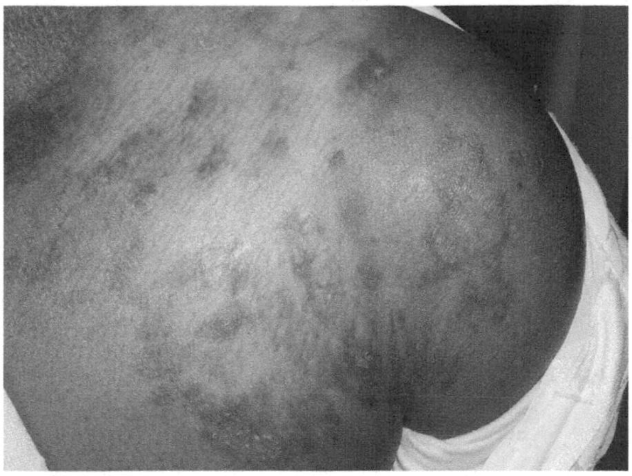

Fig. 30.32 Scaling, erythema, and pustules in tinea incognito with steroid abuse

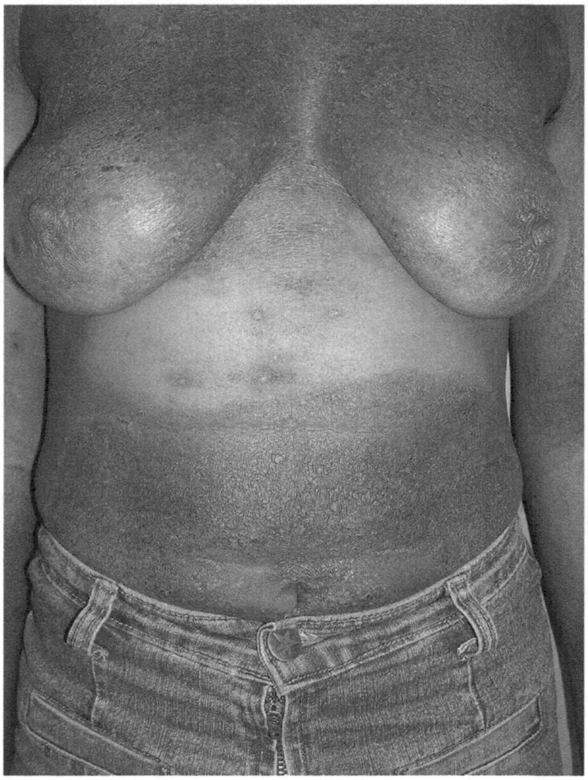

Fig. 30.33 Extensive erythema, scaling, hyperpigmentation, and active edge of tinea corporis

Diagnosis

The diagnosis can be confirmed by microscopic examination of skin scrapings, nail clippings, and hair samples treated with 20% KOH.

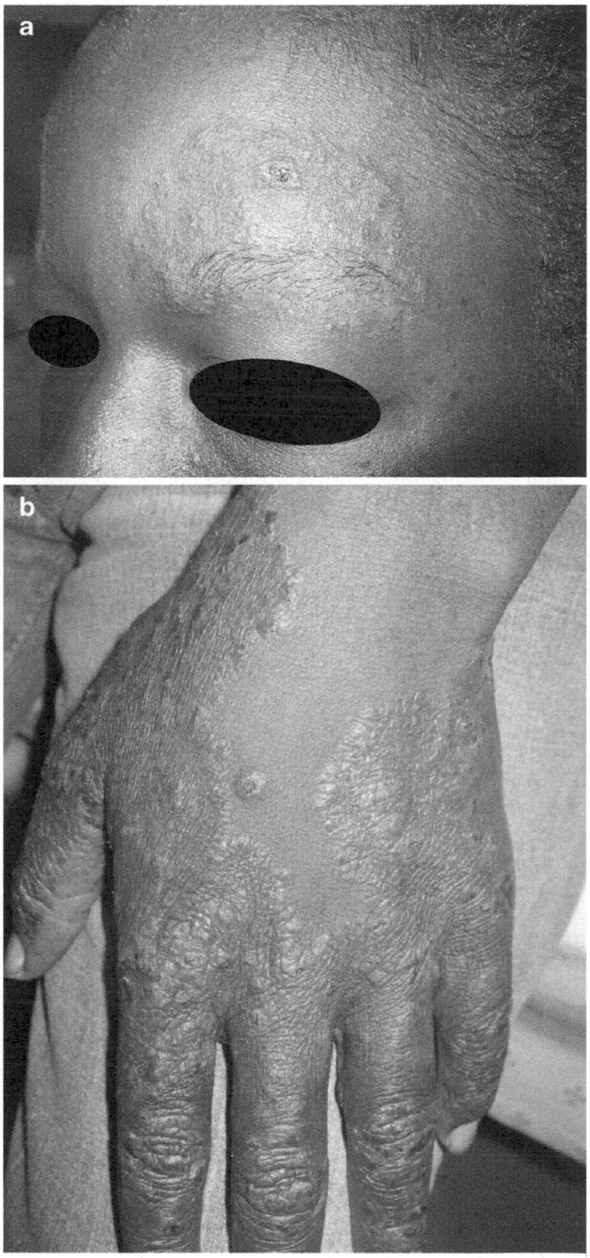

Fig. 30.34 Erythematous annular plaques with central clearing involving the face and hands

Treatment

Topical whitfields ointment, zinc undecenoate ointment, imidazoles or terbinafine creams, lotions, or sprays can be used for localized lesions. Early recognition and systemic therapy are important in HIV-infected patients to prevent severe infection [61].

First-line therapy in widespread cases includes oral griseofulvin 1 g daily for 4–6 weeks. More expensive antifungals – ketoconazole, itraconazole, fluconazole, and terbinafine – can also be prescribed, if available. For onychomycosis, griseofulvin should be administered for 12–18 months, Itraconazole 200 mg twice daily for 7 days, repeated after 3 weeks (pulse therapy) for 2 months for finger nails and 4 months for toe nails, and terbinafine 250 mg daily for 3 months for finger nails and 4 months for toe nails. If the patient is on HAART, terbinafine is favored as there are fewer drug interactions compared to itraconazole. The dose of both terbinafine and itraconazole for children is 5 mg/kg body weight. Tinea infections can recur as a manifestation of immune reconstitution syndrome.

30.4.4 Systemic Fungal Infections

30.4.4.1 Cryptococcosis (Figs. 30.35 and 30.36)

The yeast *Cryptococcus neoformans* causes this common systemic infection. Cutaneous cryptococcosis usually occurs with severe immunosuppression (CD4 < 100 cells/mm^3) and is AIDS defining. Skin involvement occurs in 10% of patients with systemic disease and may be the first sign of systemic involvement. Lesions may be umbilicated, hemorrhagic, ulcerated nodules and papules often resembling molluscum contagiosum. They have a predilection for the face and scalp. Headache, confusion, and neck stiffness indicate meningitis and a lumbar puncture is indicated.

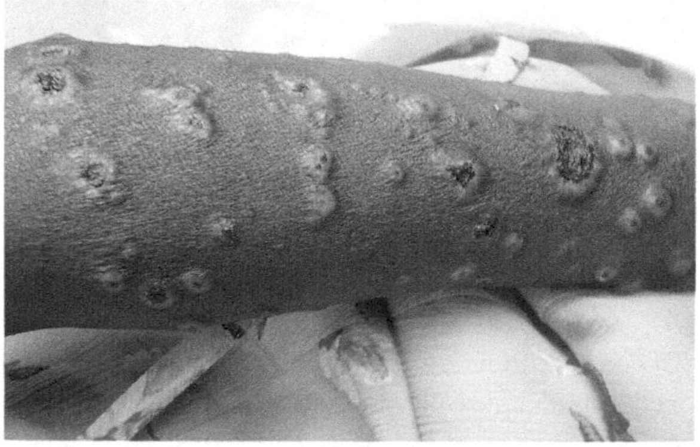

Fig. 30.35 Umbilicated papules and nodules with central hemorrhagic crusting in cryptococcosis

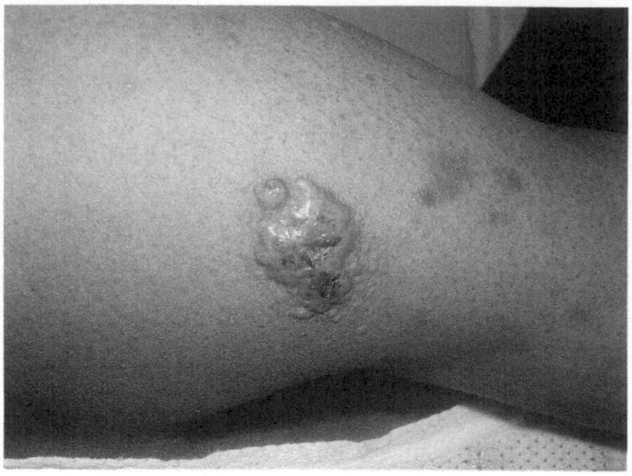

Fig. 30.36 Skin-colored nodule with hemorrhagic crusting centrally

Diagnosis

Diagnosis can be confirmed by skin biopsy and culture.

Treatment

All patients should be administered amphotericin B IVI for the first 14 days; thereafter, oral fluconazole 200 mg twice daily until clinical and mycological resolution. Fluconazole prophylaxis 200 mg daily should continue as long as the CD4 count remains below 200 cells/mm^3. Cryptococcosis recurs as a manifestation of IRIS.

30.4.4.2 Histoplasmosis (Fig. 30.37)

This is caused by the yeast *Histoplasma capsulatum* and is associated with severe immunosuppression (CD4 < 100 cells/mm^3) and is AIDS defining. Up to 10% present with skin manifestations. The skin lesions are polymorphic: papules, nodules, plaques, abscesses, and oral ulcers. Patients are often misdiagnosed with tuberculosis as they are ill with fever, anemia, respiratory symptoms, lymphadenopathy, and hepatosplenomegaly.

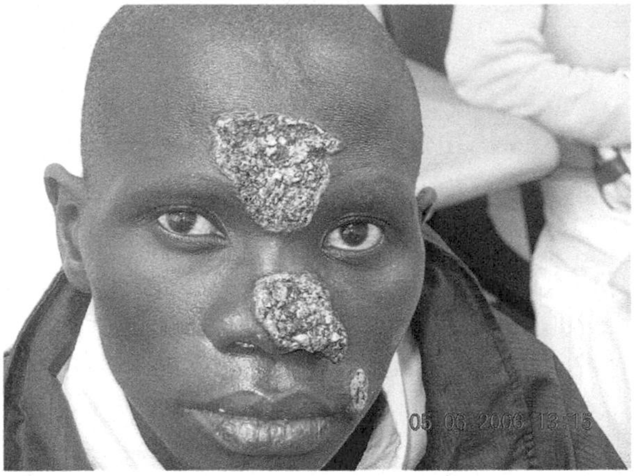

Fig. 30.37 Large ulcers with exuberant crusting involving the face in histoplasmosis

Diagnosis

Diagnosis can be confirmed by biopsy and culture.

Treatment

All patients should be administered amphotericin B IVI for the first 14 days; thereafter, oral fluconazole 200 mg twice daily until clinical and mycological resolution. Fluconazole prophylaxis 200 mg daily should continue as long as the CD4 count remains below 200 cells/mm^3.

30.4.5 Parasitic Infestations

30.4.5.1 **Scabies** (Fig. 30.38)

Although scabies is an extremely common parasitic infestation in Africa, it is often widespread and severe with intense pruritus in HIV. It is caused by *Sarcoptes scabiei* var. *hominis*. Other members of the family are very often affected. The common sites are the web spaces and the sides of the hands and feet, wrists, axillae, abdomen, groin, and the buttocks and gluteal cleft. There may be burrows, papules, and vesicles 1–2 mm in size. Some may be infected presenting as impetigo. In severe immunodeficiency, the lesions may be thickly crusted (Norwegian scabies) with secondary impetigo and is often misdiagnosed as psoriasis.

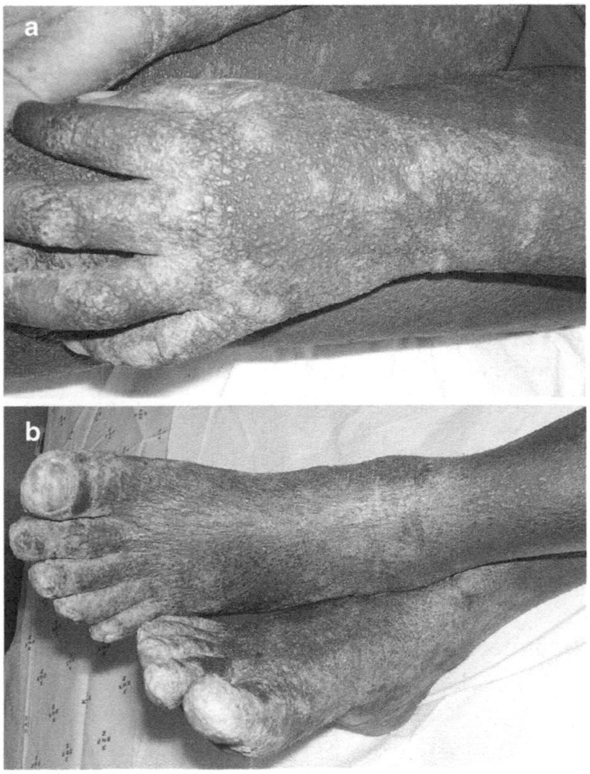

Fig. 30.38 (**a**, **b**) Extensive crusting accentuated on the extensors and web spaces of the hands and feet with nail changes indicating crusted scabies

Diagnosis

The differential diagnosis is papular urticaria or papular pruritic eruption which is commonly seen in HIV. Microscopic examination of skin scrapings and crusts treated with 20% KOH will reveal mites, ova body parts, and feces.

Treatment

Twenty-five percent benzyl benzoate applied from neck to the body consecutively for three nights or sulfur 10% (5% for children) for ten nights is a cost-effective way of treating scabies. Gamma benzene hexachloride applied overnight also helps (not in young children or pregnant females because of neurotoxicity). Crusted scabies can be treated with a single dose of oral ivermectin 200μg /kg. A repeat dose two weeks later improves the cure rate. Antihistamines for pruritus and antibiotics for secondary infection may be prescribed. All members of the family are to be treated.

Clothing and bed linen have to be thoroughly washed.

30.4.5.2 Papular Urticaria (Insect bites)

This is also common especially among children in Africa. In HIV, the lesions are intensely pruritic with erythematous papules, nodules, with or without a central punctum and some with secondary infection. The distribution may be grouped or linear usually on the exposed areas of the face, arms, and legs.

Diagnosis

A history of insect bites or having pets will help in the diagnosis.

Treatment

Oral antihistamines like phenergan 25 mg twice daily, hydroxyzine 25 twice a day or chlorpheniramine 4 mg three times a day will help relieve the pruritus

Topical steroids creams or lotions are useful.

Take-Home Pearls

- Patients with extensive dermatoses should be tested for HIV infection.
- Dermatoses highly suggestive of HIV are: Seborrhoeic dermatitis, papular pruritic eruptions, herpes zoster, extensive molluscum contagiosum, verrucae, chicken pox, and disseminated cryptococcosis and histoplasmosis.
- Dermatoses may be altered in HIV/AIDS, appearing more severely than in immune competent individuals.
- In addition to the above, a number of dermatoses may coexist, more so as the CD4 declines.
- A high index of clinical suspicion is required to diagnose multiple conditions.
- This should be supported by invaluable investigations, for example, KOH, Tzanck smear, pus swab, WR, skin biopsy, and culture.
- Low threshold to obtain skin biopsy and culture is essential and can be lifesaving, since it will allow for timeous therapy.
- Pulmonary and cutaneous tuberculosis should alert one to underlying HIV/AIDS.
- A high index of suspicion is necessary to diagnose drug reactions and to differentiate them from immune reconstitution phenomena related to successful HAART; both occurring in the first 6 weeks of therapy.
- Nevirapine and Trimethoprim-sulfamethoxazole are notorious for drug reaction in the first 4 weeks of therapy, while antituberculous agents can be delayed up to 6 weeks after therapy.

30.5 Conclusion

The introduction of HAART has been associated with the dramatic decline in the prevalence of mucocutaneous conditions associated with HIV/AIDS [62]. However, the incidence of adverse cutaneous drug reactions has increased 100-fold and many infectious and noninfectious skin conditions recur as a manifestation of immune reconstitution. A thorough working knowledge of skin conditions affecting those who are HIV infected will assist the healthcare professional to improve the quality of life of patients in Africa.

References

1. Lim, W., Sadick, N., Gupta, A., et al.: Skin diseases in children with HIV infection and their association with degree of immunosuppression. Int. J. Dermatol. **29**, 24–29 (1990)
2. Aftergut, K., Cockerell, C.J.: Update on the cutaneous manifestations of HIV infection. Dermatol. Clin. **17**, 445–447 (1999)
3. Dlova, N.C., Mosam, A.: Inflammatory noninfectious dermatoses of HIV. Dermatol. Clin. **24**, 439–448 (2006)
4. Dlova, C.N., Mosam, A.: A Clinical Atlas of Skin Conditions in HIV/AIDS: An Illustrated Management Guide for Health Care Professionals. HMPG, Claremont, South Africa (2005). 2005 and 2009
5. Goh, B.K., Chan, R.K., Sen, P., Theng, C.T., Tan, H.H., Wu, Y.J., Paton, N.I.: Spectrum of skin disorders in human immunodeficiency virus-infected patients in Singapore and the relationship to CD4 lymphocyte counts. Int. J. Dermatol. **46**(7), 695–9 (2007 Jul)
6. Morar, N., Dlova, N., Mosam, A., Aboobaker, J.: Cutaneous manifestations of HIV in KwaZulu Natal, South Africa. Int. J. Dermatol. **45**(8), 1006–7 (2006)

7. Mosam, A., Irusen, E.M., Kagoro, H., et al.: The impact of HIV/AIDS on skin disease in Kwa- Zulu Natal, South Africa. Int. J. Dermatol. **43**(10), 782–783 (2004)
8. Nnoruka, E.N., Chukwuka, J.C., Anisuiba, B.: Correlation of mucocutaneous manifestations of HIV/AIDS infection with CD4 counts and disease progression. IJD **46**(Suppl 2), 14–8 (2007 Oct)
9. Gupta, A.K., Nicol, K., Batra, R.: Role of antifungal agents in the treatment of seborrheic dermatitis. Am. J. Clin. Dermatol. **5**(6), 417–22 (2004)
10. Colebunders, R., Mann, J.M., Francis, H., et al.: Generalised papular pruritic eruptions in African patients with HIV infection. AIDS **1**, 117–121 (1987)
11. Goh, B.K., Chan, R.K., Sen, P., Theng, C.T., Tan, H.H., Wu, Y.J., Paton, N.I.: Spectrum of skin disorders in human immunodeficiency virus-infected patients in Singapore and the relationship to CD4 lymphocyte counts. Int. J. Dermatol. **46**(7), 695–9 (2007 Jul)
12. Bason, M.M., Berger, T.G., Nesbit Jr., L.T.: Pruritic papular eruption of HIV disease. Int. J. Dermatol. **32**, 784–789 (1993)
13. Dlova, N.C., Mosam, A.: Inflammatory noninfectious dermatoses of HIV. Dermatol. Clin. **24**, 439–448 (2006)
14. Freedberg, I.M., Eisen, A.Z., Wolff, K., et al.: Fitzpatrick's Dermatology in General Medicine, 6th edn. McGraw-Hill Profession, New York (2003)
15. Lim, H.W., et al.: UVB phototherapy is an effective treatment for pruritus in patients infected with HIV. J. Am. Acad. Dermatol. **37**(3 pt 1), 414–417 (1997)
16. Castelnuovo, B., Byakwaga, H., Menten, J., Schaefer, P., Kamya, M., Colebunders, R.: Can response of a pruritic papular eruption to antiretroviral therapy be used as a clinical parameter to monitor virological outcome? AIDS **22**(2), 269–73 (2008 Jan 11)
17. Handa, S., Narang, T., Wanchu, A.: Dermatologic immune restoration syndrome: report of five cases from a tertiary care center in north India. J. Cutan. Med. Surg. **12**(3), 126–32 (2008 May-Jun)
18. Smith, K.J., Skelton, H.G., Yeager, J., et al.: Pruritus in HIV-1 disease therapy with drugs which may modulate the pattern of immune dysregulation. Dermatology **195**, 353–358 (1997)
19. Rodwell, G.E., Berger, T.G.: Pruritus and cutaneous inflammatory conditions in HIV disease. Clin. Dermatol. **18**, 479–484 (2000)
20. Rigopoulos, D., Paparizos, V., Katsambas, A.: Cutaneous markers of HIV infection. Clin. Dermatol. **22**, 487–498 (2004)
21. Singh, F., Rudikoff, D.: HIV associated pruritus aetiology and management. Am. J. Clin. Dermatol. **4**(3), 177–88 (2003)
22. Rivard, J., Lim, H.W.: Ultraviolet therapy for pruritus. Dermatol. Ther. **18**(4), 344–54 (2005)
23. Garman, M.E., Ruring, S.K.: The cutaneous manifestations of HIV infection. Dermatol. Clin. **20**, 193–208 (2002)
24. Goodman, D.S., Teplitz, E.D., Wishner, A., et al.: Prevalence of cutaneous disease in patients with acquired immunodeficiency syndrome (AIDS) or AIDS-related complex. J. Am. Acad. Dermatol. **17**, 220–223 (1987)
25. Bilu, D., Mamelak, A.J., Nguyen, R.H., et al.: Clinical and epidemiologic characterisation of photosensitivity in HIV positive individual. Photodermatol. Photoimmunol. Photomed. **20**(4), 175–83 (2004)
26. Lim, H.M., Morrisson, W.L., Kamide, R., et al.: Chronic actinic dermatitis. An analysis of 51 patients evaluated in the United States and Japan. Archiv. Dermatol. **130**, 1284–9 (1994)
27. Duvic, M., Johnson, T.M., Rapini, R.P., Freese, T., Brewton, G., Rios, A.: Acquired immunodeficiency syndrome-associated psoriasis and Reiter's syndrome. Arch. Dermatol. **123**(12), 1622–32 (1987 Dec)
28. Arnett, F.C., Reveille, J.D., Duvic, M.: Psoriasis and psoriatic arthritis associated with human immunodeficiency virus infection. Rheum. Dis. Clin. North Am. **17**(1), 59–78 (1991 Feb)
29. Mallon, E.: Retroviruses and psoriasis. Curr. Opin. Infect. Dis. **13**(2), 103–107 (2000)
30. Carr, A., Cooper, D.A.: Adverse effects of antiretroviral therapy. Lancet **356**, 1423 (2000)
31. Dlova, C.N., Mosam, A.: Drug reactions and the skin in HIV/AIDS. S. Afr. J. HIV Med. March: 19–22 (2006)
32. Battegay, M., Opravil, M., Wuthrich, B., Luthy, R.: Rash with amoxycillin-clavulanate therapy in HIV-infected patients. Lancet **ii**, 1100 (1989)
33. Coopman, S.A., Stern, R.S.: Cutaneous drug reactions in Human Immunodeficiency Virus infection. Arch. Dermatol. **127**, 714–7 (1991)
34. Vilar, F., Naisbett, D., Park, B., Pirmohamed, M.: Mechanisms of drug hypersensitivity in HIV infected patients: the role of the immune system. J HIV Ther. **8**, 42–47 (2003)
35. Phillips, E., Mallal, S.: Drug hypersensitivity in HIV. Curr. Opin. Allergy Clin. Immunol. **7**(4), 324–30 (2007 Aug)
36. Bigby, M.: Rates of cutaneous reactions to drugs. Arch. Dermatol. **113**, 832–836 (2001)
37. Bigby, M., Jick, S., Jick, H., et al.: Drug-induced cutaneous reactions. A report from the Boston Collaborative Drug Surveillance Program on 15,438 consecutive inpatients, 1975 to 1982. JAMA **256**(24), 3358–3363 (1986)
38. Shelburne, S.A., Montes, M., Hamill, R.J.: Immune reconstitution inflammatory syndrome: more answers, more questions. J. Antimicrob. Chemother. **57**(2), 167–170 (2006)
39. Shelburne III, S.A., Hamil, R.J., Rodriguez-Barradas, M.C., et al.: Immune reconstitution inflammatory syndrome: emergence of a unique syndrome during highly active antiretroviral therapy. Medicine (Baltimore) **81**(3), 213–227 (2002)
40. Lehloenya, R., Meintjies, G.: Dermatologic manifestations of the immune reconstitution inflammatory syndrome. Dermatol. Clin. **24**, 549–57 (2006)
41. Mosam, A., Hurkchand, H.P., Cassol, E., Page, T., Cassol, S., Bodasing, U., Aboobaker, J., Dawood, H., Friedland, G.H., Coovadia, H.M.: Characteristics of HIV-1-associated Kaposi 's sarcoma among men and women in South Africa. Int. J. STD AIDS **19**, 400–405 (2008)
42. Weiss, H.: Epidemiology of Herpes simplex virus type 2 infection in the developing world. Herpes **11**(supp 1), 24A–34A (2004)
43. Ratnam, I., Chiu, C., Kandala, N.B., Easterbrook, P.J.: Incidence and risk factors for immune reconstitution inflammatory syndrome in an ethnically diverse HIV type-1 infected cohort. Clin. Infect. Dis. **42**(3), 418–427 (2006)

44. Yudin, M.H., Kaul, R.: Progressive hypertrophic genital herpes in an HIV-infected woman despite immune recovery on antiretroviral therapy. Infect. Dis. Ostet. Gynecol. (2008). doi: 10.1155/2008/592532
45. Gershon, A.A.: Prevention and treatment of VZV infections in patients with HIV. Herpes **8**(2), 32–6 (Jul 2001)
46. Armenian, S.H., Han, J.Y., Dunaway, T.M., Church, J.A.: Safety and immunogenicity of live varicella virus vaccine in children with human immunodeficiency virus type 1. Pediatr. Infect. Dis. J. **25**(4), 368–70 (2006 Apr)
47. Wood, S.M., Shah, S.S., Steenhoff, A.P., Rutstein, R.M.: Primary varicella and herpes zoster among HIV-infected children from 1989 to 2006. Pediatrics **121**(1), e150–6 (2008 Jan)
48. Levin, M.J., Anderson, J.P., Seage, G.R., Williams, P.L.: PACTG/IMPAACT 219C Team. Short-term and long-term effects of highly active antiretroviral therapy on the incidence of herpes zoster in HIV-infected children. J. Acquir. Immune Defic. Syndr. **50**(2), 182–91 (2009 Feb 1)
49. Skerlev, M., Husar, K., Sirotkovi -Skerlev, M.: Mollusca contagiosa. From paediatric dermatology to sexually transmitted infection. Hautarzt **60**(6), 472–6 (2009 Jun)
50. van der Wouden, J.C., van der Sande, R., van Suijlekom-Smit, L.W., Berger, M., Butler, C., Koning, S.: Interventions for cutaneous molluscum contagiosum. Cochrane database Syst. Rev. Oct 7, **4**, CD004767 (2009)
51. Sadick, N., Sorhaindo, L.: A comparative split-face study of cryosurgery and trichloroacetic acid 100% peels in the treatment of HIV-associated disseminated facial molluscum contagiosum. Cutis **83**(6), 299–302 (2009 Jun)
52. Yoshinaga, I.G., Conrado, L.A., Schainberg, S.C., Grinblat, M.: Recalcitrant molluscum contagiosum in a patient with AIDS: combined treatment with CO(2) laser, trichloroacetic acid, and pulsed dye laser. Laser Surg Med **27**(4), 291–4 (2000)
53. Gormley, R.H., Kovarik, C.L.: Dermatologic manifestations of HPV in HIV-infected individuals. Curr. Opin. HIV/AIDS Rep. **6**(3), 130–8 (2009 Aug)
54. Kojic, E.M., Cu-Uvin, S.: Update: human papillomavirus infection remains highly prevalent and persistent among HIV-infected individuals. Curr. Opin. Oncol. **19**(5), 464–9 (2007 Sep)
55. Palefsky, J.: Human papillomavirus-related tumors in HIV. **18**(5), 463–8 (2006 Sep)
56. Muller, E.E., Chirwa, T.F., Lewis, D.A.: Human papillomavirus (HPV) infection in heterosexual South African men attending sexual health services: associations between HPV and HIV serostatus. Sex Transm. Infect. Nov 1 (2009) (Epub ahead of print)
57. Cutler, K., Kagen, M.H., Don, P.C., McAleer, P., Weinberg, J.M.: Treatment of facial verrucae with topical imiquimod cream in a patient with human immunodeficiency virus. Acta Derm. Venereol. **80**(2), 134–5 (2000 Mar-Apr)
58. Walzman, M.: Successful treatment of profuse recalcitrant extra-genital warts in an HIV-positive patient using 5% imiquimod cream. Int. J. STD AIDS **20**(9), 657–8 (2009 Sep)
59. Meys, R., Gotch, F.M., Bunker, C.B.: Human papillomavirus in the era of highly active antiretroviral therapy for human immunodeficiency virus: an immune reconstitution-associated disease? Br. J. Dermatol. Jun 22 (2009) (Epub ahead of print)
60. Ghanem, K.G., Moore, R.D., Rompalo, A.M., Erbelding, E.J., Zenilman, J.M., Gebo, K.A.: Antiretroviral therapy is associated with reduced serologic failure rates for syphilis among HIV-infected patients. Clin. Infect. Dis. **47**(2), 258–65 (2008 Jul 15)
61. Burkhart, C.N., Chang, H., Gottwald, L.: Tinea corporis in human immunodeficiency virus-positive patients: case report and assessment of oral therapy. Int. J. Dermatol. **42**(10), 839–43 (2003 Oct)
62. Calista, D., Morri, M., Stagno, A., Boschini, A.: Changing morbidity of cutaneous diseases in patients with HIV after the introduction of highly active antiretroviral therapy including a protease inhibitor. Am. J. Clin. Dermatol. **3**(1), 59–62 (2002)

Kaposi's Sarcoma

31

Erwin Tschachler

Core Messages

- Kaposi's sarcoma is a multifocal tumor of endothelial cell origin.
- Human herpesvirus 8 infection is invariably linked with the all clinical variants of Kaposi's sarcoma.
- Despite the viral origin of this tumor, antiviral treatments are not available.
- Treatment options for Kaposi's sarcoma range from Excision of single lesions to systemic chemotherapy in progressive disease.

31.1 Clinics

31.1.1 Classic KS

This variant was first described by the Austro-Hungarian dermatologist Moriz Kaposi in 1872 [1] as "idiopathic multiple pigment sarcoma." A preponderance of male patients with a male:female ratio of about 3:1 is found in large surveys of most regions [2, 3]. The annual incidence rates for classic KS are different in different geographic regions with ranges from 0.14 per million inhabitants in Great Britain to 10.5 per million in Italian men [2]. Typically, a patient with classic KS is an elderly Caucasian male of Mediterranean or Jewish descent. The tumors frequently start on the distal lower extremities as unilateral or bilateral bluish-red (hematoma-like) macules and progress to firm plaques (Fig. 31.1) and nodules. The tumor surroundings frequently show a pitting edema; the surface is frequently hyperkeratotic. Classic KS usually progresses only slowly [2–4]. After several years, the tumor may start to involve other body sites as well as lymph nodes, mucous membranes, and inner organs, in particular, the gastrointestinal tract [2, 4].

31.1.2 African Endemic KS

An increased incidence of Kaposi's sarcoma in Central Africa was reported in the 1950s [5] and in several countries of this region KS accounts for up to 10% of all neoplasms in men [6]. Also in this variant, a

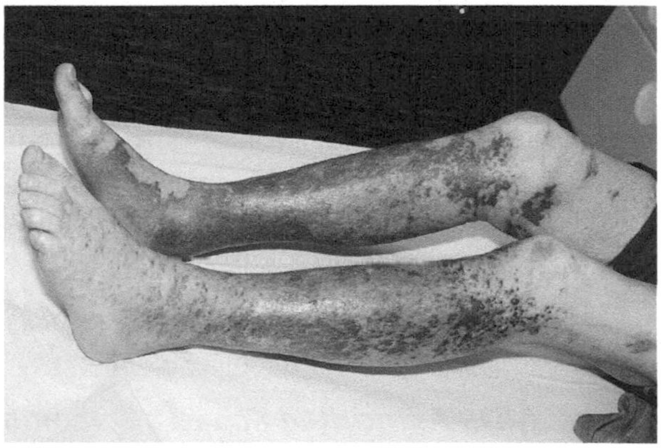

Fig. 31.1 Extensive involvement of both legs in a patient with classical KS

E. Tschachler
Research Division for skin Biology and Pathobiology, Department of Dermatology, Medical University of Vienna, Waehringer Guertel 18–20, A-1090, Vienna, Austria
e-mail: erwin.tschachler@meduniwien.ac.at

G. Gross and S.K. Tyring (eds.), *Sexually Transmitted Infections and Sexually Transmitted Diseases*,
DOI: 10.1007/978-3-642-14663-3_31, © Springer-Verlag Berlin Heidelberg 2011

prevalence of male patients with ratios ranging up to 18:1 is observed [2]. The age at onset is lower than in classic KS – around 35–39 years for males and 25–39 for females [2]. Clinically, African endemic KS occurs as nodular-, florid-, infiltrative-, and lymphadenopathic types [7, 8]. The florid/vegetating and infiltrative variants show aggressive biologic behavior and lesions may extend deeply into the skin reaching underlying muscle and bones. The lymphadenopathic variant predominantly affects children and young adults and may show rapid progression [9]. The reasons for the different courses observed in African KS are not clear and potential cofactors have not yet been unequivocally identified.

31.1.3 KS in Patients Receiving Immunosuppressive Therapies

During the 1970s KS was found to occur 500 times more frequently in organ-transplant recipients under immunosuppressive therapy as compared to control populations [10, 11]. Predominantly kidney allograft recipients were affected and only rarely in other solid organ and bone marrow allografts [10–12] or patients receiving immunosuppressive therapy for other reasons such as the treatment of autoimmune diseases.

The course of KS in immunosuppressed patients may mimic that of the classic variant but may also be rapidly disseminating like in AIDS KS. The skin is involved in more than 85% of the patients whereas less than 15% show visceral (gastrointestinal, lungs, lymph nodes) disease without skin involvement [12]. First lesions can occur as early as 1 month as well as more than 10 years after transplantation. The clinical course appears to be dependent on the dose and type of the immunosuppressive drug used [12], i.e., the risk is higher and the disease onset is earlier with cyclosporin A than with other drugs such as glucocorticoids and azathioprine [12]. Also in transplantation-associated KS, a preponderance of male patients with a ratio of about 3:1 is observed [12].

31.1.4 AIDS-Associated Kaposi's Sarcoma

In 1981, the occurrence of rapidly progressing, multifocal KS was noted in young homosexual men [13] and has since then been an emblematic disease of the AIDS pandemic. During the 1980s, KS has been diagnosed as AIDS-defining disease in more than 20% of HIV-1 infected patients in Europe [14]. Despite a decline in recent years KS is still the most frequent AIDS-associated tumor in homosexual patients to date whereas other patient groups at risk for AIDS are far less affected [15]. By contrast, in Africa KS is the most frequent tumor arising in HIV-1 infected patients independently of their risk group and occurs also in children suffering from AIDS [16].

AIDS KS differs from Classic KS by its more rapid course and its rapid multifocal dissemination and in contrast to other KS variants, initial lesions in AIDS patients frequently occur on the face and on the trunk (Fig. 31.2). The oral mucosa is frequently involved and represents a site of first manifestation in up to 15% of AIDS KS (Fig. 31.3) and progressive disease may result in difficulties of eating, speaking, and breathing [17]. Besides, on the skin KS lesions frequently are

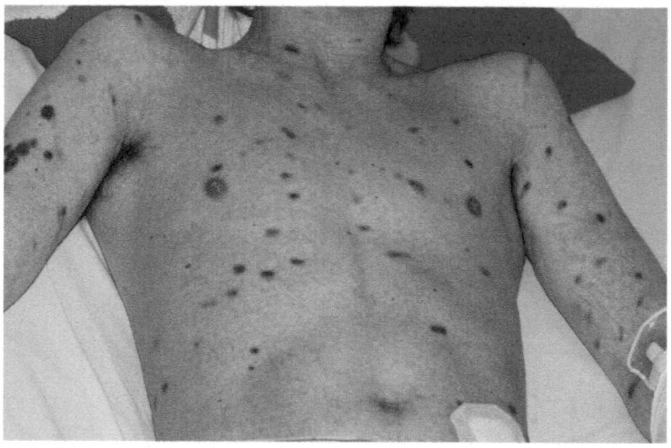

Fig. 31.2 Multifocal lesions on the trunk in a patient with AIDS KS

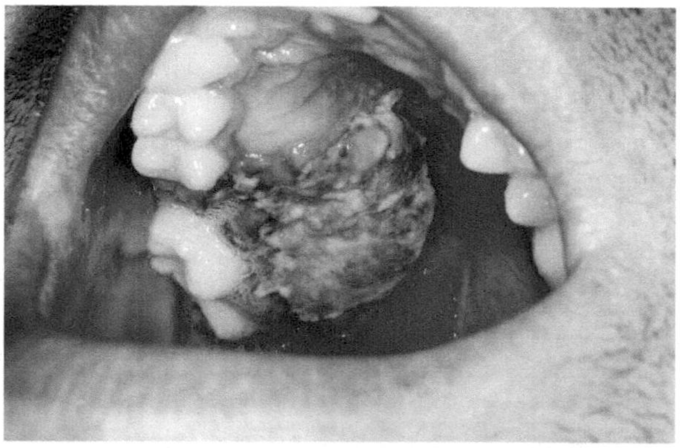

Fig. 31.3 KS lesion on the hard palate in a patient with AIDS KS

present in lymph nodes, in the gastrointestinal tract, and the lungs [18] and these organs may be involved even when skin lesions are absent.

31.2 Pathogenesis of KS

In 1994 Chang and colleague reported the discovery of DNA of an unknown virus in Kaposi's sarcoma lesions [19]. Subsequent cloning established that this DNA belonged to a novel human herpesvirus now referred to as Kaposi's sarcoma-associated herpesvirus (KSHV) or alternatively as human herpesvirus (HHV)-8 [20]. HHV-8 belongs to the γ-herpesviridae subfamily, genus rhadinovirus [20]. Its 165 kb DNA genome contains approximately 90 open reading frames [20] and several genes within the viral genome are homologous to human genes involved in regulation of apoptosis, cell proliferation, and angiogenesis [20]. Like in other herpesviruses, HHV-8 expresses genes which are associated either with viral latency such as LANA-1, V cyclin, and vFLIP or with lytic viral replication such as vGPCR, vIL 6, and v-bcl-2 [20]. Several of these gene products have the ability to transform cells in vitro and in animal models [20]. In patients with KS, the HHV-8 viral genome is detectable in all KS lesions of all stages regardless of the clinical variant [20, 21] and within the lesions latent HHV-8 is found in virtually all tumor cells [22] where it shows monoclonal integration [20]. It is therefore generally accepted that HHV-8 is a transforming herpesvirus and that it plays a direct role in the development of KS.

The time span from infection with HHV-8 to KS development is different in different clinical types: disease manifestation in organ transplant recipients occurs within 1–2 years, in HIV-1 infected patients 5–10 years after infection (reviewed in 6). For classic KS this time span is not determined but appears to be far longer, i.e., several decades. In contrast to the two other types, immunosuppression is not present in the latter patients and precipitating host-related or environmental factors remain to be established [6].

Besides with KS, HHV-8 is also associated with pleural effusion lymphoma, a rare B cell neoplasm seen primarily in AIDS patients where it is found in all reported cases, and multicentric Castleman's disease [6, 20, 23]. In the latter, HHV-8 is present in >95% cases occurring in HIV-infected patients but only in about 40% of HIV-negative patients [23].

In contrast to other herpes viruses HHV-8 is not ubiquitous but shows seroprevalences within the general population ranging from 0.1% in Scandinavian countries to over 10% in Italy to up to 70% in certain countries of Central Africa. In HIV-1-infected patients in developed countries, the prevalence is higher in homosexual and bisexual men than in the general population [6]. Thus the seroprevalence of HHV-8 is largely congruent with the incidence of KS in the different regions and different populations. In several epidemiological studies it was confirmed that sexual activities are a route for HHV-8 transmission in low-prevalence countries and that the transmission risk increases with the numbers of sexual partners [6] as well as the engagement with certain practices in particular oral/genital and oral/anal sex [6]. By contrast, in areas where the virus is widespread such as in Mediterranean countries and Africa, strong evidence exists, that nonsexual transmission among family members [6] plays a major role. The oropharynx is a site of viral replication and high HHV-8 copy numbers are detectable in saliva of infected individuals [24]. Therefore, the nonsexual transmission via saliva may play an important role in childhood transmission in endemic areas [25]. Vertical transmission from mother to child during pregnancy or birth seems not to play an important role [6]. In the hospital setting it is important to remember that HHV-8 is also transmitted by blood and blood products as well as by donor organs during transplantations [6].

The histogenetic origin of the KS tumor cells has been intensively studied over the last 2 decades and the immunophenotype of these cells, (i.e., vWF+/–, PAL-E-, CD31+, CD34+, VEGFR3+) characterizes them as part of the lymphatic endothelial differentiation lineage [26]. The recent demonstration that HHV-8 replicates better in lymphatic than in blood vascular endothelial cells is a further argument for this assumption [27]. However, the finding that infection of blood vascular endothelial cells with HHV-8 leads to a phenotypic switch toward lymphatic endothelial cells [27, 28] suggests that also immature angioblasts able to differentiate into both endothelial cell lineages might represent precursors of KS tumor cells. As to the question whether KS is a reversible proliferative disorder or a true neoplasm, analyses of the methylation pattern of the human androgen receptor gene have shown that lesions with both clonal and polyclonal proliferations can be identified [5, 29, 30]. Studies of HHV-8 terminal repeat sequences which show monoclonality in nodular KS lesions [31] indicate that KS might start as a polyclonal disease with subsequent evolution to a monoclonal process.

31.3 Diagnosis and Differential Diagnoses

Differential diagnoses for cutaneous KS depend on the clinical stages and include Hematoma and statis dermatitis (pseudo-KS) for early lesions and Melanoma, pyogenic granuloma, spindle cell hemangioendothelioma, arteriovenous malformations, bacillary angiomatosis, angiosarcoma, cavernous hemangioma, angiokeratoma, and nodal myofibromatoma for more advanced lesions. Histopathology together with the demonstration of the presence of HHV-8 within the lesions should allow to establish the diagnosis.

31.4 Treatment of Kaposi's Sarcoma

Treatment of KS depends on the clinical type, the extent of the lesions, and on the extent of the involvement of organs other than the skin. For localized cutaneous KS therapies aimed at eliminating individual lesions can be used as initial treatment [32, 33] regardless of the clinical variant. However, in nonclassical KS it is imperative that local therapy is complemented by additional measures such as change of the immune suppressive therapy in transplantation-associated KS and initiation of highly active antiretroviral therapy (HAART) in patients with AIDS KS. The most commonly used local therapies include surgical excision [34], local destruction with liquid nitrogen, laser or photodynamic therapy [35], and topical therapy with 9cis-retinoic acid [36]. Although recurrence rates are high, local therapies might be satisfactory for several years in slowly progressing classical KS.

When patients present with progressive KS, therapeutic different measures need to be taken for the different clinical types.

Due to the low incidence of classic KS, large comparative, prospective therapeutic studies are not available. Different chemotherapies including vinblastine (6 mg IV once a week) doxorubicin, bleomycin, vincristine as monotherapies or in combination (Doxorubicin/Bleomycin/Vincristine – 20–30 mg/m^2//10 mg/m^2//1–2 mg//every 2–4 weeks) have been used for patients with rapidly progressive and/or widespread disease [37] and liposomal anthracyclines (see below) have been reported to be efficient [38] and superior to low-dose interferon alpha.

For AIDS-associated Kaposi's sarcoma which progresses under a HAART regimen, liposomal anthracyclines have been shown to be more efficient and better tolerated than combination therapies such as bleomycin combined with vincristine or both combined also with doxorubicin [39]. A typical drug regimen consists of 20 mg/m^2 liposomal anthracyclines given intravenously every 2–4 weeks [40]. Liposomal anthracyclines show therapeutic efficacy also in patients previously treated by other forms of chemotherapy. For patients with anthracycline-refractory AIDS KS paxicatel (100 mg/m^2 given every 2 weeks) has been added as potential rescue therapy [40]. Interferon alpha which has been the first-line therapeutic approach for AIDS KS during the 1980s and early 1990s still could be tried in AIDS patients with early disseminated KS, of course, together with HAART.

KS in transplant patients responds well to a reduction of immunosuppressive therapy and the replacement of calcineurin inhibitors by rapamycin has recently been shown to lead to a dramatic therapeutic effect with complete remission even of advanced KS lesions [41]. This effect seems to be not only due to the modulation of the immune response by the change of therapy but also to direct antitumor effects of the drug [41].

In addition to these therapies, several experimental therapies ranging from VEGF antisense to antiherpetic drugs are currently evaluated in clinical trials [32].

Take-Home Pearls

- The confirmation of the diagnosis of Kaposi's sarcoma should be based on both the typical histopathology and the demonstration of HHV-8 in tumor tissue.
- Treatment of Kaposi's sarcoma in patients with AIDS should always be combined with antiretroviral i.e. anti-HIV-1 therapy.

References

1. Kaposi, M.: Idiopathisches multiples Pigmentsarkom der Haut. Arch. Dermatol. Syphil. **4**, 265 (1872)
2. Iscovich, J., et al.: Classic Kaposi's sarcoma: epidemiology and risk factors. Cancer **88**, 500 (2000)

3. Brenner B, et al.: Classical Kaposi sarcoma: prognostic factor analysis of 248 patients. Cancer. **95**,1982 (2002)
4. Franceschi, S., et al.: Survival of classic Kaposi's sarcoma and risk of second cancer. Br. J. Cancer **74**, 1812 (1996)
5. Dukers, N.H., Rezza, G.: Human herpesvirus 8 epidemiology: what we do and do not know. AIDS **17**, 1717 (2003)
6. Thijs, A.: L'angiosarcomatose de Kaposi au Congo belge et au Ruanda-Urundi. Ann. Soc. Belge Méd. Trop. **37**, 295 (1957)
7. Taylor, J.F., et al.: Kaposi's sarcoma in Uganda: a clinico-pathological study. Int. J. Cancer **8**, 122 (1971)
8. Templeton, A.C., Bhana, D.: Prognosis in Kaposi's sarcoma. J. Natl Cancer Inst. **55**, 1301 (1975)
9. Dutz, W., Stout, A.P.: Kaposi's sarcoma in infants and children. Cancer **13**, 684 (1960)
10. Harwood, A.R., et al.: Kaposi's sarcoma in recipients of renal transplants. Am. J. Med. **67**, 759 (1979)
11. Penn, I.: Kaposi's sarcoma in organ transplant recipients: report of 20 cases. Transplantation **27**, 8 (1979)
12. Penn, I.: Kaposi's sarcoma in organ transplant recipients. Transplantation **64**, 669 (1997)
13. Centers for Disease Control: Kaposi's sarcoma and Pneumocystis carinii pneumonia among homosexual men – New York City and California. MMWR Morb. Mortal Wkly Rep. **25**, 305 (1981)
14. Hermans, P., et al.: Epidemiology of AIDS-related Kaposi's sarcoma in Europe over 10 years. AIDS **10**, 911 (1996)
15. Renwick, N., et al.: Seroconversion for human herpesvirus 8 during HIV infection is highly predictive of Kaposi's sarcoma. AIDS **12**, 2481 (1998)
16. Ziegler, J.L., Katongole-Mbidde, E.: Kaposi's sarcoma in childhood: an analysis of 100 cases from Uganda and relationship to HIV infection. Int. J. Cancer **65**, 200 (1996)
17. Ficarra, G., et al.: Kaposi's sarcoma of the oral cavity: a study of 134 patients with a review of the pathogenesis, epidemiology, clinical aspects, and treatment. Oral Surg. Oral Med. Oral Pathol. **66**, 543 (1998)
18. Ioachim, H.L., et al.: Kaposi's sarcoma of internal organs: a multiparameter study of 86 cases. Cancer **75**, 1376 (1995)
19. Chang, Y., et al.: Identification of herpesvirus-like DNA sequences in AIDS-associated Kaposi's sarcoma. Science **266**, 1865 (1994)
20. Dourmishev, L.A., et al.: Molecular genetics of Kaposi's sarcoma-associated herpesvirus (human herpesvirus-8) epidemiology and pathogenesis. Microbiol. Mol. Biol. Rev. **67**, 175 (2003)
21. Huang, Y.Q., Li, J.J., Kaplan, M.H., et al.: Human herpesvirus-like nucleic acid in various forms of Kaposi's sarcoma. Lancet **345**, 759 (1995)
22. Sturzl, M., et al.: Expression of K13/v-FLIP gene of human herpesvirus 8 and apoptosis in Kaposi's sarcoma spindle cells. J. Natl Cancer Inst. **91**, 1725 (1999)
23. Cathomas, G.: Kaposi's sarcoma-associated herpesvirus (KSHV)/human herpesvirus 8 (HHV-8) as a tumour virus. Herpes **10**, 72 (2003)
24. Pauk, J., et al.: Mucosal shedding of human herpesvirus 8 in men. N Engl J. Med. **343**, 1369 (2000)
25. Cattani, P., et al.: Human herpesvirus 8 seroprevalence and evaluation of nonsexual transmission routes by detection of DNA in clinical specimens from human immunodeficiency virus-seronegative patients from central and southern Italy, with and without Kaposi's sarcoma. J. Clin. Microbiol. **37**, 1150 (1999)
26. Weninger, W., et al.: Expression of vascular endothelial growth factor receptor-3 and podoplanin suggests a lymphatic endothelial cell origin of Kaposi's sarcoma tumor cells. Lab. Invest. **79**, 243 (1999)
27. Wang, H.W., et al.: Kaposi sarcoma herpesvirus-induced cellular reprogramming contributes to the lymphatic endothelial gene expression in Kaposi sarcoma. Nat. Genet. **36**, 687 (2004)
28. Hong, Y.K., et al.: Lymphatic reprogramming of blood vascular endothelium by Kaposi sarcoma-associated herpesvirus. Nat. Genet. **36**, 683 (2004)
29. Rabkin, C.S., et al.: Monoclonal origin of multicentric Kaposi's sarcoma lesions. N Engl J. Med. **336**, 988 (1997)
30. Gil, P.S., et al.: Evidence for multiclonality in multicentric Kaposi's sarcoma. Proc. Natl Acad. Sci. USA **95**, 8257 (1998)
31. Judde, J.G., et al.: Monoclonality or oligoclonality of human herpesvirus 8 terminal repeat sequences in Kaposi's sarcoma and other diseases. J. Natl Cancer Inst. **92**, 729 (2000)
32. Aoki, Y., Tosato, G.: Therapeutic options for human herpesvirus-8/Kaposi's sarcoma-associated herpesvirus-related disorders. Expert Rev. Anti Infect Ther. **2**, 213 (2004)
33. Hengge, U.R., et al.: Update on Kaposi's sarcoma and other HHV8 associated diseases. Part 1: epidemiology, environmental predispositions, clinical manifestations, and therapy. Lancet Infect. Dis. **2**, 281 (2002)
34. Levine, A.M., Tulpule, A.: Clinical aspects and management of AIDS-related Kaposi's sarcoma. Eur. J. Cancer **37**, 1288 (2001)
35. Karrer, S., et al.: Role of lasers and photodynamic therapy in the treatment of cutaneous malignancy. Am. J. Clin. Dermatol. **2**, 229 (2001)
36. Walmsley, S., et al.: Treatment of AIDS-related cutaneous Kaposi's sarcoma with topical alitretinoin (9-cis-retinoic acid) gel. Panretin Gel North American Study Group. J. Acquir. Immune Defic. Syndr. **22**, 235 (1999)
37. Safai, B.: Kaposi's sarcoma: an overview of classical and epidemic forms. In: Broder, S. (ed.) AIDS, Modern Concepts and Therapeutic Challenges, p. 205. Marcel Dekker, New York (1987)
38. Gottlieb, J.J., et al.: Treatment of classic Kaposi's sarcoma with liposomal encapsulated doxorubicin. Lancet **350**, 1363 (1997)
39. Northfelt, D.W., et al.: Pegylated-liposomal doxorubicin versus doxorubicin, bleomycin, and vincristine in the treatment of AIDS-related Kaposi's sarcoma: results of a randomized phase III clinical trial. J. Clin. Oncol. **16**, 2445 (1998)
40. Hengge, U.R., et al.: Long-term chemotherapy of HIV-associated Kaposi's sarcoma with liposomal doxorubicin. Eur. J. Cancer **37**, 878 (2001)
41. Stallone, G. et al: Sirolimus for Kaposi's sarcoma in renal-transplant recipients. N. Engl. J. Med. **352,** 1317, 20 (2005)

Biology of Sexually Transmitted Human Papillomaviruses

32

Massimo Tommasino

Core Messages

- A large number of human papillomavirus types have been isolated so far, and according to their tissue tropism can be divided in mucosal or cutaneous types.
- Approximately 15 mucosal HPV types are the etiological factors of cervical cancers and other ano-genital cancers.
- HPV infection is a common event in sexually-active women, only in a minority of women the infection can persist, leading to the development of cervical lesions.
- The products of two early genes, E6 and E7, play a key role in the life cycle of the virus and cellular transformation via interaction with several cellular proteins.

32.1 The Human Papillomavirus Family

Human papillomaviruses (HPV) are double-stranded circular DNA viruses with an icosahedral capsid, capable of infecting epithelial cells. More than 90 HPV types have been isolated and fully sequenced, but independent studies indicate that many more exist. An HPV phylogenetic tree has been designed based on the homologous nucleotide sequence of the major capsid protein L1 that groups the different HPV types in genera [1]. The Alpha genus comprises approximately 30 HPV types that infect the mucosa of the genital tract and several benign cutaneous HPV types, e.g., HPV2, that cause common skin warts. The mucosal HPV types are divided into two groups: low-risk HPVs (e.g., types 6 and 11), which are mainly associated with benign genital warts, and high-risk HPVs, which are the etiological agents of cervical cancer [2]. Epidemiological studies indicate that 15 different HPVs, namely 16, 18, 31, 33, 35, 39, 45, 51, 52, 56, 58, 59, 68, 73, and 82, are associated with cervical cancer, while an additional three HPV types of the same genus can be classified as probable high-risk types, i.e., 26, 53, and 66 [3]. HPV16 and HPV18 are the most frequently found HPV types in cervical cancers worldwide, being detected in approximately 50% and 20% of the cases, respectively [3, 4]. For this reason, the majority of the biological studies were focused on these two HPV types.

Genus beta is another HPV subgroup that includes a large number of types. These viruses were first isolated in skin-cancer-prone patients suffering from a rare autosomal recessive genetic disorder called Epidermodysplasia Verruciformis (EV), but it is now clear that they are very common in the skin of immunocompromised and healthy individuals [5]. Twenty-five HPV types within the genus beta have been fully characterized so far, namely 5, 8, 9, 12, 14, 15, 17, 19–25, 36–38, 47, 49, 75, 76, 80, 92, 93, 96. However, additional beta HPV types have been identified by different sensitive HPV detection methods, but are not yet fully characterized. Although the involvement of beta HPV types in the development of non-melanoma skin

M. Tommasino
Infections and Cancer Biology Group, International Agency for Research on Cancer - World Health Organization,
150 Cours Albert-Thomas, 69372 Lyon cedex 08, France
e-mail: tommasino@iarc.fr

G. Gross and S.K. Tyring (eds.), *Sexually Transmitted Infections and Sexually Transmitted Diseases*,
DOI: 10.1007/978-3-642-14663-3_32, © Springer-Verlag Berlin Heidelberg 2011

cancers in EV patients is well accepted, their role in skin carcinogenesis in the general population is still under debate.

The additional genera, gamma, mu, and nu, include cutaneous HPV types that are normally associated with the development of cutaneous papillomas and verrucas.

32.2 Genomic Organization of HPV and Viral Gene Products

The circular double-strand DNA genome of all HPV contains approximately 8,000 bp. The molecular cloning and sequencing of the papillomaviruses have revealed a genomic organization typical of all the members of the HPV family, with eight or nine open reading frames (ORFs) found on the same DNA strand. The HPV genome can be divided into three different regions: (1) a coding region containing the early genes, E1, E2, E4, E5, E6, and E7; (2) a region containing the late genes encoding the major (L1) and minor (L2) capsid proteins; and (3) a non-coding region, termed long control region (LCR), which is localized between open reading frames (ORF) L1 and E6 and contains most of the regulatory elements involved in viral DNA replication and transcription. The length of LCR can vary in different HPV genomes and ranges between 650 and 900 nucleotides. The genome of HPV 16 is shown in Fig. 32.1.

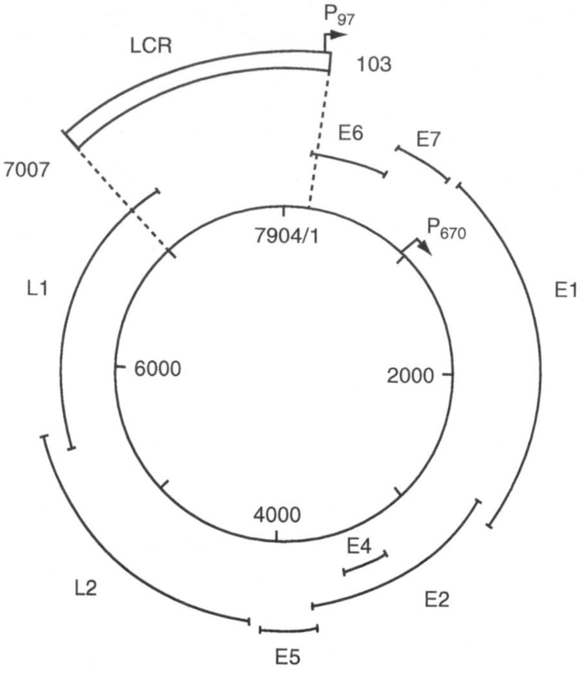

Fig. 32.1 The double-strand DNA HPV genome is represented by a *black circle* with the nucleotide numbers. The position of the long control region (LCR) and the early and late genes are also shown. The early and late promoters, P_{97} and P_{670}, respectively, are indicated by the *arrows*

32.3 HPV Life Cycle

The HPV cycle is tightly linked to the differentiation program of stratified epithelia. In fact, the temporal window of early and late gene expression is dependent on specific cellular events occurring during cellular differentiation. HPV infects cells of the basal layer, where it is maintained at relatively low copy number. When cells leave the basal layer of the epithelium, HPV initiates the productive phase of the life cycle, characterized by vegetative viral DNA replication. During this phase, the HPV genome is amplified up to more than 1,000 copies per cell. Immediately after, the expression of late genes starts. Finally, viral particles are produced and released. The different events of the HPV life cycle are illustrated in Fig. 32.2 and will be described in greater detail in the following paragraphs.

32.3.1 *Infection of Epithelium Basal Layer Cells*

The first step in HPV infection is the reaching of the undifferentiated cells of the basal layer of the epithelia. This may occur due to micro-lesions of the skin or mucosa. Binding of the cellular membrane is mainly mediated by the major capsid protein L1, which interacts with cell surface heparin sulfate proteoglycan [6, 7]. It is also possible that the viral particles bind another component of the cellular membrane. In fact, it has been proposed that α6 integrin may act as a secondary cellular receptor for HPV particles [8]. However, other studies have shown that cells that do not express α6 integrin can be still infected by animal or human PV [6, 9].

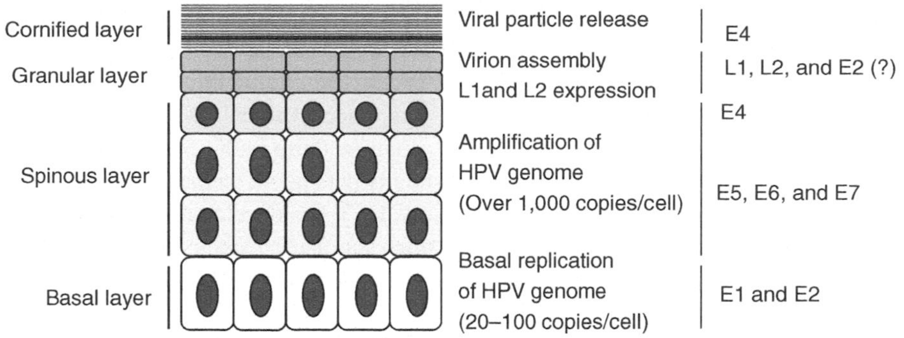

Fig. 32.2 HPV infects the cells of basal layer of the epithelium, in which its genome is maintained at low copy number/cell (20–100). Vegetative HPV replication occurs during the differentiation (Spinous layer), and more than 1,000 copies of HPV genome are amplified in each cell. Immediately after, late genes are expressed and HPV DNA is encapsidated. The release of the viral particle occurs in the last layer of the epithelium. The different layers of the epithelium are indicated on the left. The viral proteins involved in the different events of the HPV life cycle are listed on the right. The question mark in front of E2 indicates that its role in virion assembly is not clear

After HPV16 particles bind to the cellular membrane, their internalization is mediated by a clathrin-dependent endocytic pathway [10]. However, there is evidence that other HPV types may use different endocytosis pathways [11]. It is also highly likely that the minor L2 capsid protein plays a role in membrane binding and cellular internalization. In fact, anti-L2 antibodies against specific linear epitopes are able to block the internalization of L1/L2 virus-like particles in *in vitro* assays [12, 13].

32.3.2 HPV DNA Replication in Epithelium Basal Layer Cells

After cell entry, viral particles are disassembled in late endosome, and the viral DNA is transported into the nucleus. L2 appears to play an important role in endosome escape, traverse of the cytoplasm, and nuclear transport of viral DNA. In agreement with this model, L2 and viral genome have been detected in the same nuclear compartments [14]. In the cells of the basal layer, HPV DNA replicates together with the cellular DNA during S phase and is maintained as an extrachromosomal plasmid in the nucleus at relatively low copy number, i.e., 20–100. In addition to the cellular DNA replication machinery, the products of the early E1 and E2 genes are required for replication and maintenance of HPV DNA.

E2 is the initiating factor of viral DNA replication. This viral protein has an approximate molecular weight of 45 kDa and consists of three different domains: (1) the trans-acting domain located at the N-terminus (TA), (2) a central flexible hinge of approximately 100 amino acids, and (3) a C-terminus region that comprises the dimerization and the DNA-binding domain (DBD) [15]. E2 binds 12bp palindromic sequences (E2BS) in HPV origin replication (ori) that is located within the LCR, immediately before the E6 gene. The E2BS are close to an E1 binding site (E1BS). Due to the ability to complex with E1, E2 facilitates the recruitment of the E1 monomeric form to ori and its interaction with the E1BS. After DNA binding, E1 assembles in a hexamer/dihexamer complex and recruits several components of the DNA replication machinery to the ori, e.g., polymerase α-primase complex, the single-stranded DNA-binding protein replication protein A, and topoisomerase I (Topo I). The C-terminal domain of E1 possesses a helicase/ATPase activity that is responsible for the unwinding of the viral DNA during replication. There are several mechanisms that influence the E1 activity. For instance, E1 interacts with and is phosphorylated by the kinase complexes cyclin E/CDK2 and cyclin A/CDK2. Their kinase activity fluctuates during the cell cycle, being critical for the G1/S transition and S phase, respectively. As HPV DNA replication is entirely dependent on the host machinery, the CDK-mediated E1 phosphorylation is most likely a way to synchronize cellular and viral DNA replication. The mutation of E1 CDK phosphorylation sites resulted in a reduction of HPV DNA replication, highlighting the importance of E1 phosphorylation in the viral life cycle [16].

In addition to initiation of viral DNA replication, E2 plays a key role in HPV DNA segregation into daughter cells during cell division, acting as a bridge between viral and host genome. Studies on bovine papillomavirus (BPV) E2 have shown that the N-terminus binds the mitotic chromatin, while the C-terminus interacts with the viral genome [17–20]. The cellular protein Brd4 appears to mediate the E2 association with the mitotic chromatin [21]. Although HPV16 E2 is also able to interact with Brd4, it has been suggested that HPV DNA segregation occurs via mechanisms different from those of BPV. During mitosis HPV E2 was not found to be associated with mitotic chromatin, but instead with centrosomes and mitotic spindle [22]. A recent study has shown that BPV and HPV E2 bind another cellular protein, ChlR1, a DNA helicase that plays a role in sister chromatid cohesion [23].

32.3.3 Genome Amplification

HPV DNA amplification occurs in cells of the suprabasal layer of the epithelium. This step of the virus life cycle leads to the production of over 1,000 copies of HPV genome/cell. In a physiological situation, cells of the suprabasal layer withdraw from the cell cycle and undergo commitment to differentiation. Therefore, all components of the DNA replication machinery are not active in these cells. Since HPV DNA replication is totally dependent on the host DNA replication machinery, HPV has developed several mechanisms to maintain suprabasal cells in a proliferative state and reactivate the cellular DNA replication machinery. It is now well established that the early gene products E5, E6, and E7 are directly involved in the stimulation of cellular proliferation in the suprabasal layers of the epithelium.

Among these early HPV proteins, E7 appears to be a most efficient cell cycle deregulator. HPV16 E7 is an acidic phosphoprotein of 98 amino acids, which is structurally and functionally related to a gene product of another DNA tumor virus, the Adenovirus E1A protein. Based on the similarity in primary structure between the two viral proteins, they can be divided into three domains: conserved regions 1–3 (CR1–3) (Fig. 32.3). CR2 contains an LXCXE (amino acids 22–26) domain involved in binding to the tumor suppressor protein retinoblastoma (pRb1) and its related proteins p107 and p130, also termed pocket proteins. All three proteins are deeply involved in cell cycle regulation. pRb1 negatively regulates, via direct association, the activity of several transcription factors, including members of the E2F family (E2F1 to 3), which are associated with their partners, DPs [24, 25]

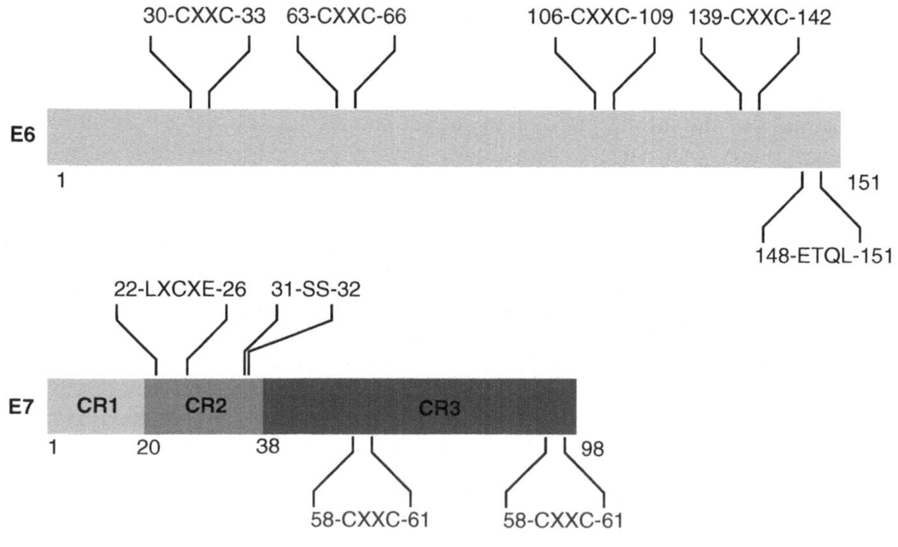

Fig. 32.3 E6 and E7 are the main transforming proteins of the high-risk HPV types. Both proteins contain CXXC motifs (two in E7 and four in E6) that are able to complex with the zinc. E6 also contains at the C-terminus a consensus PDZ-binding motif (ETQL). E7 includes three regions that are homologous to Adenovirus E1A (conserved regions 1–3, CR1–3). CR2 comprises the pRb-binding motif (LXCXE) and two serines (31 and 32) that phosphorylated by Casein Kinase II (CKII). The numbers indicate the position of motifs in each protein

(Fig. 32.4). Under normal cell cycle regulation, phosphorylation of pRb, which is mediated by cyclin-dependent kinase (CDK) activity, leads to the disruption of pRb/E2F complexes, with consequent activation of E2Fs. HPV16 E7 binds the pocket proteins and, analogously to CDK-mediated phosphorylation, results in the release of active E2F1 to 3, which in turn activate the transcription of a group of genes encoding proteins essential for cell cycle progression, such as cyclin E and cyclin A (Fig. 32.4).

The other two members of the pocket protein family, p107 and p130, associate with E2F4 or E2F4 and E2F5, respectively, and are involved in controlling additional cell cycle checkpoints. p130 exerts its transcriptional regulatory function during the G0/G1 transition, while p107 is active in the G1/S transition and in the G2 phase [24, 25]. In contrast to E2F1-3, E2F4 and E2F5 play a negative role in gene expression. They form co-repressor complexes together with p107 or p130 and histone deacetylase enzymes that bind specific E2F elements resulting in inhibition of gene expression. HPV16 E7, by binding 107 and p130, may lead to inhibition of the repressing activity of the E2F4 and E2F5 complexes. Thus, the interaction of HPV16 E7 with the three pocket proteins results in the inactivation of (1) pRb/E2F1-3 complexes and a consequent release of active transcription factors and (2) p107 or p130/E2F4-5 complexes and release of the transcriptional repression.

Besides targeting the pocket proteins, E7 can alter the cell cycle via additional mechanisms. The HPV16 E7 protein is able to associate with the CDK inhibitors $p21^{WAF1/CIP1}$ and $p27^{KIP1}$, causing neutralization of their inhibitory effects on the cell cycle. Cells co-expressing HPV16 E7 and $p21^{WAF1/CIP1}$ or $p27^{KIP1}$ are still able to enter S phase, while in the absence of E7, cells are arrested in G1 phase [26–28].

HPV16 E7 can also directly and/or indirectly interact with the cyclin A/CDK2 complex [29–31]. The biological function of this interaction is not entirely understood. A recent study has shown that HPV16 E7 strongly stimulates the histone H1 kinase activity of CDK2 complexed with either cyclin A or cyclin E. In addition, cross-linking experiments have indicated that HPV16 E7 interacts mainly with cyclin A [32]. It is possible that E7 may also act by redirecting the kinase complexes to a different set of substrates important for the progression/completion of the viral life cycle.

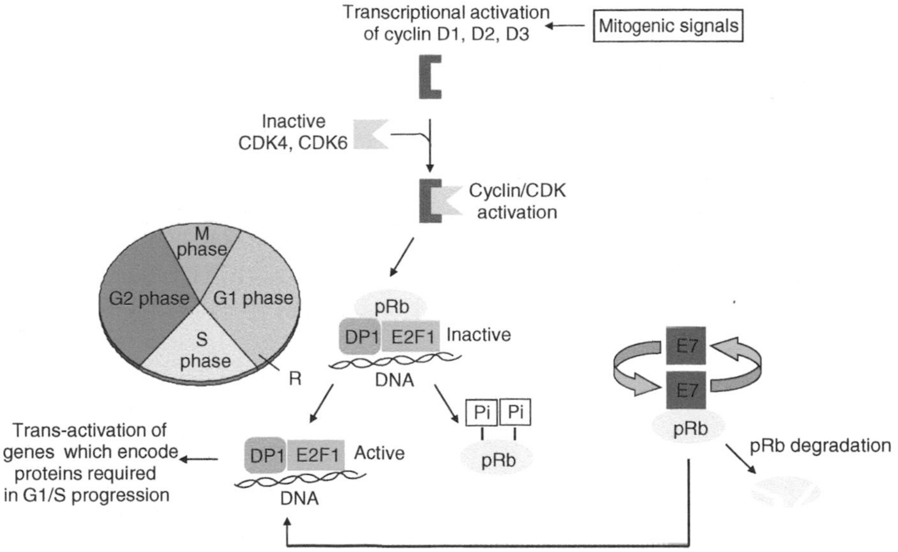

Fig. 32.4 HPV16 E7 deregulates the cell cycle restriction point (R). E2F transcription factors form heterodimer complexes with members of the DP family and regulate the transcription of several genes during the cell cycle. In quiescent cells, pRb is present in a hypophosphorylated form and associates with E2F molecules, thereby inhibiting their transcriptional activity. When quiescent cells are exposed to mitogenic signals, genes encoding the G1-specific D-type cyclins (D1, D2, and D3) are activated. Subsequently, cyclins associate with a catalytic subunit, CDK4 or 6, and after transport into the nucleus the kinase complexes phosphorylate pRb in mid-G1 phase, causing release of active E2F/DP1 heterodimer complexes and progression through the restriction point (R). E7 binding to pRb mimics its phosphorylation. Thus, E7 expressing cells can enter S phase in the absence of a mitogenic signals

Like E7, HPV16 E6 has also developed several mechanisms to promote cellular proliferation. HPV16 E6 is a small basic protein of 151 amino acids. The major structural characteristic of E6 is the presence of two atypical zinc fingers. At the base of these zinc fingers are two motifs containing two cysteines (Cys-X-X-Cys), which are conserved in all E6 HPV types (Fig. 32.3).

The best-characterized HPV16 E6 activity is its ability to induce degradation of the tumor suppressor protein p53 via the ubiquitin pathway (reviewed in [33]). This cellular protein is a transcription factor that can trigger cell cycle arrest or apoptosis in response to a large variety of cellular stresses, such as hypoxia or DNA damages. Overall, the role of p53 is to ensure the integrity of the cellular genome, preventing cell division after DNA damage or delaying it until the damage has been repaired. Alternatively, if replication of damaged DNA has already occurred or is too large, p53 can divert the cell into apoptosis, thus preventing the production of potentially transformed progeny. HPV16 E6 binds to a 100 kDa cellular protein, termed E6 associated protein (E6AP), which functions as an ubiquitin protein ligase (E3). The E6/E6AP complex then binds the central region (also termed the core domain) of p53, which becomes rapidly ubiquitinated and is targeted to proteasomes [34–36] (Fig. 32.5). Recent data, however, have shown that HPV16 and 18 E6 can also promote p53 degradation in epithelial cells derived from E6AP-null mice, implying that additional ubiquitin ligases may be involved in HPV-mediated p53 degradation [37].

It is likely that HPV16 E6-mediated p53 degradation is required to fully guarantee viral replication under any circumstances and cellular stresses. Studies of *in vitro* and *in vivo* experimental models have shown that, in addition to cellular proliferation, HPV16 E7 is able to promote apoptosis [38, 39]. This event appears to be dependent, at least in part, on p53 and is most likely a cellular defense elicited by E7-induced unscheduled proliferation. Thus, in this scenario, it is obvious that the p53 inactivation mediated by HPV16 is an essential requirement to keep the infected cells in a proliferative state.

Low-risk and high-risk mucosal HPV E6 proteins, as well as E6 from certain cutaneous HPV types, can also interfere with the apoptotic pathways independently of p53, but via its association with Bak, a member of the Bcl-2 family [40, 41]. Early apoptotic signals lead Bak to form pores in the mitochondrial membrane, resulting in release of cytochrome C from the mitochondria, followed by induction of caspase apoptotic cascades [42]. Analogously to its effect on p53, E6 induces Bak degradation via the ubiquitin-mediated pathway. In normal epithelium, the Bak protein is highly expressed in the upper layers during differentiation. It is possible that neutralization of Bak by mucosal HPV types is necessary for the progression/completion of the viral life cycle. Regarding the cutaneous HPV types, Bak degradation may be required to antagonize the anti-proliferative effects of UV irradiation in skin. In fact, Bak is highly stabilized and activated throughout the entire epidermis in response to UV irradiation. However, in the presence of HPV E6 protein, neither stabilization of the Bak protein nor detection of the apoptotic process occurs in regenerated human epidermis following UV-B irradiation [41].

Another feature of HPV16 E6 is to activate the transcription of the hTERT (human Telomerase Reverse Transcriptase) gene encoding the catalytic subunit of the

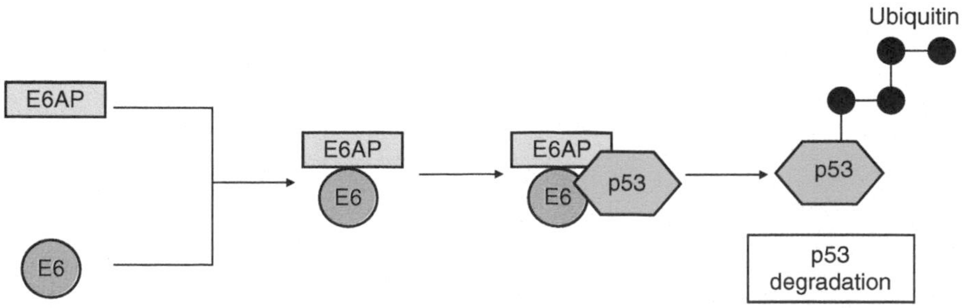

Fig. 32.5 HPV16 E6 targets p53 for degradation via the ubiquitin/proteasome pathway. The E6 oncoprotein associates with the ubiquitin-protein ligase E6AP. The dimeric complex then binds p53, and E6AP catalyzes multiubiquitination of p53 in presence of ubiquitin and additional enzymes of the ubiquitin pathway, e.g., E1 and E2

telomerase complex [43]. Somatic cells are characterized by very little or no telomerase activity, and telomeres shorten as a function of cellular division to finally reach a critical size, leading to replicative senescence (reviewed in [44]). By contrast, HPV16-infected cells harbor a very high level of telomerase activity, allowing telomere length maintenance and indefinite proliferation. Independent studies have shown that several mechanisms may be implicated in HPV-induced hTERT transcriptional activation. HPV16 E6 is able, through its association with E6AP, to promote the degradation of the transcriptional repressor NFX1-91 and, consequently, to activate hTERT transcription [45]. Another study has shown that HPV16 E6, via direct binding, increases Myc efficiency in activating the hTERT promoter [46]. It is possible that this HPV-mediated hTERT transcriptional activation is not dependent on E6/E6AP interaction. In agreement with this model, it has been recently shown that HPV16 E6 mutants deficient for E6AP binding are still able to stimulate the expression of hTERT. In addition, chromatin immunoprecipitation assays have revealed the presence of E6AP binding-defective E6 mutants and Myc, but not E6AP, on the endogenous hTERT promoter [47]. In contrast to HPV16 E6, E7 alone is not able to modulate hTERT expression. However, it has been recently shown that E7, when expressed together with E6, significantly augments E6-induced hTERT transcription [48]. In summary, the virus uses multiple mechanisms to activate hTERT and prevent senescence.

As shown for E7, E6 also appears to directly act on the G1/S transition [49, 50]. Overexpression of E6 from cutaneous benign HPV1 or HPV16 in rodent immortalized fibroblasts and primary human fibroblasts induces cellular proliferation, retinoblastoma (pRb) phosphorylation, and accumulation of products of genes that are negatively regulated by pRb, such as CDC2, E2F-1, and cyclin A [50].

In addition to what has been described above, a large number of interactions between the E6 or E7 and cellular proteins have been reported (for review see [51, 52]). However, in most cases their biological significance is not yet entirely understood. In particular, it is not clear which of these viral/cellular protein complexes are only involved in the viral life cycle and which also contribute to the malignant transformation of the infected cell.

E5 is a small hydrophobic protein located in the endoplasmatic reticulum (ER), nuclear membrane, and cytoplasmic vesicles. Two recent studies have provided convincing evidence that E5 plays a role in HPV16 and HPV31 vegetative replication [53, 54]. In these studies, the replication efficiency of wild-type or E5-mutated HPV genomes was analyzed in monolayer or organotypic keratinocyte cultures. Although the absence of E5 did not significantly affect the HPV genome replication in keratinocytes cultured under undifferentiated conditions (monolayer), a strong reduction of HPV genome amplification was observed in the upper layers of the epithelium in the organotypic cultures. How E5 influences the productive phase of the HPV life cycle is still unclear. Independent studies have shown that HPV16 E5 is able to enhance growth factor-mediated signal transduction to the nucleus. HPV16 E5 associates with and inhibits the 16 kDa subunit c of the vacuolar H+-ATPase [55–58], which is responsible for the acidification of membrane-bound organelles, such as Golgi, endosomes, and lysosomes. The HPV16 E5-mediated loss of pH gradients in the endosomes inhibits degradation of internal growth factor receptors that are recycled onto the plasma membrane.

E4 also appears to play a positive role in the vegetative HPV DNA replication. E4 is a late protein expressed by the promoter located in the early coding region (P_{670} for HPV16) in the suprabasal layer of the infected epithelium. In HPV, infected E4 is present at very high levels, and several E4-derived proteins have been detected. The primary product is a 17 kDa protein, which is expressed from E1^E4 transcript. Mutations in HPV18 or 31 genome that disrupt the E4 expression, but do not alter the E2 gene, strongly impaired genome amplification in the suprabasal layers of the epithelium in keratinocyte organotypic cultures [59, 60]). The contribution of E4 on vegetative HPV replication may be explained by its ability to interfere with cell cycle regulation. E4 from cutaneous and mucosal HPV types induces a G2 arrest [61–63]. This E4 activity appears to be mediated by inactivation of the cyclin B/cdc2 complex that plays a key role in G2/M transition [64]. Ectopic expression of cyclin B in HPV1 E4-expressing cells overrides the inhibitory function of E4 on cell cycle [63]. It is highly likely that the E4-induced G2 arrest positively impacts the productive viral life cycle, creating favorable conditions for HPV genome amplification without progress into mitosis.

In addition to the HPV oncoproteins E4, E5, E6, and E7, E2 may also indirectly interfere with HPV genome amplification. In fact, E2, via its ability to act as transcription factor, can modulate the expression of E6 and E7. The E2 DBD binds four cis elements (ACCN6GGT) in the LCR of the HPV16 genome in front of the p97 promoter. E2 may lead to repression or activation of the promoter of the early genes depending on the binding of specific cis elements and its intracellular levels. E2 binding to the promoter-distal or promoter-proximal elements leads to a positive or negative regulation of the promoter, respectively (reviewed in [65]).

32.3.4 Production and Release of Viral Particles

The final events of the productive phase of the HPV life cycle are the expression of the late genes E1^E4, L1, and L2, encapsidation of viral DNA, and release of newly assembled infectious virions. The icosahedral HPV capsid is formed by the 72 capsomers, which are made of five L1 molecules and one L2 molecule. Several polycistronic transcripts containing the three late genes E4, L1, and L2 in different combinations are generated by a differentiation-specific promoter located within the E7 gene (P_{670} for HPV16 or P_{742} for HPV31). This promoter uses different transcription start sites that are distributed in a region of approximately 200 bp [66–68].

Studies with a cell line (CIN612-9E) established from biopsies of low-grade cervical lesions containing the episomal form of HPV31 genome [69] have revealed that the late P_{742} promoter is strongly activated in the upper layers of the epithelium of organotypic cultures [66]. DNase I hypersensitivity analysis of HPV-31 chromatin in CIN612-9E cell lines revealed that the region surrounding the P_{742} promoter became accessible to DNase I during differentiation. These findings indicate that this region becomes accessible to transcription factor binding upon differentiation to initiate the transcription of the late genes. Activators of protein kinase C (PKC) have been shown to strongly stimulate the transcription of the late genes [70]. Interestingly, specific forms of PKC are highly expressed in the epithelium and are intimately linked to induction of differentiation (reviewed in [71, 72]). Thus, PKC may be at least partly responsible for the link between viral late gene expression and differentiation. However, the molecular mechanisms of PKC in up-regulating the HPV promoter are not well understood, but it is possible that PKC directly phosphorylates and activates specific transcription factors involved in the regulation of HPV late promoter.

Expression of the late genes is also regulated by short elements present in the 3' end in the uncoding and coding regions of L1 and L2 [73–77]. Several cellular factors, e.g., splicing or adenylation factors, are able to bind these elements in L1 and L2 transcripts, which favors their degradation or nuclear sequestration [74, 77–79]. Findings suggest that E4 may interfere with the stability of L1 and/or L2 transcripts. It has been shown that E4 interacts with a novel DEAD-box protein, E4-DBP [80]. Members of the DEAD-box protein family are implicated in a number of RNA-related cellular events, including RNA splicing and degradation [81]. The functions of E4-DBP are still unknown. However, the high similarity of E4-DBP to bacterial and yeast proteins implicated in RNA stability supports its involvement in these events. Thus, it can be speculated that E4-DBP may directly or indirectly associate with viral transcripts, and its ability to modulate RNA stability may be altered by the association with E4.

HPV DNA encapsidation and release of viral particles are the last steps of the HPV life cycle. The former event appears to be highly dependent on L2 [82, 83]. Deletion of the L2 gene in the HPV31 genome strongly affects HPV DNA encapsidation and virus particle infectivity [83]. It has also been suggested that the nonstructural E2 protein may play a role in virion production by favoring the recruitment of HPV DNA to the sites of assembly [82] . However, recent findings obtained in an experimental *in vitro* model for artificial production of BPV particles did not support this hypothesis [84].

HPV is not a lytic virus, and the molecular events involved in the release of virus particles from the desquamating keratinocyte are not entirely understood. It has been proposed that E4 may facilitate the escape of HPV particles from cornified layers of the epithelium by inducing a number of cellular events, disruption of keratin network, apoptosis, and modification of cornified cell envelopes [85–88].

32.4 HPV and Cervical Cancer

The mucosal HPV types preferentially infect the cervical transformation zone, which is the junction point of the endocervix columnar cells and the ectocervix stratified squamous epithelial cells. The transformation zone epithelium is subject to continuous changes during a woman's life, and it is believed that the specific features of this region facilitate the development of cervical cancer. However, the majority of HPV infections do not lead to cytological anomalies or cancer, but they are cleared by the immune system in a relatively short time (6–12 months). A small percentage of infections persist and promote the development of low- and/or high-grade cervical intraepithelial neoplasia (CIN), which may regress or progress to an invasive cervical carcinoma after a period of latency [89] (Fig. 32.6). Several epidemiological studies have identified additional risk factors that play a role in the progression of HPV-induced disease, most likely influencing the immune surveillance system or acting as additional carcinogens. These include sexual habits, cigarette smoking, oral contraceptives, parity and host genetic predisposition [90–95].

More than 99% of cervical cancers resulted in HPV DNA positivity [96], and it is highly likely that the few apparent HPV-negative cancers contain rare HPV types or subtypes. From a rational point of view, it is not easy to understand why the high-risk HPV types have to induce cancer, which results in the disruption of the viral life cycle. The only interest of a virus is to generate its progeny. Since synthesis of viral components is totally dependent on host cellular machineries, HPV has developed several mechanisms to maintain infected cells in a constant active and proliferative state. In addition to the activation of cellular machineries, HPV

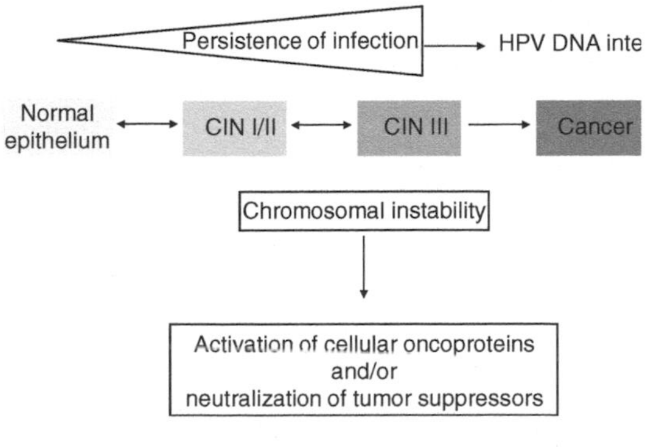

Fig. 32.6 In cervical cancer cells, HPV DNA is often integrated. This event appears to occur randomly throughout the host genome, although a possible preference may be the fragile sites of the chromosomes. Regarding the viral genome, integration always occurs in E1/E2 region. After HPV DNA integration, the majority of the HPV genes are not expressed, with the exception of E6 and E7. The loss of E2 can lead to an up-regulation of E6 and E7 expression, facilitating cellular transformation

must efficiently evade the immune system. The longer a virus is able to persist in the host, the more progeny are generated and transmitted to other hosts. It is plausible to imagine that the combination of these two HPV-mediated events, stimulation of cellular proliferation, and neutralization of the immune system, may facilitate the malignant transformation of infected cells. Based on this model, it should be predicted that the low-risk HPV types are less efficient than the high-risk HPV types in subverting the normal life of infected cells. A large number of studies demonstrated that this is the case indeed. The difference between these two groups of HPVs is determined by the intrinsic biological properties of the E6 and E7, which are also considered the main oncoproteins of HPV types.

32.5 The Role of E6 and E7 in Cellular Transformation

The first indication of the role of E6 and E7 in carcinogenesis came from the analysis of cervical cancer-derived cells, e.g., SiHa and CaSki [97], in which viral DNA was found randomly integrated in the host genome. It was also shown that the viral DNA integration resulted in the disruption of several viral genes with preservation of only the E6 and E7, which were actively transcribed (Fig. 32.7). Analysis of the HPV DNA status in low- and high-grade premalignant lesions and in cervical cancer have revealed that the frequency of viral DNA integration increases with the severity of the cervical disease (reviewed in [98]). In fact, the majority of cervical cancers, if not all, have few or several copies of viral DNA integrated into the genome. As the integration of viral DNA often results in a loss of E5 gene expression, its activity in deregulation of proliferation may be involved only in early events during the multistep process of cervical cancinogenesis, and not after cancer development. In contrast, continuous E6 and E7 expression is necessary for the maintenance of the malignant phenotype. Silencing of both viral genes in cervical cancer-derived cell lines resulted in rapid cellular death (reviewed in [99]).

The discovery that both proteins display transforming activities in *in vitro* and *in vivo* experimental models provides further lines of evidence for their involvement in cancer development. Immortalized rodent fibroblasts, e.g., NIH3T3, are fully transformed by expression of HPV 16 E6 or E7 protein and acquire the ability to grow

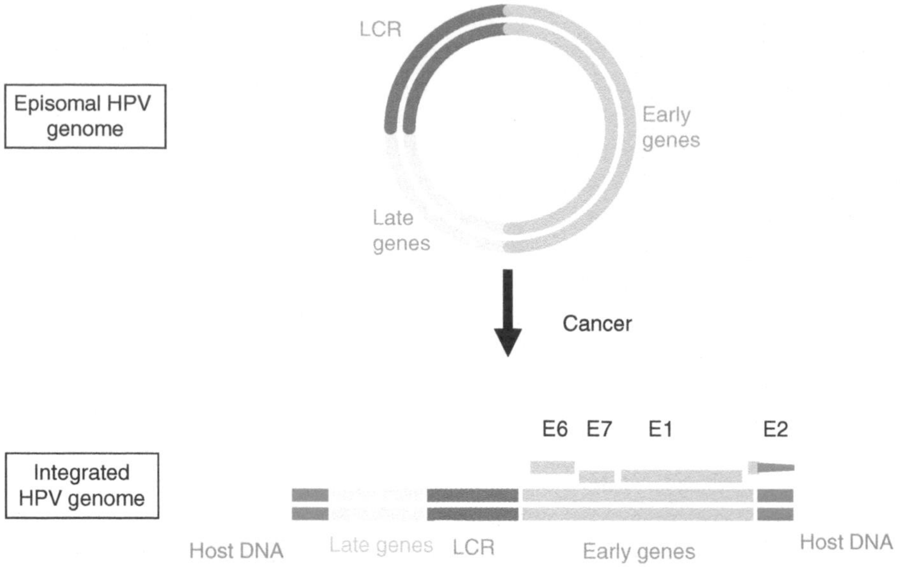

Fig. 32.7 HPV-induced cervical cancer is a multistep process. Most of the high-risk HPV infections spontaneously regress without generating any pathological condition. In a small percentage of cases, persistency of the viral infection leads to the development of low-grade disease, termed low-grade cervical intraepithelial neoplasia (CIN I), which is characterized by abnormal differentiation in the lower third of the epithelium. The lesion may regress or progress to severe dysplasia, high-grade CIN (CIN II/III). CINII/III can still regress or evolve to invasive cervical carcinoma. The latter stage is associated with accumulation of damages in the chromosomes of the host cells that lead to activation of cellular oncoproteins and/or neutralization of tumor suppressors. The frequency of HPV DNA integration increases with the severity of the cervical lesion. The majority of cancer cells have integrated viral DNA

in an anchorage-independent manner and to form tumors when injected into nude mice. In addition, HPV 16 E6 and E7 together are able to immortalize primary human keratinocytes, the natural cellular host of the virus. In agreement with the *in vitro* assays, transgenic mice that co-express both viral genes under the control of keratinocyte-specific promoters exhibit epidermal hyperplasia and are susceptible to cancer development promoted by different means, e.g., chemical carcinogens or estrogen treatment (reviewed in [100]).

Biochemical studies have clarified E6 and E7 mechanisms in cellular transformation. In particular, comparative analysis of E6 and E7 from noncarcinogenic and carcinogenic HPV types has led to the discovery that, while some properties are shared between the two groups of viruses, others are exclusively associated with the carcinogenic HPV types.

An excellent example of the difference between low- and high-risk HPV types is given by the ability of the different E6 and E7 proteins to target p53 and pRb, respectively.

All E7 proteins from mucosal HPV types contain the pRb-binding domain LXCXE, but their affinity for the tumor suppressor can differ considerably. E7 from the low-risk HPV types 6 and 11 binds pRb with a weak affinity compared with HPV16 E7 [101]. Analysis of the primary structure of the pRb-binding region of the low- and high-risk HPV E7 proteins revealed a difference in one amino acid, aspartic acid 21 in HPV16 E7 versus glycine 22 in HPV6 and 11 E7. Substitution of glycine 22 with an aspartic acid in HPV6 E7 confers greater Rb1 binding affinity and ability to cooperate with activated ras in the transformation of primary rodent cells [102, 103]). The correlation between pRb-binding efficiency and transforming activity does not hold, however, for all E7 proteins. In fact, the E7 protein from certain noncarcinogenic HPV types, i.e., the cutaneous HPV1 and the mucosal HPV32, strongly associates with pRb [104–107]). In spite of this, however, these E7 proteins do not display any *in vitro* transforming activities [104, 105, 107]. It is possible that although HPV1, 32 and 16 E7s associate with pRb with similar affinity, the consequences of these interactions can be different. In agreement with this hypothesis, it has been shown that HPV16 E7 is able to induce pRb degradation via a ubiquitin/proteasome-dependent mechanism [108, 109], while HPV1 and 32 E7 proteins do not display this activity [110, 111]. Thus, the ability to promote pRb degradation appears to be an exclusive property of the high-risk HPV types. Two recent studies have provided further insights into the mechanisms involved in HPV16 E7-mediated pRb degradation, which appears to be mediated by the cullin 2 ubiquitin ligase complex and calcium-activated cysteine protease, calpain [112, 113].

In addition to genetic alterations, cellular alkalinization appears to be a phenotype common to all cancer cells. This cytoplasmic alkalinization is the consequence of a stimulation of a member of the Na^+/H^+ exchanger protein family, NHE-1, a ubiquitously expressed transporter in the plasma membrane having the main function of extruding H^+ from the cytoplasm (for more details see [114] and references therein). It has been shown that HPV16 E7 induces cytoplasmic alkalinization in NIH3T3 cells and primary human keratinocytes by a stimulation of NHE-1 activity. Annulment of the HPV16 E7-induced cytoplasmic alkalinization by specific NHE-1 inhibitors prevented the development of the transformed phenotype [114], supporting the importance of this event in HPV-mediated carcinogenesis.

As in the HPV16 E7 and pRb association, HPV16 E6 interaction with p53 leads to degradation of the tumor suppressor protein p53 via the ubiquitin pathway (reviewed in [34]). Due to the key role of p53 in safeguarding the genome integrity, HPV16-infected cells tend to accumulate chromosomal abnormalities, greatly increasing the probability of these cells to evolve toward malignancy. The induction of p53 degradation appears to be an exclusive feature of E6 proteins from the high-risk HPV types. A recent study analyzed the p53 degradation ability of E6 from the high-risk HPV types 16, 18, 33, 35, 39, 45, 51, 52, 53, 56, 58, 66, 70, and 82. All these E6 proteins showed a similar efficiency in degrading p53 in an *in vitro* assay. In contrast, no p53 degradation was observed in keratinocytes expressing E6 from the low-risk HPV6, 11, 44, 54, and 61 [115, 116]. Thus, HPV-mediated p53 degradation represents a key step in cervical carcinogenesis, as in other human cancers in which the p53 gene is frequently mutated. A recent study has further corroborated this conclusion, providing direct evidence for the active role of E6-mediated p53 degradation in the survival of HPV-positive neoplastic cells [117]. Expression of E6-binding peptide aptamers in HPV16-positive cells resulted in abrogation of p53 degradation and induction of apoptosis [117]. Thus, therapeutic approaches aiming to inhibit the biological functions of the E6 protein may represent a successful strategy to induce regression of an HPV-positive lesion.

Recently, new members of the p53 family have been identified, e.g., p63 and p73 [118]. It is not yet clear whether E6 has an effect on these p53-related proteins. Park et al. [119] have reported that p73 can be functionally inactivated by the E6 protein of low- and high-risk HPV types via direct binding, but without inducing its degradation [119]. In contrast, another investigation found no interaction between E6 and p73 [120].

Another characteristic of E6 from the high-risk HPV types is the ability to target several members of the membrane-associated guanylate kinase (MAGUK) family, e.g., the human homologues of the Drosophila discs large protein (DLG) hDLG and Scribble, MUPP1 and MAG1-3 [52]. MAGUK family members, large proteins localized in the cytoplasmic membrane, regulate the cell–cell contact via the tight junction and cell polarity [121]. They contain various protein/protein interaction domains, including PDZ motifs. Due to this characteristic, MAGUKs associate with various membrane and cytoplasmic proteins acting, therefore, as scaffolds for the formation of multi-protein complexes. The high-risk HPV16 E6 oncoproteins have a four amino acid PDZ-binding motif at the C-terminus that mediates the interaction with the MAGUK family members (Fig. 32.3). The E6/MAGUK association leads to degradation of the cellular protein with consequent loss of cell–cell contact and cell polarity. Deletion of the carboxy terminus of HPV16 E6 abolishes its binding to hDLG without influencing its ability to promote p53 destabilization. However, loss of the PDZ-binding domain results in a strong reduction of the HPV16 E6 transforming protein in *in vitro* and *in vivo* experimental models [122, 123]. The key role of the E6/MAGUK complex in HPV-induced carcinogenesis is also supported by the fact that the E6 proteins from the low-risk HPV types do not contain the PDZ-binding site at the C-terminus.

32.6 Conclusions

The possible association between HPV infection and cervical carcinogenesis was proposed more than three decades ago. Since then, clinical, epidemiological and biological studies have constantly provided substantial lines of evidence, leading to the conclusive demonstration of the carcinogenic properties of the high-risk HPV types. The biological studies have not only clarified the molecular mechanisms of HPV proteins, but also contributed to our understanding of the fundamental cellular pathways involved in the life of a normal cell. Studies on other DNA tumor viruses, such as SV40 and Adenovirus, have led to the identification of two very important tumor suppressors, pRb and p53 [124, 125, 126]. Characterization of the HPV16 E6 and E7 properties has provided further insights into the cellular pathways controlled by these two tumor suppressors and the mechanisms involved in their regulation. It is now clear that investigation of the potential role of infectious agents in human carcinogenesis represents a very important topic in cancer research. The establishment of a link between a specific infection and cancer development is an extremely important step as it will allow the generation of novel therapeutic and prophylactic strategies. The recently-generated HPV prophylactic vaccine fully supports these concepts.

Take-Home Pearls

› Chronic mucosal high-risk HPV infections lead to cervical cancer
› E6 and E7 are main viral oncoproteins
› Studies on these two oncoproteins resulted in the discovery of mechanisms involved in fundamental events in normal cells
› The association of HPV with human carcinogenesis led to the development of a prophylactic vaccine that will have a profound impact on HPV-induced cancers

References

1. de Villiers, E.M., Fauquet, C., Broker, T.R., Bernard, H.U., zur Hausen, H.: Classification of papillomaviruses. Virology **324**, 17–27 (2004)
2. zur Hausen, H.: Papillomaviruses and cancer: from basic studies to clinical application. Nat. Rev. Cancer **2**, 342–350 (2002)
3. Munoz, N., Bosch, F.X., de Sanjose, S., Herrero, R., Castellsague, X., Shah, K.V., Snijders, P.J., Meijer, C.J.: Epidemiologic classification of human papillomavirus types associated with cervical cancer. N. Engl. J. Med. **348**, 518–527 (2003)
4. Smith, J.S., Lindsay, L., Hoots, B., Keys, J., Franceschi, S., Winer, R., Clifford, G.M.: Human papillomavirus type distribution in invasive cervical cancer and high-grade cervical lesions: a meta-analysis update. Int. J. Cancer **121**, 621–632 (2007)
5. Pfister, H.: Chapter 8: human papillomavirus and skin cancer. J. Natl. Cancer Inst. Monogr. **31**, 52–56 (2003)
6. Shafti-Keramat, S., Handisurya, A., Kriehuber, E., Meneguzzi, G., Slupetzky, K., Kirnbauer, R.: Different heparan sulfate proteoglycans serve as cellular receptors for human papillomaviruses. J. Virol. **77**, 13125–13135 (2003)
7. Joyce, J.G., Tung, J.S., Przysiecki, C.T., Cook, J.C., Lehman, E.D., Sands, J.A., Jansen, K.U., Keller, P.M.: The L1 major capsid protein of human papillomavirus type 11 recombinant virus-like particles interacts with heparin and cell-surface glycosaminoglycans on human keratinocytes. J. Biol. Chem. **274**, 5810–5822 (1999)
8. Evander, M., Frazer, I.H., Payne, E., Qi, Y.M., Hengst, K., McMillan, N.A.: Identification of the alpha6 integrin as a candidate receptor for papillomaviruses. J. Virol. **71**, 2449–2456 (1997)
9. Sibbet, G., Romero-Graillet, C., Meneguzzi, G., Campo, M.S.: alpha6 integrin is not the obligatory cell receptor for bovine papillomavirus type 4. J. Gen. Virol. **81**, 327–334 (2000)
10. Day, P.M., Lowy, D.R., Schiller, J.T.: Papillomaviruses infect cells via a clathrin-dependent pathway. Virology **307**, 1–11 (2003)
11. Bousarghin, L., Touze, A., Sizaret, P.Y., Coursaget, P.: Human papillomavirus types 16, 31, and 58 use different endocytosis pathways to enter cells. J. Virol. **77**, 3846–3850 (2003)
12. Gambhira, R., Karanam, B., Jagu, S., Roberts, J.N., Buck, C.B., Bossis, I., Alphs, H., Culp, T., Christensen, N.D., Roden, R.B.: A protective and broadly cross-neutralizing epitope of human papillomavirus L2. J. Virol. **81**, 13927–13931 (2007)
13. Kawana, Y., Kawana, K., Yoshikawa, H., Taketani, Y., Yoshiike, K., Kanda, T.: Human papillomavirus type 16 minor capsid protein l2 N-terminal region containing a common neutralization epitope binds to the cell surface and enters the cytoplasm. J. Virol. **75**, 2331–2336 (2001)
14. Day, P.M., Baker, C.C., Lowy, D.R., Schiller, J.T.: Establishment of papillomavirus infection is enhanced by promyelocytic leukemia protein (PML) expression. Proc. Natl. Acad. Sci. USA **101**, 14252–14257 (2004)
15. McBride, A.A., Byrne, J.C., Howley, P.M.: E2 polypeptides encoded by bovine papillomavirus type 1 form dimers through the common carboxyl-terminal domain: transactivation is mediated by the conserved amino-terminal domain. Proc. Natl. Acad. Sci. USA **86**, 510–514 (1989)
16. Ma, T., Zou, N., Lin, B.Y., Chow, L.T., Harper, J.W.: Interaction between cyclin-dependent kinases and human papillomavirus replication-initiation protein E1 is required for efficient viral replication. Proc. Natl. Acad. Sci. USA **19**(96), 382–387 (1999)
17. Lehman, C.W., Botchan, M.R.: Segregation of viral plasmids depends on tethering to chromosomes and is regulated by phosphorylation. Proc. Natl. Acad. Sci. USA **95**, 4338–4343 (1998)

18. Ilves, I., Kivi, S., Ustav, M.: Long-term episomal maintenance of bovine papillomavirus type 1 plasmids is determined by attachment to host chromosomes, which Is mediated by the viral E2 protein and its binding sites. J. Virol. **73**, 4404–4412 (1999)
19. Bastien, N., McBride, A.A.: Interaction of the papillomavirus E2 protein with mitotic chromosomes. Virology **270**, 124–134 (2000)
20. Skiadopoulos, M.H., McBride, A.A.: Bovine papillomavirus type 1 genomes and the E2 transactivator protein are closely associated with mitotic chromatin. J. Virol. **72**, 2079–2088 (1998)
21. You, J., Croyle, J.L., Nishimura, A., Ozato, K., Howley, P.M.: Interaction of the bovine papillomavirus E2 protein with Brd4 tethers the viral DNA to host mitotic chromosomes. Cell **117**, 349–360 (2004)
22. Van Tine, B.A., Dao, L.D., Wu, S.Y., Sonbuchner, T.M., Lin, B.Y., Zou, N., Chiang, C.M., Broker, T.R., Chow, L.T.: Human papillomavirus (HPV) origin-binding protein associates with mitotic spindles to enable viral DNA partitioning. Proc. Natl. Acad. Sci. USA **101**, 4030–4035 (2004)
23. Parish, J.L., Bean, A.M., Park, R.B., Androphy, E.J.: ChlR1 is required for loading papillomavirus E2 onto mitotic chromosomes and viral genome maintenance. Mol. Cell **24**, 867–876 (2006)
24. Dimova, D.K., Dyson, N.J.: The E2F transcriptional network: old acquaintances with new faces. Oncogene **24**, 2810–2826 (2005)
25. Cobrinik, D.: Pocket proteins and cell cycle control. Oncogene **24**, 2796–2809 (2005)
26. Zerfaß-Thome, K., Zwerschke, W., Mannhardt, B., Tindle, R., Botz, J., Jansen-Dürr, P.: Inactivation of the cdk inhibitor p27KIP1 by the human papillomavirus type 16 E7 oncoprotein. Oncogene **13**, 2323–2330 (1996)
27. Funk, J.O., Waga, S., Harry, J.B., Espling, E., Stillman, B., Galloway, D.A.: Inhibition of CDK activity and PCNA-dependent DNA replication by p21 is blocked by interaction with the HPV-16 E7 oncoprotein. Genes Dev. **11**, 2090–2100 (1997)
28. Jones, D.L., Alani, R.M., Munger, K.: The human papillomavirus E7 oncoprotein can uncouple cellular differentiation and proliferation in human keratinocytes by abrogating p21Cip1-mediated inhibition of cdk2. Genes Dev. **11**, 2101–2111 (1997)
29. Tommasino, M., Adamczewski, J.P., Carlotti, F., Barth, C.F., Manetti, R., Contorni, M., Cavalieri, F., Hunt, T., Crawford, L.: HPV16 E7 protein associates with the protein kinase p33CDK2 and cyclin A. Oncogene **8**, 195–202 (1993)
30. Davies, R., Hicks, R., Crook, T., Morris, J., Vousden, K.: Human papillomavirus type-16 E7 associates with a histone H1 kinase and with p107 through sequences necessary for transformation. J. Virol. **67**, 2521–2528 (1993)
31. Arroyo, M., Bagchi, S., Raychaudhuri, P.: Association of the human papillomavirus type-16 E7 protein with the S-phase-specific E2F-cyclin-A complex. Mol. Cell. Biol. **13**, 6537–6546 (1993)
32. He, W., Staples, D., Smith, C., Fisher, C.: Direct activation of cyclin-dependent kinase 2 by human papillomavirus E7. J. Virol. **77**, 10566–10574 (2003)
33. Tommasino, M., Accardi, R., Caldeira, S., Dong, W., Malanchi, I., Smet, A., Zehbe, I.: The role of TP53 in Cervical carcinogenesis. Hum. Mutat. **21**, 307–312 (2003)
34. Huibregtse, J.M., Scheffner, M., Howley, P.M.: A cellular protein mediates association of p53 with the E6 oncoprotein of human papillomavirus types 16 or 18. EMBO J. **10**, 4129–4136 (1991)
35. Scheffner, M., Huibregtse, J.M., Vierstra, R.D., Howley, P.M.: The HPV-16 E6 and E6-AP complex functions as a ubiquitin-protein ligase in the ubiquitination of p53. Cell **75**, 495–505 (1993)
36. Scheffner, M., Werness, B.A., Huibregtse, J.M., Levine, A.J., Howley, P.M.: The E6 oncoprotein encoded by human papillomavirus types 16 and 18 promotes the degradation of p53. Cell **63**, 1129–1136 (1990)
37. Massimi, P., Shai, A., Lambert, P., Banks, L.: HPV E6 degradation of p53 and PDZ containing substrates in an E6AP null background. Oncogene **27**, 1800–1804 (2008)
38. Pan, H.C., Griep, A.E.: Temporally distinct patterns of p53-dependent and p53-independent apoptosis during mouse lens development. Genes Dev. **9**, 2157–2169 (1995)
39. White, A.E., Livanos, E.M., Tlsty, T.D.: Differential disruption of genomic integrity and cell cycle regulation in normal human fibroblasts by the HPV oncoproteins. Genes Dev. **8**, 666–677 (1994)
40. Thomas, M., Banks, L.: Inhibition of Bak-induced apoptosis by HPV-18 E6. Oncogene **17**, 2943–2954 (1998)
41. Jackson, S., Harwood, C., Thomas, M., Banks, L., Storey, A.: Role of Bak in UV-induced apoptosis in skin cancer and abrogation by HPV E6 proteins. Genes Dev. **14**, 3065–3073 (2000)
42. Sorenson, C.M.: Bcl-2 family members and disease. Biochim. Biophys. Acta **1644**, 169–177 (2004)
43. Klingelhutz, A.J., Foster, S.A., McDougall, J.K.: Telomerase activation by the E6 gene product of human papillomavirus type 16. Nature **380**, 79–82 (1996)
44. Shay, J.W., Wright, W.E.: Senescence and immortalization: role of telomeres and telomerase. Carcinogenesis **26**, 867–874 (2005)
45. Gewin, L., Myers, H., Kiyono, T., Galloway, D.A.: Identification of a novel telomerase repressor that interacts with the human papillomavirus type-16 E6/E6-AP complex. Genes Dev. **18**, 2269–2282 (2004)
46. Veldman, T., Liu, X., Yuan, H., Schlegel, R.: Human papillomavirus E6 and Myc proteins associate *in vivo* and bind to and cooperatively activate the telomerase reverse transcriptase promoter. Proc. Natl. Acad. Sci. USA **100**, 8211–8216 (2003)
47. Sekaric, P., Cherry, J.J., Androphy, E.J.: Binding of human papillomavirus type 16 E6 to E6AP is not required for activation of hTERT. J. Virol. **82**, 71–76 (2008)
48. Liu, X., Roberts, J., Dakic, A., Zhang, Y., Schlegel, R.: HPV E7 contributes to the telomerase activity of immortalized and tumorigenic cells and augments E6-induced hTERT promoter function. Virology **375**, 611–623 (2008)
49. Malanchi, I., Caldeira, S., Krutzfeldt, M., Giarre, M., Alunni-Fabbroni, M., Tommasino, M.: Identification of a novel activity of human papillomavirus type 16 E6 protein in deregulating the G1/S transition. Oncogene **21**, 5665–5672 (2002)
50. Malanchi, I., Accardi, R., Diehl, F., Smet, A., Androphy, E., Hoheisel, J., Tommasino, M.: Human papillomavirus type 16 E6 promotes retinoblastoma protein phosphorylation and cell cycle progression. J. Virol. **78**, 13769–13778 (2004)

51. Mantovani, F., Banks, L.: The human papillomavirus E6 protein and its contribution to malignant progression. Oncogene **20**, 7874–7887 (2001)
52. Munger, K., Basile, J.R., Duensing, S., Eichten, A., Gonzalez, S.L., Grace, M., Zacny, V.L.: Biological activities and molecular targets of the human papillomavirus E7 oncoprotein. Oncogene **20**, 7888–7898 (2001)
53. Fehrmann, F., Klumpp, D.J., Laimins, L.A.: Human papillomavirus type 31 E5 protein supports cell cycle progression and activates late viral functions upon epithelial differentiation. J. Virol. **77**, 2819–2831 (2003)
54. Genther, S.M., Sterling, S., Duensing, S., Munger, K., Sattler, C., Lambert, P.F.: Quantitative role of the human papillomavirus type 16 E5 gene during the productive stage of the viral life cycle. J. Virol. **77**, 2832–2842 (2003)
55. Conrad, M., Bubb, V.J., Schlegel, R.: The human papillomavirus type 6 and 16 E5 proteins are membrane-associated proteins which associate with the 16-kilodalton pore-forming protein. J. Virol. **67**, 6170–6178 (1993)
56. Valle, G.F., Banks, L.: The human papillomavirus (HPV)-6 and HPV-16 E5 proteins co-operate with HPV-16 E7 in the transformation of primary rodent cells. J. Gen. Virol. **76**, 1239–1245 (1995)
57. Straight, S.W., Hinkle, P.M., Jewers, R.J., McCance, D.J.: The E5 oncoprotein of human papillomavirus type 16 transforms fibroblasts and effects the downregulation of the epidermal growth factor receptor in keratinocytes. J. Virol. **67**, 4521–4532 (1993)
58. Straight, S.W., Herman, B., McCance, D.J.: The E5 oncoprotein of human papillomavirus type 16 inhibits the acidification of endosomes in human keratinocytes. J. Virol. **69**, 3185–3192 (1995)
59. Wilson, R., Fehrmann, F., Laimins, L.A.: Role of the E1–E4 protein in the differentiation-dependent life cycle of human papillomavirus type 31. J. Virol. **79**, 6732–6740 (2005)
60. Wilson, R., Ryan, G.B., Knight, G.L., Laimins, L.A., Roberts, S.: The full-length E1E4 protein of human papillomavirus type 18 modulates differentiation-dependent viral DNA amplification and late gene expression. Virology **362**, 453–460 (2007)
61. Davy, C.E., Jackson, D.J., Wang, Q., Raj, K., Masterson, P.J., Fenner, N.F., Southern, S., Cuthill, S., Millar, J.B., Doorbar, J.: Identification of a G(2) arrest domain in the E1 wedge E4 protein of human papillomavirus type 16. J. Virol. **76**, 9806–9818 (2002)
62. Nakahara, T., Nishimura, A., Tanaka, M., Ueno, T., Ishimoto, A., Sakai, H.: Modulation of the cell division cycle by human papillomavirus type 18 E4. J. Virol. **76**, 10914–10920 (2002)
63. Knight, G.L., Grainger, J.R., Gallimore, P.H., Roberts, S.: Cooperation between different forms of the human papillomavirus type 1 E4 protein to block cell cycle progression and cellular DNA synthesis. J. Virol. **78**, 13920–13933 (2004)
64. Davy, C.E., Jackson, D.J., Raj, K., Peh, W.L., Southern, S.A., Das, P., Sorathia, R., Laskey, P., Middleton, K., Nakahara, T., Wang, Q., Masterson, P.J., Lambert, P.F., Cuthill, S., Millar, J.B., Doorbar, J.: Human papillomavirus type 16 E1 E4-induced G2 arrest is associated with cytoplasmic retention of active Cdk1/cyclin B1 complexes. J. Virol. **79**, 3998–4011 (2005)
65. Hebner, C.M., Laimins, L.A.: Human papillomaviruses: basic mechanisms of pathogenesis and oncogenicity. Rev. Med. Virol. **16**, 83–97 (2006)
66. Ozbun, M.A., Meyers, C.: Temporal usage of multiple promoters during the life cycle of human papillomavirus type 31b. J. Virol. **72**, 2715–2722 (1998)
67. Grassmann, K., Rapp, B., Maschek, H., Petry, K.U., Iftner, T.: Identification of a differentiation-inducible promoter in the E7 open reading frame of human papillomavirus type 16 (HPV-16) in raft cultures of a new cell line containing high copy numbers of episomal HPV-16 DNA. J. Virol. **70**, 2339–2349 (1996)
68. del Mar Pena, L.M., Laimins, L.A.: Differentiation-dependent chromatin rearrangement coincides with activation of human papillomavirus type 31 late gene expression. J. Virol. **75**, 10005–10013 (2001)
69. Meyers, C., Frattini, M.G., Hudson, J.B., Laimins, L.A.: Biosynthesis of human papillomavirus from a continuous cell line upon epithelial differentiation. Science **257**, 971–973 (1992)
70. Hummel, M., Lim, H.B., Laimins, L.A.: Human papillomavirus type 31b late gene expression is regulated through protein kinase C-mediated changes in RNA processing. J. Virol. **69**, 3381–3388 (1995)
71. Dlugosz, A.A., Yuspa, S.H.: Coordinate changes in gene expression which mark the spinous to granular cell transition in epidermis are regulated by protein kinase C. J. Cell Biol. **120**, 217–225 (1993)
72. Kashiwagi, M., Ohba, M., Chida, K., Kuroki, T.: Protein kinase C eta (PKC eta): its involvement in keratinocyte differentiation. J. Biochem. **132**, 853–857 (2002)
73. Kennedy, I.M., Haddow, J.K., Clements, J.B.: Analysis of human papillomavirus type 16 late mRNA 3' processing signals *in vitro* and *in vivo*. J. Virol. **64**, 1825–1829 (1990)
74. Dietrich-Goetz, W., Kennedy, I.M., Levins, B., Stanley, M.A., Clements, J.B.: A cellular 65-kDa protein recognizes the negative regulatory element of human papillomavirus late mRNA. Proc. Natl. Acad. Sci. USA **94**, 163–168 (1997)
75. Cumming, S.A., McPhillips, M.G., Veerapraditsin, T., Milligan, S.G., Graham, S.V.: Activity of the human papillomavirus type 16 late negative regulatory element is partly due to four weak consensus 5' splice sites that bind a U1 snRNP-like complex. J. Virol. **77**, 5167–5177 (2003)
76. Collier, B., Oberg, D., Zhao, X., Schwartz, S.: Specific inactivation of inhibitory sequences in the 5' end of the human papillomavirus type 16 L1 open reading frame results in production of high levels of L1 protein in human epithelial cells. J. Virol. **76**, 2739–2752 (2002)
77. Oberg, D., Collier, B., Zhao, X., Schwartz, S.: Mutational inactivation of two distinct negative RNA elements in the human papillomavirus type 16 L2 coding region induces production of high levels of L2 in human cells. J. Virol. **77**, 11674–11684 (2003)
78. Kennedy, I.M., Haddow, J.K., Clements, J.B.: A negative regulatory element in the human papillomavirus type 16 genome acts at the level of late mRNA stability. J. Virol. **65**, 2093–2097 (1991)
79. Koffa, M.D., Graham, S.V., Takagaki, Y., Manley, J.L., Clements, J.B.: The human papillomavirus type 16 negative regulatory RNA element interacts with three proteins that

act at different posttranscriptional levels. Proc. Natl. Acad. Sci. USA **97**, 4677–4682 (2000)
80. Doorbar, J., Elston, R.C., Napthine, S., Raj, K., Medcalf, E., Jackson, D., Coleman, N., Griffin, H.M., Masterson, P., Stacey, S., Mengistu, Y., Dunlop, J.: The E1E4 protein of human papillomavirus type 16 associates with a putative RNA helicase through sequences in its C terminus. J. Virol. **74**, 10081–10095 (2000)
81. Rocak, S., Linder, P.: DEAD-box proteins: the driving forces behind RNA metabolism. Nat. Rev. Mol. Cell Biol. **5**, 232–241 (2004)
82. Day, P.M., Roden, R.B., Lowy, D.R., Schiller, J.T.: The papillomavirus minor capsid protein, L2, induces localization of the major capsid protein, L1, and the viral transcription/replication protein, E2, to PML oncogenic domains. J. Virol. **72**, 142–150 (1998)
83. Holmgren, S.C., Patterson, N.A., Ozbun, M.A., Lambert, P.F.: The minor capsid protein L2 contributes to two steps in the human papillomavirus type 31 life cycle. J. Virol. **79**, 3938–3948 (2005)
84. Buck, C.B., Pastrana, D.V., Lowy, D.R., Schiller, J.T.: Efficient intracellular assembly of papillomaviral vectors. J. Virol. **78**, 751–757 (2004)
85. Doorbar, J., Medcalf, E., Napthine, S.: Analysis of HPV1 E4 complexes and their association with keratins *in vivo*. Virology **218**, 114–126 (1996)
86. Bryan, J.T., Brown, D.R.: Association of the human papillomavirus type 11 E1()E4 protein with cornified cell envelopes derived from infected genital epithelium. Virology **277**, 262–269 (2000)
87. Raj, K., Berguerand, S., Southern, S., Doorbar, J., Beard, P.: E1 empty set E4 protein of human papillomavirus type 16 associates with mitochondria. J. Virol. **78**, 7199–7207 (2004)
88. Lehr, E., Jarnik, M., Brown, D.R.: Human papillomavirus type 11 alters the transcription and expression of loricrin, the major cell envelope protein. Virology **298**, 240–247 (2002)
89. Ostor, A.G.: Natural history of cervical intraepithelial neoplasia: a critical review. Int. J. Gynecol. Pathol. **12**, 186–192 (1993)
90. Jones, N.: Transcriptional regulation by dimerization: two sides to an incestuous relationship. Cell **61**, 9–11 (1990)
91. Magnusson, P.K., Sparen, P., Gyllensten, U.B.: Genetic link to cervical tumours. Nature **400**, 6729–6730 (1999)
92. Moreno, V., Bosch, F.X., Munoz, N., Meijer, C.J., Shah, K.V., Walboomers, J.M., Herrero, R., Franceschi, S.: Effect of oral contraceptives on risk of cervical cancer in women with human papillomavirus infection: the IARC multicentric case-control study. Lancet **359**, 1085–1092 (2002)
93. Moreno, V., Munoz, N., Bosch, F.X., de Sanjose, S., Gonzalez, L.C., Tafur, L., Gili, M., Izarzugaza, I., Navarro, C., Vergara, A., et al.: Risk factors for progression of cervical intraepithelial neoplasm grade III to invasive cervical cancer. Cancer Epidemiol. Biomarkers Prev. **4**, 459–467 (1995)
94. Munoz, N., Franceschi, S., Bosetti, C., Moreno, V., Herrero, R., Smith, J.S., Shah, K.V., Meijer, C.J., Bosch, F.X.: Role of parity and human papillomavirus in cervical cancer: the IARC multicentric case-control study. Lancet **359**, 1093–1101 (2002)
95. Schiffman, M.H., Haley, N.J., Felton, J.S., Andrews, A.W., Kaslow, R.A., Lancaster, W.D., Kurman, R.J., Brinton, L.A., Lannom, L.B., Hoffmann, D.: Biochemical epidemiology of cervical neoplasia: measuring cigarette smoke constituents in the cervix. Cancer Res. **47**, 3886–3888 (1987)
96. Walboomers, J.M., Jacobs, M.V., Manos, M.M., Bosch, F.X., Kummer, J.A., Shah, K.V., Snijders, P.J., Peto, J., Meijer, C.J., Munoz, N.: Human papillomavirus is a necessary cause of invasive cervical cancer worldwide. J. Pathol. **189**, 12–19 (1999)
97. Schwarz, E., Freese, U.K., Gissmann, L., Mayer, W., Roggenbuck, B., Stremlau, A., zur Hausen, H.: Structure and transcription of human papillomavirus sequences in cervical carcinoma cells. Nature **314**, 111–114 (1985)
98. Wentzensen, N., Vinokurova, S., von Knebel, D.M.: Systematic review of genomic integration sites of human papillomavirus genomes in epithelial dysplasia and invasive cancer of the female lower genital tract. Cancer Res. **64**, 3878–3884 (2004)
99. Alvarez-Salas, L.M., DiPaolo, J.A.: Molecular approaches to cervical cancer therapy. Curr. Drug Discov. Technol. **4**, 208–219 (2007)
100. Lambert, P.F., Balsitis, S.J., Shai, A., Simonson, S.J.S., Williams, S.M.G.: Transgenic mouse models for the *in vivo* analysis of papillomavirus oncogene function. In: Saveria Campo, M. (ed.) Papillomavirus Research: From Natural History to Vaccine and Beyond, pp. 213–228. Caister Academic Press, Norfolk (2006)
101. Munger, K., Werness, B.A., Dyson, N., Phelps, W.C., Harlow, E., Howley, P.M.: Complex formation of human papillomavirus E7 proteins with the retinoblastoma tumor suppressor gene product. EMBO J. **20**(8), 4099–4105 (1989)
102. Heck, D.V., Yee, C.L., Howley, P.M., Munger, K.: Efficiency of binding the retinoblastoma protein correlates with the transforming capacity of the E7 oncoproteins of the human papillomaviruses. Proc. Natl. Acad. Sci. USA **89**, 4442–4446 (1992)
103. Sang, B.C., Barbosa, M.S.: Single amino acid substitutions in "low-risk" human papillomavirus (HPV) type 6 E7 protein enhance features characteristic of the "high-risk" HPV E7 oncoproteins. Proc. Natl. Acad. Sci. USA **89**, 8063–8067 (1992)
104. Ciccolini, F., Di Pasquale, G., Carlotti, F., Crawford, L., Tommasino, M.: Functional Studies of E7 proteins from different HPV types. Oncogene **9**, 2342–2348 (1994)
105. Schmitt, A., Harry, J.B., Rapp, B., Wettstein, F.O., Iftner, T.: Comparison of the properties of the E6 and E7 genes of low- and high-risk cutaneous papillomaviruses reveals strongly transforming and high Rb-binding activity for the E7 protein of the low-risk human papillomavirus type 1. J. Virol. **68**, 7051–7059 (1994)
106. Dong, W.L., Caldeira, S., Sehr, P., Pawlita, M., Tommasino, M.: Determination of the binding affinity of different human papillomavirus E7 proteins for the tumour suppressor pRb by a plate-binding assay. J Virol Methods **98**, 91–98 (2001)
107. Caldeira, S., Dong, W., Tomakidi, P., Paradiso, A., Tommasino, M.: Human papillomavirus type 32 does not display *in vitro* transforming properties. Virology **301**, 157–164 (2002)
108. Boyer, S.N., Wazer, D.E., Band, V.: E7 protein of human papilloma virus-16 induces degradation of retinoblastoma protein through the ubiquitin-proteasome pathway. Cancer Res. **56**, 4620–4624 (1996)

109. Jones, D.L., Munger, K.: Analysis of the p53-mediated G1 growth arrest pathway in cells expressing the human papillomavirus type 16 E7 oncoprotein. J. Virol. **71**, 2905–2912 (1997)
110. Giarre, M., Caldeira, S., Malanchi, I., Ciccolini, F., Leao, M.J., Tommasino, M.: Induction of pRb degradation by the human papillomavirus type 16 E7 protein is essential to efficiently overcome p16INK4a-imposed G1 cell cycle Arrest. J. Virol. **75**, 4705–4712 (2001)
111. Gonzalez, S.L., Stremlau, M., He, X., Basile, J.R., Munger, K.: Degradation of the retinoblastoma tumor suppressor by the human papillomavirus type 16 E7 oncoprotein is important for functional inactivation and is separable from proteasomal degradation of E7. J. Virol. **75**, 7583–7591 (2001)
112. Huh, K., Zhou, X., Hayakawa, H., Cho, J.Y., Libermann, T.A., Jin, J., Harper, J.W., Munger, K.: Human papillomavirus type 16 E7 oncoprotein associates with the cullin 2 ubiquitin ligase complex, which contributes to degradation of the retinoblastoma tumor suppressor. J. Virol. **81**, 9737–9747 (2007)
113. Darnell, G.A., Schroder, W.A., Antalis, T.M., Lambley, E., Major, L., Gardner, J., Birrell, G., Cid-Arregui, A., Suhrbier, A.: Human papillomavirus E7 requires the protease calpain to degrade the retinoblastoma protein. J. Biol. Chem. **282**, 37492–37500 (2007)
114. Reshkin, S.J., Bellizzi, A., Caldeira, S., Albarani, V., Malanchi, I., Poignee, M., Alunni-Fabbroni, M., Casavola, V., Tommasino, M.: Na+/H+ exchanger-dependent intracellular alkalinization is an early event in malignant transformation and plays an essential role in the development of subsequent transformation-associated phenotypes. FASEB J. **14**, 2185–2197 (2000)
115. Lechner, M.S., Laimins, L.A.: Inhibition of p53 DNA binding by human papillomavirus E6 proteins. J. Virol. **68**, 4262–4273 (1994)
116. Hiller, T., Poppelreuther, S., Stubenrauch, F., Iftner, T.: Comparative analysis of 19 genital human papillomavirus types with regard to p53 degradation, immortalization, phylogeny, and epidemiologic risk classification. Cancer Epidemiol. Biomarkers Prev **15**, 1262–1267 (2006)
117. Butz, K., Denk, C., Ullmann, A., Scheffner, M., Hoppe-Seyler, F.: Induction of apoptosis in human papillomavirus-positive cancer cells by peptide aptamers targeting the viral E6 oncoprotein. Proc. Natl Acad. Sci. USA **97**, 6693–6697 (2000)
118. Moll, U.M., Erster, S., Zaika, A.: p53, p63 and p73–solos, alliances and feuds among family members. Biochim. Biophys. Acta **1552**, 47–59 (2001)
119. Park, J.S., Kim, E.J., Lee, J.Y., Sin, H.S., NamKoong, S.E., Um, S.J.: Functional inactivation of p73, a homolog of p53 tumor suppressor protein, by human papillomavirus E6 proteins. Int. J. Cancer **91**, 822–827 (2001)
120. Marin, M.C., Jost, C.A., DeCalprio, I.M.S., JA, C.D., Kaelin Jr., W.G.: Viral oncoproteins discriminate between p53 and the p53 homolog p73. Mol. Cell. Biol. **18**, 6316–6324 (1998)
121. Funke, L., Dakoji, S., Bredt, D.S.: Membrane-associated guanylate kinases regulate adhesion and plasticity at cell junctions. Annu. Rev. Biochem. **74**, 219–245 (2005)
122. Watson, R.A., Thomas, M., Banks, L., Roberts, S.: Activity of the human papillomavirus E6 PDZ-binding motif correlates with an enhanced morphological transformation of immortalized human keratinocytes. J. Cell Sci. **116**, 4925–4934 (2003)
123. Nguyen, M.L., Nguyen, M.M., Lee, D., Griep, A.E., Lambert, P.F.: The PDZ ligand domain of the human papillomavirus type 16 E6 protein is required for E6's induction of epithelial hyperplasia *in vivo*. J. Virol. **77**, 6957–6964 (2003)
124. Linzer, D.I., Levine, A.J.: Characterization of a 54K dalton cellular SV40 tumor antigen present in SV40-transformed cells and uninfected embryonal carcinoma cells. Cell **17**, 43–52 (1979)
125. Lane, D.P., Crawford, L.V.: T antigen is bound to a host protein in SV40-transformed cells. Nature **278**, 261–263 (1979)
126. Whyte, P., Williamson, N.M., Harlow, E.: Cellular targets for transformation by the adenovirus E1A proteins. Cell **56**, 67–75 (1989)

Epidemiology of Genitoanal HPV Infections and Associated Cancer

33

F. Xavier Bosch, Silvia de Sanjose, and Xavier Castellsagué

Core Messages

- Epidemiological studies have firmly established the causality of Human papillomavirus (HPV) infections and cervical cancer, cancers of the vulva and vagina, anal cancer in both sexes and penile cancer in men. HPV 16 is also involved in a fraction of cancers of the oral cavity.
- The viral types involved are limited to some 15 types of which HPV 16 and 18 predominate. They transmit and persist more efficiently and have a higher progression rate that any of the other high risk types. Cervical adenocarcinoma is restricted to three HPV types namely 16, 18 and 45.
- Currently available HPV vaccines have the potential to reduce cervical cancer incidence in an estimated range of 70% to 85% in properly vaccinated cohorts.

F.X. Bosch (✉)
Unit of Infections and Cancer (UNIC), Cancer Epidemiology Research Program (CERP), Catalan Institute of Oncology (Institut Català d'Oncologia – ICO)/IDIBELL, Avda. Gran Via 199-203, 08907 L'Hospitalet de Llobregat Barcelona, Spain
e-mail: admincerp@iconcologia.net

S. de Sanjose and X. Castellsagué
Unit of Infections and Cancer (UNIC), Cancer Epidemiology Research Program (CERP), Catalan Institute of Oncology (Institut Català d'Oncologia – ICO)/IDIBELL, Avda. Gran Via 199-203, 08907 L'Hospitalet de Llobregat Barcelona, Spain and CIBER en Epidemiología y Salud Pública (CIBERESP), Spain
e-mail: admincerp@iconcologia.net

33.1 The Oncogenic Potential of Human Papillomavirus

33.1.1 Epidemiological Evidence for the Causal Link Between HPV and Cervical Cancer

In 1995, the International Agency for Research on Cancer (IARC) monograph working group concluded that there was sufficient evidence for the carcinogenicity of Human Papillomavirus (HPV) types 16 and 18 and limited evidence for the carcinogenicity of HPV types 31 and 33 [1].

An updated revision of the monograph concluded that there was sufficient evidence in humans for the carcinogenicity of HPV types 16, 18, 31, 33, 35, 39, 45, 51, 52, 56, 58, 59, and 66 in the cervix [2]. HPV types 26, 68, 73, and 82 were found to be associated with cervical cancer in some case control studies, but were rarely found in case series and there are no prospective studies of enough size or follow-up length to assess their risk [3]. For some rare types (HPV 26, 53, 68, 73, and 82), the odds ratios observed are of similar magnitude to that of HPV-66, but given the low prevalence observed in cases, these types were temporarily classified as probably carcinogenic, and additional studies were encouraged. The consensus and the evidence to date is that HPV is the central and necessary cause of cervical cancer and that at least 15 HPV types are capable of inducing an invasive cancer. Two of the types – HPV 16 and 18 – are consistently found associated with at least 70% of the cases on a worldwide estimate [4].

G. Gross and S.K. Tyring (eds.), *Sexually Transmitted Infections and Sexually Transmitted Diseases*,
DOI: 10.1007/978-3-642-14663-3_33, © Springer-Verlag Berlin Heidelberg 2011

33.1.2 HPV DNA Prevalence in Clinical Series of Specimens of Cervical Cancer

The largest series of cases of invasive cervical cancer investigated with a standard protocol has been assembled by the IARC. About 1,000 women with histologically verified invasive cervical cancer were recruited from 22 countries around the world. Frozen biopsies from the tumors were analyzed in a central laboratory for the detection of HPV DNA, using strict controls for the presence of malignant cells in sections adjacent to the sections used for polymerase chain reaction (PCR)-based assays.

In the first results published, the HPV DNA prevalence was reported as 93% [5].

On a careful reanalysis of the initially HPV-negative cases, HPV DNA was detected in 99.7% of the tumors, leading to the conclusion that HPV is a necessary cause of cervical cancer [6,7]. Subsequently, the distribution of HPV types in cervical cancer has been published in a pooled analysis of about 3,000 cases from the IARC studies [4] and in a meta-analysis of about 10,000 cases [5,8]. The eight most common HPV types detected in both series, in descending order of frequency, were HPV 16, 18, 45, 31, 33, 52, 58, and 35, and these are responsible for about 90% of all cervical cancers worldwide. The results have recently been confirmed by a large international survey on HPV-related cancers, using centralized laboratory strategies coordinated by the Catalan Institute of Oncology [3].

33.1.3 Case Control Studies

At least ten case control studies with histological diagnosis of cancer and with HPV DNA detected by PCR-based methods have been completed, and these studies have estimated the risk of cancer to additional HPV types. The largest report corresponds to a pooled analysis of 11 case control studies of invasive cervical cancer conducted by the IARC in 11 countries [9]. The pooled data include about 2,500 women with cervical cancer and about 2,500 control women (women from the same socioeconomic location and strata without cervical cancer). The main advantage of these studies is the use of a common study protocol and of well-validated PCR assays for the detection of 33 HPV types carried out in a central laboratory.

Figures 33.1 and 33.2 summarize the prevalence of HPV DNA among cases and controls and the corresponding adjusted odds ratios for squamous cell carcinoma (SCC) and for adenocarcinomas (ADC)/adenosquamous carcinoma (ADSC) of the cervix, respectively. HPV 16 and 18 were the two most common types in both histological types, but the prevalence of SCCs attributable to HPV 16 and 18 was 70% while that for ADC was 86% [9,10].

Figure 33.3 summarizes the odds ratios for invasive cervical cancer, for SCC, and for ADC associated with the 15 most common HPV types. Their magnitude ranges from 3.6 for HPV 6 to 573 for HPV 33 [9].

33.1.4 Cohort Studies

Cohort studies have the advantage of clearly establishing the temporal association between exposure and disease, but have the inherent clinical limitation of interrupting observations at the CIN 2, CIN 3 stages. Therefore, extrapolation of findings to invasive cervical cancer requires some level of speculation, particularly when CIN 2 is used as endpoint. It is known that variability in the diagnosis is significant, and that a sizable fraction of CIN 2 are not true cancer precursors and tend to follow a benign CIN 2 clinical course with high rates of spontaneous regression, particularly among young women [11].

Several prospective studies have shown that women who are HPV DNA-positive at baseline have a higher risk of developing CIN 3 or invasive cervical cancer during the follow-up than women who are HPV DNA-negative, but many of the early studies did not provide results on HPV type-specific carcinogenicity. Results from these studies are sometimes difficult to interpret and compare because the HPV type detected in the cervical smears at study entry may not be the same HPV type detected in the subsequent CIN-2/3 lesions diagnosed years later.

Few studies have evaluated the HPV type-specific risk of developing CIN 2/3 and they have consistently reported an increased risk for CIN 2/3 linked to the baseline detection of HPV 16. A few of them have reported increased risks associated with the presence of HPV 18 and of HPV types phylogenetically related

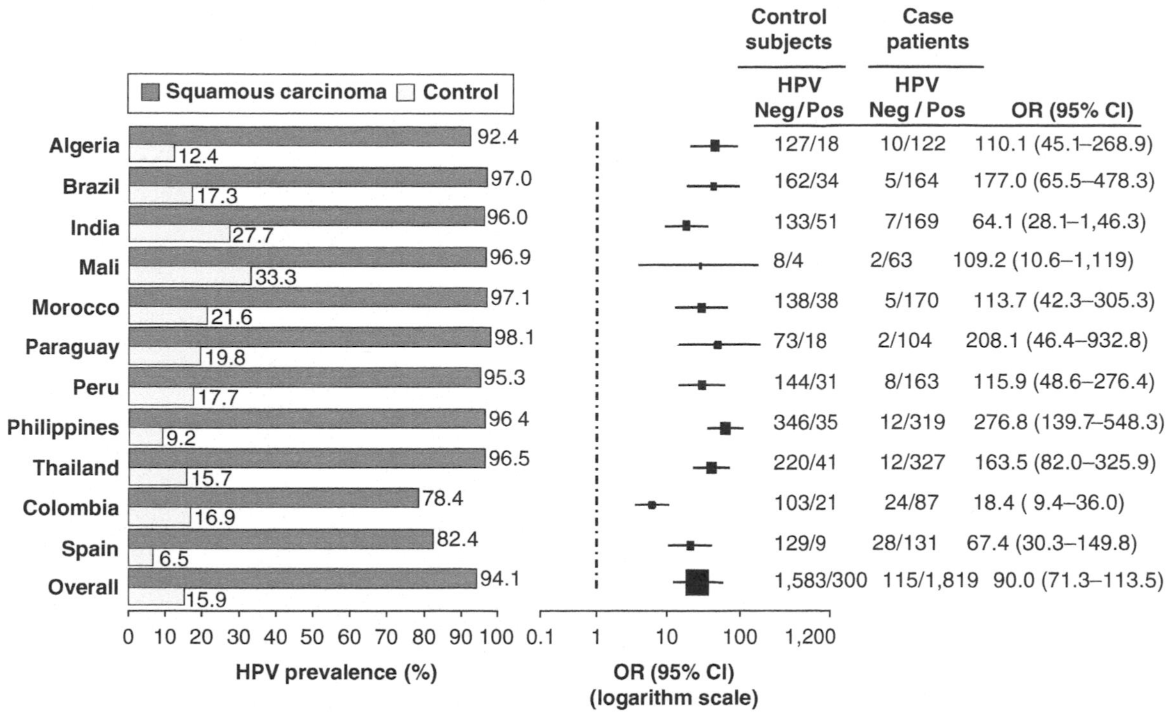

Fig. 33.1 *Left panel*: prevalence of HPV DNA by country among women with squamous cell carcinoma (SCC) and among control women. *Right panel*: odds ratio (OR) for cervical SCC with 95% confidence intervals (CI). ORs are adjusted by center and age (Adapted and expanded from [9])

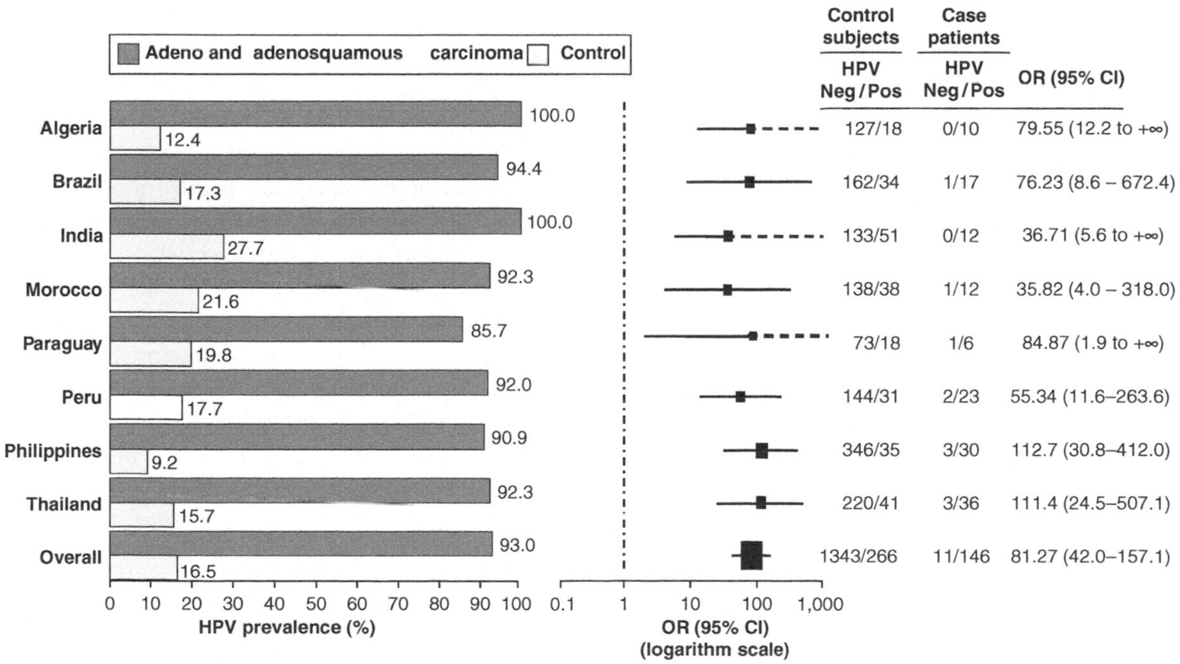

Fig. 33.2 *Left panel*: prevalence of HPV DNA by country among women with cervical adenocarcinoma (ADC) and among control women. *Right panel*: odds ratio (OR) for cervical ADC with 95% confidence interval (CI). ORs are adjusted by age group, years of schooling, age at first sexual intercourse, and number of pap smears before 12 months before enrollment (Adapted from [10])

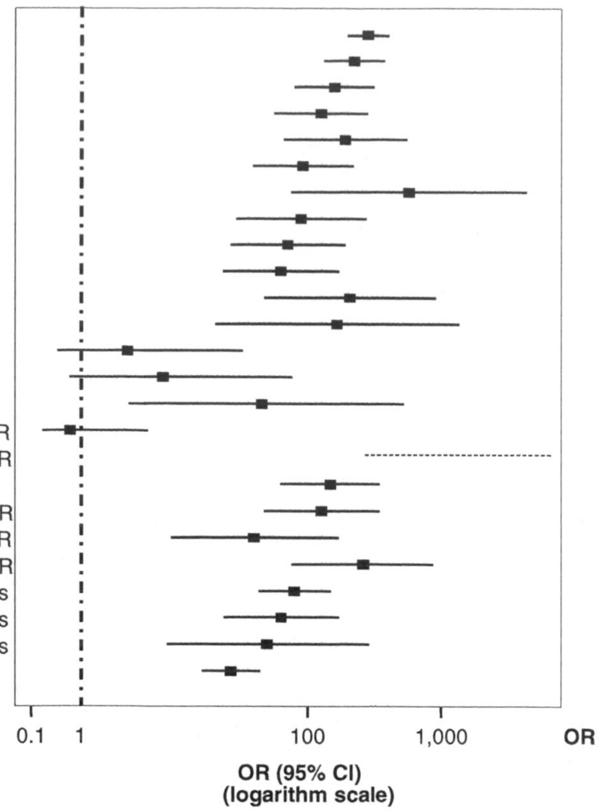

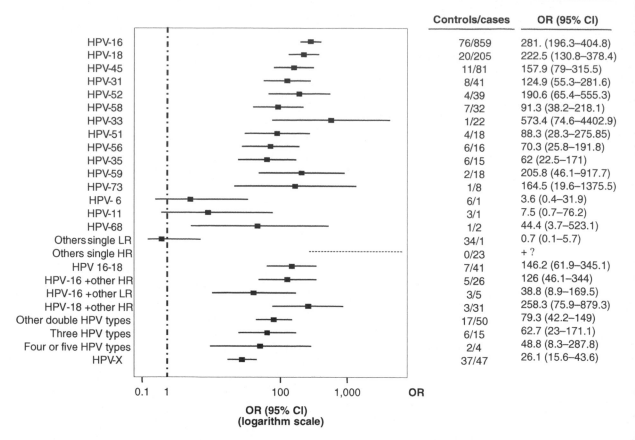

	Controls/cases	OR (95% CI)
HPV-16	76/859	281. (196.3–404.8)
HPV-18	20/205	222.5 (130.8–378.4)
HPV-45	11/81	157.9 (79–315.5)
HPV-31	8/41	124.9 (55.3–281.6)
HPV-52	4/39	190.6 (65.4–555.3)
HPV-58	7/32	91.3 (38.2–218.1)
HPV-33	1/22	573.4 (74.6–4402.9)
HPV-51	4/18	88.3 (28.3–275.85)
HPV-56	6/16	70.3 (25.8–191.8)
HPV-35	6/15	62 (22.5–171)
HPV-59	2/18	205.8 (46.1–917.7)
HPV-73	1/8	164.5 (19.6–1375.5)
HPV- 6	6/1	3.6 (0.4–31.9)
HPV-11	3/1	7.5 (0.7–76.2)
HPV-68	1/2	44.4 (3.7–523.1)
Others single LR	34/1	0.7 (0.1–5.7)
Others single HR	0/23	+ ?
HPV 16-18	7/41	146.2 (61.9–345.1)
HPV-16 +other HR	5/26	126 (46.1–344)
HPV-16 +other LR	3/5	38.8 (8.9–169.5)
HPV-18 +other HR	3/31	258.3 (75.9–879.3)
Other double HPV types	17/50	79.3 (42.2–149)
Three HPV types	6/15	62.7 (23–171.1)
Four or five HPV types	2/4	48.8 (8.3–287.8)
HPV-X	37/47	26.1 (15.6–43.6)

Fig. 33.3 Type-specific odds ratios (OR) and 95% confidence intervals (CI) for cervical carcinoma (squamous cell and adenocarcinoma). Subjects with HPV-DNA-negative results were used as the reference category. ORs are adjusted by country and age-group. HR: high risk; LR: low-risk. HPV type X denotes undetermined type (i.e., specimens that were positive with the GP5+/6+ system but that did not hybridize with any of the 33 type-specific probes) (Adapted and expanded from [9])

to HPV 16 and HPV 18. In some of these studies, CIN 2/3 developed within 2 years of first HPV DNA detection, thus indicating that, as an exception to the generalized observation that prolonged HPV infection is necessary for progression to CIN 2/3, a fraction of these lesions can be an early manifestation of HPV infection, particularly in young women [12].

Several nested case control studies within cohorts have examined the archival smears of women with invasive cervical cancer and of control women. In all of them, a higher prevalence of HPV 16 DNA was detected in the smears and diagnostic biopsies of women who subsequently developed cervical cancer as compared to the selected control group of women of similar age and place of residence without cervical cancer. The risk of types other than HPV 16 was difficult to assess.

The progression rate linked to HPV 16 and 18 is about 20% at 10 years, whereas the progression rate of any other HPV type is significantly lower. The graph strongly suggests that relatively small studies with up to 10 years of follow-up are highly informative on events related to these two HPV types but relatively less on events (CIN 2+) that are related to any other HPV types (Fig. 33.4). This is particularly important for HPV vaccine trials in which type-specific allocation of lesions is critical for the interpretation of the vaccine efficacy studies.

Cohort studies reaching at least 5 years of follow-up and using repeated testing at frequent intervals have been useful to understand outstanding issues in relation to HPV natural history and prognostic factors. The information is particularly informative if type-specific testing is performed to clearly identify type-specific persistency from a generic group of HPV DNA-positive. However, even using the most appropriate study designs, it is difficult to distinguish between persistent type-specific infections from a second infection with the same type or even to differentiate a new incident infection from the reactivation of a latent

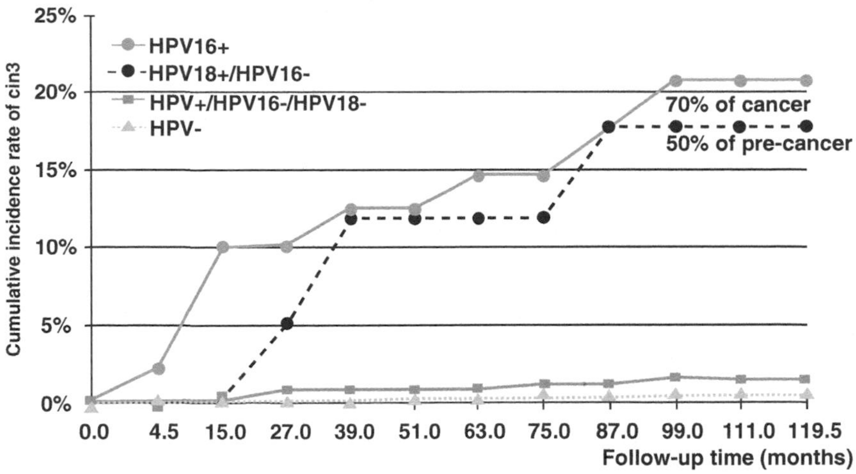

Fig. 33.4 Example of a 10-year follow-up study [12]

infection that was silent to the follow-up procedure for some time. These are all areas in which additional studies are warranted.

33.1.5 Research Areas in the HPV and Cervical Cancer Natural History

Viral load: Methodologies are still being validated to adequately assess viral load from clinical specimens. High viral load for most high-risk HPV genotypes is associated with prevalent cervical cancer precursors, but only HPV 16 load predicts the development of incident high-grade disease [13]. The risk stratification afforded by viral load is not clear-cut enough to be used clinically.

Cytology and pathology diagnostic methods: Globally and for a given HPV type, the finding of a low squamous intraepithelial lesion (LSIL) conveys a similar prognosis as the diagnosis of an abnormal squamous cell of undetermined significance (ASCUS) HPV-positive [14]. The histopathology finding of CIN 1 is not predictive of risk of CIN 3 in prospective follow-up. Colposcopy-directed biopsy is a weaker prognostic tool than previously assumed, because of the combination of error in biopsy placement and limited reproducibility of CIN 1 (and to a lesser extent CIN 2) [11,14]. CIN 2 is a much less reproducible diagnosis than CIN 3, as shown by the results of a histological review of population-based cervical samples [11].

Multiple HPV types: Systemic pathology examination of cervical cones or biopsies often reveals multiple HPV types, particularly in young women. Less often reported is the coexistence in a clinical specimen of more than one histological confirmed lesion, e.g., areas of CIN 1 and CIN 3 or invasive cancer. In these instances, causal allocation of individual viral types and lesions remains elusive and biomarkers are still under development. Literature studies are largely non-informative in this respect as routinely only the highest level lesions are reported for clinical purposes. As a consequence, the frequency and the nature of the coexistence of lesions of variable severity are not readily available from screening studies. The issue of multiple types in a given specimen has been a major issue in the HPV vaccination trials in which type-specific HPV testing and pathology was carefully done, and type-specific allocation of CIN 2/3 was critical in the estimation of vaccine efficacy. In the trials, a few such cases occurred and in the absence of more specific biomarkers, the clinical record of previous HPV types was used as the best option to allocate causality [15].

Duration of type-specific HPV infections and clinical implications: Results from the ASCUS and LISL Triage Study (ALTS) study have provided evidence of the rate of clearance of high-risk HPV types in women with initial diagnoses of ASCUS. The time to clearance of ASCUS patients by HPV type is rather similar for all types and, remarkably, most infections have cleared in an interval of 6–12 months. After that there is a plateau indicating that clearance is inversely related to duration and that management decisions should be based on at least 12–16 months' documented persistency [16].

Additional studies in the general screening population might provide evidence on the time intervals with confirmed HPV persistency required to recommend for referral to diagnostic procedures.

33.2 The Role of HPV in Genital Cancers Other Than Cervical

The number of studies on the role of HPV in other genital cancers is limited, and in most, the search for HPV DNA has been done for a limited number of HPV types in fixed tissue. The available epidemiological studies indicate that cancers of the vagina and of the anus resemble cancer of the cervix with respect to the role of HPV. In both cases, HPV DNA is detected in the great majority of tumors and their precursor lesions. Between 64% and 91% of vaginal cancer cases and 82% and 100% of vaginal intraepithelial neoplasia of grade 3 (VAIN 3) lesions are HPV DNA-positive. In anal cancers, HPV-DNA is detected in 88–94%. Cancers of the vulva have also been associated with HPV. The tumors diagnosed in young individuals are usually of basaloid or warty histological types. The majority (60–90%) are positive for HPV DNA, and their pre-neoplastic lesions are also strongly associated with HPV. In contrast, in older subjects, the tumors are usually keratinizing SCCs and are rarely (less than 10%) associated with HPV.

In all HPV-positive anogenital cancers, HPV 16 is the most common HPV type detected, followed by HPV types 18, 31, and 33. The most recent IARC monograph concluded that there was sufficient evidence for the carcinogenicity of HPV 16 in the vulva, penis (basaloid and warty tumors), vagina, and anus. It also concluded that there was limited evidence for the carcinogenicity of HPV 18 in the vulva, penis (basaloid and warty tumors), vagina, and anus and limited evidence for the carcinogenicity of HPV 6 and 11 in the vulva, penis, and anus (verrucous carcinomas) [2]. Table 33.1 summarizes a recent literature review on the HPV DNA prevalence in series of clinical cases.

33.2.1 Interaction of HPV and Human Immunodeficiency Virus (HIV) in Anal Carcinoma

Studies on special populations at high-risk of anal cancer, notably males that have sex with males (MSM) have provided important information on the interaction of joint HPV and HIV viral infections in the carcinogenic process. Table 33.2 shows that HIV-positive MSM with anal intraepithelial lesions have a higher prevalence of HPV DNA, more frequent multiple infections, and a wider range of HPV types than subjects with anal lesions who were HIV-negative. Moreover, the incidence of anal cancer among MSM is in the range of 12–35 per 100,000 among HIV-negative subjects and of 70–100 per 10,000 among HIV-positive subjects. These estimates parallel the incidence of cervical cancer in women before the widespread introduction of Pap

Table 33.1 Prevalence of HPV DNA in genital cancers. Literature review [2,17]

	Vulvar Cancer	VIN	Vaginal Cancer	VAIN	Anal Cancer	AIN
Number of subjects	1,873	1,197	136	289	955	1,280
HPV DNA	40.4%	84%	69.9%	93.6%	84.3%(male and female)	92.7%

AIN anal intraepithelial neoplasia, *VAIN* vaginal intraepithelial neoplasia, *VIN* vulvar intraepithelial neoplasia

Table 33.2 HPV and type distribution in anal intraepithelial lesions by HIV status [17]

	HIV-positive		HIV-negative	
HPV Type	N	%	N	%
HPV DNA	215	96.7	161	90.1
Multiple	208	65.9	128	13.3
16	208	55.3	145	76.6
18	182	25.5	127	6.3
31/33	182	13.2/19.2	113	2.7/6.7
Range of up to 11 other types	168–208	2–22	109–117	0–0.9

HIV human immunodeficiency virus, *HPV* human papillomavirus

smears [18,19]. The literature strongly suggests that this interaction among HPV and immunosuppression in the induction of neoplastic changes also occurs in the cervix and possibly in other locations.

33.3 The Role of HPV in Non-Anogenital Cancers

33.3.1 Evidence Linking HPV to Head and Neck Squamous Cell Carcinoma (HNSCC)

Over the last 15 years, evidence implicating HPV as a carcinogenic agent in a subset of HNSCCs (cancers of the oral cavity, pharynx, and larynx) has been accumulating.

The most recent systematic review included 5046 HNSCC specimens from 60 studies that employed PCR-based methods to detect and genotype HPV DNA [20]. The estimated summary prevalence of HPV DNA was of 25.9%, although this was significantly higher in oro-pharyngeal SCCs (35.6%; range: 11–100%) than in oral (23.5%; range: 4–80%) or laryngeal SCCs (24%; range: 0–100%). HPV 16 accounted for a larger majority of HPV-positive oro-pharyngeal SCCs (86.7%) than HPV-positive oral (68.2%) and laryngeal SCCs (69.2%). HPV 18 was the second most frequent type detected: 2.8% in oro-pharyngeal, 34.1% in oral, and 17% in laryngeal SCCs. Other oncogenic HPVs were rarely detected in HNSCC (Table 33.3).

Results from several case control studies, including a large multicentre case control study conducted by the IARC [21], have consistently identified positive and statistically significant associations between markers of HPV (DNA and/or serology) and HNSCC risk, thereby pointing to a likely role of HPV in cancers of the oro-pharynx, tonsil, and to a lesser extent, the oral cavity and larynx. As in genital cancers, HPV 16 is also the most common type in these tumors.

The 2005 IARC evaluation on the carcinogenicity of HPV in humans concluded that there is sufficient evidence for the carcinogenicity of HPV 16 in the oral cavity and in the oro-pharynx, limited evidence for HPV 18 in the oral cavity, inadequate evidence for other HPV types in the oral cavity and in the oro-pharynx, limited evidence for HPV 6, 11, 16, and 18 in the larynx, and inadequate evidence for the carcinogenicity of HPV in the esophagus [2].

Recent literature on oro-pharyngeal cancer has recently shown (1) a high prevalence of HPV DNA in paraffin preserved biopsies of oro-pharyngeal cancer; (2) a strong association with several biomarkers of exposure to HPV, notably to HPV 16; (3) a strong correlation of HPV-positive cases with sexual behavior patterns consistent with multiple partners and oral sex practices; and (4) a remarkable difference in the epidemiological profile of HPV-positive and HPV-negative cases by which the HPV-negative cases were strongly related to alcohol and tobacco consumption, whereas the HPV-positive cases showed no clear association with these recognized human carcinogens [22,23].

33.4 Epidemiology of HPV Infections in Men and Women

33.4.1 The Burden of HPV Infections in Women and HPV Type-Specific Distribution in Cervical Lesions

33.4.1.1 HPV Prevalence and Age-Specific Prevalence in Women with Normal Cytology

Most women in the world will be infected with HPV at sometime during their lifetime. The World Health Organization (WHO)/Catalan Institute of Oncology

Table 33.3 HPV DNA prevalence and type-specific relative frequency in cancers of the head and neck [20]

HPV Type	Oral (N = 2.642)	Oropharynx (N = 969)	Larynx (N = 1.435)
HPV	23.5%	35.6 %	24%
16	68.2%	86.7 %	69.2%
18	34.1%	2.8 %	17%
Any other	<1%	<1%	<1%

HPV human papillomavirus

(ICO) Information Centre on HPV and Cervical Cancer (http://www.who.int/hpvcentre/en/) [24,25] reports on the prevalence of HPV DNA in women with normal cytology worldwide. The 2007 edition includes publications from 1999 up to early 2005 on 157,897 women with normal cytology and specifically excludes data on women with any abnormality. The estimated prevalence is model-adjusted and takes into account the variability in study design and in HPV detection assays across the studies.

Furthermore, the variability in inclusion criteria is significant and impacts the estimates of HPV infections worldwide. Only women with reported normal cytology were included in the analysis in an effort to homogenize the comparison across published literature. The net impact of including all women reported in the studies (usually combining women from the general population and from referral clinics) would result in a slight increase of the global estimates of the prevalence.

The results indicate that at a given point in time, 10.4% (95% confidence interval [CI]: 10.2–10.7) of the women worldwide are positive for HPV DNA in the cervix. HPV prevalence is higher in the less developed world (13.4%; 95% CI: 13.1–13.7) than in more developed regions (8.4%; 95% CI: 8.3–8.6). African women (22.1%; 95% CI: 20.9–23.4), in particular women in Eastern Africa, have the highest HPV prevalence rates (31.6%; 95% CI: 29.5–33.8), while the lowest estimates are identified in South-Eastern Asia (6.2%; 95% CI: 5.5–7.0). Similar results were observed in an IARC population-based survey conducted with 15,613 women aged 15–74 years from eleven countries. The study benefited from standardized methods of sampling and HPV testing. Women in these surveys are also part of the global meta-analyses describing the age-specific prevalence patterns in different populations [26].

In all continents, HPV 16 is the most common HPV type with an estimated point prevalence of 2.6% (95% CI: 2.5–2.8) worldwide, ranging from 3.5% (95% CI: 2.8–4.3) in Northern America to 2.3% (95% CI: 2.0–2.5) in Europe [24]. HPV 18 is the second most frequently detected type after HPV 16 in the world estimate, in Europe and Central and South America. In Africa, HPV 52 is the second most frequent type and HPV 18 the third. In Asia, HPV 18 is the fourth most frequent type after HPV 16, 52, and 58. In Northern America, HPV 18 is also the fourth most common type, after HPV 16, 53, and 52. In Europe, Asia, and Northern America, all individual types other than HPV 16 have prevalence estimates below 1%. Conversely, in Africa and Central and South America several other types show prevalence over or equal to 1%. In Africa HPV types 58, 31, 35, 42, 66, 53, 45, 56, and 33 are frequently observed, while HPV 51, 71, 70, and 62 are frequently identified in other world regions. It should be noticed that HPV 45, a very common type in invasive cervical cancer (ICC), is the ninth most frequently found type among women with normal cytology in the overall world estimate.

Figure 33.5 shows HPV DNA prevalence by continent and age groups including both high- and low-risk

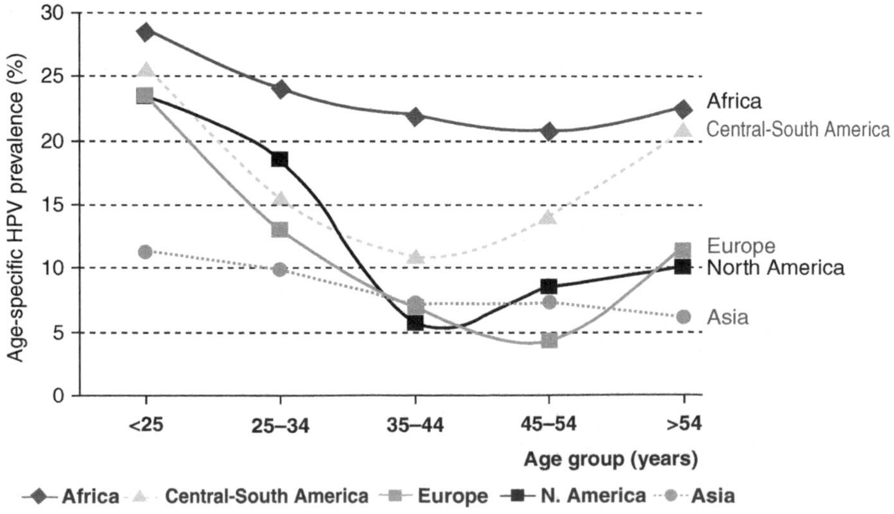

Fig. 33.5 Age-specific HPV prevalence, both low- and high-risk types, in five world regions among women with normal cytology (Adapted from [24])

types. The prevalence of HPV DNA is high (up to 30%) in young women in all regions except in Asia [24]. The prevalence declines in the middle-age groups and a second rise in prevalence rates is observed in women in the 35–44-year or 45–54-year age groups. Again this second increase is less clearly observed in the populations in Asia. It is unclear at this stage if the second increase in the peri-menopausal years is largely due to increase in the low-risk types as suggested by some studies [14,26].

Although research continues to be conducted, current understanding favors a combination of three possibilities to explain the second increase in HPV prevalence: (1) new HPV infections acquired by middle-aged women due to changes in sexual behavior, (2) reactivation of latent infection following immune senescence, and/or (3) a cohort effect translating high exposures throughout lifetime in elderly generations. The difference of close to 10 years in the age intervals in which the second mode is observed in the USA (35–44 years) *versus* Europe (45–54 years), suggests a behavioral factor rather than a biological effect linked to menopause or immune senescence. Latency of HPV infections in cervical tissue is an elusive concept, which is perhaps best illustrated by the studies on recurrent respiratory papillomatosis (RRP) in which HPV 6/11-related lesions continue to recur from apparently normal tissue, even in the absence of obvious external reinfection. Finally, the possibility of a significant cohort effect cannot be ignored although retrospective assessment of the prevalence of HPV exposure remains difficult to describe.

33.4.1.2 HPV Age-Specific Incidence in Women with Normal Cytology

Follow-up studies have shown that HPV DNA can be newly detected in all age groups (Fig. 33.6) and behavioral surveys report a high rate of new sexual partners in the 40 years and older age groups in many developed populations [27,28]. A study in a high-risk population in Colombia showed very high rates of new infection in the 15–19 age groups (over 40% at 5 years), but significant numbers of new infections in the 45+ age groups as well.

33.4.2 HPV Prevalence and Type Distribution in Women with High-Grade and Invasive Cervical Lesions

Cross-sectional studies of the natural history of cervical cancer indicate that the contribution of HPV DNA in high-grade squamous intraepithelial lesions (HSIL),

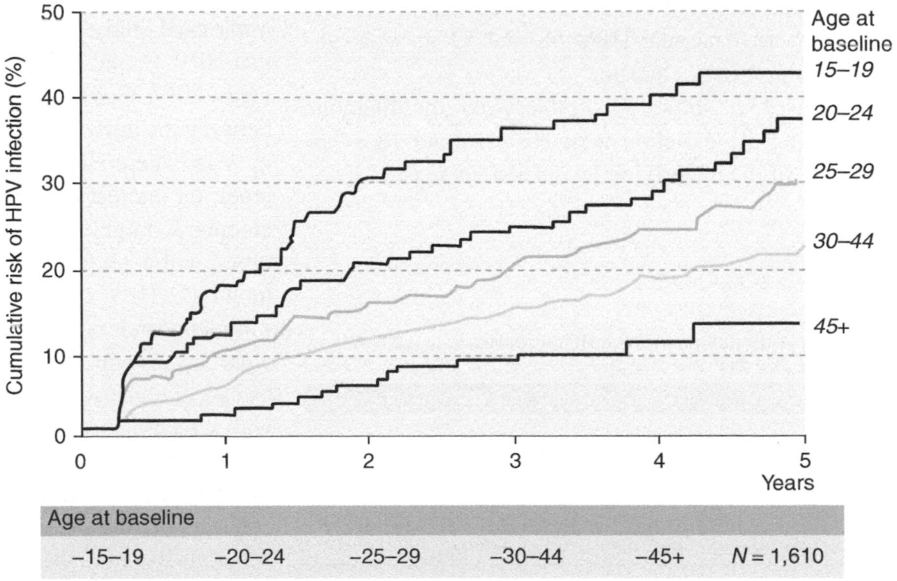

Fig. 33.6 Cumulative risk of newly detected HPV infection (any type) by age groups in women in a cohort study in Bogotá, Colombia (Adapted from [27])

which represent morphological precursors for ICC, is estimated to be over 85% [6]. This is less clear for CIN 2, which has substantial variability in diagnosis and prognosis. HPV is found in virtually 100% of ICC cases [7].

Deviations from these estimates are largely explained by variations in the quality of the specimens tested and in the sensitivity of the HPV detection assays. Interpretation of any putative geographical variations of HPV type distribution in any given lesion requires careful consideration of differences in sampling and in the sensitivity of the HPV detection assays. For example, MY09/11 probes have been more extensively used in American studies as compared to European studies, where GP5+/6+ assays have been more often used. It has been reported that the sensitivity of MY09/11-based assays was greater for HPV 52 than GP5+/6+ [29]. A validation panel organized by WHO showed that there were no differences in DNA detection for HPV 16, 18, 33, and 45 across different laboratories and assays. Conversely, HPV 31, 35, 52, and 6 did show assay differences in sensitivity and specificity that should be considered when interpreting results from different laboratories [30].

Worldwide estimates showed that HPV 16 accounted for 45.4% of all high-grade lesions. Greater variability can be seen in the other HPV type ranking positions. While worldwide, in Africa and Europe, HPV 31 and 33 were the second and the third commonest types, these ranking positions corresponded to HPV 58 and 18 in Latin America and the Caribbean, HPV 6 and 18 in Northern America, HPV 58 and 52 in Asia, and HPV 31 and 18 in Oceania.

Table 33.4 shows a summary on the literature describing the enrichment of HPV 16 and 18 as the severity of the underlying lesion also increases.

Table 33.4 Enrichment of the HPV prevalence in the cervix by diagnosis [3,9,31]

Diagnosis	HPV-DNA+	HPV 16/18
Normal	9–10%	(2–3%)
Preinvasive lesions	80–90%	(50%)
Cervical cancer	95–100%	(70%)

33.4.3 HPV Type Distribution in Women with Invasive Cervical Cancer

Table 33.5 shows the rank order of the HPV type distribution in ICC based on the data available from three different sources: (1) the IARC pooled studies on over 3,000 ICC cases [4], (2) an updated meta-analysis including 14,500 cases [6,8,25], and (3) an ongoing international survey coordinated by ICO, including close to 9,000 cases [3]. The IARC pooled study and the ICO international epidemiologic study have the advantage over the meta-analysis that both have centralized sensitive methods for HPV detection and typing, and use standardized protocols for sample processing to avoid contamination. In contrast, the meta-analyses while offering a greater international representation and a robust sample size include studies with different designs, inclusion criteria, and laboratory techniques (albeit a predefined threshold of quality). Moreover, the number of HPV types tested for in individual studies confers additional variability, particularly when multiple HPV types are concurrently found in a given specimen.

Among women with ICC, there is a consistent frequency ranking between the three studies for the first positions, with the most common types being HPV 16, 18, 45, 33, 31, 58, 52, and 35. These series are very robust in identifying that HPV 16 and 18 contribute approximately 70% of all ICC cases.

Table 33.6 shows the corresponding distributions by histology as found in the ICO international epidemiological study. In addition to the consistent finding that HPV 16 and 18 were the major types in all continents, HPV 33, 45, and 31 were consistently identified between the third and fifth positions with the exception of Asia, where HPV 58, 33, and 52 were the common types. Of interest is the finding that cervical adenocarcinoma is largely a condition related to three HPV types, with a tenfold gap between the third most common type (HPV 45) and any of the followers.

Adenocarcinomas comprise around 10% of all cervical cancers which is consistent with the range reported by cancer registries [33]. However, developed countries with screening programs tend to report increasing incidence rates and relative frequencies of ADC (up to 20% of the registered cervical cancer cases). The increased contribution of these cancers to the cervical cancer burden is attributed to the lower efficacy of cytology-based

Table 33.5 The eight most common HPV types in cervical cancer – world [6,8]

Ranking	HPV Type		
	IARC Data $N = 3,085$	Meta-Analysis $N = 14,500$	ICO Survey $N = 8,785$
1st	HPV 16	HPV 16	HPV 16
2nd	HPV 18	HPV 18	HPV 18
3rd	HPV 45	HPV 33	HPV 45
4th	HPV 31	HPV 45	HPV 31
5th	HPV 33	HPV 31	HPV 33
6th	HPV 52	HPV 58	HPV 52
7th	HPV 58	HPV 52	HPV 58
8th	HPV 35	HPV 35	HPV 35

HPV human papillomavirus

Table 33.6 The most relevant single HPV types (% over HPV + specimens) in cervical cancer by histology – ICO survey [32]

Cervical Cancer		Squamous Cell Carcinoma		Adeno Carcinoma	
10,365 8,792 HPV+		9,292 8,077 HPV+		748 463 HPV+	
16	56.6	16	57.7	16	45.9
18	9.6	18	7.8	18	30.5
45	5.3	45	4.9	45	10.6
33	3.5	33	3.7	31	0.6
31	3.5	31	3.7	51	0.6
Total	78.5		77.8		88.2
(): % of multiple infections	(6.3)		(6.3)		(7.8)

screening programs to identify its precursors, paired with a genuine increase in HPV exposure in younger generations following significant changes in sexual behavior in many populations.

33.5 Conclusion

Worldwide, HPV 16 is the most common HPV type across the spectrum of HPV-related cervical lesions. The increase in the relative contribution of HPV 16 from 2–4% in women with normal cytology to 50–55% in ICC supports the notion of its biological advantage for transmission and transformation. The same phenomenon is observed at a lower level for HPV 18 and 45. In women with ICC, the most common HPV types are HPV 16, 18, 33, 45, 31, and 58. HPV 16, 18, and 45 are the three most relevant types in cervical adenocarcinoma. The geographical variation in type distribution is of minor significance with the exception of Asia where HPV 58 and 52 are particularly relevant.

Sexual behavioral patterns across age groups and populations are central to the description of the HPV circulation and risk of infection.

Rates of HPV infections in young women are high and often include multiple types. There is a spontaneous and rapid decrease of the DNA detection rates in the middle-age groups, followed by a second rise in the postmenopausal age groups. The interpretation of this second rise has been related to sexual behavior. However, the hypothesis that a period of HPV latency can partially explain the second rise remains difficult to prove.

Following HPV infection, prognosis is significantly linked to the HPV type. HPV 16 and 18 show the clearest pattern of progression *versus* regression as compared to the rest of the high-risk types. Viral load – particularly of HPV 16 – seems to convey an additional prognostic value, but clinical validation is still lacking.

Some of the key remaining issues continue to include the prognostic value of multiple infections for HSIL and cervical cancer, the establishment of threshold time intervals that discriminate for persistency and that are of clinical utility, and the diagnosis of HPV latency that would help to explain the second mode in the age-specific HPV prevalence worldwide.

Acknowledgment F. Xavier Bosch's, Xavier Castellsague's, and Silvia de Sanjose's work was partially supported by Spanish public grants from the Instituto de Salud Carlos III (grants RCESP C03/09, RTICESP C03/10 and RTIC RD06/0020/0095 and CIBERESP) and from the Agència de Gestió d'Ajuts Universitaris i de Recerca (AGAUR 2005 SGR 00695).

The contribution of Maria Jesus Vázquez and Cristina Rajo in the preparation of the manuscript is deeply recognized.

Take-Home Pearls

- Cervical cancer is always caused by non resolved infections by a high risk human papillomavirus (HPV). Up to 12 types have been labeled as oncogenic. HPV 16 and 18 account for 70% of the types involved.
- Most anogenital tract cancers in men and women are also caused by HPV, mostly by HPV 16 and 18.
- A fraction of cases of the oro-pharyngeal (some 30%) and oral cavity region (some 10–15%) are also caused by HPV, largely HPV 16.
- The predominant types involved in carcinogenesis are largely constant across geographical regions.
- Sexual intercourse is the predominant mode of transmission of genital and oral HPV infections.

References

1. IARC monograph on the evaluation of carcinogenic risks to human. IARC, Lyon (1995)
2. IARC Monographs on the Evaluation of Carcinogenic Risks to Humans Volume 100B. A Review of Human Carcinogens: Biological Agents IARC press (2011)
3. de Sanjose, S., Quint, W., Klaustenmeier, J. et al.: HPV type distribution in invasive cervical cancer: the worldwide perspective. Proceedings of the 24th International Papillomavirus Conference and Clinical Workshop, Beijing, China, 2007. Abstracts Book
4. Munoz, N., Bosch, F.X., Castellsague, X., et al.: Against which human papillomavirus types shall we vaccinate and screen? The international perspective. Int J Cancer **111**(2), 278–285 (2004 Aug 20)
5. Bosch, F.X., Manos, M.M., Munoz, N., et al.: Prevalence of human papillomavirus in cervical cancer: a worldwide perspective. International biological study on cervical cancer (IBSCC) Study Group. J Natl Cancer Inst **87**(11), 796–802 (1995 Jun 7)
6. Smith, J.S., Lindsay, L., Hoots, B., et al.: Human papillomavirus type distribution in invasive cervical cancer and high-grade cervical lesions: a meta-analysis update. Int J Cancer **121**(3), 621–632 (2007 Aug 1)
7. Walboomers, J.M., Jacobs, M.V., Manos, M.M., et al.: Human papillomavirus is a necessary cause of invasive cervical cancer worldwide. J Pathol **189**(1), 12–19 (1999 Sep)
8. Clifford, G.M., Smith, J.S., Plummer, M., Munoz, N., Franceschi, S.: Human papillomavirus types in invasive cervical cancer worldwide: a meta-analysis. Br J Cancer **88**(1), 63–73 (2003 Jan 13)
9. Munoz, N., Bosch, F.X., de Sanjose, S., et al.: Epidemiologic classification of human papillomavirus types associated with cervical cancer. N Engl J Med **348**(6), 518–527 (2003 Feb 6)
10. Castellsague, X., Diaz, M., de Sanjose, S., et al.: Worldwide human papillomavirus etiology of cervical adenocarcinoma and its cofactors: implications for screening and prevention. J Natl Cancer Inst **98**(5), 303–315 (2006 Mar 1)
11. Carreon, J.D., Sherman, M.E., Guillen, D., et al.: CIN2 is a much less reproducible and less valid diagnosis than CIN3: results from a histological review of population-based cervical samples. Int J Gynecol Pathol **26**(4), 441–446 (2007 Oct)
12. Khan, M.J., Castle, P.E., Lorincz, A.T., et al.: The elevated 10-year risk of cervical precancer and cancer in women with human papillomavirus (HPV) type 16 or 18 and the possible utility of type-specific HPV testing in clinical practice. J Natl Cancer Inst **97**(14), 1072–1079 (2005 Jul 20)
13. Gravitt, P.E., Kovacic, M.B., Herrero, R., et al.: High load for most high risk human papillomavirus genotypes is associated with prevalent cervical cancer precursors but only HPV16 load predicts the development of incident disease. Int J Cancer **121**(12), 2787–2793 (2007 Dec 15)
14. Castle, P.E., Jeronimo, J., Schiffman, M., et al.: Age-related changes of the cervix influence human papillomavirus type distribution. Cancer Res **66**(2), 1218–1224 (2006 Jan 15)
15. Paavonen, J., Jenkins, D., Bosch, F.X., et al.: Efficacy of a prophylactic adjuvanted bivalent L1 virus-like-particle vaccine against infection with human papillomavirus types 16 and 18 in young women: an interim analysis of a phase III double-blind, randomised controlled trial. Lancet **369**(9580), 2161–2170 (30 June 2007)
16. Plummer, M., Schiffman, M., Castle, P.E., Maucort-Boulch, D., Wheeler, C.M.: A 2-year prospective study of human papillomavirus persistence among women with a cytological diagnosis of atypical squamous cells of undetermined significance or low-grade squamous intraepithelial lesion. J Infect Dis **195**(11), 1582–1589 (2007 Jun 1)

17. De Vuyst, H., Clifford, G.M., Nascimento, M.C., Madeleine, M.M., Franceschi, S.: Prevalence and type distribution of human papillomavirus in carcinoma and intraepithelial neoplasia of the vulva, vagina and anus: a meta-analysis. Int J Cancer **124**(7), 1626–1636 (1 Apr 2009)
18. Chiao, E.Y., Krown, S.E., Stier, E.A., Schrag, D.: A population-based analysis of temporal trends in the incidence of squamous anal canal cancer in relation to the HIV epidemic. J Acquir Immune Defic Syndr **40**(4), 451–455 (2005 Dec 1)
19. Bowers, N.A., Gromada, K.K.: Pregnancy after age 35. AWHONN Lifelines **8**(2), 99–100 (2004 Apr)
20. Kreimer, A.R., Clifford, G.M., Boyle, P., Franceschi, S.: Human papillomavirus types in head and neck squamous cell carcinomas worldwide: a systematic review. Cancer Epidemiol Biomarkers Prev **14**(2), 467–475 (2005 Feb)
21. Herrero, R., Castellsague, X., Pawlita, M., et al.: Human papillomavirus and oral cancer: the International Agency for Research on Cancer multicenter study. J Natl Cancer Inst **95**(23), 1772–1783 (3 Dec 2003)
22. D'Souza, G., Kreimer, A.R., Viscidi, R., et al.: Case-control study of human papillomavirus and oropharyngeal cancer. N Engl J Med **356**(19), 1944–1956 (2007 May 10)
23. Gillison, M.L., D'Souza, G., Westra, W., et al.: Distinct risk factor profiles for human papillomavirus type 16-positive and human papillomavirus type 16-negative head and neck cancers. J Natl Cancer Inst **100**(6), 407–420 (2008 Mar 19)
24. de Sanjose, S., Diaz, M., Castellsague, X., et al.: Worldwide prevalence and genotype distribution of cervical human papillomavirus DNA in women with normal cytology: a meta-analysis. Lancet Infect Dis **7**(7), 453–459 (2007 Jul)
25. Castellsague, X., de Sanjose, S., Aguado, T., et al.: HPV and Cervical Cancer in the World. 2007 Report. WHO/ICO Information Centre on HPV and Cervical Cancer (HPV Information Centre). Vaccine 25(Suppl 3) (2007)
26. Franceschi, S., Herrero, R., Clifford, G.M., et al.: Variations in the age-specific curves of human papillomavirus prevalence in women worldwide. Int J Cancer **119**(11), 2677–2684 (2006 Dec 1)
27. Munoz, N., Mendez, F., Posso, H., et al.: Incidence, duration, and determinants of cervical human papillomavirus infection in a cohort of Colombian women with normal cytological results. J Infect Dis **190**(12), 2077–2087 (15 Dec 2004)
28. Wellings, K., Collumbien, M., Slaymaker, E., et al.: Sexual behaviour in context: a global perspective. Lancet **368**(9548), 1706–1728 (11 Nov 2006)
29. Chan, P.K., Cheung, T.H., Tam, A.O., et al.: Biases in human papillomavirus genotype prevalence assessment associated with commonly used consensus primers. Int J Cancer **118**(1), 243–245 (1 Jan 2006)
30. Quint, W.G., Pagliusi, S.R., Lelie, N., de Villiers, E.M., Wheeler, C.M.: Results of the first World Health Organization international collaborative study of detection of human papillomavirus DNA. J Clin Microbiol **44**(2), 571–579 (Feb 2006)
31. Clifford, G.M., Smith, J.S., Aguado, T., Franceschi, S.: Comparison of HPV type distribution in high-grade cervical lesions and cervical cancer: a meta-analysis. Br J Cancer **89**(1), 101–105 (7 July 2003)
32. De Sanjose, S., et al.: Worldwide HPV Genotype Distribution in 10,365 Cases of Cervical Cancer, 2009 p. Poster 30.13
33. Parkin, D., Whelan, S., Teppo, L., Thomas, D.: Cancer Incidence in Five Continents. IARC Press, Lyon (2003)

34 Immune Responses to Sexually Transmitted HPV Infection

Margaret Stanley

Core Messages

- Genital HPV infection, is very common in young sexually active individuals, most mount an effective immune response and control the infection by generating a Th1 dominated cell mediated immune response.
- Both antibody and cell mediated responses are protective against subsequent viral challenge in natural infections in animals.
- About 10% of individuals develop a persistent infection and it is this cohort that is at risk for progressive or recurrent disease.
- The infectious cycle of HPV is one in which viral replication and release is not associated with inflammation and effective evasion of innate immune recognition is the hallmark of HPV infections.
- HPV infections disrupt cytokine expression and signalling with the E6 and E7 oncoproteins particularly targeting the type I interferon (IFN) pathway.
- Prophylactic vaccines consisting of HPV L1 VLPs generate a strong antibody response and prevent disease associated with vaccine HPVs.
- These vaccines are delivered intra-muscularly circumventing HPV immune evasion strategies.

M. Stanley
Department of Pathology, Tennis Court Road, Cambridge, Cb2 1QP, UK
e-mail: mas@mole.bio.cam.ac.uk

34.1 Introduction

Papillomaviruses are extraordinarily successful infectious agents. The human papillomavirus (HPV) branch of the Papillomavirideae includes more than 100 of these small double-stranded DNA viruses that infect the skin and internal squamous mucosae. The majority of the HPV family members coexist comfortably with their hosts, establishing long-term residence in their epithelial locales with little disturbance. If clinically detectable HPV infections develop, they are mostly self-limiting benign proliferations, cosmetically unattractive, but rarely life-threatening, i.e., warts and low-grade intraepithelial neoplasms. Only a subset of HPVs has significant oncogenic potential and cancer is a rare outcome of infection with one of this subset. However, the common thread in HPV infections is that they induce chronic and persistent infection that remain undetected, or perhaps tolerated, by the host for long periods of time. All viruses attempt to evade host defenses and HPVs are particularly effective at this. However, eventually pathogenic HPVs are detected by the host and its defenses, the viruses are effectively contained, and the lesions regress. The details of the mechanisms by which HPV evades host defenses and how these are eventually overcome are imperfectly understood, but are central for the design of rational therapies for these agents.

34.2 Host Defense to Viral Infections

Host defense is a partnership between innate immunity (phagocytes, soluble proteins, e.g., cytokines complement and epithelial barriers) together with adaptive immunity (antibody cytotoxic effector cells). In simple

G. Gross and S.K. Tyring (eds.), *Sexually Transmitted Infections and Sexually Transmitted Diseases*,
DOI: 10.1007/978-3-642-14663-3_34,

terms, the innate immune system detects the pathogen and acts as the first line of defense clearing estimated, it is up to 90% of microbial infections alone. Innate immunity has no specific memory but crucially activates the appropriate adaptive immune response that generates both lethal effector responses of exquisite specificity for, and long-lived cells with, memory for the insult. Thus, the adaptive responses of antibody-mediated humoral immunity clear free virus particles from body fluids and can prevent reinfection. Those of cell-mediated immunity (CMI) are essential for the clearance of virus-infected cells. Innate immunity is alerted by cell injury and stress and cell death; phenomena that activate the innate sensors such as toll-like receptors (TLRs) and nucleotide oligomerization domain proteins (NODs) and manifested by inflammation. In the inflammatory process soluble and cellular innate immune effectors are recruited and local parenchymal cells such as keratinocytes and phagocytes, the latter both recruited and local, are activated to secrete pro-inflammatory cytokines and other defense molecules that in turn recruit more cytotoxic effectors to the inflammatory focus. Crucially, in this process antigen presenting cells (APC) in the periphery are activated to kick start the adaptive immune response by presenting processed antigen to naive T cells in the draining lymph node. The innate immune system, therefore, is the first line of host defense against pathogens and acquired immunity is involved in the elimination of pathogens in the late phase of infection as well as the generation of immunological memory [1]. How this marvelous defense system is activated and recruited to respond to HPV infections and how the virus ducks and weaves to avoid it is the subject of the following brief discussion.

34.3 HPVs Are Exclusively Intraepithelial Infections

The exclusively intraepithelial life cycle of HPVs is central to understanding the host response. Virus infects primitive basal keratinocytes, probably by microabrasions of the epithelial surface that leave the basal lamina intact [2]. All the subsequent events in the viral life cycle are tightly linked to the differentiation program of the keratinocyte as it progresses up through the epithelium [3]. The terminal events that result in viral genome encapsidation, viral assembly, and maturation of infectious virus occur in the most superficial differentiated cells of squamous epithelium. This intraepithelial life cycle has some key features that are important in the recognition and response of the host immune system to these viral infections. No inflammation accompanies viral infection, viral replication, viral assembly and release, and thus there is no danger signal to alert the innate immune senses. HPVs are not lytic viruses. The life cycle is played out in the keratinocyte as it progresses from the basal layer up through to the most superficial layers of the epithelium, ending up in the terminally differentiated keratinocyte, a cell destined for death from natural causes. High-level viral replication and viral assembly occur, therefore, in cells that have already undergone a regulated death program. Although HPVs appear to be able to bind to and enter cells other than keratinocytes, as far as is known, viral gene expression and viral protein synthesis in natural infections are confined to keratinocytes. There is no synthesis or expression of viral protein in antigen presenting cells (APC) such as the dendritic cells (DC) or Langerhans cells (LC) in the epithelium. Finally there is no, or very little, viremia and virus is shed from mucosal or cutaneous surfaces far from vascular and lymphatic channels. Thus there is poor access of virus and virus proteins to the draining lymph nodes where adaptive immune responses will be initiated [4].

34.4 Immune Responses to HPV

Genital HPVs fall into two groups:

- Low-risk types that cause benign self-limiting proliferations, anogenital warts, and low-grade squamous intraepithelial lesions (LGSIL). The most common viral types associated with these lesions in the genital tract are HPV 6 and HPV 11.
- High-risk HPV types are associated with the obligate precancerous lesions (high-grade squamous intraepithelial lesions (HGSIL) and adenocarcinoma in situ (AIS) of the cervix) and invasive cancer. The key players here are HPV 16 and HPV 18.

It is important to recognize that there are two distinct biologies occurring concomitantly in high-grade disease: HPV infection and neoplasia. In terms of immune responses the events in genital warts and LGSIL represent the response to HPV infection uncomplicated by the genetic instability of neoplasia. HGSIL in contrast are aneuploid, genetically unstable lesions in which both viral and host gene expression is deregulated.

34.4.1 Immune Responses in Regressing Genital Warts

The chronicity and duration of the HPV life cycle raises the question of whether there is an immune response to HPV, but evidence from a range of sources shows that, indeed, there is. Spontaneous regression is a feature of both cutaneous and anogenital warts and immunohistological analysis of this phenomenon is informative. Non-regressing genital warts are characterized by a lack of immune cells, both intraepithelial and stromal. The few intraepithelial lymphocytes present are CD8+ T cells; mononuclear cells are present mainly in the stroma. Histological examination of regressive genital warts reveals a large infiltrate into the wart stroma and epithelium, principally T cells, both CD4+ and CD8+, and macrophages [5]. The infiltrating lymphocytes express activation markers, the cytokine milieu is dominated by pro-inflammatory cytokines such as interleukin 12 (IL-12), tumor necrosis factor alpha (TNF-α), interferon gamma (IFNγ) [6] and there is upregulation of the adhesion molecules required for lymphocyte trafficking on the endothelium of the wart capillaries [7]. These appearances are characteristic of the cell-mediated Th_1 biased immune response to a viral infection (Fig. 34.1a).

34.4.2 Natural Animal Infections

Cross-sectional studies of regressing warts provide only a snapshot of what is a dynamic process occurring over a period of weeks and months. The natural history of HPV infections for both low- and high-risk HPVs is erratic, and ethical and practical considerations inhibit longitudinal studies in humans. However, in animal

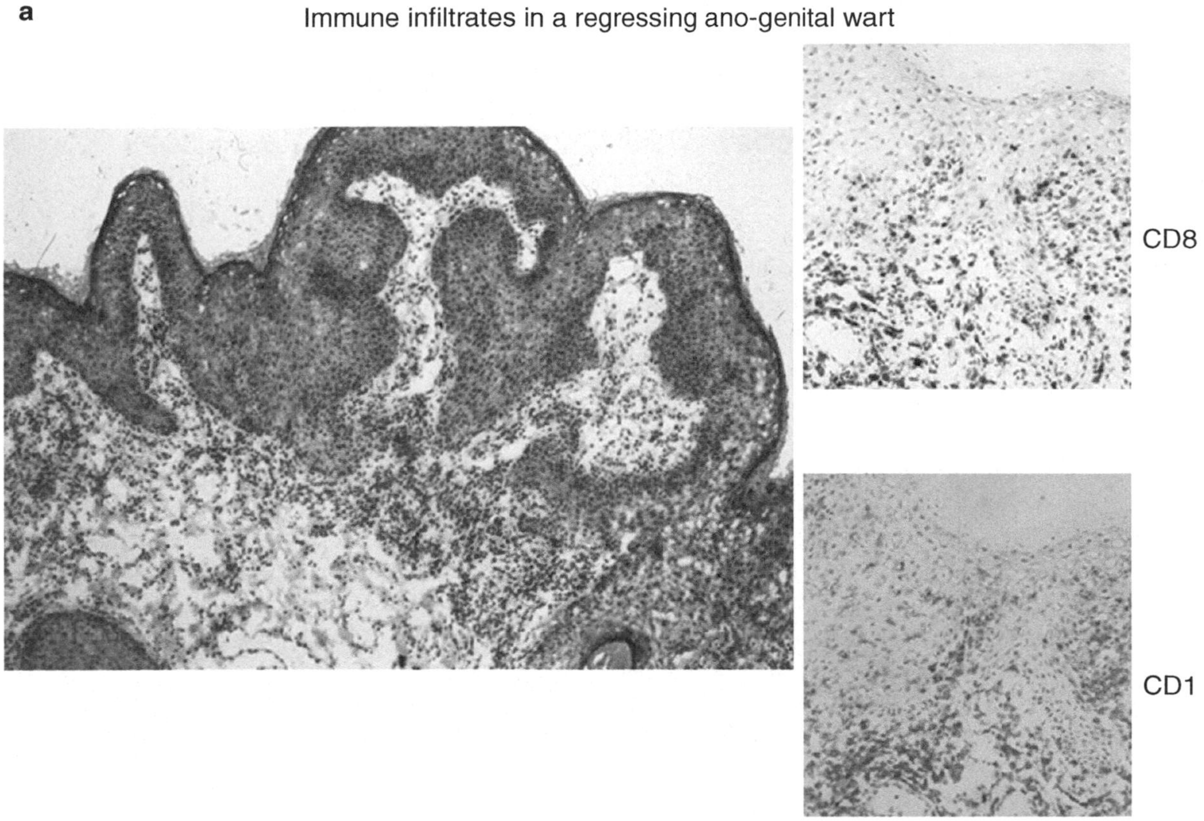

Fig. 34.1 Immune infiltrates in spontaneously regressing anogenital warts (**a**) and regressing COPV warts (**b**). In both the canine [8] and human lesions [5] the infiltrates are dominated by CD4 and CD8 T cells

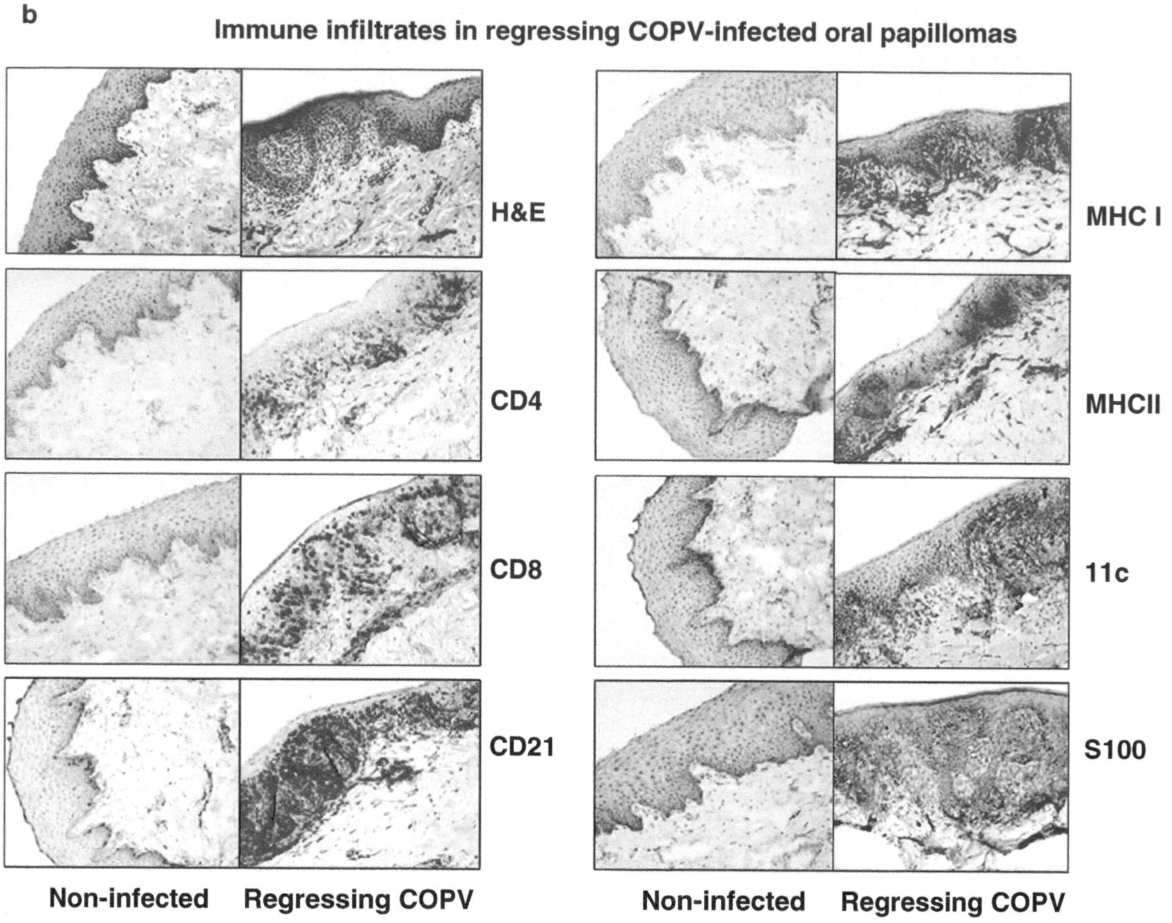

Fig. 34.1 (continued)

models of mucosal papillomavirus infection such as the canine oral papillomavirus (COPV), the immunological events of the entire wart cycle from infection to regression can be followed. COPV is a mucosal infection of dogs inducing warts in the oral cavity comparable to those seen on the human anogenital skin. In COPV infections wart regression is accompanied by an intense local cellular infiltrate (Fig. 34.1b) similar to that seen in regressing cutaneous and genital warts [8]. Despite the florid local response, systemic T-cell responses occur at low frequency; they are directed to the E2 and E6 proteins and can be detected at distinct time points during the infectious cycle [9]. These responses occur in narrow time windows that coincide with periods of viral DNA application and are maximal at the time of wart regression, thereafter declining quite rapidly. Serum-neutralizing antibody to the major capsid protein L1 can be detected at or just after wart regression (Fig. 34.2) with peak antibody concentrations at 2–3 weeks post wart regression [10]. Serum antibody concentrations even at peak are modest and slowly decline in the following weeks and months, but the animals remain resistant, even in the absence of detectable serum antibody, to challenge to the oral epithelium with large doses of infectious virus [11]. Although these animals remain resistant to challenge apparently throughout their remaining life, COPV is not cleared from the epithelium but remains in a latent state in rare cells in the basal epithelium [12]. Latency is a poorly understood aspect of papillomavirus biology but is clearly of importance for therapeutic and prophylactic intervention strategies.

34.4.3 Epidemiological and Natural History Studies

Epidemiological and natural history studies strongly suggest that the course of events in HPV infections in the genital tract in women follows a similar pattern to

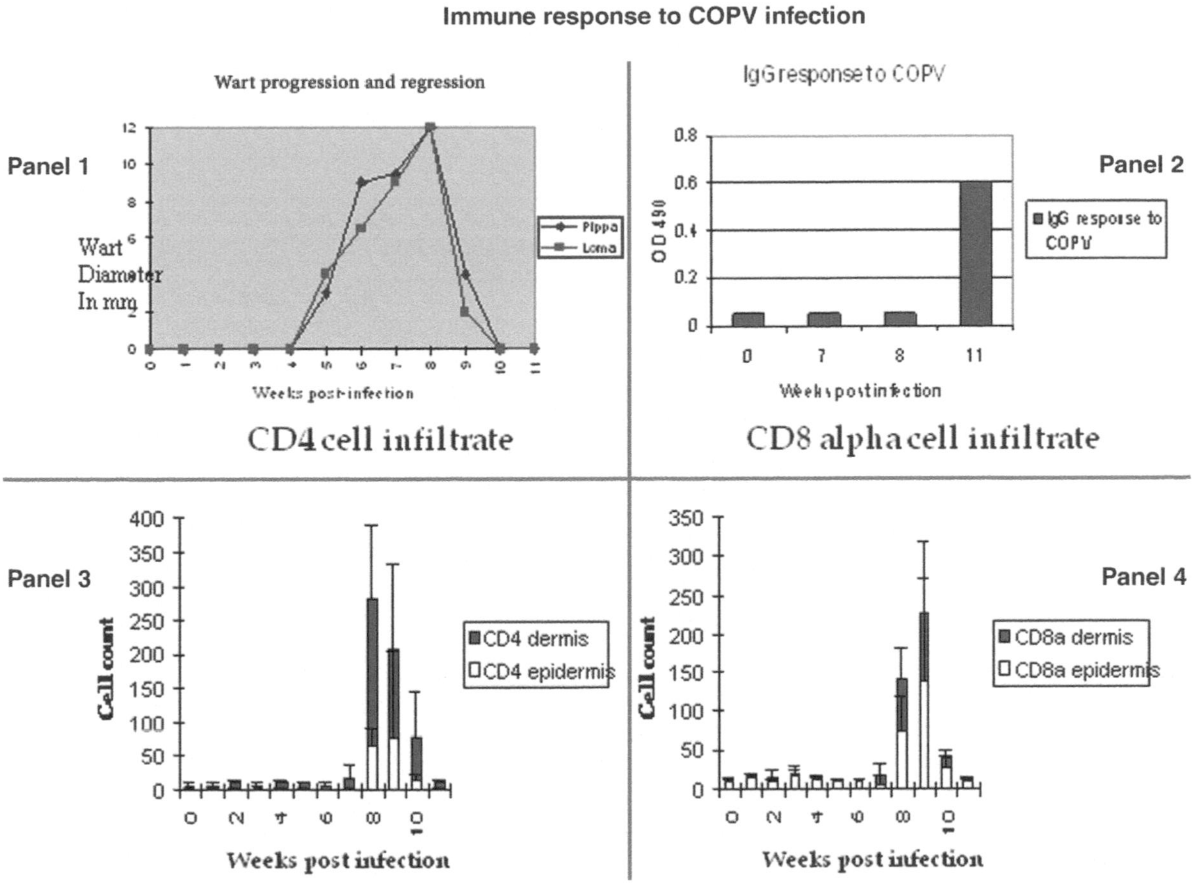

Fig. 34.2 After infection of the oral mucosa with canine oral papillomavirus, there is a lag of 4 weeks before warts can be detected. The subsequent growth and regression of these lesions is shown in *panel 1*. Antibody to L1, the major capsid protein is not detected until 11 weeks post-infection when the warts have regressed – *panel 2*. CD4 and CD8 lymphocytes infiltrate the stroma and epithelium of the warts at weeks 8–10 – *panels 3* and *4*, respectively. Maximal infiltration of CD4 cells is seen at week 8 with CD8 cell infiltrates peaking at week 9. These events coincide with wart regression [10]

that seen in animal infections [13]. Virtually all the natural history studies show that genital HPV infection as determined by detection of HPV DNA in cervico-vaginal lavages is extremely common in young, sexually active women, with a cumulative prevalence of 60–80% [14]. Most of these infections clear, i.e., DNA for that specific time HPV type can no longer be detected in the exfoliated cells. The time taken to clearance for the high-risk HPVs, particularly HPV 16, seems to be on average 8–16 months after the first detection of DNA, considerably longer than the 4–8 months reported for the low-risk HPVs [15]. However, if the immune response, in this case the cell-mediated cytotoxic response, fails to clear or control the infection, then a persistent viral infection is established (Fig. 34.3). It is this cohort of individuals with persistent infection with a high-risk HPV that has an increased probability of progression to HGSIL and, therefore, invasive cancer [13]. Those who fail to clear a low-risk HPV experience recurrence of genital warts that are usually refractory to treatment [16].

34.5 Cell-Mediated Immunity to HPV

The increased incidence and progression of HPV infections in immunosuppressed individuals illustrates the critical importance of the CD4 T-cell-regulated cell-mediated immune response in the resolution and

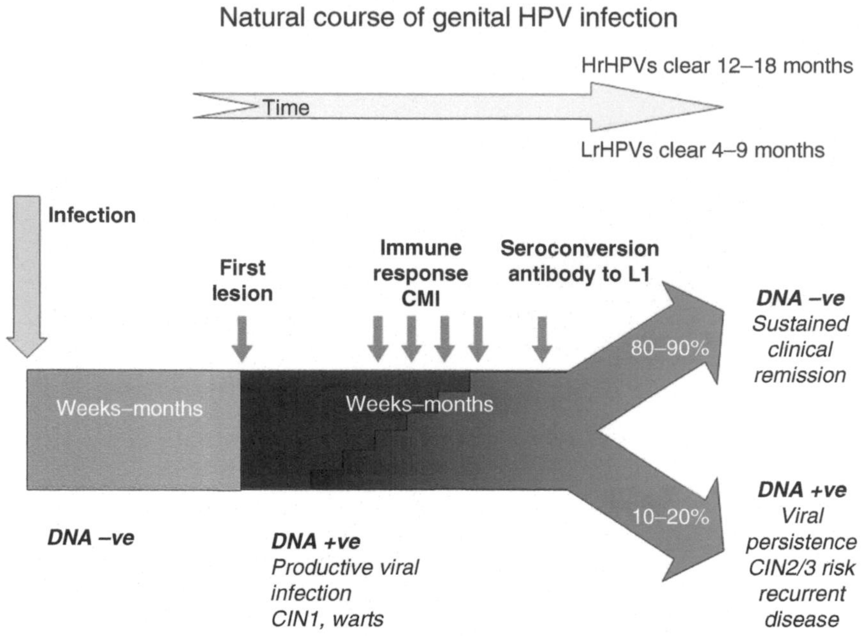

Fig. 34.3 HPV is highly infectious, with an incubation period of 3 weeks to 8 months. The majority of individuals who develop genital warts, do so about 2–3 months after infection. Spontaneous regression occurs in 10–30% of patients within 3 months [16]. This is associated with an appropriate cell-mediated immune response [5]. After regression, subclinical infection may persist for life. Evidence for this is the recurrence of HPV disease in immunocompromised patients such as those with AIDS [18–20]. Recurrence may also occur in patients with normal immune function. Infection with "high risk" HPV, such as types 16 and 18, follows the same pattern as "low risk" HPV types 6 and 11. Unfortunately, those lesions that progress and those that recur, and then progress, are associated with CIN and invasive cancers [13]

control of HPV infections [17, 18]. HIV-infected patients show multiple recurrences of cervical HPV infections [19] and an increased incidence of both cutaneous and genital warts [20] that appears to reflect an increased risk of progression from subclinical to clinical disease. Prospective studies show prolonged persistence of high-risk HPV DNA in HIV-infected 13–18-year-old girls who are otherwise healthy [21] and a high incidence of HGSIL in this group [22]. Importantly, the risk for incident HGSIL in these HIV-infected girls appears to be due primarily to the persistence of LGSIL rather than persistence of high-risk HPV DNA without a detectable lesion, implying that florid gene expression in a persistent active infectious cycle is important in progression.

34.5.1 CD4 T-Cell Responses

There is increasing evidence that as in COPV infections, CD4 T-cell responses to E2 [23] and probably E6 but not E7 [24] or L1 [25] are important for the clearance of HPV 16 and 18 infections. A nonintervention follow-up study of women with cytological evidence of LGSIL (CIN1) showed that HPV 16 E2-specific T-cell responses as measured by IL-2 release in vitro occurred frequently at the time of lesion clearance [26]. Good Th_1-type immunity against the E2 and E6 protein has been detected in healthy individuals with no clinical signs of HPV 16 infection [24]. Importantly, these Th_1-type responses were found only occasionally in patients with HGSIL (CIN2/3) and were impaired in those with invasive cervical cancer [27]. In a longitudinal study extending over 12 months of women with histologically diagnosed CIN1, E2-specific CD4 T-cell responses were detected in HPV-16-positive histological regressors but were absent in women with lesions that showed progression and were infected with HPV 16. No E2 specific responses were found in patients with high-grade CIN2/3 at the time of recruitment now published [87]. These data suggest that a hallmark of effective immune control of HPV 16 infection in the cervix is the generation of CD4+ T cells specific for E2.

34.5.2 Cytotoxic Effectors

Cell-mediated cytotoxicity is the most important effector mechanism for the control and clearance of viral infections and is implemented by a range of cells which include both antigen-specific cytotoxic T lymphocytes (CTL) and the so-called innate lymphocytes, a heterogeneous group that includes natural killer (NK) cells, gamma delta T cells (γδT), and invariant natural killer T cells (iNKT).

HPV antigen-specific CTL can be detected in patients with previous or ongoing HPV infection; both CD4+ and CD8+ cytotoxic effectors have been shown to be involved in these responses. In a longitudinal study of women with PCR-determined cervical HPV 16 infection, lack of CD8+ responses to E6 but not E7 correlated with persistent HPV infection, suggesting that an antigen-specific CTL response to HPV 16 E6 is important for viral clearance and, by implication, neoplastic progression [28]. Memory T cells specific for HPV E6 CD8 epitopes have been detected in women previously infected but currently HPV-16-negative [29]. Potential antigenic CD8+ T-cell epitopes have been identified [30] and interestingly one study has shown considerable HLA class I binding promiscuity with the same viral peptide being bound by HLA-A0201, -B48, and -B61 [31].

Natural killer cells are key components of the antiviral defenses controlling viral replication in the interval between infection and the induction of adaptive immunity [32]. They are a subset of lymphocytes activated via soluble mediators and direct cell-to-cell contact, and kill infected cells directly by cytolysis and the secretion of pro-inflammatory cytokines. There is increasing evidence that NK cells are important in the response to HPV infections. NK activation is complex and regulated via the integration of signals from a number of inhibitory and activating receptors, many of which employ MHC class I (HLA) or class-I-like proteins as their ligands. The NK receptors human killer cell immunoglobulin-like receptor (KIR) family are highly polymorphic molecules utilizing MHC 1 molecules as their ligands. It has been reported that combinations of KIR/HLA affect the risk of developing cervical neoplasia with specific pairs associated with a decreasing risk, whereas the expression of the KIR3DS1-activating receptor increases susceptibility to cervical progression [33].

Investigation of patients with anogenital warts [34] and small numbers of individuals with HPV-associated anogenital intraepithelial neoplasia [35] and verrucous carcinoma [36] has revealed poor NK cell activity. Peripheral blood mononuclear cells (PBMCs) from patients with active HPV 16 induced neoplastic disease display reduced NK cell activity against HPV 16 infected keratinocytes[36]. In vitro expression of the E7 protein of HPV 16 or 18 precludes the lysis of HPV transformed cells by interferon-activated NK cells and the HPV 16 E6 or E7 proteins inhibit IL18 expression by NK cells binding to both IL18 and its receptor [37, 38]. Long-term follow-up of patients with severe combined immunodeficiency (SCID) following hemopoietic stem cell transplantation has shown that a subset of these patients exhibits a severe cutaneous papillomatosis associated either with a common γ C receptor cytokine unit or defects in the Janus Kinase-3 (JAK3) signaling pathway. A common consequence of such signaling defects is NK cell deficiency and NK cell counts are very much lower in these patients [39]. Patients with Fanconi's Anemia have marked defects both in NK cell number and activity and a fraction of these individuals develop severe HPV infection with associated malignant change [40]. Finally, the rare inherited disorder, epidermodysplasia verruciformis in which widespread infection with cutaneous HPV types that do not normally cause warts is associated with subtle immune defects include abnormalities of NK cell activation [41].

Gamma delta T cells (γδT) are a small subset of T cell that possess a distinct T-cell receptor (TCR) comprising a gamma and delta T chain rather than an alpha and beta chain. The antigenic molecules that activate γδT cells are still largely unknown but these cells are unusual in that the γδTCR does not seem to require antigen processing and presentation of peptide epitopes via MHC, although some γδT cells recognize HLA-B molecules. Gamma deltas are believed to have a prominent role in recognition of lipid antigens and they may be important in the recognition of 'stress-related molecules on cells. They are part of the bridge between innate and adaptive immunity and play an early role in sensing danger by invading pathogens, expanding extensively in many acute infections in the early phase [42]. Large numbers of gamma delta T cells migrate into regressing papillomas induced by Bovine papillomavirus type 4 (BPV-4) [43]. In COPV infections statistically significant increases in gamma delta cells in early regressing COPV warts could not be identified [8].

NKT cells are a subset of lymphocytes that co-express cell surface markers of both the NK and T cell lineage. These cells that can be either CD4+/CD8−, CD4/CD8+, or CD4−/CD8−, express a very restricted T-cell repertoire consisting of an invariant V chain. The T-cell receptor (TCR) on NKT cells recognizes glycolipids presented by the CD1d molecule that is expressed on (amongst others) dendritic cells. On ligation of the TCR, NKT cells do have the capacity to rapidly produce large amounts of pro-inflammatory cytokines including IFN-γ and TNF-α, in addition to immunoregulatory cytokines including IL-4 and IL-10. The function of NKT cells is not well understood but there is increasing evidence to suggest a role in both the regulation and development of the adaptive immune response. There is very little information about the role of NKT cells in the response to HPV lesions. An early quantitative immunocytochemical study of large granular lymphocytes (LGLs) in the normal cervix and in HPV-associated CIN, detected an intra-epithelial lymphocyte population expressing both T cell and NK markers, i.e., CD3+, CD8+, CD56+, and CD16+ [44]. These cells were detected in CIN 3 but absent from CIN 1 and normal cervix.

34.6 Humoral Immune Responses

Numerous serological studies using HPV virus-like particles (VLPs) have shown that infection with a genital HPV is followed in most women, eventually, by seroconversion and type-specific antibody to the major viral code protein L1 [45]. Antibody to the minor viral coat protein L2 is not detectable in natural infections in animals or humans. Seroconversion most frequently occurs between 6 and 18 months after the first detection of HPV DNA in subjects who have a persistent genital HPV infection, i.e., the detection of HPV DNA of the same type on two occasions at least 6 months apart [46, 47] and very rarely in subjects with incident HPV infection, i.e., detection of HPV DNA on only one occasion [48]. However, as in animal infections, antibody concentrations are low, even at the time of seroconversion. Furthermore, not all HPV-infected subjects seroconvert and 20–50% of women with HPV DNA or who have had detectable persistent HPV DNA infections do not have detectable type-specific anti-HPV antibodies [46, 47, 49] but it must be recognized that the serological assays used in these studies are relatively insensitive. This modest humoral response is not surprising since there is no blood-borne phase of infection or viremia and with this exclusively intraepithelial infection, free virus particles are shed from the surface of squamous epithelia. Virus has poor access to vascular and lymphatic channels and therefore to lymph nodes where humoral and cell-mediated immune responses would be initiated. Nonetheless, in seropositive women, anti-HPV L1 antibodies persist for many years and 10 years post the first detection of HPV DNA approximately 20–25% of women who seroconverted remain antibody-positive [50].

A controversial issue is whether these low levels of anti-L1 antibody protect against reinfection with the same HPV type [51]. This question is not easy to address. In animal infections with COPV [52], CRPV [53], and BPV [54] after lesion regression the virus remains in a latent state in a few basal keratinocytes. The repeated recurrences in recurrent respiratory papillomatosis are considered to be reactivation of latent virus rather than reinfection and latent virus can be detected in the trachea and larynx of many subjects [55, 56]. The evidence is accumulating, with recent data from the large randomized clinical trials for the prophylactic HPV vaccines that a similar situation exists for HPV in the genital tract [57]. The detection of HPV DNA of the same type in a seropositive individual after apparent clearance may therefore reflect reactivation of latent virus rather than reinfection. Only if the (new) HPV DNA can be shown to be distinct in sequence from the HPV DNA originally detected can reinfection rather than reactivation be proven.

34.7 Immune-Evasion Mechanisms for HPV

HPV infection is clearly ignored and undetected by the immune system for extended periods of time and the mechanisms that underlie this remain a central question. HPV infections are exclusively intraepithelial and

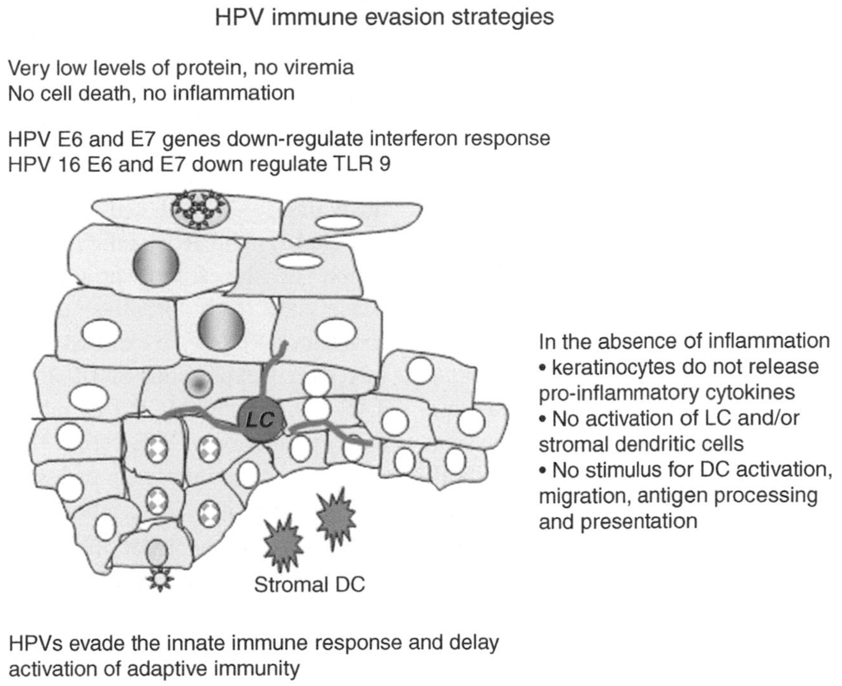

HPV immune evasion strategies
Very low levels of protein, no viremia
No cell death, no inflammation
HPV E6 and E7 genes down-regulate interferon response
HPV 16 E6 and E7 down regulate TLR 9
LC
Stromal DC
In the absence of inflammation
• keratinocytes do not release pro-inflammatory cytokines
• No activation of LC and/or stromal dendritic cells
• No stimulus for DC activation, migration, antigen processing and presentation
HPVs evade the innate immune response and delay activation of adaptive immunity

Fig. 34.4 HPV infections are not lytic infections; the cell in which virus particles are assembled and released is a terminally differentiated squame undergoing cell death as part of the normal process. There is therefore no danger signal to the immune system and no inflammation. HPV downregulates interferon responses and disables a key antiviral defense. HPV early genes also downregulate at least one of the intracellular stress and injury sensors, TLR9 receptors. HPV evades the innate immune response and delays the activation of adaptive immunity [4]

theoretically HPV attack should be detected by the professional antigen-presenting cell of squamous epithelia, the Langerhans cell (LC). The activated LC should then migrate to the draining lymph node, processing HPV antigens on route, present antigen in the context of MHC to naive T cells in the node that would then differentiate into armed effector cells, migrate back to the infected site, and destroy the infected keratinocytes (Fig. 34.4).

This cycle is certainly deflected in a number of ways. The infectious cycle of HPV is in itself an immune-evasion mechanism inhibiting detection by the host defenses of virus. HPV replication and release does not cause cell death. The differentiating keratinocyte is already programmed to die and this "death by natural causes" does not act as a danger signal in the infected site. Thus for most of the duration of the HPV infectious cycle, there is little or no release into the local milieu of pro-inflammatory cytokines, important for antigen-presenting cell or dendritic cell, activation, and migration and the central signals to kick start the immune response are absent. There is no viremia, no blood-borne phase of the HPV life cycle and only minimal amounts of replicating virus are exposed to immune defenses. In effect, the virus is practically invisible to the host, a viral strategy that results in persistent chronic infections as the host remains ignorant of its presence for long periods.

Virus capsid entry is usually an activating signal for dendritic cells, but there is evidence that Langerhans cells are not activated by the uptake of HPV capsids. LC, when incubated with L1 virus-like particles (VLPs) of HPV 16 does not initiate epitope-specific immune responses against L1-derived antigens [58]. In contrast, stromal dendritic cells are activated by VLPs and stimulate HPV-specific T cells [59, 60]. Studies in TLR4 (toll-like receptor 4)-deficient mice suggest that TLR4 contributes to the recognition of HPV 16 VLPs by stromal DCs but not for Langerhans cells [61, 62].

34.7.1 Inhibition of the Interferon Response

For most of the duration of the HPV infectious cycle there is little or no release into the local milieu of pro-inflammatory cytokines, important for dendritic cell activation and migration and the essential signals to kick start the immune response in the epithelium are absent. However, even in the absence of viral-induced cytolysis and death, HPV-infected keratinocytes should release stress activated cytokines, the most important of which would be the type 1 interferons which represent a powerful generic antiviral defense system. Interferon alpha (IFN-α) and interferon beta (IFN-β), the type 1 interferons, have antiviral, anti-proliferative, anti-angiogenic, and immunostimulatory properties acting as a bridge between innate and adaptive immunity and activating immature dendritic cells [63]. It has in fact been known for more than 40 years that nucleic acids are strong inducers of type 1 interferons and most viruses, both RNA and DNA, have mechanisms for inhibiting interferon induction and signaling; the papillomaviruses are no exception reviewed in [64]. Toll-like receptor 9 has been identified as the pattern recognition receptor for unmethylated CpG oligonucleotides. Unmethylated CpG sequences occur in HPV DNA and keratinocytes infected with recombinant retroviruses expressing HPV 16 E7 inhibit TLR9 transcription [65]. Interestingly, this inhibition was not observed with the low-risk virus HPV 6 and was less efficient with HPV 18. The latter is a less persistent virus than HPV 16.

However, there is evidence that double-stranded (ds) but not single-stranded (ss) DNA can induce production of type 1 interferons in a range of cells including epithelial cells, without need for specific unmethylated CpG motifs, activating signaling pathways independently of TLR9 [66]. It is now becoming clear that several distinct molecules are involved in immune recognition of microbial or viral DNA inside the cell and a key research question is how HPV evades these intracellular surveillance systems, inhibiting the release of the activating pro-inflammatory cytokines.

HPV infection also deregulates interferon signaling; high-risk HPV infection downregulates IFN-α-induced gene expression and the HPV 16 E6 and E7 oncoproteins directly interact with components of the interferon signaling pathways. Thus E7 inhibits IFN-α-mediated signal transduction by binding to P48/IRF9 preventing translocation to the nucleus thereby inhibiting the formation of the ISG3 transcription complex that binds ISRE (interferon-specific response element) in the nucleus [67]. E7 interferes with immediate interferon-mediated signals also by physically associating with IRF1-inhibiting IRF1-mediated activation of the IFN-β promoter recruiting histone deacetylase to the promoter thereby preventing transcription [68]. In vivo expression of HPV 18 E7 results in reduced expression of IRF1 target genes such as TAP-1 IFN-β and MCP-1 by inhibition of the transactivating function of IRF-1 [69]. The E6 protein of HPV also targets the interferon pathway. E6 binds to IRF3 and inhibits its transcriptional activation function, thereby preventing transcription of IFN-α mRNA [70]. E6 binds to TYK2 preventing binding to the cytoplasmic portion of the IFN receptor inhibiting phosphorylation of TYK-2 STAT-1/STAT-2 impairing JAK STAT activation and therefore inhibiting specifically IFN-α-mediated signaling [71]. DNA microarray analysis of gene expression shows that HPV 16 alters expression of three groups of genes – interferon response genes, NF κ B stimulated genes, and cell cycle regulation genes ([72] and references therein). E6 decreases expression of IFN-α and IFN-β, downregulates nuclear STAT-1 protein and decreases binding in STAT1 to the ISRE. E6 and E7 therefore directly alter expression of genes that enable host resistance to infection and both innate and adaptive immune function.

34.8 Immune Responses in High-Grade Disease

One can conclude that HPV very efficiently evades the innate immune response (Fig. 34.4), delaying the activation of the adaptive immune response, but eventually the defenses are activated, the infection is controlled, and immune memory to that specific HPV type is established. There are risks to the host of such a strategy since host DCs are exposed to low levels of viral proteins in a noninflammatory milieu for a protracted time period and local immune nonresponsiveness to these antigens may be established in the infected mucosa. In this milieu that is operationally tolerant to HPV antigens such as E6 or E7 or E2, host defenses could become irrevocably compromised. HPV antigen-specific effector cells may either not be recruited to the infected focus or their activity could be downregulated or both. Thus, if during a persistent high-risk HPV infection there was deregulation of E6 and E7 with the consequent increased protein expression in dividing cells, this might not result in an armed effector CMI response and the progression to high-grade disease and invasive carcinoma would not be impeded. There is accumulating evidence that this is indeed the scenario in progressive high-risk HPV infection of the cervix. There are two biological processes in such an infected epithelium, HPV infection and neoplasia. The local immune environment in low-grade and high-grade lesions would be influenced by the events of neoplastic progression. Low-grade SIL (CIN1) reflect in the main HPV infection in contrast to HGSIL (CIN2/3) that are neoplastic, aneuploid, genetically unstable, exhibiting heterogeneity in the expression of immunological relevant molecules. In low-grade disease the virus is present as episome, there is a complete infectious cycle, and viral gene expression is tightly regulated particularly expression of the oncoproteins E6 and E7 in dividing cells. High-grade lesions, CIN2/3, do not support a complete viral infectious cycle. Late gene expression is either lost or significantly reduced, viral DNA sequences may be integrated into the host genome, and overexpression of the E6 and E7 oncogenes occurs. Immunohistochemical studies of low-grade cervical disease suggests overall that these lesions are immunologically quiescent with few infiltrating T cells and a decreased number of Langerhans cells compared to normal cervical ectocervical epithelium [5]. A decreased number of LC are also seen at HGSIL but this phenomenon may be related to neoplasia since there is in vitro evidence that immortalized HPV-infected cervical cells actually inhibit LC recruitment [73]. In addition overexpression of HPV 16 E6 in keratinocytes inhibits the expression of E cadherin, a molecule that mediates Langerhans cell keratinocyte adhesion, and this could reduce LC retention in squamous epithelia [74]. Immature stromal dendritic cells that express the immunosuppressive cytokines IL10 and TGF-β have been shown to be resident throughout the normal cervical stroma but increased in a high-grade disease [75]. These DC have been implicated in inducing immunotolerance and their increased density in the stroma of high-grade lesions would support the notion that the immune milieu in these lesions is immunosuppressive or immunoregulatory.

Paradoxically, strong pro- and anti-inflammatory responses can be detected in a high-grade disease. In particular, a robust Th_1 response with abundant expression of interferon gamma by both CD4+, CD8+, and natural killer cells exist, but despite this the HPV-infected lesion persists. The evidence is that progression of HPV-infected cervical neoplasia is accompanied by an increasingly immunosuppressive environment with recruitment and dominance of regulatory T cells [76] and a cytokine milieu in which IL-10 and TGF-β dominate. At the same time, responses to the pro-inflammatory antiviral cytokines such as TNF-α, IFN-α, and IFN-β are lost and the key immune defenses that would induce apoptosis and death of the infected neoplastic cell are lost.

34.9 Prophylactic HPV Vaccines

It might well have been thought that since the antibody response to natural infections was so modest that vaccines generating serum-neutralizing antibody to the major capsid protein L1 would not be very effective. However, some of the very earliest experimental work from Shope in rabbits using the cottontail rabbit papillomavirus (CRPV) showed very clearly that neutralizing antibodies were protective. In these experiments, if rabbits were infected systemically with CRPV by direct injection of virus into the muscle or blood stream, papillomas did not arise on the skin of the challenged animals but serum-neutralizing antibodies were generated. The immunized animals were completely resistant to viral challenge by abrasion of the epithelium, the route of infection that would normally generate papillomas [77]. This and other subsequent data suggested very strongly that generating neutralizing antibodies to the virus coat proteins would be an effective prophylactic vaccine strategy and this, of course, has proven to be so.

Two HPV L1 VLP vaccines have been developed by major pharmaceutical companies: Cervarix, a bivalent HPV 16/18 VLP vaccine from GSK, and Gardasil, also known as Silgard, a quadrivalent HPV 16/18 6/11 vaccine from Merck vaccines. These products are delivered in a three-dose immunization schedule lasting over 6 months and induce, at their peak after the third immunization, high concentrations of neutralizing antibodies to L1. Virtually all subjects in the vaccine trials have seroconverted and no vaccine breakthroughs have been demonstrated to date. As in the original Shope experiments these vaccines are delivered intramuscularly; this results in rapid access of antigen to the local lymph nodes and thus circumvents the immune avoidance strategies of the viral intraepithelial infectious cycle. Furthermore, HPV L1 VLPs are highly antigenic, inducing potent antibody responses in the absence of adjuvant due to their ability to activate both innate and adaptive immune responses. VLPs are rapidly bound by myeloid dendritic cells and B cells and signal via the toll-like receptor dependent pathway MyD88 [61, 62]. The activation of this pathway is essential for B-cell activation and antibody generation in mice and probably also in humans.

These vaccines have been shown to be highly efficacious in large phase III randomized control trials achieving, over a 4-year period, at least 98% protection against HPV 16/18-caused high-grade cervical intraepithelial disease and adenocarcinoma in situ in 15–26-year-old women, naive for these virus types at entry to the trials reviewed in [78]. Currently, the best assumption is that the mechanism of protection elicited by VLP immunization is the generation of neutralizing antibody. The mostly unequivocal evidence for this notion comes from experiments in rabbits and dogs in which it was shown that naive animals passively immunized with purified serum IgG from VLP-immunized animals were completely protected against high viral challenge [79, 80]. Interestingly, dogs immunized with purified serum IgG from naturally infected but recovered animals were also completely protected against high viral challenge, suggesting that the low antibody levels acquired in natural infection are also protective [81].

The mechanism by which neutralizing antibodies to HPV L1 protein prevent viral entry is speculative at present. However, new data on HPV infection suggest different stages at which neutralizing antibodies could be effective. Recent studies have shown that HPV infection requires a micro-abrasion of the squamous epithelium that results in epithelial denudation but retention of the epithelial basal lamina [2]. HPV initially binds by a primary receptor to the exposed basal lamina before entering the keratinocyte, presumably as the keratinocyte migrates along the basement membrane to repair the small wound. This appears to be a protracted process extending up to 24 and possibly 48 h, during which the virus capsid undergoes conformational changes that expose the secondary receptor by which the virus binds to and enters the keratinocyte [82]. Virus-neutralizing antibodies could therefore act by binding to the receptors or by binding to the capsid and preventing the conformational distortion essential for successful viral entry. Probably both types of antibodies are generated after VLP immunization, but in general higher concentrations blocking antibodies (anti-receptors) are needed for neutralization compared with those preventing conformational change. This is of interest since it implies that relatively low concentrations of the latter would be needed for protection and is consistent from the observations from the animal papillomavirus studies. For example, in the dog and the rabbit, low concentrations of anti-L1 antibodies provide long-term protection against high doses of challenge virus [11].

Immune memory has been shown to be generated to these vaccines. The quadrivalent vaccine has shown an impressive recall response to antigen challenge [83], the functional readout from memory 5 years post-immunization and circulating B memory cells can be detected 1 month after third and final immunization with the bivalent vaccine [84]. Furthermore, the persistence of antibody levels in excess of that found in natural infection strongly suggests both robust B and T memory cell induction. Immune memory is fundamental to successful immunization and the observations of persistence of antibody and robust recall from the VLPs in the RCTs leads to optimism that duration of protection might be measured in decades as, for example, has been shown for hepatitis B subunit vaccines [85].

34.10 Cross-Protection

In natural infections the detectable neutralizing antibody responses are type-specific but the HPV L1 vaccines generate not only type-specific, but cross-reactive and cross-neutralizing antibodies. Both commercial prophylactic vaccines have now shown some evidence of cross-protection, or protection against non-vaccine types reviewed in [78]. The high antibody concentrations generated by the vaccines probably explain this phenomenon. In general, the population of antibodies produced in response to a particular antigenic stimulus such as a protein VLP is heterogeneous. Protein antigens are structurally complex containing many different epitopes and the immune system responds to the antigen by producing antibodies to most of the accessible epitopes. Thus, in any response to a specific protein there will be several populations of antibodies, the overall antibody response therefore is polyclonal or heterogeneous and it comprises the output of all the individual stimulated B cells. Epitopes recognized by B cells are usually conformational and these B-cell epitopes are only displayed by proteins folded in the native or tertiary structure. Complex proteins such as L1 contain multiple overlapping epitopes, some of which are immunodominant, i.e., they produce a more profound and stronger response in the host than other epitopes and therefore dominate the polyclonal response. This can be seen quite clearly in the antibody response to HPV L1 VLPs, the immunodominant antibodies are type-specific antibodies, but there are subpopulations of antibodies, some of which will lead to epitopes shared by other HPV types. In natural infections, the antibody concentrations generated are low so that only the immunodominant species is detected, but in VLP immunized individuals antibody concentrations at least at peak are high, and the subpopulations with cross-reactive and cross-neutralizing antibodies can therefore be detected in serological assays. These subpopulations, however, are present at antibody concentrations one to two logs lower than the dominant type-specific response [86]. Not every individual will generate cross-neutralizing antibodies since immunodominance is a complex phenomenon and the MHC haplotype of the individual may play a part.

34.11 Summary

HPV infection in the genital tract is common in young, sexually active individuals, most of whom clear the infection without overt clinical disease. However, most of those who develop lesions eventually mount an effective cell-mediated immune response with lesion regression. Regression of anogenital warts is accompanied histologically by a CD4+ T-cell-dominated Th_1-biased response. Animal models support this and provide evidence that the response is modulated by CD4+ T-cell-dependent mechanisms, although the effectors important in lesion clearance are still not known. Emerging evidence implicates both conventional and unconventional cytotoxic T cells in these responses. Failure to develop an effective cell-mediated immune response and to clear or control the infection results in a persistent viral infection and, in the case of the high-risk HPVs, a very much increased probability of progression to CIN3 and the risk then of further progression to invasive carcinoma. The central importance of the CD4+ T-cell population in the control of HPV infection is shown by the increased prevalence of HPV infection and the high-grade lesions they induce in individuals immunosuppressed as a consequence of HIV infection. The prolonged duration of infection associated with HPV appears to be associated with an effective evasion of innate immunity as reflected in the absence of inflammation during virus replication assembly and release with the downregulation of secretion of pro-inflammatory cytokines, particularly type 1 interferons and thus delaying the activation of adaptive immunity. Serum-neutralizing antibody to the major capsid protein L1 usually develops after the induction of successful cell-mediated immunity and these antibody and cell-mediated responses are protective against subsequent viral challenge in natural infections in animals. Prophylactic vaccines consisting of HPV L1 VLPs generate high anti-L1 serum-neutralizing antibody concentrations and clinical trials have shown a remarkable efficacy against both benign and neoplastic-associated disease caused by the vaccine HPV types. These vaccines are delivered intramuscularly and therefore circumvent the immune-evasion strategies of the virus.

Take-Home Pearls

- Regression of HPV caused lesions is mediated by Th1 dominated cell mediated immune responses
- The cellular effectors in this are not known unequivocally by both conventional and unconventional cytotoxic T cells are implicated
- Failure to develop an effective cell mediated immune response and to clear or control the infection results in a persistent viral infection and,

in the case of the high risk HPVs, a very much increased probability of progression to CIN3

- The prolonged duration of infection associated with HPV associated with an effective evasion of innate immunity due to absence of inflammation during virus replication assembly and release together with downregulation of secretion of pro-inflammatory cytokines, particularly type 1 inteferons
- Serum neutralising antibody to the major capsid protein L1 usually develops after the induction of successful cell mediated immunity
- Both antibody and cell mediated responses are protective against subsequent viral challenge in natural infections in animals
- Prophylactic HPV L1 vaccines are delivered intramuscularly and evade HPV immune evasion strategies

References

1. Medzhitov, R., Janeway Jr., C.A.: Decoding the patterns of self and nonself by the innate immune system. Science **296**, 298–300 (2002)
2. Roberts, J.N., Buck, C.B., Thompson, C.D., et al.: Genital transmission of HPV in a mouse model is potentiated by nonoxynol-9 and inhibited by carrageenan. Nat. Med. **13**, 857–861 (2007)
3. Doorbar, J.: The papillomavirus life cycle. J. Clin. Virol. **32**(suppl 1), S7–S15 (2005)
4. Stanley, M.: Immune responses to human papillomavirus. Vaccine **24**(suppl 1), S16–S22 (2006)
5. Coleman, N., Birley, H.D., Renton, A.M., et al.: Immunological events in regressing genital warts. Am. J. Clin. Pathol. **102**, 768–774 (1994)
6. Stanley, M.A., Scarpini, C., Coleman, N.: Cell mediated immunity and lower genital tract neoplasia. In: McLean, A.B., Singer, A., Critchley, H. (eds.) Lower Genital Tract Neoplasia. RCOG Press, London (2003)
7. Coleman, N., Stanley, M.A.: Characterization and functional analysis of the expression of vascular adhesion molecules in human papillomavirus related disease of the cervix. Cancer **74**, 884–892 (1994)
8. Nicholls, P.K., Moore, P.F., Anderson, D.M., et al.: Regression of canine oral papillomas is associated with infiltration of CD4+ and CD8+ lymphocytes. Virology **283**, 31–39 (2001)
9. Jain, S., Moore, R.A., Anderson, D.M., et al.: Cell-mediated immune responses to COPV early proteins. Virology **356**, 23–34 (2006)
10. Nicholls, P.K., Klaunberg, B.A., Moore, R.A., et al.: Naturally occurring, nonregressing canine oral papillomavirus infection: host immunity, virus characterization, and experimental infection. Virology **265**, 365–374 (1999)
11. Stanley, M.A., Moore, R.A., Nicholls, P.K., et al.: Intraepithelial vaccination with COPV L1 DNA by particle-mediated DNA delivery protects against mucosal challenge with infectious COPV in beagle dogs. Vaccine **19**, 2783–2792 (2001)
12. Moore, R.A., Nicholls, P.K., Santos, E.B., et al.: COPV DNA absence following prophylactic L1 PMID vaccination. J. Gen. Virol. **83**, 2299–2301 (2002)
13. Moscicki, A.B., Schiffman, M., Kjaer, S., et al.: Chapter 5: Updating the natural history of HPV and anogenital cancer. Vaccine **24**(suppl 3), S42–S51 (2006)
14. Burchell, A.N., Winer, R.L., de Sanjose, S., et al.: Chapter 6: Epidemiology and transmission dynamics of genital HPV infection. Vaccine **24**(suppl 3), S52–S61 (2006)
15. Trottier, H., Franco, E.L.: The epidemiology of genital human papillomavirus infection. Vaccine **24**(suppl 1), S1–S15 (2006)
16. Lacey, C.J., Lowndes, C.M., Shah, K.V.: Chapter 4: Burden and management of non-cancerous HPV-related conditions: HPV-6/11 disease. Vaccine **24**(suppl 3), S35–S41 (2006)
17. Purdie, K.J., Surentheran, T., Sterling, J.C., et al.: Human papillomavirus gene expression in cutaneous squamous cell carcinomas from immunosuppressed and immunocompetent individuals. J. Invest. Dermatol. **125**, 98–107 (2005)
18. Palefsky, J.M., Gillison, M.L., Strickler, H.D.: Chapter 16: HPV vaccines in immunocompromised women and men. Vaccine **24**(suppl 3), S140–S146 (2006)
19. Fruchter, R.G., Maiman, M., Sedlis, A., et al.: Multiple recurrences of cervical intraepithelial neoplasia in women with the human immunodeficiency virus. Obstet. Gynecol. **87**, 338–344 (1996)
20. Fennema, J.S.A., Van Ameijden, E.J.C., Coutinho, R.A., et al.: HIV, sexually transmitted diseases and gynaecologic disorders in women: Increased risk for genital herpes and warts among HIV-infected prostitutes in Amsterdam. AIDS **9**, 1071–1078 (1995)
21. Moscicki, A.B., Ellenberg, J.H., Farhat, S., et al.: Persistence of human papillomavirus infection in HIV-infected and -uninfected adolescent girls: risk factors and differences, by phylogenetic type. J. Infect. Dis. **190**, 37–45 (2004)
22. Moscicki, A.B., Ellenberg, J.H., Crowley-Nowick, P., et al.: Risk of high-grade squamous intraepithelial lesion in HIV-infected adolescents. J. Infect. Dis. **190**, 1413–1421 (2004)
23. de Jong, A., van der Burg, S.H., Kwappenberg, K.M., et al.: Frequent detection of human papillomavirus 16 E2-specific T-helper immunity in healthy subjects. Cancer Res. **62**, 472–479 (2002)
24. Welters, M.J., de Jong, A., van den Eeden, S.J., et al.: Frequent display of human papillomavirus type 16 E6-specific memory t-Helper cells in the healthy population as witness of previous viral encounter. Cancer Res. **63**, 636–641 (2003)
25. van Poelgeest, M.I., Nijhuis, E.R., Kwappenberg, K.M., et al.: Distinct regulation and impact of type 1 T-cell immunity against HPV16 L1, E2 and E6 antigens during HPV16-induced cervical infection and neoplasia. Int. J. Cancer **118**, 675–683 (2006)

26. Bontkes, H.J., de Gruijl, T.D., Bijl, A., et al.: Human papillomavirus type 16 E2-specific T-helper lymphocyte responses in patients with cervical intraepithelial neoplasia. J. Gen. Virol. **80**, 2453–2459 (1999)
27. Welters, M.J.P., van der Logt, P., van den Eeden, S.J.F., et al.: Detection of human papillomavirus type 18 E6 and E7-specific CD4+ T-helper 1 immunity in relation to health versus disease. Int. J. Cancer **118**, 950–956 (2006)
28. Nakagawa, M., Stites, D.P., Patel, S., et al.: Persistence of human papillomavirus type 16 infection is associated with lack of cytotoxic T lymphocyte response to the E6 antigens. J. Infect. Dis. **182**, 595–598 (2000)
29. Wang, X., Moscicki, A.B., Tsang, L., et al.: Memory T-cells specific for novel HPV 16 E6 epitopes in women whose HPV 16 infection has become undetectable. Clin. Vaccine Immunol. **15**, 937–945 (2008)
30. Nakagawa, M., Kim, K.H., Moscicki, A.B.: Patterns of CD8 T-cell epitopes within the human papillomavirus type 16 (HPV 16) E6 protein among young women whose HPV 16 infection has become undetectable. Clin. Diagn. Lab. Immunol. **12**, 1003–1005 (2005)
31. Nakagawa, M., Kim, K.H., Gillam, T.M., et al.: HLA class I binding promiscuity of the CD8 T-cell epitopes of human papillomavirus type 16 E6 protein. J. Virol. **81**, 1412–1423 (2007)
32. Moretta, L., Moretta, A.: Unravelling natural killer cell function: triggering and inhibitory human NK receptors. EMBO J. **23**, 255–259 (2004)
33. Carrington, M., Wang, S., Martin, M.P., et al.: Hierarchy of resistance to cervical neoplasia mediated by combinations of killer immunoglobulin-like receptor and human leukocyte antigen loci. J. Exp. Med. **201**, 1069–1075 (2005)
34. Cauda, R., Tyring, S.K., Grossi, C.E., et al.: Patients with condyloma acuminatum exhibit decreased interleukin-2 and interferon gamma production and depressed natural killer activity. J. Clin. Immunol. **7**, 304–311 (1987)
35. Malejczyk, J., Majewski, S., Jablonska, S., et al.: Abrogated NK-cell lysis of human papillomavirus (HPV)-16-bearing keratinocytes in patients with pre-cancerous and cancerous HPV-induced anogenital lesions. Int. J. Cancer **43**, 209–214 (1989)
36. Malejczyk, J., Malejczyk, M., Majewski, S., et al.: NK cell activity in patients with HPV16 associated anogenital tumors: defective recognition of HPV16 harboring keratinocytes and restricted unresponsiveness to immunostimulatory cytokines. Int. J. Cancer **54**, 917–921 (1993)
37. Lee, S.J., Cho, Y.S., Cho, M.C., et al.: Both E6 and E7 oncoproteins of human papillomavirus 16 inhibit IL-18-induced IFN-gamma production in human peripheral blood mononuclear and NK cells. J. Immunol. **167**, 497–504 (2001)
38. Cho, Y.S., Kang, J.W., Cho, M., et al.: Down modulation of IL-18 expression by human papillomavirus type 16 E6 oncogene via binding to IL-18. FEBS Lett. **501**, 139–145 (2001)
39. Laffort, C., Le Deist, F., Favre, M., et al.: Severe cutaneous papillomavirus disease after haemopoietic stem-cell transplantation in patients with severe combined immune deficiency caused by common gammac cytokine receptor subunit or JAK-3 deficiency. Lancet **363**, 2051–2054 (2004)
40. Lebbe, C., Rybojad, M., Ochonisky, S., et al.: Extensive human papillomavirus-related disease (bowenoid papulosis, Bowen's disease, and squamous cell carcinoma) in a patient with hairy cell leukemia: clinical and immunologic evaluation after an interferon alfa trial. J. Am. Acad. Dermatol. **29**, 644–646 (1993)
41. Majewski, S., Malejczyk, J., Jablonska, S., et al.: Natural cell-mediated cytotoxicity against various target cells in patients with epidermodysplasia verruciformis. J. Am. Acad. Dermatol. **22**, 423–427 (1990)
42. Pennington, D.J., Vermijlen, D., Wise, E.L., et al.: The integration of conventional and unconventional T cells that characterizes cell-mediated responses. Adv. Immunol. **87**, 27–59 (2005)
43. Knowles, G., O'Neil, B.W., Campo, M.S.: Phenotypical characterization of lymphocytes infiltrating regressing papillomas. J. Virol. **70**, 8451–8458 (1996)
44. McKenzie, J., King, A., Hare, J., et al.: Immunocytochemical characterization of large granular lymphocytes in normal cervix and HPV associated disease. J. Pathol. **165**, 75–80 (1991)
45. Dillner, J.: The serological response to papillomaviruses. Semin. Cancer Biol. **9**, 423–430 (1999)
46. Carter, J.J., Koutsky, L.A., Wipf, G.C., et al.: The natural history of human papillomavirus type 16 capsid antibodies among a cohort of university women. J. Infect. Dis. **174**, 927–936 (1996)
47. Carter, J.J., Wipf, G.C., Hagensee, M.E., et al.: Use of human papillomavirus type 6 capsids to detect antibodies in people with genital warts. J. Infect. Dis. **172**, 11–18 (1995)
48. Wideroff, L., Schiffman, M.H., Nonnenmacher, B., et al.: Evaluation of seroreactivity to human papillomavirus type 16 virus-like particles in an incident case-control study of cervical neoplasia. J. Infect. Dis. **172**, 1425–1430 (1995)
49. Kirnbauer, R., Hubbert, N.L., Wheeler, C.M., et al.: A virus-like particle enzyme-linked immunosorbent assay detects serum antibodies in a majority of women infected with human papillomavirus type 16. J. Natl. Cancer Inst. **86**, 494–499 (1994)
50. af Geijersstam, V., Eklund, C., Wang, Z., et al.: A survey of seroprevalence of human papillomavirus types 16, 18 and 33 among children. Int. J. Cancer **80**, 489–493 (1999)
51. Viscidi, R.P., Schiffman, M., Hildesheim, A., et al.: Seroreactivity to human papillomavirus (HPV) types 16, 18, or 31 and risk of subsequent HPV infection: results from a population-based study in Costa Rica. Cancer Epidemiol. Biomarkers Prev. **13**, 324–327 (2004)
52. Moore, R.A., Nicholls, P.K., Santos, E.B., et al.: Absence of canine oral papillomavirus DNA following prophylactic L1 particle-mediated immunotherapeutic delivery vaccination. J. Gen. Virol. **83**, 2299–2301 (2002)
53. Amella, C.A., Lofgren, L.A., Ronn, A.M., et al.: Latent infection induced with cottontail rabbit papillomavirus. A model for human papillomavirus latency. Am. J. Pathol. **144**, 1167–1171 (1994)
54. Campo, M.S., Jarrett, W.F., O'Neil, W., et al.: Latent papillomavirus infection in cattle. Res. Vet. Sci. **56**, 151–157 (1994)
55. Maran, A., Amella, C.A., Di Lorenzo, T.P., et al.: Human papillomavirus type 11 transcripts are present at low abundance in latently infected respiratory tissues. Virology **212**, 285–294 (1995)

56. Abramson, A.L., Nouri, M., Mullooly, V., et al.: Latent Human Papillomavirus infection is comparable in the larynx and trachea. J. Med. Virol. **72**, 473–477 (2004)
57. Paavonen, J., Jenkins, D., Bosch, F.X., et al.: Efficacy of a prophylactic adjuvanted bivalent L1 virus-like-particle vaccine against infection with human papillomavirus types 16 and 18 in young women: an interim analysis of a phase III double-blind, randomised controlled trial. Lancet **374**, 301–314 (2009)
58. Fausch, S.C., Da Silva, D.M., Rudolf, M.P., et al.: Human papillomavirus virus-like particles do not activate Langerhans cells: a possible immune escape mechanism used by human papillomaviruses. J. Immunol. **169**, 3242–3249 (2002)
59. Lenz, P., Lowy, D.R., Schiller, J.T.: Papillomavirus virus-like particles induce cytokines characteristic of innate immune responses in plasmacytoid dendritic cells. Eur. J. Immunol. **35**, 1548–1556 (2005)
60. Da Silva, D.M., Fausch, S.C., Verbeek, J.S., et al.: Uptake of human papillomavirus virus-like particles by dendritic cells is mediated by Fc{gamma} receptors and contributes to acquisition of T cell immunity. J. Immunol. **178**, 7587–7597 (2007)
61. Yang, R., Murillo, F.M., Cui, H., et al.: Papillomavirus-like particles stimulate murine bone marrow-derived dendritic cells to produce alpha interferon and Th1 immune responses via MyD88. J. Virol. **78**, 11152–11160 (2004)
62. Yan, M., Peng, J., Jabbar, I.A., et al.: Activation of dendritic cells by human papillomavirus-like particles through TLR4 and NF-kappaB-mediated signalling, moderated by TGF-beta. Immunol. Cell Biol. **83**, 83–91 (2005)
63. Le Bon, A., Tough, D.F.: Links between innate and adaptive immunity via type I interferon. Curr. Opin. Immunol. **14**, 432–436 (2002)
64. Kanodia, S., Fahey, L.M., Kast, W.M.: Mechanisms used by human papillomaviruses to escape the host immune response. Curr. Cancer Drug Targets **7**, 79–89 (2007)
65. Hasan, U.A., Bates, E., Takeshita, F., et al.: TLR9 expression and function is abolished by the cervical cancer-associated human papillomavirus type 16. J. Immunol. **178**, 3186–3197 (2007)
66. Takeshita, F., Ishii, K.J.: Intracellular DNA sensors in immunity. Curr. Opin. Immunol. **20**, 383–388 (2008)
67. Arany, I., Goel, A., Tyring, S.K.: Interferon response depends on viral transcription in human papillomavirus-containing lesions. Anticancer Res. **15**, 2865–2869 (1995)
68. Park, J.S., Kim, E.J., Kwon, H.J., et al.: Inactivation of interferon regulatory factor-1 tumor suppressor protein by HPV E7 oncoprotein. Implication for the E7-mediated immune evasion mechanism in cervical carcinogenesis. J. Biol. Chem. **275**, 6764–6769 (2000)
69. Um, S.J., Rhyu, J.W., Kim, E.J., et al.: Abrogation of IRF-1 response by high-risk HPV E7 protein in vivo. Cancer Lett. **179**, 205–212 (2002)
70. Ronco, L.V., Karpova, A.Y., Vidal, M., et al.: Human papillomavirus 16 E6 oncoprotein binds to interferon regulatory factor-3 and inhibits its transcriptional activity. Genes Dev. **12**, 2061–2072 (1998)
71. Li, S., Labrecque, S., Gauzzi, M.C., et al.: The human papilloma virus (HPV)-18 E6 oncoprotein physically associates with Tyk2 and impairs Jak-STAT activation by interferon-alpha. Oncogene **18**, 5727–5737 (1999)
72. Stanley, M.A., Pett, M.R., Coleman, N.: HPV: from infection to cancer. Biochem. Soc. Trans. **35**, 1456–1460 (2007)
73. Hubert, P., Caberg, J.H., Gilles, C., et al.: E-cadherin-dependent adhesion of dendritic and Langerhans cells to keratinocytes is defective in cervical human papillomavirus-associated (pre)neoplastic lesions. J. Pathol. **206**, 346–355 (2005)
74. Matthews, K., Leong, C.M., Baxter, L., et al.: Depletion of Langerhans cells in human papillomavirus type 16-infected skin is associated with E6-mediated down regulation of E-cadherin. J. Virol. **77**, 8378–8385 (2003)
75. Kobayashi, A., Greenblatt, R.M., Anastos, K., et al.: Functional attributes of mucosal immunity in cervical intraepithelial neoplasia and effects of HIV infection. Cancer Res. **64**, 6766–6774 (2004)
76. Adurthi, S., Krishna, S., Mukherjee, G., et al.: Regulatory T cells in a spectrum of HPV-induced cervical lesions: cervicitis, cervical intraepithelial neoplasia and squamous cell carcinoma. Am. J. Reprod. Immunol. **60**, 55–65 (2008)
77. Shope, R.E.: Immunization of rabbits to infectious papillomatosis. J. Exp. Med. **65**, 607–624 (1937)
78. Stanley, M.: Human papillomavirus vaccines versus cervical cancer screening. Clin. Oncol. (R. Coll. Radiol.) **20**, 388–394 (2008)
79. Breitburd, F., Kirnbauer, R., Hubbert, N.L., et al.: Immunization with viruslike particles from cottontail rabbit papillomavirus (CRPV) can protect against experimental CRPV infection. J. Virol. **69**, 3959–3963 (1995)
80. Suzich, J.A., Ghim, S.J., Palmer Hill, F.J., et al.: Systemic immunization with papillomavirus L1 protein completely prevents the development of viral mucosal papillomas. Proc. Natl. Acad. Sci. USA **92**, 11553–11557 (1995)
81. Ghim, S., Newsome, J., Bell, J., et al.: Spontaneously regressing oral papillomas induce systemic antibodies that neutralize canine oral papillomavirus. Exp. Mol. Pathol. **68**, 147–151 (2000)
82. Day, P.M., Gambhira, R., Roden, R.B., et al.: Mechanisms of human papillomavirus type 16 neutralization by 12 cross-neutralizing and 11 type-specific antibodies. J. Virol. **82**, 4638–4646 (2008)
83. Olsson, S.E., Villa, L.L., Costa, R.L., et al.: Induction of immune memory following administration of a prophylactic quadrivalent human papillomavirus (HPV) types 6/11/16/18 L1 virus-like particle (VLP) vaccine. Vaccine **25**, 4931–4939 (2007)
84. Giannini, S.L., Hanon, E., Moris, P., et al.: Enhanced humoral and memory B cellular immunity using HPV16/18 L1 VLP vaccine formulated with the MPL/aluminium salt combination (AS04) compared to aluminium salt only. Vaccine **24**, 5937–5949 (2006)
85. Van Damme, P., Van Herck, K.: A review of the long-term protection after hepatitis A and B vaccination. Travel Med. Infect. Dis. **5**, 79–84 (2007)
86. Smith, J.F., Brownlow, M., Brown, M., et al.: Antibodies from women immunized with Gardasil ((R)) cross-neutralize HPV 45 pseudovirions. Hum. Vaccines **3**, 109–115 (2007)
87. Woo, Y.L., van den Hende, M., Sterling, J.C., Coleman, N., Crawford, R.A., Kwappenberg, K.M., Stanley, M.A., van der Burg, S.H.: A prospective study on the natural course of low-grade squamous intraepithelial lesions and the presence of HPV16 E2-, E6- and E7-specific T-cell responses. Int. J. Cancer **136,** 133–141 (2010)

HPV-Infection and Squamous Cell Cancer of the Lower Female Genital Tract

35

Karl Ulrich Petry

Core Messages

- HPV play an essential role in the genesis of almost all cervical cancer, all CIN3, the majority of VaIN, vaginal cancers and VIN, while approximately 60% of squamous cell cancers of the vulva are not linked to HPV.
- For an individual to be HPV positive at one point of time is nothing peculiar. Not to get rid of HPV is the important step towards malignancy. Important risk factors for HPV persistency are age over 30, smoking, high parity, HPV-type 16, immunodeficiency and long-term use of oral contraceptives.
- The full cycle of HPV-induced genesis of cervical cancer from initial infection to invasive disease is typically extended over decades with a minimum latency of 7–8 years.
- HPV vaccination is a primary prevention method of HPV16/18-associated cancers of the lower female genital tract. It prevents the full cycle of carcinogenesis with almost 100% efficacy in HPV 16/18-naïve individuals. However, current vaccines will at best prevent some but not all cervical cancers that are associated with other high-risk HPV-types.
- Although Pap smear screening significantly reduced the incidence of cervical cancer, organized screening based on HPV-testing is more efficient in detecting high-grade precursors and cancer, reducing incidence and mortality from cervical cancer and allows for an extension of screening intervals.

35.1 The Role of Human Papillomavirus in the Genesis of Cancer of the Female Lower Genital Tract

Invasive cancers of the lower genital tract develop from intraepithelial precursor lesions. These precursors were called dysplasia in the past; recent classifications favour the terms intraepithelial neoplasia or intraepithelial lesions. The model of a successive carcinogenesis is best established for invasive squamous cell carcinoma of the uterine cervix. Cervical intraepithelial neoplasia (CIN) "begins as well differentiated intraepithelial neoplasm, which is classified as a mild dysplasia, and ends with invasive cancer" [1]. Infection with so-called high-risk types of human papillomavirus is the driving force behind the development of almost all invasive cervical cancers and CIN grade 2 and 3, the majority of vaginal and anal neoplasms and finally a distinguished subgroup of neoplasms of the vulva. However, while genital HPV infections are very common, development of HPV-related cancer is a rare endpoint of these infections. Less than 10% of HR-HPV infected women without any access to screening facilities will finally suffer from cervical cancer [2] and the risk for other HPV-related cancers is even smaller.

K.U. Petry
Frauenklinik im Klinikum Wolfsburg, Sauerbruchstr. 7, 38440 Wolfsburg, Germany
e-mail: gyn@klinikum.wolfsburg.de

G. Gross and S.K. Tyring (eds.), *Sexually Transmitted Infections and Sexually Transmitted Diseases*,
DOI: 10.1007/978-3-642-14663-3_35,

Typically, the genesis of HPV-associated cancers needs much more than a decade from initial infection to invasive disease. This reliably slow progression of HPV-induced tumour development is the key to a successful prevention of these cancers. Although the success of cervical cancer prevention is unique, it created a number of new problems and questions. What is the best algorithm to identify and manage women at risk, what are the co-factors of papillomavirus infection, how can we optimise screening within the peculiarities of different national screening systems, is there any way to offer cervical cancer prevention to women in the third world and how will HPV vaccination change screening are just some examples of not yet completely answered questions in this field.

As it is not possible to address all questions about state-of-the-art prevention and management of pre-invasive and invasive neoplasia of the female genital tract, this chapter will focus on the management of squamous intraepithelial neoplasia and atypical smears of the uterine cervix and the prevention of cervical cancer.

In 1977, Harald zur Hausen postulated a causal role for human papillomavirus (HPV), and in 1983, his group discovered a new HPV type in invasive cervical tumours that was finally listed as HPV type 16. and coined the term HPV 16 [3]. Since then, more than 20 different HPV types were found to be associated with cervical cancer. Papillomaviruses consist of an icosahedric capsid with a diameter of 55 nm and a double stranded viral DNA with a length of approximately 8 kb. The viral DNA of all HPV types contains so-called open reading frames (ORF) that encode for specific proteins. The ORF E6 and E7 of high-risk HPV encode for oncoproteins that are able to neutralize and destroy important proteins of cell regulation such as p53 and pRb with high affinity. As a result cells are immortalized and transformed [4, 5].

HPV 16 is the most important high-risk HPV type because it is associated with approximately 50% of all invasive tumours of the uterine cervix. HPV 16/18/45 and 31 account for more than 80% of all cervical cancers. Overall, 99.7% of invasive cervical cancers were associated with HPV in one large study that included more than 1,000 tumours from five continents [6] Other groups confirmed that all true CIN grade III (severe dysplasia and carcinoma in situ) are associated with HPV-DNA [7]. A final proof for the HPV-induced genesis of cervical neoplasia came from the vaccine trials. HPV 16/18 as well as HPV 6/11/16/18 vaccines effectively prevented development of HPV-type specific CIN [8, 9] HPV-induced carcinogenesis is a rather slow process with at least four important steps:

- Incident infection with a high-risk HPV type
- Establishment of a persistent HPV infection
- Transformation of human keratinocytes in pre-invasive neoplastic cells
- Malignant transformation of intraepithelial neoplasia into invasive cancer

The process is reversible at any pre-invasive stage. The majority of genital HPV infections are transient and more than 90% will be cleared spontaneously within 18 months in women younger than 25 [10]. Older age, smoking, high parity, cellular immunodeficiency and long-term use of oral contraceptives significantly favour persistence of HPV infections as well as development of CIN and cancer [11–13]. The HPV-type matters too. The risk of development of CIN3 is increased significantly in women infected with HPV 16 or 18 compared with other high-risk HPV types [14–16].

35.2 Natural History of Cervical Intraepithelial Neoplasia

In 1886, Williams described intraepithelial lesions adjacent to cervical cancers that resembled the invasive tumour but did not infiltrate the stroma [17].

Persistent HPV-infections and low-grade intraepithelial neoplasia will regress without any treatment within 2–5 years in 60–80% of all cases. The risk factors for progression of low-grade SIL resemble very much those for HPV persistency. Spontaneous resolution is observed even among at least 40% of lesions with biopsy-proven moderate dysplasia (CIN grade II) and only a 20% minority of CIN 2 will progress to CIN 3 and less than 5% to invasive cancer [18]. Although the natural history of CIN 2 resembles that of low-grade lesions, it is regarded as a high-grade lesion in most clinical management guidelines for practical and legal reasons.

The presence of high-risk HPV is essential for progression to invasive disease, but the individual risk of progression depends on the presence of risk factors such as smoking or cellular immunodeficiency and the HPV-type. Lesions associated with HPV 16 are significantly more likely to progress to CIN 3 than lesions related to other HPV types, and while spontaneous regression of

CIN 1 is very common in young women, the risk of progression is significantly increased in patients over 30 [15, 19]. As cervical neoplasia depends on a viral infection, cervical cancer is not an inherited disease. However, an increased risk for CIN 3 and invasive cancer was observed in the daughters of women suffering from cervical neoplasm probably because of an inherited dysfunction in the immune response to HPV [20].

It is well established that even CIN3 lesions may regress spontaneously [21]. But there is little information on the risk of progression of CIN 3 to invasive disease. Most of the literature is based on an unethical clinical study at the National Women's Hospital, Auckland, New Zealand. Treatment of CIN 3 was withheld from a substantial number of women between 1965 and 1974. In a careful long-term analysis of 143 women managed only by punch or wedge biopsy, cumulative incidence of invasive cancer of the cervix or vaginal vault was 31.3% (95% CI 22.7–42.3) at 30 years and 50.3% (37.3–64.9) in the subset of 92 such women who had persistent disease within 24 months [22]. The true risk of progression should be even higher because biopsies were taken in all patients and the removal of neoplastic tissue may change the natural course of disease.

Figure 35.1 summarizes the natural history of HPV infection, CIN and cervical cancer. The full cycle from initial HPV infection to invasive cervical cancer needs decades in most cases. Rapid-onset cervical cancers may occur within less than 10 years following initial HPV infection, but there is no published case with a latency period of less than 8 years between HPV infection and the diagnosis of invasive cervical cancer. However, it is important to notice that some rare types of cervical cancers such as clear cell adenocarcinoma or serous-papillary adenocarcinoma are not linked to HPV and may occur even in school-aged virgins [23].

35.3 Diagnosis

35.3.1 Diagnosis of Cervical Intraepithelial Neoplasia

35.3.1.1 Colposcopy

Intraepithelial neoplasia of the uterine cervix is virtually never visible to the naked eye. Usually it is detected by colposcopy following atypical Pap smears and/or positive HPV testing in cervical screening programs.

For a colposcopic examination, a suitably sized speculum is used to expose the cervix. Any excess mucus or blood should be removed using dry or saline-soaked cotton wool ball. Presence of gross lesions or leucoplakia should be then identified. Then acetic acid (3–5%) is gently applied to the cervix with saturated cotton wool balls and left for 10 s in contact with the cervix. Lugol´s iodine may be used

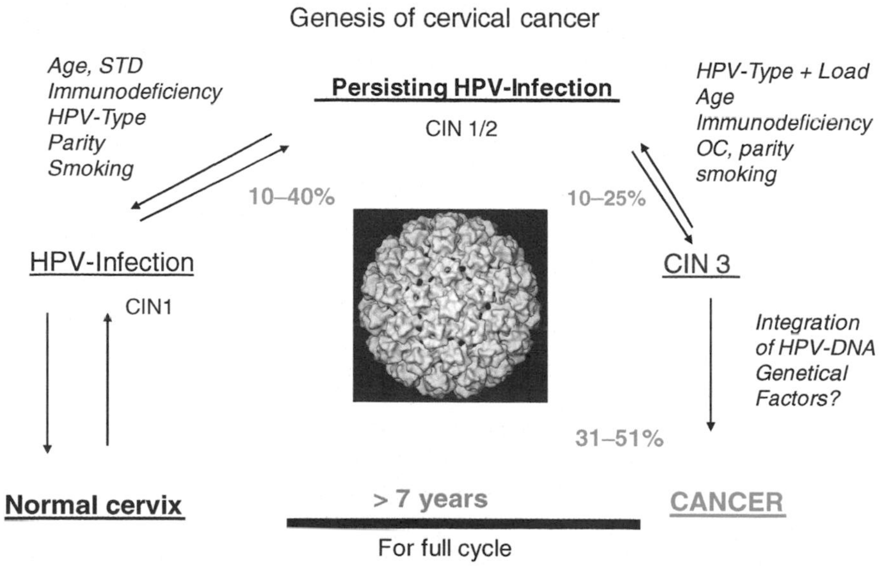

Fig. 35.1 The full cycle of carcinogenesis from the initial HPV infection to invasive cancer occurs only in a minority of infected individuals. Even in affected patients the full cycle needs decades in most cases, development of invasive cancer within 19 years after initial HPV infection is rare and never happens within less than 7 years

to further distinguish atypical epithelium which contains little or no glycogen and therefore fails to take up the iodine stain.

The focus of the colposcopic examination is the so-called transformation zone. The peripheral ectocervix is covered with squamous epithelium and the deeper endocervical canal is lined with mullerian glandular epithelium in most women. The location of the squamous-columnar junction (SCJ) depends on endocrine factors but differs individually. Usually, the junction is situated in the endocervix during childhood and everted onto the ectocervix during puberty; the variable extent of columnar epithelium onto the ectocervix is described as columnar ectopy. The original SCJ is the most external line to which the glandular epithelium has been extended. In most individuals, the columnar epithelium is replaced by metaplastic epithelium. The original SCJ therefore becomes a sort of squamous–squamous junction and is colposcopically detectable only if the metaplastic process is not completely achieved. The actual SCJ is the junction between metaplastic/squamous and columnar epithelium. The area between actual and original SCJ is defined as transformation zone (TZ). The TZ and especially, the actual SCJ is prone to the development of HPV-induced neoplasia for a number of reasons. Basal cells seem to be the target cell of primary HPV infection. These cells are exposed only to the surface of the tissue at the actual SCJ. Furthermore, only basal cells of the SCJ are capable to differentiate into different cell types. It is very likely that the existence of multiple programs for differentiation within one cell is a key for HPV-induced malignant transformation. Almost all cervical high-grade neoplasms occur within the TZ and the incidence of CIN by far outnumbers the incidence of vaginal intraepithelial neoplasia although both vagina and cervix are exposed to HPV at identical risks.

After application of acetic acid, the original squamous epithelium is pink, translucent, flat and smooth. The columnar epithelium appears deep pink and its folds have a grape-like morphology after acetic acid application. The normal TZ includes areas of immature squamous metaplasia that become more opaque after acetic acid application than the differentiated squamous epithelium. The most frequent abnormality seen with the colposcope is acetowhite epithelium. Areas with high nuclear density appear white after acetic acid application. Generally, the faster and the denser the change, the more severe the lesion may be. However, acetowhite epithelium is not diagnostic for CIN; immature metaplasia, regenerating epithelium, inflammation and congenital transformation are other conditions that may display acetowhiteness.

Other important colposcopic findings are vascular patterns. New vessel formation may appear as a rectangular pattern resembling a mosaic. Regular and gentle mosaics are found in metaplasia or CIN1. When coarser, wider and more irregular, the more likely the lesions are to be of high grade (see Figs. 35.2 and 35.3). Similarly, regular looped fine capillaries within the stromal papilla may appear as a fine punctuation in metaplastic tissues while high-grade CIN display capillaries with increased calibre, malformation and irregular spacing.

Colposcopy can only be considered satisfactory if the complete TZ is visualized. Kogan´s endocervical forceps will allow a vision up to about 10 mm in the cervical canal if the TZ extends into the endocervix. Colposcopy is the diagnostic tool to identify the most suspicious areas, but the final diagnosis needs to be based on histopathology. In case of a fully visible TZ, colposcopically guided punch biopsies can be taken directly from areas with major changes. The ectocervix lacks nociceptors; therefore, no anaesthesia is required to take cervical biopsies. Haemostasis is achieved by the application of Monsell´s solution. In cases of unsatisfactory colposcopy and a need for a definite diagnosis, either endocervical curettage or complete excision of the transformation zone may be necessary.

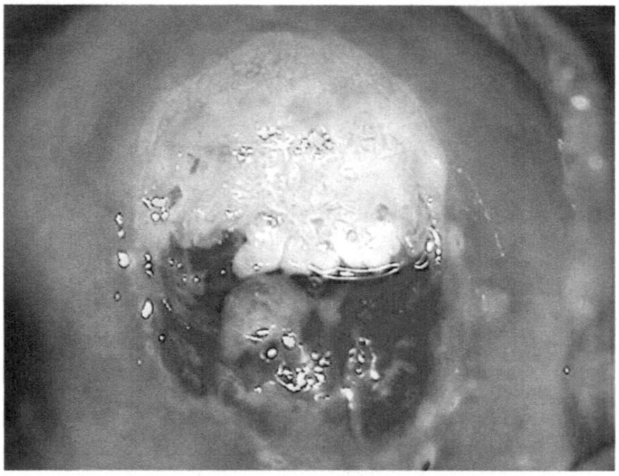

Fig. 35.2 Colposcopy figure of CIN3 after application of 3% acetic acid. The transformation zone extends just 2 mm into the endocervical canal (type II transformation zone). Atypical acetowhite epithelium is found clockwise from 9 to 3′. A mosaic with discrete irregularities is seen at the periphery from 10 to 12′, the punch biopsy showed CIN1. The dense acetowhite epithelium at 2′ directly situated at the external os corresponds to CIN3 on histology

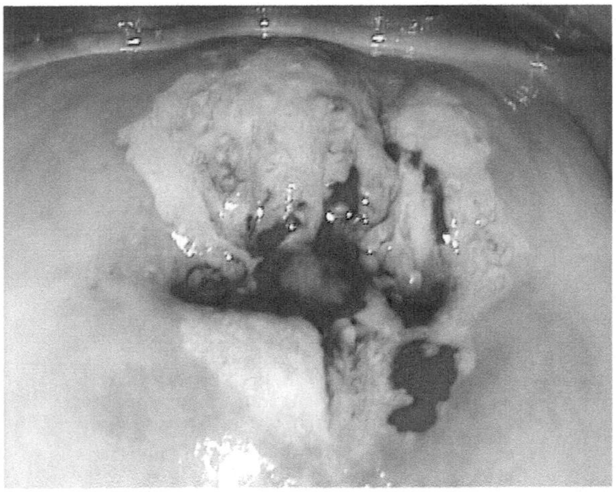

Fig. 35.3 Colposcopy figure of Carcinoma in situ after application of 3% acetic acid with dense greyish epithelium and coarse mosaic. The upper limit of the atypical transformation zone is located in the deep endocervix and cannot be identified on colposcopy (type III transformation zone)

It has been questioned if colposcopy with biopsies is really the diagnostic gold standard in women with atypical smears or if a reasonable number of high-grade lesions will be missed. However, the TOMBOLA study, a large randomized controlled trial, could confirm that immediate resection of the complete transformation zone in women with mild abnormal smears did not result in a higher rate of CIN2/3 diagnoses when compared to colposcopy plus biopsies, but led to unnecessary operations in healthy women and more after effects [24]. As any ablative treatment of the uterine cervix results in increased risks of late abortion, premature labour and infant mortality for subsequent pregnancies, immediate resection of the transformation zone should be discouraged in women with mild abnormal smears [25].

35.3.2 HPV, Squamous Intraepithelial Lesion of the Vulva and Cancer of the Vulva

In contrast to high-grade CIN and invasive cancer of the cervix which are almost exclusively associated with HPV the genesis of vulva neoplasms is more heterogenous. Malignant melanoma, pre-invasive and invasive Paget carcinoma, adenocarcinoma of the different vulva glands are obviously not related to papillomavirus, while squamous cell cancers can be divided in at least two different entities, the undifferentiated and the differentiated squamous cell carcinoma (SCC) [26]. Undifferentiated SCC are associated with HPV 16 and to a lesser extent with other high-risk HPV types. The genesis is very much similar to the development of cervical cancer. HPV will lead to the development of vulvar intraepithelial neoplasia (VIN) only in a minority of infected women. Overall, the prevalence of VIN is much lower than the prevalence of CIN. But the incidence of VIN3 increased by 400% during the last 3 decades in the USA and other industrialised countries. It is especially high in immunocompromised women and heavy smokers [27]. On histology, HPV-associated precursor lesions show a basaloid or verrucous morphology very similar to the undifferentiated invasive SCC.

Differentiated keratinizing squamous cell cancers of the vulva are not linked to HPV. They are frequently associated with Lichen sclerosus (see Fig. 35.4). The ISSVD distinguishes between differentiated and undifferentiated VIN as two different precursor lesions

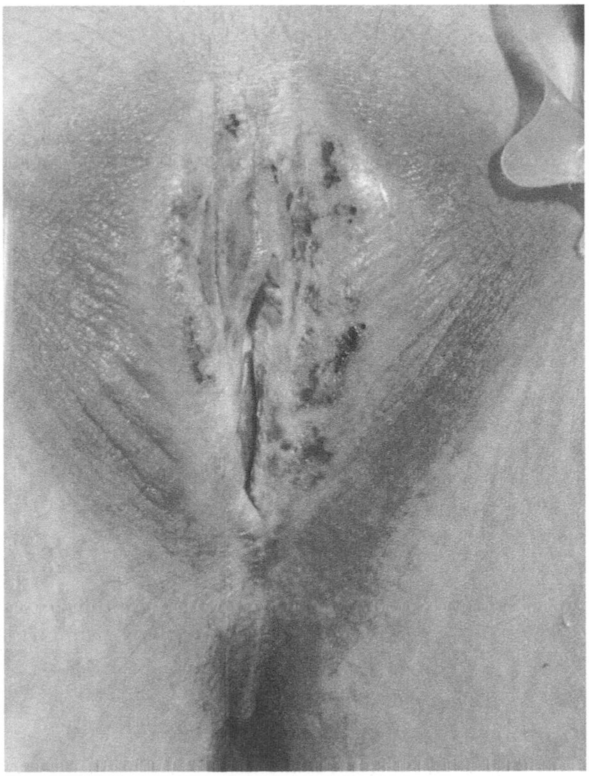

Fig. 35.4 Lichen sclerosus with atrophy of the labia minora, synechie of the praeputium clitoris and skin irritations due to severe itching

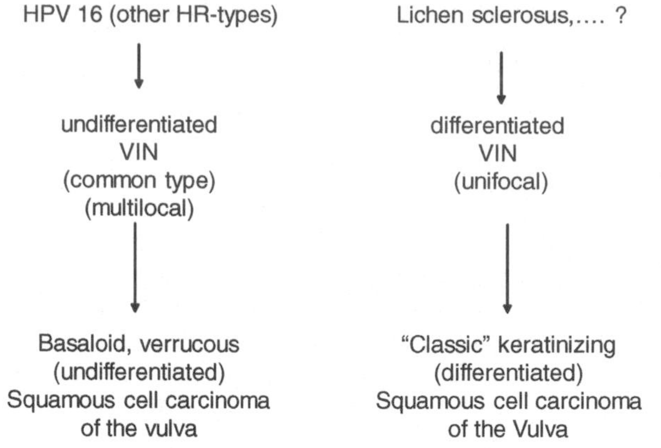

Fig. 35.5 The two entities of squamous VIN/vulvar cancer

of two different SCC types of the vulva (Fig. 35.5). While the concept of two different entities of invasive SCC is generally accepted and the genesis of undifferentiated VIN and cancer undisputed, there are many doubts about the role of differentiated VIN as a true precursor. Differentiated VIN are frequently found adjacent to differentiated invasive SCC of the vulva, but they are rarely detected as isolated pre-invasive lesions. This could be explained by the fact that they are very difficult to identify on colposcopy, because they do not necessarily react on application with acetic acid (see Fig. 35.6). While this type of vulva neoplasia is usually an isolated lesion and invasive cancers occur mainly in older women (see Fig. 35.7), HPV-associated cancers and precursors are typically multifocal and may be observed in very young women (Fig. 35.8).

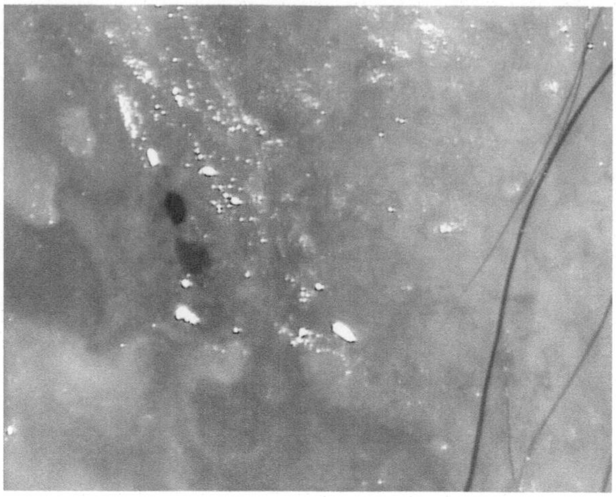

Fig 35.6 High magnification of differentiated VIN3 which is not associated with HPV. This rare lesion does not change its appearance after application of acetic acid. On histology VIN is only found in the small area with atypical vessels in the centre of the figure but not in the neighbouring leukoplacic areas

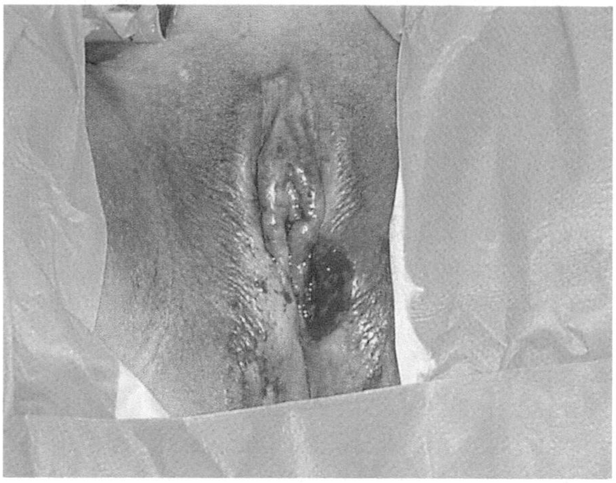

Fig. 35.7 Differentiated squamous cell cancer of the vulva which is *not* linked to HPV

35.3.2.1 Diagnosis of VIN

Cytology shows a poor sensitivity and specificity in the detection of VIN. Its use in the diagnosis of vulval lesions should be discouraged. The best diagnostic approach is to refer any suspicious clinical lesion of the vulva and high-risk populations to colposcopy. The majority of patients with VIN will present with simultaneous CIN or have a history of cervical neoplasia. Therefore, women referred for colposcopy because of cervical, vaginal or vulval lesions should always undergo a careful colposcopic examination of the complete lower genital tract and anus.

VIN3 may present as flat condyloma-like lesions of different colours including white areas with hyperkeratosis, pigmented tissue and reddish patches with increased vascularization (see Fig. 35.9). Other VIN3, especially those located in the wet epithelium of the vaginal introitus may be invisible to the naked eye and show up only after application of acetic acid (Fig. 35.10). In contrast to cervical lesions which are never associated with clinical symptoms, VIN may result in itching and dysparaesthesia.

Biopsies need to be taken either under local or general anaesthesia. Keyes punch forceps is a suitable method. It removes a round skin area 3–6 mm in diameter and allows for a full skin thickness examination on

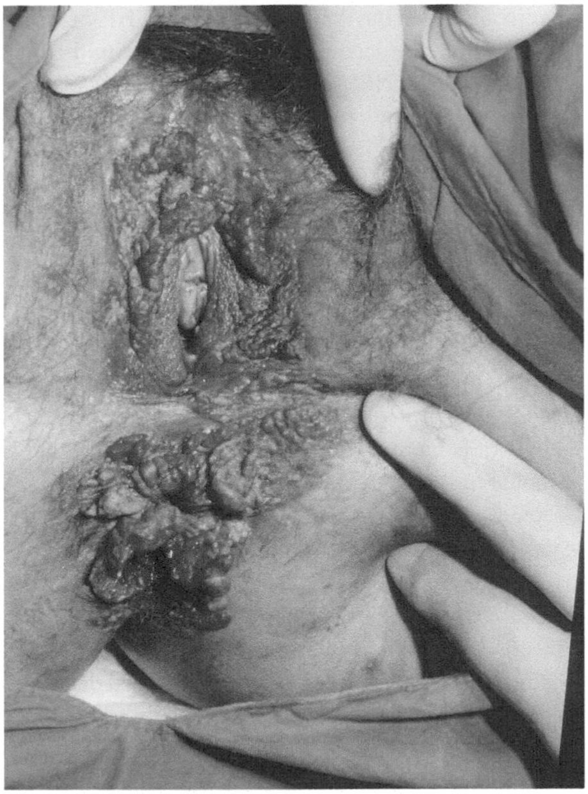

Fig. 35.8 Microinvasive undifferentiated squamous cell carcinoma of the vulva, multiple VIN3 lesions and invasive anal cancer. All neoplastic lesions were associated with HPV 16

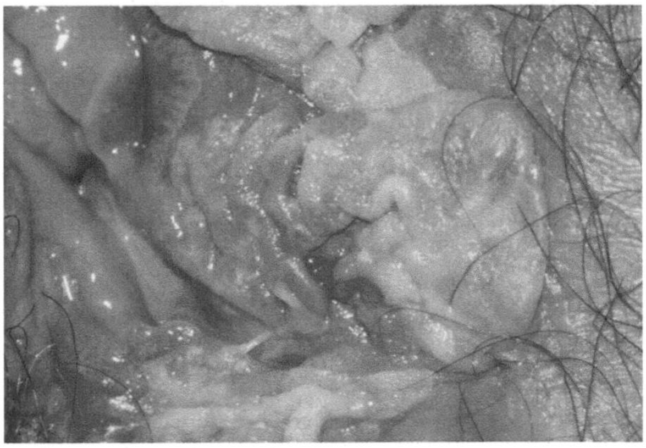

Fig. 35.9 Magnified figure of undifferentiated VIN3 associated with HPV16. These clinical lesions may look white, reddish or pigmented

histology. In most cases, haemostasis can be achieved by compression of the biopsy sites for 3 min; sutures are rarely needed.

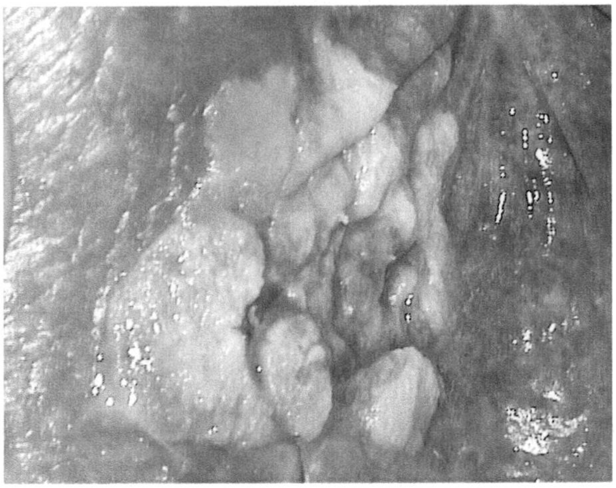

Fig. 35.10 Magnified figure of undifferentiated VIN3 associated with HPV16. The lesions of the wet squamous cell epithelium are only visible after application of acetic acid

35.3.3 HPV-Infection, Vaginal Intraepithelial Neoplasia and Cancer of the Vagina

Cancer of the vagina and high-grade intraepithelial neoplasia of the vagina (VaIN2/3) are rare diseases and the published knowledge about the aetiology and epidemiology is therefore based on small numbers. In one ongoing pilot project with 19,081 women attending routine screening, we diagnosed CIN3 in 134 participants, another 18 suffered from invasive cervical cancer, while just 7 women were diagnosed with VIN3 and a single patient with VaIN3. In this screening project, participants had to be 30 years or older. Women with a history of CIN and/or those who had undergone hysterectomy were excluded.

The risk of VaIN and vaginal cancer is increased in immunocompromised hosts and in women with HPV-induced neoplasia of cervix and/or vulva.

Vaginal adenocarcinoma is a rare entity that is not linked to HPV. The majority but not all squamous cell cancers of the vagina and VaIN are associated with HPV. A meta-analysis concluded that 90,1% of VaIN2/3 and 69,9% of invasive cancers of the vagina can be linked to HPV. HPV16 was the most important type and was found in 57,6% of VaIN2/3 and 53,7% of invasive cancers which is almost identical with the established prevalence rates of HPV 16 in high-grade lesions of the uterine cervix [28]. In our own population of patients with SCC of the vagina, 16.5% tested negative for HR-HPV using Hybrid Capture 2 and 9.1% of VaIN2/3 had a negative HC2 test result which is very much in line with the meta-analysis.

Frank invasive cancer of the vagina is a clinical diagnosis, but micro-invasive and pre-invasive disease are invisible to the naked eye and can be detected only with the use of a colposcope. Vaginal lesions very much resemble cervical lesions after application of acetic acid. In contrast to cervical lesions which are almost exclusively situated in the transformation zone, VaIN is frequently multilocal and may be spread over large areas of the vagina. Iodine staining with Lugoll´s solution is helpful only to distinguish some cases of CIN from metaplasia, but it is mandatory to detect multifocal vaginal intraepithelial neoplasia. The histological diagnosis is obtained by punch biopsies taken from all suspicious vaginal lesions. Usually, anaesthesia is not needed for punch biopsies in the upper third of the vagina due to the scarce distribution of nociceptors, but local anaesthesia will be necessary for biopsies taken from other parts of the vagina. Haemostasis can be achieved by application of Monsell's solution.

35.4 Prevention of Cancer and Pre-cancer of the Lower Female Genital Tract

35.4.1 Primary Prevention with HPV Vaccination

HPV vaccination is explained in detail in a separate chapter by Lutz Gissmann; therefore, only a few aspects concerning prevention of genital lesions are addressed here.

The immunogenicity of HPV involves presentation to the immune system of conformational epitopes displayed on viral capsids composed of the so-called L1 protein. This major capsid protein can be synthesized with the use of microbial or cellular expression systems. L1 proteins will self-assemble to empty viral capsids, termed "virus like particles" (VLP). VLP do not contain DNA and they are not live or attenuated viruses. Vaccination with L1-VLPs derived from type-specific papillomaviruses induces high titres of specific neutralizing antibodies [29]. Two prophylactic vaccines based on VLP have been developed and licensed in 2010. One, Gardasil (Merck & Co.) is a quadrivalent vaccine that protects against HPV 6,11,16 and 18, while the second Cervarix (GlaxoSmithKline) protects against HPV 16 and 18 (bivalent). Several double-blinded and placebo-controlled clinical trials of both prophylactic HPV vaccines have being conducted in different countries including about 60,000 individuals. Safety and tolerability of the vaccines were excellent in all trials. No increase in systemic side effects was observed between individuals in vaccine and placebo study arms. The per-protocol populations included women who were naïve to HPV 6, 11, 16 and 18 at baseline as determined by serology testing for presence of HPV type-specific antibodies or polymerase chain reaction (PCR) testing of genital samples for the presence of HPV DNA [30]. For both vaccines, results of different trials allow for the examination of broad trends in efficacy in preventing HPV 6/11/16/18-related disease in several groups of patients categorized according to their HPV status at baseline. The quadrivalent vaccine was 100% effective in reducing the incidence of HPV 6/11/16/18-related disease in HPV-naïve women as well as in women who had been previously exposed to at least one vaccine HPV type at enrolment, but had no ongoing HPV infection (i.e. seropositive but HPV DNA negative by PCR) [9, 31]. However, VLP-vaccines had no therapeutic effect and did not improve spontaneous regression rates of prevalent infections with HPV types 16 or 18 [32].

A full course of HPV vaccination requires three intramuscular injections at months 0, 1 (Cervarix) or 2 (Gardasil) and 6.

HPV vaccination is highly effective in protecting against HPV 16 and 18 infections and associated intraepithelial neoplasia, including CIN3, adenocarcinoma in situ, VaIN2/3 and VIN2/3 in HPV16/18-naïve women [9, 31, 33, 34]. Although some cross-protection was observed against HPV31 which is closely related to HPV16 and against HPV45 which is closely related to HPV 18, vaccinated individuals are still at risk from HPV-infections with other high-risk types that may result in the development of cancer of the lower female genital tract [35].

Most guidelines recommend vaccination of school girls or adolescents prior to sexual debut at the age of 9–14 years, the American Cancer society favours the age of 11–12 years. Vaccination of young women in the age group of 15–18 years is recommended to catch up or complete vaccination. For women at the age of 19–26 years, there is neither a recommendation for nor against vaccination. Decisions should be based on individual counselling [36]. Although one randomized controlled trial could demonstrate that women aged 25–45 years were protected from persisting HPV 16/18 infections and associated diseases as well, the effect was much lower in the intention to treat population because one third of the participants had already an infection or a history of infection with at least one of the HPV vaccine types [37]. Furthermore, the incidence of HPV 16/18 infections declines significantly in older populations. While the annual incidence among women 15–25 years was 4.77% in the PATRICIA trial, it dropped to just 0.7 in the 35–45 years age group [35, 38]. In conclusion, women aged 25–45 years will profit from HPV vaccination, but this will be cost efficient only when prices for HPV vaccination drop significantly.

The exact duration of vaccine protection is unknown; based on the available data from ongoing trials, both vaccines showed no decline in effectiveness after 4.5–6.5 years and even more than 8 years in a monovalent HPV16 vaccine [39]. It seems very likely that the final duration will exceed 10 years or might even last for decades.

HPV vaccination is a so-called primary prevention method, because it prevents the full cycle of carcinogenesis including HPV infection, intraepithelial lesions and cancer. Under best conditions, the current bivalent and quadrivalent HPV vaccines offer a 100% protection against HPV 16 and 18-associated cancers and some cross-protection to related HPV types. This would correspond to a protection against 70–80% of all cervical cancers, approximately 40% of squamous cell cancers (SCC) of the vulva and 60–80% of SCC of vagina and anus. As SCC of vulva and vagina are relatively rare cancers and the incidence of cervical cancer is low in populations with sufficient screening programmes under socioeconomic aspects, the impact of HPV vaccination on the burden of pre-invasive disease will be much more important. The cost of treating CIN as well as the management of atypical Pap smears exceeds the cost of treating cervical cancer in many countries [40, 41].

35.4.2 *Prevention of Cervical Cancer with Primary Screening Programmes*

35.4.2.1 Introduction

Pap smear screening programmes significantly reduced the incidence of cervical cancer in most industrialized countries. It is a so-called secondary prevention method because it does not prevent the full cycle of carcinogenesis. The central concept of this exceptionally successful cancer prevention is the identification and treatment of women with high-grade intraepithelial lesions (CIN 2 and CIN 3). Excision of these lesions interrupts the genesis of cervical cancer at a pre-invasive stage.

Although future HPV vaccines may offer complete protection from all diseases caused by HPV [42], screening will be needed to prevent cervical cancer in non-vaccinated women and not per protocol-vaccinated individuals for the next decades. Even women who were vaccinated per protocol will need to participate in screening programmes as the current vaccines will prevent only 70–80% of all high-grade CIN and invasive cancer. This reduction is equivalent to the effect of the established Pap smear programmes. Combining vaccination and screening will offer best protection from cervical cancer.

35.4.2.2 Is HPV Testing the Better Screening Test Than Pap Smear?

The full process of carcinogenesis from HPV infection to malignant growth is typically extended over 15–30 years; intervals shorter than 10 years seem to be extremely rare. As CIN 3 lesions typically persist for years before progressing to malignancy, chances of an early detection within the screening programme are high [43–46]

The implementation of a Pap smear-based primary screening for cervical cancer and its precursors in the second half of the twentieth century was one of the greatest success stories in cancer prevention. While in countries without such screening programmes 3–5% of the female population will develop cervical cancer, the corresponding risk is 1% in areas with Pap smear screening [2]. Although the Pap smear is still the undisputed screening test in almost all programmes to prevent cervical cancer, numerous studies could demonstrate that the sensitivity of a single Pap smear for CIN2/3 is much lower than conceived previously. In a meta-analysis that included six different controlled studies with more than 60,000 women attending for primary cancer screening, just 53% of high-grade lesions were detected by cytology compared to a sensitivity of 96% of HPV-DNA testing [47].

Based on several large randomized controlled trials, there is now a high level of evidence that under certain conditions, HPV testing is the better screening strategy in women above an age of 30 years. In organized screening programmes HPV testing will:

- Detect CIN3 and cancer with significantly higher sensitivity than cytology
- Be more efficient in preventing invasive cervical cancer than cytology
- Be better in reducing mortality from cervical cancer than cytology
- Have a better negative predictive value and allow for longer screening intervals than cytology

Randomised population-based studies in Italy, Canada, UK, Finland, Sweden and The Netherlands confirmed that HPV-DNA testing detects CIN3 lesions with significantly better sensitivity than Pap smear screening [48–53]. Earlier arguments that CIN3 detected by HPV testing would be irrelevant and regress spontaneously over time could be cleared by the Swedish and the Dutch trials. During a 6 years follow-up, the number of CIN3 and invasive cancers was identical in intervention group with HPV testing and the control group with conventional Pap smear screening. But in the intervention group, significantly more cases were found at study entry, while most cases in the Pap smear cohort were detected at the second screening round 5–6 years later. This improvement in earlier detection of CIN3/cancer was achieved although referral rates to colposcopy were only slightly higher in the intervention group (3.6% vs. 3.2% within 6 years).

The Italian screening trial could demonstrate that the better sensitivity of HPV-testing for CIN3+ finally results in a lower incidence of cervical cancer. While no decline in cervical cancer incidence was observed in the cytology arm (nine cases of cancer at each screening round), no case of invasive cancer was diagnosed in the HPV screening cohort at the second screening round [51].

In an Indian primary screening trial that compared the efficacy of HPV-testing, cytology and VIA (visual inspection of the cervix with acetic acid) performed once in a lifetime, only primary HPV screening showed a significant drop in mortality from cervical cancer within an 8 years follow-up.

Surprisingly, the best clinical HPV-DNA test is not the most sensitive one. Studies that used very sensitive tests based on polymerase chain reaction (PCR) found very high HPV prevalence rates in healthy individuals, but failed to detect HPV-DNA in some cancers and CIN3 [54]. The latter can be explained by DNA deletions in malignant cells that might disable PCR primers to hybridise with the target DNA. Clinical state of art in the year 2008 was either Hybrid Capture 2 (HC2) or PCR with GP5+/GP6+ primers.

Almost all HPV-DNA screening trials examined women who were 30 years or older. Due to the high prevalence of HPV in younger populations, the specificity of HPV-testing is too low and referral rates to colposcopy would be too high in the younger age groups to make HPV testing a cost-efficient alternative to Pap smear screening. This might change in HPV-vaccinated populations within the next 10 years, but for the near future, primary HPV screening will have no place in this age group.

Besides the high sensitivity for CIN3+, the extraordinarily high negative predictive value is another advantage of HPV testing. HPV-negative women cannot develop cervical cancer within the next 5–7 years even if they get infected the next day because the minimum latency from infection to cancer is in the range of 8 years [23]. HPV testing will identify the minority of women at risk of having or developing CIN3+ with very high precision while excluding any risk for the majority of participants with a reliability that is unmatched in oncology.

However, primary HPV screening will be cost efficient only in organised screening programmes with an extension of screening intervals to 5–7 years. Primary HPV testing followed by cytology in all HPV-positive cases will be an attractive concept in the future. One unsolved problem in such an HPV-based screening program is the still missing algorithm of how to identify CIN3+ cases among women with positive HPV tests but normal cytology [55]. HPV genotyping with referral of all HPV 16 or 18-positive cases or triage with p16INK4a as a marker of HPV-induced cell transformation might be good options but this needs to be determined.

35.4.3 Management of Abnormal Smears

Even if HPV testing will replace cytology in the future, the Pap smear will continue to be the primary screening test for some time and it will continue to be the standard of primary screening in women younger than 30 years. HPV testing and other new methods are already used to overcome some pitfalls of Pap smear screening. Cytology as an efficient method of cancer prevention should detect all true precursor lesions of cervical cancer with a high accuracy. But this expectation is not fulfilled for at least three reasons:

1. The accuracy of cytology is far from perfect. While the definitive diagnosis of cervical neoplasia depends on the histological identification of neoplastic cells in tissue sections, cytology uses the degree of dyskaryosis in single cells or clumps of cells recovered from the cervix to interpret the grade of the underlying neoplastic lesions. Even under best conditions, this methodological difference must result in disagreement between the cytological diagnoses of cervical neoplasia and the histological confirmation of disease. Further, in routine practice, the performance of the Pap smear is flawed by sampling and interpretation errors which are inherent to cytology as a diagnostic method; menstruation, ovulation, inflammation, pregnancy are just a few of many more frequent conditions that regularly influence Pap smear screening results even in the absence of technical sampling or interpretation errors. All these factors contribute to a reduction in accuracy of Pap smear screening by increasing the likelihood of false-positive as well as false-negative smears and by increasing the number of equivocal results.
2. No consensus on what a true precursor of cancer is. The role of cervical intraepithelial neoplasia grade III (CIN 3) as a true cancer precursor with a confirmed high risk of progression to invasive disease is undisputed. In contrast, significant controversy exists over the management of borderline atypia, CIN 1 and even CIN 2 lesions. It is well known that the majority of CIN 1/2 will regress spontaneously with only a minority progressing to CIN 3 or invasive cancer [56]. Borderline atypia, mild and moderate dysplasia are common in young women of reproductive age and as incidence rates are rising in many countries, conservative management of such lesions could help to reduce the significant costs of surgery and avoid the complications associated with invasive treatment of the uterine cervix [57]. While this would appear to be an attractive option, it has been established that a significant proportion of women with a cytological diagnosis of mild or moderate dysplasia have underlying disease of a more severe nature and those women followed with cytology alone, have a 16–47 fold increased risk of developing invasive cervical cancer [58]. In conclusion, there is little agreement on how severe a cellular atypia needs to be to justify a definition as precursor and even less consensus on the appropriate management of borderline atypia as well as mild and even moderate dysplasia.
3. The number of equivocal Pap smear results by far exceeds the number of women with clinically relevant disease.

Pap smears classified as high-grade neoplasia are associated with CIN 2/3 in most cases and therefore should be referred to colposcopy immediately. However, between 6% and 7% of the estimated 50 million Pap smears taken each year in the USA are reported as abnormal; however, the majority of the approximately three million women will be diagnosed with equivocal cytological abnormalities (atypical squamous cells of undetermined significance = ASCUS) and low-grade squamous intraepithelial lesions (LSIL). In thc USA, $2.5 billion are spent on the management of ASCUS per year which exceeds the cost of treating all women with high-grade neoplasia. Although equivalent data are missing from some countries, it is reasonable to assume that the situation in most member states of the European community is similar.

Importantly, participants in screening programmes expect results either to exclude disease by normal findings or to prove the presence of disease by atypical findings. Equivocal results are not readily understood and are often perceived as cancer until proven otherwise. Equivocal Pap smears can therefore cause in the women involved severe psychological stress and significant costs in the absence of appropriate counselling and management strategies.

Any effective management strategy of equivocal cytology needs to address the heterogeneity of epithelial changes that may result in borderline atypia, the high rate of spontaneous remission of these minor cellular changes and finally the increased risk of underlying high-grade neoplasia that accompanies this result. Kinney and colleagues demonstrated that the majority of histologically confirmed high-grade neoplasia was not diagnosed as high-grade lesion on cytology [59]. Rather, approximately 2/3 of high-grade neoplasia was classified as either ASCUS or LSIL on cytology. Other investigators confirmed that an equivocal result corresponds to a greater than background risk for incident or prevalent invasive cervical carcinoma.

For the attending clinician, the problem associated with equivocal cytology is to efficiently identify the minority of women with either prevalent CIN 3/cancer or a high risk of developing them during follow-up. Therefore, to be clinically useful, any management strategy for equivocal Pap smears must be able to assist with the identification of women with underlying disease while not unduly increasing either patient stress or patient management costs. The currently available options are repeat Pap smear, immediate colposcopy or HPV testing. Other options are under investigation and these include microsatellite instability, $p16^{INK4a}$ and telomerase immunostaining.

35.4.3.1 Repeat Pap Smear

Theoretically, equivocal Pap smears without neoplasia should return to normal cytology on follow-up, while those with underlying high-grade neoplasia should result either in persisting equivocal or obviously atypical smears when controlled by repeat cytology 3–6 months after the initial Pap smear. If this were true, then repeat cytology would be an inexpensive and attractive option for secondary screening, but most studies have found high rates of false positives and negatives together with persisting equivocal results for women without colposcopically identifiable neoplasia. A number of studies have looked at the performance of repeat cytology for the follow-up of women with equivocal Pap smears and the sensitivity rate for the detection of underlying clinically relevant disease was in the range of 60–85% together with specificities in the range of 77–96% [41, 60, 61].

One option to achieve a reduction of equivocal cytology findings is the implementation of stricter definitions of borderline atypia that resets very mild cellular changes in the category 'normal'. However, as high-grade disease may underlie even minimal cellular changes, such an approach will increase the overall false-negative rate of cytology within the mass screening. The magnitude of reduction of equivocal cytology by stricter definitions will correlate with the increase of false-negative smears [62].

35.4.3.2 Colposcopy

Colposcopy with histological assessment by directed punch biopsies is the gold standard procedure for the evaluation of cytological diagnoses of high-grade neoplasia and for the further investigation of persistent LSIL in North America and some, but not all member states of the European Community. However, referral to colposcopy is associated with anxiety in a reasonable proportion of patients and the method is relatively expensive. To reduce the number of referrals to colposcopy among women with equivocal smears, a second or more tests are used to identify women with underlying high-grade neoplasia. The process to screen again an already screened group of individuals is defined either as secondary screening or triaging.

Cervicography, repeat Pap smear, HPV-testing, HPV-DNA-integration, aneuploidy measuring, Polar Probe, immunohistochemistry to detect p16 or other potential markers of cervical neoplasia are methods that were used and evaluated in the triage of equivocal cytology.

35.4.3.3 HPV-DNA Testing

Genital HPV types are very common among young women although the majority of these infections are transient and will resolve spontaneously within 2 years. Only persisting HPV infections are capable to induce the transforming steps within the host cell that may finally lead to carcinogenesis.

HPV-DNA is a unique risk marker as its absence virtually excludes any risk of developing high-grade pre-invasive and invasive cervical neoplasia, because HR-HPV negative individuals lack the necessary cause of this disease. As such, HR-HPV testing has been established for the triage of women with equivocal cytology on the basis that those testing negative are at virtually no risk of having underlying clinically relevant lesions and could be returned to routine screening pool, while those testing positive could be referred to colposcopy for further follow-up.

A number of trials compared the efficacy of HPV testing and repeat Pap smear for the triage of women with equivocal smears.

The ASCUS/LSIL Triage Study (ALTS) was a multicentre, randomised trial that compared three different management strategies to detect underlying CIN3 among 3,488 women with a diagnosis of ASCUS:

1. Immediate colposcopy
2. Triaging for colposcopy based on HPV-testing (HC-2) and thin layer cytology
3. Triaging for colposcopy based on repeat cytology alone

The highest number of underlying CIN3 was detected in the HR-HPV testing arm ($n=77$) followed by 59 cases in the immediate colposcopy arm and 44 cases among women with conservative (repeat Pap smear) management. Compared to immediate colposcopy, triaging based on HPV testing reduced the number of referrals to colposcopy by 44%. Overall, the sensitivity of HR-HPV testing for CIN 3 was 96.3%, while repeat Pap smears showed a sensitivity of 44.1% for HSIL+, 64.0% for LSIL and 85.3% for ASCUS+cytology [41].

Based on the ALTS-trial findings as well as on the meta-analysis of five more published trials on the management of women with ASCUS, the ASCCP Consensus Conference in Bethesda recommended in 2001 and 2006: "A program of repeat cervical cytological testing, colposcopy, or DNA testing for high-risk types of HPV are all acceptable methods for managing women with ASC-US (rating A1). When liquid-based cytology is used or when co-collection for HPV DNA testing can be done, reflex HPV DNA testing is the preferred approach"[63, 64]. The consensus recommendation for ASC-H (atypical squamous cells, high-grade lesion cannot be ruled out) was immediate colposcopy.

The efficacy of HPV testing depends on a number of factors that vary between different health systems. The 44% reduction in colposcopy numbers seen in the ALTS trial saves money in the US health system with its high cost of colposcopy, but to make up for the cost of HPV testing, a larger reduction may be needed in most European countries.

However, in a primary screening trial in Germany, 167 out of 8,101 (2.1%) participants had equivocal (Pap IIw) smears. This number is far lower than that seen in the ALTS trial and the Pap IIw category is not a direct correlate of ASCUS. This view is supported by the prevalence of HR-HPV in the Pap IIw category which was only 10.8% as compared with an HR-HPV prevalence of 56% in the ASCUS category in the ALTS trial. No cases were observed among 149 (89.2%) women with equivocal smears and a negative HPV test result and all women with underlying CIN2/3 were HR-HPV positive [62]. Importantly, this indicates that over three fourth of the women in Germany with a Pap IIw result would be HR-HPV-negative and could be returned to routine screening without further follow-up. It is likely that HPV testing would be able to provide a positive cost benefit within the German healthcare system while providing a substantial degree of reassurance for the vast majority of women with an equivocal Pap smear [65].

It is important to note that the German trial was restricted to women over the age of 30 and this is likely to be one reason for the lower prevalence of HR-HPV compared to the ALTS trial. However, regardless of the prevalence of HPV in the respective populations, the negative predictive value of HPV testing in both studies was virtually identical and this characteristic of HPV testing appears to be independent of age (Fig. 35.11).

35.5 Therapy

35.5.1 Therapy of CIN

35.5.1.1 Conservative Treatment

In case of satisfactory colposcopy, a biopsy-proven CIN1 can be followed without invasive treatment. The rate of spontaneous regression is high (50–80%), especially in young women. In some countries, even CIN2 lesions can be followed conservatively for 6–12 months.

During pregnancy, invasive treatment of any grade of CIN should be postponed until 2 months after delivery. Invasive disease must be excluded by colposcopy. If biopsies need to be taken at the 18th week of gestation or later in pregnancy, loop biopsies are more appropriate than standard punch biopsies to get a histological specimen with sufficient stroma. When invasive cancer can be excluded with high reliability, the remaining risk for CIN3 lesions to progress to malignancy during pregnancy is very small, while the foetal and maternal risks related to invasive treatment of the cervix are high and complete excision of lesions cannot be achieved in almost half of the cases [21].

35.5.1.2 Surgical Treatment

Surgical treatment of CIN3 is an accepted standard of care with conization and loop electric excisional

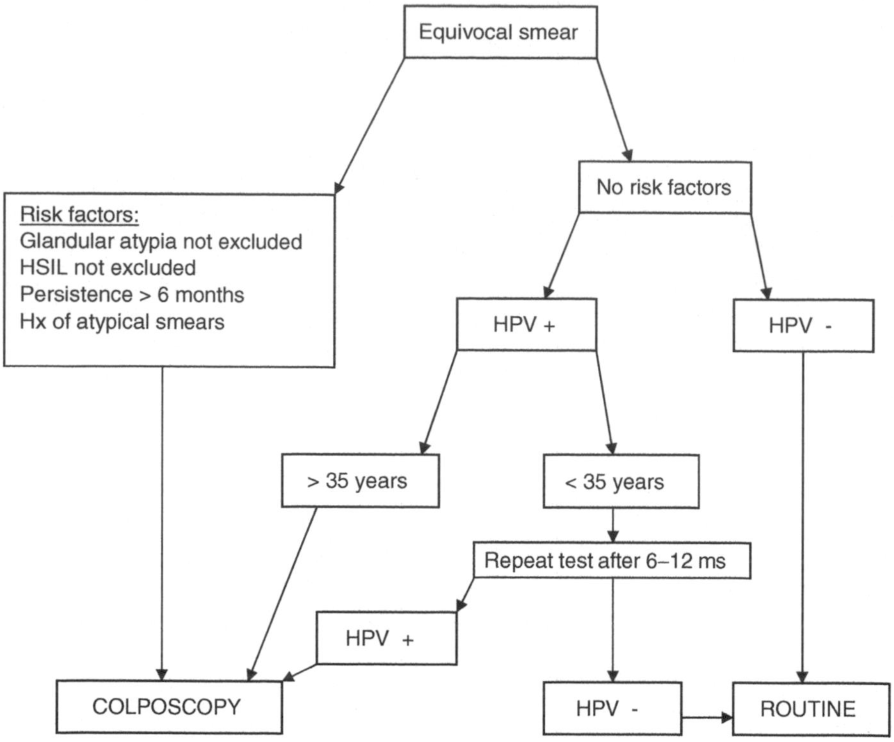

Fig. 35.11 Management of equivocal smears

procedure (LEEP) being the most common surgical method. In many countries, invasive treatment is obligatory for CIN2 and CIN3, although the risk of progression to invasive disease is low in CIN2 and many CIN2 lesions will regress spontaneously in younger women.

The primary goal in the management of CIN 2/3 is to prevent the development of invasive cancer by complete surgical destruction of all neoplastic tissue. To achieve this with as little loss of cervical function as possible is an important secondary goal.

The healthy uterine cervix protects the uterine and abdominal cavities from ascending infections and plays an important role in the regulation of fertility and during pregnancy. As the mean age of women with CIN 3 is around 30 years in most populations, destructive therapy of the cervix may affect fertility and increase the number of abortions, premature labour and perinatal mortality in following pregnancies [25, 66].

Colposcopy is the single method to identify the exact topography of cervical lesions and thus plays a crucial role in selecting the appropriate surgical treatment of individual CIN 3. The target host cells of primary human papillomavirus infection are the basal cells which are exposed superficially along the squamo-columnar junction. This explains the long-known observation that almost all high-grade neoplasias are located within the transformation zone and that the maximum findings are typically adjacent to the junction. To achieve high cure rates in the treatment of pre-malignant disease of the cervix, it is necessary to destroy the complete transformation zone and any neighbouring lesions. As the extension of individual CIN3 lesions and transformation zones differ significantly, colposcopically guided surgical treatment will remove neoplastic tissue with high accuracy and avoid unnecessary destruction of neighbouring healthy tissue.

35.5.1.3 Principals of Surgery: Recommended Primary Treatment

Any method of treatment of CIN 3 carries a small risk of the subsequent development of invasive cancer. Although this event appears to occur as frequently after excisional treatment with cold knife-, needle-, laser-cone biopsy or large loop excision of the transformation zone (LLETZ) as after destructive therapy using laser vaporization, electrocoagulation diathermy, cryotherapy or cold coagulation, excisional methods are the standard treatment of CIN because of the better histological evaluation [67, 68]. The use of destructive techniques should be applied only for extended and multifocal lesions.

No single excisional method could ever prove superior cure rates in randomized multicentre trials and the multiple smaller observational or single centre studies differ significantly in study design and do not allow for a general recommendation of one method of surgical treatment of CIN 3. But it is possible to recommend the best surgical method for each individual CIN 3 based on the colposcopical categorization of the transformation zone and the evidence-based risk/benefit profile of available surgical methods.

Surgical treatment of CIN requires the complete removal of the transformation zone (TZ). The International Society for Colposcopy defined three different types of TZ:

Type 1 The TZ is completely located on the ectocervix
Type 2 The TZ extends into the endocervical canal, but the upper border is visible on colposcopy
Type 3 The TZ extends into the endocervix and the upper border is not visible on colposcopy

In all types of TZ, the ectocervical or vaginal border of the lesion, and in types 1 and 2, even the endocervical can be identified by colposcopy. To achieve a full thickness resection of a type 1 TZ with clear basal margins, the cutting depth for the external os must be 8 mm while 5 mm may be sufficient for the periphery of the TZ.

Large loop excision of the transformation zone (LLETZ) [69] is the best suited treatment for CIN located in TZ type 1 and 2. The loops are tailored for an optimal bowl-like resection of the TZ. The cutting effect is achieved by light arches that spark between the 0.2 mm thin wire and the tissue. Modern high-frequency generators regulate electronically the needed optimal cutting currency. Properly performed LLETZ causes only minimal thermonecrosis; the obtained samples allow a full histopathological review. The out-patient procedure is safe, easy, can be done under local anaesthesia, and causes little bleeding and complications. TZ type 1 and TZ type 2 with minimal extension to the endocervix can be resected completely with a loop in one piece. TZ type 2 that extend 7–10 mm into the endocervix may require a second resection of the adjacent canal with a smaller loop to achieve clear endocervical margins.

For a complete excision of type 3 TZs, the relatively flat 5–7 mm ectocervical TZ and the endocervical canal involved must be resected. The form of the correctly removed sample resembles more that of a hat or an Indian pagode than a cone. Although a complete resection can be achieved with all excisional methods, laser- or needleconization are the recommended methods of treatment. Cold-knife conization of type 3 TZ has the disadvantages that it should be done under general anaesthesia, is an in-patient procedure and causes significantly more bleeding and scarring than laser- or needleconization [70, 71]. Loops are not designed for the removal of type 3 TZ. Either very large loops with 20–25 mm diameter need to be used which will unnecessarily remove not involved tissue of the cervical stroma or the excision will be done in multiple pieces. Frequently, a histological evaluation of such specimens is difficult. Furthermore, deep endocervical resection causes reasonable bleeding and precise cutting with a loop will not be possible in some circumstances.

Laser- and needleconization are out-patient treatments and may be done under local anaesthesia and colposcopic guidance. The cones obtained show almost no thermonecrosis and do not disturb histological assessment. As the equipment for needleconization is much cheaper than for laserconization, it is very likely that it will become the standard treatment of CIN 3 located in type3 TZ in most places.

Following the resection of the transformation zone by any of the above-mentioned excisional and destructive methods, residual endocervical disease needs to be excluded either by endocervical curettage or brush. Haemostasis can be achieved by application of Monsell´s solution onto the wound surface.

35.5.2 Therapy of VIN

The ISSVD proposed to use the term vulvar intraepithelial neoplasia only for high-grade lesions and to group the former VIN1 together with HPV infection and reactive changes. This move is based on the observation that there is no evidence that an isolated VIN1 carries an increased risk for progression to malignancy. The corresponding risk of progression in VIN2 is very low too. Therefore, the standard of care is an observational management.

VIN3 lesions are true precursors of SCC of the vulva. Even under adequate treatment, the risk of malignant progression is high; 9% of VIN3 will progress to invasive disease within 12 months and 3% of patients will develop cancer of the vulva following operative therapy of VIN3. Although Imiquimod proved to be a safe and effective treatment of VIN3 in one placebo-controlled trial [72], state-of-the-art treatment is still either excisional or destructive therapy. Clinical lesions of the haired skin of the vulva may involve hair follicles or glands. Wide excision of the full thickness skin with free margins is the standard of care. However, in cases of extended or multilocal disease, excisional treatment will result in severe mutilation. CO2 laser vaporization still has a place as an adjunct to surgery especially in young women to limit surgical damage. It is especially useful to treat peri-urethral and peri-clitoral VIN3 lesions. Colposcopically guided superficial laser excision has the advantages of laser vaporisation and offers the possibility of a specimen for histological examination but is a relatively difficult technique.

The risk of recurrent disease after any kind of treatment is high. The management of multilocal VIN3 lesions is a challenging search for the best individual concept with the need to balance the danger of unnecessary mutilation with the risk of development of invasive disease. Patients should be transferred to specialised clinics with a sufficient expertise.

35.5.3 Therapy of VaIN

35.5.3.1 Conservative Management

Low-grade neoplasia (VaIN1) has a low risk of progression and a high rate of spontaneous regression. Conservative management with colposcopic follow-up every 6–12 months is therefore recommended when high-grade lesions are excluded.

35.5.3.2 Surgical Treatment

Destructive or excisional therapy is the standard treatment of high-grade neoplasia. We prefer carbon dioxide laser vaporisation in younger women when invasive disease is excluded. A 2–3 mm depth of destruction is usually sufficient because vaginal tissue lacks adjacent glands and hair follicles. In women who underwent hysterectomy and suffer from high-grade neoplasia of the vaginal vault as well as in cases when invasive disease is not excluded, we recommend a colposcopically guided excision of the entire lesion to allow for a histological assessment of the basal resection margin and for exclusion of invasive growth.

Women with CIN who underwent hysterectomy are at increased risk of developing invasive cancer of the vaginal vault. Some of these tumours may develop from intraepithelial neoplasia of the vaginal surface epithelium, but in other cases, tumour growth will start in the scar under intact epithelium. Typically, these squamous cell cancers develop in the left or right corner of the scar after abdominal hysterectomy when VaIN lesions were buried under scar tissue due to deep stitching of the vagina (see Fig. 35.12). Correct suturing of the vaginal stroma will leave the squamous epithelium completely at the vaginal surface and allow for colposcopic detection and treatment of VaIN before invasive cancer can develop.

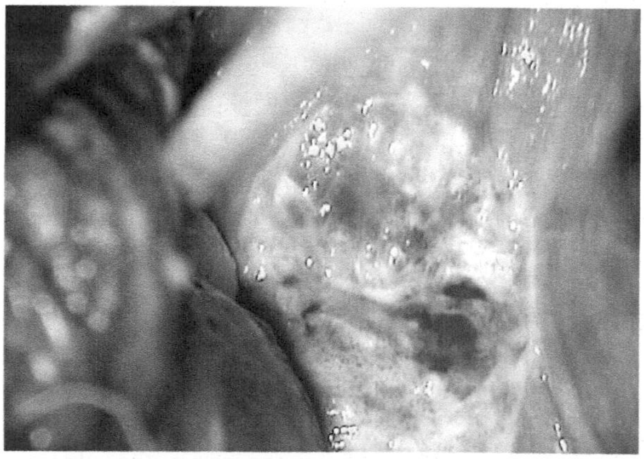

Fig. 35.12 Cancer of the vaginal vault 8 years after abdominal hysterectomy because of CIN3. The complete diameter of the tumour is 4 cm, the bulk of disease is situated in the deeper part of the scar, only a small ulcer penetrated into vaginal cavity

Take-Home Pearls

- HPV is the cause of all CIN3 and almost all cervical cancers.
- HPV is linked only to one entity of squamous cell cancer of the vulva.
- HPV-negative and HPV-positive cancers of the vulva show different clinical and histological figures and risk factors.
- HPV vaccination prevents the complete cycle of carcinogenesis.
- Screening interrupts the cycle of carcinogenesis by detecting and treating precursors.
- HPV screening is significantly more sensitive in detecting CIN3/cancer.
- HPV screening is significantly more efficient in reducing cervical cancer incidence and mortality.
- The diagnosis of VaIN, CIN and the majority of VIN is based on colposcopy with biopsies.
- Triaging of borderline atypia with HPV-testing became a standard of care.
- HPV-vaccination and screening provide complete protection from cervical cancer and a significant reduction in other HPV-related cancers.
- For CIN3, the standard of therapy is the resection of the entire transformation zone.
- CIN2 lesions can be managed conservatively in younger women, but should undergo surgical treatment in women who are 30 years or older.
- CIN1, VaIN1 and VIN1 have a very low risk of progression and should be managed conservatively.
- The standard of care in high-grade VaIN and VIN is surgical treatment. Distinct unifocal lesion should be excised with clear margins. Multifocal disease should be transferred to specialized clinics.

References

1. Ferenczy, A., Winkler, B.: Cervical intraepithelial neoplasia. In: Kurman, R. (ed.) Blaustein´s Pathology of the Female Genital Tract, 3rd edn, pp. 184–191. Springer Verlag, New York (1987). Ref ID: 389
2. Siebert, U., Sroczynski, G., Hillemanns, P., Engel, J., Stabenow, R., Stegmaier, C., et al.: The German cervical cancer screening model: development and validation of a decision-analytic model for cervical cancer screening in Germany. Eur. J. Public Health **16**(2), 185–192 (2006 April). Ref ID: 416
3. Dürst, M., Gissmann, L., Ikenberg, H., zur Hausen, H.: A papillomavirus DNA from a cervical carcinoma and its prevalence in cancer biopsy samples from different geographic regions. Proc. Natl Acad. Sci. USA **80**, 3812–3815 (1983). Ref ID: 65
4. Vousden, K.H.: Interactions between papillomavirus proteins and tumor suppressor gene products. Adv. Cancer Res. **64**, 1–24 (1994). Ref ID: 181
5. Crook, T., Vousden, K.H.: HPV oncoprotein function. In: Lacey, C. (ed.) Papillomavirus Reviews: Current Research on Papillomaviruses, 1st edn, pp. 55–60. Leeds University Press, Leeds, UK (1996). Ref ID: 182
6. Walboomers, J.M.M., Jacobs, M.V., Manos, M.M., Bosch, F.X., Kummer, J.A., Shah, K.V., et al.: Human Papillomavirus is a necessary cause of invasive cervical cancer worldwide. J. Pathol. **189**, 12–19 (1999). Ref ID: 69
7. Böhmer, G., van den Brule, A.J., Brummer, O., Meijer, C.J., Petry, K.U.: No confirmed case of human papillomavirus DNA negative cervical intraepithelial neoplasia grade III (CIN 3) or invasive primary cancer of the uterine cervix among 511 patients. Am. J. Obstet. Gynecol. **189**, 118–120 (2003). Ref ID: 360
8. Harper, D.M., Franco, E.L., Wheeler, C.M., Moscicki, A.B., Romanowski, B., Roteli-Martins, C.M., et al.: Sustained efficacy up to 4.5 years of a bivalent L1 virus-like particle vaccine against human papillomavirus types 16 and 18: follow-up from a randomised control trial. Lancet **367**, 1247–1255 (2006). Ref ID: 384
9. Group, F.I.S.: Quadrivalent vaccine against human papillomavirus to prevent high-grade cervical lesions. N Engl J. Med. **356**(19), 1915–1927 (2007). Ref ID: 403
10. Ho, G.Y.F., Bierman, R., Beardsley, L., Chang, C.J., Burk, R.D.: Natural history of cervicovaginal papillomavirus infection in young women. N Engl J. Med. **338**, 423–428 (1998). Ref ID: 77
11. Moreno, V., Bosch, F.X., Munoz, N., Meijer, C.J., Shah, K.V., Walboomers, J.M.M., et al.: Effect of oral contraceptives on risk of cervical cancer in women with human papillomavirus infection: the IARC multicentric case-control study. Lancet **359**, 1085–1092 (2002). Ref ID: 374
12. Munoz, N., Franceschi, S., Bosetti, C., Moreno, V., Herrero, R., Smith, J.S., et al.: Role of parity and human papillomavirus in cervical cancer: the IARC multicentris case-control study. Lancet **359**, 1093–1101 (2002). Ref ID: 373
13. Petry, K.U., Scheffel, D., Bode, U., Gabrysiak, T., Köchel, H., Kupsch, E., et al.: Cellular immunodeficiency enhances the progression of human papillomavirus-associated cervical lesions. Int. J. Cancer **57**, 836–840 (1994). Ref ID: 218
14. Khan, M.J., Castle, P.E., Lorincz, A., Wacholder, S., Sherman, M., Scott, D.R., et al.: The elevated 10-year risk of cervical precancer and cancer in women with human papillomavirus (HPV) Type 16 or 18 and the possible utility of type-specific hpv testing in clinical practice. J. Natl Cancer Inst. **97**, 1072–1079 (2005). Ref ID: 396
15. Kjaer, S.K., Hogdall, E., Frederiksen, K., Munk, C., van den Brule, A.J., Svare, E., et al.: The absolute risk of cervical abnormalities in high-risk human papillomavirus-positive,

cytologically normal women over a 10-year period. Cancer Res. **66**(21), 10630–10636 (2006). Ref ID: 390

16. Petry, K.U., Böhmer, G., Iftner, T., Davies, P., Brummer, O., Kühnle, H.: Factors associated with an increased risk of prevalent and incident grade III cervical intraepithelial neoplasia and invasive cervical cancer among women with Papanicolaou tests classified as grades I or II cervical intraepithelial neoplasia. Am. J. Obstet. Gynecol. **186**, 28–34 (2002). Ref ID: 332
17. Williams, J.: Cancer of the Uterus: Harveian Lectures for 1886. London: H.K. Lewis; 1888. Ref ID: 42
18. Östör, A.G.: Natural history of cervical intraepithelial neoplasia: a critical review. Int. J. Gynecol. Pathol. **12**(2), 186–192 (1993). Ref ID: 361
19. Brummer, O., Stegner, H.E., Bohmer, G., Kuhnle, H., Petry, K.U.: HER-2/neu expression in Paget disease of the vulva and the female breast. Gynecol. Oncol. **95**(2), 336–340 (2004 November). Ref ID: 413
20. Magnusson, P.K.E., Sparen, P., Gyllenstein, U.B.: Genetic link to cervical tumours. Nature **400**, 29–30 (1999). Ref ID: 365
21. Silverman, M.H., Hedley, M.L., Petry, K.U., Weber, J.S.: Clinical trials in cervical intraepithelial neoplasia: balancing the need for efficacy data with patient safety. J. Low. Genit. Tract Dis. **6**(4), 206–211 (2002 October). Ref ID: 419
22. McCredie, M.R., Sharples, K.J., Paul, C., Baranyai, J., Medley, G., Jones, R.W., et al.: Natural history of cervical neoplasia and risk of invasive cancer in women with cervical intraepithelial neoplasia 3: a retrospective cohort study. Lancet Oncol. **9**(5), 425–434 (2008 May). Ref ID: 418
23. Liebrich, C., Brummer, O., von Wasielewski, R., et al.: Primary cervical cancer truly negative for high-risk human papillomavirus is a rare but distinct entity that can affect virgins and young adolescents, Eur. J. Gynaecol. Oncol. **30**, 45–48 (2009).
24. TOMBOLA Group: Biopsy and selective Biopsy and selective recall compared with immediate large loop excision in management of women with low grade abnormal cervical cytology referred for colposcopy: multicentre randomised controlled trial. BMJ 2009;339:b2548. Ref ID: 59
25. Arbyn, M., Kyrgiou, M., Simoens, C., Raifu, A.O., Koliopoulos, G., Martin-Hirsch, P., et al.: Perinatal mortality and other severe adverse pregnancy outcomes associated with treatment of cervical intraepithelial neoplasia: meta-analysis. BMJ **337**, a1284 (2008). Ref ID: 433
26. Ansink, A.C., Krul, M.R.L., De Weger, R.A., Kleyne, J.A.F.W., Pijpers, H., Van Tinteren, H., et al.: Human Papillomavirus, lichen sclerosus, and squamous cell carcinoma of the vulva: detection and prognostic significance. Gynecol. Oncol. **52**, 180–184 (1994). Ref ID: 86
27. Petry, K.U., Köchel, H., Bode, U., Schedel, I., Niesert, S., Glaubitz, M., et al.: Human papillomavirus is associated with the frequent detection of warty and basaloid high-grade neoplasia of the vulva and cervical neoplasia among immunocompromised women. Gynecol. Oncol. **60**, 30–34 (1996). Ref ID: 295
28. De, V.H., Clifford, G.M., Nascimento, M.C., Madeleine, M.M., Franceschi, S.: Prevalence and type distribution of human papillomavirus in carcinoma and intraepithelial neoplasia of the vulva, vagina and anus: a meta-analysis. Int. J. Cancer **124**(7), 1626–1636 (2009 April 1). Ref ID: 452
29. Block, S.L., Nolan, T., Sattler, C., Barr, E., Giacoletti, E.D., Marchant, C.D., et al.: Comparison of the immunogenicity and reactogenicity of a prophylactic quadrivalent human papillomavirus (Types 6, 11, 16, 1nd 18) L1 virus-like particle vaccine in male and female adolescents and young adult women. Paediatrics **118**, 2135–2145 (2006). Ref ID: 395
30. Harper, D.M., Franco, E.L., Wheeler, C.M., et al.: Efficacy of a bivalent L1 virus-like particle vaccine in prevention of infection of human papillomavirus type 16 and 18 in young women: a randomised controlled trial. Lancet **364**, 1757–1765 (2004). Ref ID: 393
31. Garland, S.M., Hernandez-Avila, M., Wheeler, C.M., Perez, G., Harper, D.M., Leodolter, S., et al.: Quadrivalent vaccine against human papillomavirus to prevent anogenital diseases. N Engl J. Med. **356**(19), 1928–1943 (2007). Ref ID: 402
32. Hildesheim, A., Herrero, R., Wacholder, S., Rodriguez, A.C., Solomon, D., Bratti, C., et al.: Effect of human papillomavirus 16/18 l1 viruslike particle vaccine among young women with preexisting infection. JAMA **298**(7), 743–753 (2007). Ref ID: 400
33. Paavonen, J., Jenkins, D., Bosch, F.X., Naud, P., Salmeron, J., Wheeler, C.M. et al.: Efficacy of a prophylactic adjuvanted bivalent L1 virus-like-particle vaccine against infection with human papillomavirus types 16 and 18 in young women: an interim analysis of a phase III double-blind, randomised controlled trial. Lancet 2008;369(9580):2161–70; (9580):2161–70. Ref ID: 404.
34. Joura, E., Leodolter, S., Hernandez-Avila, M., Perez, G., Koutsky, L.A., Garland, S.M., et al.: Efficacy of a quadrivalent prophylactic human papillomavirus (types 6, 11, 16, and 18) L1 virus-like-particle vaccine against high-grade vulval and vaginal lesions: a combined analysis of three randomised clinical trials. Lancet **369**(9574), 1693–1702 (2008). Ref ID: 405
35. Paavonen, J., Naud, P., Salmeron, J., Wheeler, C.M., Chow, S.N., Apter, D., et al.: Efficacy of human papillomavirus (HPV)-16/18 AS04-adjuvanted vaccine against cervical infection and precancer caused by oncogenic HPV types (PATRICIA): final analysis of a double-blind, randomised study in young women. Lancet **374**(9686), 301–314 (2009 July 25). Ref ID: 431
36. Pathirana, D., Hillemanns, P., Petry, K.U., Becker, N., Brockmeyer, N.H., Erdmann, R., et al.: Short version of the German evidence-based guidelines for prophylactic vaccination against HPV-associated neoplasia. Vaccine **27**(34), 4551–4559 (2009 July 23). Ref ID: 436
37. Munoz, N., Manalastas Jr., R., Pitisuttithum, P., Tresukosol, D., Monsonego, J., Ault, K., et al.: Safety, immunogenicity, and efficacy of quadrivalent human papillomavirus (types 6, 11, 16, 18) recombinant vaccine in women aged 24–45 years: a randomised, double-blind trial. Lancet **373**(9679), 1949–1957 (2009 June 6). Ref ID: 448
38. Poppe, W.A.: Rates of HPV-16/18 persistent infection and associated cervical lesions in relation to initial serostatus in the control arm of the Patricia trial. EUROGIN 2010, Monte Carlo EP-7[17–20 FEB 2010]. 2010. Ref Type: Abstract Ref ID: 449.
39. Rowhani-Rahbar, A., Mao, C., Hughes, J.P., Alvarez, F.B., Bryan, J.T., Hawes, S.E., et al.: Longer term efficacy of a prophylactic monovalent human papillomavirus type 16 vaccine. Vaccine **27**(41), 5612–5619 (2009 September 18). Ref ID: 444

40. Petry, K.U., Breugelmans, J.G., Benard, S., Lamure, E., Littlewood, K.J., Hillemanns, P.: Cost of screening and treatment of cervical dyskaryosis in Germany. Eur. J. Gynaecol. Oncol. **29**(4), 345–349 (2008). Ref ID: 417
41. Solomon, D., Schiffman, M., Tarone, R.: Comparison of three management strategies for patients with atypical squamous cells of undetermined significance: baseline results from a randomized trial. J. Natl Cancer Inst. **93**, 293–299 (2001). Ref ID: 327
42. Jagu, S., Kwak, K., Garcea, R.L., Roden, R.B.: Vaccination with multimeric L2 fusion protein and L1 VLP or capsomeres to broaden protection against HPV infection. Vaccine **28**(28), 4478–4486 (2010 June 17). Ref ID: 454
43. Hildesheim, A., Hadjmichael, O., Schwartz, P., Wheeler, C.M., Barnes, W., Lowell, D.M., et al.: Risk factors for rapid onset cervical cancer. Am. J. Obstet. Gynecol. **180**, 571–577 (1999). Ref ID: 335
44. Kottmeier, H.L.: Evolution et traitment des epitheliomas. Rev. Fr. Gynec. Obstet. **56**, 821 (1961). Ref ID: 61
45. Koss, L.G., Stewart, F.W., Foote, F.W.: Some histological aspects of behaviour of epidermoid carcinoma in situ and related lesions of the uterine cervix. Cancer **16**, 1160–1164 (1963). Ref ID: 60
46. Kolstad, P., Klem, V.: Long-term follow-up of 1121 cases of carcinoma in situ. Obstet. Gynecol. **48**, 125 (1976). Ref ID: 58
47. Cuzick, J., Clavel, C., Petry, K.U., Meijer, C.J., Hoyer, H., Ratnam, S., et al.: Overview of the European and North American studies on HPV testing in primary cervical cancer screening. Int. J. Cancer **119**(5), 1095–1101 (2006). Ref ID: 388
48. Bulkmans, N.W., Berkhof, J., Rozendaal, L., van Kermenade, F.J., Boeke, A.J.P., Bulk, S., et al.: Human papillomavirus DNA testing for the detection of cervical intraepithelial neoplasia grade 3 and cancer: 5-year follow-up of a randomised controlled implementation trial. Lancet **370**, 1764–1772 (2007). Ref ID: 401
49. Mayrand, M.H., Duarte-Franco, E., Rodrigues, I., Walter, S.D., Hanley, J., Ferenczy, A., et al.: Human papillomavirus versus papanicolaou screening tests for cervical cancer. N Engl J. Med. **357**(16), 1579–1588 (2007). Ref ID: 407
50. Naucler, P., Ryd, W., Törnberg, S., Strand, A., Wadell, G., Elfgren, K., et al.: Human papillomavirus and papanicolaou tests to screen for cervical cancer. N Engl J. Med. **357**, 1589–1597 (2007). Ref ID: 410
51. Ronco, G., Giorgi-Rossi, P., Carozzi, F., Confortini, M., Palma, P.D., Del, M.A., et al.: Efficacy of human papillomavirus testing for the detection of invasive cervical cancers and cervical intraepithelial neoplasia: a randomised controlled trial. Lancet Oncol. **11**, 249–257 (2010 January 18). Ref ID: 441
52. Leinonen, M., Nieminen, P., Kotaniemi-Talonen, L., Malila, N., Tarkkanen, J., Laurila, P., et al.: Age-specific evaluation of primary human papillomavirus screening vs conventional cytology in a randomized setting. J. Natl Cancer Inst. **101**(23), 1612–1623 (2009 December 2). Ref ID: 442
53. Kitchener, H.C., Almonte, M., Thomson, C., Wheeler, P., Sargent, A., Stoykova, B., et al.: HPV testing in combination with liquid-based cytology in primary cervical screening (ARTISTIC): a randomised controlled trial. Lancet Oncol. **10**(7), 672–682 (2009 July). Ref ID: 451
54. Schiffman, M., Wheeler, C.M., Dasgupta, A., Solomon, D., Castle, P.E.: A comparison of a prototype PCR assay and hybrid capture 2 for detection of carcinogenic human papillomavirus DNA in women with equivocal or mildly abnormal papanicolaou smears. Am. J. Clin. Pathol. **124**, 722–732 (2005). Ref ID: 406
55. Luyten, A., Theiler, K.G., Pietralla, M., Braun, B.E., Reinecke-Lüthge, A., Petry, K.U.: Primary HPV screening in Wolfsburg, German. Experience of 18 months. Geburtshilfe Frauenheilkd 2008;68:1–6. Ref ID: 421.
56. Richart, R.M., Wright, T.C.: Controversies in the management of low-grade cervical intraepithelial neoplasia. Cancer **71**, 1413–1421 (1993). Ref ID: 16
57. Singer, A.: Screening for CIN. In: Monsonego, J. (ed.) Screening for Cervical Cancer. For Whom, Why and How? pp. 54–57. (1994). Ref ID: 132
58. Soutter, W.P., Fletcher, A.: Invasive cancer of the cervix in women with mild dyskaryosis followed up cytologically. BMJ **308**, 1421–1423 (1994). Ref ID: 1
59. Kinney, W.K., Manos, M.M., Hurley, L.B., Ransley, J.E.: Where´s the high-grade cervical neoplasia? The importance of minimally abnormal Papanicolaou diagnoses. Obstet. Gynecol. **91**(973), 976 (1998). Ref ID: 320
60. Cox, J.T., Lörincz, A., Schiffman, M.H., Sherman, M., Cullen, A., Kurman, R.J.: Human paillomavirus testing by hybrid capture appears to be useful in triaging women with a cytologic diagnosis of atypical squamous cells of undetermined significance. Am. J. Obstet. Gynecol. **172**, 946–954 (1995). Ref ID: 117
61. Manos, M.M., Kinney, W.K., Hurley, L.B., Sherman, M., Shieh-Ngai, J., Kurman, R., et al.: Identifying women with cervical neoplasia. JAMA **281**(17), 1605–1610 (1999). Ref ID: 262
62. Petry, K.U., Menton, S., Menton, M., van Lonen-Frosch, F., de Carvalho Gomes, H., Holz, B., et al.: Inclusion of HPV testing in routine cervical cancer screening for women above 29 years in Germany: results for 8466 patients. Br. J. Cancer **88**, 1570–1577 (2003). Ref ID: 333
63. Wright, T.C., Cox, J.T., Massad, L.S., Twiggs, L.B., Wilkinson, E.J.: 2001 consensus guidelines for the management of women with cervical cytological abnormalities. JAMA **287**(16), 2120–2129 (2002). Ref ID: 312
64. Wright Jr., T.C., Massad, L.S., Dunton, C.J., Spitzer, M., Wilkinson, E.J., Solomon, D.: 2006 consensus guidelines for the management of women with abnormal cervical cancer screening tests. Am. J. Obstet. Gynecol. **197**(4), 346–355 (2007 October). Ref ID: 453
65. Sheriff, S.K., Petry, K.U., Ikenberg, H., Crouse, G., Mazonson, P.D., Santas, C.C.: An economic analysis of human papillomavirus triage for the management of women with atypical and abnormal Pap smear results in Germany. Eur. J. Health Econ. **8**(2), 153–160 (2007 June). Ref ID: 411
66. Kyrgiou, M., Koliopoulos, G., Martin-Hirsch, P., Arbyn, M., Prendiville, W., Paraskevaidis, E.: Obstetrics outcomes after conservative treatment for intraepithelial or early invasive cervical lesions: systematic review and meta-analysis. Lancet **367**, 489–498 (2006). Ref ID: 382
67. Bigrigg, A., Haffenden, D.K., Sheehan, A.L., Codling, B.W., Read, M.D.: Eficacy and safety of the large-loop excision of the transformation zone. Lancet **343**, 32–34 (1994). Ref ID: 103
68. Kennedy, A.W., Belinson, J.L., Wirth, S., Taylor, J.: The role of the loop electrosurgical excision procedure in the

diagnosis and management of early invasive cervical cancer. Int. J. Gynecol. Cancer **5**, 117–120 (1995). Ref ID: 104
69. Prendiville, W., Cullimore, J., Norman, S.: Large loop excision of the transformation zone (LLETZ). A new method of management for women with cervical neoplasia. Br. J. Obstet. Gynaecol. **96**, 1054 (1989). Ref ID: 362
70. Mathevet, P., Dargent, D., Roy, M., Beau, G.: A randomized prospective study comparing three techniques of conization: cold knife, laser, and LEEP. Gynecol. Oncol. **54**, 175–179 (1994). Ref ID: 106
71. Oyesanya, O.A., Amerasinghe, C.N., Manning, E.A.D.: Outpatient excisional management of cervical intraepithelial neoplasia. Am. J. Obstet. Gynecol. **168**, 485–488 (1993). Ref ID: 108
72. van Seters, M., van Beurden, M., ten Kate, F.J., Beckmann, I., Ewing, P.C., Eijkemans, M.J., et al.: Treatment of vulvar intraepithelial neoplasia with topical imiquimod. N Engl J. Med. **358**(14), 1465–1473 (2008 April 3). Ref ID: 412

Tumor Surgery–Cervical Cancer Treatment

36

Achim Schneider and Christhardt Köhler

Core Messages

> Today there is a broad spectrum of treatment modalities (surgery, radiotherapy, chemotherapy and combined approaches) available for patients with invasive cervical cancer. Knowledge of tumor stage, lymph node involvement and tumor extend to adjacent organs is essential to tailor appropriate therapy individually. Surgical staging, best done by laparoscopy, can exactly provide this information with minimal morbidity. Early stage cervical cancer can successfully be treated by radical hysterectomy. Laparoscopic and robotic-assisted techniques are beneficial for the patient with adequate oncologic outcome compared to open radical hysterectomy.

> In young patients with tumors less than 2 cm radical trachelectomy can be performed in order to preserve fertility.

> Locally advanced and/or nodal positive tumors should be treated by primary platinum-based chemoradiation. In stage IVa and in recurrent diseases individual therapy after interdisciplinary tumor board decision and careful counseling of the patient should be done. DFS and OS are the most important oncologic parameters in the treatment of cervical cancer patients, however, quality of life and possible side effects of various treatment modalities must be taken in consideration.

36.1 Introduction

Cervical cancer is the seventh most common malignancy among women in Western Europe comprising 3.5% of all new cancer cases and about 3% of all tumor-related deaths. Incidence rates vary worldwide between 3/100,000 women (Syria) and 94/100,000 women (Haiti) [1]. Germany has an incidence of 12/100,000 women. The number of new cases of cervical cancer decreased continuously from 9,200 to 6,400 between the years 1980 and 2002 [2] (Fig. 36.1). During the same period of time, deaths also decreased in Germany from 2,200 to 1,800. Worldwide, cervical cancer causes approximately 500,000 new cases and about 35,000 deaths each year, particularly in third world countries.

The mean age at diagnosis is 52 with age peaks at 35–39 and 60–64. Histologically, the majority of cases (80%) involve squamous cell carcinomas; 20% are adenocarcinomas. The pathogenetic role of the (high-risk) papilloma viruses in the development of cervical cancer is now regarded as proven and is the basis for new preventive vaccination strategies. Sexual and reproductive factors such as early first intercourse and numerous sexual partners are associated with an increased probability of HPV infection. Multiparae, women with a low socioeconomic status, and smokers have an increased risk of developing cervical cancer.

A. Schneider (✉) and C. Köhler
Department of Gynecology and Interdisciplinary Breast Center, Charité Universitätsmedizin Berlin, Charité Campus Mitte, Charitéplatz 1, D – 10117 Berlin, Germany
e-mail: achim.schneider@charite.de

G. Gross and S.K. Tyring (eds.), *Sexually Transmitted Infections and Sexually Transmitted Diseases*,
DOI: 10.1007/978-3-642-14663-3_36, © Springer-Verlag Berlin Heidelberg 2011

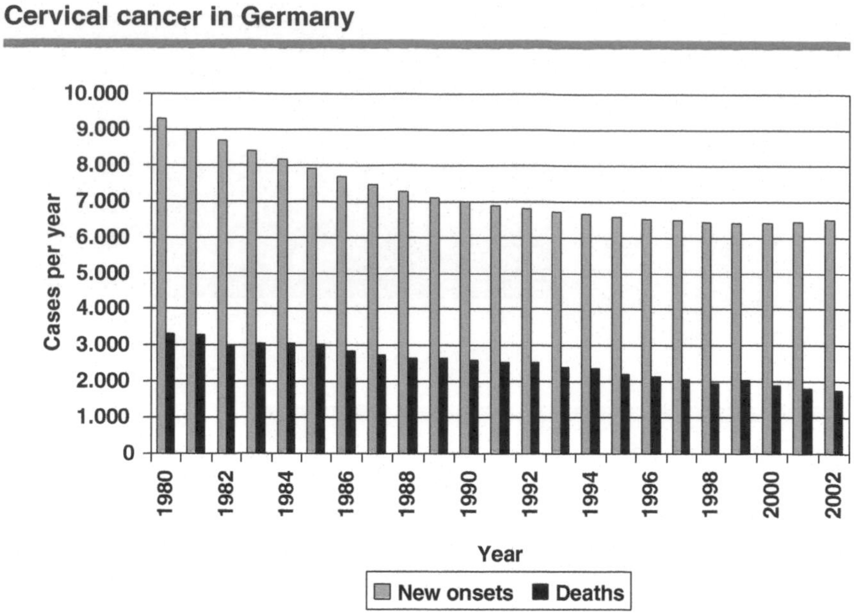

Fig. 36.1 Incidence and mortality of cervical cancer in Germany. Cases per year. New onsets – deaths. (Robert Koch Institute [new cases], Federal Statistical Office 2006 [deaths])

36.2 Diagnostics

Cervical cancer is thus far the only gynecological tumor that is clinically classified, which of course leads to a high rate (30–50%) of over- and underestimations of the tumor stage. The local tumor spread estimated by an experienced examiner for the FIGO classification cannot confirm or exclude intraabdominal tumor dissemination, tumor-invaded pelvic and/or para-aortic lymph nodes, or possible spread to adjacent organs (bladder, rectum).

36.2.1 Clinical Diagnostics

Clinical examination of the portio by endoscopy and colposcopy, palpation (vaginal and rectovaginal), possibly under anesthesia, and biopsy confirm the diagnosis of visible cancer and determine the tumor stage. Cytologically suspicious findings with no sign of a macroscopically recognizable tumor call for further clarification by endocervical curettage and, if necessary, conization with examination in serial sections. For the FIGO classification (Table 36.1), it is permissible to perform a cystoscopy and rectoscopy as well as an x-ray of the chest and efferent urinary ducts (i.v. urogram). Instead of excretory urography, renal ultrasound is usually performed to detect obstruction.

36.2.2 Tumor Markers

The tumor markers SCC (for squamous cell carcinoma) and CA 125 (for adenocarcinoma) are suitable for follow-up but not for primary diagnostics.

36.2.3 Imaging Diagnostics

Pelvic and para-aortic lymph nodes as well as the primary tumor size can be assessed by MRI, CT, PET, and ultrasound. The once frequently applied technique of lymph scintigraphy is now obsolete because of its low sensitivity [3].

CT is helpful for guided puncture of retroperitoneal structures. Since it cannot reliably detect microscopic lymph node invasion or distinguish between reactive and malignant lymph node enlargement, its sensitivity in the literature is only 12–72% for detecting lymph node metastases. It also has low sensitivity for detecting an invasion of adjacent organs [4].

Table 36.1 TNM and FIGO staging

TNM classification Tx	FIGO stages	Primary tumor cannot be assessed
T0		No evidence of primary tumor
Tis	0	Carcinoma in situ (preinvasive cancer)
T1	I	Cervical cancer confined to uterus (extension to corpus should be disregarded)
T1a	Ia	Invasive carcinoma diagnosed only by microscopy All macroscopically visible lesions – even with superficial invasion – are classified as T1b/stadium IB
T1a1	Ia1	Tumor with stromal invasion 3 mm or less in depth and 7 mm or less in maximum horizontal spread
T1a2	Ia2	Tumor with stromal invasion between 3 and 5 mm in depth and 7 mm or less in maximum horizontal spread
T1b	Ib	Clinically (macroscopically) visible lesion confined to the cervix or microscopic lesion > stage T IA2/1A2
T1b1	Ib1	Clinically (macroscopically) visible lesion 4 cm in maximum dimension
T1b2	Ib2	Clinically (macroscopically) visible lesions >4 cm in maximum dimension
T2	II	Cervical carcinoma infiltrated beyond the uterus but not to the pelvic wall or to the lower third of the vagina
T2a	IIa	Without infiltration of the parametrium
T2b	IIb	With infiltration of the parametrium
T3	III	Cervical carcinoma extends to the pelvic wall and/or invades the lower third of the vagina and/or causes hydronephrosis or nonfunctioning kidney
T3a	IIIa	Tumor invades lower third of the vagina, no extension to the pelvic wall
T3b	IIIb	Tumor extends to the pelvic wall and/or causes hydronephrosis or nonfunctioning kidney
T4	IVa	Tumor infiltrates bladder or rectal mucosa and/or extends beyond the true pelvis
M1	IVb	Distant metastases

MRI accurately demonstrates the primary tumor size with a significant correlation to the size measured in the surgical specimen. MRI is limited for assessing incipient infiltration of adjacent organs. Its detection sensitivity is 38–97% for parametric infiltration and 82–90% for vaginal infiltration. Problematic is the low sensitivity of 31–86% reported for MRI in detecting lymph node metastases, particularly micrometastases [4]. Transvaginal ultrasound can reliably evaluate the size of tumors limited to the cervix but is not suitable for estimating parametric infiltration, invasion of adjacent organs, or lymph node metastases.

PET can visualize tumor-invaded lymph nodes better than MRI (38–91% sensitivity), though here too the detection of micrometastases is problematic. PET is also more sensitive than MRI for detecting tumor recurrence. Altogether, it must be stressed that PET data partly derive from very small patient populations and therefore require further evaluation.

36.2.4 Surgical Staging

Only surgical staging (see below) enables the precise detection and histological confirmation of tumor spread, particularly the proof or exclusion of intraabdominal tumor dissemination, pelvic and/or para-aortic lymph node involvement, and invasion of adjacent organs. In the last 30 years, surgical staging of cervical cancer has been the topic of more than 40 publications, and the vast majority cast a positive or indifferent vote. Only three studies find no benefit from surgical staging, and one of them is also the only prospective randomized study [5]. Although this study in a small group of patients involves considerable methodological problems, its results nevertheless underscore the fact that no prospective study thus far has been able to demonstrate a survival advantage for surgical staging.

36.3 Surgical Strategies

Invasive cervical cancer is treated by surgery, radiotherapy, chemotherapy, or a combination of these procedures. Early tumor stages (IA2 to IIa/b) are usually treated by surgery, while advanced tumors are mostly managed by chemoradiation.

In surgical stages IB and II, surgery and irradiation basically yield the same long-term results with a different recurrence pattern and side-effect profile. This has been demonstrated in randomized studies [3]. Combining the two treatment modalities (surgery followed by adjuvant (chemo-)radiation or neoadjuvant tele-brachytherapy followed by radical hysterectomy) does not improve the oncological prognosis but significantly increases the complication rate [6].

Interdisciplinary treatment planning should be done by a team of pathologists, medical oncologists, radiotherapists, radiologists, and gynecologists. The histomorphological, clinical, and imaging findings are used to evaluate the disease extension, including prognostic factors, and to decide what procedure seems to be most suitable for the respective patient. Neoadjuvant and adjuvant treatment concepts should also be considered.

36.3.1 Surgical Staging with Debulking of Tumor-Invaded Lymph Nodes

Surgical staging comprises complete exploration of the abdominal cavity for peritoneal tumor dissemination, including Douglas lavage for cytological examination, para-aortic and pelvic lymphadenectomy, and inspection and dissection of the vesicocervical and rectovaginal septum, with biopsy if necessary (Figs. 36.2 and

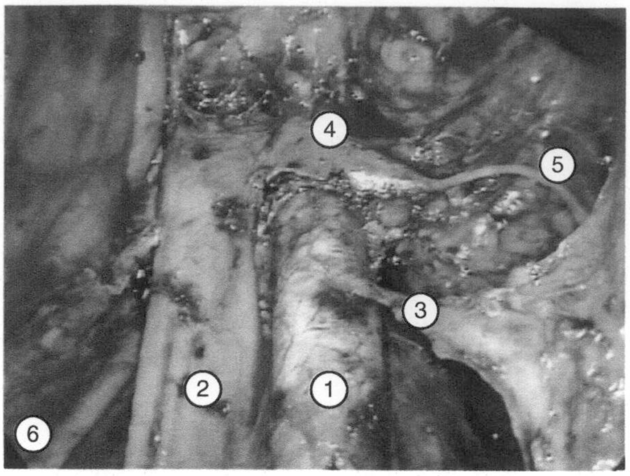

Fig. 36.2 Sites after laparoscopic transperitoneal infrarenal lymphadenectomy. Visualization of the abdominal aorta (*1*), inferior vena cava (*2*), inferior mesenteric artery (*3*), left renal vein (*4*), left ovarian vein (*5*), and right ureter (*6*)

36.3). Basically, staging (including lymphadenectomy) can be performed by transperitoneal or extraperitoneal laparotomy or laparoscopy. The oncological equivalence of laparoscopic and open lymphadenectomy has been demonstrated in a number of large retro- and prospective studies [7–9] (Fig. 36.4). Depending on the frozen section diagnosis of excised lymph nodes or biopsies, the further treatment concept can be established or modified intraoperatively in a single session or in two sessions.

A significant survival advantage has been retrospectively demonstrated for patients submitted to removal of

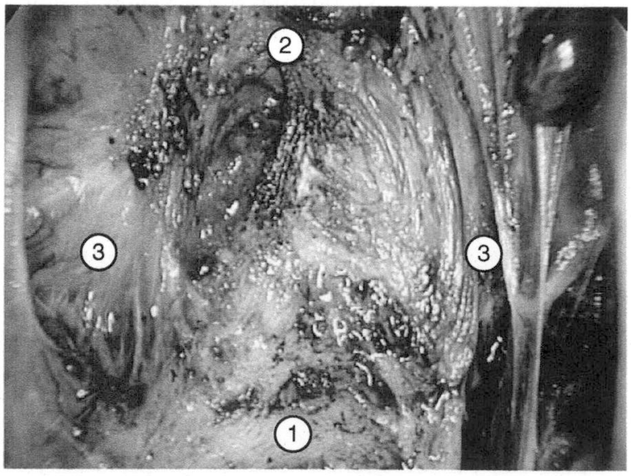

Fig. 36.3 Dissection of the vesicocervical and vesicovaginal septum for laparoscopic staging. Visualization of anterior cervical wall (*1*), posterior bladder wall (*2*), and both bladder pillars (*3*)

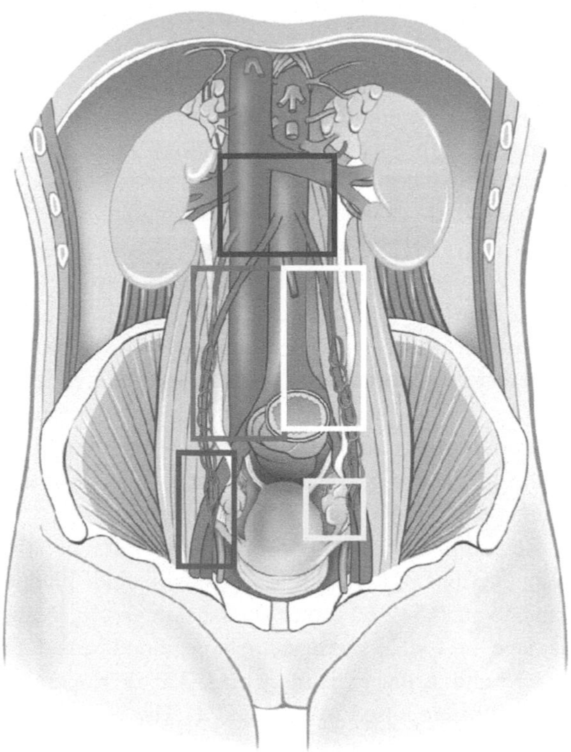

Fig. 36.4 Areas of laparoscopic lymphadenectomy (*red* = infrarenal; *green* = right paraaortic; *white* = left para-aortic inframesenteric; *violet* = pelvic; *yellow* = parametric)

tumor-invaded lymph nodes in terms of debulking and subsequent radiochemotherapy [10] (Fig. 36.5). The initiation of primary radiochemotherapy was not delayed due to minimal morbidity of laparoscopic staging.

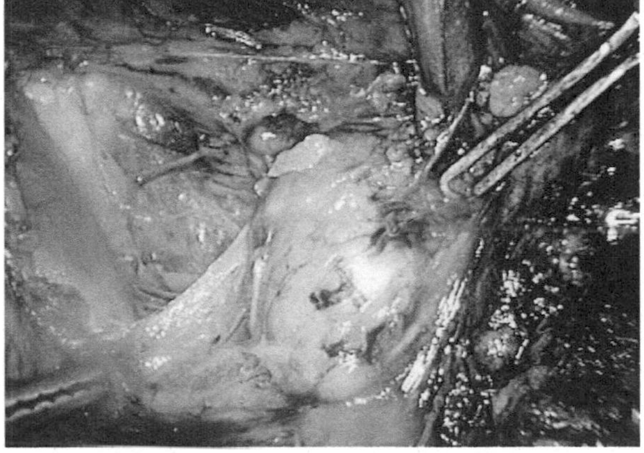

Fig. 36.5 Tumor-infiltrated left-pelvic lymph node

36.3.2 Radical Hysterectomy

Radical hysterectomy for cervical cancer was introduced 100 years ago in Vienna. The vaginal approach was inaugurated by Friedrich Schauta, while Ernst Wertheim chose the abdominal approach [11,12]. Since lymphadenectomy is not possible by the vaginal route, radical vaginal hysterectomy was thrust far into the background by Wertheim's operation (with its modifications and further developments). Schauta's operation only experienced a renaissance when reliable laparoscopic lymphadenectomy became possible.

Radical hysterectomy with pelvic lymphadenectomy is the standard therapy for early invasive cervical cancer. The radicality of parametrial resection depends on the size of the primary tumor. The parametria include parts of the cardinal ligament, the uterosacral ligament (rectal pillar), and the vesicocervical ligament (bladder pillar). The radicality of parametrial resection is based on the Rutledge–Piver classification [13]. Surgical treatment of cervical cancer is mainly performed by type II radical hysterectomy, which corresponds to the original method applied by Wertheim for the abdominal approach or by Schauta for the vaginal approach, or the type III technique (according to Latzko, Meigs, and Mackenrodt) (Figs. 36.6–36.8). An obligatory part of the operation is lymphadenectomy in the pelvis. The indication and extent of para-aortic lymphadenectomy (inframesenteric/infrarenal) is not

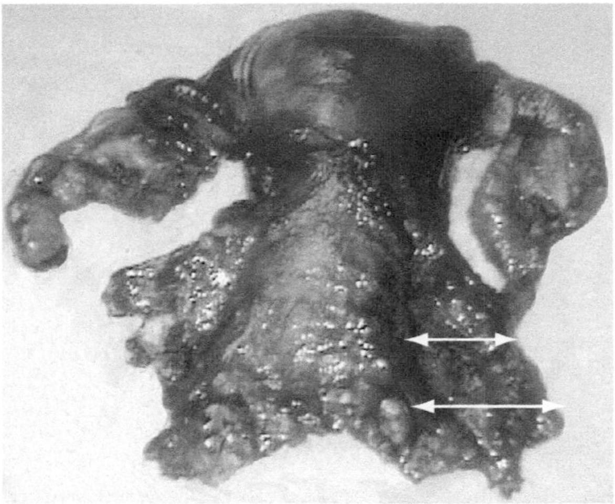

Fig. 36.6 Type II radical hysterectomy (with adnexae) with resection of half of the parametrium (Fig. 36.3). Arrows mark length of the attached parametrium

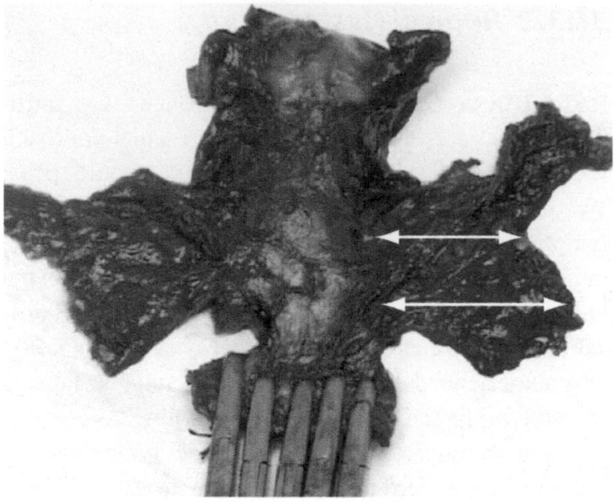

Fig. 36.7 Type III radical hysterectomy (without adnexae) with extensive parametrial resection. The vaginal cuff is held with five clamps; arrows mark the resected parametria

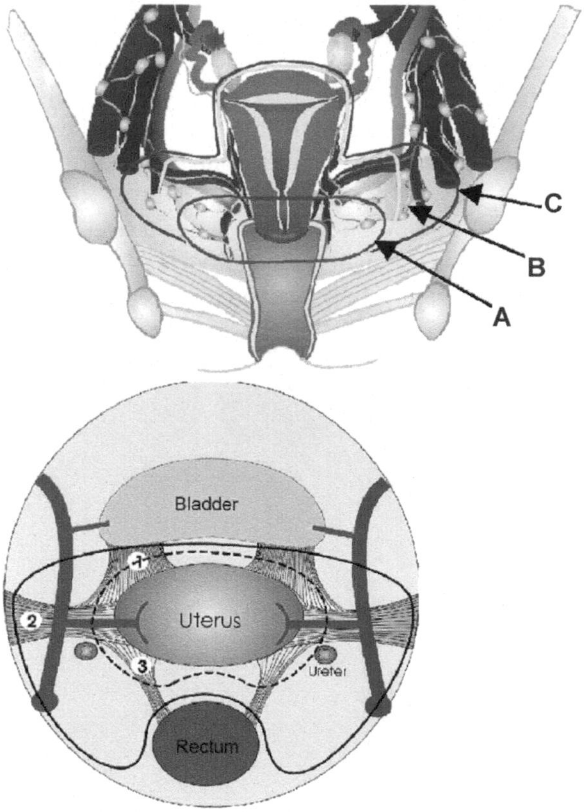

Fig. 36.8 Different degrees of radicality in the treatment of cervical cancer. *A*, radical trachelectomy; *B*, Type II radical hysterectomy; *C*, Type III radical hysterectomy (*1* Bladder pillar, *2* Cardinal ligament, *3* Rectal pillar)

precisely defined and must be individually determined with special reference to the frozen section examination of pelvic lymph nodes.

With the standardization of laparoscopic lymphadenectomy in gynecological oncology, laparoscopic-assisted vaginal hysterectomy has recently become an established alternative to radical abdominal hysterectomy (e.g., [14]). Total laparoscopic radical hysterectomy with pelvic lymphadenectomy is also possible for early invasive cervical cancer (e.g., [15]). The first studies have been published on robot-assisted radical hysterectomy. Common to all these procedures is the fact that they involve minimal blood loss (laparoscopic vs. open transfusion rate: 19% vs. 92%), faster mobilization, a shorter hospitalization, and better cosmetic results with comparable oncological safety.

Regardless of the approach route, intraoperative complications of radical hysterectomy include bladder damage in 0.5–7%, ureter damage in 3–4%, bowel damage in 1–2%, damage to large blood vessels in 2–3%, and urinary fistulas in 1–3%. Perioperative mortality is reported to be 0.7–1%. The most important late complications are lymphoceles as well as persistent bladder and bowel emptying disorders. The morbidity of bladder and rectal function are essentially determined by the radicality of the parametrial resection: the more extensive the tumor resection volume, the more serious the chronic intestinal constipation and the changes in bladder sensitivity, detrusor instability, bladder capacity, and bladder compliance. The anatomic structures in the bladder pillar, cardinal ligament, and rectal pillar consist mainly of autonomic nerves of the sympathetic (inferior hypogastric plexus) and parasympathetic (pelvic splanchnic nerves) nervous system (Fig. 36.9). There are basically only two ways to reduce the immanent mortality of radical hysterectomy:

1. Type III radical hysterectomy is performed as a nerve-sparing procedure by preserving parts of the parasympathetic and sympathetic innervation of the bladder and intestine, mainly in the lower part of the rectal pillar and cardinal ligament, which significantly reduces postoperative morbidity associated with the pelvic organs [16–18] (Fig. 36.9).
2. Smaller tumors (<2 cm) are treated only by a type II operation, thus preserving the lateral part of the parametrium. An argument against reducing radicality is provided by greater sections of surgical

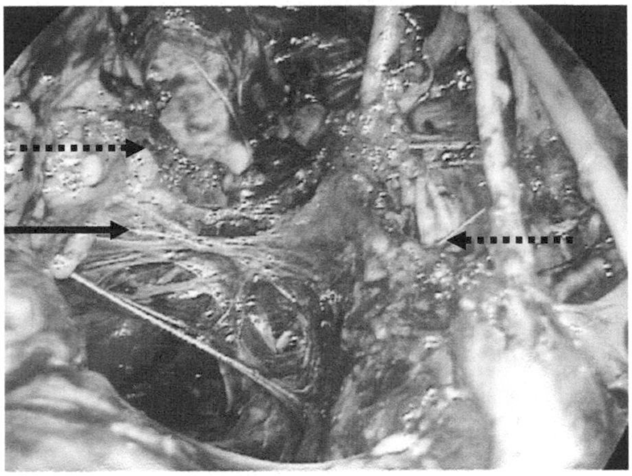

Fig. 36.9 Laparoscopic demonstration and preservation of the right-pelvic splanchnic nerves (*solid line arrow*) after severing the vascular part of the cardinal ligament (*broken line arrow*)

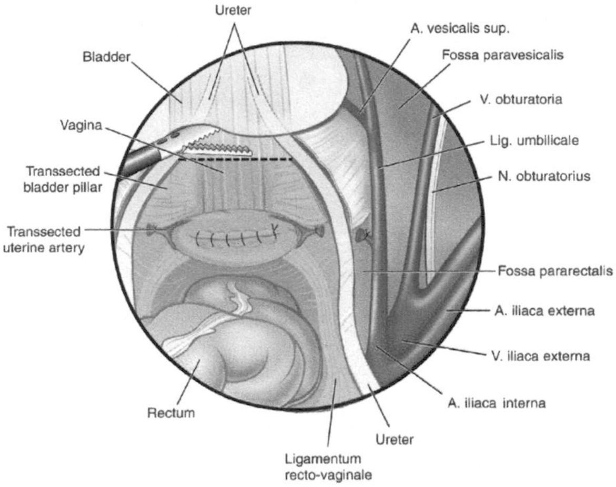

Fig. 36.10 Diagram of the resection figure (*green*) for radical parametrectomy

specimens that showed discontinuous tumor growth in parametrial structures as well as tumor-involved lymph nodes in the parametrium of patients with tumor-free pelvic lymph nodes [19].

Radical hysterectomy can be performed at any time interval after conization, if adequate perioperative thrombosis and antibiotic prophylaxis is performed.

36.3.3 Radical Parametrectomy

The unexpected finding of invasive cervical cancer during a simple hysterectomy is rare and accounts for about 1% of all tumors. Such cases require an individual decision between primary radiochemotherapy and radical parametrectomy combined with lymphadenectomy, since oncologically important risk factors like parametrial or lymph node involvement are not known. On the other hand, we are dealing here mostly with early tumor stages that have an excellent prognosis after adjuvant radiochemotherapy if no residual tumor remains in situ. If this is uncertain, radical parametrectomy should involve removal of the remaining parts of the parametria in combination with the pelvic and/or para-aortic lymph nodes. This intervention can basically be performed by open surgery ("Wertheim sine utero") or by the laparoscopic-assisted vaginal approach ("Schauta sine utero") [20] (Fig. 36.10).

36.3.4 Fertility-Preserving Surgery for Early Cervical Cancer

Based on the excellent prognosis of node-negative early invasive cervical cancer, Daniel Dargent inaugurated fertility-preserving surgery at the end of the last century. During the procedure, designated as radical trachelectomy, the pelvic lymph nodes are first removed by laparoscopy and examined by frozen section. Detection of tumor-free lymph nodes is followed by resection of the lower 2/3 of the cervix uteri with an adequate vaginal cuff as well as the median part of the sacrouterine ligaments and the parametria. A permanent cerclage is only placed in cases with tumor-free resection margins and a residual cervix length of 7–8 mm, and the vagina is adapted to the residual cervix. Thus, cesarean section is the only mode of delivery (see Fig. 36.8). Strict indications must be applied for radical trachelectomy to achieve an oncological safety comparable to or higher than that provided by radical hysterectomy (Table 36.2). Results obtained in the meantime from more than 800 operations describe a recurrence rate of 2.7–4% with a low complication rate [21,22]. The cumulative pregnancy rate after radical trachelectomy is 53% with a higher early abortion rate than in the normal population [23]. Radical trachelectomy with pelvic lymphadenectomy is a valid and oncologically safe mode of fertility preservation for young patients with early invasive cervical cancer.

Table 36.2 Criteria for performing fertility-preserving surgery in early cervical cancer (trachelectomy according to DARGENT)

• Planned pregnancy
• pT1A1 L1
• pT1A2
• pT1B1<2 cm
• No vascular space invasion
• Tumor-free lymph nodes
• Endocervical resection with a resection margin of 0.5 cm
• Length of residual cervix 1 cm

36.3.5 Primary Exenteration for Locally Advanced Cervical Cancer

Patients with clinically or surgically confirmed stage IVa cervical cancer usually receive primary radiochemotherapy, although exenteration (anterior/posterior/total) would also be suitable for locally advanced cervical cancer. This radical surgery is internationally accepted only for tumor-related urogenital or intestinogenital fistulas, since exenterative operations are interventions with high morbidity (30–70%), a perioperative mortality of up to 7%, a high blood loss (2,000–4,000 ml), and a long hospitalization period (25–30 days).

The favorable data obtained for primary radiochemotherapy cannot be applied to stage IVa, however, since the percentage of these patients in randomized studies is minimal (3–20% of the patients in the respective randomized studies), and their survival rate was not analyzed separately. However, the results of exenterative surgery also originate mostly from inhomogeneous patient populations. Data obtained by Marnitz in patients who had stage IVa primary cervical cancer with a 5-year survival of 52.5% demonstrate that preference of radiochemotherapy is not justified in this stage [24].

Only the detection of positive para-aortic lymph nodes and intraabdominal or peritoneal dissemination must be regarded as a contraindication for exenteration. This can be laparoscopically confirmed with high sensitivity and specificity prior to a planned exenteration. Thus, primary exenteration is a valid alternative to primary radiochemotherapy in patients with surgically (laparoscopically) confirmed stage IVa cervical cancer.

36.3.6 Surgery for Recurrence

The indications for surgery in cases of proven recurrence always depend on the previous primary therapy and the localization of the finding. All treatment decisions in a recurrence situation must be individually discussed with the patient after being presented at the interdisciplinary tumor board. Apart from curative-intent therapy, the patient's quality of life is always a primary consideration.

36.4 Radiotherapy and Chemotherapy

36.4.1 Primary Radiochemotherapy

Combined percutaneous and intracavitary radiotherapy together with chemotherapy is an effective treatment modality for primary management of patients with invasive cervical cancer. Selection of the treatment method depends not only on patient-related criteria like tumor stage, age, and general condition but also on the personal expertise and experience of the physicians who participate in making the therapy decision. As summarized in the meta-analysis by Green [25], prospective randomized studies have demonstrated that, in the presence of risk factors, irradiation combined with chemotherapy (radiochemotherapy) is superior to radiotherapy alone for both primary treatment and adjuvant therapy. Simultaneous application of platinum-containing substances significantly improves the local recurrence-free and disease-free survival as well as the overall survival. The potential absolute survival advantage is 12% for platinum-containing radiotherapy compared to radiotherapy alone.

In the potentially operable tumor stages (up to stage Ib2 or IIb), surgery should only be performed if the tumor tissue can be removed with an adequate safety margin and there is no predictable need for adjuvant therapy due to risk factors. If this is not the case, surgery should not be performed or the intervention should be terminated as a staging operation with systematic para-aortic and pelvic lymphadenectomy, and primary combined radiochemotherapy should be carried out.

Identical disease-specific and overall survival rates were achieved in a randomized study examining

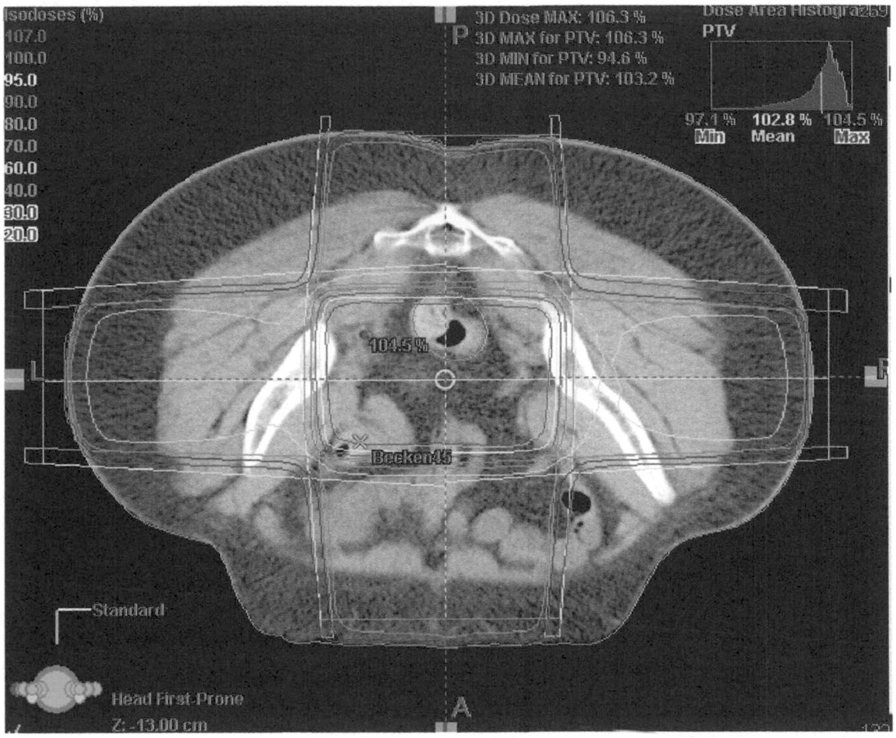

Fig. 36.11 Axial section of the planning CT of a patient with cervical cancer. Positioning on a belly board, prone position for optimal bowel protection. Conformal dose distribution in the planning target volume (*red*)

primary irradiation versus radical hysterectomy (Piver III) in stage Ib and IIA patients [6]. Both groups had a 5-year overall survival of 83%, but the incidence of late side effects was twice as high in patients who had undergone radical surgery combined with adjuvant irradiation than in those submitted to either surgery or radiotherapy. Higher tumor stages (Ib2 or higher) are internationally managed exclusively by primary radiochemotherapy. Primary radiotherapy of cervical cancer comprises percutaneous irradiation of the pelvis, simultaneous chemotherapy with cisplatin, intracavitary brachytherapy, and on detection of positive para-aortic lymph nodes, extended-field irradiation of the para-aortic region (Fig. 36.11). For radiochemotherapy of cervical cancer, cisplatin is administered as a weekly intravenous infusion of 40 mg/qm of body-surface area with a total of 5–6 applications. Carboplatin can be used if cisplatin is contraindicated. Combinations with other chemotherapeutic agents increase the toxicity, particularly through simultaneous application without confirmed improvement of the response rates. The total treatment time should not exceed 60 days.

Routine secondary hysterectomy after primary radiochemotherapy yielded an improved local control rate, but the overall survival was not improved by the hysterectomy. The situation is different for very large primary tumors or a poor treatment response in cases with a residual tumor. Here an individual treatment decision must be made, taking into account the patient's clinical condition and the expected toxicity.

36.4.2 Adjuvant Radiochemotherapy

Positive resection margins and other risk factors for locoregional recurrence (tumor-invaded lymph nodes, parametrial involvement, poorly differentiated tumors, or lymphovascular space invasion) are an indication for adjuvant radiochemotherapy, if the patient's condition permits. The irradiation volume must include the former tumor region and the internal iliac, external iliac and common iliac, as well as the presacral lymph nodes up to S2/3.

36.4.3 Neoadjuvant Chemotherapy

The data on neoadjuvant chemotherapy prior to radiotherapy or radical hysterectomy have thus far shown no improvement of overall survival, disease-free survival, or recurrence-free survival. Moreover, a comparison of results is limited by the heterogeneity of the treatment schemes and application techniques.

36.4.4 Palliative Chemotherapy

Chemotherapy alone is indicated for treating cancer that has developed distant metastases or recurred after surgery and/or radio(chemo)therapy. Patients in this therapy situation have a median survival of about 6–9 months.

Various substances are effective for treating cervical carcinoma patients with metastases or recurrence (cisplatin, carboplatin, ifosfamide, taxol, taxotere, irinotecan, topotecan, gemcitabine, vinorelbine). Selection of the substance(s) depends on previous therapies and administered drugs. It has basically been established that two- and three-drug combinations are more effective but also more toxic than single-drug therapy.

36.5 Follow-Up Recommendation

The aim of follow-up in tumor diseases is physical, psychic, and social rehabilitation. While the concepts of psychic and social rehabilitation are similar for all tumor diseases, physical care has organ-specific aspects.

Follow-up in cervical cancer patients should be tailored to the individual. Detailed structured history and a symptom-oriented examination are obligatory. It is important to note that tumor regression can take up to 3 months and that the majority of recurrences are seen within the first 2 years after primary therapy. Besides early recognition of recurrences and metastases, the main tasks of follow-up include continuation of hormonal or cytostatic therapy, treatment of therapy-related side effects, and tumor documentation.

The vagina is often shortened after radical hysterectomy, and the patient should be asked specifically about postoperative bladder emptying disorders. Gynecological examinations after irradiation usually reveal progressive cervical atrophy as well as vaginal stenosis in the upper third. The rectal pillar and parametria can be explored during the rectovaginal examination. Any palpable pelvic node is suspicious and should be histologically clarified either by fine-needle biopsy or by high-speed punch biopsy. The cytological smear is of limited value after irradiation. Endocervical curettage can be used to detect vital tumor tissue in patients with status post-irradiation. Renal ultrasound should always be performed. New-onset urinary retention is just as suspicious as leg vein thrombosis, anemia, discharge of blood from the bladder or rectum, or new-onset fistulation. The tumor markers SCC and CA 125 can only be used for follow-up control if they were primarily elevated. The supraclavicular or inguinal lymph nodes must always be examined as well.

Additional technical examinations like CT or MRI, bone scintigraphy, IV urography, thoracic CT, cysto- and rectoscopy or laparoscopy should only be performed if there is well-grounded suspicion (symptoms, abnormal findings).

36.6 Benchmark

The most important outcome parameters for cervical cancer as well as for most other gynecological tumors are disease-free and overall survival. Of decisive importance is the choice of the primary treatment modality, if surgery and radiochemotherapy are basically suitable for the tumor stage in question. In view of the significantly increased morbidity, the combination of radical hysterectomy and adjuvant radiochemotherapy should be avoided, if possible [6]. Surgical (laparoscopic) staging enables this differentiation based on the histopathological findings. Purely surgical therapy is ideal for patients with a small tumor, tumor-free lymph nodes, and no lymphatic or vascular carcinosis, since their healing rate without subsequent irradiation is above 90% [14]. The centralization of cervical cancer surgery appears to be more important than the surgical approach route: oncological surgeons must have suitable equipment (surgical, diagnostic, radiotherapeutic) and conduct a large number of interventions each year in order to meet the necessary quality standards [26].

Primary and especially recurrence therapy is complex in patients with invasive cervical cancer and should be tailored to the individual after the specialist consultation of all disciplines involved (gyneco-oncology, medical oncology, radiotherapy, gynecopathology, and psycho-oncology). Special emphasis should be placed on the quality of life in making all treatment decisions.

36.7 Open Questions, Future Prospects

The introduction of vaccines against oncogenic HPV types will revolutionize the primary prevention of cervical cancer. It will markedly reduce the incidence of cervical cancer in 20–30 years. However, vaccination is not currently able to prevent all HPV types. Thus, the value of prevention remains unchallenged.

In surgical therapy, the sentinel node procedure will gain general clinical acceptance, particularly for early invasive cervical cancer. Surgical staging and debulking of enlarged lymph nodes will also gain increasing importance. The various surgical procedures of radical hysterectomy (open surgical, combined laparoscopic-vaginal, totally laparoscopic, robot-assisted, TMMR) will be compared with regard to their oncological and morbidity-related results in order to ensure tumor-tailored individualized therapy.

The value of modern radiotherapy concepts like IMRT (intensity-modulated radiotherapy) or helical tomotherapy must be assessed. Therapeutic vaccines, novel chemotherapy concepts, and the application of tyrosine kinase and angioneogenesis inhibitors (targeted therapies) must be clinically evaluated for treatment of recurrent and/or metastatic cervical cancer.

Acknowledgment We thank Dr. Joanne Weirowski for the excellent support in translating and editing the manuscript.

References

1. Ferlay, J., Pisani, P., Parkin, D.M.: GLOBOCAN 2000: Cancer Incidence, Mortality and Prevalence worldwide. IARC press, Lyon (2001)
2. Krebs in Deutschland. Häufigkeiten und Trends (2006) Gesellschaft der epidemiologischen Krebsregister in Deutschland e.V. in Zusammenarbeit mit dem Robert – Koch – Institut. 5. überarbeitete Ausgabe.
3. Beckmann, M.W.: Interdisziplinäre S2-Leitlinie für die Diagnostik und Therapie des Zervixkarzinoms. M.Zuckschwerdt Verlag, München, Wien, New York (2004)
4. Hertel, H., Kohler, C., Elhawary, T., Michels, W., Possover, M., Schneider, A.: Laparoscopic staging compared with imaging techniques in the staging of advanced cervical cancer. Gynecol. Oncol. **87**(1), 46–51 (2002)
5. Lai, C.H., Huang, K.G., Hong, J.H., Lee, C.L., Chou, H.H., Chang, T.C., Hsueh, S., Huang, H.J., Ng, K.K., Tsai, C.S.: Randomized trial of surgical staging (extraperitoneal or laparoscopic) versus clinical staging in locally advanced cervical cancer. Gynecol. Oncol. **89**, 160–167 (2003)
6. Landoni, F., Maneo, A., Colombo, A., Placa, F., Milani, R., Perego, P., Favini, G., Ferri, L., Mangioni, C.: Randomised study of radical surgery versus radiotherapy for stage Ib-IIa cervical cancer. Lancet **350**, 535–540 (1997)
7. Köhler, C., Klemm, P., Schau, A., Possover, M., Krause, N., Tozzi, R., Schneider, A.: Introduction of transperitoneal lymphadenectomy in a gynecologic oncology center: analysis of 650 laparoscopic and /or paraaortic transperitoneal lymphadenectomies. Gynecol. Oncol. **95**, 52–61 (2004)
8. Schlaerth, J.B., Spirtos, N.M., Carson, L.F., Boike, G., Adamec, T., Stonebraker, B.: Laparoscopic retroperitoneal lymphadenectomy followed by immediate laparotomy in women with cervical cancer: a gynecologic oncology group study. Gynecol. Oncol. **85**(1), 81–88 (2002)
9. Catron, G., Leblanc, E., Ferron, G., Martel, P., Narducci, F., Querleu, D.: Complications of laparoscopic lymphadenectomy in gynecologic oncology. A series of 1102 procedures in 915 patients. Gynécol. Obstét. Fertil. **33**(5), 304–314 (2005)
10. Marnitz, S., Köhler, C., Roth, C., Füller, J., Hinkelbein, W., Schneider, A.: Is there a benefit of pretreatment laparoscopic transperitoneal surgical staging in patients with advanced cervical cancer? Gynecol. Oncol. **99**, 536–544 (2005)
11. Schauta, F.: Die erweiterte vaginale Totalexstirpation des Uterus bei Kollumkarzinom. J. Safar, Wien, Leipzig (1908)
12. Wertheim, E.: Die erweiterte abdominale Operation bei Carcinoma colli uteri. Urban & Schwarzenberg, Berlin, Wien (1911)
13. Piver, M.S., Rutledge, F., Smith, J.P.: Five classes of extended hysterectomy for women with cervical cancer. Obstet. Gynecol. **44**, 265–272 (1974)
14. Hertel, H., Kohler, C., Michels, W., Possover, M., Tozzi, R., Schneider, A.: Laparoscopic-assisted radical vaginal hysterectomy (LARVH): prospective evaluation of 200 patients with cervical cancer. Gynecol. Oncol. **90**, 505–511 (2003)
15. Gil-Morena, A., Puig, O., Perez-Benavente, M.A., Diaz, B., Verges, R., De la Torre, J., Martinez-Palones, J.M., Xercavins, J.: Total laparoscopic radical hysterectomy (type II–III) with pelvic lymphadenectomy in early invasive cervical cancer. J. Minim. Invasive Gynecol. **12**(2), 113–120 (2005)
16. Höckel, M., Wolff, W., Schmid, W., Spanel-Borowski, K.: Nervenschonende radikale Hysterektomie. I. Anatomische Grundlagen und Operationstechnik. Geburtsh. Frauenheilk. **60**, 314–319 (2000)
17. Yabuki, Y., Asamoto, A., Hoshiba, T., Nishimoto, H., Nishikawa, Y., Nakajima, T.: Radical hysterectomy: An

anatomic evaluation of parametrial dissection. Gynecol. Oncol. **77**(1), 155–163 (2000)
18. Possover, M., Stober, S., Plaul, K., Schneider, A.: Identification and preservation of the motoric innervation of the bladder in radical hysterectomy type III. Gynecol. Oncol. **79**(2), 154–157 (2000)
19. Winter, R., Haas, J., Reich, O., Koemetter, R., Tamussino, K., Lahousen, M., Petru, E., Pickel, H.: Parametrial spread of cervical cancer in patients with negative pelvic lymph nodes. Gynecol. Oncol. **84**(2), 252–257 (2002)
20. Köhler, C., Tozzi, R., Klemm, P., Schneider, A.: "Schauta sine utero": technique and results of laparoscopic-vaginal radical parametrectomy. Gynecol. Oncol. **91**(2), 359–368 (2003)
21. Hertel, H., Köhler, C., Grund, D., Hillemanns, P., Possover, M., Michels, W.: Schneider A (2006) Radical vaginal trachelectomy (RVT) combined with laparoscopic pelvic lymphadenectomy: Prospective multicenter study of 100 patients with early cervical cancer. Gynecol. Oncol. **103**(2), 506–511 (2006)
22. Plante, M., Renaud, M.C., Francois, H., Roy, M.: Vaginal radical trachelectomy: an oncologically safe fertility-preserving surgery. An updated series of 72 cases and review of the literature. Gynecol. Oncol. **94**, 614–623 (2004)
23. Shepherd, J.H., Spencer, C., Herod, J., Ind, T.E.D.: Radical vaginal trachelectomy as a fertility-sparing procedure in women with early-stage cervical cancer-cumulative pregnancy rate in a series of 123 women. BJOG **113**, 719–724 (2006)
24. Marnitz, S., Köhler, C., Müller, M., Behrens, K., Hasenbein, K., Schneider, A.: Indications for primary and secondary exenterations in patients with cervical cancer. Gynecol. Oncol. **103**(3), 1023–1030 (2006)
25. Green, J., Kirwan, J., Tierney, J., Vale, C., Symonds, P., Fresco, L., Williams, C., Collingwood, M.: Concomitant chemotherapy and radiation therapy for cancer of the uterine cervix. Cochrane Database Syst. Rev. CD002225, 2005
26. Trimbos, J.B., Hellebrekers, B.W.J., Kenter, G.G., Peters, L.A.W., Zwinderman, K.H.: The long learning curve of gynaecological cancer surgery: an argument for centralisation. BJOG **107**, 19–23 (2000)

Links

www.asco.org: American Society of Clinical Oncology (ASCO)

www.esgo.org: European Society of Gynaecological Oncology (ESGO)

www.krebsgesellschaft.de: Deutsche Krebsgesellschaft

www.krebsinfo.de: Krebsinfo des Tumorzentrums München

www.nih.gov: National Institutes of Health

www.oeggg.at: Österreichische Gesellschaft für Gynäkologie und Geburtshilfe

Genitoanal HPV Infection and Associated Neoplasias in the Male

37

Gerd Gross

Core Messages

- › HPVs associated with lesions on the male genitoanal areas have been divided into low-risk and high-risk HPV types.
- › Manifestations of genitoanal HPV infection in the male as in the female present as latent infections, subclinical infections and clinically benign lesions such as genital warts (condylomata acuminata) related to low-risk HPVs. Penile and particularly anal cancer as well as the precursor lesions, penile intraepithelial neoplasias and intraepithelial neoplasias of perianal and anal sites are closely associated with high-risk HPVs.
- › Genitoanal HPV infections in men are widespread in communities, not generally restricted to core-groups.
- › Genital warts harbour in about 90 % HPV 6 or HPV 11. About 20–44 % of genital warts show coinfections of HPV 6 or HPV 11 and high-risk HPV types, with HPV 16 the most frequently detected type.
- › Early diagnosis and consequent treatment of genital warts in males will contribute to reduce the burden of anogenital HPV infection and associated disease.
- › Men experience a longer duration of genital warts and incur higher treatment costs than women.
- › In analogy to vulvar cancer two different pathogenic pathways seem to exist for squamous cell cancer of the penis. About 40%–50% of penile cancer are associated with high-risk HPV (mainly HPV 16).

37.1 Introduction

HPV is one of the most common sexually transmitted infections among men. It contributes to men's burden of genitoanal diseases such as penile, anal cancer, and genitoanal warts [35].

The majority of genitoanal HPV infections are asymptomatic, unrecognized, or subclinical (Center for Disease Control and Prevention – Treatment Guidelines for Prevention – Sexually Transmitted Diseases, MMWR 2006; 55: No. RR-11:38) [20].

There are approximately 40 HPV types out of about 150 genotypes which have been shown to infect the epithelia of the genitoanal region. Some of these have been considered to be high-risk or oncogenic types.

Depending on their preferential association with benign or malignant lesions, "mucosal" HPV types have been classified as low-risk (LR) or high-risk (HR) HPV types [26,33]. Low-risk types (HPV6, 11, 26, 30, 34, 40, 42-44, 53, 55, 57, 61, 62, 63, 69, 70, 72, 73, 77, 79–82) are almost regularly encountered in genital warts. These LR HPV types however, have been only very rarely found in high-grade dysplasias and invasive cancers of the genitoanal region [83]. High-risk HPV types (HPV16, 18, 31, 33, 35, 39, 45, 51, 52, 54, 56, 58, 59, 65, 67, 68) have been recovered from

G. Gross
Department of Dermatology and Venereology, University of Rostock, Strempelstraße 13, 18057 Rostock, Germany
e-mail: gerd.gross@med.uni-rostock.de

G. Gross and S.K. Tyring (eds.), *Sexually Transmitted Infections and Sexually Transmitted Diseases*,
DOI: 10.1007/978-3-642-14663-3_37, © Springer-Verlag Berlin Heidelberg 2011

high-grade dysplasias, in situ carcinomas, and invasive cancers of the cervix uteri, the vagina, the vulva but also of the anus, the perianal skin, and the penis [96].

The concept of the "male factor" refers to characteristics of the male sexual behavior which were shown to contribute to the risk of HPV infection and subsequent HPV-associated disease in women, mainly at the cervix [5]. Rates of HPV DNA detection in women are increasing with increasing numbers of sexual partners [143]. According to data from Bosch and colleagues [15] the risk of cervical cancer is threefold higher in women whose regular partner has detectable HPV DNA on the penis.

The increasing incidence of cervical dysplasia, anal cancer, and HPV-related vulvar cancer in the countries of the western hemisphere, implies the importance of HPV not only in women but also in men. Apparently men serve both as vectors and possibly as reservoirs of HPV.

So far we have learned by far more about HPV infections in women than in men [35,111]. This chapter reviews genitoanal HPV infections and associated neoplasias in men, focusing on diagnosis, treatment, and prevention of penile, anal, and perianal lesions including HPV-related cancers and precursor lesions.

37.2 Penile HPV Infection

37.2.1 Epidemiology and Pathogenesis

Genitoanal HPV infection is predominantly transmitted by sexual contacts. In both sexes a transient course is regularly seen. Male-to-female transmission of HPV influences the outcome of infection in the females [1,15,18,149]. HPV prevalence in men varies widely, depending on the type of population studied [34].

[6,12] showed independently that more than 60% of male partners of women with cervical intraepithelial neoplasia are HPV DNA positive. Ninety percent of these infections are of HR-HPV type. [35] reported that HPV prevalence was typically $\geq$ 20% and infection rates of up to 72.9% have been documented. So far, few studies have addressed the age-specific prevalence estimates of HPV in men. Only recently a high prevalence of HPV infections in men has been observed in a study across three countries evaluated (Brazil, Mexico, and USA) [48]. In samples from coronal sulcus, glans penis, penile shaft, and scrotum of 1,100 men, overall HPV prevalence was 65.2% with 12% oncogenic types only, 20.7% non-oncogenic types, 17.8% both oncogenic and non-oncogenic, and 14.7% unclassified HPV infections. HPV prevalence was higher in Brazil (72.3%) than in the USA (61.3%) and Mexico (61.9%) [48].

Risk factors for genital HPV DNA detection in men resemble those found in women and consist in lifetime and recent number of sexual partners, age, lack of condom use, and smoking [48,50,100,130]. According to Giuliano and colleagues [50] circumcision is associated with a reduced risk of HPV detection from penile sites (coronal sulcus, glans penis, penile shaft). In addition to transmission by sexual contacts, nonsexual (vertical) transmission of HPV can also occur. HPV DNA is detectable in smears from the buccal mucosa in 30–80% of children born to genital HPV DNA positive women [119]. These mostly asymptomatic HPV infections may be either transient or lead to laryngeal papillomas (see Syrjänen S, chapter). Less frequently, genital warts may develop during childhood. Thus, genital warts in children are not always evidence of sexual abuse [77]. Some data suggest in general that HPV may be transmitted to some extent also via nonsexual routes, fomites, undergarments, surgical gloves, and contaminated instruments [39,120].

In a large percentage of children with genital warts HPV is likely to be transmitted by autoinoculation or heteroinoculation from genital lesions or from cutaneous warts mainly located at the fingers [64]. Whenever sexual abuse is suspected, cooperation with a pediatrician and child psychologist is mandatory.

37.2.2 Categories of Genitoanal HPV Infections

In general, three different categories of genitoanal HPV infection have been known to exist: latent infections, subclinical infections, and visible manifestations [131].

Primarily, HPV infections of genitoanal epithelial sites result in local, mostly latent infections. In these cases, HPV DNA and RNA are detectable only by molecular biologic means. There are no macroscopic or histological features indicating the presence of HPV. The vast majority of infections with HR-HPV genotypes are latent and subclinical or very flat.

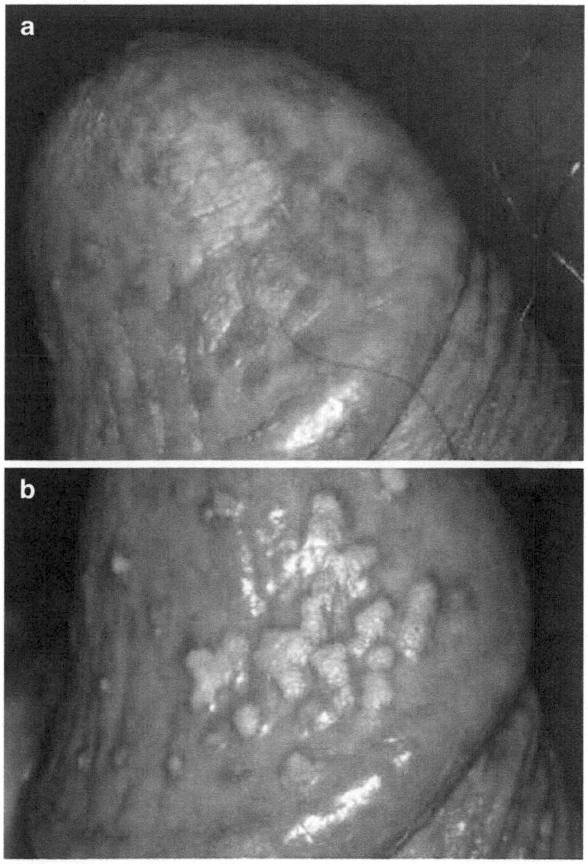

Fig. 37.1 (**a**) Subclinical papillomavirus infection of the glans penis. (**b**) The lesions become apparent after the application of 3% acetic acid

By definition in subclinical HPV infection, HPV DNA is present in epithelia from macroscopically unsuspicious areas. Subclinical infections are particularly caused by HR HPV types. The majority of these remain undetected and may regress spontaneously. Subclinical lesions are detectable using acetic acid application (3% or 5% acetic acid during 5 min). A positive aceto-white test result is defined as a clearly marked grayish-white area with visible atypical vessels (Fig. 37.1). Subclinical lesions are mainly found on mucous parts of the genitoanal area. A series of different conditions may mimic HPV-associated whitening such as erosions, fresh scars, balanitis, lichen planus, lichen sclerosus, psoriasis, eczema, and others. This may cause diagnostic problems.

HPVs associated with lesions in the male genital areas have been divided into LR- and HR-HPV types, based on each genotypes' association with benign or malignant lesions such as genital warts, penile intraepithelial neoplasia (PIN), and penile cancer.

37.2.3 Genital Warts

Genital warts are the most common sexually transmitted genitoanal tumors of viral origin worldwide. The benign tumors contain mature HPV virions. This is in contrast to severely dysplastic epithelia that are unable to produce virus. Genital warts are recognized as the main clinical manifestation of genital HPV infection in men as they are in women. They are highly infectious with an incubation period between 3 weeks and 8 months [105]. This may explain their early occurrence in life at an age around 20 years [147]. Evidence exists that transmission of HPV from men with genital warts to their female consorts is high [46]. Furthermore, HPV infection in men has been shown to contribute to subsequent cervical disease in women. Some data exist that males experience a longer duration of genital warts and incur higher treatment costs than women [47].

Gissmann and colleagues detected in 1983 HPV6 and HPV11 in genital warts and laryngeal papillomas [45]. About 90% of genital warts are caused by these LR HPV types [138]. As a rule these types cause genitoanal cancer only very rarely. However, women with a history of genital warts have been shown to have an increased risk of cervical intraepithelial neoplasia and also cancer [42,82]. According to another large cohort study on hospitalized patients with genital warts, a strong association is likely to exist with an increased risk of cancers of the vulva, vagina, penis, and anus, but not invasive cervical cancer [102].

The existence of both genital warts and simultaneous infections with HR "oncogenic" HPV types in different genitoanal epithelia may explain these data. According to reports of [2,16,55], about 20–44% of genital warts show coinfections of HPV6 or 11 and HR-HPV types, with HPV16, the most frequently detected type. The overall incidence of external genital warts is high in males and females with an estimated lifetime risk of about 10% [80, 81]. The incidence rate of genital warts in privately insured patients in the USA is 1.7/1,000 in males and 1.5/1,000 in females. In contrast the incidence in Australia is 2.2/1,000 [29]. Demographic data from USA have shown that the number of new cases of genital warts is

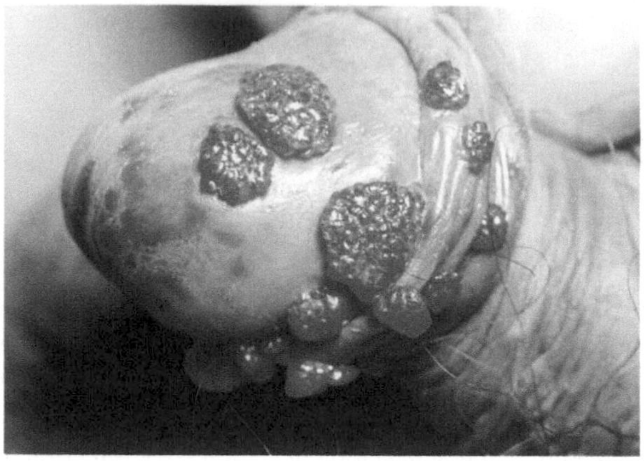

Fig. 37.2 Penile condylomata acuminata (glans and inner part of the prepuce)

about 1 million per year [129] and the incidence seems to be increasing. The highest rates of genital warts are observed in males 20–24 years of age, which is in contrast to females with a peak in the ages 16–24 years.

Clinically, genital warts appear as fleshy, sometimes brownish pigmented painless papules with a verrucous surface. They grow preferentially in warm, moist areas of the skin. There is consensus that there are four different types of genital warts [62,64]: Condylomata acuminata and flat lesions, which grow on moist areas of non-keratinized epithelia. Furthermore, there are papular as well as keratotic genital warts which are typically located on dry skin with a keratinized epidermis [62] (Fig. 37.2). The most common sites of genital warts in uncircumcised men are the prepucial cavity, the glans, the coronal sulcus, the frenum, and parts of the prepuce. Genital warts in circumcised men are found preferentially on the penile shaft [136]. Histologically, genital warts either caused by HPV6 or HPV11 consist in a cauliflower-like growth, composed of an epithelial hyperplasia with acanthosis, papillomatosis, and koilocyte present in the upper portions of the epidermis (Fig.37.3). By definition atypical keratinocytes are absent. The underlying stroma is fibrous and rich of dilated vessels as well as varying numbers of inflammatory cell infiltrates [56].

In nearly 50% of patients, genital warts are found at multiple sites. Recently, warts have been detected increasingly at the pubic skin in both genders (Fig. 37.4). This is probably due to shaving habits in Western countries realized in the past years. The role

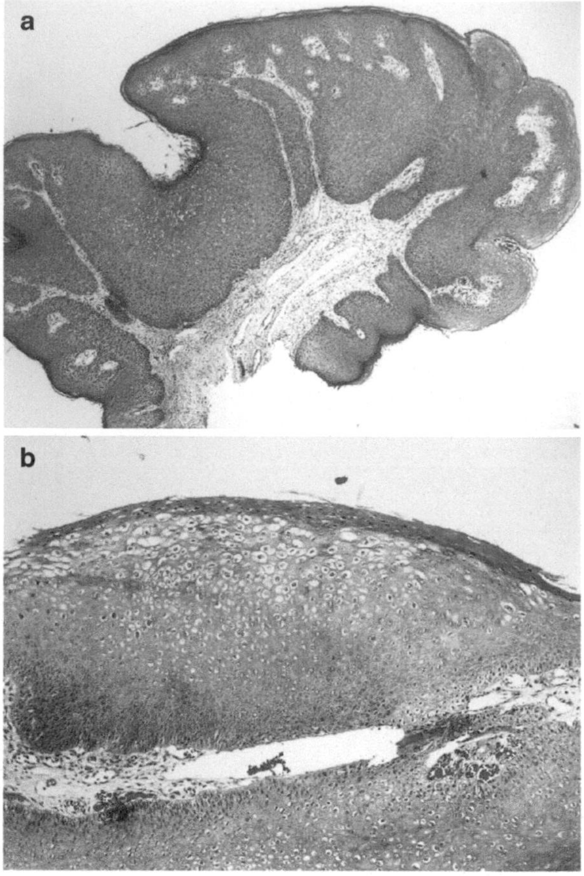

Fig. 37.3 (**a**) Histology of condylomata acuminata showing acanthosis, papillomatosis, elongated dermal papillae, and sharp border with the dermis. (**b**) Numerous koilocyte in the upper spinous layer (H & E stain)

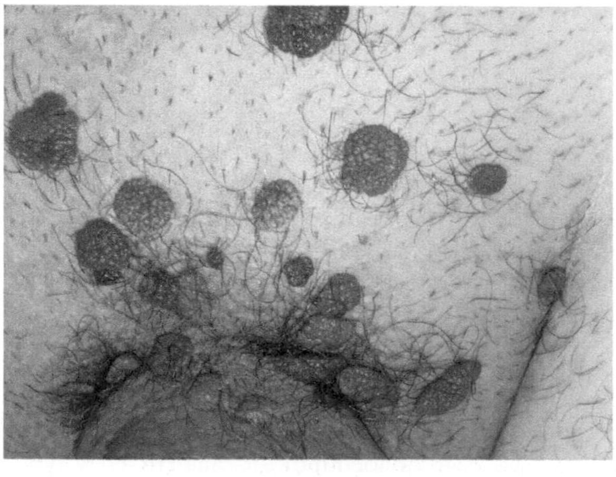

Fig. 37.4 Multiple papular warts of pubic skin

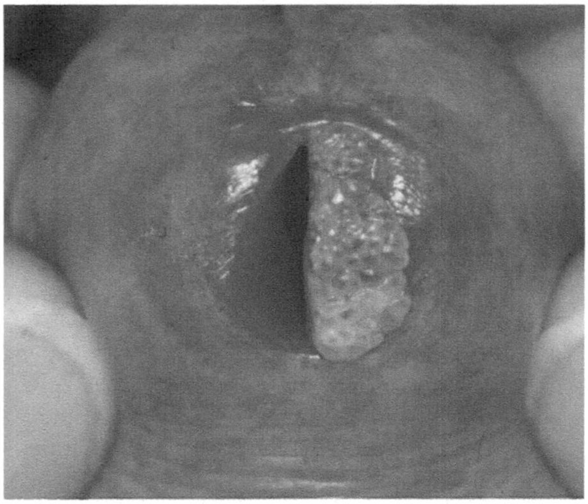

Fig. 37.5 Meatal warts

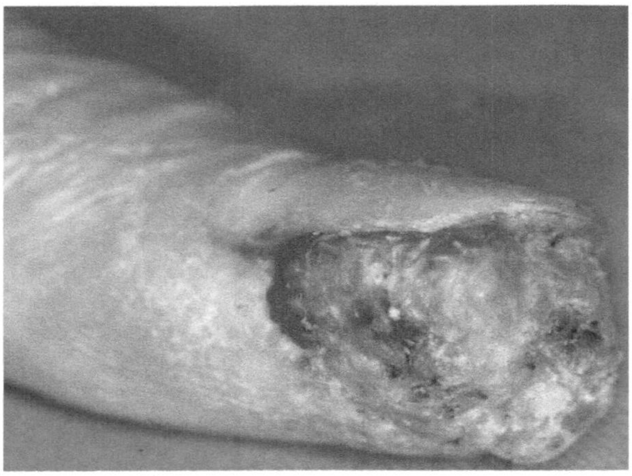

Fig. 37.6 Subungual squamous cell carcinoma associated with HPV 6 in a 64-year-old male heart transplant recipient

of genitoanal hair as a possible reservoir of mucosal HPV types has been postulated by Poljak and colleagues [116]. Recently, three cases of condylomata acuminata of the pannus and the inguinal folds in obese patients have been described [127]. It seems likely that the abdominal pannus provides a further suitable environment for disseminating genital warts. In about 20% of males the urethra is affected (Fig. 37.5). Most frequently, distal urethral warts are observed in the meatus urethrae and in the fossa navicularis [122]. Perianal warts occur only occasionally in heterosexual men, whereas they are common findings in men with receptive anal intercourse [106].

Long-lasting genital warts may grow exuberantly and giant condylomata may develop. These lesions harbor preferentially HPV 6 and HPV 11 as do genital warts. Their vertical growth pattern is characterized by both exophytic and endophytic proliferations destroying underlying dermal and other structures. Some overlap exists with the Buschke–Loewenstein tumor, which has been classified as a verrucous carcinoma [83,124]. Histology of giant condyloma is that of a condyloma acuminatum with areas of atypical cells that may require thorough investigation to rule out invasive carcinoma [124].

Increasingly, genitoanal HPV types have been detected at extragenital sites such as the nail bed of the fingers [94], the lips, the oral cavity, the oropharynx, and the larynx (see Chapter 39) and even the conjunctivae as well as the nipples [92]. At these sites papillomatous and macular lesions may arise. At periungual and subungual sites, high-grade HPV-associated precancerous lesions and squamous cell cancer were described [94,97], especially in severely immunosuppressed patients (Fig. 37.6).

37.2.4 Diagnosis and Differential Diagnosis

Diagnosis of subclinical HPV infections and clinical manifestations should always include diagnosis of other sexually transmitted infections such as HIV, *Treponema pallidum*, *Chlamydia trachomatis*, *Mycoplasma genitalis*, *Trichomonas*, *Neisseria gonorrhoeae*, genital herpes, and *Candida albicans* as well as hepatitis B and hepatitis C.

Accurate diagnosis is an essential step in the management of external genital warts. Requisites are bright light and magnification by a lens or a peniscope [8, 9]. An otoscope and a small spreader may be helpful for inspection of the male urinary meatus and the fossa navicularis. Proctoscopy should be performed only after all visible perianal HPV lesions have been removed. This is done to avoid inoculation of viral material to more proximal parts of the anus [136].

In analogy to women, differential diagnosis of genital warts in men includes a large variety of conditions such as condylomata lata (syphilis stage 2), mollusca contagiosa, pearly penile papules, seborrheic keratoses (see Table 37.1). Even bullous disease such as pemphigus

Table 37.1 Differential diagnosis of external warts

Anatomic variants	
Pearly penile papules (Papillomatosis penis)	
Syringomas	
Fox-Fordyce disease	
Benign skin tumors and inflammatory dermatoses	
Melanocytic nevi/ epidermal nevi	Balanitis/Vulvitis
Fibromas	Psoriasis
Angiokeratomas	Darier's disease
Seborrheic warts	Acanthosis nigricans
Lichen planus	Lymphangioma
Lichen sclerosus	Pemphigus familiaris benignus (M. Hailey-Hailey)
Other STDs	
Condylomata lata (secondary Syphilis)	
Mollusca contagiosa	
Genital herpes	
Candida infection	
Malignant tumors	
Intraepithelial neoplasias (external genitalia, perianal skin, anus)	
Bowenoid papulosis (Penile intraepithelial neoplasia grade 3 (PIN 3))	
Bowen's disease, Erythroplasia of Queyrat (PIN 3)	
Squamous cell carcinoma, verrucous carcinoma	
Malignant melanoma	

familiaris benignus (Hailey-Hailey's disease) [36] may pose problems in differentiating genital warts. Dysplastic nevi, high-grade intraepithelial lesions, and invasive cancer may also mimic genital warts. In immunocompromised individuals it is always indicated taking a biopsy for histological workup. The same is true if a large verrucous or wart-like atypical lesion is present. But also lesions refractory to treatment and lesions in patients older than 40 years should be biopsied and thoroughly investigated by histologic means [96]. Pigmented lesions have to be strictly removed entirely. In such cases histology is absolutely mandatory in order to rule out malignant melanoma.

37.2.5 Clinical Course and Economic Burden

Genital warts may persist for months and even years. Spontaneous regression may occur in about one-third of cases. Obviously genital warts are under control of the cellular immunity [27]. Smoking seems to lower local immunity and may contribute to development of genital warts as well as recurrent and long-lasting disease [38]. In immunosuppressed individuals remission has been observed when immunosuppressive therapy was dropped. Similarly genital warts in pregnant women are known to regress to a great deal after giving birth (Petry, personal communication). One of the main problems of genital warts, however, is their recurrent nature after initial successful therapy.

There is a substantial burden of disease from genital warts in terms of their chronic nature and their impact on health-related quality of life [148]. According to a study of a cohort of 357 men, clearance of HPV infection including infection with HR-HPV types was slower at the glans and coronal sulcus of the penis of uncircumcised men compared to that of circumcised men [71]. Apparently, circumcision may protect against HPV-associated disease by enhancing the resolution of infection.

Burning, itching, and discharge are rarely reported symptoms particularly in patients with urethral warts and warts of the anal canal. Especially giant condylomas may cause bleeding. In rare cases obstruction of anus or urethra may result [88,92,124]. Most of the associated morbidity is thought to be psychological. Emotionally genital warts may be very stigmatizing. Guilt, fear of cancer, cancerophobia, fear of loss of fertility, and decrease of self-esteem may develop. Also in men the psychosocial distress of warty lesions is higher and similar to that caused by lesions of high-grade dysplasia. There is a clear need for counseling also because of a possible negative influence of genital warts on the partnership.

HPV infection and particularly genital warts carry a high financial burden given their recalcitrant response to conventional therapies [84]. According to [46,79] males experience not only a longer duration of genital warts but also incur greater treatment cost than women. Data from Germany implicate considerable costs of managing and treating genital warts [72]. The total societal costs in Germany were estimated at €54.1 million, which correspond to an average cost per patient with new genital warts of €378 and for recurrent warts of €607, respectively. Average costs in USA were estimated to US$477 per episode treated in males in contrast to US$404 per episode treated in females [76].

37.2.6 Treatment

Genitoanal warts may follow varying courses that are possibly due to individual genetic or immunological factors. Warts may spontaneously regress. They may remain unchanged during months and even years. Furthermore, they may increase in size and number or very rarely they may undergo malignant conversion [150].

The primary goal of treatment is to ameliorate symptoms, and to remove visible warts permanently when they cause physical and psychologic distress. The influence of gender on clearance and recurrence has not been clearly addressed in studies. Whether external genital warts located on moist tissues respond better than warts on dry and cornified tissues has not been evaluated either so far. According to studies with separate analyses of warts of the meatus urethrae, it seems likely that clearance rates correspond to the affected tissue type.

No one treatment is ideal for all kinds of HPV-induced lesions. Treatment of external genital warts can induce wart-free periods. However, HPV infection may or may not persist. So far, no HPV-specific antiviral compound exists that is able to eliminate HPV completely. There is no therapy that clearly eradicates genital warts permanently. So, current treatment has been suboptimal, with recurrence rates generally high, at least 20–30%. No therapy is without local side effects such as burning, itching, pain, or even erosions. In view of the self-limiting character of a large number of genital warts, therapies leading to long-term sequelae such as scars should be generally avoided.

37.2.7 Recommended Therapies

There is a wide variety of therapies available for the treatment of external genital warts [60, 61]. These include surgical and nonsurgical therapies (Table 37.2), which have been recommended by several national and international guidelines established over the past years [19,25,63,113,138]. Therapies of genital warts have been divided into physician–applied and patient-applied therapies. Surgical therapies comprise electrocauterization, surgical excision (scissor-snip excision),

Table 37.2 Recommended therapies for genital warts according to International Guidelines

Patient-applied therapy	Physician-applied therapy
Podophyllotoxin cream/ solution	Scissor-snip excision
Imiquimod 5% cream	Electrocauterization CO_2-laser Cryotherapy[b] Trichloroacetic (<85%)[b]
Polyphenon® E 10% cream[a]	PDT (investigational) Podophyllin
Not (yet) recommended therapies	
Cidofovir (investigational)	5-flourouracil Interferon alpha il Interferon alpha s.c.

[a]According to three trials

[b]Efficacious and safe treatment in first half of pregnancy

cryotherapy, and laser surgery. Both CO_2 laser and electrocauterization produce smoke which must be evacuated by vacuum devices with specialized filters. Furthermore special laser masks have to be used and protective lenses are mandatory for patients and personnel [60].

Nonsurgical physician-applied therapies include application of bi- and trichloroacetic acid (≤85%), which should be administered only to small warty lesions. It is advantageous that these therapies can be used also during pregnancy. Patient-applied therapies are podophyllotoxin gel, podophyllotoxin solution, and imiquimod. The latter is an immunomodulator which works by inducing cytokines such as interferon alpha and tumor-necrosis-factor alpha by activating toll-like receptor 7 [95]. The optimal application schedule of imiquimod 5% cream for external anogenital warts is three times per week (8 h overnight) for up to 16 weeks [53]. Podophyllotoxin is a safe and more effective treatment for primary condylomata acuminata than Podophyllin. It has a significant advantage in being suitable for home use, resulting in more convenience for the patient. Most recently Polyphenon® E, a defined extract of catechines of green tea leaves of *Camellia sinensis* has been established as a further active and safe local treatment modality [65,128,132]. In contrast to podophyllotoxin and imiquimod Polyphenon® E has an extremely low recurrence rate of 6.5% and a very good safety profile. It is given three times a day for a maximum of 16 weeks. The biological properties of Polyphenon® E are immunomodulatory and antioxidant.

37.2.8 Therapies Not Currently Recommended

According to European Guidelines for primary care physicians for the diagnosis and management of anogenital warts [138], the following therapies are not generally recommended for treatment of genital warts (Table 37.2): interferons, 5-fluorouracil, and podophyllin.

5-fluorouracil is a mutagen and teratogen. It is contraindicated in pregnancy. 5-fluorouracil (5%-cream) has some place (off-label use) in local therapy of urethral warts and intraepithelial neoplasia in problem cases. Intralesional interferon alpha and local interferon beta is sometimes used as adjuvant to surgery under special circumstances [138]. Cidofovir which is a nucleoside analog used systemically as an antiviral against cytomegalovirus has shown some activity against HPV lesions when used intralesionally or as topical preparation [123,125]. Cidofovir is still an investigational preparation and cannot be generally recommended. Podophyllin has an only moderate efficacy and seems to possess mutagenic properties. Systemic toxicity of podophyllotoxin is described especially if applied in larger volumes [60].

Choice of therapy, either patient-administered or physician-administered, is a decision that should be made by both the clinician and the patient. It is based on the morphology and extent of the warts, the experience of the physician, and the preference of the patient [138] (Table 37.3).

37.2.9 Penile Intraepithelial Neoplasia

Genitoanal HPV infection can cause intraepithelial neoplasias in the whole genitoanal tract.

HPV-associated penile intraepithelial neoplasias (PIN) mostly present clinically as unsuspicious flat lesions (Fig. 37.6). In analogy to intraepithelial neoplasia of other genitoanal sites (cervix uteri, vagina, vulva, and anus) PIN lesions exhibit histologically low, moderate, or severe dysplasia (PIN grades 1, 2, or 3). In PIN 3 atypical cells are found in all layers of the affected epithelium. It has been clearly shown that these higher-grade PIN lesions are precursor lesions of penile cancer. Cell differentiation is completely absent, no or only very small amounts of virus are produced, and thus infectivity of these lesions is extremely low or absent. This is in contrast to genital warts and PIN1 and PIN2. Studies by Malek and coworkers [91] and

Table 37.3 Algorithm for the treatment of external warts in the primary care setting

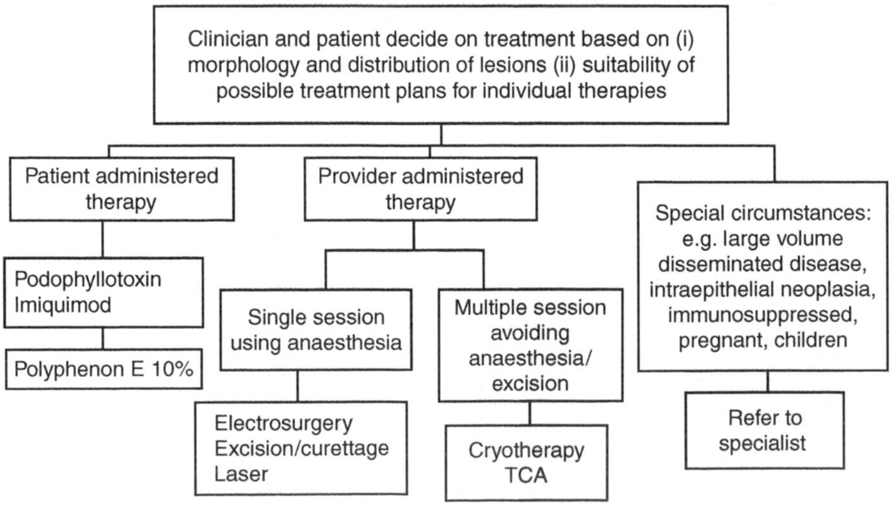

Source: [138]

by [3] have shown that the mean age of patients with lesions histologically characterized as PIN is 35.8 years for patients with either PIN1 or PIN2, 56.1 years for patients with PIN3 and 65.3 years for patients suffering from invasive squamous cell carcinoma of the penis. This allows the suggestion that it takes at least 15–20 years for penile HPV infection to develop into invasive cancer. HPV types discovered in PIN2 and PIN3 lesions belong to the HR-HPV types with HPV 16 and 18 the most frequently detectable types. In contrast both LR and to a lesser extent HR-HPV types have been isolated from PIN-1 lesions.

Penile intraepithelial neoplasias present differently in young men (25–40 years of age) and in men older than 40 years [6,41]. Differentiation between PIN in men of young and older age groups is only possible on clinical grounds [7,41]. Histology alone is not helpful. There are three clinical entities, fulfilling the histologic criteria of PIN 3: erythroplasia of Queyrat, penile Bowen's disease, and bowenoid papulosis. The latter is seen almost always in younger men [3]. While Bowen's disease and erythroplasia of Queyrat were described 100 years ago bowenoid papulosis (syn: multicentric (pigmented) Bowen's disease) was initially described in 1970 by Lloyd and colleagues [86]. Wade et al. were the first to use the term bowenoid papulosis [140, 141] for multiple papular lesions with histologic features of high-grade dysplasia. In the early 1980s HPV 16 DNA was repeatedly identified in biopsies from bowenoid papulosis [57–59,75]. In the late 1980s HPV16 and 18 and other HR-HPV types were detected coincidentally in PIN3, VIN3, CIN3 of sexual partners [66,104], implicating transmission of HR HPV between sexual partners.

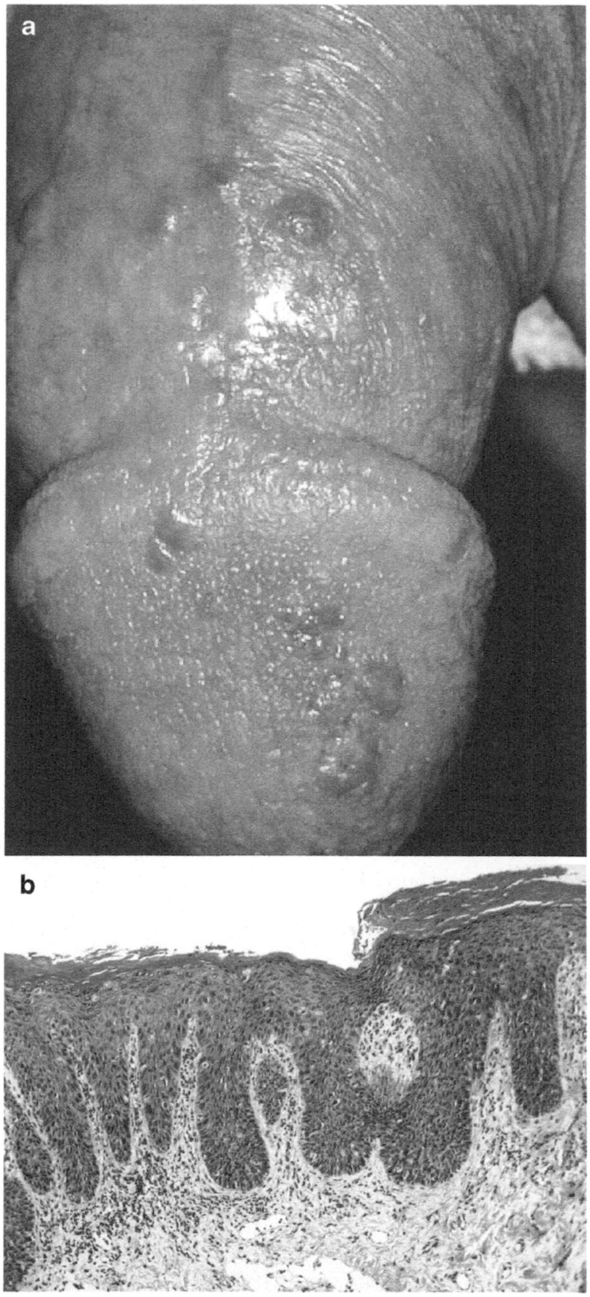

Fig. 37.7 (**a**) So-called bowenoid papulosis (**b**) Histology: severe penile intraepithelial neoplasia (PIN grade 3) (HPV 16 DNA-positive)

37.2.10 PIN in Young Men

HPV-associated lesions in young men with histologic features of PIN grade 1–3, manifest macroscopically as multiple brownish or red papules, or macules as well as leukoplakia-like lesions. Rarely mixtures of these may occur [62]. PIN lesions in young men tend to be multiple (Fig. 37.7). They grow multifocally at the entire genitoanal skin and the adjacent mucosal sites and show a tendency to confluence. Severe PIN (PIN3-lesions) occurring in young men have been known as bowenoid papulosis [140]. Spontaneous regression has been noticed. The same is known from VIN 3 lesions in young females [104]. However, malignant conversion of bowenoid papulosis may also occur [110], particularly in immunodeficient and HIV-positive individuals as well as in transplant recipients.

Smoking seems to be a risk factor for the persistence of PIN and for cancer development [38]. The same holds true for the development of HPV-associated VIN and vulvar carcinoma. Bowenoid papulosis and other PIN lesions in the young male have to be differentiated from a large number of dermatologic disorders located in the genitoanal area. This is done by taking a biopsy and by histologic workup. For instance, pigmented lesions such as benign genitoanal warts, melanocytic nevi, seborrheic keratoses, lichen sclerosus, resolving lesions of lichen planus, angiokeratoma, and even malignant melanoma may mimic pigmented PIN lesions. Red lesions with features of PIN have to be differentiated from lichen planus and psoriasis. Leukoplakia-like HPV-associated PIN in young men are usually multifocal. This enables to distinguish them from invasive cancer and lichen sclerosus. The latter appear regularly as solitary plaques.

Red areas with histologic features of PIN can be easily distinguished from simple balanitis or erosive lichen planus by missing symptoms as burning or itching. Polymorphous and polychromatous lesions always are suspicious of invasive cancer and should be removed by scalpel excision followed by a thorough histologic workup of the material.

37.2.11 PIN in Older Men

HR-HPV types have been regularly detected in PIN lesions of the elderly [3,57,59,75]. In older men PIN lesions comprise Bowen's disease and erythroplasia of Queyrat. The manifestation of Bowen's disease at the genitoanal skin is a velvet-red solitary area or a whitish plaque with a smooth or verrucous surface. Lesions of Bowen`s disease grow centrifugally, leading to large areas involving the pubes, perineal, and perianal skin sites.

Lesions of erythroplasia of Queyrat often are erosive and affect mainly the glans, the coronal sulcus, and the inner aspect of the foreskin. In older men PIN lesions have to be differentiated from other genitoanal conditions such as an atypical genital wart or lichen sclerosus. Histology is mandatory to distinguish reddish PIN lesions from psoriasis, lichen ruber, eczema (lichen simplex chronicus) or Paget's disease. The same is true to distinguish erythroplasia of Queyrat from Zoon's plasmacellular balanitis, erosive lichen planus or even simple balanitis. Treatment of HR-HPV-associated intraepithelial neoplasia is primarily surgical. In PIN of young adults, however, local immunotherapy with imiquimod has become an option [52, 137]. However, it is a goal that PIN in old men has to be completely excised and thoroughly investigated by histological means [63] in order to exclude malignant conversion.

37.3 Penile Cancer

37.3.1 Epidemiology and Pathogenesis

Penile cancer usually appears in the adult population with a peak incidence in the sixth decade [68]. Invasive cancer of the penis is an uncommon diagnosis in developed countries with an annual incidence of 0.1–0.9/100,000 inhabitants [40] in Europe and the USA. Penile cancer accounts only for 0.3–0.5% of all malignancies detected in the male population of the USA. It is the cause of less than 1–2% of all deaths from cancer in men [99]. In some developing countries of Africa, South America, and Asia, however, the prevalence is much higher than in Europe and in USA, reaching 10–20% of all malignancies in males [91]. In Uganda and Paraguay the yearly incidence is as high as 4.4 and 4.2 per 100,000 inhabitants, respectively [74,139].

There is evidence that HR HPV have a role in a subclass of penile squamous cell cancer [34,40,68,121]. Most likely the pathogenesis reflects several steps of events over some decades from precursor lesions to squamous cell cancer. Risk factors for invasive penile carcinomas are phimosis and poor hygiene [34,43,89,90]. Other risk factors for the development of penile cancer include injury to the penis, cigarette smoking, and to a lesser extent, history of genital warts as well as other infectious or chronic inflammatory diseases of the penis. Recently Bleeker and colleagues claimed flat penile lesions a special risk of penile carcinoma [11].

The risk of UV light and photo-chemotherapy (psoralen with UVA, PUVA) in this context have not been clearly addressed and clarified so far. Circumcision performed neonatally but not after the neonatal period was associated with a threefold decreased risk of penile cancer [89]. Again, Maden and coworkers, however, showed that 20% of penile cancer patients had been circumcised neonatally [89]. In contrast, circumcision is associated with a reduced risk of penile HPV infection and in the case of high-risk men, having a history of numerous sexual partners, also with a lowered risk of cervical cancer in their current female consort [18].

The role of sexual behavior in the development of penile cancer still remains unclear. Already 20 years ago, HPV has been implicated as a causal agent, suggesting penile cancer to be a sexually transmitted disease [93,135].

But probably other microbial agents, chemical factors such as smoking, and immunosuppression may also contribute to the carcinogenesis of carcinoma of the penis [31,69]. In contrast to detection of "oncogenic" HPV in almost all invasive cervical cancers investigated [142], penile cancer biopsies showed regularly less frequently positive HPV results in a series of investigations. A systematic review of the HPV prevalence in 1,266 invasive penile squamous cell carcinoma cases from 30 studies showed a HPV prevalence of 47.9% [4]. Interestingly the HPV prevalence was clearly higher in basaloid/warty subtypes of penile cancer (66.3%) than in verrucous penile cancers (22.4%). The most prevalent types in penile cancer found are HPV 16 and HPV 18. So there is evidence that a subset of penile carcinomas is caused by infection with HR HPV. The incidence rate and the prevalence of the different subtypes seem to depend largely on the geographical area [21,22].

Being similar to the pathogenesis of vulvar cancer there may be two etiologies for penile cancer: one being HPV-related and the other due to other HPV-unrelated factors [121]. Penile carcinomas are heterogeneous and include different histological subtypes [34]. The majority of the tumors are well-differentiated keratinizing squamous cell carcinomas. The second most common tumor subtype is verrucous carcinoma. The less prevalent variants are basaloid carcinomas and warty carcinomas [30].

It is noteworthy that PIN3 comprising Bowen's disease, erythroplasia of Queyrat, and bowenoid papulosis, the latter being the papular variant of PIN3 in young men, are precursor lesions to only the subset of basaloid and warty carcinomas of the penis. The precursor lesions of keratinizing squamous cell carcinoma and verrucous carcinoma of the penis have not well established yet. In this context it is known that lichen sclerosus and squamous cell hyperplasia frequently coexist with keratinizing penile cancer [117]. Penile squamous cell carcinoma seems to be frequently associated with histological changes of lichen sclerosus and especially with phimosis. As with vulvar squamous cell carcinoma, non-lichen sclerosus-associated penile cancer tends to be frequently associated with HPV infection. Lichen sclerosus-associated penile squamous cell carcinoma, however, is not regularly HPV-associated [112,118]. Long-lasting giant condylomata acuminata may precede verrucous carcinoma (Buschke–Loewenstein tumor). Both conditions have been simultaneously detected [64,88]. Sometimes they have been difficult to differentiate. Penile Buschke–Loewenstein tumors occur mainly in uncircumcised men [17]. This tumor has been described in men between 18 and 80 years of age. About two-thirds of the affected men were younger than 50 years. Histologically, Buschke–Löwenstein tumor is a low-grade well-differentiated verrucous carcinoma with local invasion but minimal dysplasia and a low tendency to metastasize [83,88,124]. Since HR HPVs are more frequently detected in verrucous carcinomas than in giant condylomas, HPV typing seems to be a helpful diagnostic step to differentiate giant condyloma from verrucous carcinoma [65,67,101].

As a rule, cancer of the penis appears clinically as a solitary, indurated, sometimes exulcerated tumor (Fig. 37.8). Excessive hyperkeratosis and a verrucous surface are suspicious clinical findings. The main differential diagnoses of penile carcinoma are solitary

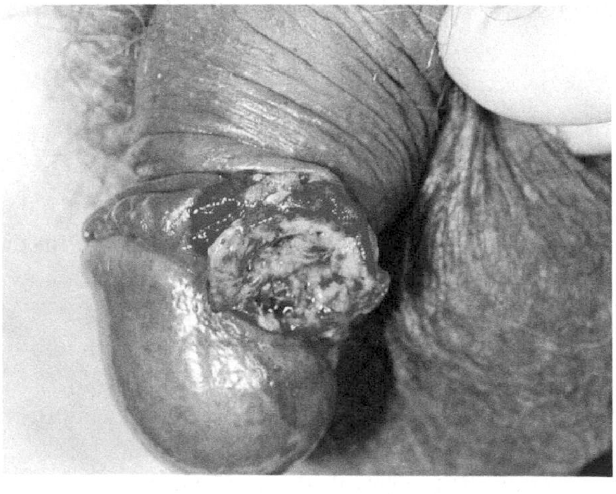

Fig. 37.8 Ulcerated penile cancer (HPV 16 DNA-positive)

benign condyloma acuminatum, giant condyloma, precursor lesions of PIN3 as Bowen's disease, erythroplasia of Queyrat, as well as lichen sclerosus. Rarely melanocytic nevi, seborrheic warts, basal cell carcinoma, and malignant melanoma pose problems in this context. The first diagnostic step is to take a biopsy or in case of a pigmented lesion to completely excise the tumor and to have a complete histology workup.

37.3.2 Treatment

Therapy of squamous cell carcinoma of the penis depends on the stage of the neoplasia. Amputation, either partial or total, has been the therapy of choice to locally control deeply invasive disease. Recurrences have been detected in about 19% [91]. A recent investigation on HPV DNA presence in 176 patients with squamous cell cancer of the penis led to new prognostic data. Patients with penile carcinoma in which HR HPV DNA (HPV16 and others) is detected by PCR seem to have a more favorable outcome in survival [87].

Lymph node metastasis is the most important prognostic factor in penile cancer. The role of HPV DNA detection in normal appearing lymph nodes as shown by [23,114], however, has not been generally accepted [10]. Prevention of penile cancer comprises neonatal circumcision, prevention of chronic HPV infection, prevention of phimosis, and smoking cessation. Chronic inflammatory conditions have to be treated consequently and UV-exposition and dermatologic PUVA treatment have to be minimized.

37.4 Perianal and Anal HPV Infection

HPV infections at anal and perianal sites are detectable in heterosexual men as well as in women at about the same frequency. However, most frequently such infections occur in men who have receptive anal intercourse. Natural history of HPV in the anal region should be probably similar to genital HPV infection [126].

The method by which HPV transfers to and infects the anus of heterosexual men, however, has been unknown. The clinical features of HPV-associated lesions of perianal and anal sites resemble those located on the external genitalia. The morphologic differences between cutaneous and mucosal lesions are comparable as are the differences between non-oncogenic and oncogenic HPV-associated lesions.

37.4.1 Non-Oncogenic LR-HPV-Associated Lesions

As at genital sites, exophytic warts are the most frequent manifestations at anal and perianal sites. According to Goorney and colleagues, anal warts have been detected in 30–45% of men with penile warts with about one-third of men being unaware of their presence. Perianal and anal warts have been almost never been detected as precursors of anal cancer. Flat warts and subclinical infections, the latter being detectable in the anal canal only after application of 3% acetic acid, often are not diagnosed by simple inspection. Warts above the dentate line have been rarely seen and usually in small numbers. Anal warts may coexist especially in immunodeficient patients with other benign lesions, such as fungal infections, herpetic lesions, fissures, mollusca contagiosa, rectal prolapse, haemorrhoids, skin tags, and eczema. Differentiation of perianal and anal warts from these conditions and from condylomata lata is of special importance. Thus in all cases screening for other sexually transmitted diseases and infections is mandatory as it is in genital warts at other sites.

Anal and perianal warts may regress spontaneously as shown in placebo-controlled studies [145]. However, anal warts may progress to exophytic partially giant lesions with the need for immediate therapy. Present treatment options comprise conservative procedures such as topical application of cytotoxic agents (podophyllotoxin) and immunomodulators such as imiquimod or intralesional injection of interferon. Additionally ablative therapies used are excision, cryosurgery, electrocautery, and laser surgery. Another option is the use of ultrasound-driven scalpel [28] which may, however, produce some sort of fume or bioaerosols [107] as do CO_2-laser and electrocauter [138]. Thus special safety measures during therapy are required as in CO_2 laser therapy [60, 61].

Conservative treatment and cryosurgery are the methods of choice for limited disease with circumscribed anal and perianal warts. Disseminated exophytic lesions need ablative therapies, sometimes in general systemic anesthesia.

37.4.2 Oncogenic HR-HPV-Associated Lesions and Anal Cancer

Anal cancer is an uncommon malignancy occurring in middle-aged adults and representing 4% of all cancers of the lower gastrointestinal tract. There is a slight female predominance of 1.5–2.0 times in USA and up to 3–6 times in Europe [24].

The annual incidence is approximately 1 case per 100,000 in the heterosexual population. Anal cancer accounts for about 500 new cases per year in the UK and about 3,500 in the USA [54]. There is a significantly higher (up to 35 per 100,000) incidence in men who practice anal receptive sexual intercourse. HIV-positive men have twice the risk of those are not. Rates of anal cancer have been increasing among men and women in the USA for more than three decades. Between 1973 and 2004 the incidence of anal cancer in US men increased from 0.5 to 1.3 per 100,000 [98]. Although the cause of this increase is uncertain, it is remarkable that the incidence of anal cancer among men in the USA is lower than that among women [78].

The most important etiological agent is the sexually transmitted infection of oncogenic HPV. Predominantly HR HPV types as HPV 16 and others have been detected in about 80% of squamous cell cancers of the anus, which accounts for the majority of anal cancers in the USA and in Europe [73]. [44] have shown that about 58% of anal cancers among heterosexual men and 100% among homosexual men were positive for HR HPV DNA. The most frequent HPV types detected in invasive anal cancer were HPV types 16 (87%), 18 (7.1%), 31 (1%), and 33 (6%) [44]. Although HPV is known to be the primary cause of anal cancer [32,44], little has been known about risk factors of HPV infection at anal sites of healthy heterosexual men until recently. In 2008, Nyitray et al. described these risk factors as lifetime number of female sexual partners and frequency of sexual contacts with females during the preceding month [103]. It was assumed that probably nonsexual HPV transmission via hand carriage may also play a role. Further alternative routes of transmission seem to exist including nonpenetrative sex or inoculation through fomites and contaminated objects [115].

37.4.3 Pathology

There is a fundamental distinction between epithelia of the skin-like anal margin and the mucosa-lined anal canal. The distal anal canal is lined with squamous epithelium which alters to a transitional epithelium near the dentate line (squamocolumnar junction) and ultimately to non-squamous rectal mucosa [133]. Thus, the histology of the anal canal shares essential parallels with that of the cervix uteri (transformation zone). Distal anal tumors have a keratinizing squamous morphology. However, the more proximal tumors are less likely to be keratinized [146]. Adenocarcinomas and other rare tumors of the anal canal, such as anal melanomas and sarcomas, having a bad prognosis, have to be differentiated. The same is also true for rare neuroendocrine tumors of the anal canal [24].

37.4.4 Clinical Features and Diagnosis

The morphology of HR-HPV-related intraepithelial neoplastic lesions at perianal sites (perianal intraepithelial neoplasia) is identical to intraepithelial neoplasia lesions at other external genital sites and at the perineum, presenting as flat pigmented lesions, red lesions, or leukoplakia-like lesions. Oncogenic (HR) HPV types have been shown to cause anal intraepithelial neoplasia (AIN) which can progress from low-grade to high-grade dysplasia (AIN1 to AIN2 and AIN3) and ultimately to invasive anal cancer. This is likely to suggest a biological continuum as it exists for the cervix uteri.

AIN grade 3 is regarded as the precursor lesion of anal cancer. Some HPV subtypes, preferentially HPV16 have been associated with a high risk of malignant transformation [109]. The natural histories of HPV-associated neoplasias of the anus and cervix begin with viral infection and progress to a dysplastic precursor lesion (intraepithelial neoplasia) followed by cancer [108]. Histologic features of intraepithelial neoplasia are found in flat or slightly papular lesions of the anal canal which strongly react to acetic acid as it is similarly seen in PIN or VIN. Some evidence exists that AIN in HIV-positive men who have sex with men is more likely to progress to anal cancer and that such progression occurs more rapidly than in heterosexual men. Low-grade AIN lesions frequently resolve but high-grade lesions are much more stable and often persist. Diagnostic methods available for AIN are inspection by a proctoscope or anoscope, digital rectal examination, high-resolution anoscopy, cytology (anal Pap smears), biopsy, and histology. In view of recent data it is advisable to use high-resolution anoscopy (similar to colposcopy) to identify areas of AIN and to take a biopsy. Appropriate screening with high-resolution anoscopy can be easily done in a primary care practice. Male individuals that would benefit are MSM, HIV-infected men, as well as immunosuppressed men [85].

Symptoms of anal cancer are bleeding (in about half of the affected patients) and anal pain. Less than 15% of patients have no symptoms at all. Clinically almost always a mass is detectable. Inguinal and perirectal lymph nodes are often palpable. Sonography, endocanal sonography, CT, and/or MRT are used to verify the diagnosis.

37.4.5 Treatment

Actual treatments for AIN are electrocautery, CO_2 laser, and infrared coagulator treatment. All of these are associated with a relatively high recurrence rate [51]. The most effective treatment known for CIN2 and CIN3 is excision of the transformation zone of the cervix with a conization procedure. This, however, is no option for treatment of anal lesions. Excision of large sections of the anal canal would be associated with anal stenosis and other severe complications. Circumscribed AIN are easily treated using trichloroacetic acid. An additional therapeutic possibility is liquid nitrogen ablation. More recently, topical application of imiquimod administered in form of anal tampons has shown some effect [144]. However, large studies evaluating the efficacy and safety of these methods have not been published yet. Another promising topical agent seems to be cidofovir A 1% gel. It has been used 5 days a week for up to 6 weeks. Cidofovir A 1% gel has led to complete clearance of benign anal warts and there was some clearance of high-risk HPV lesions [125] in a small clinical study.

Anal cancer can be cured by synchronous chemotherapy. This treatment enables anal continence and reserves abdominoperineal resection of the rectum and anal canal (with formation of permanent colostomy) for recurrent or residual disease after primary chemoradiotherapy. Overall survival from anal cancer is now around 70–80% at 5 years [24].

37.4.6 Prevention

Information, preferably in written form, and counseling are essential for the patient to understand the natural history, diagnosis and treatment, outcome, and possible complications of genitoanal HPV infection as well as of other sexually transmitted diseases [70].

Patients should be encouraged to use barrier protection with new sexual contacts. This not only since many sexually transmitted infections, including HIV infection, chlamydia, gonorrhoea, and syphilis are effectively prevented by condom use, but also to prevent or at least to reduce HPV infections and clinical manifestations [13]. Current sexual partners should be assessed for the presence of lesions and for education and counseling about STDs and their prevention. Smokers affected by genital warts should be encouraged to stop smoking since a correlation seems to exist with wart development and delayed clearance of warts [38].

37.4.7 Vaccination of Males

The burden of disease and costs of managing and treating genitoanal warts and intraepithelial neoplasias in men are considerable. A vaccination program using the quadrivalent HPV vaccine also for male adults could provide a substantial health benefit and reduce the costs associated with genitoanal warts and penile as well as anal cancer (see Chapter 51, page 686).

The impact of prophylactic quadrivalent HPV vaccination on men is protection against vaccine HPV type intraepithelial neoplasia and cancer as well as genitoanal warts. Studies in males (16–24-year-old) clearly showed prophylactic efficacy of the quadrivalent HPV vaccine against HPV 6, 11, 16, 18 external genitoanal lesions including genital warts [48]. There is clear evidence for safety and immunogenicity of HPV vaccines in men aged 10–15 years [14].

The impact of quadrivalent HPV vaccination in Australia 1 year after the implementation in women younger than 28 years of age resulted in a 25% reduction of genital warts and other diseases appearing early after HPV acquisition in women younger than 28 years of age. Such a high level of success clearly needs a high vaccination coverage of more than 65% as shown in Australia [37]. Since the quadrivalent HPV vaccine has shown efficacy in males, vaccination strategies that include both sexes may be also more cost-effective in reducing female disease burden than a gender-targeted strategy [47].

In addition to the prophylactic effect in genital wart development early data published suggest possible additional therapeutic effects of the quadrivalent HPV vaccine administration to otherwise healthy individuals with multiple viral warts [134]. In view of these and other observations, placebo-controlled studies of the vaccine should be performed also to prevent recurrence of warts after ablation and even to eliminate manifest warts.

37.5 Conclusion

HPV is one of the most common sexually transmitted infections among men. In contrast to other venereal infections HPV is widespread in communities and not restricted to core groups.

Low-risk HPV types cause genital warts which have been continuously on the rise since years. High-risk HPVs, such as HPV16 and other types are associated with penile and anal cancer as well as with precursor lesions. The proportion of HPV-associated penile cancer is at most 40–50% while more than 80% of anal cancers are caused by HPV.

There is substantial burden of disease from genital warts in terms of their chronic nature and their impact on health-related quality of life. Despite some recent developments current therapies are not satisfactory.

In view of the recently published data it is highly mandatory to emphasize non-gender quadrivalent HPV vaccination. Primary prevention of genitoanal HPV infection in the male enables reduction of HPV infection and of HPV-associated morbidity in both genders.

Take-Home Pearls

- Genitoanal HPV infection in men is equally common as in women.
- The highest rates of genital warts are observed in males 20 – 24 years of age, whereas in females the peak is in the age between 16 – 24 years.
- Genitoanal warts are highly infectious with an incubation period between 3 weeks and 8 months.
- Current treatment of genitoanal warts has been not optimal since high recurrence rates have been noticed.
- Diagnosis of genitoanal warts should include exclusion of other sexually transmitted conditions, simple anatomic variants, genitoanal dermatoses and malignant squamous cell neoplasias including cancer precursor lesions.
- Every atypic lesion has to be biopsied. Pigmented lesions have to be excised entirely and histologically investigated.
- The histology of the anal canal shows parallels with that of the cervix uteri (transformation zone).
- Anal intraepithelial neoplasia (AIN) is a precursor lesion for squamous cell carcinoma of the anus.
- There is a clear etiological association between AIN and high-risk HPV subtype infection.
- The proportion of HPV-associated anal cancer is about 90 % and that of penile cancer 40 – 50 %.
- In order to prevent the development of anal cancer high-risk individuals have to be identified.

References

1. Agarwal, S.S., Sehgal, A., Sardana, S., Kumar, A., Luthra, U.K.: Role of male behavior in cervical carcinogenesis among women with one lifetime sexual partner. Cancer **72**(5), 1666–1669 (1993)
2. Aubin, F., Prétet, J.L., Jacquard, A.C., Saunier, M., Carcopino, X., Jaroud, F., Pradat, P., Soubeyrand, B., Leocmach, Y., Mougin, C., Riethmuller, D., EDiTH Study Group: Human papillomavirus genotype distribution in

external acuminata condylomata: a Large French National Study (EDiTH IV). Clin. Infect. Dis. **47**(5), 610–615 (2008)
3. Aynaud, O., Ionesco, M., Barrasso, R.: Penile intraepithelial neoplasia. Specific clinical features correlate with histlogic and virologic findings. Cancer **74**, 1762–1767 (1994)
4. Backes, D.M., Kurman, R.J., Pimenta, J.M., Smith, J.S.: Systematic review of human papillomavirus prevalence in invasive penile cancer. Cancer Causes Control **20**(4), 449–457 (2009)
5. Baldwin, S.B., Wallace, D.R., Papenfuss, M.R., Abrahamsen, M., Vaught, L.C., Giuliano, A.R.: Condom use and other factors affecting penile human papillomavirus detection in men attending a sexually transmitted disease clinic. Sex. Transm. Dis. **31**(10), 601–607 (2004)
6. Barrasso, R., De Brux, J., Croissant, O., Orth, G.: High prevalence of papillomavirus-associated penile intraepithelial neoplasia in sexual partners of women with cervical intraepithelial neoplasia. N Engl J. Med. **317**, 916–923 (1987)
7. Barrasso, R., Gross, G.: Male HPV-associated lesions. Epidemiology and diagnostic criteria. In: Gross, G., Jablonska, S., Pfister, H., Stegner, H.E. (eds.) Genital papillomavirus infections. Springer, Berlin, Heidelberg, New York (1990)
8. Barrasso, R., Gross, G.: External genitalia: diagnosis. In: Gross, G., Barrasso, R. (eds.) Human papillomavirus infection. A clinical atlas. Ullstein-Mosby, Wiesbaden (1997)
9. Beutner, K.R., Reitano, M.V., Richwald, G.A., Wiley, D.J.: External genital warts: report of the American Medical Association Consensus Conference. AMA Expert Panel on External Genital Warts. Clin. Infect. Dis. **27**(4), 796–806 (1998)
10. Bezerra, A.I.R., Lopez, A., Santiago, G.A., et al.: Human papillomavirus as a prognostic factor in carcinoma of the penis. Cancer **91**, 2315–2321 (2000)
11. Bleeker, M.C., Snijders, P.F., Voorhorst, F.J., Meijer, C.J.: Flat penile lesions: the infectious "invisible" link in the transmission of human papillomavirus. Int. J. Cancer **119**(11), 2505–2512 (2006)
12. Bleeker, M.C., Hogewoning, C.J., Van Den Brule, A.J., Voorhorst, F.J., Van Andel, R.E., Risse, E.K., Starink, T.M., Meijer, C.J.: Penile lesions and human papillomavirus in male sexual partners of women with cervical intraepithelial neoplasia. J. Am. Acad. Dermatol. **47**(3), 351–357 (2002)
13. Bleeker, M.C., Hogewoning, C.J., Voorhorst, F.J., van den Brule, A.J., Snijders, P.J., Starink, T.M., Berkhof, J., Meijer, C.J.: Condom use promotes regression of human papillomavirus-associated penile lesions in male sexual partners of women with cervical intraepithelial neoplasia. Int. J. Cancer **107**(5), 804–810 (2003)
14. Block, S.L., Nolan, T., Sattler, C., Barr, E., Giacoletti, K.E., Marchant, C.D., Castellsagué, X., Rusche, S.A., Lukac, S., Bryan, J.T., Cavanaugh Jr., P.F., Reisinger, K.S., Protocol 016 Study Group: Comparison of the immunogenicity and reactogenicity of a prophylactic quadrivalent human papillomavirus (types 6, 11, 16, and 18) L1 virus-like particle vaccine in male and female adolescents and young adult women. Pediatrics **118**(5), 2135–2145 (2006)
15. Bosch, F.X., Castellsagué, X., Muñoz, N., de Sanjosé, S., Ghaffari, A.M., González, L.C., Gili, M., Izarzugaza, I., Viladiu, P., Navarro, C., Vergara, A., Ascunce, N., Guerrero, E., Shah, K.V.: Male sexual behavior and human papillomavirus DNA: key risk factors for cervical cancer in Spain. J. Natl Cancer Inst. **88**(15), 1060–1067 (1996)
16. Brown, D.R., Schroeder, J.M., Bryan, J.T., Stoler, M.H., Fife, K.H.: Detection of multiple human papillomavirus types in Condylomata acuminata lesions from otherwise healthy and immunosuppressed patients. J. Clin. Microbiol. **37**, 3316–3322 (1999)
17. Buschke, A., Löwenstein, L.: Über carcinomähnliche Condylomata acuminata. Klin. Wochenschr. **4**, 1726–1728 (1925)
18. Castellsagué, X., Bosch, F.X., Muñoz, N., Meijer, C.J., Shah, K.V., de Sanjose, S., Eluf-Neto, J., Ngelangel, C.A., Chichareon, S., Smith, J.S., Herrero, R., Moreno, V., Franceschi, S.: Male circumcision, penile human papillomavirus infection, and cervical cancer in female partners. N Engl J. Med. **346**(15), 1105–1112 (2002)
19. Centers for Disease Control and Prevention: Sexually transmitted disease treatment guidelines 1998. US Department of Health Service. Public Health Service. Centers for Disease Control and Prevention, Atlanta. MMWR 2006; 47: No. RR-11: 1–111 (1998).
20. Centers for Disease Control and Prevention: Sexually transmitted disease treatment guidelines 2006. US Department of Health Service. Public Health Service. Centers for Disease Control and Prevention, Atlanta. MMWR 2006; 55: No. RR-11: 1–100 (2006).
21. Chaux, A., Tamboli, P., Lezcano, C., Ro, J., Ayala, A., Cubilla, A.L.: Comparison of subtypes of penile squamous cell carcinoma from high and low incidence geographical regions. Int. J. Surg. Pathol. **18**(4), 268–277 (2009)
22. Chaux, A., Reuter, V., Lezcano, C., Velazquez, E.F., Torres, J., Cubilla, A.L.: Comparison of morphologic features and outcome of resected recurrent and nonrecurrent squamous cell carcinoma of the penis: a study of 81 cases. Am. J. Surg. Pathol. **33**(9), 1299–1306 (2009)
23. Chaux, A., Caballero, C., Soares, F., Guimarães, G.C., Cunha, I.W., Reuter, V., Barreto, J., Rodríguez, I., Cubilla, A.L.: The prognostic index: a useful pathologic guide for prediction of nodal metastases and survival in penile squamous cell carcinoma. Am. J. Surg. Pathol. **33**(7), 1049–1057 (2009)
24. Clark, M.A., Hartley, A., Geh, J.I.: Cancer of the anal canal. Lancet Oncol. **5**(3), 149–157 (2004)
25. Clinical Effectiveness Group (Association of Genitourinary Medicine and the Medical Society for the Study of Venereal Diseases: National guideline for the management of anogenital warts. Sex Transm. Inf. **75**(Suppl 1), S71–S75 (1999)
26. Cogliano, V., Baan, R., Straif, K., Grosse, Y., Secretan, B., El Ghissassi, F., WHO International Agency for Research on Cancer: Carcinogenicity of human papillomaviruses. Lancet Oncol. **6**(4), 204 (2005)
27. Coleman, N., Birley, H.D., Renton, A.M., Hanna, N.F., Ryait, B.K., Byrne, M., Taylor-Robinson, D., Stanley, M.A.: Immunological events in regressing genital warts. Am. J. Clin. Pathol. **102**(6), 768–774 (1994)
28. Colombo-Benkmann, M., Tübergen, D., Buchweitz, O., Senninger, N.: Ultrasonic technology: a new treatment option for anal condylomata acuminata. Dis. Colon Rectum **51**(11), 1681–1685 (2008)

29. Conway, E.L., Stein, A.N., Pirotta, M., Garland, S.: Genital warts and associated health care use in general practice in Australia. Sex. Health **4**(4), 305 (2007)
30. Cubilla, A.L., Reuter, V.E., Gregoire, L., Ayala, G., Ocampos, S., Lancaster, W.D., Fair, W.: Basaloid squamous cell carcinoma: a distinctive human papilloma virus-related penile neoplasm: a report of 20 cases. Am. J. Surg. Pathol. **22**(6), 755–761 (1998)
31. Daling, J.R., Sherman, K.J.: Relationship between human papillomavirus infection and tumours of anogenital sites other than the cervix. IARC Sci. Publ. (119):223–241 (1992). Review.
32. Daling, J.R., Madeleine, M.M., Johnson, L.G., Schwartz, S.M., Shera, K.A., Wurscher, M.A., Carter, J.J., Porter, P.L., Galloway, D.A., McDougall, J.K.: Human papillomavirus, smoking, and sexual practices in the etiology of anal cancer. Cancer **101**(2), 270–280 (2004)
33. de Villiers, E.M., Fauquet, C., Broker, T.R., Bernard, H.U., zur Hausen, H.: Classification of papillomaviruses. Virology **324**(1), 17–27 (2004)
34. Dillner, J., von Krogh, G., Horenblas, S., Meijer, C.J.: Etiology of squamous cell carcinoma of the penis. Scand J Urol Nephrol Suppl. (205):189–193 (2000).
35. Dunne, E.F., Nielson, C.M., Stone, K.M., Markowitz, L.E., Giuliano, A.R.: Prevalence of HPV infection among men: A systematic review of the literature. J. Infect. Dis. **194**(8), 1044–1057 (2006)
36. Ewald, K., Gross, G.: Perianal Hailey-Hailey disease: an unusual differential diagnosis of condylomata acuminata. Int. J. STD AIDS **19**(11), 791–792 (2008)
37. Fairley, C.K., Hocking, J.S., Gurrin, L.C., Chen, M.Y., Donovan, B., Bradshaw, C.S.: Rapid decline in presentations of genital warts after the implementation of a national quadrivalent human papillomavirus vaccination programme for young women. Sex. Transm. Infect. **85**(7), 499–502 (2009)
38. Feldman, J.G., Chirgwin, K., Dehovitz, J.A., Minkoff, H.: The association of smoking and risk of condyloma acuminatum in women. Obstet. Gynecol. **89**(3), 346–350 (1997)
39. Ferenczy, A., Bergeron, C., Richart, R.M.: Human papillomavirus DNA in fomites on objects used for the management of patients with genital human papillomavirus infections. Obstet. Gynecol. **74**(6), 950–954 (1989)
40. Ferreux, E., Lont, A.P., Horenblas, S., Gallee, M.P., Raaphorst, F.M., von Knebel, D.M., Meijer, C.J., Snijders, P.J.: Evidence for at least three alternative mechanisms targeting the p16INK4A/cyclin D/Rb pathway in penile carcinoma, one of which is mediated by high-risk human papillomavirus. J. Pathol. **201**(1), 109–118 (2003)
41. Franceschi, S., Castellsagué, X., Dal Maso, L., Smith, J.S., Plummer, M., Ngelangel, C., Chichareon, S., Eluf-Neto, J., Shah, K.V., Snijders, P.J., Meijer, C.J., Bosch, F.X., Muñoz, N.: Prevalence and determinants of human papillomavirus genital infection in men. Br. J. Cancer **86**(5), 705–711 (2002)
42. Friis, S., Kjaer, S.K., Frisch, M., Mellemkjaer, L., Olsen, J.H.: Cervical intraepithelial neoplasia, anogenital cancer, and other cancer types in women after hospitalization for condylomata acuminata. J. Infect. Dis. **175**(4), 743–748 (1997)
43. Frisch, M., Friis, S., Kjaer, S.K., Melbye, M.: Falling incidence of penis cancer in an uncircumcised population (Denmark 1943–90). BMJ **311**(7018), 1471 (1995)
44. Frisch, M., Glimelius, B., van den Brule, A.J., Wohlfahrt, J., Meijer, C.J., Walboomers, J.M., Goldman, S., Svensson, C., Adami, H.O., Melbye, M.: Sexually transmitted infection as a cause of anal cancer. N Engl J. Med. **337**(19), 1350–1358 (1997)
45. Gissmann, L., Wolnik, L., Ikenberg, H., Koldovsky, U., Schnürch, H.G., zur Hausen, H.: Human papillomavirus types 6 and 11 DNA sequences in genital and laryngeal papillomas and in some cervical cancers. Proc. Natl Acad. Sci. USA **80**(2), 560–563 (1983)
46. Giuliano, A.R.: Human papillomavirus vaccination in males. Gynecol. Oncol. **107**(2 Suppl 1), S24–S26 (2007). Review
47. Giuliano, A.R., Salmon, D.: The case for a gender-neutral (universal) human papillomavirus vaccination policy in the United States: Point. Cancer Epidemiol. Biomarkers Prev. **17**(4), 805–808 (2008)
48. Giuliano, A., Palefsky, J., on behalf of the male quadrivalent HPV vaccine efficacy trial study group: The efficacy of quadrivalent HPV (types 6/11/16/18) vaccine in reducing the incidence of HPV infection and HPV-related genital disease in young men. Abstract of presentation at the European Research Organization on Genital Infection and Neoplasia (EUROGIN) International Multidisciplinary Conference, Nov 13. Nice, France, SS17–19 (2008).
49. Giuliano, A.R., Lazcano-Ponce, E., Villa, L.L., Flores, R., Salmeron, J., Lee, J.H., Papenfuss, M.R., Abrahamsen, M., Jolles, E., Nielson, C.M., Baggio, M.L., Silva, R., Quiterio, M.: The human papillomavirus infection in men study: human papillomavirus prevalence and type distribution among men residing in Brazil, Mexico, and the United States. Cancer Epidemiol. Biomarkers Prev. **17**(8), 2036–2043 (2008)
50. Giuliano, A.R., Lazcano, E., Villa, L.L., Flores, R., Salmeron, J., Lee, J.H., Papenfuss, M., Abrahamsen, M., Baggio, M.L., Silva, R., Quiterio, M.: Circumcision and sexual behavior: factors independently associated with human papillomavirus detection among men in the HIM study. Int. J. Cancer **124**(6), 1251–1257 (2009)
51. Goldstone, S.E., Kawalek, A.Z., Huyett, J.W.: Infrared coagulator: a useful tool for treating anal squamous intraepithelial lesions. Dis. Colon Rectum **48**(5), 1042–1054 (2005)
52. Goorney, B.P., Polori, R.: A case of Bowenoid papulosis of the penis successfully treated with topical imiquimod cream 5%. Int. J. STD AIDS **15**(12), 833–835 (2004)
53. Gotovtseva, E.P., Kapadia, A.S., Smolensky, M.H., Lairson, D.R.: Optimal frequency of imiquimod (Aldara) 5% cream for the treatment of external genital warts in immunocompetent adults: a meta-analysis. Sex. Transm. Dis. **35**(4), 346–351 (2008)
54. Greenlee, R.T., Murray, T., Bolden, S., Wingo, P.A.: Cancer statistics, 2000. CA Cancer J. Clin. **50**(1), 7–33 (2000)
55. Greer, C.E., Wheeler, C.M., Ladner, M.B., Beutner, K., Coyne, M.Y., Liang, H., Langenberg, A., Yen, T.S., Ralston, R.: Human papillomavirus (HPV) type distribution and serological response to HPV type 6 virus-like particles in patients with genital warts. J. Clin. Microbiol. **33**(8), 2058–2063 (1995)

56. Gross, G., Ikenberg, H., Gissmann, L., Hagedorn, M.: Papillomavirus infection of the anogenital region: correlation between histology, clinical picture, and virus type. Proposal of a new nomenclature. J. Invest. Dermatol. **85**(2), 147–152 (1985)
57. Gross, G., Hagedorn, M., Ikenberg, H., Rufli, T., Dahlet, C., Grosshans, E., Gissmann, L.: Bowenoid papulosis. Presence of human papillomavirus (HPV) structural antigens and of HPV 16-related DNA sequences. Arch. Dermatol. **121**, 858–863 (1985)
58. Gross, G., Ikenberg, H., de Villiers, E.M., Schneider, A., Wagner, D., Gissmann, L.: Bowenoid papulosis: a venereally transmitted disease as reservoir for HPV 16. In: Zur Hausen, H., Peto, P. (eds.) Origins of female genital cancer: virological and epidemiological aspects. (Banbury Report), pp. 140–165. Cold Spring Harbor Laboratories, Cold Spring Harbor (1986)
59. Gross, G., Jablonska, S., Pfister, H., Stegner, H.E.: Genital papillomavirus infections. In: Modern Diagnosis and Treatment. Springer-Verlag, Berlin, Heidelberg, New York, London, Paris, Tokyo, Hon Kong, Barcelona (1990)
60. Gross, G.: Treatment of human papillomavirus infection. In: Mindel, A. (ed.) Genital warts. Human papillomavirus infection, pp. S.148–S.236. Edward Arnold, London, Boston, Melbourne, Auckland (1995)
61. Gross, G., Tyring, S.K., von Krogh, G., Barrasso, R.: External genitalia treatment. In: Gross, G., Barrasso, G. (eds.) Human Papillomavirus Infections. A Clinical Atlas. Ullstein-Mosby, Wiesbaden, Berlin (1997)
62. Gross, G., Barrasso, R.: Human Papillomavirus Infection. A Clinical Atlas. Ullstein-Mosby, Wiesbaden, Berlin (1997)
63. Gross, G., Korting, H.C., Schöfer, H., Szeimies, R.M., Ebisch, M.A., Ikenberg, H., Petry, K.U., Schneede, P., Pfister, H.: Condylomata acuminata und andere HPV-assoziierte Krankheitsbilder des Genitale und der Harnröhre, Leitlinie der Deutschen STD-Gesellschaft. Hautarzt **52**, 405–410 (2001)
64. Gross, G., Pfister, H.: Role of human papillomavirus in penile cancer, penile intraepithelial squamous cell neoplasias and in genital warts. Med. Microbiol. Immunol. **193**(1), 35–44 (2004)
65. Gross, G., Meyer, K.G., Pres, H., Thielert, C., Tawfik, H., Mescheder, A.: A randomized, double-blind, four-arm parallel-group, placebo-controlled phase II/III study to investigate the clinical efficacy of two galenic formulations of Polyphenon® E in the treatment of external genital warts. J. Eur. Acad. Dermatol. Vernereol. **21**(10), 1404–1412 (2007)
66. Hauser, B., Gross, G., Schneider, A., Ikenberg, H., Gissmann, L.: HPV-16-related Bowenoid papulosis. Lancet **2**(8446), 106 (1985)
67. Haycox, C.L., Kuypers, J., Krieger, J.N.: Role of human papillomavirus typing in diagnosis and clinical decision making for a giant verrucous genital lesion. Urology **53**(3), 627–630 (1999)
68. Heideman, D.A., Waterboer, T., Pawlita, M., Delis-van Diemen, P., Nindl, I., Leijte, J.A., Bonfrer, J.M., Horenblas, S., Meijer, C.J., Snijders, P.J.: Human papillomavirus-16 is the predominant type etiologically involved in penile squamous cell carcinoma. J. Clin. Oncol. **25**(29), 4550–4556 (2007)
69. Hellberg, D., Valentin, J., Eklund, T., Nilsson, S.: Penile cancer: is there an epidemiological role for smoking and sexual behaviour? Br. Med. J. (Clin Res Ed) **295**(6609), 1306–1308 (1987)
70. Henderson, Z., Irwin, K.L., Montaño, D.E., Kasprzyk, D., Carlin, L., Greek, A., Freeman, C., Barnes, R., Jain, N.: Anogenital warts knowledge and counseling practices of US clinicians: results from a national survey. Sex. Transm. Dis. **34**(9), 644–652 (2007)
71. Hernandez, B.Y., Shvetsov, Y.B., Goodman, M.T., Wilkens, L.R., Thompson, P., Zhu, X., Ning, L.: Reduced clearance of penile human papillomavirus infection in uncircumcised men. J. Infect. Dis. **201**(9), 1340–1343 (2010)
72. Hillemanns, P., Breugelmans, J.G., Gieseking, F., Bénard, S., Lamure, E., Littlewood, K.J., Petry, K.U.: Estimation of the incidence of genital warts and the cost of illness in Germany: a cross-sectional study. BMC Infect. Dis. **8**, 76 (2008)
73. Hoots, B.E., Palefsky, J.M., Pimenta, J.M., Smith, J.S.: Human papillomavirus type distribution in anal cancer and anal intraepithelial lesions. Int. J. Cancer **124**(10), 2375–2383 (2009)
74. IARC, WHO: IARC monographs on the evolution of carcinogenic risks to humans. Human Papillomaviruses, vol. 64. IARC, Lyon (1995)
75. Ikenberg, H., Gissmann, L., Gross, G., Grussendorf-Conen, E.I., zur Hausen, H.: Human papillomavirus type-16-related DNA in genital Bowen's disease and in Bowenoid papulosis. Int. J. Cancer **32**(5), 563–565 (1983)
76. Insinga, R.P., Dasbach, E.J., Myers, E.R.: The health and economic burden of genital warts in a set of private health plans in the United States. Clin. Infect. Dis. **36**(11), 1397–1403 (2003)
77. Jayasinghe, Y., Garland, S.M.: Genital warts in children: what do they mean? Arch. Dis. Child. **91**(8), 696–700 (2006)
78. Joseph, D.A., Miller, J.W., Wu, X., Chen, V.W., Morris, C.R., Goodman, M.T., Villalon-Gomez, J.M., Williams, M.A., Cress, R.D.: Understanding the burden of human papillomavirus-associated anal cancers in the US. Cancer **113**(10 Suppl), 2892–2900 (2008)
79. Koshiol, J.E., Laurent, S.A., Pimenta, J.M.: Rate and predictors of new genital warts claims and genital warts-related healthcare utilization among privately insured patients in the United States. Sex. Transm. Dis. **31**(12), 748–752 (2004)
80. Koutsky, L.A., Galloway, D.A., Holmes, K.K.: Epidemiology of genital human papillomavirus infection. Epidemiol. Rev. **10**, 122–163 (1988). Review
81. Koutsky, L.: Epidemiology of genital human papillomavirus infection. Am. J. Med. **102**(5A), 3–8 (1997)
82. Kjaer, S.K., Tran, T.N., Sparen, P., Tryggvadottir, L., Munk, C., Dasbach, E., Liaw, K.L., Nygård, J., Nygård, M.: The burden of genital warts: a study of nearly 70, 000 women from the general female population in the 4 Nordic countries. J. Infect. Dis. **196**(10), 1447–1454 (2007)
83. Lacey, C.J.N., Roman, A., Brown, D.R.: Low oncogenic risk anogenital HPV infection. Papillomavirus Rep. **13**, 103–109 (2002)
84. Lacey, C.J., Lowndes, C.M., Shah, K.V.: Burden and management of non-cancerous HPV-related conditions: HPV-6/11 disease. Vaccine **24**(Suppl 3), 35–41 (2006)

85. Lindsey, K., DeCristofaro, C., James, J.: Anal Pap smears: should we be doing them? J. Am. Acad. Nurse Pract. **21**(8), 437–443 (2009). Review
86. Lloyd, K.M.: Multicentric pigmented Bowen's disease of the groin. Arch. Dermatol. **101**, 48–51 (1970)
87. Lont, A.P., Kroon, B.K., Horenblas, S., Gallee, M.P., Berkhof, J., Meijer, C.J., Snijders, P.J.: Presence of high-risk human papillomavirus DNA in penile carcinoma predicts favorable outcome in survival. Int. J. Cancer **119**(5), 1078–1081 (2006)
88. Lu, S., Bodemer, W., Ostwald, C., Barten, M., Zimmermann, R., Seipp, C., Gross, G.: Anal verrucous carcinoma and penile condylomata acuminata. Dermatology **200**(4), 320–323 (2000)
89. Maden, C., Sherman, K.J., Beckmann, A.M., Hislop, T.G., Teh, C.Z., Ashley, R.L., Daling, J.R.: History of circumcision, medical conditions, and sexual activity and risk of penile cancer. J. Natl Cancer Inst. **85**(1), 19–24 (1993)
90. Madsen, B.S., van den Brule, A.J., Jensen, H.L., Wohlfahrt, J., Frisch, M.: Risk factors for squamous cell carcinoma of the penis–population-based case-control study in Denmark. Cancer Epidemiol. Biomarkers Prev. **17**(10), 2683–2691 (2008)
91. Malek, R.S., Goellner, J.R., Smith, T.F., Espy, M.J., Cupp, M.R.: Human papillomavirus infection and intraepithelial, in situ, and invasive carcinoma of penis. Urology **42**(2), 159–170 (1993)
92. Majewski, S., Jablonska, S.: Human papillomavirus-associated tumors of the skin and mucosa. J. Am. Acad. Dermatol. **36**, 659–685 (1997)
93. McCance, D.J., Kalache, A., Ashdown, K., Andrade, L., Menezes, F., Smith, P., Doll, R.: Human papillomavirus types 16 and 18 in carcinomas of the penis from Brazil. Int. J. Cancer **37**, 55–59 (1986)
94. Mc Hugh, R.W., Hazen, P., Eliezri, Y.D., et al.: Metastatic periungual squamous cell carcinoma: detection of human papillomavirus type 35 RNA in the digital tumor and axillary lymphnodes metastases. J. Am. Acad. Dermatol. **34**, 1080–1082 (1996)
95. Miller, R.L., Gerster, J.F., Owens, M.L., Slade, H.B., Tomami, M.A.: Imiquimod applied topically: a novel immune response modifier and new class of drug. Int. J. Immunopharmacol. **21**, 1–14 (1999)
96. Monk, B.J., Tewari, K.S.: The spectrum and clinical sequelae of human papillomavirus infection. Gynecol. Oncol. **107**(2 Suppl. 1), S6–S13 (2007)
97. Moy, R.L., Eliezri, Y.D., Nuovo, G.J., Zitelli, J.A., Bennett, R.G., Silverstein, S.: Human papillomavirus type 16 DNA in periungual squamous cell carcinomas. JAMA **261**(18), 2669–2673 (1989)
98. National Cancer Institute. The Cancer Trends Progress Report: 2007 Update. http://www.cancer.gov/newscenter/pressreleases/ProgressReport2007 (2007).
99. Narayana, A.S., Olney, L.E., Loening, S.A., Weimar, G.W., Culp, D.A.: Carcinoma of the penis: analysis of 219 cases. Cancer **49**(10), 2185–2191 (1982)
100. Nielson, C.M., Harris, R.B., Dunne, E.F., Abrahamsen, M., Papenfuss, M.R., Flores, R., Markowitz, L.E., Giuliano, A.R.: Risk factors for anogenital human papillomavirus infection in men. J. Infect. Dis. **196**(8), 1137–1145 (2007)
101. Noel, J.C., Vandenbossche, M., Peny, M.O., Sassine, A., de Dobbeleer, G., Schulman, C.C., Verhest, A.: Verrucous carcinoma of the penis: importance of human papillomavirus typing for diagnosis and therapeutic decision. Eur. Urol. **22**(1), 83–85 (1992)
102. Nordenvall, C., Chang, E.T., Adami, H.O., Ye, W.: Cancer risk among patients with condylomata acuminata. Int. J. Cancer **119**(4), 888–893 (2006)
103. Nyitray, A., Nielson, C.M., Harris, R.B., Flores, R., Abrahamsen, M., Dunne, E.F., Giuliano, A.R.: Prevalence of and risk factors for anal human papillomavirus infection in heterosexual men. J. Infect. Dis. **197**(12), 1676–1684 (2008)
104. Obalek, S., Jablonska, S., Beaudenon, S., Walczak, L., Orth, G.: Bowenoid papulosis of the male and female genitalia: risk of cervical neoplasia. J. Am. Acad. Dermatol. **14**(3), 433–444 (1986)
105. Oriel, J.D.: Natural history of genital warts. Br. J. Vener. Dis. **47**, 1–13 (1971)
106. Oriel, J.D.: HPV infections of the urethra. In: Gross, G., Jablonska, S., Pfister, H., Stegner, H.E. (eds.) Genital papillomavirus infections, pp. 181–187. Springer, Berlin, Heidelberg, New York (1990)
107. Ott, D.E., Moss, E., Martinez, K.: Aerosol exposure from an ultrasonically activated (Harmonic) device. J. Am. Assoc. Gynecol. Laparosc. **5**(1), 29–32 (1998)
108. Palefsky, J.M., Holly, E.A., Ralston, M.L., Da Costa, M., Greenblatt, R.M.: Prevalence and risk factors for anal human papillomavirus infection in human immunodeficiency virus (HIV)-positive and high-risk HIV-negative women. J. Infect. Dis. **183**(3), 383–391 (2001)
109. Palmer, J.G., Scholefield, J.H., Coates, P.J., Shepherd, N.A., Jass, J.R., Crawford, L.V., Northover, J.M.: Anal cancer and human papillomaviruses. Dis. Colon Rectum **32**(12), 1016–1022 (1989)
110. Park, K.C., Kim, K.H., Youn, S.W., Hwang, J.H., Park, K.H., Ahn, J.S., Kim, Y.G., Kim, S.D., Lee, D.Y., Choe, J.H., Chung, J.H., Cho, K.H.: Heterogeneity of human papillomavirus DNA in a patient with Bowenoid papulosis that progressed to squamous cell carcinoma. Br. J. Dermatol. **139**(6), 1087–1091 (1998)
111. Partridge, J.M., Koutsky, L.A.: Genital human papillomavirus infection in men. Lancet Infect. Dis. **6**(1), 21–31 (2006)
112. Perceau, G., Derancourt, C., Clavel, C., Durlach, A., Pluot, M., Lardennois, B., Bernard, P.: Lichen sclerosus is frequently present in penile squamous cell carcinomas but is not always associated with oncogenic human papillomavirus. Br. J. Dermatol. **148**(5), 934–938 (2003)
113. Petzoldt, D., Gross, G. (eds.): Diagnostik und Therapie sexuell übertragbarer Krankheiten. Springer-Verlag, Berlin, Heidelberg, New York (2001)
114. Picconi, M.A., Eiján, A.M., Distéfano, A.L., Pueyo, S., Alonio, L.V., Gorostidi, S., Teyssié, A.R., Casabé, A.: Human papillomavirus (HPV) DNA in penile carcinomas in Argentina: analysis of primary tumors and lymph nodes. J. Med. Virol. **61**(1), 65–69 (2000)
115. Piketty, C., Darragh, T.M., Da Costa, M., Bruneval, P., Heard, I., Kazatchkine, M.D., Palefsky, J.M.: High prevalence of anal human papillomavirus infection and anal cancer precursors among HIV-infected persons in the absence

of anal intercourse. Ann. Intern. Med. **138**, 453–459 (2003)
116. Poljak, M., Kocjan, B.J., Potocnik, M., Seme, K.: Anogenital hairs are an important reservoir of alpha-papillomaviruses in patients with genital warts. J. Infect. Dis. **199**(9), 1270–1274 (2009)
117. Powell, J., Robson, A., Cranston, D., Wojnarowska, F., Turner, R.: High incidence of lichen sclerosus in patients with squamous cell carcinoma of the penis. Br. J. Dermatol. **145**(1), 85–89 (2001)
118. Renaud-Vilmer, C., Cavelier-Balloy, B., Verola, O., Morel, P., Servant, J.M., Desgrandckamps, F., Dubertret, L.: Analysis of alterations adjacent to invasive squamous cell carcinoma of the penis and their relations with associated carcinoma. J. Am. Acad. Dermatol. **62**(2), 284–290 (2010)
119. Rice, P.S., Mant, C., Cason, J., Bible, J.M., Muir, P., Kell, B., Best, J.M.: High prevalence of human papillomavirus type 16 infection among children. J. Med. Virol. **61**(1), 70–75 (2000)
120. Roden, R.B., Lowy, D.R., Schiller, J.T.: Papillomavirus is resistant to desiccation. J. Infect. Dis. **176**(4), 1076–1079 (1997)
121. Rubin, M.A., Kleter, B., Zhou, M., Ayala, G., Cubilla, A.L., Quint, W.G., Pirog, E.C.: Detection and typing of human papillomavirus DNA in penile carcinoma: evidence for multiple independent pathways of penile carcinogenesis. Am. J. Pathol. **159**(4), 1211–1218 (2001)
122. Schneede, P., Münch, P., Wagner, S., Meyer, T., Stockfleth, E., Hofstetter, A.: Fluorescence urethroscopy following instillation of 5-aminolevulinic acid: a new procedure for detecting clinical and subclinical HPV lesions of the urethra. J. Eur. Acad. Dermatol. Venereol. **15**(2), 121–125 (2001)
123. Schürmann, D., Bergmann, F., Temmesfeld-Wollbrück, B., Grobusch, M.P., Suttorp, N.: Topical cidofovir is effective in treating extensive penile condylomata acuminata. AIDS **14**(8), 1075–1076 (2000)
124. Schwartz, R.A.: Verrucous carcinoma of the skin and mucosa. J. Am. Acad. Dermatol. **32**, 1–18 (1995)
125. Snoeck, R., Van Ranst, M., Andrei, G., De Clercq, E., De Wit, S., Poncin, M., Clumeck, N.: Treatment of anogenital papillomavirus infections with an acyclic nucleoside phosphonate analogue. N Engl J. Med. **333**(14), 943–944 (1995)
126. Sonnex, C., Scholefield, J.H., Kocjan, G., Kelly, G., Whatrup, C., Mindel, A., Northover, J.M.: Anal human papillomavirus infection in heterosexuals with genital warts: prevalence and relation with sexual behaviour. BMJ. **303**(6812), 1243 (1991)
127. Staples, C.G., Henderson, D., Tsongalis, G.J., Fernandez, M., Krejci-Manwaring, J.: Condylomata of the pannus in 3 obese patients: a new location for a common disease. Arch. Dermatol. **146**(5), 572–574 (2010)
128. Stockfleth, E., Beti, H., Orasan, R., Grigorian, F., Mescheder, A., Tawfik, H., Thielert, C.: Topical Polyphenon E in the treatment of external genital and perianal warts: a randomized controlled trial. Br. J. Dermatol. **158**(6), 1329–1338 (2008)
129. Stone, K.M.: Epidemiologic aspects of genital HPV infection. Clin. Obstet. Gynecol. **32**(1), 112–116 (1989)
130. Svare, E.I., Kjaer, S.K., Worm, A.M., Osterlind, A., Meijer, C.J., van den Brule, A.J.: Risk factors for genital HPV DNA in men resemble those found in women: a study of male attendees at a Danish STD clinic. Sex. Transm. Infect. **78**(3), 215–218 (2002)
131. Syrjänen, K.J.: Association of human papillomavirus with penile cancer. In: Mindel, A. (ed.) Genital Warts. Human Papillomavirus Infection, pp. 163–197. Edward Arnold, Kent, London, Boston, Melbourne, Auckland (1995)
132. Tatti, S., Stockfleth, E., Beutner, K.R., Tawfik, H., Elsasser, U., Weyrauch, P., Mescheder, A.: Polyphenon E: a new treatment for external anogenital warts. Br. J. Dermatol. **162**(1), 176–184 (2010)
133. Thompson-Fawcett, M.W., Warren, B.F., Mortensen, N.J.: A new look at the anal transitional zone with reference to restorative proctocolectomy and the columnar cuff. Br. J. Surg. **85**, 1517–1521 (1998)
134. Venugopal, S.S., Murrell, D.F.: Recalcitrant cutaneous warts treated with recombinant quadrivalent human papillomavirus vaccine (types 6, 11, 16, and 18) in a developmentally delayed, 31-year-old white man. Arch. Dermatol. **146**(5), 475–477 (2010)
135. Villa, L.L., Lopez, A.: Human papillomavirus DNA sequences in penile carcinomas in Brazil. Int. J. Cancer **37**(6), 853–855 (1986)
136. Von Krogh, G., Gross, G., Barrasso, R.: Warts and HPV-related squamous cell tumors of the genitoanal area in adults. In: Gross, G., Von Krogh, G. (eds.) Human Papillomavirus Infections in Dermatovenereology, pp. 259–304. CRC Press, Boca Raton (1997)
137. Von Krogh, G., Horenblas, S.: The management and prevention of premalignant penile lesions. Scand. J. Urol. Nephrol. Suppl. **205**, 220–229 (2000)
138. Von Krogh, G., Lacey, C.I.N., Gross, G., Barrasso, R., Schneider, A.: European Course on HPV Associated Pathology (ECHPV): guidelines for primary care physicians for the diagnosis and management of anogenital warts. Sex. Transm. Infect. **76**, 162–168 (2000)
139. Wabinga, H.R., Parkin, D.M., Wabwire-Mangen, F., Nambooze, S.: Trends in cancer incidence in Kyadondo County, Uganda, 1960–1997. Br. J. Cancer **82**(9), 1585–1592 (2000)
140. Wade, T.R., Kopf, A.W., Ackerman, A.B.: Bowenoid papulosis of the penis. Cancer **42**(4), 1890–1903 (1978)
141. Wade, T.R., Kopf, A.W., Ackermann, A.B.: Bowenoid papulosis of the genitalia. Arch. Dermatol. **115**, 306–308 (1979)
142. Walboomers, J., Jacobs, M., Manos, M., et al.: Human papillomavirus as a necessary cause of invasive cervical cancer world wide. J. Pathol. **189**, 12–19 (1999)
143. Wheeler, C.M., Parmenter, C.A., Hunt, W.C., Becker, T.M., Greer, C.E., Hildesheim, A., Manos, M.M.: Determinants of genital human papillomavirus infection among cytologically normal women attending the University of New Mexico student health center. Sex. Transm. Dis. **20**(5), 286–289 (1993)
144. Wieland, U., Brockmeyer, N.H., Weissenborn, S.J., Hochdorfer, B., Stücker, M., Swoboda, J., Altmeyer, P., Pfister, H., Kreuter, A.: Imiquimod treatment of anal intraepithelial neoplasia in HIV-positive men. Arch. Dermatol. **142**(11), 1438–1444 (2006)

145. Wiley, D.J., Douglas, J., Beutner, K., Cox, T., Fife, K., Moscicki, A.B., Fukumoto, L.: External genital warts: diagnosis, treatment, and prevention. Clin. Infect. Dis. **35**(Suppl 2), S210–S224 (2002)
146. Williams, G.R., Talbot, I.C.: Anal carcinoma – a histological review. Histopathology **25**(6), 507–516 (1994)
147. Winer, R.L., Koutsky, L.A.: Human papillomavirus through the ages. J. Infect. Dis. **191**(11), 1787–1789 (2005)
148. Woodhall, S.C., Jit, M., Cai, C., Ramsey, T., Zia, S., Crouch, S., Birks, Y., Newton, R., Edmunds, W.J., Lacey, C.J.: Cost of treatment and QALYs lost due to genital warts: data for the economic evaluation of HPV vaccines in the United Kingdom. Sex. Transm. Dis. **36**(8), 515–521 (2009)
149. Zunzunegui, M.V., King, M.C., Coria, C.F., Charlet, J.: Male influences on cervical cancer risk. Am. J. Epidemiol. **123**(2), 302–307 (1986)
150. Zur Hausen, H.: Human papillomaviruses and their possible role in squamous cell carcinoma. Curr. Top. Microbiol. Immunol. **78**, 1–30 (1977)

38 HPV-Infection in HIV-Positive Men Who Have Sex with Men (MSM)

Ulrike Wieland, Alexander Kreuter, and Herbert Pfister

Core Messages

- Persistent anogenital infections with high- and low-risk HPV types are very frequent in HIV-positive men who have sex with men (MSM).
- Genital warts are frequently observed in HIV-positive men.
- Anal intraepithelial neoplasia (AIN) is very frequent in HIV-positive MSM.
- HAART does not seem to reduce the prevalence of AIN or anal cancer in HIV-positive MSM.
- The diagnosis of AIN includes cytology, high resolution anoscopy (HRA) and HRA-guided biopsy for histological evaluation.
- Anal cancer incidence is drastically increased in HIV-positive MSM compared to the general population.
- In the HAART era, outcome of anal cancer treatment is similar in HIV-negative and in HIV-positive patients.
- Penile intraepithelial neoplasia (PIN) seems to be more frequent in HIV-positive MSM and occurs at a younger age than in the general male population.
- All HIV-positive men should be screened for PIN/penile cancer in addition to anal screening.
- A physical examination of HIV-positive patients should include an inspection of the oral cavity to detect HPV-induced warts, dysplasias, or cancers.

U. Wieland (✉) and H. Pfister
Institute of Virology, University of Cologne, Fuerst-Pueckler-Strasse 56, 50935 Koeln, Germany
e-mail: ulrike.wieland@uni-koeln.de; herbert.pfister@uk-koeln.de

A. Kreuter
Department of Dermatology, Ruhr University Bochum, Gudrunstrasse 56, 44791 Bochum, Germany
e-mail: a.kreuter@derma.de

38.1 Introduction

More than 110 different human papillomavirus (HPV) types have been completely classified so far (http://www.ncbi.nlm.nih.gov/Taxonomy/ > Viruses > Papillomaviridae). The majority of alpha-HPV infects the anogenital mucosa and the adjacent anogenital skin. Alpha-HPV are further subdivided into high-risk (HR) and low-risk (LR) types. HR types as HPV16 or HPV18 are regularly found in anogenital cancers, whereas LR types as HPV6 or HPV11 are regularly detected in benign lesions or low-grade anogenital dysplasias, but rarely in cervical or anal cancers [1, 2]. Most alpha-HPV are sexually transmitted and their prevalence in the anogenital region of young, sexually active males and females is high [3, 4]. In immunocompetent persons most anogenital HPV infections are transient and less than 1% of women eventually develop cervical cancer due to persistent infections with HR-HPV types and even fewer men develop anal or penile cancer [1, 5]. In immunosuppressed individuals as HIV-infected men and women the rate of persistent HPV infection is much higher than in immunocompetent persons, and consequently, these patients have a considerably increased risk for HPV-induced cancers as cervical or anal cancer [6–9].

DOI: 10.1007/978-3-642-14663-3_38,

Recently, two prophylactic vaccines against HPV16/18 (Cervarix®) or HPV6/11/16/18 (Gardasil®) have been introduced and are recommended for girls and young women before the first sexual intercourse in most Western countries [10–12]. These vaccines were shown to prevent persistent infection with the vaccine types and cervical, vulvar, or vaginal intraepithelial neoplasia induced by the types included in the vaccine in HPV-naive women [13, 14]. In women with prevalent HPV infection, the HPV vaccines had no effect and did not influence HPV clearance [13, 15]. In young men that were HPV-negative at study entry, the efficacy of the quadrivalent vaccine against persistent infection with the vaccine types was recently reported to be 86% and the efficacy against external genital lesions (condyloma, penile/perianal/perineal intraepithelial neoplasia) induced by the vaccine types was 90% [16, 17]. These data give hope that the burden of HPV-induced diseases described below could possibly decrease sometime in the future.

38.2 Anal HPV-Infection in HIV-Positive MSM

38.2.1 Prevalence of Anal HPV-Infection and Anal HPV-Associated Disease in HIV-Positive MSM

Anal HPV prevalence, measured by the detection of HPV DNA by PCR in anal swabs, is high in men who have sex with men (MSM). HIV-positive MSM have an increased anal HPV prevalence (around or above 90%) compared to HIV-negative MSM (around 60%) and heterosexual men (around 25%) [18–22]. In HIV-positive MSM most anal HPV infections are persistent and infections with multiple HPV types are seen in the majority of patients. As in HIV-negative persons, HPV16 is the most frequent type in HIV-positive MSM found in more than 50% of patients [18–23]. Due to the high rate of persistent infections with HR-HPV types, HIV-infected MSM have a strongly increased risk for the development of anal cancer and its precursor lesion, anal intraepithelial neoplasia (AIN) [6, 21, 24–26]. Furthermore, peri- or intraanal condylomata (benign genital warts) are frequently observed in HIV-positive men. The majority of them are HPV6- or HPV11-induced. In 450 German HIV-positive MSM who underwent HRA-screening, 53% had anal condyloma. More than three quarters were asymptomatic and located intraanally (unpublished own data). On the other hand, extensive condylomata can be seen in HIV-infected individuals (Fig. 38.1). All genital warts in HIV-positive patients should be histologically evaluated, since 78% of condylomata removed from HIV-positive men showed signs of (focal) dysplasia [27].

The pathophysiology of AIN and cervical intraepithelial neoplasia (CIN) is very similar. Both can progress to the respective cancers due to expression of HR-HPV oncogenes (E6, E7) leading to genomic instability and suppression of apoptosis [28, 29]. Cells of the transformation zone, where monolayered columnar epithelium transforms into multilayered squamous epithelium, are particularly susceptible to HPV infection. Therefore, AIN and anal cancer are

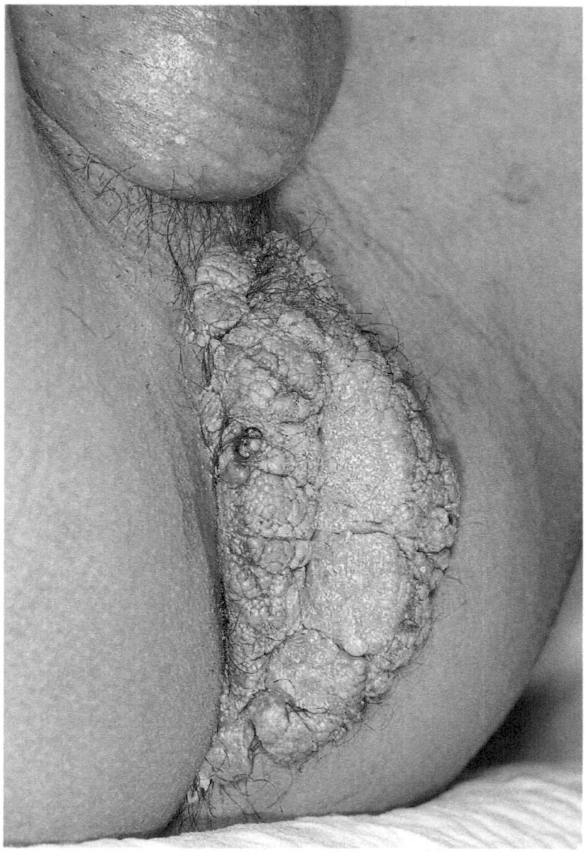

Fig. 38.1 Perianal condylomata acuminata (genital warts). Extensive verrucous lesions (about 12 cm in diameter) at the perianal area of an HIV-infected MSM

predominantly located intraanally (anal canal, linea dentata), but perianal AIN/anal cancer originating from keratinized skin also occur regularly. In analogy to CIN, AIN is histologically classified in grades 1–3 (see below). AIN2 and AIN3 are considered as true cancer precursors (high-grade AIN). In HIV-positive men, progression of normal, HR-HPV-positive anal epithelium or low-grade AIN (AIN1) to high-grade AIN can occur very fast. Palefsky et al. have reported progression from normal cytology to high-grade anal lesions in 20% and from low-grade to high-grade lesions in 62% of HIV-positive men within 2 years, compared to 8% and 36% in HIV-negative males [30]. Lacey et al. found progression from normal or low-grade to high-grade anal lesions within 17 months in 54% of their patients [23]. In recent studies, AIN of any grade has been found in 21–81% and high-grade AIN (AIN2/3) in 3% up to 52% of HIV-positive MSM [21, 31–35]. Smoking, infections with multiple HPV types, and low CD4-counts have been identified as risk factors for AIN in HIV-positive individuals [21, 26, 36–38]. In contrast to diseases caused by opportunistic infections with human herpesviruses as cytomegalovirus (e.g., retinitis, colitis) or human herpesvirus 8 (Kaposi sarcoma), highly active antiretroviral therapy (HAART) has no effect on HPV-induced AIN. Palefsky et al. found that HAART was not associated with a reduced prevalence of AIN in 357 HIV-positive MSM and Piketty et al. reported a high prevalence of AIN in 45 HIV-infected MSM, despite immune restoration under HAART [21, 35, 39].

Anal cancer is a rare disease in the general population (1/100, 000) [1]. In analogy to the increased risk for AIN, HIV-positive MSM also have a strongly increased risk for anal cancer compared to the general population [6]. In recent years, the incidence rates of anal cancer in HIV-positive MSM in Western countries (92/100,000–224/100,000) have exceeded those of cervical cancer in women in developing countries (40/100,000 for Southern Africa) without screening programs [40, 41]. Standardized incidence ratios (SIR) of 13.4–50.0 or standardized rate ratios (SRR) of 42.9 have been reported for anal cancer of people with HIV/AIDS compared to the general population [8, 9, 42, 43]. As reported for AIN, HAART does not seem to have an effect on the incidence of anal cancer in HIV-infected MSM, since increased incidence rates have been reported in the HAART era (after 1995) compared to the pre-HAART era [9, 43–45]. Compared to HIV-negative individuals, HIV-positive patients with anal cancer are more than 10 years younger at cancer diagnosis. Chiao et al. have reported a median age of 63 years in HIV-negative and 49 years in HIV-positive anal cancer patients [46]. The respective numbers published by Abbasakoor and Boulos were 63 and 37 years [47]. Prolonged survival of HIV-infected individuals due to HAART in the absence of widespread screening for and early treatment of AIN will probably lead to a further increase of anal cancer incidence in HIV-positive MSM in the future.

38.2.2 Diagnosis of Anal HPV-Associated Disease in HIV-Positive MSM

External HPV-associated lesions as perianal genital warts (condylomata acuminata) can usually be diagnosed clinically [48]. Perianal AIN can present clinically as single or multiple, well-demarcated, brownish or reddish, slightly elevated papules or plaques resembling bowenoid papulosis (bowenoid AIN), as erythematous, slightly erosive or scaly macules resembling erythroplasia of Queyrat (erythroplakic AIN), as flat, well-demarcated, acetowhite lesions (leukoplakic AIN), or as white or grayish exophytic lesions with irregular and hyperkeratinized surface (verrucous AIN) [19]. Differential diagnosis should include psoriasis inversa, lichen simplex chronicus, epidermal nevi, flat condyloma, nummular eczema, extra mammary Paget's disease, malignant melanoma, and basal cell carcinoma. Intraanal AIN (mostly located at the transformation zone) is much more common than perianal AIN, often asymptomatic and in most cases only detectable by high resolution anoscopy (HRA). In contrast to CIN screening, formalized and widely distributed AIN screening programs for HIV-infected MSM have not been established yet. The diagnosis of AIN comprises anal cytology, clinical diagnosis by HRA, and histology of suspicious lesions. Anal cytology is the primary screening test for AIN and cytologic screening should be performed for all HIV-infected MSM, in analogy to Pap-screening recommended for women for the detection of CIN [24, 25, 49]. The clinical value and the cost-effectiveness of anal cytologic screening in HIV-positive men have been shown [32, 50, 51]. Compared to histology, the sensitivity of anal cytology to detect AIN ranges between 69% and 93%

and the specificity between 32% and 59% [52]. The sensitivity to detect histologically confirmed AIN is higher for intraanal brush samples than for perianal brush samples (91% vs. 79%), probably due to lower cellularity in the latter material [53]. In order to obtain sufficient cells, patients should not have receptive anal intercourse or an enema 24 h before sample collection. As cervical cytology, anal cytology is graded according to the Bethesda classification as normal, ASCUS (atypical squamous cells of undetermined significance), LSIL (low-grade squamous intraepithelial lesion), HSIL (high-grade squamous intraepithelial lesion), or invasive cancer [54]. HRA (and HRA-guided biopsy) must follow after an abnormal cytology result has been obtained. Ideally, all HIV-positive MSM should be screened annually by HRA and cytology [55, 56]. HRA is similar to colposcopy used in gynecology for the diagnosis of CIN. To perform HRA, the patient should be placed in the left lateral decubitus or in the dorsal recumbent position. A disposable anoscope is inserted in the anal canal and mucous membranes are inspected at 30-fold magnification (Figs. 38.2 and 38.3). A few minutes after application of 3% acetic acid subclinical lesions become apparent (Fig. 38.2). Normal mucosa has a light red, shiny appearance. A granular surface, pronounced keratinization, or flat or elevated leukoplakic areas are suspicious for anal dysplasia. Neovascularization with vessel interruption and caliber variation are further signs of dysplasia or invasive growth. Typical HPV-associated vascular changes pointing to high-grade AIN are "punctuation" and "mosaicism" [56, 57]. In addition to 3% acetic acid, Lugol's (iodine) solution can be used for visualization of AIN. After application of iodine, normal mucosa (that stores glycogen) stains dark brown and dysplastic epithelium appears yellow or unstained. A recent study showed that about half of intraanal AIN would be missed without HRA [58]. In our patients, 5.8% of AIN were subclinical, i.e., only detectable by HRA after application of acetic acid [33]. Any suspicious lesions seen in HRA require the collection of biopsies for histological evaluation. Histologically, AIN is graded AIN1–AIN3, depending on the extent of the dysplastic changes. The lower third, the lower two-thirds, or the entire epithelium is affected in AIN1, AIN2, or AIN3, respectively [59]. The cytological classification of LSIL corresponds to AIN1 (low-grade AIN), and HSIL corresponds to AIN2/AIN3 (high-grade AIN).

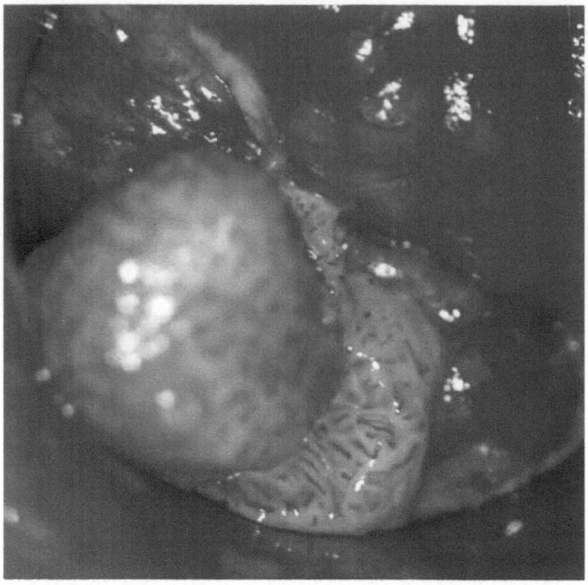

Fig. 38.3 Intraanal condylomata acuminata as seen with HRA. Terminal capillaries are typical for condylomata acuminata, whereas neovascularization, vessel interruption, and caliber variation are suspicious for anal dysplasia/malignant disease

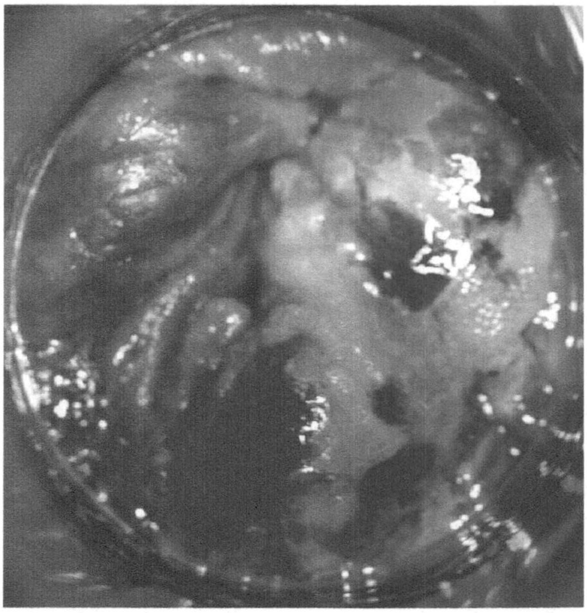

Fig. 38.2 AIN as seen with HRA after application of 3% acetic acid. Widespread, irregularly shaped leukoplakic lesions are present in an HIV-positive MSM

$P16^{INK4a}$ is an indirect marker of high-risk HPV-E7-oncogene expression and has been proven useful for the detection and grading of cervical intraepithelial neoplasia [60]. P16^{INK4a} immunohistochemistry was also shown to be helpful for diagnosis, grading, and evaluation of treatment response in AIN [61–63]. p16 ^{INK4a}-staining has also been used in anal cytology specimens. The positive predictive value for anal dysplasia was good (93%), but compared to histology, sensitivity and specificity were only 72% and 71%, respectively [64].

38.2.3 Treatment of Anal HPV-Associated Disease in HIV-Positive MSM

Treatment options for perianal or intraanal condylomata acuminata are numerous and comprise cytotoxic agents such as podophyllotoxin (0.5% solution or 0.15% cream), trichloroacetic acid (50–85% TCA), 5′-fluorouracil (5-FU) cream or injectable 5-FU/adrenalin gel, and immunotherapies as imiquimod (5% cream or suppositories), interferon (topical, intralesional, systemic), polyphenon E (green tea extracts), and surgical treatment with knife or scissor excision, electrosurgery, laser vaporization, infrared coagulation (IRC), cryotherapy with liquid nitrogen, or photodynamic therapy [65, 66]. Efficacy of all treatment options is less than optimal and multiple therapies are often necessary to achieve complete cure. In HIV-positive patients relapse rates after condyloma treatment are very high, especially at intraanal location.

Concerning treatment of AIN, generally accepted guidelines are missing and controlled studies have not yet been performed. Nevertheless, several pilot studies dealing with AIN therapy have been published in recent years. All high-grade lesions must be treated and it is advisable to treat also low-grade AIN to avoid enlargement and progression of lesions [25, 67]. Similar to condyloma management, treatment modalities for AIN can be grossly divided in topical or ablative therapies. The former group comprises imiquimod treatment, application of 85% TCA, photodynamic therapy, liquid nitrogen, podophyllotoxin, and the latter group includes surgical excision, electrocautery, laser evaporation, and IRC. Recently, (staged) HRA-guided surgical destruction with needle-tip cautery was reported as an effective office-based method for controlling high-grade AIN. Recurrent high-grade AIN was observed in 57%, but after retreatment 78% of patients had no signs of high-grade AIN at their last visit [68]. Using mainly laser ablation for AIN-treatment in HIV-positive and HIV-negative males, Nathan et al. reported a disease-free state in 63% of the patients 12 months after treatment. Median time to cure was significantly affected by HIV-status and was 39 months in the group of HIV-positive patients [69]. Newer technical developments are IRC and imiquimod treatment of AIN [70–72]. IRC is usually well tolerated, leads to less post-procedure discomfort, and fewer complications than surgery, and, in contrast to laser, does not produce smoke plume. Recently, clearance rates of 64% and 62.5% were reported for IRC-treatment of high-grade AIN in HIV-positive patients in two different studies [73, 74]. Imiquimod is a topical immune response modifier licensed for the treatment of anogenital warts, superficial basal cell carcinoma, and actinic keratoses. In a pilot study with 28 HIV-positive MSM, we recently showed that patient-applied imiquimod treatment for a total of 16 weeks led to a complete clearance of AIN in 61% of all patients and in 77% of compliant patients [72]. The successfully treated patients were followed for a mean of 30 months and 74% remained free of AIN at the site previously treated, accompanied by a reduction in the number of infecting HPV types and a drop in HPV-DNA load. However, 58% of patients developed new high-grade AIN in previously untreated anal sites [75]. Two phase I/II studies on therapeutic vaccination for the treatment of AIN in HIV-positive and in HIV-negative men have been published, but the results were not too promising. In 75% of the HIV-negative [76] and in 67% of the HIV-positive individuals AIN persisted; only 1 of 15 HIV-infected patients showed complete clearance and 4 of 15 regression of high-grade AIN 48 weeks after therapeutic vaccination with HPV16 E7 mycobacterium bovis heat shock protein 65 [77].

Invasive anal cancer in HIV-positive individuals is treated in the same way as in HIV-negative patients with combined chemo-radiotherapy (CRT). Advanced anal cancer that has spread to the lymph nodes and/or nearby organs may require surgery in addition to CRT. CRT consists of 5-fluorouracil and mitomycin C (or cisplatin) plus radiation (45–70 Gy) [1, 57, 78–81]. In the HAART era, outcome of CRT in HIV-positive patients is comparable to HIV-negative patients. Two-year survival rates of 77%, 5-year anal-cancer-specific survival of 75%, and 5-year overall survival rates of 61–65% have been recently reported for HIV-positive patients [46, 82, 83]. However, long-term local disease control is lower and therapy-related toxicity higher than in HIV-negative patients [82, 83]. Possibly, intensity-modulated radiation therapy could help to reduce radiation-associated toxicity also in HIV-infected anal cancer patients [84].

38.3 Penile HPV Infection in HIV-Positive MSM

38.3.1 *Prevalence of Penile HPV Infection and Penile HPV-Associated Disease in HIV-Positive MSM*

Penile HPV prevalence in males is high and prevalence rates recently published for heterosexual males ranged between 50% and more than 70%, mainly depending on sexual behavior and circumcision status [3, 85, 86]. In immunocompetent men most penile HPV infections are transient [87]. For HIV-positive men, only two smaller studies on penile HPV prevalence have been published so far. In one of the studies penile HPV-prevalence rates of 38% (HIV-positive MSM) and 32% (HIV-positive heterosexual men) were reported [88]. The other study found HPV at the coronal sulcus in 23.5% of HIV-positive compared to 15.8% of HIV-negative men [89]. In contrast to collection of swabs from mucous membranes as oral cavity, cervix, or anal canal, collection of penile swabs is usually less efficient concerning cellular input. This may lead to an underestimation of penile HPV prevalence. Some investigators have suggested penile brushing or pretreatment of penile skin with sandpaper or emery paper for this reason [90, 91].

Penile intraepithelial neoplasia (PIN) and penile cancer are rare diseases in HIV-negative heterosexual men in Europe and North America and mostly elderly patients are affected [92]. High-risk HPV-associated PIN is considered a precursor lesion of basaloid and warty penile cancer. Concerning PIN and penile cancer in HIV-positive men, only few studies exist. Compared to HIV-negative men, high-grade PIN seems to be more frequent in HIV-positive men [93]. We recently found PIN in 4.2% of 263 HIV-positive MSM and most of them also had AIN in the observation period. Mean CD4 counts were lower in PIN-patients compared to the rest of the cohort [33]. Clinically, different types of PIN as bowenoid papulosis, erythroplasia of Queyrat, Bowen's disease, and leukoplakic PIN have been described [33, 94, 95]. The most frequent HPV type found in all types of PIN of HIV-negative and HIV-positive men is HPV16 [33, 94, 96, 97]. The same applies to penile cancer [98, 99]. Compared to the general population, the risk of penile cancer is increased in HIV-positive men, although not to the extent reported for anal cancer [6, 8, 100]. Grulich et al. have calculated SIRs of 4.42 for penile cancer and 28.75 for anal cancer in HIV/AIDS patients [8]. The respective SIRs reported by Engels et al. were 5.6 (penile cancer) and 20.7 (anal cancer) in the pre-HAART era, and 8.0 and 19.6 in the HAART era [100].

38.3.2 *Diagnosis of Penile HPV-Associated Disease in HIV-Positive MSM*

Similar to perianal genital warts, penile condylomata acuminata can usually be diagnosed clinically [48]. In contrast to cervical (and anal) cytology, penile cytology is not a well-established method for the detection of PIN [101]. Three to five percent of acetic acid helps to detect subclinical and early lesions (acetowhitening). However, many, not HPV-associated conditions as superficial erosions, fresh scars, inflammation, eczema, lichen sclerosus, or genital herpes can lead to false-positive acetic acid test results [81, 94]. Similar to HRA, peniscopy has been used to improve detection of PIN compared to naked-eye inspection [102, 103]. Alternatively, a handheld magnifying lens can be used [81]. Suspicion of PIN always requires histological confirmation of the diagnosis. In a recent study of HIV-positive MSM, immunohistochemical detection of p16-expression was positive in all of 11 cases of PIN and correlated both with the histological PIN grade and with high-risk HPV-DNA loads [33].

Since HIV-infected men have an increased risk for penile cancer and since explosive courses of penile cancer in AIDS patients have been described [6, 8,

104, 105], all HIV-positive men should be screened for PIN/penile cancer in addition to anal screening.

38.3.3 Treatment of Penile HPV-Associated Disease in HIV-Positive MSM

All PIN lesions and penile condylomata should be treated, irrespective of the HIV status. Treatment options for penile genital warts are like those described for anal condylomata acuminata (see above). Similar to AIN, controlled studies for the management of PIN in HIV-negative or HIV-positive men do not exist and numerous treatment modalities comprising topical 5-fluorouracil, imiquimod, local cidofovir, local or systemic interferons, cryotherapy, electrocautery, hyfrecation (cold cautery), laser vaporization, superficial radiotherapy, photodynamic therapy, curettage, surgical excision, and circumcision have been reported. The choice of therapy depends on lesion type, size and location, age, immune-status, and expected compliance [33, 94, 95, 106, 107]. HIV-infected men receiving HAART with CD4-counts above 200/μL showed good treatment efficacy. For patients with more extended disease as frequently seen in erythroplasia of Queyrat, sequential therapy with circumcision followed by topical 5-FU has been described [95]. In all cases, a histological diagnosis ruling out invasive cancer should be obtained before therapy of PIN [94]. Invasive penile cancer is treated with surgical excision, Mohs micrographic surgery, circumcision, or partial or total penectomy, depending on tumor size and stage. For smaller cancers (T1) laser or radiotherapy may be used alternatively. In addition to penectomy, lymph node removal, radiation, and chemotherapy may be required for advanced or metastasized penile cancer [81, 107].

38.4 Oral HPV Infection in HIV-Positive MSM

Oral HPV infection is more frequent in HIV-positive than in HIV-negative individuals. Oral HPV-DNA has been found in 14–46% of HIV-positive men or women, with about half of the detected HPV types being high-risk types, especially HPV 16 [88, 108–113]. The majority of oral HPV infections in HIV-positive individuals are asymptomatic [114, 115]. Recently, increases in the incidence of HPV-associated oral squamous cell carcinomas (especially tonsil and base of the tongue carcinomas) have been observed for the population of the USA. This is mainly attributed to changes in sexual behavior (more widespread acceptance of oral sex) [116, 117]. Concerning oral HPV-related cancers in HIV-infected individuals, Grulich et al. and Hessol et al. reported SIRs of 2.32 and 2.6 for oral cavity and pharyngeal cancers, compared to the general population, respectively [8, 9].

An increase of oral warts has been described in HIV-positive patients on HAART [118–121]. Others, however, could not confirm these findings [122]. HPV types found in oral warts of HIV-positive patients comprised the low-risk types HPV2, 6, 7, 11, 13, 32, 55, 69, 72, and in some cases the high-risk types 18, 59, and 73. The clinical spectrum of oral warts in HIV-infected patients includes condylomata acuminata, verrucae vulgaris, and focal epithelial hyperplasia. Signs of dysplasia can occasionally be found in these lesions [118, 123, 124]. We recently reported the case of a rapidly developing multifocal HPV72-associated high-grade oral intraepithelial neoplasia in an MSM, whose HIV infection was well controlled by HAART [115].

For all the above-mentioned reasons, a physical examination of HIV-positive patients should always include an inspection of the oral cavity.

Take-Home Pearls

› Persistent anogenital and oral HPV infections are widespread in HIV-positive MSM. For this reason all HIV-positive MSM should regularly be screened for AIN to prevent a further increase of anal cancer incidence in this patient population by early treatment of AIN. Clinical screening for HPV-associated disease should include the penis and the oral cavity as well. Ideally, anal screening should consist of cytology, HRA, and histology of suspicious lesions.

Abbreviations

ASCUS	Atypical squamous cells of undetermined significance
AIN	Anal intraepithelial neoplasia
CIN	Cervical intraepithelial neoplasia
CRT	Chemo-radiotherapy
5-FU	5′-Fluorouracil
LR	Low-risk
HAART	Highly active antiretroviral therapy
HIV	Human immunodeficiency virus
HPV	Human papillomavirus
HR	High-risk
HRA	High resolution anoscopy
HSIL	High-grade squamous intraepithelial lesion
IRC	Infrared coagulation
LSIL	Low-grade squamous intraepithelial lesion
MSM	Men who have sex with men
PIN	Penile intraepithelial neoplasia
SIR	Standardized incidence ratio
TCA	Trichloroacetic acid

References

1. Clark, M.A., Hartley, A., Geh, J.I.: Cancer of the anal canal. Lancet Oncol. **5**, 149–157 (2004)
2. Munoz, N., Bosch, F.X., de Sanjose, S., et al.: Epidemiologic classification of human papillomavirus types associated with cervical cancer. N. Engl. J. Med. **348**, 518–527 (2003)
3. Nielson, C.M., Harris, R.B., Dunne, E.F., et al.: Risk factors for anogenital human papillomavirus infection in men. J. Infect. Dis. **196**, 1137–1145 (2007)
4. Schiffman, M., Castle, P.E., Jeronimo, J., et al.: Human papillomavirus and cervical cancer. Lancet **370**, 890–907 (2007)
5. Schiffman, M., Kjaer, S.K.: Chapter 2: Natural history of anogenital human papillomavirus infection and neoplasia. J. Natl. Cancer Inst. Monogr. 14–19 (2003)
6. Frisch, M., Biggar, R.J., Goedert, J.J.: Human papillomavirus-associated cancers in patients with human immunodeficiency virus infection and acquired immunodeficiency syndrome. J. Natl. Cancer Inst. **92**, 1500–1510 (2000)
7. Frisch, M., Smith, E., Grulich, A., et al.: Cancer in a population-based cohort of men and women in registered homosexual partnerships. Am. J. Epidemiol. **157**, 966–972 (2003)
8. Grulich, A.E., van Leeuwen, M.T., Falster, M.O., et al.: Incidence of cancers in people with HIV/AIDS compared with immunosuppressed transplant recipients: a meta-analysis. Lancet **370**, 59–67 (2007)
9. Hessol, N.A., Pipkin, S., Schwarcz, S., et al.: The impact of highly active antiretroviral therapy on non-AIDS-defining cancers among adults with AIDS. Am. J. Epidemiol. **165**, 1143–1153 (2007)
10. Kahn, J.A., Burk, R.D.: Papillomavirus vaccines in perspective. Lancet **369**, 2135–2137 (2007)
11. Rogers, L.J., Eva, L.J., Luesley, D.M.: Vaccines against cervical cancer. Curr. Opin. Oncol. **20**, 570–574 (2008)
12. Schiller, J.T., Castellsague, X., Villa, L.L., et al.: An update of prophylactic human papillomavirus L1 virus-like particle vaccine clinical trial results. Vaccine **26**(suppl 10), K53–K61 (2008)
13. Garland, S.M., Hernandez-Avila, M., Wheeler, C.M., et al.: Quadrivalent vaccine against human papillomavirus to prevent anogenital diseases. N. Engl. J. Med. **356**, 1928–1943 (2007)
14. Paavonen, J., Jenkins, D., Bosch, F.X., et al.: Efficacy of a prophylactic adjuvanted bivalent L1 virus-like-particle vaccine against infection with human papillomavirus types 16 and 18 in young women: an interim analysis of a phase III double-blind, randomised controlled trial. Lancet **369**, 2161–2170 (2007)
15. Hildesheim, A., Herrero, R., Wacholder, S., et al.: Effect of human papillomavirus 16/18 L1 viruslike particle vaccine among young women with preexisting infection: a randomized trial. JAMA **298**, 743–753 (2007)
16. Giuliano, A., Palefsky, J., group obotmqHvets: The efficacy of quadrivalent HPV (types 6/11/16/18) vaccine in reducing the incidence of HPV infection and HPV-related genital disease in young men. Eurogin2008 Nice, France. Abstract SS 19–17 (2008)
17. Palefsky, J., Giuliano, A., group obotmqHvets (2008) Efficacy of the quadrivalent HPV vaccine against HPV 6/11/16/18-related genital infection in young men. Eurogin2008 Nice, France. Abstract TC 2-11
18. Kiviat, N.B., Critchlow, C.W., Holmes, K.K., et al.: Association of anal dysplasia and human papillomavirus with immunosuppression and HIV infection among homosexual men. AIDS **7**, 43–49 (1993)
19. Kreuter, A., Brockmeyer, N.H., Hochdorfer, B., et al.: Clinical spectrum and virologic characteristics of anal intraepithelial neoplasia in HIV infection. J. Am. Acad. Dermatol. **52**, 603–608 (2005)
20. Nyitray, A., Nielson, C.M., Harris, R.B., et al.: Prevalence of and risk factors for anal human papillomavirus infection in heterosexual men. J. Infect. Dis. **197**, 1676–1684 (2008)
21. Palefsky, J.M., Holly, E.A., Efirdc, J.T., et al.: Anal intraepithelial neoplasia in the highly active antiretroviral therapy era among HIV-positive men who have sex with men. AIDS **19**, 1407–1414 (2005)
22. Palefsky, J.M., Holly, E.A., Ralston, M.L., et al.: Prevalence and risk factors for human papillomavirus infection of the anal canal in human immunodeficiency virus (HIV)-positive and HIV-negative homosexual men. J. Infect. Dis. **177**, 361–367 (1998)
23. Lacey, H.B., Wilson, G.E., Tilston, P., et al.: A study of anal intraepithelial neoplasia in HIV positive homosexual men. Sex. Transm. Infect. **75**, 172–177 (1999)
24. Fox, P.A.: Human papillomavirus and anal intraepithelial neoplasia. Curr. Opin. Infect. Dis. **19**, 62–66 (2006)

25. Palefsky, J.: Human papillomavirus and anal neoplasia. Curr. HIV/AIDS Rep. **5**, 78–85 (2008)
26. Palefsky, J.M., Holly, E.A., Ralston, M.L., et al.: High incidence of anal high-grade squamous intra-epithelial lesions among HIV-positive and HIV-negative homosexual and bisexual men. AIDS **12**, 495–503 (1998)
27. McCloskey, J.C., Metcalf, C., French, M.A., et al.: The frequency of high-grade intraepithelial neoplasia in anal/perianal warts is higher than previously recognized. Int. J. STD AIDS **18**, 538–542 (2007)
28. IARC: IARC monographs on the evaluation of carcinogenic risks to humans - Human Papillomaviruses. International Agency for Research on Cancer (IARC) Lyon, France (2007)
29. zur Hausen, H.: Papillomaviruses and cancer: from basic studies to clinical application. Nat. Rev. Cancer **2**, 342–350 (2002)
30. Palefsky, J.M., Holly, E.A., Ralston, M.L., et al.: Anal squamous intraepithelial lesions in HIV-positive and HIV-negative homosexual and bisexual men: prevalence and risk factors. J. Acquir. Immune Defic. Syndr. Hum. Retrovirol. **17**, 320–326 (1998)
31. Abramowitz, L., Benabderrahmane, D., Ravaud, P., et al.: Anal squamous intraepithelial lesions and condyloma in HIV-infected heterosexual men, homosexual men and women: prevalence and associated factors. AIDS **21**, 1457–1465 (2007)
32. Cranston, R.D., Hart, S.D., Gornbein, J.A., et al.: The prevalence, and predictive value, of abnormal anal cytology to diagnose anal dysplasia in a population of HIV-positive men who have sex with men. Int. J. STD AIDS **18**, 77–80 (2007)
33. Kreuter, A., Brockmeyer, N.H., Weissenborn, S.J., et al.: Penile intraepithelial neoplasia is frequent in HIV-positive men with anal dysplasia. J. Invest. Dermatol. **128**, 2316–2324 (2008)
34. Pereira, A., Lacerda, H.R., Barros, R.R.: Prevalence and factors associated with anal lesions mediated by human papillomavirus in men with HIV/AIDS. Int. J. STD AIDS **19**, 192–196 (2008)
35. Piketty, C., Darragh, T.M., Heard, I., et al.: High prevalence of anal squamous intraepithelial lesions in HIV-positive men despite the use of highly active antiretroviral therapy. Sex. Transm. Dis. **31**, 96–99 (2004)
36. Critchlow, C.W., Surawicz, C.M., Holmes, K.K., et al.: Prospective study of high grade anal squamous intraepithelial neoplasia in a cohort of homosexual men: influence of HIV infection, immunosuppression and human papillomavirus infection. AIDS **9**, 1255–1262 (1995)
37. Durante, A.J., Williams, A.B., Da Costa, M., et al.: Incidence of anal cytological abnormalities in a cohort of human immunodeficiency virus-infected women. Cancer Epidemiol. Biomarkers Prev. **12**, 638–642 (2003)
38. Etienney, I., Vuong, S., Daniel, F., et al.: Prevalence of anal cytologic abnormalities in a French referral population: a prospective study with special emphasis on HIV, HPV, and smoking. Dis. Colon Rectum **51**, 67–72 (2008)
39. Palefsky, J.M., Holly, E.A., Ralston, M.L., et al.: Effect of highly active antiretroviral therapy on the natural history of anal squamous intraepithelial lesions and anal human papillomavirus infection. J. Acquir. Immune Defic. Syndr. **28**, 422–428 (2001)
40. Bower, M., Powles, T., Newsom-Davis, T., et al.: HIV-associated anal cancer: has highly active antiretroviral therapy reduced the incidence or improved the outcome? J. Acquir. Immune Defic. Syndr. **37**, 1563–1565 (2004)
41. Diamond, C., Taylor, T.H., Aboumrad, T., et al.: Increased incidence of squamous cell anal cancer among men with AIDS in the era of highly active antiretroviral therapy. Sex. Transm. Dis. **32**, 314–320 (2005)
42. Clifford, G.M., Polesel, J., Rickenbach, M., et al.: Cancer risk in the Swiss HIV Cohort Study: associations with immunodeficiency, smoking, and highly active antiretroviral therapy. J. Natl. Cancer Inst. **97**, 425–432 (2005)
43. Patel, P., Hanson, D.L., Sullivan, P.S., et al.: Incidence of types of cancer among HIV-infected persons compared with the general population in the United States, 1992–2003. Ann. Intern. Med. **148**, 728–736 (2008)
44. D'Souza, G., Wiley, D.J., Li, X., et al.: Incidence and epidemiology of anal cancer in the multicenter AIDS cohort study. J. Acquir. Immune Defic. Syndr. **48**, 491–499 (2008)
45. Piketty, C., Selinger-Leneman, H., Grabar, S., et al.: Marked increase in the incidence of invasive anal cancer among HIV-infected patients despite treatment with combination antiretroviral therapy. AIDS **22**, 1203–1211 (2008)
46. Chiao, E.Y., Giordano, T.P., Richardson, P., et al.: Human immunodeficiency virus-associated squamous cell cancer of the anus: epidemiology and outcomes in the highly active antiretroviral therapy era. J. Clin. Oncol. **26**, 474–479 (2008)
47. Abbasakoor, F., Boulos, P.B.: Anal intraepithelial neoplasia. Br. J. Surg. **92**, 277–290 (2005)
48. Barrasso, R., Gross, G.: External genitalia: diagnosis. In: Gross G, Barrasso R (eds.) Human Papilloma Virus Infection – A Clinical Atlas, pp. 291–361. Ullstein Mosby Berlin/Wiesbaden, Germany (1997)
49. Chin-Hong, P.V., Palefsky, J.M.: Natural history and clinical management of anal human papillomavirus disease in men and women infected with human immunodeficiency virus. Clin. Infect. Dis. **35**, 1127–1134 (2002)
50. Goldie, S.J., Kuntz, K.M., Weinstein, M.C., et al.: Cost-effectiveness of screening for anal squamous intraepithelial lesions and anal cancer in human immunodeficiency virus-negative homosexual and bisexual men. Am. J. Med. **108**, 634–641 (2000)
51. Goldie, S.J., Kuntz, K.M., Weinstein, M.C., et al.: The clinical effectiveness and cost-effectiveness of screening for anal squamous intraepithelial lesions in homosexual and bisexual HIV-positive men. JAMA **281**, 1822–1829 (1999)
52. Chiao, E.Y., Giordano, T.P., Palefsky, J.M., et al.: Screening HIV-infected individuals for anal cancer precursor lesions: a systematic review. Clin. Infect. Dis. **43**, 223–233 (2006)
53. Garcia, F.U., Haber, M.M., Butcher, J., et al.: Increased sensitivity of anal cytology in evaluation of internal compared with external lesions. Acta Cytol. **51**, 893–899 (2007)
54. Crothers, B.A.: The Bethesda System 2001: update on terminology and application. Clin. Obstet. Gynecol. **48**, 98–107 (2005)
55. Chin-Hong, P.V., Berry, J.M., Cheng, S.C., et al.: Comparison of patient- and clinician-collected anal cytology samples to screen for human papillomavirus-associated

anal intraepithelial neoplasia in men who have sex with men. Ann. Intern. Med. **149**, 300–306 (2008)
56. Kreuter, A., Brockmeyer, N.H., Altmeyer, P., et al.: Anal intraepithelial neoplasia in HIV infection. J. Dtsch Dermatol. Ges. **6**, 925–934 (2008)
57. Berry, J.M., Palefsky, J.M., Welton, M.L.: Anal cancer and its precursors in HIV-positive patients: perspectives and management. Surg. Oncol. Clin. N. Am. **13**, 355–373 (2004)
58. Watson, A.J., Smith, B.B., Whitehead, M.R., et al.: Malignant progression of anal intra-epithelial neoplasia. ANZ J. Surg. **76**, 715–717 (2006)
59. Fenger, C., Nielsen, V.T.: Precancerous changes in the anal canal epithelium in resection specimens. Acta Pathol. Microbiol. Immunol. Scand. [A] **94**, 63–69 (1986)
60. Klaes, R., Friedrich, T., Spitkovsky, D., et al.: Overexpression of p16(INK4A) as a specific marker for dysplastic and neoplastic epithelial cells of the cervix uteri. Int. J. Cancer **92**, 276–284 (2001)
61. Bernard, J.E., Butler, M.O., Sandweiss, L., et al.: Anal intraepithelial neoplasia: correlation of grade with p16INK4a immunohistochemistry and HPV in situ hybridization. Appl. Immunohistochem. Mol. Morphol. **16**, 215–220 (2008)
62. Kreuter, A., Wieland, U., Gambichler, T., et al.: p16ink4a expression decreases during imiquimod treatment of anal intraepithelial neoplasia in human immunodeficiency virus-infected men and correlates with the decline of lesional high-risk human papillomavirus DNA load. Br. J. Dermatol. **157**, 523–530 (2007)
63. Walts, A.E., Lechago, J., Bose, S.: P16 and Ki67 immunostaining is a useful adjunct in the assessment of biopsies for HPV-associated anal intraepithelial neoplasia. Am. J. Surg. Pathol. **30**, 795–801 (2006)
64. Darvishian, F., Stier, E.A., Soslow, R.A., et al.: Immunoreactivity of p16 in anal cytology specimens: histologic correlation. Cancer **108**, 66–71 (2006)
65. Gross, G., Tyring, S., von Krogh, G., et al.: External genitalia: treatment. In: Gross G, Barrasso R (eds.) Human Papilloma Virus Infection – A Clinical Atlas, pp. 365–376. Ullstein Mosby, Berlin/Wiesbaden (1997)
66. Mayeaux Jr., E.J., Dunton, C.: Modern management of external genital warts. J. Low. Genit. Tract Dis. **12**, 185–192 (2008)
67. Kreuter, A., Wieland, U.: Human papillomavirus-associated diseases in HIV-infected men who have sex with men. Curr. Opin. Infect. Dis. **22**(2), 109–114 (2009)
68. Pineda, C.E., Berry, J.M., Jay, N., et al.: High-resolution anoscopy targeted surgical destruction of anal high-grade squamous intraepithelial lesions: a ten-year experience. Dis. Colon Rectum **51**, 829–835 (2008). discussion 835–827
69. Nathan, M., Hickey, N., Mayuranathan, L., et al.: Treatment of anal human papillomavirus-associated disease: a long term outcome study. Int. J. STD AIDS **19**, 445–449 (2008)
70. Goldstone, S.E., Hundert, J.S., Huyett, J.W.: Infrared coagulator ablation of high-grade anal squamous intraepithelial lesions in HIV-negative males who have sex with males. Dis. Colon Rectum **50**, 565–575 (2007)
71. Goldstone, S.E., Kawalek, A.Z., Huyett, J.W.: Infrared coagulator: a useful tool for treating anal squamous intraepithelial lesions. Dis. Colon Rectum **48**, 1042–1054 (2005)
72. Wieland, U., Brockmeyer, N.H., Weissenborn, S.J., et al.: Imiquimod treatment of anal intraepithelial neoplasia in HIV-positive men. Arch. Dermatol. **142**, 1438–1444 (2006)
73. Cranston, R.D., Hirschowitz, S.L., Cortina, G., et al.: A retrospective clinical study of the treatment of high-grade anal dysplasia by infrared coagulation in a population of HIV-positive men who have sex with men. Int. J. STD AIDS **19**, 118–120 (2008)
74. Stier, E.A., Goldstone, S.E., Berry, J.M., et al.: Infrared coagulator treatment of high-grade anal dysplasia in HIV-infected individuals: an AIDS malignancy consortium pilot study. J. Acquir. Immune Defic. Syndr. **47**, 56–61 (2008)
75. Kreuter, A., Potthoff, A., Brockmeyer, N.H., et al.: Imiquimod leads to a decrease of human papillomavirus DNA and to a sustained clearance of anal intraepithelial neoplasia in HIV-infected men. J. Invest. Dermatol. **128**, 2078–2083 (2008)
76. Klencke, B., Matijevic, M., Urban, R.G., et al.: Encapsulated plasmid DNA treatment for human papillomavirus 16-associated anal dysplasia: a Phase I study of ZYC101. Clin. Cancer Res. **8**, 1028–1037 (2002)
77. Palefsky, J.M., Berry, J.M., Jay, N., et al.: A trial of SGN-00101 (HspE7) to treat high-grade anal intraepithelial neoplasia in HIV-positive individuals. AIDS **20**, 1151–1155 (2006)
78. Ajani, J.A., Winter, K.A., Gunderson, L.L., et al.: Fluorouracil, mitomycin, and radiotherapy vs fluorouracil, cisplatin, and radiotherapy for carcinoma of the anal canal: a randomized controlled trial. JAMA **299**, 1914–1921 (2008)
79. Blazy, A., Hennequin, C., Gornet, J.M., et al.: Anal carcinomas in HIV-positive patients: high-dose chemoradiotherapy is feasible in the era of highly active antiretroviral therapy. Dis. Colon Rectum **48**, 1176–1181 (2005)
80. Kauh, J., Koshy, M., Gunthel, C., et al.: Management of anal cancer in the HIV-positive population. Oncology (Williston Park) **19**, 1634–1638 (2005). discussion 1638–1640, 1645 passim
81. Palefsky, J.M.: HPV infection in men. Dis. Markers **23**, 261–272 (2007)
82. Oehler-Janne, C., Huguet, F., Provencher, S., et al.: HIV-specific differences in outcome of squamous cell carcinoma of the anal canal: a multicentric cohort study of HIV-positive patients receiving highly active antiretroviral therapy. J. Clin. Oncol. **26**, 2550–2557 (2008)
83. Wexler, A., Berson, A.M., Goldstone, S.E., et al.: Invasive anal squamous-cell carcinoma in the HIV-positive patient: outcome in the era of highly active antiretroviral therapy. Dis. Colon Rectum **51**, 73–81 (2008)
84. Salama, J.K., Mell, L.K., Schomas, D.A., et al.: Concurrent chemotherapy and intensity-modulated radiation therapy for anal canal cancer patients: a multicenter experience. J. Clin. Oncol. **25**, 4581–4586 (2007)
85. Giuliano, A.R., Lazcano, E., Villa, L.L., et al.: Circumcision and sexual behavior: factors independently associated with human papillomavirus detection among men in the HIM study. Int. J. Cancer **124**, 1251–1257 (2009)
86. Giuliano, A.R., Lazcano-Ponce, E., Villa, L.L., et al.: The human papillomavirus infection in men study: human papillomavirus prevalence and type distribution among men residing in Brazil, Mexico, and the United States. Cancer Epidemiol. Biomarkers Prev. **17**, 2036–2043 (2008)

87. Giuliano, A.R., Lu, B., Nielson, C.M., et al.: Age-specific prevalence, incidence, and duration of human papillomavirus infections in a cohort of 290 US men. J. Infect. Dis. **198**, 827–835 (2008)
88. Sirera, G., Videla, S., Pinol, M., et al.: High prevalence of human papillomavirus infection in the anus, penis and mouth in HIV-positive men. AIDS **20**, 1201–1204 (2006)
89. van der Snoek, E.M., Niesters, H.G., Mulder, P.G., et al.: Human papillomavirus infection in men who have sex with men participating in a Dutch gay-cohort study. Sex. Transm. Dis. **30**, 639–644 (2003)
90. Giovannelli, L., Migliore, M.C., Capra, G., et al.: Penile, urethral, and seminal sampling for diagnosis of human papillomavirus infection in men. J. Clin. Microbiol. **45**, 248–251 (2007)
91. Weaver, B.A., Feng, Q., Holmes, K.K., et al.: Evaluation of genital sites and sampling techniques for detection of human papillomavirus DNA in men. J. Infect. Dis. **189**, 677–685 (2004)
92. Dillner, J., von Krogh, G., Horenblas, S., et al.: Etiology of squamous cell carcinoma of the penis. Scand. J. Urol. Nephrol. **205**(suppl), 189–193 (2000)
93. Gomousa-Michael, M., Gialama, E., Gomousas, N., et al.: Genital human papillomavirus infection and associated penile intraepithelial neoplasia in males infected with the human immunodeficiency virus. Acta Cytol. **44**, 305–309 (2000)
94. Gross, G., Pfister, H.: Role of human papillomavirus in penile cancer, penile intraepithelial squamous cell neoplasias and in genital warts. Med. Microbiol. Immunol. **193**, 35–44 (2004)
95. Porter, W.M., Francis, N., Hawkins, D., et al.: Penile intraepithelial neoplasia: clinical spectrum and treatment of 35 cases. Br. J. Dermatol. **147**, 1159–1165 (2002)
96. Backes, D.M., Kurman, R.J., Pimenta, J.M., et al.: Systematic review of human papillomavirus prevalence in invasive penile cancer. Cancer Causes Control **100**, 405–407 (2008)
97. Rubin, M.A., Kleter, B., Zhou, M., et al.: Detection and typing of human papillomavirus DNA in penile carcinoma: evidence for multiple independent pathways of penile carcinogenesis. Am. J. Pathol. **159**, 1211–1218 (2001)
98. Heideman, D.A., Waterboer, T., Pawlita, M., et al.: Human papillomavirus-16 is the predominant type etiologically involved in penile squamous cell carcinoma. J. Clin. Oncol. **25**, 4550–4556 (2007)
99. Madsen, B.S., van den Brule, A.J., Jensen, H.L., et al.: Risk factors for squamous cell carcinoma of the penis–population-based case-control study in Denmark. Cancer Epidemiol. Biomarkers Prev. **17**, 2683–2691 (2008)
100. Engels, E.A., Pfeiffer, R.M., Goedert, J.J., et al.: Trends in cancer risk among people with AIDS in the United States 1980–2002. AIDS **20**, 1645–1654 (2006)
101. de Lima Rocha, M.G., Faria, F.L., Souza Mdo, C., et al.: Detection of human papillomavirus infection in penile samples through liquid-based cytology and polymerase chain reaction. Cancer **114**, 489–493 (2008)
102. Cardamakis, E., Kotoulas, I.G., Relakis, K., et al.: Peoscopic diagnosis of flat condyloma and penile intraepithelial neoplasia. Clinical manifestation. Gynecol. Obstet. Invest. **43**, 255–260 (1997)
103. Nicolau, S.M., Martins, N.V., Ferraz, P.E., et al.: Importance of peniscopy, oncologic cytology and histopathology in the diagnosis of penile infection by human papillomavirus. São Paulo Med. J. **115**, 1330–1335 (1997)
104. Aboulafia, D.M., Gibbons, R.: Penile cancer and human papilloma virus (HPV) in a human immunodeficiency virus (HIV)-infected patient. Cancer Invest. **19**, 266–272 (2001)
105. Theodore, C., Androulakis, N., Spatz, A., et al.: An explosive course of squamous cell penile cancer in an AIDS patient. Ann. Oncol. **13**, 475–479 (2002)
106. Markos, A.R.: The management of penile intraepithelial neoplasia in genitourinary medicine. Int. J. STD AIDS **14**, 314–319 (2003)
107. Micali, G., Nasca, M.R., Innocenzi, D., et al.: Penile cancer. J. Am. Acad. Dermatol. **54**, 369–391 (2006). quiz 391–364
108. Cameron, J.E., Mercante, D., O'Brien, M., et al.: The impact of highly active antiretroviral therapy and immunodeficiency on human papillomavirus infection of the oral cavity of human immunodeficiency virus-seropositive adults. Sex. Transm. Dis. **32**, 703–709 (2005)
109. Coutlee, F., Trottier, A.M., Ghattas, G., et al.: Risk factors for oral human papillomavirus in adults infected and not infected with human immunodeficiency virus. Sex. Transm. Dis. **24**, 23–31 (1997)
110. D'Souza, G., Fakhry, C., Sugar, E.A., et al.: Six-month natural history of oral versus cervical human papillomavirus infection. Int. J. Cancer **121**, 143–150 (2007)
111. Fakhry, C., D'Souza, G., Sugar, E., et al.: Relationship between prevalent oral and cervical human papillomavirus infections in human immunodeficiency virus-positive and -negative women. J. Clin. Microbiol. **44**, 4479–4485 (2006)
112. Kreimer, A.R., Alberg, A.J., Daniel, R., et al.: Oral human papillomavirus infection in adults is associated with sexual behavior and HIV serostatus. J. Infect. Dis. **189**, 686–698 (2004)
113. Marais, D.J., Passmore, J.A., Denny, L., et al.: Cervical and oral human papillomavirus types in HIV-1 positive and negative women with cervical disease in South Africa. J. Med. Virol. **80**, 953–959 (2008)
114. Hagensee, M.E., Cameron, J.E., Leigh, J.E., et al.: Human papillomavirus infection and disease in HIV-infected individuals. Am. J. Med. Sci. **328**, 57–63 (2004)
115. Kreuter, A., Brockmeyer, N.H., Altmeyer, P., et al.: Rapid onset of multifocal human papillomavirus 72-associated oral intraepithelial neoplasia in a human immunodeficiency virus-infected patient. Br. J. Dermatol. **157**, 826–828 (2007)
116. Chaturvedi, A.K., Engels, E.A., Anderson, W.F., et al.: Incidence trends for human papillomavirus-related and -unrelated oral squamous cell carcinomas in the United States. J. Clin. Oncol. **26**, 612–619 (2008)
117. Ryerson, A.B., Peters, E.S., Coughlin, S.S., et al.: Burden of potentially human papillomavirus-associated cancers of the oropharynx and oral cavity in the US, 1998–2003. Cancer **113**, 2901–2909 (2008)
118. Cameron, J.E., Hagensee, M.E.: Oral HPV complications in HIV infected patients. Curr. HIV/AIDS Rep. **5**, 126 131 (2008)

119. Greenspan, D., Canchola, A.J., MacPhail, L.A., et al.: Effect of highly active antiretroviral therapy on frequency of oral warts. Lancet **357**, 1411–1412 (2001)
120. King, M.D., Reznik, D.A., O'Daniels, C.M., et al.: Human papillomavirus-associated oral warts among human immunodeficiency virus-seropositive patients in the era of highly active antiretroviral therapy: an emerging infection. Clin. Infect. Dis. **34**, 641–648 (2002)
121. Leigh, J.: Oral warts rise dramatically with use of new agents in HIV. HIV Clin. **12**, 7 (2000)
122. Ramirez-Amador, V., Esquivel-Pedraza, L., Sierra-Madero, J., et al.: The changing clinical spectrum of human immunodeficiency virus (HIV)-related oral lesions in 1, 000 consecutive patients: a 12-year study in a referral center in Mexico. Medicine (Baltimore) **82**, 39–50 (2003)
123. Greenspan, D., de Villiers, E.M., Greenspan, J.S., et al.: Unusual HPV types in oral warts in association with HIV infection. J. Oral Pathol. **17**, 482–488 (1988)
124. Volter, C., He, Y., Delius, H., et al.: Novel HPV types present in oral papillomatous lesions from patients with HIV infection. Int. J. Cancer **66**, 453–456 (1996)

Sexually Transmitted HPV-Infections of the Oral Mucosa and Upper Respiratory Tract in Adults and Children

39

Stina Syrjänen

Core Messages

> Human papillomaviruses can infect mouth mucosa and upper respiratory tract both in children and adults. HPV infections have been regarded as sexually transmitted disease but recent evidence also support the mouth-to-mouth transmission of HPV. Most of the infants' HPV infections are acquired vertically from the mother at the delivery or even intrauterinelly. Part of the oral HPV infections might persist. HPV has been assoicated with a subset of head and neck cancers. Especially, the link between HPV and oropharyngeal cancer has become firm. Patients with HPV-positive tumours have significantly improved response to chemo- and radiotherapy as compared to HPV-negative tumours.

39.1 Introduction

Human papillomavirus (HPV) infections have been regarded as sexually transmitted disease (STD). Mucosal HPV types can infect oral mucosa and upper respiratory tract similarly as the genital tract in both sexes. However, the acquisition of HPV into these sites is still incompletely understood. Traditionally, oral condylomas have been regarded as an HPV lesion transmitted via oral sex. Currently, however, there is increasing amount of evidence suggesting that part of these HPV infections are maternally acquired during delivery or even during the intrauterine period. Evidence is also emerging to support the horizontal transmission of HPV via saliva or other contacts. This chapter summarizes the current knowledge on asymptomatic HPV infections and significance of HPV in the development of benign, pre-cancer, and cancer lesions of the oral mucosa and upper respiratory tract. Most recent data implicate that HPV-positive oral, oro-pharyngeal, and laryngeal cancers might have better disease outcome, which has made HPV testing an important part of the diagnostic setup of these patients to tailor the treatment options on individual basis. This communication starts with a short overview on current concepts of HPV transmission modes, before entering the discussion of individual HPV-related pathology in oral mucosa and upper respiratory tract.

39.2 Potential Transmission Modes of HPV

Sexual transmission is by far the most common route of spreading the virus. However, detection of HPV in virgins, infants, and children suggests that vertical transmission also exists, but the exact rates and routes have not been well established [1–5]. Possible nonsexual transmission modes include vertical or horizontal transmission and auto-inoculation. Vertical transmission can

S. Syrjänen
Department of Oral Pathology and Oral Radiology, Institute of Dentistry and MediCity Research Laboratory, University of Turku, Finland and
Department of Pathology, Institute of Dentistry, University of Turku, Lemminkäisenkatu 2, FI-20520, Turku, Finland
e-mail: stina.syrjanen@utu.fi

G. Gross and S.K. Tyring (eds.), *Sexually Transmitted Infections and Sexually Transmitted Diseases*,
DOI: 10.1007/978-3-642-14663-3_39, © Springer-Verlag Berlin Heidelberg 2011

be divided into three categories, according to the assumed time of HPV transmission: (1) peri-conceptual transmission (time around fertilization), (2) prenatal (during pregnancy), and (3) perinatal (during birth and immediately thereafter).

39.2.1 Sexual Transmission

Oral sex is a common practice in both heterosexuals and homosexuals. In our Kuopio cohort (1981–1998) assessing the natural history of cervical HPV infections, 44% of the women had practiced cunnilingus, 51% fellatio, and 7.2% had anal sex [6]. In the more recent Finnish Family HPV Study on HPV dynamics within family, 11% and 26% of the women and their husbands reported regular practice of oral sex, respectively [7]. However, we failed to establish any significant association between oral sex and carriage of HPV in the oral mucosa [7]. This is contradictory to the data reported by D'Souza and coworkers, who studied in a case-control setting, whether sexual behavior that increased the odds of oro-pharyngeal cancer would similarly increase the risk of oral HPV infections among the control patients [8]. HPV infection was detected in 4.8% of 332 control patients (from an outpatient clinic) and in 2.9% of 210 college-aged men. Among control patients, the odds of HPV infection developing independently increased with increased lifetime number of oral ($p = 0.007$, for trend) or vaginal sex partners ($p = .003$, for trend). Among college-aged men, there was an association between oral HPV and deep kisses ($p = 0.023$, for trend) and oral sex ($p = 0.046$, for trend) [8]. The importance of sexual transmission is confused by the fact that the HPV-type concordance in oral and genital infections seems to be poor between the sexual couples and even in the same person [9–12].

Sexual habits of the mother might have some effect on her infant's oral HPV status. In the Finnish Family HPV Study, 10% of the infants had persistent oral HPV infections during the follow-up [13, 14]. HPV persistence was significantly associated with several mother-related variables: mother's oral HPV, her hand warts, young age at the onset of sexual activity, and history of using oral contraceptives [13, 14]. Interestingly, father's sexual habits were not related to persistent oral HPV infections in the infant, whereas father's oral HPV carriage increased this risk. In the light of these data, it seems that sexual transmission might explain only a minority of all oral HPV infections [13, 14].

39.2.2 Peri-Conceptual Transmission

Peri-conceptual transmission could theoretically occur via infected oocytes or spermatozoa. HPV DNA has been detected in 8–64% of the semen samples from asymptomatic men [15–23]. Both seminal plasma and spermatozoa have been shown to contain HPV DNA [18].

39.2.3 Pre-natal Transmission

There are also data favoring intrauterine transmission, because HPV-induced lesions are occasionally present at birth [24–28]. HPV-DNA-positive infants have been born to HPV-negative mothers [1, 29–31]. However, hospital contamination in these cases cannot be always excluded. Caesarean section does not completely protect newborns against HPV [26, 31–34]. Further evidence has been provided by studies reporting HPV DNA in amniotic fluid, placenta, and cord blood samples [35–42]. Intrauterine HPV transmission could be an ascending HPV infection from the maternal genital tract through micro-tears in fetal membranes or with blood through the placenta [43, 44].

39.2.4 Perinatal Transmission

Vertical transmission is thought to result mainly from a close contact of the neonate with infected cervical and vaginal cells of the mother during the delivery. Confirmation of virus acquisition from the mother has been obtained in several studies by detecting HPV DNA in cervical samples of the mother immediately prior to delivery and in the nasopharyngeal aspirates or genital swabs from the neonate. However, the debate continues on the detection rate of HPV, and whether HPV positivity reflects passive contamination or true infection of the infant [1, 4, 5, 45–48]. The average concordance in HPV carriage (i.e., testing HPV+)

between the mother and the infant is 39%, ranging between 0.2% and 73% [5, 49–51].

39.3 Oral Mucosa

39.3.1 *Asymptomatic HPV Carriage*

39.3.1.1 Adults

The detection rate of asymptomatic oral HPV infection in adults (i.e., presence of HPV DNA) varies among different studies from 0% to 81%. The mean prevalence rate is approximately 11% [50–53]. Kreimer and coworkers recently made a meta-analysis on HPV detection in oral mucosa concluding that only 4.5% (95% CI: 3.9–5.1) of 4,070 subjects were positive for any HPV and 3.5% (95% CI: 3.0–4.1) of 4,441 subjects had carcinogenic mucosal HPV [54]. HPV16 was detected in 1.3% (95% CI: 1–1.7%) of 3,977 healthy subjects accounting for 28% of all HPV positive cases of the oral region (2010). Detection rate of any HPV varied widely in individual studies from 2.6% to 20.7%, even when the same primers were used for PCR [54].

39.3.1.2 Children

HPV prevalence rate in children aged from 0.3 to 11.6 years varies from 0% to 47% [13, 32, 45, 47, 55–58]. There is limited amount of data on age and asymptomatic oral HPV carriage but the current evidence suggests a bimodal age distribution, similar as found in skin warts, oral papillomas, and recurrent respiratory papillomas (RRP). The highest prevalence is found before 1 year of age, and the second peak at the age of 13–20 years [12, 59, 60]. It seems that the risk is increasing by 3–5% with each year of age [61, 62].

39.3.1.3 Gender and Oral HPV Infection

Only few studies have addressed the gender aspects of asymptomatic oral HPV. In their review, Miller and White in 1996 found a slight female-to-male preponderance; 1.5:1 [63]. Kreimer and coworkers have made two confusing meta-analyses; in the first one (from 2004) they reported that there might be a threefold higher risk for oral HPV infection in men than in women (OR = 3.0, 95% CI, 1.3–7.0) [62]. Contradictory to that, in 2010 they reported that both men and women have the same prevalence of any HPV detected in oral mucosa (4.6% vs. 4.4%, respectively) [54].

39.3.2 *Wide Range in Oral HPV Prevalence, Why?*

This wide variation in the detection rates of asymptomatic oral HPV can be explained by the sampling site, sampling method, and HPV-testing methods. In most studies, the exact anatomic sites of the samples are not given, and thus, the origin of HPV infection (whether oral or oro-pharyngeal) is impossible to trace. The samples are taken either as mucosal scrapings, oral rinses, or tissue biopsies. There are two types of normal oral mucosa: keratinized and non-keratinized. When a scraping is taken from an ortho-keratinized mucosa (similar as the skin), the sample is frequently inadequate due to the lack of nucleated cells. Overall, the HPV detection rate is higher in oral rinse samples (12–51%) and oral scrapings (45%) than in brush samples from the tonsils (3%) or biopsies (12%) [11, 61, 64, 65]. In oral rinse, however, the majority of HPV-positive cells might origin from the oro-pharynx and tonsils. A recent meta-analysis on oral and oro-pharyngeal cancers showed that a representative biopsy from the lesion resulted in the highest HPV detection rates especially when PCR was used (29.8% vs. 38.1%) [66]. Not only the sampling itself, but also the technical aspects in sample processing are of importance, e.g., the sample transport media, storage time, and temperature. For example in saliva, there are some 10 million bacteria/mL which might compromise HPV testing. The media used for HPV testing of oral scrapings include the same transport media as used also for cervical samples (usually slightly alkaline buffers with antibiotics), ethanol [7, 13, 14, 31, 32], or mouth wash [66].

The sensitivity and specificity of the HPV-testing method as well as the expertise of the researchers in interpreting these results are of key importance in addition to sampling site and sample processing. Based on our early experience on HPV testing from 309 scrapings, we found that three sequential swabs from the buccal mucosa will result in approx. 100,000 cells, which is optimal for HPV testing [64]. In these samples, HPV detection rate was related to the sensitivity of the HPV testing method; HPV DNA was found in 3.8%, 15.6%, and 23.1% with dot blot hybridization, Southern blot hybridization, and PCR, respectively [11, 64]. An important aspect frequently neglected is the quality of DNA for PCR, particularly because the microbe load is so high in saliva. A purified DNA will result in much higher HPV detection rate than non-purified DNA, as shown by us already in 1997 [31, 32], and confirmed by D'Souza and coworkers in 2005 [66]. Nested PCR will increase HPV detection rate and should be used especially when the cell count in the sample is not optimal. In our Finnish Family HPV Study, we have used nested PCR with subsequent hybridization. With this method, we found high-risk HPVs in 16–27% of the oral scrapings taken in 80% ethanol. DNA extraction was made with the high salt method [7, 13, 14]. Similarly, Kay et al. 2002 reported that HPV detection rate in buccal swabs increased from 19% to 74% when single PCR with MY09/11 primers was replaced by nested PCR with MY09/11 and GP05+/06+ primers [67].

39.3.3 Follow-Up Studies on Asymptomatic Oral HPV Infection in Adults

A few prospective follow-up studies have been conducted only recently to understand the natural history of oral HPV infections. Kurose and coworkers (in 2004) collected oral buccal scrapings from 662 volunteers during a 2-year follow-up. At baseline, only 0.6% (4/662) samples tested HPV-positive in PCR. The detected HPV types were 12, 16, 53, 71. After 2 years, two subjects remained still positive for HPV12 and HPV71 [68].

D'Souza and coworkers evaluated natural history of oral HPV by collecting oral rinse samples on two occasions at 6-month interval from 136 HIV-positive and 63 HIV-negative participants [69]. The 6-month cumulative prevalence of oral HPV infection was significantly less than for cervical infection ($p < 0.0001$). HIV-positive women were more likely than HIV-negative women to have an oral (33% vs. 15%, $p = 0.016$) or cervical (78% vs. 51%, $p < 0.001$) infection. Oral HPV infections detected at baseline were as likely as cervical infections to persist for 6 months among HIV-negative (60% vs. 51%, $p = 0.70$) and HIV-positive (55% vs. 63%, $p = 0.27$) women. Factors that independently increased the odds for oral HPV persistence differed from cervical infection and included current smoking (OR = 8, 95% CI = 1.3–53), age above 44 years (OR = 20, 95% CI = 4.1–83), CD4 < 500 (OR = 6, 95% CI = 1.1–26), use of HAART therapy (OR = 12, 95% CI = 1.0–156) [69].

39.3.4 Finnish Family HPV Study

Finnish Family HPV Study was started in 1998 to understand the dynamics of HPV infection within regular Finnish families designed as a continuation to our previous studies on HPV in oral mucosa and its transmission modes [11, 31, 32, 64, 70]. We initially followed up 331 women (mean age 25.5 ± 3.4 years) pregnant at their baseline visit, their 131 spouses (mean age 28.8 ± 5 years) and 333 newborns for 36 months. Subsequently, the follow-up was extended to 6 years, over 50% of the cohort being compliant with that. The study protocol includes a detail medical history and questionnaire on sexual habits, in addition to extensive serial sampling starting from the baseline visit before delivery, at delivery, and at month 2, 6, 12, 24, 36, and 72, including samples of sera, saliva, placenta, breast milk, and semen. The study has progressed to the stage of active reporting by now [7, 13, 14, 22, 41, 71–74].

39.3.4.1 Adults

In spouses, oral high-risk (HR) HPV detection rate varied from 16% to 27% at different time points [7, 14]. Of the baseline-negative spouses, 10% had an incident oral HPV infection. Among those who tested HR–HPV+ at baseline, none of the fathers and only 5% of the mothers cleared their HPV within 2 years. Persistent oral HPV infection was detected in 9% of the adults. One can speculate that persistent oral HR-HPV could present a risk for precancer or oral cancer [7, 14].

We also reported that HPV seropositivity was common among mothers, being most frequent for HPV6, followed by HPV16, 11, 18, and 45 [74]. Importantly, testing HPV-DNA-positive in the oral mucosa was not associated with HPV seropositivity for HPV types 6, 11, 16, 18, or 45.

39.3.4.2 Infants

In the infants, the prevalence of HPV DNA in oral mucosa fluctuated from 14% at delivery to 21% at 6 months, and down to 12% at 36 months [13, 14]. These figures present oral HPV infections and not oropharyngeal HPV, because all scrapings were taken only from the oral mucosa avoiding the posterior part of the tongue. During the 3-year follow-up, 42% of the infants acquired incident HPV infection, while 11% cleared their HPV, and 10% had persistent oral HPV infection [13]. This HPV persistence was associated with oral HPV of both parents, hand warts in mothers, young age at the onset of sexual activity by the mother, and use of oral contraceptives [13]. Interestingly, father's sexual habits were not related to infant's persistent oral HPV infection, whereas father's oral HPV increased the risk.

In the above-cited Kuopio cohort, we showed several years ago that vertically transmitted HPV was detectable from 2 days up to 3 years in 44% of the infants whose nasopharyngeal aspirate fluid tested HPV-positive at birth. The overall concordance between HPV types found in mother's genital sample and her infants nasopharyngeal aspirate fluid was 69% [31]. Among 98 children (aging from 0.3 to 11.6 years) born to 66 mothers of this same cohort, HPV was detected in 32% of the oral scrapings, of which 52% had the same HPV types as in the genital sample of the mother at the time of delivery [32].

39.3.5 Acetic Acid Application is of No Diagnostic Use in Oral Mucosa

Application of acetic acid has been widely used to identify cervical HPV lesions on colposcopy. We tested the specificity of acetic acid application in detection of oral HPV among 334 women in the prospective (1981–1998) Kuopio cohort [11, 64, 70]. Acetowhiteness on oral mucosa was seen significantly more frequently in smokers, but the staining did not show any correlation with alcohol consumption, histological and cytological findings, or presence of HPV DNA. In oral epithelia, vacuolated cells are frequently seen and some of them mimic the cytopathic effect of HPV (koilocytes). These vacuolated cells were found significantly more often in periodic acid-Shiff (PAS)-positive biopsies, indicating that the clear zone (peri-nuclear halo) contained glycogen. No correlation was seen between vacuolated cells and acetowhite staining, however. Thus, in oral mucosa, vacuolization is most probably related to degenerative changes in the epithelial cells. To conclude, positive acetic acid staining in oral cavity should not be regarded as a diagnostic criteria of HPV infection [70].

39.3.6 Pregnancy and Oral HPV Infection

In addition to our recent report [7, 73], there is only one previous study on oral HPV infection in pregnant women. Smith and coworkers detected HPV DNA in 2.5% of the oral samples of pregnant women [12]. In the Finnish Family HPV Study, we found HPV in 16% of the 329 oral samples of mothers at their third trimester [7]. In the same cohort, 78 mothers became pregnant for the second time during the follow-up. This allowed us to study the effects of the second pregnancy more closely using age-matched, nonpregnant women as controls. There was no statistically significant difference in HR-HPV detection in oral mucosa between the first and second pregnancy. However, the HR-HPV detection rate in oral mucosa was significantly higher during the inter-pregnancy period, i.e., before the second pregnancy than during the second pregnancy (OR = 3.19, 95% CI 1.4–7.0) [73].

39.3.7 The Effect of Menopause and Hormone Replace Therapy

According to the scanty existing data, hormone replacement therapy had no effect on oral HPV detection rate [75].

39.3.8 Simultaneous HPV Detection in Both Oral and Genital Mucosa

We were one of the first to report oral and genital HPV prevalence, while analysing 309 women of the Kuopio cohort, prospectively followed up between 1981 and 1998. Of the oral samples, 3.8%, 16%, and 23% tested

HPV-positive with dot blot hybridization, Southern blot hybridization, and PCR, respectively. HPV 16/11 and 16/18 were the most common types. However, only four women had the same HPV types in both sites [11, 70]. Nine male partners had anogenital HPV infection, but all with different HPV types than their female partners in oral samples. In an Italian study, 5/29 women had an infection in the oral cavity concomitantly with genital HPV infection, but only in three patients, HPV types were the same [76]. Multiple infections were common. Giraldo and coworkers reported that the overall prevalence of HPV in the oral cavity of patients with and without genital HPV was 37.1% and 4.3%, respectively ($p < 0.0001$). The presence of oral HPV was unrelated to the practice of fellatio (22% vs. 19%) [37]. Among Spanish female sex workers, HPV DNA was detected in 8% of oral samples and the concordance of HPV16 was 5% between the oral cavity and the cervix. Over 80% of HPV infections in genital sites were high-risk types while the low-risk types predominated in the oral mucosa [9]. D'Souza et al. collected both oral and cervical samples from the controls and cases with HIV or head and neck cancers, followed-up for 6 months [69]. The rate of newly detected oral HPV infection was lower than for cervical infection (10% vs. 23%).

Taken together, cervical infection does not seem to predispose to oral transmission, even in the presence of oral-genital sexual habits, thus suggesting independence of HPV infection at these two mucosal sites.

39.3.9 Risk Factors Associated with Oral HPV Detection

39.3.9.1 Adults

The risk factors of oral HPV infection are incompletely studied. In our Kuopio cohort, hand warts were encountered significantly more frequently in women with concomitant oral HPV infection [11, 70], as later confirmed by Terai and coworkers in 1999 [77]. This might signify some kind of impaired immunity, e.g., a specific defect in rejecting HPV.

As discussed before, it is nearly a common dogma that oral sex is the main transmission mode of oral HPV infection. In our cohort, however, oral sex had no association to oral transmission of HPV infection between spouses, but a persistent oral HPV infection of one spouse increased the risk of persistent oral HPV infection in the other spouse by tenfold (OR = 10.0; 95% CI 1.5–68.7; $p = 0.005$) [14]. Similarly, D'Souza and coworkers reported that deep kissing was associated with asymptomatic oral HPV infection, but contrary to our data, they also found oral sex (but not genital sex) to be such risk factors [8, 69].

39.3.9.2 Infants

In the Finnish Family HPV Study, there was a subgroup of the infants (10%) who had persistent HPV infection in oral mucosa. The determinants of such persistent oral HR-HPV in infants pointed toward maternal transmission, including mothers' younger age at onset of sexual activity, early age at start of oral contraception, and mother's hand warts [13, 14]. Interestingly, we also found HPV DNA in 4.2% of the 306 placental samples and HPV6 and HPV16 DNA could be localized in syncytiotrophoblasts by ISH. HPV-positivity of the placenta increased the risk of an offspring to be HPV-carrier in the oral mucosa (OR = 8.2, 95% C1 2.6–26.0, $p = 0.001$). Also 3.5% of the 311 core blood samples tested HPV-positive. This HPV positivity also increased the risk of an offspring to be HPV-carrier in the oral mucosa (OR = 4.3, 95% CI, 1.2–16, $p = 0.039$) as well as in the genitals (OR = 4.1, 95% CI 1.1.–15.2, $p = 0.045$) at delivery [41].

So far there is only one systematic review on vertical transmission of HPV. This review included 2,111 pregnant women and their 2,113 newborns [49]. Pooled mother-to-child HPV transmission was 6.5% and higher after vaginal delivery than after caesarean section (18.3% vs. 8%) (RR = 1.8; 95% CI 1.3–2.4). The combined relative risk (RR) of mother-to-child HPV transmission was RR = 7.3 (95% CI, 2.4–22.2). However, there was extensive clinical heterogeneity in study designs like in most meta-analyses [49].

39.3.10 Benign Oral HPV Lesions

There are no population-based studies on the incidence or prevalence of oral papilloma or condyloma. The largest cohort comprises 20,000 Swedish citizens, of whom 0.1% had oral warty lesions [78]. Squamous cell papillomas (SCP) are the most common benign tumors of oral epithelium. However, in some textbooks, papillomas are clumped together with benign epithelial neoplasia, which represent a reaction to injury rather than true tumors. SCPs are reported to be most frequent in children and adults in their 4th and 5th decades. There are also some rare syndromes which are known to be associated with multiple oral papillomas, e.g., focal dermal hypoplasia syndrome, acrodermatitis enteropathica, Cowdens's syndrome, nevus unius lateralis, Costello syndrome, and Down's syndromes (OMIM data base, http://www.ncbi.nlm.nih.gov/omim OMIM).

Oral condylomas (OC) have been traditionally associated with oral sex, in contrast to oral SCP. However, no reliable differential diagnosis can be made between oral SCP and OC either clinically or in histological examination. In the literature published by 1998, the author found a total of 481 SCPs and 284 OCs, of which 50% and 75% tested HPV-positive. HPV6 and 11 were the major HPV types in these lesions [51, 79–83]. The role of HPV in other benign epithelial hyperplasia is unknown. Recently, some evidence was presented that the majority of white oral mucosal lesions – flat, exophytic, wart-like, or papillary proliferations – could be considered as clinical manifestations of oral HPV infection [84].

In our cohort of children born to mothers with genital HPV infection, we correlated HPV DNA status (PCR and oral scrapings) with the clinical appearance of oral mucosa [32]. Clinically, minor hyperplastic growths were found in 22.4% of the 98 children, with mean age of 4 years (range 0.6–11.6 years). Eight of these children with clinical findings tested HPV-positive (36.4%). Interestingly, a 7-year-old girl had an HPV16-positive oral SCP, and the same HPV type was also detected in the genital tract of her mother at delivery [32].

39.4 Oro-Pharynx

In adults, HPV has been detected in 50–80% of oropharyngeal cancers, mostly attributed to HPV in tonsillar carcinomas [85]. This makes it important to clarify the natural history of HPV infections in the tonsils, prevalence of HPV in children, and the time when tonsillar HPV infections are acquired. Unfortunately, only few studies on HPV infection in tonsillar and adenoid hyperplasia exist, with HPV detection rates varying from 0% to 8.5% [86–89]. Chen and coworkers found HPV in 6.3% of tonsillitis and hypertrophic tonsillar tissues, and in 0.6% of exfoliated cells from normal tonsillar tissues. Importantly, they found only HPV16, but it did appear to lead to L1 antibody response [21]. Similarly, also Sisk and associates detected predominantly HPV16 in tonsillar samples that tested HPV-positive [89]. In one study, swabs were taken from four sites of healthy mucosa in the oropharynx (tonsils, soft palate, base of the tongue, and back wall of the pharynx). HPV DNA was present in 14% of the individuals, and the identified genotypes were 16, 18, 52, and 61. Base of the tongue and soft palate were the two most frequent sites of HPV [90].

39.5 Larynx

39.5.1 Asymptomatic HPV Carriage

Only a few studies have addressed asymptomatic HPV carriage in the larynx. Using the short fragment PCR (SPF_{10}) Morshed et al. detected HPV DNA in 8.2% of 49 normal mucosa samples representing surgical margins in patients with laryngeal carcinoma, but none of the samples from healthy control group was HPV-DNA-positive [63]. Brandsma et al. reported an HPV prevalence of 4% in normal laryngeal mucosa of healthy subjects [91]. Nunez et al. [92] found that 25% of the samples were positive for HPV11. No other HPV types were found [92].

39.5.2 Recurrent Respiratory Papillomatosis

Recurrent respiratory papillomatosis (RRP) has a bimodal age distribution which forms the basis of their classification as juvenile- (JO) or adult-onset (AO). Recently, a comprehensive review on RRP literature was published [93]. Juvenile onset RRP (JO-RRP) is presented in prepubertal children usually before 5 years of age, while in adults, the typical age is 20–40 years. The younger the age of onset, the more severe is the disease [93, 94]. RRP presents with multiple SCPs on the vocal cords, followed by spread to the false cords, epiglottis, and sub-glottic area, and more rarely into the trachea and even bronchi [80, 93, 95–97]. JO-RRP is a potentially life-threatening disease, because it shows a tendency to grow in size and number of lesions causing total respiratory obstruction.

The symptoms include hoarseness, chronic dyspnea, and cough, present from 2 months to >2 years before definitive diagnosis has been settled [93]. The incidence figures of laryngeal papillomas are not accurate and are subject to wide variation in different countries. This is because small papillomas are asymptomatic and not easy to detect. In a Danish population, the incidence and prevalence of JO-RRP were 0.6 and 0.8/100,000, respectively [96, 98]. In a pediatric population from the USA, the incidence is approximately 1.7–4.3/100,000 [3, 99]. JO-RRP is almost invariably associated with HPV type 6 or 11, and HPV11 is more likely to cause a more severe disease with earlier onset [99–101]. Persistence of HPV DNA in the adjacent normal epithelium is consistent with the frequent recurrence of these lesions [102].

39.5.3 Risk Factors of RRP

In 1956, Hajek [24] wrote: "Multiple laryngeal papillomata are found in small children and adolescents. They are not hereditary, but in 20% of cases can be found at birth" [24]. Since then, several studies have demonstrated a relationship between JO-RRP and maternal genital condylomata in 30–50% of the patients [95, 103–105]. However, the prevalence of genital condylomata among women at childbearing age far exceeds the reported number of new cases of JO-RRP. The risk of transmission from an HPV-infected mother to her newborn has been estimated to range from 1:80 to 1:1,500 [106]. In a retrospective cohort of Danish births between 1974 and 1993 by Silverberg and colleagues [107], seven out of every 1,000 births with maternal history of genital warts during pregnancy resulted in laryngeal lesions. In women with genital warts, delivery exceeding 10 h was associated with a twofold risk of disease.

The majority of children who subsequently developed JO-RRP have been born to mothers with no history of genital warts during pregnancy, and these mothers might have HPV as a subclinical infection. Children whose mothers had a history of genital warts have been reported to develop JO-RRP at an earlier median age than children without such a history (4.3 vs. 5.9 years) [107]. Other risk factors associated with JO-RRP include maternal age <20 years, first-order births, and vaginal delivery [108]. Recently, the susceptibility to AO-RRP was associated with DRB1*0301 while HLA-DRB1*14 increases the risk of JO-RRP [109]. A prospective study of Stern and coworkers [110] brought new evidence that cellular immunity is compromised in children with JO-RRP. However, it remained unclear whether HPV causes this impaired response or whether children with impaired immunity will develop JO-RRP. Interestingly, there are no documented cases of RRP occurring among siblings, marital partners, or family members, suggesting the importance of impaired mucosal or systemic immunity in the development of RRP.

Malignant transformation of laryngeal SCP to carcinoma has been reported in 3–5% of the RRP patients, but nearly all cases are associated with previous irradiation of these papillomas and/or history of heavy smoking [111, 112].

The presence of HPV infection in premalignant and hyperplastic laryngeal lesions other than RRP is controversial. Poljak et al. [113] analyzed HPV prevalence in laryngeal epithelial hyperplastic lesions using PCR and ISH methods. HPV was present in only 2 of 88 specimens and the authors suggested that most of the hyperplastic lesions in the larynx are not associated with HPV infection.

39.6 Nasal Cavity and Paranasal Sinuses

39.6.1 Sino-Nasal Papillomas

Papillomas of the nasal mucosa have been recognized since 1854 when initially described by the name "warted papillomas". A comprehensive review on these sino-nasal lesions was published in 2003 [114]. Sino-nasal papilloma is a rare disease and males seem to be more frequently affected than females with an M:F ratio of 3:1. Typical for these lesions is their high recurrence rate; 32%. Based on the literature, approximately 3–8% has a malignant potential. By 2003, 1,401 sino-nasal papillomas have been subjected to HPV detection and HPV DNA has been reported in 33%, HPV6 and 11 being the two most common viral types [114].

39.6.2 Cancer of Nasal Cavity and Paranasal Sinuses

Cancer of nasal cavity and paranasal sinuses is a rare disease. Squamous cell carcinoma is the most frequent histological type of sino-nasal carcinoma. In a recent review from 2003, the number of cases tested for HPV was 322 and the detection rate was 22%. The single predominant HPV type was HPV16, but well-documented cases of sino-nasal carcinomas with HPV 6 or 11 DNA have been reported as well [114].

39.7 Oral, Oro-Pharyngeal and Laryngeal Cancer

The first evidence linking oral carcinomas to HPV was reported in 1983 by us [115]. Recently, several meta-analyses and case-control studies have been published on HPV involvement in head and neck tumors [79, 116–127]. HPV has been detected in oral cancers but the detection rate is less than in oro-pharyngeal cancers [54, 116, 120, 128]. In many studies, it is nearly impossible to trace the results separately for oral and oro-pharyngeal cancers. Small sample size and publication bias complicate the assessment of HPV prevalence in head and neck sites beyond the oro-pharynx.

39.7.1 Oral Cancer

One of the most cited works is the systematic review on HPV types in head and neck squamous cell carcinomas (HNSCC) worldwide done by Kreimer and coworkers in 2005 [121]. In 5,046 HNSCC specimens from 60 studies, the overall HPV prevalence was 25.9% [95% CI, 24.7–27.2]. HPV prevalence was significantly higher in oro-pharyngeal SCCs (35.6% of 969; 95% CI, 32.6–38.7) than in oral SCCs (23.5% of 2,642; 95% CI, 21.9–25.1) or laryngeal SCCs (24% of 1,435; 95% CI, 21.8–26.3). HPV16 accounted for a larger majority of HPV-positive cases in oro-pharyngeal SCCs (86.7%; 95% CI, 82.6–90.1) as compared with HPV-positive oral SCCs (68.2%; 95% CI, 64.4–71.9) and laryngeal SCCs (69.2%; 95% CI, 64.0–74.0). Conversely, HPV18 was rare in HPV-positive oro-pharyngeal SCCs (2.8%; 95% CI, 1.3–5.3) as compared with other head and neck sites (34.1%; 95% CI, 30.4–38.0) of oral SCCs and 17.0% (95% CI, 13.0–21.6) of laryngeal SCCs. Aside from HPV16 and HPV18, other oncogenic HPVs were rarely detected in HNSCC. Tumor site-specific HPV prevalence was higher among studies from North America as compared with Europe and Asia. High HPV16 prevalence and lack of HPV18 in oro-pharyngeal cancer as compared with other HNSCCs may point to specific virus–tissue interactions. Importantly, HPV6 and 11 were also found in a small minority of these cancers, implicating that these benign HPV types are not entirely benign while in oral, oro-pharyngeal, or upper respiratory sites [57]. However, It is still too early to confirm, whether the eight most common HR-HPV types in cervical cancer (16, 18, 31, 33, 35, 45, 53, 58) are also the most prevalent types in oral, oro-pharyngeal, and laryngeal cancers, because of the lack of studies using HPV-testing methods covering most of the mucosal types, e.g., the Luminex-based multiplex genotyping which can detect 100 different HPV genotypes simultaneously [129].

39.7.2 Oro-Pharyngeal Cancer

The incidence of both tonsillar cancer and the base of tongue cancer is increasing [130–132]. This increase has been attributed to increased HPV infections. In Sweden, an overall increase in the incidence of base of tongue cancer from 0.15/100,000 person-years during 1970–1974 to 0.47/100,000 during 2005–2007 was found [130]. In the meantime, prevalence of HPV in base of tongue cancer in Stockholm county increased from 58% during 1998–2001 to 84% during 2004–2007 ($p < 0.05$). In HPV-positive tumors, HPV16 dominated (86%) but interestingly, HPV33 was detected in as many as 10% of the cases. E6 and/or E7 RNA were found in 85% of the samples tested. This concomitant increase in incidence of base of tongue cancer and proportion of HPV-positive tumors suggests that HPV may contribute to this increase [130].

According to SEER data (U.S. National Cancer Institute) also in USA the incidence of HNSCCs that are potentially related to HPV infection (base of tongue, lingual and palatine tonsil, pharynx) significantly increased between 1973 and 2004, with an annual increase of 0.8% [131]. Thus, clinicians should be aware of the risk of oro-pharyngeal cancer in young people to avoid unnecessary delay in diagnosis and treatment.

39.7.3 Laryngeal Cancer

The first evidence linking laryngeal carcinomas to HPV was reported in early 1982 by us [133]. Since then, a large number of studies have been published. In the literature published until 1998, there were 1,252 laryngeal cancers tested for HPV, of which 25% were HPV-positive. As expected, HPV16 is the single most common HPV type detected in these lesions, with other HR-HPV types 18, 31, and 33 reported occasionally. In a small number of cases, HPV types 6 and 11 have been found as well. During the last 10 years, the literature on this subject has increased rapidly, but no significant changes have occurred in HPV prevalence in laryngeal carcinoma. The overall HPV detection rate varies from 17% to 25% [51, 121].

39.7.4 Risk Factors of HNSCC

Numerous case-control studies have identified several risk factors for HPV-associated oral cancer. According to the current literature, the risk factors are partly the same as in cervical cancer: number of sexual partners, younger age at first sexual intercourse, practice of oral sex, history of genital warts, and younger age [44, 119, 120, 124, 134].

D'Souza and coworkers [135] reported that a high number of lifetime vaginal-sex partners (26 or more) was associated with oro-pharyngeal cancer (OR = 3.1; 95%, 1.5–6.5), as was a high lifetime number of oral-sex partners (6 or more) (OR = 3.4; 95% CI, 1.3–8.8). The degree of association increased with the number of vaginal-sex and oral-sex partners (*p* values for trend, 0.002 and 0.009, respectively). Oro-pharyngeal cancer was significantly associated with oral HPV16 infection (OR = 14.6; 95% CI, 6.3–36.6), oral infection with any of 37 types of HPV (OR = 12.3; 95% CI, 5.4–26.4), and seropositivity for the HPV16 L1 capsid protein (OR = 32.2; 95% CI, 14.6–71.3). HPV 16 DNA was detected in 72% (95% CI, 62–81) of 100 paraffin-embedded tumor specimens, and 64% of patients with cancer were seropositive for the HPV16 oncoprotein E6, E7, or both. HPV16 L1 seropositivity was closely associated with oro-pharyngeal cancer among subjects with a history of heavy tobacco and alcohol use (OR = 19.4; 95% CI, 3.3–113.9) and among those without such a history (OR = 33.6; 95% CI, 13.3–84.8). The association was similarly increased among subjects with oral HPV16 infection, regardless of their tobacco and alcohol use [135].

In another multicenter case-control study with 5,642 HNSCC and 6,069 controls, the authors analyzed several risk factors: specific sexual behaviors, including practice of oral sex, number of lifetime sexual partners and oral sex partners, age at sexual debut, a history of same-sex contact, and a history of oral-anal contact [134]. Cancer of the oro-pharynx was associated with having a history of six or more lifetime sexual partners (OR = 1.25, 95% CI 1.01, 1.54) and four or more lifetime oral sex partners (OR = 2.25, 95% CI 1.42, 3.58). Cancer of the tonsils was associated with four or more lifetime oral sex partners (OR = 3.36, 95 % CI 1.32, 8.53), and, among men, with ever having oral sex (OR = 1.59, 95% CI 1.09, 2.33) and with an earlier age at sexual debut (OR = 2.36, 95% CI 1.37, 5.05). Cancer of the base of tongue was associated with ever having oral sex among women (OR = 4.32, 95% CI 1.06, 17.6), having two sexual partners in comparison with only one (OR = 2.02, 95% CI 1.19, 3.46) and, among men, with a history of same-sex sexual contact (OR = 8.89, 95% CI 2.14, 36.8) [134].

39.7.5 Prognosis Related to HPV Status in HNSCC

The current evidence suggests that HPV status is an important and independent predictor of overall and disease-specific survival in HNSCC [44, 119, 131, 136]. Several studies have reported that detection of HPV DNA is significantly associated with poor differentiation of the cancer, positive lymph nodes, and late-stage disease, which traditionally indicate poor prognosis. Despite this, patients with HPV-positive tumors seem to have significantly improved response to chemotherapy as compared to HPV-negative tumors, and these patients seems to have lower risk of second primary cancers as well. The mechanism is not understood but three possible explanations are: (1) the genome of HPV-positive cancer cells is less unstable, (2) HPV-positive cells due to hypoxia can be induced to apoptosis, and (3) treatment improves the local immunity.

39.8 Reservoir of HPV Infection

It has been suggested that HPV prevalence in the normal mucosa includes subclinical and/or latent infections, and that the infection with a low number of virus copies is common in the oral cavity [137–141]. The reservoirs of latent or persistent HPV infection are unknown in oral mucosa [140, 141]. Potential areas of reservoir could be the sites of quickly proliferating epithelia like tonsillar crypts or the zone between two different types of epithelia, like salivary glands where the squamous epithelium undergoes transition to the ductal epithelium or gingival pocket epithelium [5, 82]. In the larynx, it is not known whether a specific predilection site for HPV reservoir exists.

39.9 Prophylactic HPV Vaccines and Head and Neck Tumors

At present, two commercially available prophylactic HPV vaccines exist: the bivalent (HPV16/18) vaccine Cervarix® (GSK), and the quadrivalent (HPV6/11/16/18) Gardaril® (Merck). Licensed globally, these two vaccines have been loaded with great expectations in prevention of infections and tumors induced by the vaccine HPV types. At the moment, however, the accepted indications include only cervical cancer (CC) and its precursors (for Cervarix), and in addition, cancers of the vulva and vagina and their precursors (VIN, VAIN) as well as AIS (adenocarcinoma in situ) for Gardasil. In addition, Gardasil is intended to be used for prophylaxis of genital warts (condylomata) due to HPV6/11. Until now, only Gardasil has been tested in the males.

In the reported randomized controlled trials (RCT), both vaccines have proven almost 100% effective in preventing CC and CIN as well as persistent HPV16/18 infections. Similarly, Gardasil is highly effective against genital warts. There is little doubt that once shown highly effective against these viral types in one anatomic region, there is no reason why they should not work against these same viruses at other anatomic sites as well. Most likely, this would apply equally well to benign (HPV6/11) lesions, cancer, and their precursors, e.g., in head and neck region. If proven to do so, this would represent a major conceptual breakthrough, not only in prevention of these diseases, but equally importantly, by providing the "missing link" in the chain of evidence with the final proof of HPV etiology of these tumors [140].

Unfortunately, however, we are not that far yet. Although the current HPV vaccines are manufactured by two multinational global giants (GSK, Merck), the resources are limited to the extent that setting priorities is necessary. At the moment, both companies have the second generation polyvalent HPV vaccines (with seven or eight viral types) in the pipeline ready to go for global RCTs. At the same time, vaccine efficacy trials in the males are starting. As far as the author is aware, clinical trials with either Cervarix or Gardasil to extend the current indications to diseases (and infections) at extra-genital sites have not yet started. The good news is, however, that interest in all head and neck lesions has increased tremendously during the past few years [140], and it is most probably only a matter of time when the domain of HPV vaccines will be extended to head and neck lesions. RCTs in these lesions are much more difficult to design, however, and providing this required formal evidence on their efficacy in head and neck lesions will take several more years.

Take-Home Pearls

- HPV is not exclusively a sexually transmitted disease
- Asymptomatic HPV infections can be found in the oral mucosa of both children and adults
- HPV16 is the most common genotype to cause asymptomatic infections and in HNSCC
- Benign papillomas in head and neck region are caused by HPV6/11, both in children and adults
- A subset of HNSCCs are related to oncogenic HPV types
- The final proof of their HPV etiology will be obtained after widespread implementation of prophylactic HPV vaccines that should eventually lead to global decline of HPV-related HNCC incidence and mortality

References

1. Cason, J., Mant, C.A.: High-risk mucosal human papillomavirus infections during infancy & childhood. J. Clin. Virol. **32**(suppl 1), S52–S58 (2005)
2. Castellsague, X., Drudis, T., Paz Canadas, M., et al.: Human papillomavirus (HPV) infection in pregnant women and mother-to-child transmission of genital HPV genotypes: a prospective study in Spain. BMC Infect. Dis. **9**, 74–86 (2009)
3. Dillner, J., Andersson-Ellstrom, A., Hagmar, B., et al.: High risk genital papillomavirus infections are not spread vertically. Rev. Med. Virol. **9**, 23–29 (1999)
4. Syrjänen, S.: HPV infections in children Invited review. Papillomavirus Rep. **14**, 93–110 (2003)
5. Syrjänen, S., Puranen, M.: HPV infections in children: the potential role of maternal transmission. Crit. Rev. Oral Biol. Med. **11**, 259–274 (2000)
6. Kataja, V., Syrjanen, S., Yliskoski, M., et al.: Risk factors associated with cervical human papillomavirus infections: a case-control study. Am. J. Epidemiol. **138**, 735–745 (1993)
7. Rintala, M., Grénman, S., Puranen, M., et al.: Natural history of oral papillomavirus infections in spouses: a prospective Finnish HPV family study. J. Clin. Virol. **35**, 89–94 (2006)
8. D'Souza, G., Agrawal, Y., Halpern, J., et al.: Oral sexual behaviors associated with prevalent oral human papillomavirus infection. J. Infect. Dis. **199**, 1263–1269 (2009)
9. Canadas, M., Bosch, F., Junquera, M., et al.: Concordance of prevalence of human papillomavirus DNA in anogenital and oral infections in a high-risk population. J. Clin. Microbiol. **42**, 1330–1332 (2004)
10. Giraldo, P., Goncalves, A., Pereira, S., et al.: Human papillomavirus in the oral mucosa of women with genital human papillomavirus lesions. Eur. J. Obstet. Gynecol. Reprod. Biol. **126**, 104–106 (2006)
11. Kellokoski, J., Syrjänen, S., Chang, F., et al.: Southern blot hybridization and PCR in detection of oral human papillomavirus (HPV) infections in women with genital HPV infections. J. Oral Pathol. Med. **21**, 459–464 (1992)
12. Smith, E., Ritchie, J., Yankowitz, J., et al.: Human papillomavirus prevalence and types in newborns and parents. Sex. Transm. Dis. **31**, 57–62 (2004)
13. Rintala, M., Grenman, S., Jarvenkyla, M., et al.: High-risk types of human papillomavirus (HPV) DNA in oral and genital mucosa of infants during their first 3 years of life: experience from the Finnish HPV Family Study. Clin. Infect. Dis. **41**, 1728–1733 (2005)
14. Rintala, M., Grenman, S., Puranen, M., et al.: Transmission of high-risk human papillomavirus (HPV) between parents and infant: a prospective study of HPV in families in Finland. J. Clin. Microbiol. **43**, 376–381 (2005)
15. Chan, P.J., Su, B.C., Kalugdan, T., et al.: Human papillomavirus gene sequences in washed human sperm deoxyribonucleic acid. Fertil. Steril. **61**, 982–985 (1994)
16. Green, J., Monteiro, E., Bolton, V.N., et al.: Detection of human papillomavirus DNA by PCR in semen from patients with and without penile warts. Genitourin. Med. **67**, 207–210 (1991)
17. Lai, Y.M., Lee, J.F., Hy, H., et al.: The effect of human papillomavirus infection on sperm cell motility. Fertil. Steril. **67**, 1152–1155 (1997)
18. Lai, Y.M., Yang, F.-P., Pao, C.C.: Human papillomavirus deoxyribonucleic acid and ribonucleic acid in seminal plasma and sperm cells. Fertil. Steril. **65**, 1026–1030 (1996)
19. Olatunbosun, O., Deneer, H., Pierson, R.: Human papillomavirus DNA detection in sperm using polymerase chain reaction. Obstet. Gynecol. **97**, 357–360 (2001)
20. Ostrow, R.S., Sachow, K.R., Niimura, M., et al.: Detection of papillomavirus DNA in human semen. Science **31**, 731–733 (1986)
21. Pakendorf, U.W., Bornman, M.S., Du Plessis, D.J.: Prevalence of human papillomavirus in men attending the infertility clinic. Andrologia **30**, 11–14 (1998)
22. Rintala, M., Grenman, S., Pöllänen, P., et al.: Detection of high-risk HPV DNA in semen and its association with the quality of semen. Int. J. STD AIDS **15**, 740–743 (2004)
23. Rintala, M., Pöllänen, P., Nikkanen, V., et al.: Human papillomavirus DNA is found in vas deferens. J. Infect. Dis. **185**, 1664–1667 (2002)
24. Hajek, E.: Contribution to the etiology of laryngeal papilloma in children. J. Laryngol. Otol. **70**, 166–168 (1956)
25. Marcoux, D., Nadeau, K., McCuaig, C., et al.: Pediatric anogenital warts: a 7-year review of children referred to a tertiary-care hospital in Montreal, Canada. Pediatr. Dermatol. **23**, 199–207 (2006)
26. Obalek, S., Jablonska, S., Orth, G.: Anogenital warts in children. Clin. Dermatol. **15**, 369–376 (1997)
27. Rogo, K.O., Nyansera, P.N.: Congenital condylomata acuminata with meconium staining of amniotic fluid and fetal hydrocephalus: case report. East Afr. Med. J. **66**, 411–413 (1989)
28. Tang, C.K., Shermeta, D.W., Wood, C.: Congenital condylomata acuminata. Am. J. Obstet. Gynecol. **131**, 912–913 (1978)
29. Gottschling, M., Göker, M., Köhler, A., et al.: Cutaneotropic Human β-/γ-Papillomaviruses Are Rarely Shared between Family Members. J. Invest. Dermatol. **129**, 2427–2434 (2009)
30. Mazzatenta, C., Fimiani, M., Rubegni, P., et al.: Vertical transmission of human papillomavirus in cytologically normal women. Genitourin. Med. **72**, 445–446 (1996)
31. Puranen, M., Yliskoski, M., Saarikoski, S., et al.: Exposure of an infant to cervical human papillomavirus infection of the mother is common. Am. J. Obstet. Gynecol. **176**, 1039–1045 (1997)
32. Puranen, M., Yliskoski, M., Saarikoski, S., et al.: Vertical transmission of human papillomavirus from infected mothers to their newborn babies and persistence of the virus in childhood. Am. J. Obstet. Gynecol. **174**, 694–699 (1996)
33. Tseng, C.J., Liang, C.C., Soong, Y.K., et al.: Perinatal transmission of human papillomavirus in infants: relationship between infection rate and mode of delivery. Obstet. Gynecol. **91**, 92–96 (1998)
34. Tseng, C.J., Lin, C.Y., Wang, R.L., et al.: Possible transplacental transmission of human papillomaviruses. Am. J. Obstet. Gynecol. **166**, 35–40 (1992)
35. Bodaghi, S., Wood, L.V., Roby, G., et al.: Could human papillomaviruses be spread through blood? J. Clin. Microbiol. **43**, 5428–5434 (2005)

36. Boulenoua, S., Weyn, C., Van Noppen, M., et al.: Effects of HPV-16 E5, E6, E7 proteins on survival, adhesion, migration and invasion of trophoblastic cells. Carcinogenesis **31**, 473–480 (2010)
37. Eppel, W., Worda, C., Frigo, P., et al.: Human papillomavirus in the cervix and placenta. Obstet. Gynecol. **96**, 337–341 (2000)
38. Gomes, L.M., Ma, Y., Ho, C., et al.: Placental infection with human papillomavirus is associated with spontaneous preterm delivery. Hum. Reprod. **23**, 709–715 (2008)
39. Liu, Y., You, H., Chiriva-Internati, M., et al.: Display of complete life cycle of human papillomavirus type 16 in cultured placental trophoblasts. Virology **290**, 99–105 (2001)
40. Pao, C.C., Lin, S.S., Lin, C.Y., et al.: Identification of human papillomavirus DNA sequences in peripheral blood mononuclear cells. Am. J. Clin. Pathol. **95**, 540–546 (1991)
41. Sarkola, M.E., Grenman, S.E., Rintala, M.A., et al.: Human papillomavirus in the placenta and umbilical cord blood. Acta Obstet. Gynecol. Scand. **87**, 1181–1188 (2008)
42. You, H., Liu, Y., Agrawal, N., et al.: Multiple human papillomavirus types replicate in 3A trophoblasts. Placenta **29**, 30–38 (2008)
43. Armbruster-Moraes, E., Ioshimoto, L.M., Leão, E., et al.: Presence of human papillomavirus DNA in amniotic fluids of pregnant women with cervical lesions. Gynecol. Oncol. **54**, 152–158 (1994)
44. Gillison, M.L., D'Souza, G., Westra, W., et al.: Distinct risk factor profiles for human papillomavirus type 16 positive and human papillomavirus type 16 negative head and neck cancers. J. Natl. Cancer Inst. **100**, 407–420 (2008)
45. Rice, P.S., Cason, J., Best, J.M., et al.: High risk genital papillomavirus infections are spread vertically. Rev. Med. Virol. **9**, 15–21 (1999)
46. Trottier, H., Burchell, A.N.: Epidemiology of mucosal human papillomavirus infection and associated diseases. Publ. Health Genom. **12**, 291–307 (2009)
47. Watts, D.H., Koutsky, L.A., Holmes, K.K., et al.: Low risk of perinatal transmission of human papillomavirus: Results from a prospective cohort study. Am. J. Obstet. Gynecol. **178**, 365–373 (1998)
48. Winer, R.L., Koutsky, L.A.: Delivering reassurance to parents: perinatal human papillomavirus transmission is rare. Sex. Transm. Dis. **31**, 63–64 (2004)
49. Medeiros, L.R., Ethur, A.B., Hilgert, J.B., et al.: Vertical transmission of the human papillomavirus: a systematic quantitative review. Cad. Saúde Pública [serial on the Internet] **21**, 1006–1015 (2005)
50. Smith, E.M., Swarnavel, S., Ritchie, J.M., et al.: Prevalence of human papillomavirus in the oral cavity/oropharynx in a large population of children and adolescents. Pediatr. Infect. Dis. J. **26**, 836–840 (2007)
51. Syrjänen, K., Syrjänen, S.: Papillomavirus infections in human disease, pp. 1–615. Wiley, New York (2000)
52. Miller, C., Johnstone, B.: Human papillomavirus as a risk factor for oral squamous cell carcinoma: a meta-analysis, 1982–1997. Oral Surg. Oral Med. Oral Pathol. Oral Radiol. Endod. **91**, 622–635 (2001)
53. Miller, C., White, D.: Human papillomavirus expression in oral mucosa, premalignant conditions, and squamous cell carcinoma. Oral Surg. Oral Med. Oral Pathol. Oral Radiol. Endod. **82**, 57–68 (1996)
54. Kreimer, A., Bhatia, R., Messeguer, A., et al.: Oral human papillomavirus in healthy individuals: a systematic review of the literature. Sex. Transm. Dis. **14**, 2010 (Jan 2010)
55. Jenison, S.A., Yu, X.P., Valentine, J.M., et al.: Evidence of prevalent genital-type human papillomavirus infections in adults and children. Cancer Res. **162**, 60–69 (1990)
56. Koch, A., Hansen, S.V., Nielsen, N.M., et al.: HPV detection in children prior to sexual debut. Int. J. Cancer **73**, 621–624 (1997)
57. Mant, C., Kell, B., Rice, P., et al.: Buccal exposure to human papillomavirus type 16 is a common yet transitory event of childhood. J. Med. Virol. **71**, 593–598 (2003)
58. Rice, P.S., Mant, C., Cason, J., et al.: High prevalence of human papillomavirus type 16 infection among children. J. Med. Virol. **61**, 70–75 (2000)
59. Smith, E.M., Parker, M.A., Rubinstein, L.M. et al.: Evidence of vertical transmission of HPV from mothers to infants. Infect. Dis. Obstet. Gynecol. (2010) [Epub; 14 Mar 2010]
60. Summersgill, K.F., Smith, E.M., Levy, B.T., et al.: Human papillomavirus in the oral cavities of children and adolescents. Oral Surg. Oral Med. Oral Pathol. Oral Radiol. Endod. **91**, 62–69 (2001)
61. Giovannelli, L., Campisi, G., Colella, G., et al.: Brushing of oral mucosa for diagnosis of HPV infection in patients with potentially malignant and malignant oral lesions. Mol. Diagn. Ther. **10**, 49–55 (2006)
62. Kreimer, A., Alberg, A., Daniel, R., et al.: Oral human papillomavirus infection in adults is associated with sexual behaviour and HIV serostatus. J. Infect. Dis. **189**, 686–698 (2004)
63. Morshed, K., Polz-Dacewicz, M., Szyma ski, M., et al.: Short-fragment PCR assay for highly sensitive broad-spectrum detection of human papillomaviruses in laryngeal squamous cell carcinoma and normal mucosa: clinico-pathological evaluation. Eur. Arch. Otorhinolaryngol. **265**(suppl 1), S89–S96 (2008)
64. Kellokoski, J., Syrjänen, S., Yliskoski, M., et al.: Dot blot hybridization in detection of human papillomavirus (HPV) infections in the oral cavity of women with genital HPV infections. Oral Microbiol. Immunol. **7**, 19–23 (1992)
65. Saheb Jamee, M., Boorghani, M., Ghaffari, S.R., et al.: Human papillomavirus in saliva of patients with oral squamous cell carcinoma. Med. Oral Patol. Oral Cir. Bucal. **14**, e525–e528 (2009)
66. D'Souza, G., Sugar, E., Ruby, W., et al.: Analysis of the effect of DNA purification on detection of human papillomavirus in oral rinse samples by PCR. J. Clin. Microbiol. **43**, 5526–5535 (2005)
67. Kay, P., Meehan, K., Williamson, A.L.: The use of nested polymerase chain reaction and restriction fragment length polymorphism for the detection and typing of mucosal human papillomaviruses in samples containing low copy numbers of viral DNA. J. Virol. Meth. **105**, 159–170 (2002)
68. Kurose, K., Terai, M., Soedarsono, N., et al.: Low prevalence of HPV infection and its natural history in normal oral mucosa among volunteers on Miyako Island, Japan. Oral Surg. Oral Med. Oral Pathol. Oral Radiol. Endod. **98**, 91–96 (2004)
69. D'Souza, G., Fakhry, C., Sugar, E.A., et al.: Six month natural history of oral versus cervical human papillomavirus infection. Int. J. Cancer **121**, 143–150 (2007)
70. Kellokoski, J., Syrjänen, S., Kataja, V., et al.: Acetwhite staining and its significance in diagnosis of oral mucosa

lesions in women with genital HPV infections. J. Oral Pathol. Med. **19**, 278–283 (1990)
71. Louvanto, K., Syrjänen, K., Rintala, M. et al.: Human papillomavirus (HPV) and other predictors of incident CIN among young mothers prospectively followed-up for 6 years in the Finnish Family HPV Study. JID. **202**, 436–444 (2010)
72. Sarkola, M., Rintala, M., Grenman, S., et al.: Human papillomavirus DNA detected in breastmilk. Pediatr. Infect. Dis. J. **27**, 557–558 (2008)
73. Sarkola, M.E., Grenman, S.E., Rintala, M.A., et al.: Effect of second pregnancy on maternal carriage and outcome of high-risk human papillomavirus (HPV) Experience from the prospective finnish family HPV study. Gynecol. Obstet. Invest. **67**, 208–216 (2009)
74. Syrjänen, S., Waterboer, T., Sarkola, M., et al.: Dynamics of human papillomavirus serology in women followed up for 36 months after pregnancy. J. Gen. Virol. **90**, 1515–1526 (2009)
75. Leimola-Virtanen, R., Syrjänen, S.: Failure to detect human papillomavirus DNA in oral mucosa of postmenopausal women. Clin. Infect. Dis. **22**, 593–594 (1996)
76. Badaracco, G., Venuti, A., Di Lonardo, A., et al.: Concurrent HPV infection in oral and genital mucosa. J. Oral Pathol. Med. **27**, 130–134 (1998)
77. Terai, M., Hashimoto, K., Sata, T.: High prevalence of human papillomaviruses in the normal oral cavity of adults. Oral Microbiol. Immunol. **14**, 201–205 (1999)
78. Axéll, T.: A prevalence study of oral mucosal lesions in an adult Swedish population. Odontol. Revy Suppl. **36**, 1–103 (1976)
79. Castro, T., Bussoloti Filbo, I.: Prevalence of human papillomavirus (HPV) in oral cavity and oropharynx. Review **72**(2)), 272–282 (Mar–Apr 2006)
80. Chang, F., Syrjänen, S., Kellokoski, J., et al.: Human papillomavirus (HPV) infections and their associations with oral disease. J. Oral Pathol. Med. **20**, 305–317 (1991)
81. Giovannelli, L., Campisi, G., Lama, A., et al.: Human papillomavirus DNA in oral mucosal lesions. J. Infect. Dis. **185**, 833–8336 (2003)
82. Syrjänen, S.: Human papillomavirus infections and oral tumors. Med. Microbiol. Immunol. **192**, 123–128 (2003)
83. Syrjänen, S., Syrjänen, K., Happonen, R., et al.: In situ DNA hybridization analysis of human papillomavirus (HPV) sequences in benign oral mucosal lesions. Arch. Dermatol. Res. **279**, 543–549 (1987)
84. Varnai, A.D., Bollmann, M., Bankfalvi, A., et al.: The prevalence and distribution of human papillomavirus genotypes in oral epithelial hyperplasia: proposal of a concept. J. Oral Pathol. Med. **38**, 181–187 (2009)
85. Syrjänen, S.: HPV infections and tonsillar carcinoma. Clin. Pathol. **57**, 449–455 (2004)
86. Chen, R., Sehr, P., Waterboer, T., et al.: Presence of DNA of human papillmoavirus 16 but no other types in tumor-free tonsillar tissue. J. Clin. Microbiol. **43**, 1408–1410 (2005)
87. Mammas, I.N., Sourvinos, G., Michael, C., et al.: Hyman papillomavirus in hyperplastic tonsillar and adenoid tissues in children. Pediatr. Infect. Dis. **25**, 1158–1162 (2006)
88. Ribeiro, K.M.Z., Alvez, J.M., Pignatari, S.S.N., et al.: Detection of human papillomavirus in the tonsils of children undergoing tonsillectomy Barazilian. J. Infect. Dis. **10**, 165–168 (2006)
89. Sisk, J., Schweinfurth, J.M., Wang, X.T., et al.: Presence of human papillomavirus DNA in tonsillectomy specimens. Laryngoscope **116**, 1372–1374 (2006)
90. do Sacramento, P.R., Babeto, E., Colombo, J., et al.: The prevalence of human papillomavirus in the oropharynx in healthy individuals in a Brazilian population. J. Med. Virol. **78**, 614–618 (2006)
91. Brandsma, J.L., Abramson, A.L.: Association of papillomavirus with cancer of the head and neck. Arch. Otolaryngol. Head Neck Surg. **115**, 621–625 (1989)
92. Nunez, D.A., Astley, S.M., Lewis, F.A., et al.: Human papilloma viruses: a study of their prevalence in the normal larynx. J. Laryngol. Otol. **108**, 319–320 (1994)
93. Derkay, C., Watrak, B.: Recurrent respiratory papillomatosis: review. Laryngoscope **118**, 1236–1247 (2008)
94. Gallager, T.Q., Derkay, C.S.: Pharmacotherapy of recurrent respiratory papillomatosis: an expert opinion. Expert Opin. Pharmacother. **10**, 645–655 (2009)
95. Abramson, A.L., Steinberg, B.M., Winkler, B.: Laryngeal papillomatosis: clinical, histopathologic and molecular studies. Laryngoscope **97**, 678–685 (1987)
96. Bomholt, A.: Juvenile laryngeal papillomatosis: an epidemiological study from the Copenhagen region. Acta Otolaryngol. **105**, 367–371 (1988)
97. Mahnke, C.G., Frohlich, O., Lippert, B.M., et al.: Recurrent laryngeal papillomatosis. Retrospective analysis of 95 patients and review of the literature. Otolaryngol. Pol. **50**, 567–578 (1996)
98. Lindeberg, H., Elbrond, O.: Malignant tumours in patients with a history of multiple laryngeal papillomas: the significance of irradiation. Clin. Otolaryngol. **16**, 149–151 (1991)
99. Armstrong, L.R., Preston, E.J., Reichert, M., et al.: Incidence and prevalence of recurrent respiratory papillomatosis among children in Atlanta and Seattle. Clin. Infect. Dis. **31**, 107–109 (2000)
100. Mounts, P., Shah, K.V., Kashima, H.: Viral etiology of juvenile and adult onset squamous papilloma of the larynx. Proc. Natl. Acad. Sci. USA **79**, 5425–5429 (1982)
101. Wiatrak, B.J., Wiatrak, D.W., Broker, T., et al.: Recurrent Respiratory papillomas: a longitudinal study comparing severity associated with human papilloma viral types 6 and 11 and other risk factors in a large pediatric population. Laryngoscope **114**, 1–23 (2004)
102. Rihkanen, H., Peltomaa, J., Syrjänen, S.: Prevalence of human papillomavirus (HPV) DNA in vocal cords without laryngeal papillomas. Acta Otolaryngol. **114**, 348–351 (1994)
103. Cook, A., Cohn, A.M., Brunschwig, J.P., et al.: Wart viruses and laryngeal papillomas. Lancet **1**, 782 (1973)
104. Hallden, C., Majmudar, B.: The relationship between juvenile laryngeal papillomatosis and maternal condylomata acuminata. J. Reprod. Med. **31**, 804–807 (1986)
105. Quick, C.A., Krzyzek, R.A., Watts, S.L., et al.: Relationship between condylomata and laryngeal papillomata clinical and molecular virological evidence. Ann. Otol. **89**, 467–471 (1980)
106. Shah, K., Kashima, H., Polk, B.F., et al.: Rarity of cesarean delivery in cases of juvenile-onset respiratory papillomatosis. Obstet. Gynecol. **68**, 795–799 (1986)
107. Silverberg, M.J., Thorsen, P., Lindeberg, H., et al.: Condyloma in pregnancy is strongly predictive of juvenile-onset recurrent respiratory papillomatosis. Obstet. Gynecol. **101**, 645–652 (2003)
108. Shah, K.V., Stern, W.F., Shah, F.K., et al.: Risk factors for juvenile onset recurrent respiratory papillomatosis. Pediatr. Infect. Dis. J. **17**, 372–376 (1998)

109. Gelder, C.M., Williams, O.M., Hart, K.W., et al.: HLA Class II polymorphisms and susceptibility to recurrent respiratory papillomatosis. J. Virol. **77**, 1927–1239 (2003)
110. Stern, Y., Felipovich, A., Cotton, R., et al.: Immunocomptency in children with recurrent respiratory papillomatosis: prospective study. Ann. Otol. Rhinol. Laryngol. **116**, 169–171 (2007)
111. Lindeberg, H., Syrjänen, S., Kärjä, J., et al.: Human papillomavirus type 11 DNA in squamous cell carcinomas and pre-existing multiple laryngeal papillomas. Acta Otolaryngol. **107**, 141–149 (1989)
112. Zarod, A.P., et al.: Malignant progression of laryngeal papilloma associated with HPV 6 DNA. J. Clin. Pathol. **41**, 280–283 (1988)
113. Poljak, M., Gale, N., Kambic, V.: Human papillomaviruses: a study of their prevalence in the epithelial hyperplastic lesions of the larynx. Acta Otolaryngol. Suppl. **527**, 66–69 (1997)
114. Syrjänen, K.J.: HPV infections in benign and malignant sinonasal lesions. J. Clin. Pathol. **56**(3), 174–181 (2003)
115. Syrjänen, K., Syrjänen, S., Lamberg, M., et al.: Morphological and immunohistochemical evidence suggesting human papillomavirus (HPV) involvement in oral squamous cell carcinogenesis. Int. J. Oral Surg. **12**, 418–424 (1983)
116. Campisi, G., Panzarella, V., Giuliani, M., et al.: Human papillomavirus: Its identity and controversial role in oral oncogenesis, premalignant and malignant lesions (Review). Int. J. Oncol. **30**, 813–823 (2007)
117. Chaudhary, A., Singh, M., Sundaram, S., et al.: Role of human papillomavirus and its detection in potentially malignant and malignant head and neck lesions: updated review. Head Neck Oncol. **1**, 22 (Jun 2009)
118. Hansson, B., Rosenqvist, K., Antonsson, A., et al.: Strong association between infection with human papillomavirus and oral and oropharyngeal squamous cell carcinoma: a population-based case-control study in southern Sweden. Acta Otolaryngol. **125**, 1337–1344 (2005)
119. Hennessey, P.T., Westra, W.H., Califano, J.A.: Human papillomavirus and head and neck squamous cell carcinoma: recent evidence and clinical implications. J. Dent. Res. **88**, 300–306 (2009)
120. Herrero, R., Castellangue, X., Pawlita, M., et al.: Human papillomavirus and oral cancer: the international Agency for Research on cancer Multicenter Study. J. Natl. Cancer Int. **95**, 1772–1783 (2003)
121. Kreimer, A., Clifford, G., Boyle, P., et al.: Human papillomavirus types in head and neck squamous cell carcinomas worldwide: a systematic review. Cancer Epidemiol. Biomarkers Prev. **14**, 467–475 (2005)
122. Maden, C., Beckmann, A.M., Thomas, D.B., et al.: Human papillomaviruses, herpes simplex viruses, and the risk of oral cancer in men. Am. J. Epidemiol. **135**, 1093–1102 (1992)
123. Schwartz, S.M., Daling, J.R., Doody, D.R., et al.: Oral cancer risk in relation to sexual history and evidence of human papillomavirus infection. J. Natl. Cancer Inst. **90**, 1626–1636 (1998)
124. Smith, E., Hoffman, H., Summersgill, K., et al.: Human papillomavirus and risk of oral cancer. Laryngoscope **108**, 1098–1103 (1998)
125. Smith, E.M., Ritchie, J.M., Summersgill, K.F., et al.: Human papillomavirus in oral exfoliated cells and risk of head and neck cancer. J. Natl. Cancer Inst. **96**, 449–455 (2004)
126. Termine, N., Panzarella, V., Falaschini, S., et al.: HPV in oral squamous cell carcinoma vs head and neck squamous cell carcinoma biopsies: a meta-analysis (1988–2007). Ann. Oncol. **19**, 1681–1690 (2008)
127. Vidal, L., Gillison, M.: Human papillomavirus in HNSCC: recognition of a distinct disease type. Hematol. Oncol. Clin. N. Am. **22**, 1125–1142 (2008)
128. Campisi, G., Giovannelli, L.: Controversies surrounding human papilloma virus infection, head & neck vs oral cancer, implications for prophylaxis and treatment. Head Neck Oncology **1**, 8 (2009)
129. Schmitt, M., Bravo, I., Snijders, P., et al.: Bead-based multiplex genotyping of human papillomaviruses. J. Clin. Microbiol. **44**, 504–512 (2006)
130. Attner, P., Du, J., Näsman, A., et al.: The role of human papillomavirus in the increased incidence of base of tongue cancer. Int. J. Cancer **126**, 2879–2884 (2010)
131. Chaturvedi, A.K., Engels, E.A., Anderson, W.F., et al.: Incidence trends for human papillomavirus-related and -unrelated oral squamous cell carcinomas in the United States. J. Clin. Oncol. **26**, 612–619 (2008)
132. Hammarstedt, L., Lindquist, D., Dahlstrand, H., et al.: Human papillomavirus as a risk factor for the increase in incidence of tonsillar cancer. Int. J. Cancer **119**, 2620–2623 (2006)
133. Syrjänen, K., Syrjänen, S., Pyrhönen, S.: Human papilloma virus (HPV) antigens in lesions of laryngeal squamous cell carcinomas. ORL J. Otorhinolaryngol. Relat. Spec. **44**, 323–334 (1982)
134. Heck, J.E., Berthiller, J., Vaccarella, S., et al.: Sexual behaviours and the risk of head and neck cancers: a pooled analysis in the International Head and Neck Cancer Epidemiology (INHANCE) consortium. Int. J. Epidemiol. **39**, 166–181 (2009)
135. D'Souza, G., Kreimer, A.R., Viscidi, R., et al.: Case control study of human papillomavirus and oropharyngeal cancer. N. Engl. J. Med. **356**, 1944–1956 (2007)
136. Flohr, J., Lee, J.: Identical but different: mechanism of cancer development and response to treatment for human papillomavirus-related and non-related squamous cell cancer of the head and neck. S D Med **61**, 453–455 (2008)
137. Machado, J., Reis, P.P., Zhang, T., et al.: Low prevalence of Human Papillomavirus in oral cavity carcinomas. Head Neck Oncol. **2**, 6 (2010)
138. Santoro, V., Pozzuoli, M., Colella, G.: Role of human papilloma virus in precancerous and cancerous lesions of the oral cavity Review of the literature. Minerva Stomatol. **46**, 595–601 (1997)
139. Smith, E., Johnson, S., Jiang, D., et al.: The association between pregnancy and human papilloma virus prevalence. Cancer Detect. Prev. **15**, 397–402 (1991)
140. Syrjänen, K.J.: Annual disease burden due to human papillomavirus (HPV) 6 and 11 infections in Finland. Scand. J. Infect. Dis. Suppl. **107**, 3–32 (2009)
141. Syrjänen, S.: Human papillomavirus (HPV) in head and neck cancer. J. Clin. Virol. **32**, 59–66 (2005)

Laboratory Diagnosis of HPV and its Clinical Use

40

Hans Ikenberg

Core Messages

› Molecular HPV diagnostics (which means in the following always testing for high-risk HPVs) detects CIN 2+ in up to 99% compared to on average 50% for cytology in a first approach and it has the potential to predict the risk of developing CIN 2+ in the future.
› However the higher clinical sensitivity leads to a lower specificity.
› There are three main fields where HPV diagnostics is already in routine use: 1) triage of cytological borderline abnormalities 2) follow-up of patients after therapy of CIN as a test of cure 3) as an adjunct to conventional and thin-layer cytology (in women above 30 years).
› All these indications have been validated in a number of high-quality trials and are recommended by US and European guidelines.
› Meanwhile also the substitution of cytology as primary screening instrument by HPV testing is discussed.
› The balance between analytical (low) and clinical (high) sensitivity is crucial for the specificity of a routine HPV test especially in a screening approach.
› That is the reason why the hc2 test which hybridizes 13 (near) full-length stabilized RNA probes of high-risk HPV types to denatured HPV target DNA followed by detection via antibodies and chemiluminescence is still regarded as the gold standard in routine diagnostics.
› New tests for routine HPV testing must pass extensive clinical studies in screening settings in different populations. Meanwhile standards for such evaluations have been defined by leading experts on the field. Recently several new HPV detection assays have been commercialized. They all show promising data in first published studies but still await full validation according to the criteria mentioned above.
› HPV 16 and 18 confer a much higher risk for development of a CIN 2+ compared to the other HPV high risk types. It is therefore appropriate to test for these HPV types independently after a positive HPV high risk basic test.
› Apart from that testing for individual HPV types is of very limited clinical value up to now.
› HPV testing before vaccination is at present regarded by the majority of experts and major guidelines not as helpful.
› HPV RNA testing is an interesting option. Its clinical value still needs to be confirmed in adequate studies.

40.1 Laboratory

While HPV diagnostics may become of relevance also for detection or triaging of oral and larnygeal/pharyngeal [1] as well as anal [2] neoplasias, up to now it is mainly used in the diagnosis of cervical (pre)cancerous lesions.

H. Ikenberg
Bernerstr. 76, D-60437, Frankfurt, Germany
e-mail: hikenberg@gmx.de, hans.ikenberg@cytomol.de

G. Gross and S.K. Tyring (eds.), *Sexually Transmitted Infections and Sexually Transmitted Diseases*,
DOI: 10.1007/978-3-642-14663-3_40, © Springer-Verlag Berlin Heidelberg 2011

Compared with morphologic techniques (i.e., mainly cytology) which fail to detect clinically relevant cervical disease (i.e., CIN 2+) in a first approach, on average in 50% of the cases [3] molecular HPV diagnostics is able to achieve this goal in up to 99%. Probably this is mainly due to the "descending" of viral genetic material in the cervical canal which leads to the detection of lesions also in cases where no or insufficient material for cytological analysis is available. And unlike morphology, HPV testing has the potential to predict the risk of developing CIN 2+ in the future. Except in some special situations, meanwhile, only HPV high-risk testing is regarded of clinical value. In the following, HPV testing, therefore, means identification of HPV high-risk types.

There are *three main fields* where HPV diagnostics has become a routine tool within the last 10 years. First, mainly after the seminal results of the ALTS study [4] triage of cytologically borderline [5, 6] or low-grade [7, 8] abnormalities became a validated indication, thereafter recommended by US and European guidelines. Subsequently, HPV testing proved to be superior to cytology in the follow-up of patients after therapy of CIN as a test of cure [9, 10]. Finally, the use of HPV testing as an adjunct to conventional and thin-layer cytology was shown to be effective in a number of high-quality trials [7, 11–15]. This again led to recommendations in major guidelines [5, 16]. Meanwhile, the substitution of cytology as primary screening instrument by HPV testing is discussed and yet examined in scientific studies [17]. Because adenocarcinomas of the cervix are almost as closely associated with HPV as squamous carcinomas, HPV testing is an equally valuable tool for their prevention [18].

In contrast to other viral pathogens with HPV the detection of the virus is not necessarily indicative of the disease resulting from the infection. A certain amount of virus has to be present for a certain time in order to induce cervical neoplasia [19–22]. This means that transient infections with HPV and low amounts of virus are clinically irrelevant. For routine use this again requires a (clinically defined) cutoff value of a detection system to avoid nonrelevant HPV positivities which might cause unnecessary further diagnostic procedures and treatments.

As to the *methods of HPV detection*, in situ hybridization has some scientific interest due to its ability to locate the viral DNA in specific cellular structures; however, its low sensitivity and lacking suitability for high-throughput exclude a use in routine diagnostics [23]. Only a limited number of individuals DNA-positive for HPV, but also with CIN and even with invasive HPV-induced disease show a seroconversion to HPV antigens [24]. This is due to the superficiality of the infection and the scanty expression of HPV oncogenes even in carcinomas. This precludes any routine diagnostic use of HPV protein detection or serology tests. Against this background, two main groups of HPV assays are currently available for clinical applications. First, PCR techniques which can be divided into type-specific and consensus (general primer) PCRs, and second, a signal amplification technology (hc2 test, Qiagen, Gaithersburg, MD).

Several *PCRs* for HPV detection are commercially available. The most widely distributed is the Amplicor assay, a consensus PCR which covers 13 HPV high-risk types, and the linear array assay as a type-specific method detecting 37 high- and low-risk types (both Roche Molecular Diagnostics, Pleasanton, CA), followed by the SPF10 assay [25] (Immogenetics, Gent, Belgium). The most common PCR techniques for scientific applications are the GP5+/6+ [26] and the PGMY [27] general primer sets. They all target the L1 region of the HPV genome with resulting amplicons from 65 bp to 450 bp length. Enzyme immunoassays or reverse line blot assays are used as detection systems. The analytical sensitivity varies from less than 10 copies with SPF10 primers with purified DNA to around 1,000 copies with the GP5+/6+ primers in crude extracts [20].

Numerous commercial labs have made up their own PCRs, which are at best internally validated, generally have not been investigated in scientific studies, and are for these reasons, less suitable for clinical use.

The analytical sensitivity of PCR can go down to some copies of HPV DNA. Surprisingly, that is not reflected in a similar clinical sensitivity. Only a few larger studies showed an ability to identify more than 95% of CIN 2+ lesions and the median sensitivity of HPV PCR was reported to be 82% in 16 papers [28]. This can be explained by several factors. Primers usually targeting the L1 region of the HPV genome may lack to bind in up to 7% of high-grade lesions and cancers that have lost this region [29, 30]. Other reasons are random partial inhibition (which is not necessarily indicated by internal controls) and competition effects if several HPV types are present [31]. One problem with consensus HPV PCRs is the difficulty to obtain an equal and regular level of detection of different HPV types as shown by the range of sensitivity of the GP5+/6+ assay between 10 and 200 copies depending on the HPV type [26]. Another challenge is the adjustment of a reliable cutoff, which is even a major point in ultra-sensitive type-specific PCRs.

The *hc2 test* hybridizes 13 (near) full-length stabilized RNA probes of high-risk HPV types to denatured HPV target DNA followed by detection via antibodies and chemiluminescence. The threshold value of the system is 1 pg/mL which corresponds to around 5,000 copies of HPV DNA per test [28]. It is very robust in the pre-analytical phase, has a simple sample preparation and requires no separate rooms for different work steps.

The inter-laboratory variation of the hc2 test is very low [32] and its results are highly reproducible [33]. Respective data on PCR are less consistent [34, 35]. One theoretical drawback of the hc2 test is the lack of a control for the presence of human cellular material. In routine this seems to be of minor importance regarding the 99% sensitivity for CIN 2+ measured on a histology gold standard, which may be reached by the method [36, 37]. Additionally, risk estimates were hardly affected by adjusting for the amount of a housekeeping gene in a PCR system [21]. Another potential problem may be a cross-reaction with a couple of low risk HPV types. However, because some of them are regarded in fact as being of intermediate risk, finally this may even contribute to the high clinical sensitivity of the test [38]. While it is an advantage of the hc2 test that its use out of the vial of the ThinPrep™ thin-layer cytology has been approved as the only HPV test by the FDA, there are hints that the performance of the system under these conditions (which requires an elaborate transformation process) is somewhat poorer than from the standard medium [39].

The clinical sensitivity of the hc2 test is very high; in 26 trials worldwide its median was 94% [28]. More than 200,000 women have been included in screening studies with this assay published in peer-reviewed journal papers, a number which exceeds by far the data available for any single PCR method. Significant differences in performance were observed between HPV screening studies conducted in Europe and Northern America reaching up to 99% sensitivity and investigations performed in developing countries. Here regularly, the sensitivity was 20–30% lower, which might be explained by weaknesses of regional colposcopy and histology leading to deficits in gold standard definition [40, 41]. Though in "real life" the clinical sensitivity even under optimized conditions will not exceed 95–98% due to sampling errors or minor technical variations [28, 42].

An important aspect of HPV diagnostics is its ability to deliver negative results. This means that in case of a negative HPV test there is a near-zero risk for prevalent or incident cervical (pre) neoplasia for at least 3 years, the negative predictive value is 100% [7]. This is the base for lengthening the interval of cervical prevention exams without risk.

The major problem of HPV diagnostics is its relatively low *specificity* which is limited even with non-DNA-amplifying methods. This restricts its use in a screening approach to women over 30 years [5, 16]. Below this age, testing is regarded as useful in case of cytological and/or colposcopic abnormality (triage) and after therapy of CIN as a test of cure [5, 6]. But even in this triage setting the revised ASCCP guidelines in the US discourage HPV testing in the below 20s due to very high remission rates in this age group [8]. In general, HPV testing up to now is the more useful, i.e., predictive, the older the tested women are. If, however, the right test is used in the right age group, screening by HPV-DNA testing may already now reach the specificity of cytology as demonstrated by 5 of 26 studies reviewed in an HTA [43].

The specificity can be increased by further increasing the viral load cutoff. This can be achieved more easily with the hc2 than with PCR. Studies show a slightly lower [28] or an unchanged [44] sensitivity, while in either case, the specificity was raised.

In this context, a central point if HPV testing is used as an adjunct to cytological screening is the rate of women positive for high-risk HPV in the absence of cytological abnormalities. In the age group over 30 years usually this is very low. Among more than 800,000 tests in nearly 600,000 women in California tested with the hc2 system it was 3.99% with only about one-third of them remaining positive over 1 year, thus leaving less than 1.5% for colposcopy [45, 46]. An even lower rate (1.9%) was observed among cytologically normal women screened with thin-layer cytology and computer assistance [47]. That means that with even an ASCUS rate of just 3% (where at maximum half of the cases will be HPV-positive) the total number of women scheduled for colposcopy will not increase, whereas this group now comprises also all cytologically false-negatives.

The crucial criterion for the clinical value of a routine HPV test is not its analytical but its *clinical sensitivity*. The observance of a well-defined threshold must be guaranteed. Up to now this has only been proven in large-scale studies for the hc2 test. For several reasons as stated above this objective is rather complicated to achieve for PCR techniques. Beside the fact that it covers the L1 as well as the E6/7 regions of the HPV genome that point has led to the hc2 tests superior performance in a great number of studies. Therefore, up to now only the hc2 test and recently another signal-amplifying technique, the Cervista test [48] have received an approval by the FDA. Meanwhile, some more recent studies found a comparable sensitivity and specificity for hc2 and several PCRs for the detection of CIN 2+ in triage [49, 50] and screening [51] settings. However, it remains very important that considering the complexity of HPV natural history and carcinogenesis, it is indispensable that new tests for routine HPV testing must pass extensive clinical studies in screening settings in different populations. Meanwhile standards for such evaluation have been defined by leading experts on the field [52].

Recently several new HPV detection assays have been commercialized. Among them are PCR DNA assays like the Abbott Real Time High Risk HPV Test (Abbott Molecular, Wiesbaden, Germany) [53] which detects 14 HR HPV types as a group-specific test (and separately HPV 16 and 18) and a DNA chip approach for the type-specific detection of 18 high-risk and 6 low-risk HPV types (Papillocheck, greiner bio-one, Frickenhausen, Germany) [54] . Further a signal amplification test (Cervista, Hologic, Marlborough, MA) [48] which detects 14 HR HPV types as a group and in addition HPV 16 and 18 as well as a new HPV mRNA test, the APTIMA HPV test (Genprobe, San Diego, CA) which detects 14 HR HPV types as a group [55] all show promising data in first published studies but still await full validation according to the criteria mentioned above [52] .

Even though the importance of a minimal viral load for the development of HPV-induced disease is obvious, there seems to be no clear-cut association between *quantitative* (real-time PCR) or semi-quantitative (hc2) measurements of viral load and prognostic potential at a level above the detection limit of the hc2 test [20, 56, 57].

Several studies showed a significantly higher risk for development of a CIN 2+ among women positive for *HPV 16, 18, and 45* (which is closely related to HPV18) compared to positivity for other HPV high-risk types. This was valid for cytologically normal women [58] as well as in patients with borderline cytologic findings [59]. It is therefore appropriate to test for these HPV types independently. This makes only sense after a positive HPV high-risk basic test because clinically not irrelevant cases positive for high-risk types beside 16, 18, and 45 would otherwise be missed.

It is generally accepted that a diagnosis of *individual HPV types* is of great scientific importance but its clinical value is rather limited up to now. First, the risk potential of other HPV types than 16, 18, and 45 is not well-defined and seems to be rather equal, and second, even if this potential would be better defined it might be very difficult to implement the routine application of complicated "type-specific" algorithms. Even at present the follow-up in case of HPV positivity (which has for a clinical approach always to be assessed together with cytology results and age of a woman) is a rather difficult task in clinical practice. Another problem with routine HPV typing is the high analytical sensitivity and consecutively lower specificity when using the only, therefore, available PCR assays. A detection of HPV 16, 18, and 45 can be achieved by a variant of the hc2 test with the same cutoff as the basic test which is currently under FDA review. In the future type-specific testing may become more important with systems which have a defined and equal cutoff level for different HPV types.

HPV testing before vaccination seems an interesting option because HPV DNA positivity for a vaccine type is associated with low efficiency of the vaccination but is at present regarded by the majority of experts and major guidelines [60, 61] not as helpful. This is due to several factors. First, there is no HPV test commercially available which is sufficiently validated for this purpose as to cutoff and specificity. Second, only rarely more than one HPV type persists, extremely rarely more than two, which still leaves vaccination meaningful in most cases of HPV positivity. Third the irritation potential due to a high rate of (mostly not persistent) HPV positivity among younger women and finally the high costs of routine testing before vaccination which would not be equalized by respective savings.

Self-collection of samples seems to be an interesting option in HPV diagnostics. Unlike with cytology, concordance of the results with smears taken by experts reaches up to 90% [62–64]. Offering self-sampling for HPV testing in nonresponders to cervical screening programs is an attractive possibility to increase population coverage [65].

A logical approach to overcome some limitations in HPV diagnostics is testing for *HPV RNA*. Due to non-transforming activities of HPV oncogenes and subsequent transcription also in non-neoplastic lesions or instability of RNA HPV RNA analytics turned out to be more tricky than initially expected. First promising results [66, 67] of a commercial assay (pretectproofer™, norchip, Klokkarstua/Norway now Nuclisens™, Biomerieux, Marcy L'Étoile/France) could not be confirmed. In a publication of intermediate results from the PREDICTORS study [68] the sensitivity of this test for CIN 2+ was only 73%. This was amongst other reasons probably due to the fact that the system targets only five HPV types. However, it is not finally cleared whether lacking HPV mRNA expression might also indicate high-grade disease without the potential for progression. A new HPV-RNA detection system has recently been presented by Genprobe (San Diego, CA). First data point to a similar sensitivity and a slightly higher specificity of the APTIMA™ test as for DNA detection assays [68, 69]. A promising aspect of the system is that it requires no RNA isolation and can be performed in sealed vials.

Although there is a close association between HPV and male precancerous genital lesions up to now the majority of experts do not recommend routine use of HPV diagnostics in *men*. This is due to an on average 30 times lower incidence of HPV-associated disease, a lack of standardization in smear taking and testing in men, but also to a deficiency of clinical examination and follow-up in HPV-positive men, which might result in inadequate diagnostic and therapeutic procedures [70]. Equally, at present any kind of HPV diagnostics in male partners of women with HPV positivity or HPV-associated lesions is regarded as inappropriate (except clinical examination in case of condylomata acuminata).

Take-Home Pearls

- Molecular HPV diagnostics detects significantly more CIN 2+ than cytology.
- Equally valuable for the prevention of adenocarcinoma of the cervix.
- Molecular HPV diagnostics has the potential to predict the risk of future CIN 2+.
- Its higher clinical sensitivity leads to a lower specificity compared with cytology.
- Routine use of HPV diagnostics is established for triage of borderline cytology, follow-up after therapy of CIN and as an adjunct to cytology in women above 30 years.
- Primary screening by HPV testing is intensively discussed.
- Low analytical and high clinical sensitivity are important in routine HPV testing.
- Still the hc2 test is regarded as the gold standard in routine diagnostics.
- Extensive clinical studies are mandatory for new HPV tests.
- Standards for such evaluations have been defined by leading experts on the field.
- Several new HPV detection assays showed promising data in first studies.
- HPV 16 and 18 are the highest risk types.
- Only testing for those individual HPV types is of clinical value up to now.
- HPV testing before vaccination is at present not helpful.
- Self collection of samples for HPV testing is an interesting option.
- HPV RNA testing is an interesting option.
- HPV testing is men and in male partners is not recommended up to now.

References

1. D'Souza, G., Kreimer, A.R., Viscidi, R., et al.: Case-control study of human papillomavirus and oropharyngeal cancer. N. Engl. J. Med. **356**, 1944–1956 (2007)
2. Frisch, M., Glimelius, B., van den Brule, A.J., et al.: Sexually transmitted infection as a cause of anal cancer. N. Engl. J. Med. **337**, 1350–1358 (1997)

3. McCrory, D., Matchar, D., Bastian, L. et al.: Evaluation of cervical cytology. Evidence report/Technology assessment No. 5. AHCPR Publication No. 99-E010. Agency for Health Care Policy and Research, Rockville (1999)
4. Solomon, D., Schiffman, M., Tarone, R., ALTS Study group: Comparison of three management strategies for patients with atypical squamous cells of undetermined significance: baseline results from a randomized trial. J. Natl. Cancer Inst. **93**, 293–299 (2001)
5. Friese, K., Sitter, H., Anton, G., et al.: Interdisziplinäre S2k leitlinie: prävention, diagnostik und therapie der HPV-infektion und präinvasiver Läsionen des weibliche Genitale. Kramarz, Berlin (2008)
6. Wright Jr., T.C., Cox, J.T., Massad, L.S., et al.: ASCCP-Sponsored Consensus Conference. 2001 Consensus Guidelines for the management of women with cervical cytological abnormalities. JAMA **287**, 2120–2129 (2002)
7. Petry, K.-U., Menton, S., Menton, M., et al.: Inclusion of HPV testing in routine cervical cancer screening for women above 29 years in Germany: results for 8,468 patients. Br. J. Cancer **88**, 1570–1577 (2003)
8. Wright Jr., T.C., Massad, L.S., Dunton, C.J., et al.: 2006 consensus guidelines for the management of women with abnormal cervical cancer screening tests. Am. J. Obstet. Gynecol. **197**, 346–355 (2007)
9. Paraskevaidis, E., Arbyn, M., Sotiriadis, A., et al.: The role of HPV DNA testing in the follow-up period after treatment for CIN: a systematic review of the literature. Cancer Treat. Rev. **30**, 205–211 (2004)
10. Zielinski, G., Bais, A., Helmerhorst, T., et al.: HPV testing and monitoring of women after treatment of CIN 3: review of the literature and meta-analysis. Obstet. Gynecol. Surv. **59**, 543–553 (2004)
11. Bulkmans, N.W., Berkhof, J., Rozendaal, L., et al.: Human papillomavirus DNA testing for the detection of cervical intraepithelial neoplasia grade 3 and cancer: 5-year follow-up of a randomised controlled implementation trial. Lancet **370**, 1764–1772 (2007). Epub 4 Oct 2007
12. Kjaer, S.K., van den Brule, A.J., Paull, G., et al.: Type specific persistence of high risk human papillomavirus (HPV) as an indicator of high grade cervical squamous intraepithelial lesions in young women: population based prospective follow up study. BMJ **325**, 572–578 (2002)
13. Mayrand, M.H., Duarte-Franco, E., Rodrigues, I., et al.: Human papillomavirus DNA versus Papanicolaou screening tests for cervical cancer. N. Engl. J. Med. **357**, 1579–1588 (2007)
14. Naucler, P., Ryd, W., Törnberg, S., et al.: Human papillomavirus and Papanicolaou tests to screen for cervical cancer. N. Engl. J. Med. **357**, 1589–1597 (2007)
15. Ratnam, S., Franco, E.L., Ferenczy, A.: Human papillomavirus testing for primary screening of cervical cancer precursors. Cancer Epidemiol. Biomarkers Prev. **9**, 945–951 (2000)
16. Saslow, D., Runowicz, C.D., Solomon, D., et al.: American Cancer Society guideline for the early detection of cervical neoplasia and cancer. CA Cancer J. Clin. **52**, 342–362 (2002)
17. Luyten, A., Scherbring, S., Reinecke-Lüthge, A., et al.: Risk-adapted primary HPV cervical cancer screening project in Wolfsburg, Germany – experience over 3 years. J. Clin. Virol. **46** (Suppl 3), S5–S10 (2009)
18. Castellsagué, X., Díaz, M., de Sanjosé, S., et al.: Worldwide human papillomavirus etiology of cervical adenocarcinoma and its cofactors: implications for screening and prevention. J. Natl. Cancer Inst. **98**, 303–315 (2006)
19. Josefsson, A.M., Magnusson, P.K., Ylitalo, N., et al.: Viral load of human papilloma virus 16 as a determinant for development of cervical carcinoma in situ: a nested case-control study. Lancet **355**, 2189–2193 (2000)
20. Snijders, P.J., van den Brule, A.J., Meijer, C.J.: The clinical relevance of human papillomavirus testing: relationship between analytical and clinical sensitivity. J. Pathol. **201**, 1–6 (2003)
21. van Duin, M., Snijders, P.J., Schrijnemakers, H.F., et al.: Human papillomavirus 16 load in normal and abnormal cervical scrapes: an indicator of CIN II/III and viral clearance. Int. J. Cancer **98**, 590–595 (2002)
22. Ylitalo, N., Sørensen, P., Josefsson, A.M., et al.: Consistent high viral load of human papillomavirus 16 and risk of cervical carcinoma in situ: a nested case-control study. Lancet **355**, 2194–2198 (2000)
23. Hesselink, A.T., van den Brule, A.J., Brink, A.A., et al.: Comparison of hybrid capture 2 with in situ hybridization for the detection of high-risk human papillomavirus in liquid-based cervical samples. Cancer **102**, 11–18 (2004)
24. Wang, S.S., Schiffman, M., Shields, T.S., et al.: Seroprevalence of human papillomavirus-16, -18, -31, and -45 in a population-based cohort of 10,000 women in Costa Rica. Br. J. Cancer **89**, 1248–1254 (2003)
25. Kleter, B., van Doorn, L.J., Schrauwen, L., et al.: Development and clinical evaluation of a highly sensitive PCR-reverse hybridization line probe assay for detection and identification of anogenital human papillomavirus. J. Clin. Microbiol. **37**, 2508–2517 (1999)
26. Jacobs, M.V., Snijders, P.J., van den Brule, A.J., et al.: A general primer GP5+/GP6(+)-mediated PCR-enzyme immunoassay method for rapid detection of 14 high-risk and 6 low-risk human papillomavirus genotypes in cervical scrapings. J. Clin. Microbiol. **35**, 791–795 (1997)
27. Gravitt, P.E., Peyton, C.L., Alessi, T.Q., et al.: Improved amplification of genital human papillomaviruses. J. Clin. Microbiol. **38**, 357–361 (2000)
28. Lorincz, A.T., Smith, J.S.: Sexually transmissible viral pathogens: Human papillomaviruses and herpes simplex viruses. In: Lorincz, A.T., Smith, J.S. (eds.) Nucleic acid testing for human disease, pp. 244–273. Taylor & Francis, CRC Press, London (2006)
29. Karlsen, F., Kalantari, M., Jenkins, A., et al.: Use of multiple PCR primer sets for optimal detection of human papillomavirus. J. Clin. Microbiol. **34**, 2095–2100 (1996)
30. Morris, B.J.: Cervical human papillomavirus screening by PCR: advantages of targeting the E6/E7 region. Clin. Chem. Lab. Med. **43**, 1171–1177 (2005)
31. Qu, W., Jiang, G., Cruz, Y., et al.: PCR detection of human papillomavirus: comparison between MY09/MY11 and GP5+/GP6+ primer systems. J. Clin. Microbiol. **35**, 1304–1310 (1997)
32. Castle, P.E., Wheeler, C.M., Soloman, D., et al.: Interlaboratory reliability of hybrid capture 2. Am. J. Pathol. **122**, 238–245 (2004)
33. Castle, P.E., Lorincz, A.T., Mielzynska-Lohnas, I., et al.: Results of human papillomavirus DNA testing with the

hybrid capture 2 assay are reproducible. J. Clin. Microbiol. **40**, 1088–1090 (2002a)

34. Kornegay, J.R., Roger, M., Davies, P.O., et al.: International proficiency study of a consensus L1 PCR assay for the detection and typing of human papillomavirus DNA: evaluation of accuracy and intralaboratory and interlaboratory agreement. J. Clin. Microbiol. **41**, 1080–1086 (2003)
35. Quint, W.G., Pagliusi, S.R., Lelie, N., et al.: Results of the first World Health Organization international collaborative study of detection of human papillomavirus DNA. J. Clin. Microbiol. **44**, 571–579 (2006)
36. Böhmer, G., van den Brule, A.J., Brummer, O., et al.: No confirmed case of human papillomavirus DNA-negative cervical intraepithelial neoplasia grade 3 or invasive primary cancer of the uterine cervix among 511 patients. Am. J. Obstet. Gynecol. **189**, 118–120 (2003)
37. Castle, P.E., Cox, J.T., Jeronimo, J., et al.: An analysis of high-risk human papillomavirus DNA-negative cervical precancers in the ASCUS-LSIL Triage Study (ALTS). Obstet. Gynecol. **111**, 847–856 (2008)
38. Castle, P.E., Schiffman, M., Burk, R.D., et al.: Restricted cross-reactivity of hybrid capture 2 with nononcogenic human papillomavirus types. Cancer Epidemiol. Biomarkers Prev. **11**, 1394–1399 (2002b)
39. Carozzi, F.M., Del Mistro, A., Confortini, M., et al.: Reproducibility of HPV DNA Testing by Hybrid Capture 2 in a Screening Setting. Am. J. Clin. Pathol. **124**, 716–721 (2005)
40. Sankaranarayanan, R., Chatterji, R., Shastri, S.S., et al.: Accuracy of human papillomavirus testing in primary screening of cervical neoplasia: results from a multicenter study in India. Int. J. Cancer **112**, 341–347 (2004)
41. Sankaranarayanan, R., Nene, B.M., Dinshaw, K.A., et al.: A cluster randomized controlled trial of visual, cytology and human papillomavirus screening for cancer of the cervix in rural India. Int. J. Cancer **116**, 617–623 (2005)
42. Lorincz, A.T., Richart, R.: Human papillomavirus DNA testing as an adjunct to cytology in cervical screening programs. Arch. Pathol. Lab. Med. **127**, 959–968 (2003)
43. Mittendorf, T., Nocon, M., Roll, S., et al.: Assessment of effectiveness and cost-effectiveness of HPV testing in primary screening for cervical cancer. DIMDI, Köln (2007)
44. Guyot, A., Karim, S., Kyi, M.S., et al.: Evaluation of adjunctive HPV testing by Hybrid Capture II in women with minor cytological abnormalities for the diagnosis of CIN2/3 and cost comparison with colposcopy. BMC Infect. Dis. **3**, 23 (2003)
45. Kinney, W.: The prevention of cervical cancer in a changing world. Presentation at HPV, Hannover, 6–8 Dec 2007
46. Castle, P.E., Fetterman, B., Poitras, N., et al.: Five-year experience of human papillomavirus DNA and Papanicolaou test cotesting. Obstet. Gynecol. **113**, 595–600 (2009)
47. Bansal, M., Austin, R.M., Zhao, C.: High-risk HPV DNA detected in less than 2% of over 25,000 cytology negative imaged liquid-based Pap test samples from women 30 and older. Gynecol. Oncol. **115**, 257–261 (2009)
48. Day, S.P., Hudson, A., Mast, A., et al.: Analytical performance of the Investigational Use Only Cervista HPV HR test as determined by a multi-center study. J. Clip. Virol. **45**(Suppl 1), 63–72 (2009)
49. Carozzi, F., Bisanzi, S., Sani, C., et al.: Agreement between the AMPLICOR Human Papillomavirus Test and the Hybrid Capture 2 assay in detection of high-risk human papillomavirus and diagnosis of biopsy-confirmed high-grade cervical disease. J. Clin. Microbiol. **45**, 364–369 (2006). Epub 22 Nov 2006
50. Gravitt, P.E., Schiffman, M., Solomon, D., et al.: A comparison of linear array and hybrid capture 2 for detection of carcinogenic human papillomavirus and cervical precancer in ASCUS-LSIL triage study. Cancer Epidemiol. Biomarkers Prev. **17**, 1248–1254 (2008)
51. Hesselink, A.T., Bulkmans, N.W., Berkhof, J., et al.: Cross-sectional comparison of an automated hybrid capture 2 assay and the consensus GP5+/6+ PCR method in a population-based cervical screening program. J. Clin. Microbiol. **44**, 3680–3685 (2006)
52. Meijer, C.J., Berkhof, J., Castle, P.E., et al.: Guidelines for human papillomavirus DNA test requirements for primary cervical cancer screening in women 30 years and older. Int. J. Cancer **124**, 516–520 (2009)
53. Huang, S., Tang, N., Mak, W.B.: Principles and analytical performance of Abbott RealTime High Risk HPV test. J. Clin. Virol. **45**(Suppl 1), S13–S17 (2009)
54. Hesselink, A.T., Heideman, D.A., Berkhof, J., et al.: Comparison of the clinical performance of PapilloCheck human papillomavirus detection with that of the GP5+/6+-PCR-enzyme immunoassay in population-based cervical screening. J. Clin. Microbiol. **48**, 797–801 (2009)
55. Dockter, J., Schroder, A., Hill, C.: Clinical performance of the APTIMA HPV Assay for the detection of high-risk HPV and high-grade cervical lesions. J. Clin. Virol. **45**(Suppl 1), S55–S61 (2009)
56. Bory, J.P., Cucherousset, J., Lorenzato, M., et al.: Recurrent human papillomavirus infection detected with the hybrid capture II assay selects women with normal cervical smears at risk for developing high grade cervical lesions: a longitudinal study of 3,091 women. Int. J. Cancer **102**, 519–525 (2002)
57. Lorincz, A.T., Castle, P.E., Sherman, M.E., et al.: Viral load of human papillomavirus and risk of CIN3 or cervical cancer. Lancet **360**, 228–229 (2002)
58. Khan MJ, Castle PE, Lorincz AT et al. The elevated 10-year risk of cervical precancer and cancer in women with human papillomavirus (HPV) type 16 or 18 and the possible utility of type-specific HPV testing in clinical practice. J Natl Cancer Inst. 2005; 97: 1072–1079
59. Wheeler, C.M., Hunt, W.C., Schiffman. M., et al.: (ALTS Study Group): Human papillomavirus genotypes and the cumulative 2-year risk of cervical precancer. J. Infect. Dis. **194**, 1291–1299 (2006)
60. Pathirana, D., Hillemanns, P., Petry, K.U., et al.: Short version of the German evidence-based Guidelines for prophylactic vaccination against HPV-associated neoplasia. Vaccine. Epub 2009 Apr 17; **27**, 1551–1559 (2009)
61. Saslow, D., Castle, P.E., Cox, J.T., et al.: American Cancer Society Guideline for human papillomavirus (HPV) vaccine use to prevent cervical cancer and its precursors. CA Cancer J. Clin. **57**, 7–28 (2007)
62. Ogilvie, G.S., Patrick, D.M., Schulzer, M., et al.: Diagnostic accuracy of self collected vaginal specimens for human papillomavirus compared to clinician collected human papillomavirus specimens: a meta-analysis. Sex. Transm. Infect. **81**, 207–212 (2005)

63. Petignat, P., Faltin, D.L., Bruchim, I., et al.: Are self-collected samples comparable to physician-collected cervical specimens for human papillomavirus DNA testing? A systematic review and meta-analysis. Gynecol. Oncol. **105**, 530–535 (2007). Epub 28 Feb 2007
64. Stewart, D.E., Gagliardi, A., Johnston, M., et al.: Self-collected samples for testing of oncogenic human papillomavirus: a systematic review. J. Obstet. Gynaecol. Can. **29**, 817–828 (2007)
65. Bais, A.G., van Kemenade, F.J., Berkhof, J., et al.: Human papillomavirus testing on self-sampled cervicovaginal brushes: an effective alternative to protect nonresponders in cervical screening programs. Int. J. Cancer **120**, 1505–1510 (2007)
66. Molden, T., Nygard, J., Kraus, I., et al.: Predicting CIN2+ when detecting HPV mRNA and DNA by PreTect HPVproofer and consensus PCR: A 2-year follow-up of women with ASCUS or LSIL Pap smear. Int. J. Cancer **114**, 973–976 (2005a)
67. Molden T, Kraus I, Karlsen F et al. (2005) Comparison of human papillomavirus messenger RNA and DNA detection: A cross-sectional study of 4136 women >30 years of age with a 2-year follow-up of high grade squamous intraepithelial lesion. Cancer Epidemiol. Biomarkers Prev **14**, 367–372 (2005b)
68. Szarewski, A., Ambroisine, L., Cadman, L., et al.: Comparison of predictors for high-grade cervical intraepithelial neoplasia in women with abnormal smears. Cancer Epidemiol. Biomarkers Prev. **17**, 3033–3042 (2008)
69. Castle, P.E., Dockter, J., Giachetti, C., et al.: A cross-sectional study of a prototype carcinogenic human papillomavirus E6/E7 messenger RNA assay for detection of cervical precancer and cancer. Clin. Cancer Res. **13**, 2599–2605 (2007)
70. Anonymous (http://www.cdc.gov/STD/HPV/STDFact-HPV-and-men.htm#test) (2007)
71. Arbyn, M., Buntinx, F., van Ranst, M., et al.: Virologic versus cytologic triage of women with equivocal Pap smears: a meta-analysis of the accuracy to detect high-grade intraepithelial neoplasia. J. Natl. Cancer Inst. **96**, 280–293 (2004)

Mollusca Contagiosa

41

Mihael Skerlev and Karmela Husar

Core Messages

- Mollusca contagiosa (MC) are rather frequent in 1- to 5-year-old children, but their appearance in the genital area of adults is mostly regarded as sexually transmitted infection (STI).
- The extragenital appearance of MC in adults can be more typically noticed in patients with immunosuppressive conditions, especially in HIV/AIDS patients
- There is no etiological treatment of MC so far, and the majority of treatment options are mechanical, sometimes causing a certain degree of discomfort, or are not enough evidence-based.
- Adult patients with MC should be carefully screened for other STIs and counseled appropriately.

41.1 Definition

Mollusca contagiosa (MC) are defined as a common cutaneous viral infection caused by *Molluscipox* virus affecting both children and adults. MC are clinically characterized by small, waxy, dome-shaped umbilicated papules (1) (Fig. 41.1) (synonyms: epithelioma contagiosum or dimple warts). Whereas mollusca contagiosa are rather frequent in the 1- to 5-year-old children and can be localized almost anywhere on the body, their appearance in adults is mostly regarded as sexually transmitted infection (STI).

41.2 Historical Aspects

The clinical features of MC were described for the first time by Bateman in 1817 (1). Intracytoplasmic inclusion bodies ("molluscum bodies") have been described in 1841 by Henderson and Paterson (1, 2).

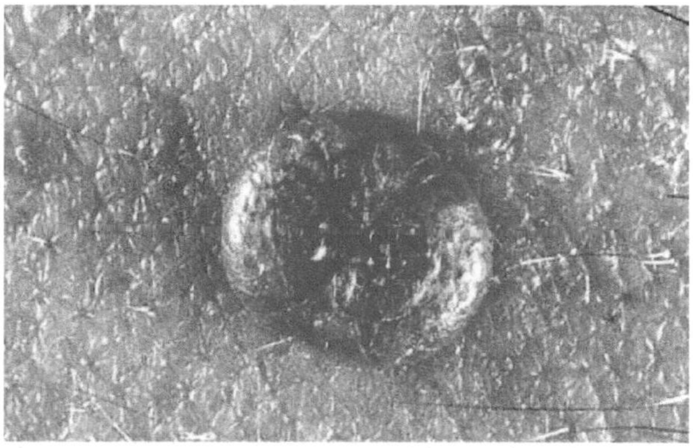

Fig. 41.1 Molluscum contagiosum – typical umbilicated (dome-shaped) papule on the healthy skin

M. Skerlev (✉) and K. Husar
Department of Dermatology and Venereology, Zagreb University Hospital Centre and Medical School of Zagreb University, Šalata 4, 10000 Zagreb, Croatia
e-mail: mskerlev@kbc-zagreb.hr

G. Gross and S.K. Tyring (eds.), *Sexually Transmitted Infections and Sexually Transmitted Diseases*,
DOI: 10.1007/978-3-642-14663-3_41, © Springer-Verlag Berlin Heidelberg 2011

In 1905, the viral nature of MC was revealed by Juliusberg as a successful "transmissibility by a filterable agent" (2) followed by the description of the Lipschütz granules within the molluscum bodies in 1911 (2).

41.3 Etiology and Pathogenesis

Molluscipox virus (MCV) (synonym – *Molluscum contagiosum virus*) is a large, double-stranded DNA orthopoxvirus belonging to the Poxviridae family (2, 3). MCV is a strictly epidermotropic (thus, not inducing scarring) and relatively large virus ranging 240–320 nm in diameter. MCV replicates in the cytoplasm of host epithelial cells, producing cytoplasmic inclusions, and may cause enlargement of infected cells. Only humans are known to be affected except for one report each of molluscum contagiosum occurring in chimpanzees and a horse (4). The virus enters the skin directly via small epithelial defects or indirectly via clothing, towels, or handkerchiefs (1).

MCV might be transmitted directly from person to person or, which seems to be more frequent, by autoinoculation – i.e., by scratching or touching a lesion and transferring the virus from one site to another on the skin of the same individual. MC in adults is most typically a sexually transmitted infection (STI), characteristically involving the genital area (5–7). However, the extragenital appearance of MC in adults can be more typically noticed in patients with immunosuppressive conditions, especially in HIV/AIDS patients (8). The onset of MC in HIV-positive individuals can be, according to the current literature data, regarded as a part of immune reconstitution inflammatory syndrome (IRIS) (9). IRIS is a recently described entity in which severely immunodepressed HIV patients, after being started on highly active antiretroviral treatment (HAART), develop inflammatory reactions to several pathogens (10). With the progression of immunoreconstitution, the lesions healed spontaneously. Molluscum contagiosum lesions are common in IRIS but presumably underreported. For example, disseminated eruptive giant mollusca contagiosa in an adult psoriasis patient during Efalizumab therapy have been very recently reported (11).

41.4 Epidemiology

The actual virus reservoir is not known. The incubation period is variable, ranging from several (2–8) weeks to one year (12). The incidence of MC and their clinical forms may somehow be different in Europe as compared with Asia (1, 13). Among children 1–5 years of age, prevalence was approximately 25% in Papua New Guinea and Fiji (14). It is most probable that MC affect both sexes equally in children's age, whereas it seems that in adult age, the incidence in males prevails. Thus, in STD clinics in England and Wales, slightly more than twice as many men as woman were diagnosed with MC (7). However, we believe that a certain number of cases of MC in both children and adults remains underreported.

41.5 Clinical Findings

Pearl-like, "discrete," smooth papules (2–5 mm in diameter), singly or in groups, occur on the healthy skin, often in a linear arrangement (pseudo-Köbner phenomenon) and are mostly skin colored or may be white, yellow, or pink. Typically, MC have a central umbilication (a small indentation or dot) at their top from which a plug of cheesy material can be expressed. As previously mentioned, in adults, mollusca contagiosa are most often sexually transmitted infections (STI); thus, their sites of involvement are usually genitals, lower abdomen, inner upper thighs, and buttocks (Fig. 41.2). Exuberant forms of MC, as well as their extragenital localization in adults (eyelids!) can be much more often observed in the immunocompromised patients, especially in HIV/AIDS (up to the 20% of patients) comparing to the HIV-negative patients (15) (Fig. 41.3).

In children, the papules may occur anywhere on the body, but the face, eyelids, neck, axillae, cubital creases and thighs are sites of predilection. MC lesions are found often as solitary (rather than confluent) lesions of varying size, and their number may be even up to

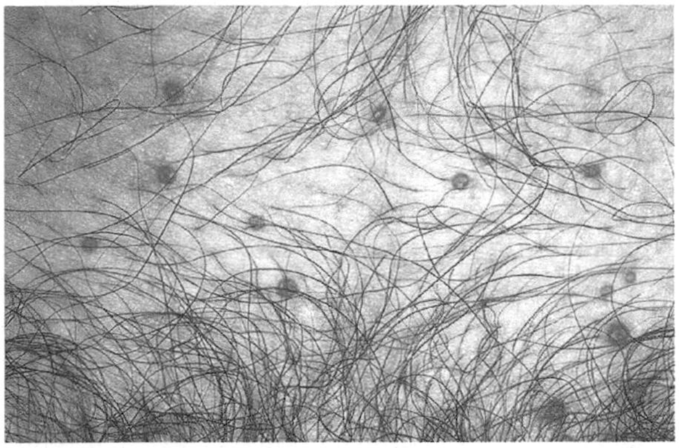

Fig. 41.2 Multiple mollusca contagiosa typically involving lower abdomen and pubic region in adults (note characteristic central dot!)

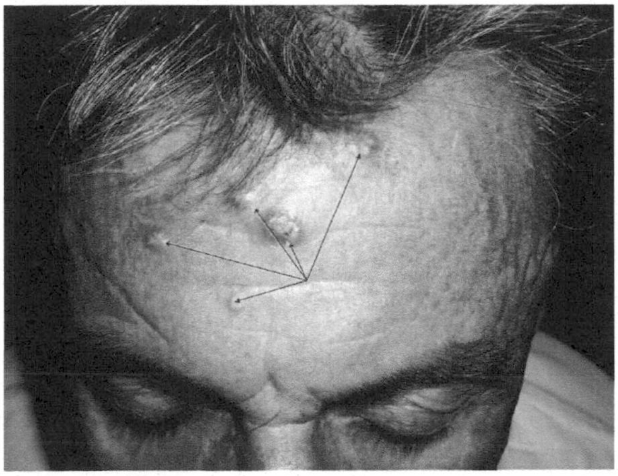

Fig. 41.3 Solitary and confluent mollusca contagiosa on the forehead of the HIV-positive patient. Extragenital localization of mollusca contagiosa in adults is not characteristic for the HIV-negative persons

several hundred. MC can become inflamed in immunologic resistance or by contamination with a pyogenic organism (12). Lesions on the eyelid margin can produce unilateral conjunctivitis; rarely, lesions may appear on the cornea (16). Lesions on patients with AIDS, in children with leukemia and other immunodeficiencies, or in children undergoing cytostatic or glucocorticosteroid therapy can be large and numerous, particularly on the face (17, 18). In patients with chronic dermatitis or even atopic dermatitis, especially in areas of skin treated with glucocorticosteroids (local immune deficiency), hundreds of MCs may develop (eczema molluscatum) (19). Unlike ordinary warts, the palms and soles are not involved (16, 18). Like all forms of warts, eventually the MC lesions disappear spontaneously in 6–9 months, but they may also last much longer. Complications include secondary impetiginization and orbital spread if the face is involved. Infection can become widespread and prolonged in children with compromised cutaneous barriers.

41.6 Diagnosis and Differential Diagnosis

Clinical findings are the most important for obtaining the diagnosis, and cytologic tests (molluscum bodies in aspirated material (17)) might be sometimes required for the confirmation. To diagnose molluscum bodies, eosinophilic viral inclusion bodies in the lower epidermis (3), punch skin biopsy is required. Abnormal keratinization process in lesional epidermis of MC can be proved by specific antibodies to filaggrin, loricrin, Ted-H-1 antigen, involucrin, cystatin A, and CD95 ligand (4, 20). Cell-mediated immunity seems to be important in host defense. The virus of MC has not been grown in tissue culture (4). Histological examination after hematoxylin and eosin staining confirmed that the proliferative lesion was due to MC, and demonstration of the presence of molluscum bodies in a section can be revealed by in situ hybridization. Sequence analysis in the polymerase chain reaction is more sensitive than in situ hybridization and in dual infection with both MCV and *Human papillomavirus* (HPV), the immunosuppressive genes of *Molluscipox* virus could enhance survival of the oncogenic types of HPV (20).

In *differential diagnosis*, papular warts in the genital region (a form of condylomata acuminata, i.e., HPV-associated lesions), ectopic sebaceous glands, trichoepithelioma, basal-cell carcinoma, syringoma, hidrocystoma, keratoacanthoma, warty dyskeratoma, common warts, varicella, milia, and cutaneous cryptococcus presenting as molluscum-like eruptions should be considered (21). We also report on our clinical observation of the Langerhans cell histiocytosis mimicking the molluscum-like lesion on the eyelid of the 4-year-old boy (22).

41.7 Treatment

MC are generally self-limited and heal after several months or years. Therapy may be beneficial in preventing transmission or autoinoculation. Unfortunately, there is no etiological treatment of MC so far, and majority of treatment options are mechanical, or are not enough "evidence-based." *Topical Applications*. Cryotherapy with liquid nitrogen (6–9 s) works best if the patient does not mind the certain discomfort and pain (23). Curettage only, or followed by either electrodessication or application of caustic agent, has been shown to be an effective treatment in children as well as adults. The papules can also be destroyed by expressing the plug with a needle, or a comedo extractor, EMLA® 5% topical anesthetic cream, a eutectic mixture of prilocaine-lidocaine, can be applied under occlusion 1–2 hours before the procedure(s). Such anesthesia before the curettage (or punch biopsy) provides effective local analgesia without serious application – site reactions in both children with atopic dermatitis and/or adults experiencing the involvement of the sensitive skin of the genital region (24). Cantharidin (single application every 3–4 weeks needs to be repeated, and the area should be washed thoroughly about 30–60 minutes after every application) is sometimes painful, and carries the risk of serious skin erosion (25, 26). Topical imiquimod 5% cream three times a week represents comparatively new and "elegant" option; however, sometimes, the irritating side effects might be significant (27, 28). Besides, this is a comparatively expansive treatment option providing the number of MC lesion; thus, it seems that imiquimod might be more appropriate for the treatment of the HPV rather than MC lesions. Tretinoin cream 0.05% or gel 0.025% applied once or twice a day to individual lesions or cidofovir 0.1% gel (29) might sometimes be beneficial. Salicylic acid applied each day (with or without tape occlusion), tincture of iodine, silver nitrate 40% paste (30), or phenol have also been described as treatment options for curing MC without scars. Trichloroacetic acid 70%, 5-fluorouracil (5-FU), bleomycin-intralesional injection, or scarification is sometimes too painful and might cause severe irritation. Some "organic" and "natural" preparations (31) have been also mentioned as "natural healing of mollusca"; however, more evidence-based studies are required. Electrosurgery, laser therapy with ultrapulsed dye or CO_2 laser, and excision are some of the treatment options, as well (32). *Systemic Agents*. Cimetidine stimulates the immune system to reject the wart (an "off-label" indication); thus, oral cimetidine, 40 mg/kg/day might be prescribed in two divided doses (23). Treatment of HIV/AIDS patients with disseminated MC with the use of HAART, intralesional interferon-alpha, and topical injection of streptococcal antigen OK-43228 is very beneficial (33). Intralesional interferon-alpha (weekly for 4 weeks) for the treatment of recalcitrant MC in AIDS patients (34), 70% trichloroacetic acid and inosiplex (35) systemically enhance underlying defective immunologic mechanisms and might be, thus, very beneficial under the circumstances (36, 37).

In general, treatment is rather effective, though sometimes causes a certain degree of discomfort, especially in small children. Overall prognosis is excellent in immunocompetent patients.

41.8 Conclusions

The appearance of mollusca contagiosa in adults is mostly regarded as sexually transmitted infection (STI) and their significance should not be underestimated. Whereas mollusca contagiosa in the immunocompetent children represent generally a benign, self-limited disease and might heal spontaneously after several months or years, in imumunocompromised patients, the clinical forms of MC may be exuberant and the lesions numerous and recalcitrant. Thus, special attention should be given to the extragenital site of involvement of MC in adults, and HIV serology testing should certainly be recommended in such patients. Both children and adults with MC should be educated to avoid skin contact with others and scratching to prevent transmission and autoinoculation. Besides, the adult patients with MC should be carefully screened for other STIs and counseled appropriately.

Take-Home Pearls

- While MC are rather frequent in 1- to 5-year-old children and can be localized anywhere on the body, their appearance in adults in the genital region is regarded as STI.
- MC in immunocompetent children represent generally a benign, self-limited disease and might heal spontaneously after several months or years.
- However, the clinical forms of MC may be exuberant and the lesions numerous and recalcitrant.
- Both children and adults with MC should be educated to avoid skin contact with others and scratching to prevent transmission and autoinoculation.
- Adult patients with MC should be carefully screened for other STIs.
- Special attention should be given to the extragenital site of involvement of MC in adults, and HIV serology testing should certainly be recommended in such patients.
- The onset of MC in HIV-positive individuals can be regarded as a part of immune reconstitution inflammatory syndrome (IRIS).

References

1. Ive, F.A., Wilkinson, D.S.: Diseases of the umbilical, perianal and genital regions. In: Rook, A., Wilkinson, D.S., Ebling, G.J.G., Champion, R.H., Burton, J.L. (eds.) Textbook of Dermatology, 4th edn. Blackwell Scientific Publications, Oxford, Edinburgh (1986). 2184
2. Nagingto, J., Rook, A., Highet, A.S.: Virus and related infections. In: Rook, A., Wilkinson, D.S., Ebling, G.J.G., Champion, R.H., Burton, J.L. (eds.) Textbook of Dermatology, 4th edn, pp. 696–700. Blackwell Scientific Publications, Oxford, Edinburgh (1986)
3. Rook, A., Wilkinson, D.S., Champion, R.H.: The principles of diagnosis. In: Rook, A., Wilkinson, D.S., Ebling, F.J.G., Champion, R.H., Burton, J.L. (eds.) Textbook of Dermatology, 4th edn, pp. 79–81. Blackwell Scientific Publications, Oxford, Edinburgh (1986)
4. Takahashi, M., Izutani, A., Tezuka, T.: An immunohistochemical study of abnormal keratinocyte differentiation in molluscum contagiosum. Br. J. Dermatol. **141**, 116–118 (1999)
5. Choong, K.Y., Roberts, L.J.: Molluscum contagiosum, swimming and bathing: a clinical analysis. Australas. J. Dermatol. **40**, 89–92 (1999)
6. Koning, S., Bruijnzeels, M.A., van Suijlekom-Smit, L.W., van der Wounden, J.C.: Molluscum contagiosum in Dutch general practice. Br. J. Gen. Pract. **44**, 417–419 (1994)
7. Lewis, E.J., Lam, M., Crutchfield, C.E.: An update on molluscum contagiosum. Cutis **60**, 29–34 (1997)
8. Husak, R., Garbe, C., Orfanos, C.E.: Mollusca contagiosa bei HIV-Infection Klinische Manifestation, Beziehung zum Immunstatus und prognostische Wertigkeit bei 39 Patienten. Hautarzt **48**, 103–109 (1997)
9. Pereira, B., Fernandes, C., Nachiambo, E., et al.: Exuberant molluscum contagiosum as a manifestation of the immune reconstitution inflammatory syndrome. Dermatol. Online J. **13**(2), 6 (2007)
10. Hirsch, H., Kaufmann, G., Sendi, P., Battegay, M.: Immune reconstitution in HIV-infected patients. Clin. Infect. Dis. **38**, 1159–1166 (2004)
11. Weisenseel, P., Kuznetsov, A.V., Flaig, M., Prinz, J.C.: Disseminated eruptive giant Mollusca Contagiosa in an adult psoriasis patient during Efalizumab therapy. Dermatology **217**, 85–86 (2008)
12. Husar, K., Skerlev, M.: Molluscum contagiosum from infancy to maturity. Clin. Dermatol. **20**(2), 170–172 (2002)
13. Jain, S., Das, D.K., Malhotra, V., et al.: Molluscum contagiosum: a case report with fine needle aspiration cytologic diagnosis and ultrastructural features. Acta Cytol. **44**, 63–66 (2000)
14. Nakamura, J., Arao, Y., Yoshida, M., Nii, S.: Molecular epidemiological study of molluscum contagiosum virus in two urban areas of western Japan by the in-gel endonuclease digestion method. Arch. Virol. **125**, 339–345 (1992)
15. Thompson, C.H., de Zwarf-Steffe, R.T., Donovan, B.: Clinical and molecular aspects of molluscum contagiosum infection in HIV-1 positive patients. Int. J. STD AIDS **3**, 101–106 (1992)
16. Matoba, A.: Ocular viral infections. Pediatr. Infect. Dis. **3**, 358–368 (1984)
17. Nieo, M.M.S., Bergonese, F.N., Godoy, A.M.: Molluscum contagiosum in herpes zoster scars. Int. J. Dermatol. **40**, 521–524 (2001)
18. Rüsch, R.: Augeninfektionen bei Aids-Patienten. Exp. Opin. Invest. Drugs **7**, 437–449 (1998)
19. Siegfried, E.C.: Warts and molluscum contagiosum on children: an approach to therapy. Dermatol. Ther. **2**, 51–67 (1997)
20. Payne, D., Yen, A., Tyring, S.: Coinfection of molluscum contagiosum with human papilloma-virus. J. Am. Acad. Dermatol. **36**, 641–644 (1997)
21. Itin, P.H., Gilli, L.: Molluscum contagiosum, mimicking sebaceous nevus of Jadassohn, ecthyma and giant condylomata acuminata in HIV-infected patients. Dermatology **189**, 396–398 (1994)
22. Husar, K., Murat-Sušić, S., Skerlev, M., Dobrić, I., Lakoš Jukić, I.: Langerhans cell histiocytosis – report of two cases. In: 4th EADV Spring Symposium, Saariselkä, Finland, 09–12 Feb 2006, Book of Abstracts: P-058.

23. Verbov, J.: How to manage warts. Arch. Dis. Child. **80**, 97–99 (1999)
24. Simonart, T., De Maertelaer, V.: Curettage treatment for molluscum contagiosum: a follow-up survey study. Br. J. Dermatol. **159**(5), 1144–1147 (2008)
25. Ronnerfalt, L., Fransson, J., Wahlgren, C.F.: EMLA cream provides rapid pain relief for the curettage of molluscum contagiosum in children with atopic dermatitis without causing serious application-site reactions. Pediatr. Dermatol. **15**, 309–312 (1998)
26. Werfel, S., Boeck, K., Abeck, D., Ring, J.: Special characteristics of topical treatment in childhood. Hautarzt **49**, 170–175 (1998)
27. Buckley, R., Smith, K.: Topical imiquimod therapy for chronic giant molluscum contagiosum in a patient with advanced human immunodeficiency virus 1 disease. Arch. Dermatol. **135**, 1–6 (1999)
28. Edwards, L.: Imiquimod in clinical practice. J. Am. Acad. Dermatol. **43**, 12–17 (2000)
29. Toro, J.R., Wood, L.V., Patel, N.K., Turner, M.L.: Topical cidofovir: a novel treatment for recalcitrant molluscum contagiosum in children infected with human immunodeficiency virus 1. Arch. Dermatol. **136**, 1–5 (2000)
30. Niizeki, K., Hashimoto, K.: Treatment of molluscum contagiosum with silver nitrate paste. Pediatr. Dermatol. **16**, 395–397 (1999)
31. Kauffman, C.L., Yoon, W. Molluscum contagiosum. eMed J 2001;2(11). Available at http://www.emedicine.com/DERM/topic270.htmsectionclinical; accessed September 1, (2002)
32. Binder, B., Weger, W., Komericki, P., Kopera, D.: Treatment of molluscum contagiosum with a pulsed dye laser: Pilot study with 19 children. J. Dtsch Dermatol. Ges. **6**(2), 121–125 (2007)
33. Horneff, G., Wahn, V.: Mollusca contagiosa in HIV-infected children receiving optimal antiretroviral therapy. Klin. Pediatr. **212**, 83–84 (2000)
34. Hourihane, J., Hodges, E., Smith, J., et al.: Interferon a treatment of molluscum contagiosum in immunodeficiency. Arch. Dis. Child. **80**, 77–79 (1999)
35. Gross, G., Jogerst, C., Schopf, E.: Systemic treatment of mollusca contagiosa with inosiplex. Acta Derm. Venereol. **66**, 76–80 (1986)
36. Conant, M.A.: Immunomodulatory therapy in the management of viral infections in patients with HIV infection. J. Am. Acad. Dermatol. **43**, S27–S30 (2000)
37. Harms, G., Blume-Peytavi, U., Bunikowski, R., et al.: Mollusca contagiosa bei einem afrikanischen Kind mit Aids. Hautarzt **46**, 799–803 (1995)

Hepatitis Viruses as Sexually Transmitted Diseases

42

Laura J. Lester and Suneal K. Agarwal

Core Messages

- HBV is a partially double stranded DNA virus of the family Hepadnaviridae that is transmitted via percutaneous and mucous membrane exposure to serum, semen and saliva. Symptomatic primary infection occurs in only 30-50% of infected adults, less often in children, and presents with fever, malaise, jaundice, anorexia, nausea and right upper quadrant pain. Ninety percent of infants and 25 to 50 percent of children aged 1 to 5 years become chronically infected, whereas 95 percent of infected adults completely recover from acute infection and do not develop chronic HBV. Non-hepatic complications include polyarteritis nodosa, glomerulonephritis and serum sickness-like syndrome. Currently there are seven approved drugs for treating HBV which include two immune modulators, interferon alpha-2b and peg interferon alpha-2a, and five antiviral medications, lamivudine, adefovir, entecavir, telbivudine and tenofovir.
- HDV is an RNA virus belonging to the genus Deltavirus that depends on hepatitis B virus for infectivity, and thus is only capable of infecting a host that is also infected with HBV. As is the case with acute HBV infection, clinical manifestations of co-infection range from asymptomatic to fulminant hepatitis. Interferon and pegylated interferon are the only treatments effective against chronic HDV.
- Hepatitis C virus is a single stranded RNA virus of the Flaviviridae family, and HCV infection is the most common chronic blood borne infection in the United States. The main form of transmission for HCV remains parenteral; however vertical transmission, sexual contact, and other forms have been reported. Hepatitis C has three main outcomes; fulminant, acute, and chronic hepatitis. Fifteen to 30% of symptomatic acute hepatitis C patients go on to spontaneous viral clearance and recovery, while the remainder of the patients go on to have chronic hepatitis. Extrahepatic manifestations of HCV include mixed cryoglobulinemia, lymphoma, porphyria cutanea tarda, lichen planus and diabetes. Patients with HCV viremia and compensated liver disease are candidates for treatment with pegylated interferon alpha and ribavirin, the current standard of care for HCV.
- Hepatitis A virus (HAV) is not traditionally considered a sexually transmitted disease, as it is transmitted via the fecal-oral route and is seen most often in travelers returning from endemic areas. In men who have sex with men (MSM) though, there is evidence that the virus

L.J. Lester (✉)
Department of Dermatology, University of Texas at Houston, 6655 Travis Street Suite 980, Houston, TX 77030, USA
e-mail: laura.j.lester@uth.tmc.edu

S.K. Agarwal
Department of Internal Medicine, Baylor College of Medicine, 4705 Caroline, Houston, TX 77004, USA
e-mail: agarwal@bcm.tmc.edu

G. Gross and S.K. Tyring (eds.), *Sexually Transmitted Infections and Sexually Transmitted Diseases*,
DOI: 10.1007/978-3-642-14663-3_42, © Springer-Verlag Berlin Heidelberg 2011

is transmitted via sexual activity. HAV does not ever lead to chronic infection and treatment is supportive and directed by clinical manifestations of the disease.

› HGV is transmitted via the same routes as HBV and HCV, including sexual contact. Anecdotal reports and non-controlled studies have associated HGV with hepatitis, but more recent studies have failed to provide convincing evidence that HGV is the causative agent in any human disease. Based on the strength of evidence that HGV does not cause human infection, the FDA does not screen donor blood for this virus. Multiple studies have demonstrated higher CD4 counts, lower HIV viral load, and increased survival in HIV infected individuals who also have HGV viremia compared to those negative for HGV viremia.

42.1 Introduction

Hepatitis viruses are a diverse group of viruses, including RNA and DNA viruses, from different families that are named alphabetically hepatitis A, B, C, D, E, G, and share in common a tropism for the liver. Four of these viruses, B, C, D, and G, also share their modes of transmission that include mucocutaneous and percutaneous exposure to infected body fluids. Because of these modes of transmission, hepatitis B, C, and D viruses can all be transmitted through sexual contact, making them part of the family of sexually transmitted diseases. Hepatitis A and E are transmitted through the fecal–oral route and are thus not traditionally considered sexually transmitted diseases; epidemiologic studies, however, have shown that hepatitis A virus can be transmitted via sexual practices, especially in men who have sex with men, and thus must also be included as a sexually transmitted disease. In this chapter hepatitis A, B, C, D, and G will be discussed including epidemiology, viral life cycle and pathogenesis, clinical manifestations, disease course, and treatment.

42.2 Hepatitis B Virus

42.2.1 The Virus

Hepatitis B virus (HBV) was identified in 1967 based on the work by Baruch Blumberg who received a Nobel Prize for his research on infectious diseases leading to the identification of the hepatitis B surface antigen.

Chronic HBV infection affects 1.25 million people in the USA, 350 million people globally, and it is estimated that 620,000 people die from liver-related complications of HBV yearly [1]. The rate of new HBV infections has declined by 80% since 1991 when a strategy was implemented for the eradication of HBV from the population, and the population with the greatest decline in incidence since this time is children because of the routine administration of HBV vaccines. In 2006, the reported number of new cases was 4,758, although the estimated number of new infections, due to asymptomatic acute infections and underreporting, is likely tenfold higher at 46,000 (Fig. 42.1) [1].

HBV is the prototypical virus of the family *Hepadnaviridae* that includes the genus *Orthohepadnavirus* which infects mammals, and the genus *Avihepadnavirus* which infects ducks and geese. *Orthohepadnaviruses*' known hosts include woodchucks and ground squirrels, but HBV only causes

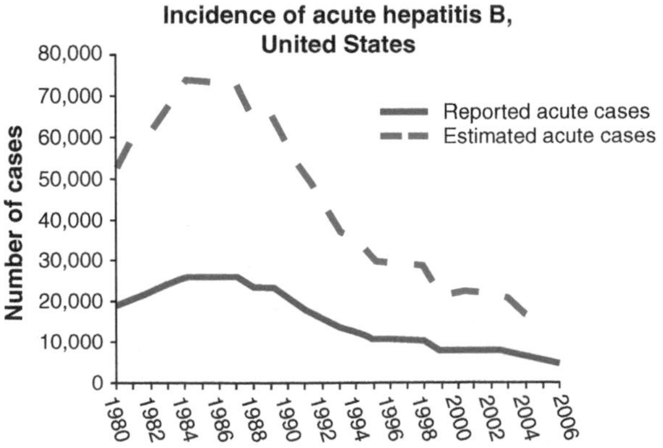

Fig. 42.1 Estimated and reported incidence of hepatitis B virus infection in the USA from 1980 through 2006 (Department of Health and Human Services, Center for Disease Control. http://www.cdc.gov/hepatitis/HBV/HBVfaq.htm#overview)

infection in humans and great apes [2]. Multiple genotypes of HBV have been described, each of which differs from the next by at least 8% of its genome, and within each genotype (except E and G) sub-genotypes have been detected, each differing by at least 4%. The genotypes thus far detected are named with letters of the alphabet A through H, and most are found in a regional distribution. For example, genotype F is found in South and Central America, genotype G in Mexico, A1 in southern Africa, A2 in Western Europe and Scandinavian countries, E in central and western Africa, B in southeastern Asia, while genotype D has a wider distribution throughout the world [3]. Coinfection with two genotypes has been described with a prevalence of 4–17% of those with HBV infection; infection with three different genotypes has even been described in intravenous drug users. The significance of coinfection lies in the demonstration of genomic changes of the virus in coinfected people thought to be due to recombination events, although the mechanism of recombination has yet to be elucidated [3].

42.2.2 Structure, Life Cycle, and Viral Genome

Hepatitis B viral particles are composed of genetic information in the form of circular, partially double-stranded DNA located inside of a nucleocapsid which is surrounded by a protein-studded envelope. The capsid is made up of the C protein which forms homodimers that assemble into an icosahedral capsid. This capsid occurs in two different forms, one made of 90 dimers of C protein measuring 30 nm, and the other consisting of 120 dimers measuring 34 nm [4]. The envelope is a phospholipid bilayer derived from the host's endoplasmic reticulum membrane and contains three membrane proteins: S, M, and L [5].

HBV is a hepatotropic virus, and while viral particles have been detected in other organs including pancreas, kidneys, and lymphocytes, hepatocytes are the only cell in which all members of the virus family have been demonstrated to replicate and thus are the main focus of viral pathogenesis [2]. Transcription, translation, and virus particle assembly have been well described for HBV, but the exact mechanism of earlier events in the viral life cycle, including hepatocyte binding and the release of the viral capsid into the cytoplasm are still not as clearly understood. Much information we have about hepatitis B virus has been obtained by studying duck hepatitis B virus. Binding of the HBV virus to the hepatocyte is known to require both hepatocyte receptor expression and viral gene expression of membrane proteins. Viral cell entry has been more extensively studied in duck hepatitis B virus infection, and carboxypeptidase D was discovered as the cellular receptor for the virus. More recently, cell binding of human HBV was found to depend on the pre-S1 region of the HBV L envelope protein (see discussion of viral genome below) and its interaction with heparin sulfate proteoglycan on the hepatocyte which acts as the primary cellular receptor for the virus [6]. Proteoglycans are fairly ubiquitous in the human body's organs and tissues, but their expression, which is determined by cell differentiation and activation, differs amongst cell types in extent of expression, length of the molecules, and the degree and position of sulfation. The particular tropism of HBV for hepatocytes has been explained by the demonstration of viral preference for the highly sulfated proteoglycans which are expressed in the liver [6]. After fusion of the viral envelope with the cellular membrane, the release of the virion from the endosome into the cytoplasm is thought to depend on proteolytic cleavage of membrane proteins to expose a fusion sequence of the viral proteins [7]. Once released, viral capsids are actively transported through the cytoplasm via microtubules, and they arrive at the nuclear envelope within 15 min [8]. At the nuclear envelope, the viral capsid associates with nuclear pore complexes; this attachment to the nuclear pore complex depends upon the phosphorylated residues of the carboxy terminus of the core protein which act as a nuclear localization signal, and is mediated by cellular proteins importing alpha and beta [9]. Following capsid attachment to the nuclear pore complex, the viral DNA is released into the nucleus along with the dissociated capsid subunits [8].

The HBV viral genome that exists inside of mature viral particles and that is delivered to the host cell nucleus is in the form of relaxed circular DNA (rcDNA). In this form, only the negative strand forms a complete circle, while the positive strand is short of being full length, making the genome mostly double-stranded with a small segment of single-stranded DNA [10]. The viral reverse transcriptase, also referred to as protein P, is covalently attached to the 5′ end of the negative strand of DNA, and an RNA oligonucleotide, a remnant of the primer for the positive strand synthesis, is attached to the 5′ end of the positive strand of DNA [10]. In order for virus replication to occur, the rcDNA must be converted to a covalently closed circular DNA (cccDNA). This entails removal of the P protein and the RNA oligonucleotide, completion of the positive strand of DNA, and covalent linkage of the ends of the two DNA strands [2]. It is thought that these processes depend on both host cell activities and the viral DNA polymerase; evidence for the action of protein P in forming cccDNA is supported by experiments showing that viral reverse transcriptase inhibitors interfere with the formation of cccDNA [11]. Insertion of HBV DNA into the host genome is not required for its replication. Rather, after cccDNA formation, host cellular RNA polymerase II functions to transcribe all hepadnaviral RNAs [10]. There are four open reading frames (ORF) in the viral genome, all of which are read from the positive strand DNA, which encode (1) the core protein, (2) the surface proteins, (3) the DNA polymerase (P protein), and (4) the X protein. After transcription, all RNAs are transported to the cytoplasm where translation occurs. An RNA transcript called the pre-genomic RNA (pgRNA) is made which encompasses the entire viral genome and a terminal redundancy. The pgRNA serves as the template for the translation of the core protein, the DNA polymerase, and reverse transcription of the viral genome [10].

The core protein, as described above, forms dimmers that assemble to create the viral capsid, and is known as the HBV core antigen (HBcAg). After the DNA polymerase is synthesized, it binds to the 5′ end of the pgRNA from which it was created at a stem-loop structure called ε which is the encapsidation signal. This binding causes the P protein and the pgRNA to become encapsulated into the newly formed viral capsid [12]. After encapsulation, the reverse transcriptase creates the viral genome, first the negative and then the positive strand of DNA, with the completed product being rcDNA. Inside of hepatocytes, viral capsids containing all forms of genomic information – RNA, single-stranded DNA, and double-stranded DNA – have been identified, but only capsids containing mature rcDNA are found in the host circulation. It is proposed that synthesis of plus strand DNA triggers phosphorylation of core proteins, which induces a conformational change in the protein structure which acts as a signal for capsid envelopment and subsequent release from the cell [13]. In addition, the carboxy terminus of the core protein that acts as the nuclear localization signal only becomes localized externally on the capsid after becoming phosphorylated, an event which coincides with maturation of the viral genome. This serves to ensure that only mature viral genomes are delivered to the nucleus. As an alternative to being released from the host cell, once the viral rcDNA is formed, the capsid can return to the nucleus to deliver the genome in order to amplify the intracellular viral load by repeating this sequence of replication (Fig. 42.2) [14].

Upstream to the core protein ORF is a sequence of 29 codons called the pre-core sequence; at this upstream location, the pre-core viral protein begins translation and continues all the way through the coding segment for the core protein [15]. Rather than being a precursor to the core protein, this peptide will become a viral protein known as the HBV e antigen. The translated pre-core protein has a hydrophobic leader sequence that directs it to the endoplasmic reticulum where it is modified by cleavage at the carboxy terminus resulting in HBeAg proteins ranging from 17 to 22 kiloDaltons (kDA) depending on site of cleavage [12]. HBeAg is then secreted from the cell as a monomeric protein. The HBeAg is referred to as an accessory protein because it is not required for acute infection in vivo or successful viral replication. Although the exact function of HBeAg is not understood, it is believed to be a modulator of host immune response such that its presence is associated with establishment of chronic HBV infection while its absence may lead to a more severe or even fulminant acute infection [16].

Orthohepadnaviridea express three surface proteins S, M, and L, each of which is produced from one ORF. The S protein is 266 amino acids long and is the shortest of the three; M and L proteins are translated from start codons upstream from the S protein and contain the S protein sequence in addition to amino-terminal extensions termed pre-S2 and pre-S1, respectively [2]. The M protein is 281 amino acids long and contains pre-S2. The L protein is the largest, consisting of either 389 or 400 amino acids, and in addition to containing the S protein and pre-S2, the L protein contains a unique upstream segment, pre-S1 [17]. These surface proteins are also known as the HBV surface antigen (HBsAg).

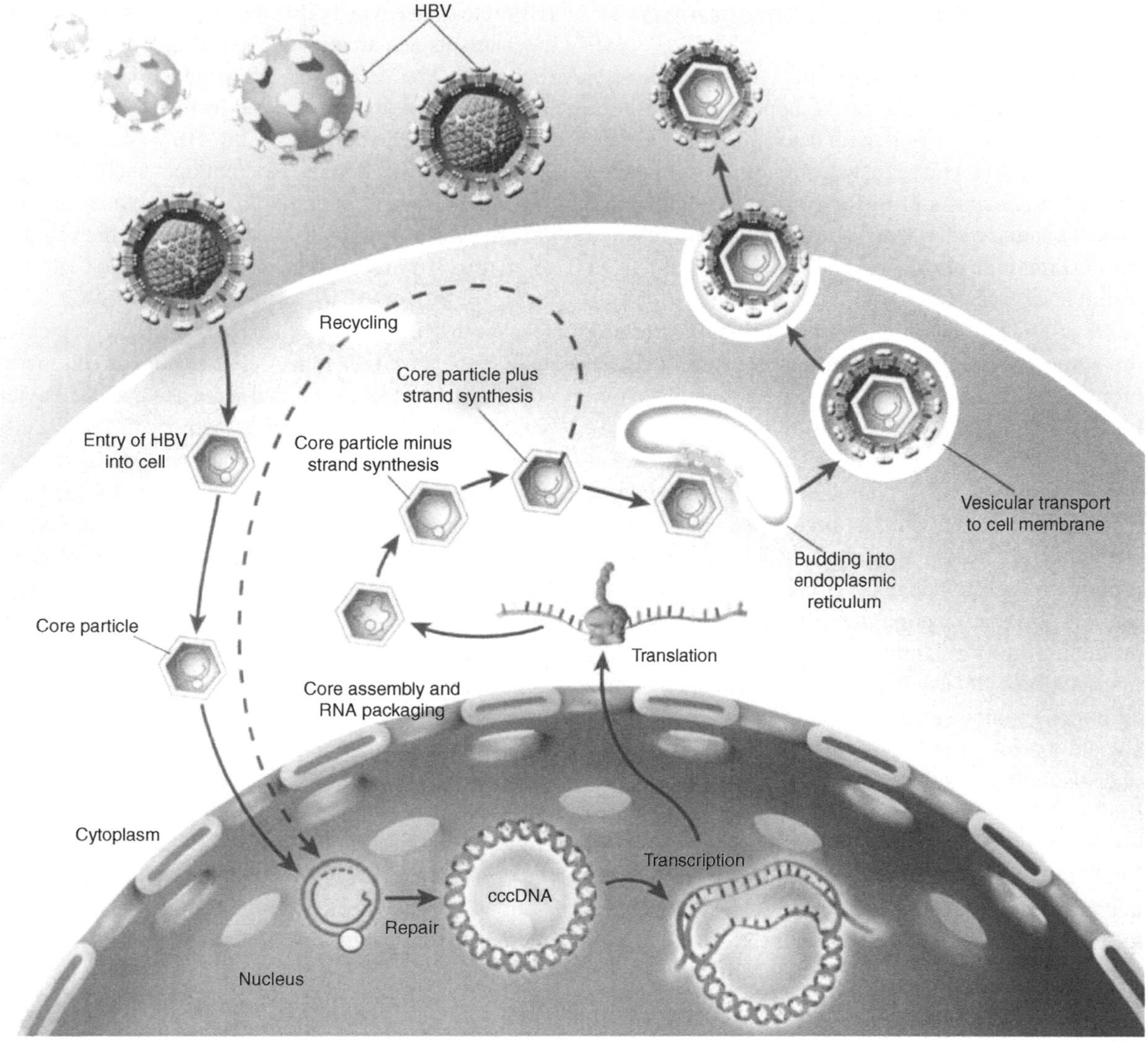

Fig. 42.2 The replication cycle of hepatitis B virus ([14]. Copyright [2004] Massachusetts Medical Society. All rights reserved)

The proteins, synthesized at the endoplasmic reticulum (ER), are phosphorylated, translocated across the ER membrane with complex transmembrane topology, and then bud from intracellular membranes located between the ER and golgi apparatus [15]. In addition to budding to form the viral envelope that surrounds the viral capsid, the surface proteins also bud from post-ER/pre-golgi membrane to form subviral particles which do not contain the viral capsid or genome. These subviral particles come in two morphologies, a 20-nm spherical particle and filamentous particles of varying lengths [18]. Viral and subviral particles all contain the same surface proteins, making them all antigenic as the HBsAg, but the spherical particles contain lower amounts of the L protein than either the filamentous or viral particles [16]. These subviral particles can be found in the serum of infected individuals at concentrations up to 10,000 times higher than the actual viral particles, and are thought to modulate the host immune response in a fashion that is advantageous for survival of the virus [16].

The last protein of the HBV genome is termed X. This protein has been shown to be necessary for initiation of infection in vivo, but its exact function and role in the viral life cycle is unclear. Proposed actions of X include activation of host and viral genes, stabilization of viral RNA, and stimulation of signal transduction [2].

42.2.3 Hepatitis B Virus Pathogenesis

Although HBV is hepatotropic, the virus is not directly cytotoxic to hepatocytes; this is supported by the large numbers of HBV carriers with detectable intra-hepatic virus replication who remain asymptomatic and do not progress to cirrhosis [19]. Rather, the liver inflammation and damage seen with HBV infection is a result of the host immune response. It is known that HBV DNA serum levels rapidly and dramatically decrease prior to onset of clinical symptoms of hepatitis [20]. Because the symptoms of hepatitis and the concurrent rise in biomarkers of liver damage, such as alanine aminotransferase (ALT), are caused by immune-mediated hepatocyte damage and lysis, this means that the clearance of viral DNA is accomplished in a non-cytotoxic fashion. To accomplish this, both innate and adaptive immune responses play a role. As part of the innate immune response, hepatocytes contain toll-like receptors (TLRs) that respond directly to viral particles by producing pro-inflammatory mediators including interleukin-6 (IL-6) and interferon alpha and beta (IFN-α/β), which serve to inhibit viral protein synthesis and recruit antigen presenting cells (APCs) in the liver including Kupfer cells (macrophages residing in the liver) and dendritic cells (DCs) [21, 22]. Antigen presenting cells then produce interleukin-12 (IL-12), interleukin-18 (IL-18), chemokine CCL3, and tumor necrosis factor α (TNF-α) that serve to activate natural killer (NK) and natural killer T cells (NKT) which produce interferon gamma (IFN-γ); IFN-γ then inhibits HBV replication and further recruits inflammatory cells to the liver [20, 23].

The adaptive immune response in acute infection involves CD4+ T lymphocytes, CD8+ lymphocytes, and B lymphocytes with antibody production. Once again, Kupfer cells and DCs are important as APCs to present foreign HBV antigen as stimulus and maturation signals for HBV-specific T cells, which are present in the serum prior to the onset of clinical symptoms of HBV infection, suggesting that they also play a role in non-cytotoxic viral clearance [19]. Platelets have also been identified as mediators of the immune response in that activated platelets recruit cytotoxic lymphocytes to the liver; in animal models, nonfunctioning platelets or platelet depletion was associated with reduction in hepatocyte death supporting platelet activation's role in recruiting cytotoxic cells [24]. Mature CD8+ T cells are the main effector cells of HBV clearance via both cytolytic and non-cytolytic mechanisms and are the main producers of IFN-γ [19]. IFN-γ and TNF-α inhibit viral replication by destabilizing or inhibiting viral capsid formation and degrading viral RNA and proteins [25]. HBV-specific CD8+ T cells recognize several viral epitopes including core protein, surface protein, and viral polymerase, and have several receptors for each epitope, which in theory helps to reduce virus escape of immune surveillance via mutation [19]. The appearance of CD8+ T cells, both specific and nonspecific for HBV coincides with an increase in serum ALT indicating T cell mediated hepatocyte damage and lysis [19]. Hepatocytes are destroyed by direct engagement by CD8+ T cells and by nonspecific anti-inflammatory response involving oxygen radicals, TNF, and proteases [14]. In chronic infections, persistent antigen stimulation of the immune system causes CD8+ T cells to produce less antiviral IFN-γ but does not decrease their cytotoxic capacities, leading to less viral clearance but continued hepatocyte destruction [24].

CD4+ T cells are more often specific to the HBV core protein than other viral proteins and are important in maintaining functional CD8+ T cells and inducing B-cell production of HBV-specific antibodies. B cells produce antibodies to core protein (HBcAg), surface protein (HBsAg), and e antigen (HBeAg) which are important in clearing circulating viral particles. Antibodies are produced from early in the infection, but their detection in the circulation by standard laboratory assays will not occur until after clearance of viral antigens because the circulating antibodies are complexed with the excess of antigen in the serum [26]. HBsAb provides protective immunity in the event of future infection and serves as the protective element in vaccinated individuals.

Development of chronic infection is due to an ineffective immune response that fails to clear the virus. In chronic infection, CD8+ T cells have been described as "partially tolerant" to the viral infection and they have a decreased ability to produce the viral-clearing IFN-γ [21]. Viral characteristics that influence immune response include presence or absence of HBeAg; when present, lower levels of expression of TLRs on hepatocytes, Kupfer cells, and peripheral monocytes were found leading to decreased production of TNF-α, while the absence of HBeAg was associated with increased expression of TLRs as compared with controls [27]. The HBV X protein has been found to up-regulate class I major histocompatibility complexes on hepatocytes which are necessary for antigen presentation and may aid in immune recognition of the virus, but they also serve to recruit immune cells to the liver to perpetuate inflammation and liver injury and perhaps lead to disease progression [28].

42.2.4 *Natural History of Hepatitis B Virus Infection*

Hepatitis B virus is transmitted via percutaneous and mucous membrane exposure to serum, semen, and saliva, although infection due to oral exposure to HBsAg-positive saliva has not been documented [29]. Mechanisms of transmission include injection with contaminated equipment, occupational needlesticks, tattooing, body piercing, intravenous drug use, transfusion of contaminated blood products (although this is rare since screening for HBsAg has become routine), perinatal exposure of mucous membranes to infected blood, sexual intercourse, and even long-term nonsexual contact among household contacts of persons chronically infected [29]. Sexual transmission is an important route of infection for homosexual men and heterosexual men and women; factors associated with increased risk of contracting the virus via sexual contact include increased number of sexual partners, number of years of sexual activity, history of other sexually transmitted diseases, and receptive anal intercourse [30]. HBV can also survive on environmental surfaces for greater than 7 days and remain viable such that exposure can occur through non-intact skin coming in contact with these surfaces [31]. The route of transmission varies depending on geography and endemicity of infection in the region. In Southeast Asia and sub-Saharan Africa, where infection rates are high, most people become infected during the perinatal period or during childhood [32]. In areas with intermediate prevalence of HBV infection including the Middle East, Russia, and Eastern Europe, infection occurs in a mixed pattern involving infants, children, and adults [32]. For regions with low endemicity of HBV infection, which include the USA, Western Europe, and Australia, HBV is most often contracted as an adult via engagement in high-risk activities including intravenous drug use, men who have sex with men (MSM), and heterosexuals with multiple partners [32]. HBV is 50–100 times more infectious than HIV, whereas hepatitis C virus is only 10 times more infectious than HIV (Fig. 42.3) [32–34].

Primary infection with HBV can be either symptomatic or asymptomatic. Symptomatic infection occurs in only 30–50% of infected adults and presents with fever, malaise, jaundice, anorexia, nausea, and right upper quadrant pain [35]. Symptomatic infection occurs more often in adults than children who are acutely infected, due to the immune immaturity of children preventing the immune-mediated liver damage that is seen in adults. After 4–10 weeks of incubation, HBsAg begins to rise in the serum 2–5 weeks prior to onset of symptoms, and peaks during or shortly after the symptoms begin [36]. Antibodies to HBsAg become detectable around the time of disease convalescence, and there is often a period of time after

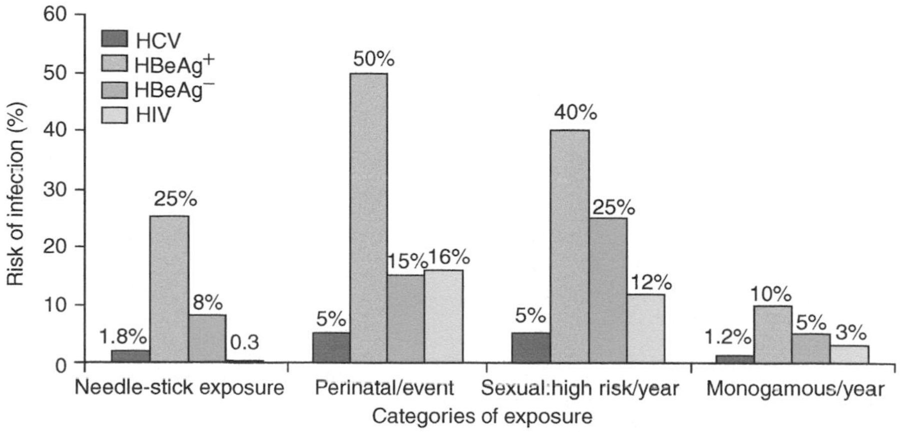

Fig. 42.3 Risk of transmission of hepatitis B virus, hepatitis C virus, and human immunodeficiency virus via different methods of exposure ([34]. Copyright [2008]. With permission from *The Lancet*)

clearance of HBsAg before HBsAb is detectable, which is referred to as the window period. The presence of HBsAb in the serum is a marker of disease recovery and immunity to future infection. IgG and IgM antibodies to the core antigen appear just before the onset of symptoms and may be the only serologic evidence of HBV infection during the window period [26]. HBsAg and IgM anti-HBcAg are the most reliable markers of acute HBV infection; IgG anti-HBcAg may persist in the serum for years [37]. HBeAg appears around the same time as HBsAg but disappears sooner, beginning around the height of clinical and biochemical evidence of hepatitis. Presence of HBeAg in the serum correlates with high viral titers and active viral replication in close to 100% of hepatocytes, and thus is associated with high rates of viral transmission, both vertically and horizontally [25, 38]. Antibodies to HBeAg arise shortly after the HBeAg disappears, which occurs during the height of clinical infection. This HBeAg seroconversion does not occur in people who progress to chronic viral hepatitis, and thus its disappearance is associated with resolution of acute infection. Amongst adults with a symptomatic acute HBV infection, 0.5–1% will develop acute liver failure, also known as fulminant hepatic failure; from any cause, this diagnosis carries a mortality rate of about one out of three patients, and liver transplantation is often the only cure [39–41]. It is postulated that clinical outcome of viral infection, including development of fulminant hepatic failure and chronic hepatitis, varies amongst viral genotypes and may be associated with mutations and variations in the pre-core gene and the promoter region for the core protein [39].

The risk of chronic infection depends on the age at the time of viral contraction; 90% of infants and 25–50% of children aged 1–5 years become chronically infected, whereas 95% of infected adults completely recover from acute infection and do not develop chronic HBV [42]. Most HBV infections in infants are contracted at the time of delivery rather than while in utero. If the mother is HBsAg and HBeAg positive, the rate of neonatal infection is about 90%, whereas if the mother has anti-HBeAg antibodies, the rate of transmission decreases to 30% but is associated with higher rates of symptomatic acute or fulminant hepatitis in the infant thought to be related to mutant HBeAg-negative virus strains [43]. The high rate of chronic infection in infants is believed to be due to immune tolerance to the viral antigens by the developing immune system; since viral clearance requires a robust immune response, which also leads to a symptomatic acute infection, infants are likely to progress to chronic infection, but they rarely experience a symptomatic acute infection [44].

Persistent or chronic infection with HBV has been divided into several phases based on immunologic markers and disease activity; evaluation of hepatitis serologies will determine the status and phase of the infection (Fig. 42.4, Table 42.1) [1, 14]. The first phase

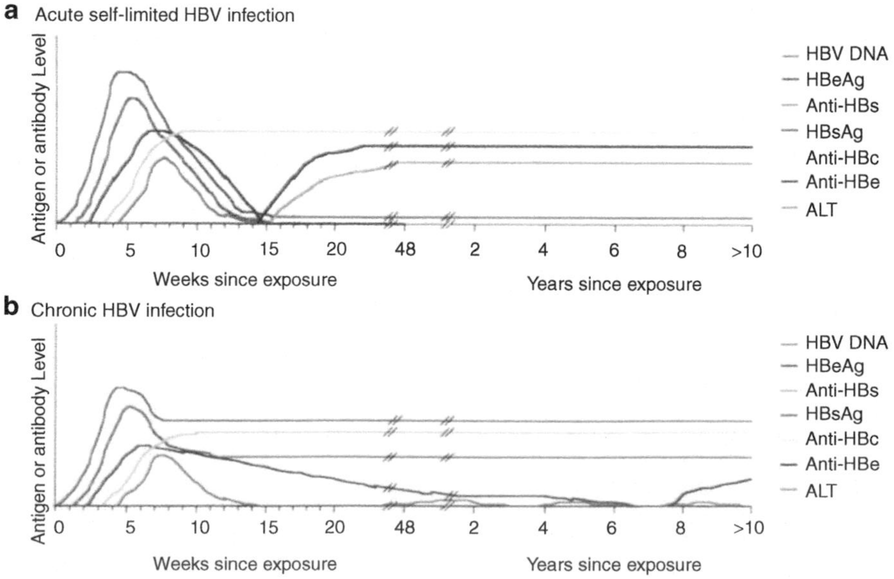

Fig. 42.4 Patterns of serologic and molecular markers in HBV infection ([14]. Copyright [2004] Massachusetts Medical Society. All rights reserved)

Table 42.1 Interpretation of hepatitis B serologic test results

Tests	Results	Interpretation
HBsAg Anti-HBc Anti-HBs	Negative Negative Negative	Susceptible
HBsAg Anti-HBc Anti-HBs	Negative Positive Positive	Immune due to natural infection
HBsAg Anti-HBc Anti-HBs	Negative Negative Positive	Immune due to hepatitis B vaccination
HBsAg Anti-HBc IgM anti-HBc Anti-HBs	Positive Positive Positive Negative	Acutely infected
HBsAg Anti-HBc IgM anti-HBc Anti-HBs	Positive Positive Negative Negative	Chronically infected
HBsAg Anti-HBc Anti-HBs	Negative Positive Negative	Interpretation unclear; four possibilities: 1. Resolved infection (most common) 2. False-positive anti-HBc, thus susceptible 3. "Low level" chronic infection 4. Resolving acute infection

(Adapted from "A comprehensive immunization strategy to eliminate transmission of hepatitis B virus infection in the United States: recommendations of the advisory committee on immunization practices. Part I: Immunization of infants, children, and adolescents. MMWR **54**(RR-16) (2005))
www.cdc.gov/hepatitis/HBV/HBVfaq.htm#general

is defined by immune tolerance, which is mostly seen in infants or young children who acquire the infection; this phase is asymptomatic and not associated with liver disease despite active viral replication [41]. The second phase is much like acute self-limited infection as described above involving immune-mediated liver injury manifest as elevation of serum aminotransferases and histologic evidence of active inflammation and fibrosis, and is referred to as HBeAg-positive chronic hepatitis [41]. Most people in this phase, as in acute self-limited infection, remain asymptomatic, but flares of hepatitis may occur with elevations of aminotransferases suggesting immune-mediated destruction of infected hepatocytes, and many times a flare will precede seroconversion to HBeAg negativity [21]. HBeAg seroconversion is an important milestone in chronic HBV infection, because after becoming negative for HBeAg, liver disease may be halted or even reversed [41]. Patients with persistently positive HBeAg are also known to progress to the development of hepatocellular carcinoma (HCC) without ever developing cirrhosis, although this occurrence is fairly rare [45]. Older age, higher levels of serum aminotransferases, and certain viral genotypes, for instance genotype B as compared with C in Asia, are all associated with higher rates of spontaneous HBeAg seroconversion; seroconversion occurs at a rate of 10–20% annually in HBeAg-positive chronically infected people [41]. Once seroconverted to anti-HBeAg status, up to 10–17% of patients revert at some time to being seropositive for HBeAg, which comes with the possibility of associated hepatitis flares [46].

After seroconversion, there are two phases that a person can enter: inactive HBsAg carrier status or HBeAg-negative chronic hepatitis. Inactive HBsAg carriers tend to have less active hepatitis with low aminotransferases, low levels of viral DNA, and low rates of progression to cirrhosis; 70–80% of these inactive carriers remain asymptomatic for their lifetime [47, 48]. Delayed spontaneous clearance of HBsAg from the serum occurs at a mean rate of 1% per year in Western countries and 0.8% in Asian countries, but this seroconversion is not completely protective from developing cirrhosis or HCC [49–51]. HBeAg-negative chronic hepatitis is defined by a fluctuating disease course involving flares and quiescence which may escape clinical recognition for years, but generally is associated with severe and progressive disease [41].

42.2.5 Non-hepatic Manifestations of Hepatitis B Virus

One of the more serious non-hepatic complications of HBV is polyarteritis nodosa (PAN). PAN occurs in 1–5% of HBV-infected people and is seen more commonly in North American and Europe where HBV tends to be contracted as an adult; in Asia where HBV infection typically occurs perinatally there is no association of HBV with PAN [52, 53]. Prior to widespread use of the vaccine for HBV in the 1980s, one-third to one-half of PAN cases were associated with HBV, but the percentage has declined to less than 10% since the 1990s [54]. PAN typically presents within 1 year of infection with HBV and has a wide range of clinical manifestations including fever, weight loss, peripheral neuropathy, arthritis, GI symptoms ranging from pain and diarrhea to bowel infarction and perforation, dermatologic symptoms such as painful subcutaneous nodules, livedo reticularis, digital gangrene and ulceration, nephrotic syndrome and glomerulonephritis, hypertension, congestive heart failure, anemia and leukocytosis; mortality rates for untreated PAN range from 30% to 50% [52, 54]. Histologically, PAN is characterized by fibrinoid necrosis of small- to medium-sized vessels leading to microaneurysms, stenosis, and occlusion [55]. The symptoms of HBV-associated PAN are similar to typical PAN (not associated with HBV), but unlike typical PAN, HBV-associated cases are rarely positive for antineutrophil cytoplasm antibodies (ANCA) [56]. The pathogenic factor in HBV-associated PAN is somewhat controversial; deposition of immune complexes (IC) is a widely accepted pathogenetic mechanism, but evidence also exists to support the role of HBeAg and correlation with fluctuating titers of HBsAg and anti-HBsAg [53].

An association between HBV and glomerulonephritis exists and is seen mostly in children from HBV endemic regions. In children it presents as nephrotic syndrome, rarely causes renal failure, and spontaneous remission occurs in 85% by 2 years and 95% by 5–7 years [55]. In contrast, as many as one-third of adults with HBV-associated glomerulonephritis have a slowly progressive disease course that can lead to renal failure and the need for hemodialysis [53]. The pathogenesis is related to immune complex deposition. Membranous glomerulonephritis (MGN) is the most common form seen, especially in children, and is associated with capillary wall deposits of HBeAg thought to result from in situ production of IC due to the formation of auto-antibodies to intrinsic glomerular antigens [55]. In adults, membranoproliferative glomerulonephritis (MPGN) is more common and occurs as a result of capillary and mesangial deposition of circulating immune complexes mostly consisting of HBsAg and anti-HBsAg complexes, although HBeAg and HBcAg have also been identified in MPGN [53, 55]. Mesangial proliferative glomerulonephritis, an immunoglobulin A-associated glomerulonephritis, has been described, but its association with HBV is controversial. The presence of ongoing chronic liver disease, HBV antigenemia, and identification of HBV antigens in glomerular deposits by immunohistochemical staining confirm the diagnosis of HBV-associated glomerulonephritis [57].

A serum sickness-like syndrome is seen in as many as 10–30% of HBV infections during the prodromal phase of infection in the 1–6 weeks preceding onset of clinical hepatitis [53]. This syndrome is also known as arthritis-dermatitis because clinically it manifests as an arthritis often mistaken for rheumatoid arthritis with bilateral, symmetrical joint swelling and pain associated with morning stiffness, and skin manifestations ranging from urticaria, maculopapular eruption, petechiae, purpura, erythema multiforme, and lichenoid dermatitis [53]. Once again, IC are implicated in the pathogenesis; relative excess of antigens creating soluble ICs correlates with disease activity and resolution of symptoms is seen as antibody titers rise making ICs less soluble and more easily cleared [58].

42.2.6 Coinfection with Hepatitis B Virus and Human Immunodeficiency Virus

It is estimated that 40 million people worldwide are infected with human immunodeficiency virus (HIV), and 2–4 million of these people (5–10%) are also chronically infected with HBV [32]. These viruses are seen infecting the same people so frequently due to their shared modes of transmission – via percutaneous and mucous membrane contact with blood or body fluids containing blood. Geographic differences in modes of transmission and endemicity of the infections are key to note when considering the epidemiology of coinfection. For instance, in sub-Saharan Africa there is a high rate of neonatal and childhood transmission of HBV leading to an increased likelihood of developing chronic HBV infection; couple this with the fact that sub-Saharan Africa accounts for greater than half of the world's HIV infections, which are mostly transmitted through heterosexual contact, and you will find a high prevalence of coinfection with HIV and HBV [32]. In contrast, in Western Europe and the USA there is low prevalence of both HIV and chronic HBV infection, and both are predominately spread through sexual contact and injection drug use. For this reason, it makes sense that in HIV-infected persons, the prevalence of chronic HBV infection is greater than tenfold that seen in persons uninfected with HIV (6–14% as compared to <1%) [32]. Because coinfection with HIV and HBV is quite frequent and both replicate by reverse transcription, there has been much interest in how the presence of one viral infection and the treatment of it affects the disease course of the other. It is believed that HBV infection has little influence over HIV disease course. Studies have shown that coinfection with HBV does not affect the incidence of developing AIDS, nor does it affect the rise in CD4 count and decline in HIV viral load (in the long-term) after institution of highly active antiretroviral therapy (HAART) [59, 60]. On the other hand, both HIV infection and HAART have an impact on the disease progression of HBV. Coinfection with HIV leads to lower rates of seroconversion from HBeAg to HBeAb positivity by 60% [61, 62]. This decreased clearance of HBV is thought to be due to the reduced immune function caused by HIV infection preventing an adequate immune response to HBV. In this same vein, some studies have shown less necro-inflammation of the liver and higher levels of HBV replication in HIV and HBV coinfected individuals; lower CD4 counts have been correlated with less serologic evidence of liver damage and higher rates of reactivation of HBV [63, 64]. Initiation of HAART causes immune reconstitution which in turn leads to improved control of HBV replication and an associated flare of hepatitis. Liver injury can also occur in HBV and HIV coinfected patients as a result of the hepatotoxicity of certain antiretroviral drugs [63]. HAART regimens containing lamivudine, a nucleoside analog reverse transcriptase inhibitor used to treat HIV and HBV independently, have been shown to reduce aminotransferases in the serum and reduce the risk of liver-related morbidity and mortality in coinfected patients as compared to HAART regimens without lamivudine [65]. Lamivudine has not been shown to prevent infection with HBV though [66].

42.2.7 Treatment of Chronic Hepatitis B Virus

Ideally, the treatment of HBV infection is aimed at decreasing progressive liver disease and the development of cirrhosis, liver failure, hepatocellular carcinoma, and death, but no randomized controlled trials of anti-HBV treatment to date have demonstrated significant impact on death or development of HCC [67]. Persons in whom treatment is indicated include those with acute liver failure, complications of cirrhosis, receiving immunosuppressive therapy, reactivation of chronic HBV, and infants born to HBsAg-positive mothers, and is perhaps indicated during the immune-active phase of infection [67]. For patients in the immune-tolerant phase of infection, who are inactive carriers with low viral replication, and those who are HBsAg-negative but with detectable viral DNA, treatment of HBV is not routinely indicated [67]. The decision to initiate treatment is guided by serum alanine aminotransferase (ALT) and HBV DNA levels. Definite indications to treat include ALT elevated at one to two times the upper limit of normal and HBV DNA levels greater than 20,000 IU/mL in HBeAg-positive patients and greater than 2,000 IU/mL in HBeAg-negative patients [68]. Patients with normal ALT levels and HBV DNA levels greater than 20,000 IU/mL often respond poorly to treatment and a liver biopsy should be considered when deciding to initiate treatment to look for histologic evidence of disease activity, especially if they are older than 35–40 years of age [68]. Regardless of the viral DNA load, patients with decompensated cirrhosis are candidates for treatment. Goals of therapy include reduction in serum levels of HBV DNA and seroconversion to absence of HBeAg and presence of anti-HBeAg.

Medications for HBV infection approach the virus in two ways: enhancement of the host immune response and inhibition of viral replication. Currently there are seven approved drugs for treating HBV which include two immune modulators, interferon alpha-2b and peg interferon alpha-2a, and five antiviral medications, lamivudine, adefovir, entecavir, telbivudine, and tenofovir [68]. Lamivudine, telbivudine, and entecavir are nucleoside analog reverse transcriptase inhibitors while tenofovir and adefovir are nucleotide analog reverse transcriptase inhibitors. The first-line agents are peg interferon alpha-2a, entecavir, and tenofovir based upon their favorable resistance profiles, efficacy, and tolerability. Peg interferon is associated with higher rates of adverse drug effects than the reverse transcriptase inhibitors that include flu-like symptoms, headache, insomnia, depression, nausea, anorexia, diarrhea, neutropenia, and thrombocytopenia. Lamivudine is associated with the highest rates of developing viral resistance, the incidence of which increases with duration of therapy and approaches

70% after 4 years of treatment [68, 69]. As other antivirals are also associated with resistance, especially telbivudine and adefovir, a rise in HBV DNA during treatment should prompt genotypic testing and adjustment of the medication regimen accordingly.

Treatment for HIV-coinfected individuals should always involve combination therapy due to the risk of resistance mutations occurring in both viruses; combination therapy options include either tenofovir and emtricitabine or tenofovir and lamivudine [70]. As emtricitabine, tenofovir, and lamivudine all have activity against both HBV and HIV, discontinuation of any of these medications as part of antiretroviral therapy can be associated with a flare of HBV activity necessitating close monitoring and possible addition of peg interferon alpha-2a, adefovir, or telbivudine as prevention [70]. If treatment of HBV is desired but it is not desired or possible to treat HIV, peg interferon alpha-2a is recommended [70]. In HBeAg-positive patients, treatment should be continued for 1 year after seroconversion of HBeAg and viral DNA is undetectable, while patients who undergo HBeAg seroconversion and have detectable but stable levels of DNA should be treated for an additional 6 months after seroconversion at which time treatment is discontinued if they remain negative for HBeAg; patients who fail to seroconvert to HBeAg negativity should receive long-term therapy because their chance for seroconversion increases with duration of treatment [68]. For HBeAg-negative patients, peg interferon treatment for 1 year versus 4–6 months is associated with improved sustained virologic response and is thus recommended [68]. Because flares of HBV are common in HBeAg-negative chronic HBV infection, long-term therapy with the antiviral reverse transcriptase inhibitors is recommended because they decrease rates of relapse [68].

42.3 Hepatitis D Virus

42.3.1 The Virus

Hepatitis D virus (HDV) was discovered in 1977 while Rizzetto and his colleagues were studying HBV antigen-antibody systems in blood and the liver [71]. HDV is an RNA virus belonging to the genus *Deltavirus* that depends on hepatitis B virus for infectivity, and thus is only capable of infecting a host that is also infected with HBV. It is estimated that approximately 5% of HBsAg carriers around the world are also infected with HDV leading to a total of 10–15 million HDV infected people worldwide [72]. There are three HDV genotypes termed I, II, and III. Type I is found worldwide and is the predominant genotype in North America and Europe, while genotype II is exclusively found in Taiwan and Japan, and genotype III is only found in South America and is associated with particularly severe disease [73].

42.3.2 Structure and Life Cycle

HDV is an enveloped spherical particle measuring 35–37 nm [74]. The outer envelope is composed of host lipid and HBsAg, and the inner viral particle consists of hepatitis D antigen (HDAg) and the viral RNA genome [74]. The HDAg is the only viral protein discovered to date, and is composed of a 27-kDA large HDAg and a 24-kDA small HDAg, both of which are translated from a single open reading frame [75].

Cellular binding and entry of HDV is mediated by HBsAg pre-S1 domain, as is the case in HBV infection [76]. Once in the cell, a 10 amino acid sequence from position 66 through 75 on the HDAg acts as the nuclear localization signal [77]. The HDV genome exists as a single strand of circular RNA that has significant Watson–Crick base-pairing internally such that it can collapse onto itself forming a linear rod in which 70% of the nucleotides are base-paired, and in this state undergoes replication in a double rolling circle [74]. The RNA replication, which does not require the aid of HBV, occurs in the host nucleus using host RNA polymerase II which normally functions to transcribe cellular mRNAs from DNA, but in the case of HDV is somehow used to create an anti-genomic copy of the viral RNA from an RNA template [78]. The anti-genomic RNA is initially linear in form but undergoes autocatalytic cleavage and ligation to form a unit length circular anti-genomic RNA; both genomic and anti-genomic RNA contain autocatalytic segments known as ribozymes [79]. The circular anti-genomic RNA serves as a template for transcription of genomic RNA that undergoes similar autocatalytic processing to take on its circular form [79]. From the genomic circular RNA a second anti-genomic RNA transcript is made. This is a linear, 800 base, polyadenylated mRNA that serves as the source of HDAg production in the cytoplasm [80]. Small HDAg is the product of translation of the unedited mRNA; editing of the mRNA by host double-strand RNA adenosine deaminase makes an adenosine-to-guanine change in the stop codon such that 19 additional amino acids are added to produce large HDAg [81, 82]. The small HDAg stabilizes the HDV RNA circle promoting viral replication while the large HDAg acts as a potent inhibitor of HDV replication [74, 83]. After the viral mRNA is edited, it can only produce large HDAg and thus viral replication ceases. The percentage of edited RNA is regulated such that approximately 30% of RNA in genotype I is edited and 15% of RNA is edited in genotype III [73]. The large HDAg is necessary for interaction with HBsAg and the formation of viral particles; this occurs via direct protein–protein interaction between HBsAg and HDAg, and only after the large HDAg has been isoprenylated [84].

42.3.3 Pathogenesis of Hepatitis D Virus Infection

The pathogenesis of liver disease in HDV infection is poorly understood despite the fact that biochemical markers of liver disease such as ALT are related to the level of viral replication [85]. A few studies have suggested that the small HDAg exerts cytotoxic effects on host hepatocytes, but the direct cytotoxicity of HDV remains unproven and is not thought to contribute to viral pathogenesis [72, 86, 87]. Just as the liver damage in HBV infection occurs via host immune response, immune-mediated liver damage is believed to account for the majority of clinical, biochemical, and histologic manifestations of HDV infection [72, 88]. The roles of cellular and humoral immune responses, and whether they are reacting to HBV antigens, HDV antigens or both, remain incompletely described.

42.3.4 Natural History of Hepatitis D Virus Infection

Hepatitis D virus infection can occur either simultaneously with HBV contraction (coinfection) or when a person with chronic HBV infection becomes exposed to HDV (superinfection) (Table 42.2) [72]. When a person becomes coinfected, HDV viremia follows shortly after the appearance of HBsAg in the serum, which reflects the dependence of HDV on HBV surface protein [72]. A bi-phasic elevation in serum ALT has been noted in coinfected individuals, but the

Table 42.2 Clinical features of hepatitis D virus coinfection and superinfection in hepatitis B virus carriers [72]

	Coinfection	Superinfection
HBV infection	Acute	Chronic
Outcomes	Recovery with seroclearance	Usually persistent infection
Markers	–	–
HBsAg	Positive, early and transient	Positive and persistent
IgM anti-HBc	Positive	Negative
Anti-HBs	Positive in recovery phase	Negative
HDV infection	Acute	Acute or chronic
Outcomes	Recovery with seroclearance	Usually persistent infection
Markers	–	–
Serum HDAg	Early and short-lived	Early and transient, undetectable later
Liver HDAg	Positive and transient	Positive, may be negative in late stages
Serum HDV RNA	Positive, early and transient	Positive, early and persistent
Anti-HDV	Late acute phase, low titer	Rapidly increasing, high titer
IgM anti-HDV	Positive, transient, pentameric	Rapidly increasing, high titers, monomeric

expression of HBsAg and HDV – whether sequentially or simultaneously – are both associated with elevation in ALT [72, 73, 89]. HDV may evoke a humoral immune response in the form of transient pentameric IgM, but because the HDAg is encapsulated and not exposed on the surface, the humoral response is likely not involved in clearing the virus and will not provide protection from future reinfection [72, 90]. The same is the case with acute HBV infection. Clinical manifestations of coinfection range from asymptomatic to fulminant hepatitis. Because HDV is dependent on HBsAg, once HBsAg is cleared, HDV also disappears from the serum. Similarly, because most acute HBV infections (in adults) do not become chronic, most acute coinfections with HDV and HBV also resolve without progressing to chronic infection. Coinfection due to HBV and HDV does not lead to higher rates of chronic infection than HBV infection alone; rather, the persistence of HDV infection may depend on the HBeAg/anti-HBeAg status of HBV infection [90].

Superinfection of HDV in a person with chronic HBV infection passes through several phases. First is the acute phase in which there is active HDV replication, HDV viremia, elevation in ALT, and suppression of HBV viremia (Fig. 42.5) [72, 85]. Chronic HDV infection, defined as hepatitis D viremia exceeding 6 months, entails a fluctuating but declining level of HDV viremia, the level of which correlates positively with levels of ALT [72]. During this period of HDV viral decline, HBV levels begin to rise. The chronic phase is followed by the late phase of infection during which development of cirrhosis and HCC can occur due to persistent viremia of either HBV, HDV or both, or else remission occurs with declining replication of both viruses [72]. Chronic HDV infection is defined serologically by the durable presence of IgM (monomeric in addition to the pentameric form seen in acute infection, a distinguishing factor of chronic infection) and IgG anti-HDAg [90]. Superinfection presents with an icteric illness and is associated with higher rates of fulminant hepatitis than in HBV-infected patients without HDV [92]. Despite this comparative increase in fulminant disease, studies have shown that it is a minority of superinfections that are rapidly progressive and severe, while the rest have a fairly stable disease course that is not significantly different from chronic HBV infection alone [73]. Following acute superinfection, 75–97% progress to a chronic HDV infection [85]. The rate of progression to cirrhosis 3 years after HDV superinfection approaches 10%, and after 5 years reaches its peak incidence at 21% [93]. Although this is faster than the rate of development of cirrhosis in patients infected with HBV only, at 10 years the total incidence of cirrhosis is not significantly different between the two groups [88]. Compared to chronic HBV infection alone and asymptomatic HBsAg carriers, patients who also have HDV infection have higher rates of clearance of HBeAg, which is thought to be due to suppression of HBV replication induced by HDV infection [94].

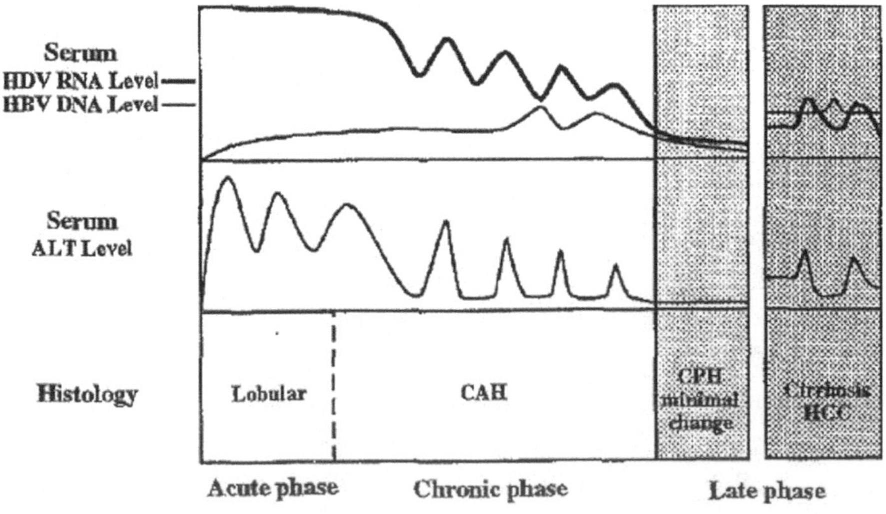

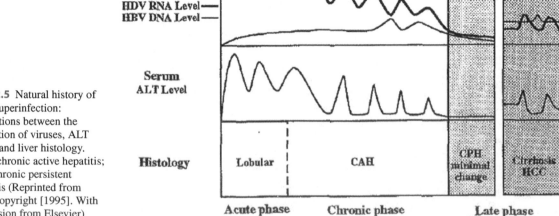

Fig. 42.5 Natural history of HDV superinfection: correlations between the replication of viruses, ALT levels, and liver histology. CAH, chronic active hepatitis; CPH chronic persistent hepatitis (Reprinted from [91]. Copyright [1995]. With permission from Elsevier)

42.3.5 Treatment of Hepatitis D Infection

Interferon and pegylated interferon are the only treatments effective against chronic HDV [72]. One study showed that high dose (nine million units) interferon alpha-2a given thrice weekly for 48 weeks induced normalization of ALT levels in 71% of patients during treatment, and was maintained in 50% of patients at six months of follow-up [95]. Other studies have shown that treatment with pegylated interferon alpha-2b induced sustained virologic response in 20–43% of patients after treatment for 53–72 weeks [96, 97]. No studies have shown any benefit in treating HDV with other medications that have been effective in treating viral hepatitis such as ribavirin or lamivudine. Current recommendations for treatment of hepatitis D, therefore, include high-dose standard interferon alpha-2a or pegylated interferon alpha-2b for at least 1 year's duration [98]. Treatment should be offered to all patients with well-compensated chronic HDV liver disease when the diagnosis is made; for patients with decompensated liver disease, transplantation is the only option [98].

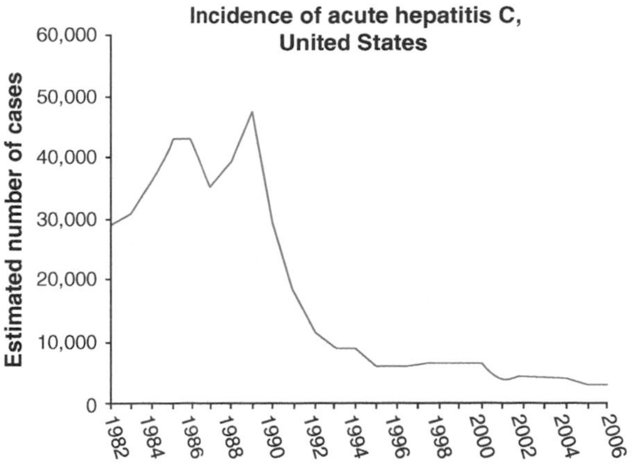

Fig. 42.6 Incidence of acute hepatitis C in the USA from 1982 through 2006 (Department of health and human services, Center for Disease Control. http://www.cdc.gov/hepatitis/Statistics.htm)

42.4 Hepatitis C Virus

42.4.1 The Virus

Hepatitis C virus (HCV) infection is the most common chronic blood-borne infection in the USA. According to the Center for Disease Control (CDC), approximately 3.2 million people are chronically infected [99]. Infection is most prevalent among those born from 1945 to 1965, the majority of whom were likely infected during the 1970s and 1980s when rates were highest. The CDC reported 802 confirmed cases of acute hepatitis C in 2006, but most patients with newly acquired hepatitis C infection actually do not present with an acute hepatic illness (Fig. 42.6) [99]. Because of this latency of the disease, it is estimated that the true number of new cases of hepatitis C was closer to 19,000 when accounting for underreporting and asymptomatic cases. Most populations in the Americas, Europe, and Southeast Asia have HCV prevalence rates of less than 2.5%, while in the Western Pacific regions and parts of South America, the prevalence rates are higher, between 2.5 and 4.9%. In contrast, in populations in the Middle East and Africa, HCV prevalence has been shown to range from 1% to 12% [100, 101]. The highest prevalence rates worldwide can be found in Egypt and Sweden. No study has found that there is an association between race, gender, age, socioeconomic background, or education for seroconversion.

HCV has been classified in the *Hepacivirus* genus within the *Flaviviridae* family, a family which also includes yellow fever and dengue viruses. HCV can be further divided into three major categories: genotypes, subtypes, and isolates, and the term quasispecies refers to the genetic heterogeneity of the HCV virus population that can coexist in one infected individual. At present, three main HCV genotypes and three to seven minor subtypes have been identified, although other genotypes have also been described. Genotype identification is particularly important for treatment options and prognosis; for instance, it has been found that patients infected with genotype 1b have a poorer response to IFN-alpha therapy than those infected with genotype 2 or 3 [99, 102]. In addition, some studies have shown an association between chronic infection, severe chronic hepatitis, and cirrhosis with subtype 1b [103]. The geographical distribution of these genotypes and subtypes varies significantly. The NHANES III study described the various genotypes found in the United States and reported that 56.7% of the current chronic HCV patients were classified as 1a, 17% as 1b,

3.5% as 2a, 11.4% as 2b, 7.4% as 3a, 0.9% as 4, and 3.2% as type 6. [104]

42.4.2 Structure and Life Cycle

HCV is a 55–65 nm spherical enveloped virus with delicate surface projections that contains a genome of a positive, single-stranded RNA molecule of about 9.6 kilobases which encodes a large polyprotein precursor of about 3,000 amino acids [105].

HCV mainly infects hepatocytes, but has also been found in B lymphocytes and dendritic cells. The envelope proteins are primarily responsible for viral entry to host cells, and several cell surface markers have been found that aid in viral entry. These surface markers, CD81, low density lipoprotein (LDL), scavenger receptor class B type I (SR-BI), DC-SIGN, L-SIGN, and heparin sulfate, interact with the envelope proteins to facilitate viral entry [106, 107]. Viral entry into host cells still remains to be fully elucidated, mainly due to the lack of technology that is able to identify when the hepatitis C virus is bound to the host cell surface. The current theory is that entry is lysosomally mediated by the interaction of the envelope proteins, mainly E2, with the various cell surface markers to trigger endocytosis of the viral particle. Viral interaction with cell surface markers is currently a subject of extensive research for they offer potential treatment options.

Once the virus has entered the cell, the virus is decapsidated, and the genomic HCV RNA is used both for polyprotein translation and replication in the cytoplasm. The virus does not contain a reverse transcriptase and the RNA does not ever integrate into the host genome [108]. Replication and posttranslational processing appear to take place in a membranous web made of the nonstructural proteins and host cell proteins. The genome is encapsulated in the endoplasmic reticulum and nucleocapsids are enveloped and matured in the Golgi apparatus before newly produced virions are released by exocytosis [109].

42.4.3 The Viral Genome

The single-stranded positive RNA genome of HCV contains three distinct regions. The first region contains a short 5′ non-coding sequence that contains two domains: a stem-loop structure involved in positive-strand priming during HCV replication, and the internal ribosome entry site (IRES) which is an RNA structure responsible for attachment of the ribosome and polyprotein translation. The second region contains a long, unique open reading frame (ORF) of more than 9,000 nucleotides which is translated into a precursor polyprotein that is secondarily cleaved to give birth to the structural proteins. The third region contains a short 3′ non-coding region principally involved in minus-strand priming during HCV replication [110].

The precursor polyprotein translated from the 9,000 nucleotide ORF undergoes processing that yields at least ten proteins: the core, envelope 1 (E1), envelope 2 (E2), p7, nonstructural (NS) 2, NS3, NS4A, NS4B, NS5A, and NS5B. The core protein is used to form the nucleocapsid around the viral genome (Fig. 42.7) [[111], [112]]. These HCV proteins not only function in viral replication but also affect a variety of cellular functions. The core protein is mainly responsible for altering various host cell functions, including causing up-regulation of various transcription factors [113]. The core protein has also been linked to changes in host immunity including down regulation of the cell regulatory cycle and antigen presentation [114]. It is also thought that the HCV core protein causes down-regulation of the host cell's ability to produce interferon, which enables viral evasion from hepatocyte response to infection. It is still unclear how specifically the core proteins and envelope proteins contribute to the overall progression to steatosis and cirrhosis.

42.4.4 Hepatitis C Virus Pathogenesis

Like hepatitis B, HCV is not considered to be directly cytotoxic. HCV infection leads to chronic inflammation of the liver and eventual fibrosis and cirrhosis, but the mechanism behind how the virus does this is still incompletely understood. It is generally accepted that liver damage in HCV infection is the result of the host immune response. Evidence to support this theory includes the temporal association of liver damage with the development of the host immune response as opposed to viral replication, the association of immunosuppression with normalization of transaminases

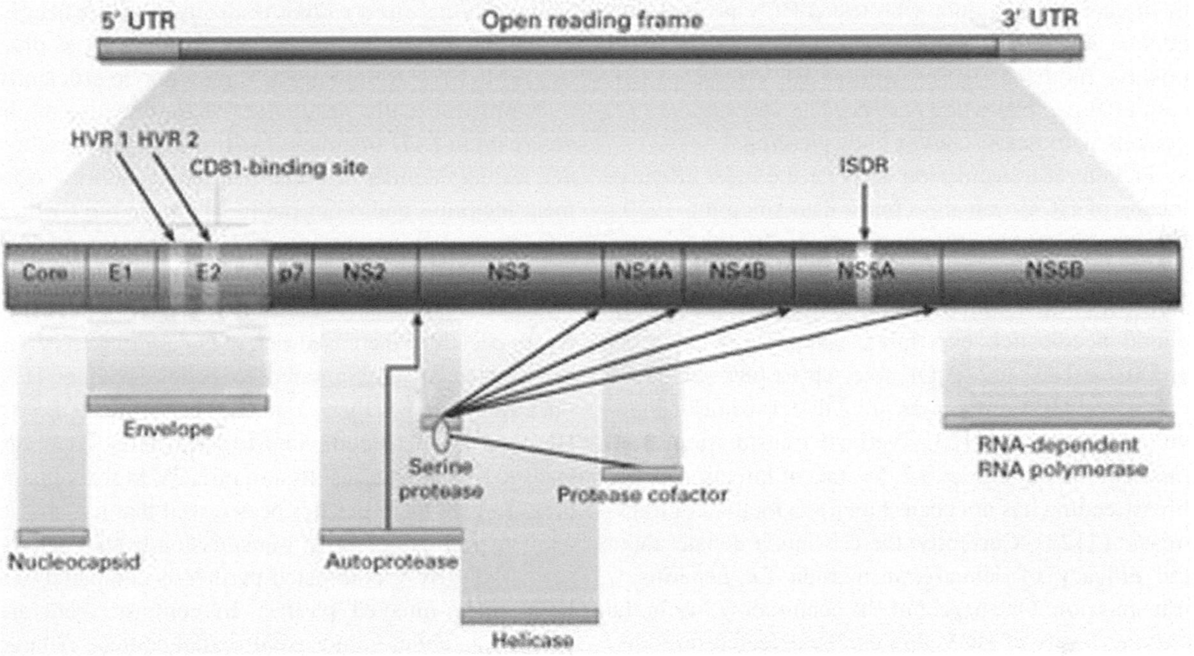

Fig. 42.7 The hepatitis C virus genome ([112]. Copyright [2001] Massachusets Medical Society. All rights reserved)

and an increase in viremia, and conversely, the removal of immunosuppression with a hepatitis flare [52]. CD8+ T lymphocytes are important mediators of cell death in viral infections, and are thought to also be an important effector of hepatocyte injury in HCV infection [52]. In response to liver injury, inflammatory processes soon ensue with neutrophil migration to the site. Chemotactant proteins, called chemokines, released from damaged cells aid in this process; these include interleukin (IL) 8 and macrophage inflammatory protein 1 (MIP-1) [115–117]. These chemokines recruit inflammatory cells including T lymphocytes, hepatocyte stellate cells (HSC), and Kupffer cells (liver specific macrophages) which in turn release more chemokines such as tumor necrosis alpha (TNF-α), interferon-gamma (IFN-γ) [118]. TNF-α leads to altered expression of cell adhesion molecules on sinusoidal endothelial cells, specifically a decrease of platelet–endothelial cell adhesion molecule and an increase of intercellular adhesion molecule-1, allowing the recruitment and sinusoidal transmigration of inflammatory cells [119, 120]. HSC are thought to be one of the main cells responsible for the fibrotic changes that occur in the liver by aiding in the activation of fibroblasts and myofibroblasts [121]. In addition, these chemokines act to induce apoptosis in the damaged cell and surrounding cells, and constant cell lysis causes a repetitive cycle of inflammatory cell recruitment and further tissue damage.

42.4.5 Natural History of Hepatitis C Virus Infection

The main form of transmission for hepatitis C virus remains parenterally; however, vertical transmission, sexual contact, and other forms have been reported. The following are populations that are at a higher risk for obtaining HCV: (1) current or former injection drug users, including those who injected only once many years ago; (2)recipients of clotting factor concentrates made before 1987, when more advanced methods for manufacturing those products were developed; (3) recipients of blood transfusions or solid organ transplants before July 1992, when better testing of blood donors became available; (4) chronic hemodialysis patients; (5) persons with known exposures to HCV, such as healthcare workers after needlesticks involving HCV-positive blood; (6) recipients of blood or organs from a donor who tested HCV-positive; (7) persons with HIV infection; (8) children born to HCV-positive mothers; (9) sex with an HCV infected person; (10) persons who share cocaine straws; and (11) persons with tattoos and/or body piercing.

Parenteral transmission is by far the most effective means of HCV transmission to date since the 1970s. Hepatitis C virus is approximately 10 times more infectious than HIV through percutaneous blood exposures. It is transmitted by 15–30 of every 1,000 accidental needlestick exposures, compared with 3 per 1,000 for HIV [122]. Of note, up to 68% of newly diagnosed HCV infections are a direct result of intravenous drug use [123]. Vertical transmission from mother to infant carries a 2–5% rate of infection, while breastfeeding has not been shown as a method of transmission [124]. Currently, there is much debate about the efficacy of sexual transmission for hepatitis C transmission. One aspect of the controversy lies in the varying levels of HCV that can be detected in bodily fluids and its role in actual infection. There have been several studies that address whether or not the virus is actually present in the bodily fluids that are exchanged during sexual contact. Some authors have not found any evidence of the virus in saliva and semen in patients that are chronically infected with HCV, while other studies have found the virus in semen [125, 126]. It is generally accepted that the HCV virion can be isolated in bodily fluids by PCR methods; however, the level of virion load can vary and to date there is no study that has accurately determined the viral load necessary to confer infectivity.

One study showed that sexual activity carries approximately 10–18% transmission rate for HCV in individuals who do not engage in intravenous drug use [127]. This study addressed individuals who had sexual contact within 6 months with a known HCV-infected individual. Studies looking at individuals who have multiple sexual partners or engage in high-risk sexual activity such as prostitution have been shown to have a higher risk of transmission, up to 18% [128]. Interestingly, this study also found that the partners of these high-risk individuals only showed a 6% HCV infectivity rate, which further confounds the effectiveness of sexual transmission. Other studies have addressed sexual transmission between stable partners and have found that sexual relations between stable partners carries no increased risk of infectivity [129, 130]. In addition, homosexual intercourse does not lead to an increased risk of transmission over heterosexual intercourse in the absence of intravenous drug use [131, 132]. Although HCV may not be efficiently transmitted sexually, persons at risk for infection might seek care in STD treatment facilities, HIV counseling and testing facilities, correctional facilities, drug treatment facilities, and other public health settings where STD and HIV prevention and control services are available.

There is still much debate about whether being HIV-positive leads to increased risk of contracting HCV via sexual contact as compared to people without HIV infection, and whether or not being coinfected with HIV and HCV, as compared to HCV monoinfection, leads to increased transmission of HCV to sexual partners. To date there has not been a trial that has shown an increased risk of HCV transmission from a heterosexual HIV/HCV coinfected partner as compared to a HCV mono-infected partner. In contrast, there are mixed data about homosexual sexual contact. A large retrospective study with over 1,800 patients found that there was a significantly increased risk of contracting HCV in patients infected with HIV as compared to patients without HIV; this was thought to be at least partially attributable to high-risk sexual activity and the increased likelihood that these patients also were infected with an ulcerative sexually transmitted infection, creating a portal of entry for HCV [133]. However, the CAESAR study suggested that there was not an increased rate of infectivity via homosexual contact in the absence of intravenous drug use [134].

Hepatitis C has predominantly three main outcomes; fulminant, acute, and chronic hepatitis. The majority of newly infected patients with hepatitis C viral infection are usually asymptomatic. As a result, very few cases of acute infection come to medical attention or are tested for HCV infection. Several estimates suggest that only 10–15% of cases present with jaundice which is the main sign that causes acute hepatitis C patients to present [135]. Symptoms other than jaundice may include mild constitutional symptoms such as nausea, loss of appetite, fatigue, and vague abdominal pain. Routine laboratory tests in acute infection may only reveal an alanine aminotransferase (ALT) which peaks below 1,000 IU/L, and the HCV RNA virus can be detected in blood within 1–3 weeks after exposure through polymerase chain reaction (PCR) (Fig. 42.8) [34], [135]. The average time from exposure to anti-HCV antibody formation, known as

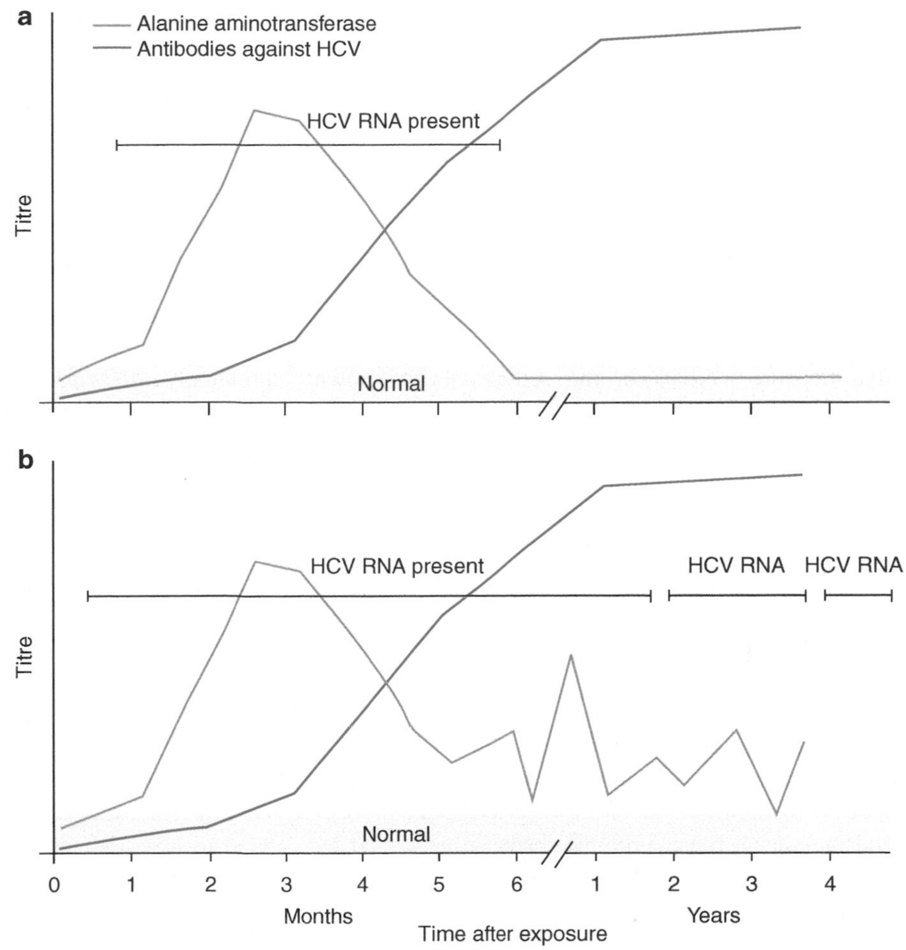

Fig. 42.8 Serologic pattern of hepatitis C virus infection with (**a**) recovery and (**b**) progression to chronic infection ([34]. With permission from *The Lancet*)

anti-HCV seroconversion, is roughly 8 weeks, with the antibody detectable in over 97% of exposed patients by 6 months after exposure. Because of the time it takes for the antibody to develop, the only reliable method to detect acute hepatitis C infection is through PCR.

Reports indicate that 15–30% of symptomatic acute hepatitis C patients go on to spontaneous viral clearance and recovery, and although there is no clear evidence as to why so few clear the infection, increased rates of spontaneous clearance have been associated with an acute infection that presents with jaundice [34]. The remainder of the patients go on to have chronic hepatitis. A vigorous immune response involving cytotoxic CD8 T lymphocytes and T-helper type 1 (Th1) CD4 lymphocytes that produce interferon-γ and interleukin 2 (IL-2) occurring within a week of infection is necessary for viral clearance, while a delayed and less robust response will lead to chronic infection [136, 137]. In contrast, a T-helper type 2 CD4 lymphocyte response with associated interleukin 4 (IL4) and interleukin 10 (IL10) is associated with viral persistence and chronic infection. Studies have shown that neutralizing antibodies to HCV epitopes are formed in patients with chronic HCV infection, but the role of these antibodies in clearing acute infection remains unclear and they have not been shown to protect from re-infection in a person who clears HCV and is then reexposed [138]. The mechanism of HCV evasion of the humoral immune response may include its extreme genetic diversity and the presence of quasispecies; some studies suggest that the viral envelope protein E2, which has a hypervariable region, may be of particular importance as an epitope for neutralizing antibodies, and via its variance explain the viral escape of humoral clearance [34, 138].

Hepatitis C induced fulminant hepatic failure is a very rare occurrence. Over 50% of fulminant hepatitis is secondary to viral causes, while the rest are mostly associated with hepatotoxic drugs [133]. To date, there are very little data that link fulminant hepatitis to hepatitis C virus, which is in contrast to the widespread data that support the association with hepatitis A and B viruses. However, there are case reports of hepatitis C-induced fulminant hepatitis, and thus HCV should be considered as a potential cause of fulminant hepatitis [139]. Fulminant hepatitis is characterized as massive hepatic necrosis in the setting of no known previous hepatic disease. Presentation of fulminant hepatitis includes jaundice, anorexia, malaise, and flu-like symptoms. Patients usually digress into fulminant hepatic failure rather quickly with bleeding diathesis, which can include hemorrhage into the gastrointestinal tract. Because the liver is also responsible for removing neurotoxic metabolites, obtundation and coma can also be present. The onset is very acute and carries a mortality of 85% and upwards. The mechanism of hepatitis C and other viral induced fulminant hepatitis still remains unknown. Two main theories have been developed as the potential pathogenic factors, the first is direct cytotoxic effect of the virus itself, and the second includes a hyper-immune response generated by the patient in response to the infection.

Chronic hepatitis C implies that an individual is infected with HCV for greater than 6 months. Persistence of infection is thought to be due to an ineffective immune response and viral evasion of immune elimination. Mechanisms of how the virus escapes immune elimination are postulated to include down-regulation of HLA gene expression necessary for viral antigen presentation, molecular mimicry, down-regulation of cytokine receptors and signaling pathways, evading cytotoxic T cell killing by reducing Fas expression or increasing genes that block apoptosis, infection of immunologically privileged sites, immune exhaustion or anergy, and mutation leading to epitope loss [111]. Chronic HCV infection develops in 70–85% of HCV-infected persons, and 60–70% of chronically infected persons have evidence of active liver disease [111]. Most of the patients with chronic hepatitis virtually never have any signs or symptoms to indicate infection unless they progress to advanced liver disease and cirrhosis, and 20–30% of people with chronic HCV infection have persistently normal levels of serum alanine aminotransferase (ALT) [140]. Because the liver is a regenerative organ, infected persons may have relatively little or no structural damage to the liver architecture in spite of persistent infection and viral replication. In fact, the only histological finding that may be present is inflammation. This is the reason why many infected patients are not diagnosed as having HCV unless specific testing is performed for some reason. The only clue that may be found to alert the clinician to the possibility of HCV infection is elevation of liver enzymes for greater than 6 months in duration. Cirrhosis is estimated to develop in 20–50% of chronically infected patients over the course of several decades [141]. Progression of cirrhosis has been found to have a significant positive correlation with elevated serum ALT levels, but having normal ALT levels does not indicate a completely benign disease course, because 5–15% of such patients are also found to have biopsy-proven cirrhosis [140].

42.4.6 Coinfection with HCV and HIV

Worldwide, about 25–30% of people with HIV are also infected with HCV [32]. HIV infection has been found to have deleterious effects on the disease progression of HCV. Serum levels of HCV RNA are significantly increased in patients with HIV/HCV coinfection compared to HCV infection alone, which is at least in part explained by the fact that in HIV-infected people, HCV replicates in lymphocytes, monocytes, and macrophages in addition to in hepatocytes [142]. A 20-year prospective study found that compared to HIV or HCV mono-infected patients, coinfected patients had significantly increased mortality from hepatitis and liver-related deaths as well as an increase in all-cause mortality [143]. Multiple studies have shown that HIV/HCV coinfected patients have a more rapid disease progression than their HCV mono-infected counterparts. One of these studies was a meta-analysis including over 7,000 patients that reported a relative risk of developing cirrhosis for coinfected individuals versus HCV mono-infected individuals of 2.5 for those not on HAART and 1.7 for those receiving HAART [144]. Other studies have noted that the increased rate of progression to liver fibrosis in coinfection is associated more specifically with a decreasing CD4 count (less than 300–500 cells/μL) [145, 146]. Explanations postulated for this association include an alteration in cytokine production caused by the relative shortage of CD4 T lymphocytes seen in HIV infection [146]. Another related finding is that in patients with cirrhosis from any cause who are HIV-seronegative, cirrhosis is also associated with a low CD4 T cell count, albeit a normal percentage of CD4 T cells [147]. This phenomenon is thought to be secondary to global sequestration of all cell lines seen in cirrhosis due to splenomegaly, and raises the question of whether the association of low CD4 count and cirrhosis in HIV/HCV coinfection is related to advanced HIV and its impact on HCV disease course, or if it is a consequence of the advanced liver disease. In addition, this brings to light an effect that advanced liver disease may have on the HIV disease course by causing a lower CD4 count, yet the interpretation of CD4 counts in patients with cirrhosis must take into account that the cirrhosis-related decrease in CD4 lymphocytes maintains a normal percentage of CD4 cells. For the most part though, studies have failed to demonstrate that HCV infection has a significant impact on the disease course of HIV. A small number of studies have shown that in HCV/HIV coinfected individuals there is faster progression to clinical AIDS or death and a blunted CD4 count response to HAART, but the majority of studies have found no significant difference in these markers of disease progression [142]. Antiretroviral medications have the potential to cause hepatotoxicity, seen most often with ritonavir; this particular side effect occurs more frequently in HIV/HCV coinfection than in those infected with HIV only, which may lead to more frequent discontinuation of HAART [142].

All patients with HIV that are found to also have HCV infection, demonstrated by HCV viremia, should be considered as candidates for anti-HCV treatment because of the increased rate of progression of liver disease seen with HIV/HCV coinfection [148]. Exceptions include patients with decompensated liver disease (which may be manifest as ascites, gastrointestinal bleed, or encephalopathy), patients with history of severe neuropsychiatric disease because of the neuropsychiatric side effects of interferon, and patients using illegal drugs or who are heavy consumers of alcohol. Patients with a CD4 count less than 350 cells/μL should first be started on HAART because of the increased risk for opportunistic infections caused by the decrease in CD4 counts and neutropenia that can be seen with interferon therapy [148]. For patients already on HAART who are to begin treatment for HCV, didanosine must be replaced with another medication because of the increased rates of didanosine-related lactic acidosis, pancreatitis, and decompensated cirrhosis in patients taking ribavirin, and AZT should be avoided because of the increased incidence of anemia seen when used in combination with ribavirin [102]. Treatment of HCV in coinfected individuals is the same as for HCV mono-infection (see below) with interferon and ribavirin, but the response rates thus far reported achieve only 15–35% sustained viral response (defined as undetectable viral load 6 months after the discontinuation of therapy) in HIV/HCV coinfected individuals as compared to 40–80% response in HCV mono-infected individuals [142, 148]. Reasons for this decreased response may include less activity of interferon and ribavirin in the setting of HIV-related immune dysfunction, more advanced liver fibrosis at initiation of treatment, higher rates of steatosis from alcohol or antiretroviral medications, lower initial HCV viral clearance, more frequent discontinuation due to side effects, and poorer medication compliance [148].

42.4.7 Non-hepatic Manifestations of Hepatitis C Virus

It is not uncommon for chronic hepatitis C to have manifestations outside of the liver. These conditions tend to occur with long-standing infection, and although symptoms may resolve with the treatment and clearance of HCV, sometimes the extra-hepatic manifestations have no correlation with viral disease activity. Certain of these manifestations, including mixed cryoglobulinemia, lymphoma, porphyria cutanea tarda, lichen planus and diabetes, have strong evidence for their association with HCV, while others such as thyroid disease, corneal ulcers, and fibromyalgia have less evidence that they are truly associated with HCV [149, 150].

One of the conditions with the best evidence for an association with HCV is mixed cryoglobulinemia. In fact, studies have found that 72–93% of individuals with cryoglobulinemia are also infected with HCV [151, 152]. This condition is caused by the presence of antibodies that precipitate at temperatures less than 37°C, and is thought to result from chronic viral stimulation of lymphocytes [151]. There are three main types of cryoglobulinemias: type I is comprised of monoclonal IgM molecules that complex with each other, type II is a combination of monoclonal IgM and polyclonal IgG antibodies, and type III is a combination of polyclonal IgM and polyclonal IgG. In type II and III, the IgM exhibits rheumatoid factor activity [150]. Hepatitis C leads to type II and III cryoglobulinemias, also called mixed cryoglobulinemias [153]. The antibodies circulate in the bloodstream, complex with one another, and deposit into small blood vessels. This leads to inflammation of the vessels known as leukocytoclastic vasculitis, and thus is recognized as one of the small vessel vasculitides. Laboratory evidence of the disease includes mixed cryoglobulins in the serum, high rheumatoid factor titer, and low levels of C4 complement [150]. Virtually any small vessels can be affected, and the most common clinical manifestations of cryoglobulinemia include glomerulonephritis, neuropathy, palpable purpura, sicca syndrome including xerophthalmia and xerostomia, arthralgias, Raynaud's phenomenon, and weakness, although asymptomatic cryoglobulinemia is also possible [151, 154]. Membranoproliferative glomerulonephritis (MPGN) is the specific type of glomerulonephritis associated with the cryoglobulinemia, which leads to complex deposition in the subendothelium. Seventy percent of the time it leads to a nephrotic-type picture; however, a mixed nephritic and nephrotic type picture can occur as well [149]. Renal involvement of cryoglobulinemia is associated with a significant decrease in survival, and renal failure due to glomerulonephritis has been reported to cause up to one-third of the deaths in patients with cryoglobulinemia [151].

Hepatitis C is also associated with non-Hodgkin's B cell lymphoma, which occurs as an evolution of cryoglobulinemia type II in about 10% of patients, as well as in patients without a history of cryoglobulinemia [149]. The reports of the percentage of non-Hodgkin's lymphoma (NHL) associated with HCV infection varies widely, ranging from 0% to 43%, and the association has a higher prevalence in southern Europe and southern USA as compared to the northern regions [149, 150]. Extra-nodal involvement is more common in HCV-associated NHL with the salivary glands, liver, and stomach being more frequently involved than in non-HCV NHL [149].

Porphyria cutanea tarda (PCT) is an uncommon extra-hepatic manifestation of HCV that is due to a deficiency of uroporphyrinogen decarboxylase; despite being uncommon, HCV is found in an average of 45% of patients with symptomatic PCT from studies conducted in different geographic locations [149]. It is thought that HCV infection triggers the clinical expression of PCT in predisposed people, the mechanism of which is unclear; clinical manifestations include increased skin fragility, ecchymosis, bullae, and blisters that may become hemorrhagic with sun exposure [149].

Lichen planus is another dermatologic manifestation of HCV infection, although its association may be stronger with liver disease in general than specifically with HCV [149]. Lichen planus is characterized by a dense lymphocytic infiltration of the upper dermis causing pruritic, polygonal, flat-topped violaceous papules and oral ulcers [155]. It is uncertain how HCV affects the development of lichen planus, but there have been reports of patients who develop lichen planus or have a flare of existing disease while receiving interferon alpha treatment [155].

Hepatitis C virus complicated by cirrhosis of the liver is associated with the development of non-insulin-dependent diabetes mellitus (NIDDM). NIDDM is seen in up to 24% of HCV-infected patients with cirrhosis, in comparison to only 9% of HBV-infected patients with cirrhosis, and there is a positive correlation of increasing severity of liver disease and the incidence of diabetes [156]. The development of NIDDM is multifactorial, and mechanisms include hyperinsulinemia and insulin resistance, decreased hepatic glucose uptake, stress response related to cirrhosis, and beta cell dysfunction [156].

42.4.8 Treatment

Patients with HCV viremia and compensated liver disease are candidates for treatment with pegylated interferon alpha and ribavirin, the current standard of care for HCV. Elevation of ALT is not requisite for initiation of therapy, nor is biopsy-proven evidence of fibrosis, although if moderate to severe fibrosis is found it should be considered a uniform indication for timely initiation of therapy [157]. Interferon causes inhibition of viral replication within host cells, activates natural killer cells, and increases antigen presentation to lymphocytes. The mechanism of action of ribavirin, a synthetic guanosine analogue, against HCV is controversial, but theories include induction of catastrophic mutations, a shift from a TH2 to a TH1 response with suppression of IL-10, depletion of intracellular guanosine triphosphate stores, and inhibition of cellular inosine monophosphate dehydrogenase activity [158]. Some of the side effects of interferon include flu-like symptoms, headache, insomnia, depression, hair loss, nausea, anorexia, diarrhea, neutropenia, and thrombocytopenia, while the side effects of ribavirin include rash, pruritus, dyspnea, dry cough, gout and hyperuricemia, nausea, diarrhea, and hemolytic anemia [157].

The current recommendation by the American Gastroenterological Association for treatment includes weekly injections of pegylated interferon, which is available in two forms (peg interferon-alpha 2b which is weight based or alpha 2a which is a fixed dose), and daily ribavirin [157]. This combination has been found to have a success rate for achieving sustained viral response (undetectable HCV RNA 6 months after the discontinuation of treatment) in 42–46% of patients with genotype 1 and in 76–82% of those with genotypes 2 and 3 [157].

The strongest predictor of response to treatment is infection with a genotype other than genotype 1, and therefore recommendations for treatment are dependent on genotype identification [159]. Duration of treatment for individuals with HCV genotype 2 and 3 is 24 weeks and includes 800 mg of ribavirin daily, while patients with genotype 1 and 4 need 48 weeks of therapy and a higher dose of ribavirin, 1,000–1,200 mg daily [158]. Other predictors of favorable response to treatment include HCV viral load less than 2 million copies/mL, absence of cirrhosis and bridging fibrosis, age less than 40 years and lighter body weight. Efficacy of treatment is monitored by checking the viral load after 12 weeks of therapy. If there is not a significant reduction in viral load, evidenced by at least a 2-$\log_{10}$ reduction of HCV RNA, there is only a 0–3% chance that sustained viral response will be achieved, while if this reduction is achieved, the likelihood of achieving sustained viral response approaches 70% [158]. Once sustained viral response has been achieved at 6 months, there is a 98% chance that response will be maintained indefinitely. For those who fail to achieve a reduction of viral load by 2-$\log_{10}$ at 12 weeks, therapy may be continued anyhow, as histologic benefit can be seen in the absence of viral clearance [158].

42.5 Complications of Chronic Hepatitis Infection

42.5.1 *Cirrhosis*

Cirrhosis is a late-stage consequence in the natural history of hepatitis B, C, or coinfection with B and D due to repeated liver injury leading to fibrosis of liver parenchyma, usually occurring after decades of chronic inflammation. Hepatic stellate cells are the main effector cell of hepatic fibrosis. They are stimulated by reactive oxygen species, apoptosis of hepatocytes, TLRs, and paracrine stimulation by Kupfer cells; once activated they transform from a quiet cell that stores vitamin A to a myofibroblast [160]. As a myofibroblast, contraction of stellate cells contributes to increases in portal resistance [160]. During the process of fibrosis, the extracellular matrix changes in composition from collagen type IV, heparin sulfate proteoglycan and laminin to being rich in fibril-forming collagen I and III; this change is driven by transforming growth factor beta (TGF-β) amongst other stimuli [160].

Although initial hepatic fibrosis can be reversible and asymptomatic, progression to cirrhosis brings a slew of clinical consequences. A small contracted liver leads to increased portal pressures which are transmitted in a retrograde manner to cause splenomegaly, gastric and esophageal varices, hemorrhoids, and caput medusa. Decreased synthetic capacity of the liver leads to hypoalbuminemia and associated decrease in oncotic pressure leading to accumulation of fluid in extravascular spaces, frequently manifest as ascites. Also a consequence of decreased synthetic function is low levels of coagulation factors and platelets leading to easy bruising and bleeding. In addition, the liver is one of the organs responsible for androgen metabolism. Consequently, cirrhotic patients have increase in basal estrogen levels that will cause gynecomastia in males, palmar erythema, and spider telangiectasias. Hepatorenal syndrome is a feared consequence caused by renal arterial vasoconstriction in response to decreased intravascular volume; this syndrome can lead to renal failure [161]. Hepatic encephalopathy is a state of altered mental status induced by the decreased clearance of metabolic encephalotoxins by the liver, including ammonia.

In chronic HBV infection, patients who are HBeAg-positive have a rate of progression to cirrhosis ranging from 2% to 5% annually while in HBeAg-negative chronic hepatitis, cirrhosis occurs at a rate of 8–10% per year [41]. High levels of viral replication and HBV DNA in the serum, regular alcohol use and coinfection with hepatitis C virus, hepatitis D virus or human immunodeficiency virus are all associated with development of cirrhosis in people infected with HBV [41]. In patients with both HBV and HDV infection, the rate of progression to cirrhosis 3 years after HDV superinfection approaches 10%, and after 5 years reaches its peak incidence at 21% [93]. Although this is faster than the rate of development of cirrhosis in patients infected with HBV only, at 10 years the total incidence of cirrhosis is not significantly different between the two groups [93]. In chronic HCV infection, increased rates of liver fibrosis are associated with elevated as compared to normal ALT levels, although patients with normal levels of ALT can also develop cirrhosis [162]. Other factors positively associated with fibrosis in HCV that may lead to cirrhosis include heavy alcohol consumption, age greater than 40 when contracting HCV infection, immunosuppression including HIV infection, and concurrent HBV infection, while viral factors including viral load and quasispecies diversity have not been found to affect disease progression [163]. In chronic HCV infection, anywhere from 3% to 20% of people will develop cirrhosis over a course of 20 years [163].

42.5.2 Hepatocellular Carcinoma

Hepatocellular carcinoma (HCC) ranks third in the most common causes of cancer death in the world, and the number of deaths from HCC each year (589,000) almost equals the number of newly reported cases (686,000), demonstrating the poor prognosis that a diagnosis of HCC carries [164]. Over 80% of cases and deaths from HCC are in developing countries with China accounting for over 50% of cases alone [164]. Together, HBV and HCV are the cause of 75–85% of cases of HCC worldwide, and because HBV is the more prevalent of the two infections, the worldwide distribution of HCC greatly parallels the distribution of HBV infection.

HBsAg carriers have an approximately 100-fold increase in risk of developing HCC as compared to non-carriers [46]. A high level of HBV DNA is the most important predictor of HCC; other factors associated with higher rates of HCC include male gender, cirrhosis, Asian or African race, alcohol or tobacco use, HBeAg positivity, genotype C as compared to B, and coinfection with hepatitis C or D virus [165]. Although the mechanism of carcinogenesis is still not completely clear, two pathways of oncogenesis have been identified. The first is an indirect pathway of chronic necroinflammation of hepatocytes inducing injury, mitosis, and regeneration leading to the accumulation of mutations [166]. The other is a direct pathway of viral genome insertion into host DNA. Although this is not requisite for the viral lifecycle, HBV genome insertion is found in many HCCs associated with HBV, and the insertions have been found to induce a variety of host genomic changes including loss of tumor suppressor genes, genomic instability, and resistance to oncogene-induced apoptosis and cell-cycle arrest [49]. In addition, the X protein of HBV is thought to contribute to carcinogenesis by its role as a transcription activator of host genes leading to deregulation of cell cycle control, interference with cellular DNA repair, and apoptosis [108]. HBV-associated HCC has been documented in patients in the absence of chronic inflammation and cirrhosis, supporting the role of the direct pathway of carcinogenesis in at least some of HBV-associated HCC [167].

In patients with HCV infection, the risk of developing HCC is 17 times that of patients without infection, and the risk is highest at 5.8% per year for those with cirrhotic HCV [167]. Because HCV does not integrate into the host genome, it leads to carcinogenesis only via the indirect pathway of chronic inflammation and the subsequent accumulation of mutations. Due to this reliance on chronic inflammation, which is similar to the pathogenesis of cirrhosis, HCV-related HCC is found almost exclusively in patients with cirrhosis [167]. Studies have compared the cumulative rates of developing HCC over time in cirrhotic patients with HBV versus HCV [167, 168]; one study found that the rates in HBV patients plateaued after about 10 years, with a peak of 27.2%, while another showed a continual gradual rise with the rate peaking at 31.9% at 15 years. For HCV, a linear relationship is consistently seen with a cumulative rate of 56.2–75.2% of HCC at the end of 15 years.

Hepatocellular carcinoma is often asymptomatic until the tumor has grown very large or has invaded or metastasized to other locations. Metastases were most often seen to the thorax, followed by abdomen and bone in one series, and another series found vascular invasion in almost half of cases reviewed at autopsy [169, 170]. Factors predictive of tumor metastasis in the previously mentioned study were tumor grade, weight loss, and portal vein obstruction, and survival rates were poorer in patients with metastasis at 395 versus 1,242 days. In accordance with these findings, smaller tumor size, early detection, and early treatment as a result of surveillance programs have been associated with improved survival [169]. Screening for hepatocellular carcinoma involves checking serum alfa-feto protein (AFP), severe and or persistent elevation of which is strongly associated with HCC, and ultrasound looking for liver masses every 6–12 months [171].

Several scoring models have been created to aid in predicting survival and selecting the optimal treatment regimen including Okuda staging, The Cancer of the Liver Italian Group Programme, and the Barcelona Clinic Liver Group system which take into account such factors as tumor size, serum bilirubin, serum albumin, serum AFP, presence of portal vein thrombosis, presence of ascites, and physical status [167]. Classically, the treatment of the hepatocellular carcinoma is surgical with either partial resection or complete liver resection with transplant. These methods remain the first-line treatments in selected patients including those with single, non-metastatic tumors and excellent functional reserve; transplantation also has the benefit of removing the cirrhotic liver at the same time it removes the cancer [172]. Due to the association of HCC with cirrhosis and the asymptomatic nature of the cancer leading to late presentation, physicians are often faced with the difficulty of treating patients who are poor surgical candidates because of little hepatic reserve, compromised liver function, and associated comorbidities. For these patients, less invasive treatments include percutaneous tumor ablation using ethanol or heat in the form of radiofrequency. The best results seen with ethanol injection lead to a 5-year survival rate of 40–50%, and while some studies have found radiofrequency ablation to have better response rates and prognosis as compared to ethanol, no survival benefit has yet been described [172]. For patients with tumor features characteristic of poor response rates, such as infiltrating or nodular tumors, non-curative measures are in order. Palliative treatments include embolization of the hepatic artery, with or without the concurrent use of intra-arterial chemotherapeutic agents. Patients who have vascular involvement or metastasis may be offered novel systemic chemotherapeutics, whereas for patients with poor functional reserve or terminal stage cancer, only symptomatic treatment is indicated [172].

42.6 Hepatitis A Virus

42.6.1 Hepatitis A Virus as a Sexually Transmitted Disease

Hepatitis A virus (HAV) is not traditionally considered a sexually transmitted disease, as it is transmitted via the fecal–oral route and is seen most often in travelers returning from endemic areas, but food-borne outbreaks also occur. In MSM though, there is evidence that the virus is transmitted via sexual activity. This is supported by epidemiologic studies that have linked outbreaks of HAV infection with MSM populations and found that MSM have higher incidence rates of HAV infection than the general population both in Europe and in the USA [173–175]. Based on these studies, HAV infection in MSM has been positively correlated with visiting gay saunas and darkrooms, which are associated with casual sex and having multiple partners in a small span of time, and oral–anal and digital–anal sexual practices. Because of these outbreaks in the MSM community, many countries and cities have implemented campaigns for educating and vaccinating against HAV in this population.

42.6.2 The Virus

HAV is the only species in the genus *Hepatovirus* which belongs to the *Picornaviridae* family that also includes *Rhinovirus* and *Enterovirus* [176]. HAV is a small, single-stranded positive-sense RNA virus of 7.5 kilobases consisting of a five prime non-coding region of approximately 740 nucleotides followed by a 6,675–6,681 nucleotide coding region and a 40–80 nucleotide non-coding region at the three prime end [176]. Viral proteins include VP1, VP2, and VP3 which make up the icosahedral viral capsid, VP4 which is necessary for the formation of the capsid, viral protease 3C that cleaves the capsid proteins from a polyprotein precursor, and VPg that initiates RNA synthesis [176].

The virus is resistant to heat, acid, ether, and because it is non-enveloped is resistant to bile lysis [159, 177]. Once ingested, the virus replicates in gastrointestinal epithelial cells and hepatocytes, and is then released into the bile and blood without causing lysis of the infected cell [176]. The liver injury in HAV infection is mediated by the immune response, including cytotoxic T lymphocytes and interferon gamma production, as in other viral hepatitis infections; this is evidenced by the peak of viral production and excretion in the stool preceding the biochemical markers of liver injury [178]. The incubation period of the virus lasts a mean of 30 days prior to the onset of a nonspecific prodrome of fever, anorexia, nausea, vomiting, abdominal pain, malaise, and headache lasting on average one week before the development of jaundice [159, 176]. Icteric illness lasts from 1 to 4 weeks, and patients may be ill for up to 2 months (Fig. 42.9) [176, 177, 179]. Up to 70% of children less than 6 years of age will have an asymptomatic infection while greater than 70% of adults will be symptomatic, reflecting the immune maturity necessary for liver damage [180]. Diagnosis of HAV infection is hinted at by elevation of transaminases and bilirubin and is confirmed by a positive test for HAV IgM, detectable 5–10 days before the onset of symptoms, which has 100% sensitivity, 99% specificity, and 88% positive predictive value [176, 177]. HAV IgG appears shortly after IgM and persists for life conferring immunity. Fulminant hepatitis occurs in 0.1% of patients, and although a prolonged, relapsing course over several months is seen in 10–20% of patients, HAV does not ever lead to chronic infection [159, 177]. Treatment is supportive and directed by clinical manifestations of the disease.

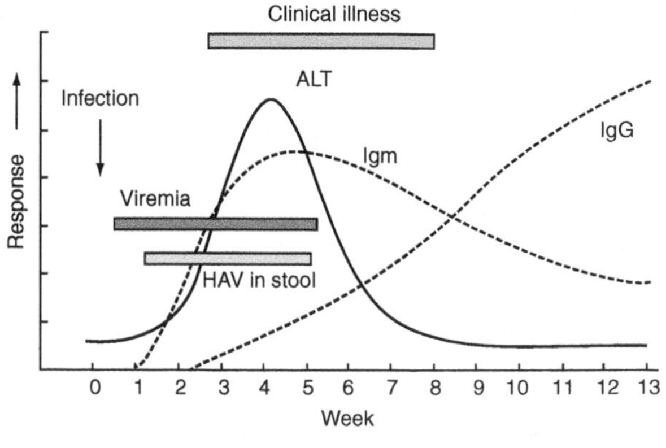

Fig. 42.9 Time course of hepatitis A virus infection [179]

42.7 Hepatitis G Virus

42.7.1 Hepatitis G Virus, Also Known as GB Virus C

Hepatitis G virus (HGV) was discovered in the mid-1990s and was classified as a member of the *Flaviviridae* family, along with HCV [181]. HGV was found to be so closely related in its genetic sequence to another virus discovered around the same time, HG virus C, that they are considered to be members of the same virus group and their names are used interchangeably [182, 183]. HGV is transmitted via the same routes as HBV and HCV, including sexual contact. Evidence to support sexual transmission of HGV includes high rates of detection in prostitutes and homosexuals, detection of HGV in sexual partners of HGV-infected hemophiliacs, and more frequent detection of HGV in people at high risk for sexually transmitted diseases compared to controls [184]. HGV replicates mainly in peripheral blood cells including B and T lymphocytes; the evidence for hepatocyte tropism and replication of the virus remains controversial [184, 185]. Anecdotal reports and noncontrolled studies have associated HGV with acute, fulminant, and chronic hepatitis, but more recent studies have failed to provide convincing evidence that HGV is the causative agent in any human disease including hepatitis, despite the fact that HGV viremia may persist for up to a decade [184, 186, 187]. Based on the strength of evidence that HGV does not cause human infection, the FDA does not screen donor blood for this virus [187]. Despite not directly causing human disease, HGV may have clinical significance when present in patients also infected with HIV. Multiple studies have demonstrated higher CD4 counts, lower HIV viral load, and increased survival in HIV-infected individuals who also have HGV viremia compared to those negative for HGV viremia (Fig. 42.10) [187, 188]. Proposed mechanisms for this effect include direct inhibition of HIV by replication of HGV in peripheral blood mononuclear cells that HIV also infect, induction of chemokines that inhibit HIV, and decreased expression of HIV co-receptor CCR5; to date though, a causal relationship between HGV and prolonged survival in HIV has yet to be proven [187, 189].

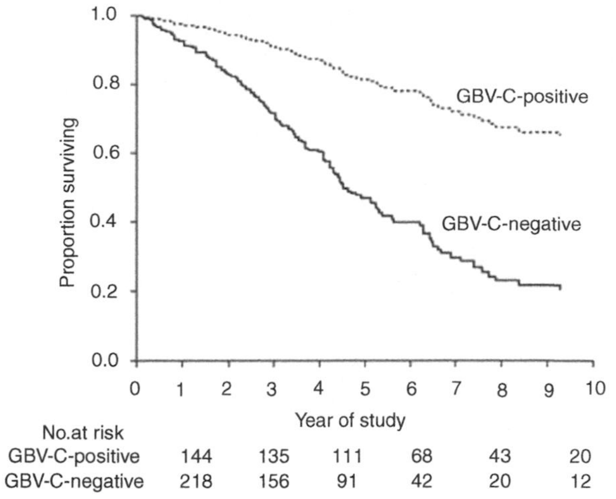

Fig. 42.10 Survival curves for HIV-infected patients with and without GBV-C ([188]. Copyright [2001] Massachusetts Medical Society. All rights reserved)

42.8 Conclusion

Hepatitis viruses A, B, C, D, and G can all be transmitted through sexual contact with an infected person, yet these are a diverse group of viruses phylogenetically, microbiologically, and clinically (Table 42.3) [112]. Sexual transmission occurs mostly via contact of mucous membranes with infected bodily fluids, but even for hepatitis A virus that is transmitted via the fecal–oral route and thus is not traditionally considered a sexually transmitted disease, sexual transmission in MSM has also been documented. They also have in common a tropism for the liver, although more recent studies of hepatitis G virus have led to significant doubt concerning the virus's pathogenicity in liver disease. The clinical manifestations range from asymptomatic infection that resolves without any residual

Table 42.3 Characteristics of hepatitis A virus, hepatitis B virus, and hepatitis C virus [112]

Characteristic	Hepatitis A virus	Hepatitis B virus	Hepatitis C virus
Type of virus	Picornavirus (RNA)	Hepadnavirus (DNA)	Flavivirus (RNA)
Mode of transmission	Fecal–oral (in some cases, parenteral)	Parenteral	Parenteral
Route of transmission	Person-to-person contact Sexual Food	Sexual Injection-drug use Perinatal (common, if mother is positive for hepatitis B early antigen)	Injection-drug use Blood products (before 1990) Sexual? Perinatal (infrequent)
Frequency of acute icteric disease	Common in adults Infrequent in children	Common in adults Infrequent in children	Uncommon
Frequency of evolution to chronic infection	Never	Infrequent in adults (<10%) Common in young children and infants	Frequent (>70%)
Estimated no. of acute infections/yr in the USA	179,000	185,000	38,000
Estimated no. of chronically infected persons in the USA	–	1,250,000	2,700,000
Estimated no. of chronically infected persons in the world	–	350,000,000	170,000,000
Treatment	None	Interferon alfa Lamivudine	Interferon alfa in combination With ribavirin
Prophylaxis	Recombinant vaccine Immune globin (postexposure)	Recombinant vaccine Hepatitis B immune globin (postexposure)	None

liver disease to chronic infection that can lead to cirrhosis and hepatocellular carcinoma.

Take-Home Pearls

- Hepatitis viruses A, B, C, D and G can all be transmitted through sexual contact with an infected person, yet these are a diverse group of viruses phylogenetically, microbiologically and clinically.
- HBV is 50 to 100 times more infectious than HIV, whereas hepatitis C virus is only 10 times more infectious than HIV.
- Sequelae of chronic hepatitis, which can be seen with HBV, HCV and co-infection with HBV and HDV, include cirrhosis and hepatocellular carcinoma.
- Co-infection with HIV is common due to shared risk factors and modes of transmission, and HIV co-infection has important implications for disease progression, treatment and mortality.

References

1. Centers for Disease Control and Prevention: Hepatitis B. http://www.cdc.gov/hepatitis/HBV/HBVfaq.htm#general. Accessed 7 Oct 2008
2. Seeger, C., Mason, W.S.: Hepatitis B virus biology. Microbiol. Mol. Biol. Rev. **64**, 51–68 (2000)
3. Schaefer, S.: Hepatitis B virus taxonomy and hepatitis B virus genotypes. World J. Gastroenterol. **13**, 14–21 (2007)
4. Crowther, R.A., Kiselev, N.A., Bottcher, B., et al.: Three-dimensional structure of hepatitis B virus core particles determined by electron cryomicroscopy. Cell **77**, 943–950 (1994)
5. Block, T.M., Guo, H., Guo, J.-T.: Molecular virology of hepatitis B virus for clinicians. Clin. Liver Dis. **11**, 685–706 (2007)
6. Schulze, A., Gripon, P., Urban, S.: Hepatitis B virus infection initiates with a large surface protein-dependent binding to heparin sulfate proteoglycans. Hepatology **46**, 1759–1768 (2007)
7. Lu, X., Block, T.M., Gerlich, W.H.: Protease-induced infectivity of hepatitis B virus for a human hepatoblastoma cell line. J. Virol. **70**, 11945–11957 (1996)
8. Kann, M., Schmitz, A., Rabe, B.: Intracellular transport of hepatitis B virus. World J. Gastroenterol. **13**, 39–47 (2007)
9. Kann, M., Sodeik, B., Vlachou, A., et al.: Phosphorylation-dependent binding of hepatitis B core particles to the nuclear core complex. J. Cell Biol. **145**, 45–55 (1999)
10. Beck, J., Nassal, M.: Hepatitis B virus replication. World J. Gastroenterol. **13**, 48–64 (2007)
11. Kock, J., Baumert, T.F., Delaney 4th, W.E., et al.: Inhibitory effect of adefovir and lamivudine on the initiation of hepatitis B viral infection in primary tupaia hepatocytes. Hepatology **38**, 1410–1418 (2003)
12. Nassal, M.: Hepatitis B viruses: reverse transcription a different way. Virus Res. **134**, 235–249 (2008)
13. Wei, Y., Travis, J.E., Ganem, D.: Relationship between viral DNA synthesis and viron envelopment in hepatitis B viruses. J. Virol. **70**, 6455–6458 (1996)
14. Ganem, D., Prince, A.M.: Hepatitis B virus infection – natural history and clinical consequences. New Engl. J. Med **350**, 1119–1129 (2004)
15. Ou, J.S.: Molecular biology of hepatitis B virus E antigen. J. Gastroenterol. Hepatol. **12**, S178–S187 (1997)
16. Milich, D., Liang, T.J.: Exploring the biological basis of hepatitis B e antigen in hepatitis B virus infection. Hepatology **38**, 1075–1086 (2003)
17. Bruss, V.: Envelopment of the hepatitis B virus capsid. Virus Res. **106**, 199–209 (2004)
18. Bruss, V.: Hepatitis B virus morphogenesis. World J. Gastroenterol. **13**, 65–73 (2007)
19. de Franchis, R., Meucci, G., Vecchi, M., et al.: The natural history of asymptomatic hepatitis B virus surface antigen carriers. Ann. Intern. Med. **118**, 191–194 (1993)
20. Webster, G.J.M., Reignat, S., Maini, M.K., et al.: Incubation phase of acute hepatitis B in man: dynamic of cellular immune mechanisms. Hepatology **32**, 1117–1124 (2000)
21. Chang, J.J., Lewin, S.R.: Immunopathogenesis of hepatitis B virus infection. Immunol. Cell Biol. **85**, 16–23 (2007)
22. Visvanathan, K., Lewin, S.R.: Immunopathogenesis: role of innate and adaptive immune responses. Semin. Liver Dis. **26**, 104–115 (2006)
23. Kimura, K., Kakimi, K., Wieland, S., et al.: Activated intrahepatic antigen presenting cells inhibit hepatitis B virus replication in the liver of transgenic mice. J. Immunol. **169**, 5188–5195 (2002)
24. Iannacone, M., Sitia, G., Ruggeri, Z.M., et al.: HBV pathogenesis in animal models: recent advances on the role of platelets. J. Hepatol. **46**, 719–726 (2006)
25. Guidotti, L.G., Morris, A., Mendez, H., et al.: Interferon-regulated pathways that control hepatitis B virus replication in transgenic mice. J. Virol. **76**, 2617–2621 (2002)
26. Chisari, F.V., Ferrari, C.: Hepatitis B virus immunopathogenesis. Annu. Rev. Immunol. **13**, 29–60 (1995)
27. Visvanathan, K., Skinner, N.A., Thompson, A.J.V., et al.: Regulation of toll-like receptor-2 expression in chronic hepatitis B by the precore protein. Hepatology **45**, 102–110 (2007)
28. Zhou, D.X., Taraboulos, A., Ou, J.H., et al.: Activation of class I major histocompatibility complex gene expression by hepatitis B virus. J. Virol. **64**, 4025–4028 (1990)
29. Alter, M.: Epidemiology of hepatitis B in Europe and worldwide. J. Hepatol. **39**, S64–S69 (2003)
30. Alter, M.: The emergence of hepatitis B as a sexually transmitted disease. Med. Clin. N. Am. **74**, 1529–1541 (1990)
31. Bond, W.W., Favero, M.S., Peterson, N.J., et al.: Survival of hepatitis B virus after drying and storage for one week. Lancet **1**, 550–551 (1981)
32. Alter, M.J.: Epidemiology of viral hepatitis and HIV co-infection. J. Hepatol. **44**, S6–S9 (2006)

33. Hepatitis B Fact Sheet. World Health Organization. August 2008. Available at http://www.who.int/mediacentre/factsheets/fs204/en/index.html. Accessed November 2, 2008
34. Maheshwari, A., Ray, S., Thuluvath, P.J.: Acute hepatitis C. Lancet **72**, 321–332 (2008)
35. McMahon, B.J., Alward, W.L., Hall, D.B., et al.: Acute hepatitis B virus infection: relation of age to the clinical expression of disease and subsequent development of the carrier state. J. Infect. Dis. **151**, 599–603 (1985)
36. Hoofnagle, J.H.: Serologic markers of hepatitis B virus infection. Annu. Rev. Med. **32**, 1–11 (1981)
37. Dufour, D.R., Lott, J.A., Nolte, F.S., et al.: Diagnosis and monitoring of hepatic injury II. Recommendations for use of laboratory tests for screening, diagnosis and monitoring. Clin. Chem. **46**, 2050–2068 (2000)
38. Kajine, K., JilbertAR, S.J., et al.: Woodchuck hepatitis virus infections: very rapid recovery after a prolonged viremia and infection of virtually every hepatocyte. J. Virol. **68**, 5792–5803 (1994)
39. Hayashi, K., Katano, Y., Takeda, Y., et al.: Association of hepatitis B subgenotypes and basal core promoter/precore region variants with the clinical features of patients with acute hepatitis. J. Gastroenterol. **43**, 558–564 (2008)
40. Ostapowicz, G., Fontana, R.J., Schiodt, F.V., et al.: Results of a prospective study of acute liver failure at 17 tertiary care centers in the United States. Ann. Intern. Med. **137**, 947–954 (2002)
41. Pungapong, S., Kim, W.R., Poterucha, J.J.: Natural history of hepatitis B virus infection: an update for clinicians. Mayo Clin. Proc. **82**, 967–975 (2007)
42. Department of Health and Human Services Center of Disease Control: Viral hepatitis FAQs for health professionals. http://www.cdc.gov/hepatitis/HBV/HBVfaq.htm#overview. Accessed 15 Oct 2008
43. Ranger-Rogez, S., Denis, F.: Hepatitis B mother-to-child transmission. Expert Rev. Anti Infective Ther. **2**, 133–145 (2004)
44. Tovo, P.A., Lazier, L., Versace, A.: Hepatitis B virus and hepatitis C virus infections in children. Curr. Opin. Infect. Dis. **18**, 261–266 (2005)
45. Liaw, Y.F., Tai, D., Chu, C.M., et al.: Early detection of hepatocellular carcinoma in patients with chronic type B hepatitis: a prospective study. Gastroenterology **90**, 263–267 (1986)
46. McMahon, B.J., Holck, P., Bulkow, S., et al.: Serologic and clinical outcomes of 1536 Alaska natives chronically infected with hepatitis B virus. Ann. Intern. Med. **153**, 759–768 (2001)
47. Hsu, Y.S., Chien, R.N., Yeh, C.T., et al.: Long-term outcome after spontaneous HBeAg seroconversion in patiens with chroinc hepatitis B. Hepatology **35**, 1522–1527 (2002)
48. McMahon, B.J.: The natural history of chronic hepatitis B virus infection. Semin. Liver Dis. **24**, 17–21 (2004)
49. Alward, W.L., McMahon, B.J., Hall, D.B., et al.: The long-term serological course of asymptomatic hepatitis B virus carriers and the development of primary hepatocellular carcinoma. J. Infect. Dis. **151**, 604–609 (1985)
50. Beasley, R.P.: Hepatitis B virus. The major etiology of hepatocellular carcinoma. Cancer **16**, 1942–1956 (1988)
51. Liaw, Y.F., Sheen, I.S., Chen, T.J., et al.: Incidence, determinants and significance of delayed clearance of serum HBsAg in chronic hepatitis B virus infection: a prospective study. Hepatology **13**, 627–631 (1991)
52. Chan, G., Kowdley, K.V.: Extrahepatic manifestations of chronic viral hepatitis. Compr. Ther. **21**, 200–205 (1995)
53. Han, S.B.: Extrahepatic manifestations of chronic hepatitis B. Clin. Liver Dis. **8**, 403–418 (2004)
54. Guillevin, L., Lhote, F., Cohen, P., et al.: Polyarteritis nodosa related to hepatitis B virus: a prospective study with long-term observation of 41 patients. Medicine **74**, 238–253 (1995)
55. Wilson, R.A.: Extrahepatic manifestations of chronic viral hepatitis. Am. J. Gastroenterol. **92**, 3–17 (1997)
56. Guillevin, L., Visser, H., Noel, L.H., et al.: Antineutrophil cytoplasm antibodies in systemic polyarteritis nodosa with and without hepatitis B virus infection and Churg–Strauss syndrome – 62 patients. J. Rheumatol. **20**, 1345–1349 (1993)
57. Lai, K.N., Li, P.K., Lui, S.F., et al.: Membranous nephropathy related to hepatitis B virus in adults. N. Engl. J. Med. **324**, 1457–1463 (1991)
58. Alpert, E., Isselbacher, K.J., Schur, P.H.: The pathogenesis of arthritis associated with viral hepatitis. N. Engl. J. Med. **285**, 185–189 (1971)
59. Konopnicki, D., Mocroft, A., de Wit, S., et al.: Hepatitis B and HIV: prevalence, AIDS progression, response to highly active antiretroviral therapy and increased mortality in the EuroSIDA cohort. AIDS **19**, 593–601 (2005)
60. Law, W.P., Duncombe, C.J., Mahanontharit, A., et al.: Impact of viral hepatitis co-infection on response to antiretroviral therapy and HIV disease progression in the HIV-NAT cohort. AIDS **18**, 1169–1177 (2004)
61. Gilson, R.J., Hawkins, A.E., Beecham, M.R., et al.: Interactions between HIV and hepatitis B virus in homosexual men: effects on the natural history of infection. AIDS **11**, 597–606 (1997)
62. Mai, A.L., Yim, C., óRourke, K., et al.: The interaction of human immunodeficiency virus infection and hepatitis B virus infection in infected homosexual men. J. Clin. Gastroenterol. **22**, 299–304 (1996)
63. Benhamou, Y.: Hepatitis B in the HIV-coinfected patient. J. Acquir. Immune Defic. Syndr. **45**, S57–S65 (2007)
64. Bodsworth, N., Donovan, B., Nightengale, B.N.: The effect of concurrent human immunodeficiency virus infection on chronic hepatitis B: a study of 150 homosexual men. J. Infect. Dis. **160**, 577–582 (1989)
65. Puoti, M., Cozzi-Lepri, A., Ancarani, F., et al.: The management of hepatitis B virus/HIV-1 coinfected patients starting their first HAART regimen. Treating two infections for the price of one drug? Antivir. Ther. **9**, 811–817 (2004)
66. Kellerman, S.E., Hanson, D.L., McNaghten, A.D., et al.: Prevalence of chronic hepatitis B and incidence of acute hepatitis B infection in human immunodeficiency virus infected subjects. J. Infect. Dis. **188**, 571–577 (2003)
67. Bolognia, E.A., Costa, J., Gareen, I.F., et al.: NIH Consensus development statement on management of hepatitis B: a draft. NIH. Consens. State. Sci. Statements **25** (2008). epub ahead of print
68. Keeffe, E.B., Dieterich, D.T., Han, S.H., et al.: A treatment algorithm for the management of chronic hepatitis B infection in the United States: 2008 update. Clin. Gastroenterol. Hepatol. **6**, 1315–1341 (2008)

69. Chang, T.T., Lai, C.L., Chein, R.N., et al.: Four years of lamivudine treatment in Chinese patients with chronic hepatitis B. Hepatology **19**, 1276–1282 (2004)
70. Panel on Antiretroviral Guidelines for Adults and Adolescents: Guidelines for the use of antiretroviral agents in HIV-1 infected adults and adolescents. Department of Health and Human Services, 29 Jan 2008, pp. 1–128. http://www.aidsinfo.nih.gov/ContentFiles/AdultandAdolescentGL.pdf. Accessed 26 Oct 2008
71. Rizzetto, M., Canese, M.G., Arico, S., et al.: Immunofluorescence detection of new antigen-antibody system (δ/anit-δ) associated to hepatitis B virus in liver and in serum of HBsAg carriers. Gut **18**, 977–1003 (1977)
72. Hsieh, T.H., Liu, C.J., Chen, D.S., et al.: Natural course and treatment of hepatitis D virus infection. J. Formos. Med. Assoc. **105**, 869–881 (2006)
73. Casey, J.L.: Hepatitis delta virus genetics and pathogenesis. Clin. Lab. Med. **16**, 451–464 (1996)
74. Rizzetto, M., Moyer, B., Canese, M.G., et al.: Delta agent: Association of δ antigen with hepatitis B surface antigen and RNA in serum of δ-infected chimpanzees. Proc. Natl. Acad. Sci USA **77**, 6124–6128 (1980)
75. Weiner, A.J., Choo, Q.L., Wang, K.S., et al.: A single antigenomic open reading frame of the hepatitis delta virus encodes the epitope(s) of both hepatitis delta antigen polypeptides p24 delta and p27 delta. J. Virol. **62**, 594–599 (1988)
76. Gudima, S., He, Y., Chai, N., et al.: Primary human hepatocytes are susceptible to infection by hepatitis delta virus assembled with envelope proteins of woodchuck hepatitis virus. J. Virol. **82**, 7276–7283 (2008)
77. Alves, C., Freitas, N., Cunha, C.: Characterization of the nuclear localization signal of the hepatitis delta virus antigen. Virology **370**, 12–21 (2008)
78. Fu, T.B., Taylor, J.: The RNAs of hepatitis delta virus are copied by RNA polymerase II in nuclear homogenates. J. Virol. **67**, 6965–6972 (2003)
79. Wu, H.N., Lin, Y.J., Lin, F.P., et al.: Human hepatitis δ virus RNA subfragments contain an autocleavage activity. Proc. Natl. Acad. USA **86**, 1831–1835 (1989)
80. Hsieh, S.Y., Chao, M., Coates, L., et al.: Hepatitis virus delta genome replication: a polyadenylated mRNA for delta antigen. J. Virol. **64**, 3192–3198 (1990)
81. Luo, G.X., Chao, M., Hsieh, S.Y., et al.: A specific base transition occurs on replicating hepatitis delta virus RNA. J. Virol. **64**, 1021–1027 (1990)
82. Polson, A.G., Bass, B.L., Casey, J.L.: RNA editing of hepatitis delta virus anitgenome by dsRNA-adenosine deaminase. Nature **380**, 544–546 (1996)
83. Chao, M., Hsieh, S.Y., Taylor, J.: Role of two forms of hepatitis delta virus antigen: evidence for a mechanism for a self-limiting genome replication. J. Virol. **64**, 5066–5069 (1990)
84. Hwang, S.B., Lai, M.M.: Isoprenylation mediates direct protein-protein interactions between hepatitis large delta antigen and hepatitis B virus surface antigen. J. Virol. **67**, 7659–7662 (1993)
85. Wu, J.C., Chen, T.Z., Huang, Y.S., et al.: Natural history of hepatitis D viral superinfection: significance of viremia detected by polymerase chain reaction. Gastroenterology **108**, 796–802 (1995)
86. Macnaughton, T.B., Gowans, E.J., Reinboth, B., et al.: Stable expression of hepatitis delta virus antigen in a eukaryotic cell line. J. Gen. Virol. **71**, 1339–1345 (1990)
87. Wang, D., Pearlberg, J., Liu, Y.T., et al.: Deleterious effects of hepatitis delta virus replication on host cell proliferation. J. Virol. **75**, 3600–3604 (2001)
88. Negro, F., Baldi, M., Bonino, F., et al.: Chronic HDV (hepatitis delta virus) hepatitis. Intrahepatic expression of delta antigen, histologic activity and outcome of liver disease. J. Hepatol. **6**, 8–14 (1988)
89. Caredda, F., d'Arminio Monforte, A., Rossi, E., et al.: Prospective study of epidemic delta infection in drug addicts. Prog. Clin. Biol. Res. **143**, 245–250 (1983)
90. Macagno, S., Smedile, A., Carreda, F., et al.: Monomeric (7s) immunoglobulin M antibodies to hepatitis delta virus in hepatitis type D. Gastroenterology **98**, 1582–1586 (1990)
91. Jaw-Ching, Wu, Chen, T.-Z., Huang, Yi-Shin, Yen, Fu-Shun, Ting, L.-T., Sheng, W.-Y., Tsay, S.-H., Lee, S.-D.: Natural history of hepatitis D: significance of viremia detected by polymerase chain reaction. Gastroenterology **108**(3), 796–802 (1995)
92. Smedile, A., Farci, P., Verme, G., et al.: Influence of delta infection on severity of hepatitis B. Lancet **2**, 945–947 (1982)
93. Liaw, Y.F., Chen, Y.C., Sheen, I.S., et al.: Impact of acute hepatitis C virus superinfection in patients with chronic hepatitis B virus infection. Gastroenterology **126**, 1024–1029 (2004)
94. Liaw, Y.F., Dong, J.T., Chiu, K.W., et al.: Why most patients with hepatitis delta virus infection are seronegative for hepatitis B e antigen. A prospective controlled study. J. Hepatol. **12**, 106–109 (1991)
95. Farci, P., Mandas, A., Coiana, A., et al.: Treatment of chronic hepatitis D with interferon alfa-2a. New Engl. J. Med. **330**, 88–94 (1994)
96. Castelnau, C., Le Gal, F., Ripault, M.P., et al.: Efficacy of peginterferon alpha-2b in chronic hepatitis delta: relevance of quantitative RT-PCR for follow-up. Hepatology **44**, 728–735 (2006)
97. Niro, G.A., Ciancio, A., Gaeta, G.B., et al.: Pegylated interferon alpha-2b as monotherapy or in combination with ribavirin in chronic hepatitis delta. Hepatology **44**, 713–720 (2006)
98. Farci, P., Chessa, L., Balestrieri, C., et al.: Treatment of chronic hepatitis D. J. Viral. Hepat. **14**, 58–63 (2007)
99. Centers for Disease Control and Prevention: Hepatitis C. http://www.cdc.gov/hepatitis/HCV.htm. Accessed 5 Nov 2008
100. Sy, T., Jamal, M.M.: Epidemiology of Hepatitis C Virus (HCV) Infection. Int. J. Med. Sci. **3**, 41–46 (2006)
101. WHO and the Viral Hepatitis Prevention Board: Global surveillance and control of hepatitis C. Report of a WHO Consultation organized in collaboration with the Viral Hepatitis Prevention Board, Antwerp, Belgium. J. Viral. Hepat. **6**, 35–47 (1999)
102. Soriano, V.: Treatment of chronic hepatitis C in HIV-positive individuals: selection of candidates. J. Hepatol. **44**, S44–S48 (2006)
103. Ogata, S., Florese, R.H., Nagano-Fujii, M., et al.: Identification of hepatitis C virus (HCV) subtype 1b strains

that are highly, or only weakly, associated with hepatocellular carcinoma on the basis of the secondary structure of an amino-terminal portion of the HCV NS3 protein. J. Clin. Microbiol. **41**, 2835–2841 (2003)
104. Alter, M.J., Kruszon-Moran, D., Nainan, O.V., et al.: The prevalence of hepatitis C virus infection in the United States, 1988 through 1994. N. Engl. J. Med. **341**, 556–562 (1999)
105. Kaito, M., Ishida, S., Tanaka, H., et al.: Morphology of hepatitis C and hepatitis B virus particles as detected by immunogold electron microscopy. Med. Mol. Morphol. **39**, 63–71 (2006)
106. Barth, H., Liang, T.J., Baumert, T.F.: Hepatitis C virus entry: molecular biology and clinical implications. Hepatology **44**, 527–535 (2006)
107. Zhang, J., Randall, G., Higginbottom, A., et al.: CD81 is required for hepatitis C virus glycoprotein-mediated viral infection. J. Virol. **78**, 1448–1455 (2004)
108. Szabo, E., Paska, C., Kaposi Novak, P., et al.: Similarities and differences in hepatitis B and C virus induced hepatocarcinogenesis. Path Oncol. Res. **10**, 5–11 (2004)
109. Penin, F., Dubuisson, J., Rey, F.A., et al.: Structural biology of hepatitis C virus. Hepatology **39**, 5–19 (2004)
110. Chevaliez, S., Pawlotsky, J.M.: Hepatitis C virus: virology, diagnosis and management of antiviral therapy. World J. Gastroenterol. **13**, 2461–2466 (2007)
111. Cerny, A., Chisari, F.V.: Pathogenesis of chronic hepatitis C: immunologic features of hepatic injury and viral persistence. Hepatology **30**, 595–601 (1999)
112. Lauer, G., Walker, B.D.: Hepatitis C virus infection. N. Engl. J. Med. **345**, 41–52 (2001)
113. Tellinghuisen, T.L., Rice, C.M.: Interaction between hepatitis C virus proteins and host cell factors. Curr. Opin. Microbiol. **5**, 419–427 (2002)
114. Wu, C.G., Budhu, A., Chen, S., et al.: Effect of hepatitis C virus core protein on the molecular profiling of human B lymphocytes. Mol. Med. **12**, 47–53 (2006)
115. Adams, D.H., Hubscher, S., Fear, J., et al.: Hepatic expression of macrophage inflammatory protein-1 alpha and macrophage inflammatory protein-1 beta after liver transplantation. Transplantation **61**, 817–825 (1996)
116. Huang, Y.S., Chan, C.Y., Wu, J.C.: Serum levels of interleukin-8 in alcoholic liver disease: relationship with disease stage, biochemical parameters and survival. J. Hepatol. **24**, 377–384 (1996)
117. Neuman, M.G.: Cytokines in alcoholic liver. Alcohol Res. Health **27**, 313–322 (2003)
118. Schwabe, R.F., Bataller, R., Brenner, D.A.: Human hepatic stellate cells express CCR5 and RANTES to induce proliferation and migration. Am. J. Physiol. Gastrointest. Liver Physiol. **285**, G949–G958 (2003)
119. Bissell, D.M., Wang, S.S., Jarnagin, W.R., et al.: Cell-specific expression of transforming growth factor-beta in rat liver. Evidence for autocrine regulation of hepatocyte proliferation. J. Clin. Investig. **96**, 447–455 (1995)
120. Neubauer, K., Ritzel, A., Saile, B., et al.: Decrease of platelet-endothelial cell adhesion molecule 1-gene-expression in inflammatory cells and in endothelial cells in the rat liver following CCl(4)-administration and in vitro after treatment with TNF-alpha. Immunol. Lett. **74**, 153–164 (2000)
121. Salmi, M., Adams, D., Jalkanen, S.: Cell adhesion and migration. IV. Lymphocyte trafficking in the intestine and liver. Am. J. Physiol. **274**, G1–G6 (1998)
122. Centers for Disease Control and Prevention: Updated U.S. Public Health Service Guidelines for the management of occupational exposures to HBV, HCV, and HIV and recommendations for postexposure prophylaxis. MMWR Recomm. Rep. **50**, 1–52 (2001)
123. Alter, M.J.: Prevention of spread of hepatitis C. Hepatology **36**, s93–s98 (2002)
124. Zanetti, A.R., Tanzi, E., Paccagnini, S., et al.: Mother-to-infant transmission of hepatitis C virus. Lancet **345**, 289–291 (1995)
125. Fried, M.W., Shindo, M., Fong, T.L., et al.: Absence of hepatitis C viral RNA from saliva and semen of patients with chronic hepatitis C. Gastroenterology **102**, 1306–1308 (1992)
126. Kotwal, G.J., Rustgi, V.K., Baroudy, B.M.: Detection of hepatitis C virus-specific antigens in semen from non-A, non-B hepatitis patients. Dig. Dis. Sci. **37**, 641–644 (1992)
127. Alter, M.J., Hadler, S.C., Judson, F.N., et al.: Risk factors for acute non-A, non-B hepatitis in the United States and association with hepatitis C virus infection. JAMA **264**, 2231–2235 (1990)
128. Kelen, G.D., Green, G.B., Purcell, R.H., et al.: Hepatitis B and hepatitis C in emergency department. N. Engl. J. Med. **326**, 1399–1404 (1992)
129. Conry-Cantilena, C., VanRaden, M., Gibble, J., et al.: Routes of infection, viremia, and liver disease in blood donors found to have hepatitis C virus infection. N. Engl. J. Med. **334**, 1691–1696 (2006)
130. Everhart, J.E., Di Bisceglie, A.M., Murray, L.M., et al.: Risk for non-A, non-B (type C) hepatitis through sexual or household contact with chronic carriers. Ann. Intern. Med. **112**, 544–545 (1990)
131. Buffington, J., Murray, P.J., Schlanger, K., et al.: Low prevalence of hepatitis C virus antibody in men who have sex with men who do not inject drugs. Public Health Rep. **122**(Suppl. 2), 63–67 (2007)
132. Osmond, D.H., Charlesbois, E., Sheppard, H.W., et al.: Comparison of risk factors for hepatitis C and hepatitis B virus infection in homosexual men. J. Infect. Dis. **167**, 66–71 (1993)
133. van de Larr, T.J., van der Bij, A.K., Prins, M., et al.: Increase in HCV incidence among men who have sex with men in Amsterdam most likely caused by sexual transmission. J. Infect. Dis. **196**, 230–238 (2007)
134. Amin, J., Kaye, M., Skidmore, S., et al.: HIV and hepatitis C coinfection within the CAESAR study. HIV Med. **5**, 174–179 (2004)
135. Blackard, J.T., Shata, M.T., Shire, N.J., et al.: Acute hepatitis C virus infection: a chronic problem. Hepatology **47**, 321–331 (2008)
136. Neuman, M.G., Sha, K., Esguerra, R., et al.: Inflammation and repair in viral hepatitis C. Dig. Dis. Sci. **53**, 1468–1487 (2008)
137. Tsai, S.L., Liaw, Y.F., Chen, M.F., et al.: Detection of type 2-like T-helper cells in hepatitis C virus infection: implications for hepatitis C virus chronicity. Hepatology **25**, 449–458 (1997)

138. Bartosch, B., Bukh, J., Meunier, J.C., et al.: In vitro assay for neutralizing antibody to hepatitis C virus: evidence for broadly conserved neutralization epitopes. Proc. Natl. Acad. Sci. USA **100**, 14199–14204 (2003)
139. Farci, P., Alter, H.J., Shimoda, A., et al.: Hepatitis C virus-associated fulminant hepatic failure. N. Engl. J. Med. **335**, 631–634 (1996)
140. Shiffman, M.L., Stewart, C.A., Hofmann, C.M., et al.: Chronic infection with hepatitis C virus in patients with elevated or persistently normal alanine aminotransferase levels: comparison of liver histology and response to interferon therapy. J. Infect. Dis. **182**, 1595–1601 (2000)
141. Afdhal, N.H.: The natural history of hepatitis C. Semin. Liver Dis. **24**, S3–S8 (2004)
142. Brau, N.: Update on chronic hepatitis C in HIV/HCV-coinfected patients: viral interactions and therapy. AIDS **17**, 2279–2290 (2003)
143. Smit, C., van den Berg, C., Geskus, R., et al.: Risk of hepatitis-related mortality among hepatitis C virus/HIV coinfected drug users compared with drug users infected only with hepatitis C virus. J. Acquir. Immune Defic. Syndr. **47**, 221–225 (2008)
144. Thein, H.H., Yi, Q., Dore, G.J., et al.: Natural history of hepatitis C virus infection in HIV-infected individuals and the impact of HIV in the era of highly active antiretroviral therapy: a meta-analysis. AIDS **22**, 1979–1991 (2008)
145. Omland, L.H., Jepsen, P., Skinhoj, P., et al.: The impact of HIV-1 co-infection on long-term mortality in patients with hepatitis C: a population-based cohort study. HIV Med. (2008) [Epub ahead of print]
146. Puoti, M., Bonacini, M., Spinetti, A., et al.: Liver fibrosis progression is related to CD4 cell depletion in patients coinfected with hepatitis C virus and human immunodeficiency virus. J. Infect. Dis. **183**, 134–137 (2001)
147. McGovern, B.H., Golan, Y., Lopez, M., et al.: The impact of cirrhosis on CD4+ T cell counts in HIV-seronegative patients. Clin. Infect. Dis. **44**, 431 (2007)
148. Soriano, V., Puoti, M., Sulkowski, M., et al.: Care of patients with hepatitis C and HIV co-infection. AIDS **18**, 1–12 (2004)
149. Mayo, M.J.: Extrahepatic manifestations of hepatitis C infection. Am. J. Med. Sci. **325**, 135–148 (2002)
150. Zignego, A.L., Craxi, A.: Extrahepatic manifestations of hepatitis C virus infection. Clin. Liver Dis. **12**, 611–636 (2008)
151. Ferri, C., Sebastiani, M., Giuggioli, M., et al.: Mixed cryoglobulinemia: demographic, clinical and serologic features and survival in 231 patients. Semin. Arthritis Rheum. **33**, 355–374 (2004)
152. Trejo, O., Ramos-Casalas, M., Garcia-Carrasco, M., et al.: Cryoglobulinemia: Study of etiologic factors and clinical and immunologic features in 443 patients from a single center. Medicine (Baltimore) **80**, 252–262 (2001)
153. Pascual, M., Perrin, L., Giostra, E., et al.: Hepatitis C virus in patients with cryoglobulinemia type II. J. Infect. Dis. **162**, 569–570 (1990)
154. Wigely, F.M.: Clincial practice. Raynaud's phenomenon. N. Engl. J. Med. **347**, 1001–1008 (2002)
155. Daoud, M., Gibson, L.E., Daoud, S., et al.: Chronic hepatitis C and skin disease: a review. Mayo Clin. Proc. **70**, 559–564 (1995)
156. Caronia, S., Taylor, K., Pagliaro, L., et al.: Further evidence for an association between non-insulin dependent diabetes mellitus and chronic hepatitis C virus infection. Hepatology **30**, 1059–1063 (1999)
157. Dienstag, J.L., McHutchison, J.G.: American Gastroenterological Association medical position statement on the management of hepatitis. Gastroenterology **130**, 225–230 (2006)
158. Dienstag, J.L., McHutchison, J.G.: American Gastroenterological Association technical review on the management of chronic hepatitis C. Gastroenterology **130**, 231–264 (2006)
159. Dienstag, J.L., Isselbacher, K.J.: Acute viral hepatitis. In: Kasper, D.J., Braunwald, E., Fauci, A.S., Hauser, S.L., Longo, D.L., Jameson, J.L. (eds.) Harrison's Principles of Internal Medicine. McGraw-Hill, New York (2005)
160. Friedman, S.L.: Mechanisms of hepatic fibrogenesis. Gastroenterology **134**, 1655–1669 (2008)
161. Roberts, L.R., Kamath, P.S.: Ascites and hepatorenal syndrome: pathophysiology and management. Mayo Clin. Proc. **71**, 874–881 (1996)
162. Hui, C.K., Belaye, T., Montegrande, K., et al.: A comparison in the progression of liver fibrosis in chronic hepatitis C between persistently normal and elevated transaminase. J. Hepatol. **38**, 511–517 (2003)
163. National Institutes of Health: NIH consensus statement on management of hepatitis C: 2002. NIH Consens. State Sci. Statements **19**, 1–46 (2002)
164. Parkin, D.M., Bray, F., Ferlay, J., et al.: Global cancer statistics, 2002. CA Cancer J. Clin. **55**, 74–108 (2005)
165. Lok, A.S.F.: Prevention of hepatitis B virus-associated hepatocellular carcinoma. Gastroenterology **127**, S303–S309 (2004)
166. Azam, F., Koulaouzidis, A.: Hepatitis B virus and hepatocarcinogenesis. Ann. Hepatol. **7**, 125–129 (2008)
167. But, D., Lai, C.L., Yuen, M.F.: Natural history of hepatitis-related hepatocellular carcinoma. World J. Gastroenterol. **14**, 1652–1656 (2008)
168. Ikeda, K., Saitoh, S., Koida, I., et al.: A multivariate analysis of risk factors for hepatocellular carcinogenesis: a prospective observation of 795 patients with viral and alcoholic cirrhosis. Hepatology **18**, 47–53 (1993)
169. Kaczynski, J., Hansson, G., Wallerstedt, S.: Metastases in cases with hepatocellular carcinoma in relation to clinicopathologic features of the tumor. An autopsy study from a low endemic area. Acta Oncol. **34**, 43–48 (1995)
170. Si, M.S., Amersi, F., Golish, S.R., et al.: Prevalence of metastasis in hepatocellular carcinoma: risk factors and impact on survival. Am. Surg. **69**, 879–885 (2003)
171. Burix, J., Sherman, M.: Management of hepatocellular carcinoma. Hepatology **42**, 1208–1236 (2005)
172. Llovet, J.P.: Updated treatment approach to hepatocellular carcinoma. J. Gastroenterol. **40**, 225–235 (2005)
173. Centers for Disease Control and Prevention, et al.: Hepatitis A vaccination of men who have sex with men – Atlanta, Georgia, 1996–1997. MMWR Morb. Mortal Wkly. Rep. **47**, 708–711 (1998)
174. Mazik, A., Howitz, M., Rex, S., et al.: Hepatitis A outbreak among MSM linked to casual sex and gay saunas in Copenhagen, Denmark. Euro Surveill. **10**, 111–114 (2005)

175. Van Rijckevorsel, G.G., Sonder, G.J., Bovee, L.P., et al.: Trends in hepatitis A, B, and shigellosis compared with gonorrhea and syphilis in men who have sex with men in Amsterdam, 1992–2006. Sex. Transm. Dis. **35**, 930–934 (2008)
176. Cuthbert, J.A.: Hepatitis A: old and new. Clin. Microbiol. Rev. **14**, 38–58 (2001)
177. Brundage, S., Fitzpatrick, A.N.: Hepatitis A. Am. Fam. Physician **73**, 162–168 (2006)
178. Fleischer, B., Fleischer, S., Maier, K., et al.: Clonal analysis of infiltrating T lymphocytes in liver tissue in viral hepatitis A. Immunology **69**, 14–19 (1990)
179. American Medical Association, et al.: Diagnosis and management of foodborne illnesses: a primer for physicians and other health care professionals. MMWR Recomm. Rep. **53**, 1–33 (2004)
180. Advisory Committee on Immunization Practices (ACIP), Fiore, A.E., Wasley, A., Bell, B.P.: Prevention of hepatitis A through active or passive immunization: recommendations of the Advisory Committee on Immunization Practices (ACIP). MMWR Recomm. Rep. **55**, 1–23 (2006)
181. Linnen, J., Wages Jr., J., Zhang-Keck, Z.-Y., et al.: Molecular cloning and disease association of hepatitis G virus: a transfusion-transmissible agent. Science **271**, 505–508 (1996)
182. Robertson, B.H.: Viral hepatitis and primates: historical and molecular analysis of human and nonhuman primate hepatitis A, B, and the GB-related viruses. J. Viral Hepat. **8**, 233–242 (2001)
183. Simons, J.N., Leary, T.P., Dawson, G.J., et al.: Isolation of novel virus-like sequences associated with human hepatitis. Nat. Med. **1**, 564–569 (1995)
184. Reshetnyak, V.I., Karlovich, T.I., Ilkchenko, L.U.: Hepatitis G virus. World J. Gastroenterol. **14**, 4725–4734 (2008)
185. Handa, A., Brown, K.E.: GB virus C/hepatitis G virus replicates in human hematopoietic cells and vascular endothelial cells. J. Gen. Virol. **81**, 2461–2469 (2000)
186. Alter, M.J., Gallagher, M., Morris, T.T., et al.: Acute non A–E hepatitis in the United States and the role of hepatitis G infection. Sentinel Counties Viral Hepatitis Study Team. N. Engl. J. Med. **336**, 741–746 (1997)
187. Stapelton, J.T.: GB virus type C/hepatitis G virus. Semin. Liver Dis. **23**, 137–148 (2003)
188. Xiang, J., Wunschmann, S., Diekema, D.J., et al.: Effect of coinfection with GB virus C on survival among patients with HIV infection. N. Engl. J. Med. **345**, 707–714 (2001)
189. Xiang, J., George, S.L., Wunschmann, S., et al.: Inhibition of HIV-1 replication by GB virus C infection through increases in RANTES, MIP-1α, MIP-1β, and SDF-1. Lancet **363**, 2040–2046 (2004)

Part IV

Ectoparasites

43 Human Lice

Sophie Bouvresse and Olivier Chosidow

Core Messages

- Pediculoses are ubiquitous parasitic dermatoses caused by human lice.
- The management of pediculoses is based on simultaneous treatment of the patient and all the patient's close infested-contacts and on environmental measures.
- As resistances are described for each group of insecticides, therapeutic alternatives for head lice have been developed.
- Body lice–infested patients should be screened for louse-borne infectious diseases: urban trench fever or endocarditis, epidemic typhus, or relapsing fever.
- Pubic lice may colonize any hairy areas of the body.

43.1 Introduction

Pediculoses are frequent ubiquitous parasitic dermatoses caused by blood-sucking insects: human lice. *Pediculus humanus* var *capitis* lives on the scalp (head lice); *P. humanus* var *corporis* stays on clothing and feeds on the body (body lice); and *Phthirus pubis* lives on the pubis and hairs around genital areas (pubic or crab lice). Lice are visible to the naked eyes and may survive a few hours outside of its host. Therefore, indirect infestation through contaminated clothes, linen, or brushes is possible even if the transmission is direct between individuals in the great majority of cases. The female louse lays approximately ten eggs, called nits, a day for a lifetime of 1–3 months. Nits hatch in 8 days into nymphs that become adults in 10 days [2]. To date, topical pediculicides are the first-line treatment of head lice and pubic lice.

S. Bouvresse and O. Chosidow (✉)
Department of Dermatology, Hôpital Henri Mondor, 51, avenue du Maréchal de Lattre de Tassigny, 94010 Créteil, France
e-mail: olivier.chosidow@hmn.aphp.fr

43.2 Head Lice

43.2.1 Etiology, Epidemiology, and Transmission

Head lice generally infest schoolchildren, especially between 4 and 11 year old, and their family. The prevalence seems to increase in many countries although longitudinal studies are lacking [2]. Pruritus is not constant. Active infestation is diagnosed by the finding of live lice in the scalp.

43.2.2 Treatments

Many pediculicidal agents are available. The most studied are *topical insecticides* [6]:

- *Natural pyrethrins and synthetic pyrethroids*, which are sometimes combined with an insecticide synergist, e.g., piperonyl butoxide. Adverse reactions are local and mild.

G. Gross and S.K. Tyring (eds.), *Sexually Transmitted Infections and Sexually Transmitted Diseases*,
DOI: 10.1007/978-3-642-14663-3_43, © Springer-Verlag Berlin Heidelberg 2011

- *Malathion* – organophosphate insecticide that inhibits cholinesterase – is contraindicated for children under 6 months. Marketed malathion preparations available in EU should be left in place for 8 h although a reduced 20-min treatment has been shown to be effective as well.
- *Lindane* was withdrawn from EU market because of neurotoxicity and/or the development of resistance.
- *Carbaryl* is available in UK. Its carcinogenicity has been demonstrated in rodents and is available on prescription only.
- Topical *crotamiton* has been used, but there are limited data to support its efficacy.
- Oral ivermectin is promising but not approved in the EU [3].

Lotions should be preferred to shampoos because they are less efficient and may facilitate the emergence of resistance. Aerosol-containing pediculicides are contraindicated for people suffering from asthma, as cases of severe bronchospasms were reported [2].

As resistances are described for each group of insecticides [3], *therapeutic alternatives* (4% or 92% dimethicone; essential oils; bug-busting, i.e., repeated meticulous combing; or electrical comb) have been developed, but further clinical trials are needed to definitively confirm their efficacy. Repellents and prophylactic use of pediculicide are not recommended.

43.2.3 Therapeutic Strategy

The management of head lice is based on simultaneous treatment of the patient and all the patient's close infested-contacts and on environmental measures. All clothes and linens should be decontaminated using either machine washing (50°C) [5] or insecticide agent for not washable items (brushes, combs, pillows, etc.). Some recommendations have been established by national institutions. Nevertheless, therapeutic strategies may evolve with emergence of insecticide resistance and development of alternatives to classical pediculicidal agents. The efficiency of these new treatments has to be more accurately estimated.

Pediculicides should be applied on dry hair for various times, specified by the manufacturer, in sufficient quantity and left for various times according to the manufacturer instructions. The product should be used again 7–11 days later because of the possible lack of ovicidal effect of the pediculicide [2]. In case of early treatment failure (24 h after application), resistance should be suspected and switch for another treatment should be performed.

43.3 Body Lice

43.3.1 Epidemiology and Diagnosis

Body lice are associated with poor hygiene condition (homeless people, refugee camp, etc.). Body louse prevalence seems to increase as well as louse-borne infectious diseases such as "urban" trench fever or endocarditis, caused by *Bartonella quintana*; epidemic typhus caused by *Rickettsia prowazekii*; or relapsing fever caused by *Borrelia recurrentis*. For note, a recent study detected head lice infected with *Bartonella quintana* in homeless people in San Francisco, California. Itching is often associated with impetiginization. Lice and nits are found in clothing seams.

43.3.2 Treatment

Decontaminating clothes and linens using either machine washing (50°C) or insecticide agent could constitute a sufficient treatment. Some authors recommend though a whole-body application of topical insecticide such as pyrethrins/pyrethroids or malathion. If associated, louse-borne bacterial diseases should be treated with adapted antibiotic regimen.

43.4 Pubic Lice

43.4.1 Epidemiology and Diagnosis

Pubic lice live on pubis and may colonize other hairy areas such as buttocks, chest, armpits, beard, eyelashes, and rarely scalp. Pubic lice are sexually transmitted in most cases, and their transmission is not prevented by condoms. HIV is not a louse-borne disease. In children, transmission is often explained by intimate – but not sexual – contact with infested parent, but the possibility of sexual abuse should be kept in mind. Indirect contamination is theoretically possible through towels or linens.

The diagnosis is suspected in case of pubic pruritus and is confirmed when finding lice in pubic hair.

43.4.2 Treatment

Family members, sexual contacts, and close companions should be examined and treated appropriately; clothes, linen, and personal items should be washed at 50°C or decontaminated with insecticide powder. Treatment is best accomplished by application of topical insecticide on every hairy infested area with the same methods as those described for head lice. Eyelashes can be treated with 1% permethrin or vaseline. Oral ivermectin has been successfully used for treatment of pubic lice in a case report [1]. Shaving hair might be necessary in case of severe infestation. Patients should also be screened for associated STD and treated as necessary. Patients should be advised to avoid close contact until they and their sexual partners have completed treatment and follow-up.

Take-Home Pearls

- The most studied pediculicides are topical insecticides: natural pyrethrins/pyrethroids and malathion.
- Pediculicide lotions should be preferred to shampoos.
- Pediculicide treatment should be systematically repeated on day 7–10.
- In case of early treatment failure, switch to another treatment should be performed.
- If associated, louse-borne bacterial diseases should be treated with antibiotic regimen.
- Pubic lice transmission is not prevented by condoms.
- Pubic lice treatment uses the same methods as those described for head lice and concerns all infested hairy areas of the body.
- Studies using oral ivermectin in head lice are promising.

References

1. Burkhart, C.G., Burkhart, C.N.: Oral ivermectin for *Phthirus pubis*. J. Am. Acad. Dermatol. **51**, 1037–8 (2004)
2. Chosidow, O.: Scabies and pediculosis. Lancet **355**, 819–26 (2000)
3. O. Chosidow, B. Giraudeau, J. Cottrell, A. Izri, R. Hoffmann, S. Mann, IF. Burgess. Oral ivermectin versus malathion lotion for difficult-to-treat head lice. *N Engl J. Med.* 2010;362:896–905
4. Chosidow, O., Chastang, C., Brue, C., Bouvet, E., Izri, M., Monteny, N., Bastuji-Garin, S., Rousset, J.J., Revuz, J.: Controlled study of malathion and d-phenothrin lotions for *Pediculus humanus* var *capitis*-infested school children. Lancet **344**, 1724–1727 (1994)
5. Izri, A., Chosidow, O.: Efficacy of machine laundering to eradicate head lice: Recommendations to decontaminate washable clothes, linens, and fomites. Clin. Infect. Dis. **42**, 9–10 (2006)
6. Vander Stichele, R.H., Dezeure, E.M., Bogaert, M.G.: Systematic review of clinical efficacy of topical treatments for head lice. BMJ **311**, 604–8 (1995)

Scabies

44

Sophie Bouvresse and Olivier Chosidow

Core Messages

- Scabies is an ubiquitous contagious parasitic dermatosis caused by the mite *Sarcoptes scabiei* var. *hominis*. It is transmitted by skin-to-skin contact, most often within couples, family or institutions. Indirect infestation is also possible.
- Clinical presentation may be atypical in infant, elderly, or immunocompromised patients. The clinical diagnosis can be confirmed by microscopical examination.
- Topical scabicides must be applied from head to toe and may cause skin irritation. The most studied topical scabicides are lindane, pyrethrins (permethrin, esdepalletrine), and benzyl benzoate.
- Oral ivermectin is an effective alternative to topical scabicides.
- The management of scabies is based on simultaneous treatment of the patient and all his close contacts and on environmental surfaces.

44.1 Etiology, Epidemiology, and Transmission

Scabies is a contagious skin infection caused by the mite *Sarcoptes scabiei* var. *hominis*, an obligate human parasite. After fertilization, female mites burrow tunnels into the stratum corneum and lay eggs (3–5 per day) for a lifetime of 1–2 months. The parasitic cycle lasts 21 days. In classic scabies, there are 5 to 15 female parasites per case, but this number can reach several hundred to several million in severe scabies and in crusted scabies. After primary infestation, the symptom-free incubation period is 2–3 weeks, but might be shortened to a few days in cases of reinfestation.

Scabies is a worldwide parasitic infection: It is endemic in many tropical countries where it occurs regardless of gender, age, or ethnicity. In northern countries, scabies occurs sporadically either in individuals or in outbreaks in institutions (nursing homes, hospitals, prisons, etc.).

Common scabies is transmitted by close skin-to-skin contact, most often within couples or families. By contrast, transmission of profuse scabies is facilitated by infestation with numerous mites with possible indirect transmission through contaminated clothes or linen. Indeed, the mite may survive a few hours outside its host.

S. Bouvresse and O. Chosidow (✉)
Department of Dermatology, Hôpital Henri Mondor, 51, avenue du Maréchal de Lattre de Tassigny, 94010 Créteil, France
e-mail: olivier.chosidow@hmn.aphp.fr

44.2 Clinical Manifestations and Diagnosis

Scabies should be suspected upon generalized itching with nocturnal predominance, especially when there is evidence for a pruritic eruption occurring in other family members or contacts. Typical topography of pruritus and inflammatory papules includes interdigital spaces of the hands, wrists, armpits, buttocks, male genitalia, and areolas. Back, neck, and face are generally spared. Specific signs: linear burrows with a small pearl-like visicile at the distal end (hands) and scabious nodules (genital organs) may be absent or hidden

G. Gross and S.K. Tyring (eds.), *Sexually Transmitted Infections and Sexually Transmitted Diseases*,
DOI: 10.1007/978-3-642-14663-3_44, © Springer-Verlag Berlin Heidelberg 2011

by nonspecific secondary lesions such as excoriations, eczematization, or impetiginization.

Clinical presentation may be atypical in infant, elderly, or immunocompromised patients, thus delaying diagnosis and increasing the risk of outbreaks.

The definitive diagnosis is microscopically confirmed when skin scrapings of external burrows or papule material reveal mites, eggs, or mite feces. Microscopical examination is recommended to confirm atypical forms of scabies, even if false-negative results are possible (especially when few lesions are found in classic scabies). New methods like epiluminiscence microscopy may increase sensitivity of skin scrapping.

There is no evidence that systematic use of scabicide therapy as a diagnostic test for unexplained pruritic eruption is a valuable strategy.

44.3 Treatment

44.3.1 Choice of Scabicide

44.3.1.1 Topical Scabicides

Topical scabicides have neurotoxic effects on mites, larvae, and eggs. Various treatments are used as topical scabicides worldwide, but there is no formal evidence for their effectiveness since randomized comparative studies are lacking. Every country has its own recommendations for topical scabicides as all treatments might not be available everywhere. The treatment of choice will depend on the existence of contraindications, expected efficacy and possible toxicity of the product, extent of the lesions, presence of eczematization or impetiginization.

The more studied products are lindane and permethrin [4].

Lindane, applied for 6 h, is a low-cost, effective treatment for scabies. It has been withdrawn from some markets, e.g., European Union, because of its potential neurotoxicity. Also, the appearance of lindane-resistant mites has been suggested.

Pyrethrins are known to be effective as scabicides. Although methodological quality varied between trials, a recent meta-analysis suggests that topical permethrin is the most effective scabicide. Pyrethrinoids as esdepallethrin (single 12-h application) are also licensed but their use with aerosols is contraindicated for people suffering from asthma as cases of severe bronchospasms were reported.

Benzyl benzoate is effective but frequently responsible for skin irritation, or even contact dermatitis. The dosing regimen is not univocal but includes at least one 24h application. Some benzyl benzoate preparations include sulfiram; therefore, drinking alcohol should be avoided during at least 48 h because of its antabuse effect.

Crotamiton cream (two consecutive applications of 24 h) seems to be less scabicidal, but it might be interesting for treatment of scabious nodules of children as it is very well tolerated. Topics with *precipitated sulfurs* are marketed, but there are limited data to support their efficacy or safety. Topical *ivermectin* is being studied as a new therapeutic approach for scabies.

44.3.1.2 Oral Ivermectin

Ivermectin is a broad-spectrum antiparasitic agent that interrupts GABA-induced neurotransmission of many parasites (including mites), leading to their paralysis and death. Drug safety surveillance is necessary, but only minor and transient side effects (gastrointestinal disorders, neurological or skin) were reported with ivermectin as scabicide treatment. An exacerbation of pruritus is possible at the beginning of treatment and the patients must be warned. Resistance to ivermectin in extensively treated patients and increasing in vitro tolerance/resistance have been reported.

It is difficult to evaluate the efficacy of ivermectin compared to the main topical treatments as significant statistical heterogeneity and methodological weaknesses should be noticed in randomized controlled trials (i.e., differences in drug regimen or length of follow up) [2, 3, 4]. Yet, ivermectin appears to be an effective oral treatment.

The presently recommended dosing regimen is one oral dose of 200 μg/kg repeated on day 14 because of the possible lack of ovicidal effect of ivermectin [2, 3] (as evidenced with treatment failure with single dose [5]). Ivermectin has received official approval for treatment of scabies in some countries (e.g., Brazil, Netherlands, and France), but the regimen is not approved for children weighting less than 15 kg or for pregnant or lactating women.

44.3.1.3 Therapeutic Strategy as First-Line Therapy

Topical treatment can be associated with treatment failures caused by poor compliance: head-to-toe application can be difficult for disabled persons, poor tolerance especially when the skin is excoriated, insufficient application of scabicide, etc. Because effective topical treatment relies on simultaneous therapy of all close physical contacts, using them on a community or institutional scale is difficult.

Oral treatment should then be preferred when topical therapy seems difficult to apply: associated excoriated dermatosis, predictable poor compliance, topical treatment failure. Ivermectin is the appropriate first-choice treatment in some special forms of scabies: severe scabies (including crusted scabies), HIV-infected patients, or scabies outbreaks in institutions necessitating a large-scale treatment [1, 2]. Ivermectin can be chosen as first-line therapy, but its cost might limit its use in developing countries.

44.3.2 Principles of Treatment

The management of common scabies is based on simultaneous treatment of the patient and all his close contacts and on environmental surfaces. Prescriptions should then be provided for all household members, as well as any sexual partner, even if they don't have any symptoms. Recently worn (3 days) clothes and linen must be decontaminated using either machine washing (50°C) or insecticide agent for not-washable items. In case of sexually acquired scabies, screening for other STD is recommended for the patient and his (her) partner (s).

Table 44.1 Persisting itching after scabicide therapy

Cutaneous irritation • Overtreatment • Eczematization • Contact dermatitis
Treatment failure • Poor compliance: Inappropriate or insufficient treatment • Resistance to scabicide • Reinfestation or relapse
Psychogenic pruritus: delusions of parasitosis
Nonparasitic dermatosis

The principles of treatments should be explained precisely to the patient in order to optimize compliance: Written instructions may be helpful. The patient should be advised that itching may persist for up to 2 weeks after an efficient treatment. Beyond this delay, persisting itching must be investigated as several diagnoses have to be discussed (Table 44.1).

In scabies outbreaks in institutions [1] topical scabicides may be difficult to handle as the number of simultaneous treatments to accomplish might be important. Indeed, an epidemiological survey is needed to identify cases and their contacts. In case of extensive spread of cases – a fortiori in case of severe scabies – a prescription has to be made for all people living, working, or visiting the institution.

The principles of treatment for *special forms of scabies* are summarized in Table 44.2.

Table 44.2 Treatment of special forms of scabies

	Topical Treatment	Oral Treatment	Associated Measures	Comments
Infants and children under 2 years old	Single 6–12 h application of esdepallethrine or benzyl benzoate Lindane is contraindicated	Ivermectin is contraindicated for children weighting less than 15 kg	Scabicide must be applied on the face, except for eyes and mouth	Crotamiton may be useful for scabious nodules Permethrin is approved for children older than 2 months
Pregnant or lactating women	Single 6–12 h application of esdepallethrine or benzyl benzoate Lindane is contraindicated	Ivermectin is contraindicated		
Severe classic scabies Scabies in HIV-positive patient	At least 2 consecutive applications of scabicide including face and scalp	Single dose of ivermectin (200 μg/kg), repeated at day 14	Isolation Hospitalization is necessary in case of severe scabies	Local treatment and ivermectin should be associated
Generalized crusted scabies	Repeated applications of scabicide and keratolytic agent (e.g., 10% salicylic acid in petrolatum) until microscopical examination becomes negative Lindane should be avoided (neurotoxicity)	Single dose of ivermectin (200 μg/kg), repeated at day 14	Hospitalization and cutaneous isolation Face and scalp must be treated Nails must be cut short and brushed with scabicide	Local treatment and ivermectin should be associated Cure is obtained after 3 weeks Screening and treatment of contacts ++
Impetiginization	Oral treatment should be preferred	Combined antiseptic and antibiotic regimen	Proteinuria should be searched 3 weeks after treatment	If topical treatment is chosen, impetiginization must be treated first
Eczematization	Intensive emollient application might avoid the use of topical steroids	Oral treatment should be preferred		

Take-Home Pearls

- Scabies should be suspected upon generalized itching with nocturnal predominance, especially when there is evidence for a pruritic eruption occurring in other family members or contacts.
- When clinical presentation is atypical (infant, elderly or immunocompromised patients), the diagnosis should be confirmed by microscopical examination.
- Topical scabicides must be applied from head-to-toe and may cause skin irritation.
- Oral ivermectin should be preferred when topical therapy seems difficult to use and in case of severe scabies (including crusted scabies), HIV-infected patients, or scabies outbreaks in institutions.
- The presently recommended dosing regimen for ivermectin is one oral dose of 200 μg/kg repeated on day 14.
- The management of scabies is based on simultaneous treatment of the patient and all his close contacts (even if asymptomatic) and on environmental surfaces.
- The principles of treatments should be explained precisely to thc patient.
- Pruritus may persist for up to 2 weeks after an effective treatment.

References

1. Bouvresse S, Chosidow O. Scabies in healthcare settings. Curr Opin Infect Dis 2010; 23:111–8
2. Chosidow, O.: Scabies. N Engl J. Med. **354**, 1718–1727 (2006)
3. Currie BJ, McCarthy JS. Permethrin and ivermectin for scabies. N Engl J. Med. 2010; 362:717–25
4. Strong, M., Johnstone, P.W.: Interventions for treating scabies. Cochrane Database Syst. Rev. **3**, CD000320 (2007)
5. Ly, F., Caumes, E., Ndaw, C.A., Ndiaye, B., Mahé, A.: Ivermectin versus benzyl benzoate applied once or twice to treat human scabies in Dakar, Senegal: a randomized controlled trial. Bull. World Health Organ. **87**, 424–430 (2009)

Part V

Protozoan Infections

45 Trichomonas

Brenda L. Pellicane and Megan Nicole Moody

Core Messages

- *Trichomonas vaginalis* is the leading causative agent of non-viral, sexually transmitted infections worldwide.
- Infection with *T. vaginalis* is a marker of high-risk sexual behavior as it is frequently seen concomitantly with other STIs.
- The natural immune response to *T. vaginalis* infection increases both transmission of and susceptibility to HIV.
- While often asymptomatic, especially in men, manifestations of infection vary from a characteristic fishy-smelling discharge with pruritus to atypical pelvic inflammatory disease with the potential for pregnancy complications.
- Given the widespread prevalence of this infection and potential for significant complications; efforts need to be directed toward increased awareness, prevention, diagnosis and treatment.
- The most common diagnostic test, is a "wet mount", which consists of simple microscopic examination of vaginal fluid in a saline preparation for organisms with characteristic quivering trichomonad motility.
- A focus on details of the interrelationship amongst causative agents of sexually transmitted infections has established that *Mycoplasma hominis* can combine forces with T. vaginalis in a symbiotic co-infection.

45.1 Introduction

Trichomonas vaginalis is a flagellated parasitic protozoan of the human urogenital tract, and remains the leading causative agent of nonviral, sexually transmitted infections worldwide [10, 13, 28, 46, 49]. While the vast majority of infected men and approximately 50% of infected women are asymptomatic [11, 34, 41], a heterogeneous array of manifestations have been documented on infection with *T. vaginalis*, which include pruritic vaginitis with a frothy, malodorous discharge [34, 41, 50], atypical pelvic inflammatory disease [18], infertility [15], as well as an increased risk for HIV sero-conversion [41] and development of cervical cancer [14, 53, 54]. Infection with *T. vaginalis* is a marker of high-risk sexual behavior as it is frequently seen concomitantly with other STIs, especially gonorrhea [34].

T. vaginalis infection has also been implicated as a source of pregnancy complications, including premature rupture of placental membranes, preterm delivery, and low birth weight infants [6, 30, 34]. Although a highly prevalent disease, trichomoniasis has not yet been designated as reportable to the Centers for Disease Control and Prevention (CDC) and often tends to be regarded as a self-limited condition. This relatively complacent outlook facilitates high rates of re-infection as well as uncontrolled primary spread, which sets

B.L. Pellicane (✉)
Department of Dermatology, Wayne State University, 540E. Canfield, 1310 Scott Hall, Detroit, MI 48201, USA
e-mail: brendaleebartlett@gmail.com

M.N. Moody
Dermatology Surgery Associates,
7515 Main Street, Suite 240, Houston, TX 77030, USA

G. Gross and S.K. Tyring (eds.), *Sexually Transmitted Infections and Sexually Transmitted Diseases*,
DOI: 10.1007/978-3-642-14663-3_45, © Springer-Verlag Berlin Heidelberg 2011

the stage for prevalence levels that border epidemic proportions. Furthermore, advances in research have indicated that infection with *T. vaginalis* is not as benign as once thought. Because infection is both easily detected and effectively treated, increased emphasis should be placed on preventative measures, public awareness, and early intervention for all infected persons and their partners.

45.2 Epidemiology

Trichomoniasis is a highly ubiquitous infection with a widespread distribution. The most recent World Health Organization report estimates an annual worldwide incidence of 174 million [52]. Given the high rate of asymptomatic infections, the true incidence is most likely underestimated. According to another WHO estimate, *T. vaginalis* is responsible for approximately half of all curable infections worldwide [4]. Despite this estimate, however, trichomoniasis is still not a reportable disease, and it is therefore difficult to obtain accurate statistical estimates of incidence and prevalence. Current statistics do show that infection is more prevalent among women, but this statistic may be inaccurate as men have an even higher rate of asymptomatic infection than do women. This is in part evidenced by the introduction of PCR testing for *T. vaginalis.* A recent cross-sectional study involving three sexually transmitted infection (STI) clinics demonstrated a 70% infection rate among asymptomatic male partners of infected women, using PCR detection [42].

Unlike other sexually transmitted infections (STIs), which tend to be more prevalent in adolescent and young adult populations, trichomoniasis appears to lack such age discrimination, as it has been found to be more equally distributed among sexually active women of all age groups [49]. In the United States, the 2001–2004 National Health and Examination Study (NHANES) collected and reported data on the first nationally representative sample of females aged 14–49 years. The prevalence of *T. vaginalis* infection in this sample was 3.1%, which is higher than that of both Chlamydia (0.33%) and gonorrhea (2.5%). Potential confounders were accounted for in the study protocol, and high-risk groups included non-Hispanic blacks, users of douche and/or feminine powders, and people with increased number of sexual partners [23].

45.3 Clinical Manifestations

When symptomatic, infected women most commonly complain of a yellowish-green, malodorous vaginal discharge, pruritus, and localized discomfort. Colpitis macularis (strawberry cervix) is a very specific clinical sign of *T. vaginalis* infection, and describes punctate hemorrhages of an infected cervix; however, it is not routinely relied on for diagnosis because it is most easily visualized by means of an invasive colposcopy. Other symptoms include lower abdominal pain of which the etiology is unclear and dysuria as the urethra is infected in the majority of women [37, 41]. Symptom severity is most likely determined by the extent of the infected host's inflammatory response to the parasite, which is influenced by hormone levels, co-existing vaginal flora components, and parasite load [41]. Symptoms tend to worsen during menstruation due to the altered vaginal environment. The increased blood flow of menstruation brings with it an increased amount of immune cells, which worsen symptoms. As the blood from the uterine lining is shed, the availability of iron, which is necessary for adhesion and pathogenesis, increases. This is discussed in more detail later.

Among males, symptoms occur only in the minority of infected individuals and consist of a clear or mucopurulent urethral discharge and/or dysuria. Possible complications include prostatitis, balanoposthitis, epididymitis, and infertility. More recently, in a large, nested, case-control study, the detection of serum antibodies to *T. vaginalis* in men has been linked with a statistically significant increase in the incidence of prostate cancer [45]. Although often considered a minor STI, significant complications have been associated with trichomoniasis. Infection with trichomonas has been associated with preterm delivery, low birth weight, and premature rupture of membranes. These cases are closely associated with high rates of mortality [6, 17, 30, 40].

Exactly how infection of the lower tract during pregnancy leads to prematurity is not entirely clear. Several studies have led to the conclusion that lower genital tract infections, including trichomoniasis and *C. trachomatis* infection, cause elevated levels of enzymes and cytokines within the vaginal and amniotic fluid. The presence of enzymes and cytokines has been linked to chorioamnionitis and premature delivery [41]. Recommended treatment regimens for trichomoniasis during pregnancy remain uncertain due to studies that showed that treatment during pregnancy resulted in an increase in preterm birth. However, these studies had significant deficits [21, 22].

Another complication of trichomoniasis is the increased risk of HIV acquisition as well as enhanced transmission of HIV in those who are infected. This relationship is discussed in detail later. Interestingly, a study from Finland showed a high relative risk of cervical cancer with *Trichomonas* infection [51].

45.4 Diagnosis

Because of the fact that trichomoniasis can present with a wide array of symptoms, none of which, alone or in combination with another, is sufficient to confirm the causative parasite's presence, it remains necessary to establish a definitive diagnosis using laboratory tests. The most common diagnostic test, known as a "wet mount," is quick and inexpensive to perform. It consists of simple microscopic examination of vaginal fluid in a saline preparation for organisms with characteristic quivering trichomonad motility. A positive test is diagnostic; however, a negative test cannot exclude trichomoniasis due to this test's low sensitivity, estimated at 60–70% [33, 53]. This method is further limited by the fact that the parasites are only viable for a maximum of 20 min once removed from the host [41].

Vaginal culture has since been deemed the "gold standard" for the diagnosis of trichomoniasis, with the results available 2–7 days postinnoculation [34]. The swab of vaginal fluid is placed in culture medium and incubated at 37°C, and subsequently, it is microscopically observed for up to 7 days. At this time, if no motile organisms are present, the culture is considered negative [33]. Diamond's microaerophilic medium has been the mainstay for culture in research settings, whereas commercially designed liquid media, such as InPouch TV, has been accepted as a less expensive, yet equally reliable alternative [28]. A study by Levi et al. showed the sensitivity for InPouch and Diamond's modified medium to be 82.4% and 87.8%, respectively. There were no significant differences in the sensitivity and negative predictive value of InPouch when compared with Diamond's modified medium [27]. A drawback to using vaginal culture for diagnosis is that it may take up to 7 days to obtain results. A delay in therapy is not desirable while awaiting results and therefore culture should be used in cases of clinical suspicion despite a negative wet mount.

Polymerase chain reaction (PCR) techniques have been developed for use on both clinic and self-collected vaginal swabs as a diagnostic tool for detection of *T. vaginalis* infection. A meta-analysis found the pooled sensitivity and specificity of PCR to be 95% and 98%, respectively. The studies had narrow confidence intervals indicating consistent results between them [33]. Studies that have performed PCR followed by a confirmatory culture on the same sample indicate that the real-time PCR has a sensitivity of 100% and a specificity of 97% [5, 41]. Advantages of this technique include the ability for patients to self-collect the specimen as well as rapid results. Other techniques, such as ELISA (enzyme-linked immunoassay) and DFA (direct fluorescence antibody assay), exist, but they are inferior tests owing to lower sensitivities when compared with PCR or culture [33].

45.5 Microbiology

T. vaginalis is a motile flagellated protozoan (see Fig. 45.1), which exists only in the trophozoite form, no cyst form being known. After coital transmission, these organisms divide via binary fission, giving rise to a population in the lumen and on mucosal surfaces of

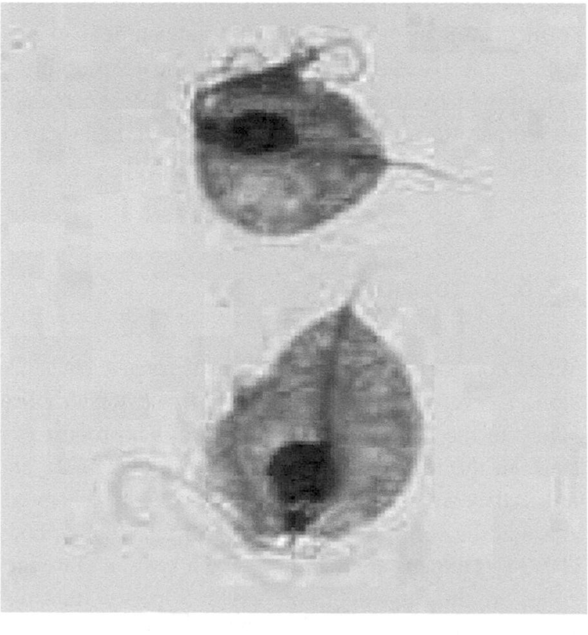

Fig. 45.1 Two trophozoites of *Trichomonas vaginalis* obtained from in vitro culture. Smear was stained with Giemsa

the urogenital tract in humans [41]. These organisms possess a total of five flagella, four of which are located anteriorly [9(2)+2 arrangement], with the fifth actually being incorporated into the parasite's undulating membrane [34, 41]. The undulating membrane gives rise to the characteristic quivering motility. Other internal organelles include the prominent nucleus and the axostyle. The axostyle is a specific, slender, hyaline, rod-like structure composed of microtubules, which appears to begin at the nucleus, and bisects the protozoan longitudinally. It has been noted to serve as an anchor for attachment to human vaginal epithelium via specific associations with the extracellular matrix basement membrane proteins, fibronectin and laminin [2].

Considered ancient eukaryotes, *T. vaginalis* organisms possess no mitochondria. For energy production, they rely instead on molecular hydrogen-producing organelles, known as hydrogenosomes. Though similar to mitochondria, hydrogenosomes lack cytochromes, mitochondrial respiratory chain enzymes, and DNA [34]. The overall process uses hydrogen as the electron acceptor, is fermentative and thus low-yield, obviating the need for *T. vaginalis* to utilize host mechanisms for supplementation [7, 34].

This protozoan can assume distinct morphologies according to specific environmental conditions. In vitro, *T. vaginalis* cultures appear almost exclusively ovoid to pear-shaped; however, on infection, transformation into a cytotoxic and cytoadherent amoeboid form occurs in order to facilitate attachment to host cells or inert surfaces [1]. Morphological variability is determined by interplay among external factors such as temperature, pH, oxygen tension, available carbohydrates, and contact with other cells [20].

45.6 Cytopathology

When considering the mechanism of parasite transmission, *T. vaginalis* is a simple protozoan, which exists solely in the trophozoite form. There is no robust cyst stage in the trichomonad life cycle(see Fig. 45.2), and unless they are protected from drying, these fragile protozoa will die very rapidly on exile from the human body [10, 34]. Humans are the only known hosts, and trophozoites are thus dependent on person-to-person transmission from one infected partner to the next. An untreated *T. vaginalis* infection lasts for an average of 3 months [49], a time period during which it can be freely transmitted on contact. Although minimal survival on fomites has been documented in vitro, *T. vaginalis* is considered to be transmitted exclusively via sexual contact [34, 41].

To establish an infection in the human female, trichomonad parasites must first gain access and subsequently adhere to vaginal epithelial cells. Studies have verified that a direct relationship exists between the level of trichomonad adhesion proteins and cytotoxicity, and that antisense genetic downregulation of specific surface proteins compromises adherence and infection by *T. vaginalis* parasites [1, 24]. In order for cell adhesion to occur, the parasite must first penetrate the protective superficial layer of mucus overlying the vaginal mucosa. *T. vaginalis* protozoa must be able to adapt to multiple environmental insults encountered within the female genital tract, including alterations in pH, mucous consistency, and carbohydrate content in addition to periodic desquamation and sloughing of surface epithelial cells and mucous. It has been postulated that these altered environmental states might actually serve as signals to alter trichomonad gene expression accordingly [12, 24].

In vitro studies have indicated that trichomonad adhesion is both contact- and iron-dependent via mechanisms that involve increased expression and redistribution of adhesion proteins from within hydrogenosomes to the surface [12, 31]. These environmental stimuli have been shown to upregulate the expression of certain trichomonad virulence genes via an iron-response element mechanism, specifically, the genes involving the following four adhesion proteins: 1- AP65, decarboxylating malic enzyme; 2- AP51, β-succinyl coA synthetase; 3- AP33, α-succinyl coA synthetase; and 4- AP120 (pyruvate:ferredoxin oxidoreductase) [31, 44].

High iron levels further enhance the virulence of *T. vaginalis* by strengthening resistance to one of the host's most valuable antiparasitic responses: activation of the antibody-independent alternative complement cascade. Specifically, iron induces the expression of genes for proteinases that degrade the C3b component [1, 44].

Once bound, a highly specific recognition cascade must ensue between corresponding ligand molecules present on both the parasite and the epithelial surface to which it has attached [3], and finally, the secretion of a variety of parasitic proteins occurs [1, 3]. Both the parasite itself and its plethora of secreted proteins influence vaginal epithelium gene expression during infection [24]. These interactions are crucial not only to the establishment of an infection, but also to the severity of clinical manifestations and long-term sequelae.

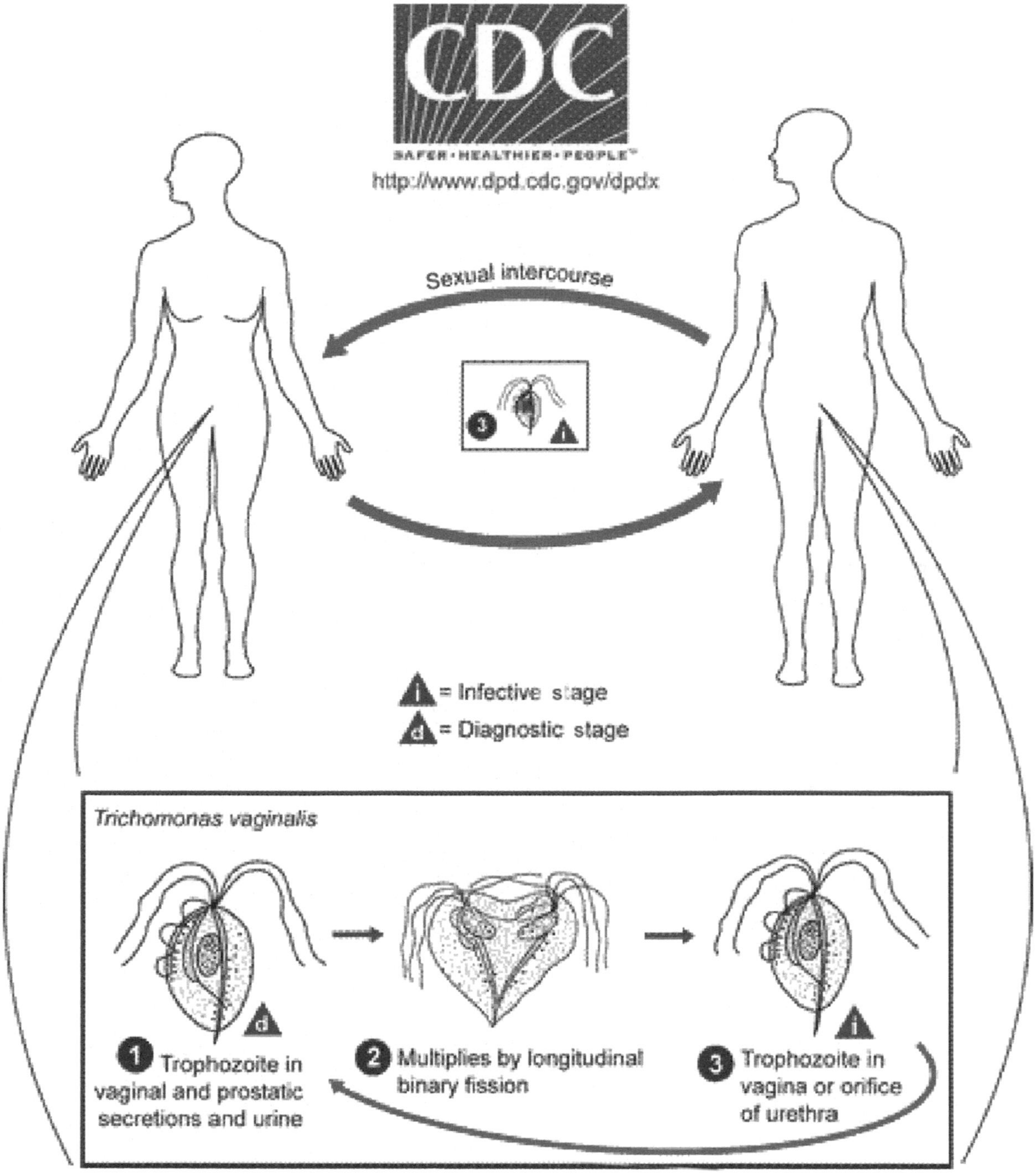

Fig. 45.2 Life cycle of *Trichomonas vaginalis*. www.dpd.cdc.gov/DPDx/HTML/ImageLibrary/S-Z/Trichomoniasis/body_Trichomoniasis_il_th.htm. Accessed 15APR08

45.7 Immunity/Host Response to *T. Vaginalis* Infection

Although minimal data exist to detail the human immune response to infection with *T. vaginalis*, it is apparent that the major antiparasitic mechanism, upregulation of cytokine production, is induced by the mere presence of the parasite within the urogenital tract, and that the natural history of disease progression is stepwise. First, parasite adhesion to vaginal epithelial cells is cytotoxic and alters gene expression. Within a few days, degeneration of infected epithelial cells causes abundant vaginal inflammation and a neutrophil-predominant response [9]. Although infection in humans does result in the production of parasite-specific antibodies, which are detectable in vaginal secretions during active infection as well as in the serum after the infection has cleared [41], previous exposure is not 100% protective, as evidenced by high rates of re-infection [3, 34]. Immunologic studies have shown that serum antibodies and monoclonal antibodies to trichomonad surface antigens are capable of blocking adhesion in vitro; however, in vivo evidence of complete protection is lacking. In fact, T. vaginalis secretes cysteine proteinases that are capable of degrading human IgG, IgM, and IgA [36].

It seems more plausible that a combination of innate, cellular, and humoral mechanisms is necessary to clear an infection with *T. vaginalis*. Samplings of vaginal discharge from symptomatic patients indicate the importance of innate immunity as they reveal high levels of neutrophils, interleukin-8 (IL-8), monocyte chemotactic protein (MPC-1), and leukotriene B4 [43]. In vitro studies went on to show that human neutrophils and monocytes did in fact respond to *T. vaginalis* with increased production of these cytokines [38, 43], a finding that was further verified at the level of quantitative gene expression levels using a cDNA library [24].

45.8 Association with HIV Transmission

An increased risk of HIV acquisition as well as enhanced transmission of HIV in those infected with *Trichomonas* has been found. Studies conducted in Africa support the association. A significant difference in the prevalence of trichomoniasis among a cohort of HIV-infected and noninfected pregnant women in Rwanda was found by Leroy et al. with 20.2% and 10.9% prevalence, respectively [26]. Another prospective study with multivariate analysis of a cohort of women in Zaire showed significant association between the incidence of trichomoniasis and HIV seroconversion [25]. The increased risk of HIV acquisition may be a result of local inflammation caused by the presence of parasite and/or increased susceptibility to HIV, resulting from breaks in mucosal barriers caused by *Trichomonas*. The parasite causes physical breaks in the protective mucosal barrier by disturbing epithelial junction complexes, thereby increasing the portal of entry for HIV to access and infect the inflammatory cells [16].

The association of *T vaginalis* infection with increased rates of HIV transmission may be due to several mechanisms [29]. First and foremost, the natural immune response to *T. vaginalis* infection increases both transmission of and susceptibility to HIV. As the parasite establishes infection, inflammatory cells (which also serve as hosts to the HIV virus) are locally recruited to the site, where they subsequently reside and multiply. If infected with HIV, this phenomenon increases transmission to partners; and if uninfected, it places a large number of host cells in the proper place to obtain a new infection. In studies that compared HIV replication in trichomonad-infected cultures to nontrichomonad-infected cultures, HIV replication was significantly higher in the former. This increased replication of HIV in the presence of *T. vaginalis* can be attributed to the previously discussed upregulation of pro-inflammatory cytokines [16]. Another study showed that the median HIV-RNA concentration in seminal fluid of men with urethritis was significantly higher in men with trichomoniasis than in those with symptomatic urethritis due to an unidentified cause [19]. A later study showed that successful treatment of trichomonal urethritis reduced seminal HIV RNA to levels similar to that found in uninfected controls [35].

45.9 Symbiotic Relationship with Mycoplasma Species

Considering the fact that sexually transmitted infections tend not to occur as isolated events, but rather as concomitant and even cooperative interactions, investigators are now focusing on details of the interrelationship among causative agents. It has recently been established that the *Mycoplasma hominis* can combine forces with *T. vaginalis* in a symbiotic co-infection. In fact, this is the first documentation of symbiosis among two obligate human pathogens [8, 48]. *M. hominis*, the smallest self-replicating bacterial organism, is a component of normal vaginal flora in some women, yet is capable of independent opportunistic infection of the human urogenital tract. After discovering that *M. hominis* was able to infect and multiply within the intracellular environment of *T. vaginalis* [8], researchers found that infections with both organisms were associated [39]. Such a relationship has implications for treatment, as well as eliciting the need for further investigation with regard to other organisms that *T. vaginalis* may carry internally.

45.10 Treatment

According to the CDC, the current standard of care for treatment of trichomoniasis is oral metronidazole in one of the three dosing regimens: (1) a single oral 2-g dose; (2) 250 mg PO tid for 7 days; or (3) 500 mg PO bid for 7 days. Reported cure rates are >95% [7, 41]. In light of the high rates of infection in asymptomatic partners and of re-infection, it is crucial to treat both infected persons and their partners.

Metronidazole is a 5-nitroimidazole compound derived from the *Streptomyces* antibiotic azomycin. Antiparasitic activity depends on hydrogenosome-mediated intracellular reduction of the nitro group at the fifth position of the imidazole ring. This reduced form of the drug targets segments of DNA rich in thymine and adenine for destruction [7]. Metabolism of the drug occurs in the liver via side-chain oxidation and glucuronidation. Side-effects are minimal, and rarely reported, but may include dizziness, nausea, vomiting, headache, and an unfavorable "metallic taste." Unfortunately, nitroimidazole therapy during pregnancy remains controversial despite the link between *T. vaginalis* infection and perinatal morbidity [32].

Metronidazole resistance is being increasingly documented; it can occur either aerobically or anaerobically [7, 47]. The most common and clinically important resistance mechanism is mediated aerobically by hydrogenosomes. Essentially, increased levels of intracellular oxygen serve to diminish hydrogenosome activity by competing for electrons (oxygen happens to be a more highly efficient electron acceptor), and decreased hydrogenosome activity translates to decreased reduction and activation of metronidazole. Fortunately, in many cases, this resistance is relative and can be overcome by larger doses of the drug. Tinidazole serves as an alternative treatment. Although its mechanism of action is quite similar to metronidazole, pharmacological features and nitroimidazole resistance patterns suggest that tinidazole may be more effective in treating patients with metronidazole treatment failure. Alternatives to nitroimidazole therapy are few, and most have limited efficacy and significant toxicity [32].

Potential drug targets to overcome resistant strains remain the subject of new research and focus on components of the parasite that differ substantially or are altogether absent from host cells. Recent studies have shown that *T. vaginalis* possesses a thioredoxin reductase that differs fundamentally from that of humans, and thus may be a promising target for innovative pharmacologic therapy [41]. Additionally, *T. vaginalis* possesses an iron superoxide dismutase enzyme, which is not a component of mammalian cells, and may therefore be a target of therapy [7].

45.11 Summary

Trichomonas vaginalis is a highly prevalent protozoan parasite that is responsible for an indeterminate, yet significant, amount of sexually transmitted infections across the globe. Manifestations of infection vary from a characteristic fishy-smelling discharge with pruritus to atypical pelvic inflammatory disease with the potential for pregnancy complications. Furthermore, infection with *T. vaginalis* increases the risk for transmission and spread of HIV. The cytopathology is highly dependent on initial adherence and alterations of gene expression, with the subsequent human response to infection involving a combination of multiple arms of the immune system. Treatment for the majority of infections is metronidazole. However, owing to the increasing emergence of resistant strains, research is being directed toward the development of alternate therapies. Given the widespread prevalence of this infection and its potential for significant complications, efforts need to be directed toward increased awareness and prevention, diagnosis, and treatment, not only of infected individuals, but also of their partners.

Take-Home Pearls

- *T. vaginalis* is a motile flagellated protozoan which exists only in the trophozoite form, as no cyst form is known.
- Trichomoniasis has not yet been designated as reportable to the Centers for Disease Control and Prevention (CDC).
- The true incidence of trichomoniasis is likely underestimated due to a high rate of asymptomatic infections.
- Symptoms in males, while occurring only in the minority of infected individuals, consist of a clear or mucopurulent urethral discharge and/or dysuria.
- Humans are the only known hosts of *T. vaginalis.*
- Infection with *T. vaginalis* increases the risk for transmission and spread of HIV.
- While less commonly used than a wet mount, vaginal culture has been deemed the "gold standard" for diagnosis of trichomoniasis.
- Colpitis macularis, or strawberry cervix, is a very specific clinical sign of *T. vaginalis* infection, and describes punctate hemorrhages of an infected cervix.
- Treatment for the majority of infections is metronidazole, however, there is an increasing emergence of resistant strains.
- High rates of infection in asymptomatic partners and of re-infection, makes the treatment of both infected persons and their partners critical.
- Infection with T. vaginalis leads to an increased risk of HIV acquisition and enhanced transmission of the virus.

References

1. Alderete, J., Demes, P., Gombosova, A., et al.: Specific parasitism of purified vaginal epithelial cells by *Trichomonas vaginalis*. Infect. Immun. **56**(10), 2558–2562 (1988)
2. Alderete, J., Nguyen, J., Mundodi, V., et al.: Heme-iron increases levels of AP65-mediated adherence by *Trichomonas vaginalis*. Microb. Pathog. **36**(5), 263–271 (2003)
3. Arroyo, R., Martinez-Palomo, A., Gonzales-Robles, A., et al.: Signalling of Trichomonas vaginalis for amoeboid transformation and adhesion synthesis follows cytoadherence. Mol. Microbiol. **7**, 299–309 (1993)
4. Cates, W., and The American Social Health Association Panel: Estimates of the incidence and prevalence of sexually transmitted diseases in the United States. Sex Transm. Dis. **26**, 52–57 (1999)
5. Caliendo, A.M., Jordan, J.A., Green, A.M., et al.: Real-time PCR improves detection of Trichomonas vaginalis infection compared with using culture self-collected vaginal swabs. Infect. Dis. Obstet. Gynecol. **13**, 145–150 (2005)
6. Cotch, M.F., Pastorek, J.G., Nugent, R.P., et al.: *Trichomonas vaginalis* associated with low birth weight and preterm delivery. Sex. Transm. Dis. **24**, 361–362 (1997)
7. Cudmore, S., Delgaty, K., Hayward, S., et al.: Treatment of infections caused by metronidazole-resistant *Trichomonas vaginalis*. Clin. Microbiol. Rev. **17**(4), 783–793 (2004)
8. Dessi, D., Delogu, G., Emonte, E., et al.: Long-term survival and intracellular replication of *Mycoplasma hominis* in *Trichomonas vaginalis* cells: potential role of the protozoan in transmitting bacterial infection. Infect. Immun. **73**(2), 1180–1186 (2004)
9. Fichorova, R., Trifonova, R., Gilbert, R., et al.: *Trichomonas vaginalis* lipophosphoglycan triggers a selective upregulation of cytokines by human female reproductive tract epithelial cells. Infect. Immun. **74**(10), 5773–5779 (2006)
10. Fiori, P., Rappelli, M.F., Addis, M.F.: The flagellated parasite Trichomonas vaginalis: new insights into cytopathogenicity mechanisms. Microb. Pathog. **1**, 149–156 (1999)
11. Fouts, A.C., Kraus, S.J.: Trichomonas vaginalis: re-evaluation of its clinical presentation and laboratory diagnosis. J. Infect. Dis. **141**, 137–143 (1980)
12. Garcia, A., Chang, T., Benchimol, M., et al.: Iron and contact with host cells induce expression of adhesions on surface of *Trichomonas vaginalis*. Mol. Microbiol. **47**(5), 1207–1224 (2003)
13. Gerbase, A.C., Rowley, J.T., Mertens, T.E.: Global epidemiology of sexually transmitted diseases. Lancet **351**, 2–4 (1998)
14. Gram, I.T., Macaluso, M., Churchill, J., et al.: Trichomonas vaginalis (TV) and human papillomavirus (HPV) infection and the incidence of cervical intraepithelial neoplasia (CIN) grade III. Cancer Causes Control **3**, 231–236 (1992)
15. Grodstein, F., Goldman, M.B., Cramer, D.W.: Relation of tubal infertility to a history of sexually transmitted diseases. Am. J. Epidemiol. **137**, 577–584 (1993)
16. Guenthner, P., Secor, D., Dezzutti, C.: *Trichomonas vaginalis*-induced epithelial monolayer disruption and human immunodeficiency virus type 1 (HIV-1) replication: implications for the sexual transmission of HIV-1. Infect. Immun. **73**(7), 4155–4160 (2005)
17. Hardy, P., Hardy, J., Nell, E., et al.: Prevalence of six sexually transmitted disease agents among pregnant inner-city adolescents and pregnancy outcome. Lancet **ii**, 333–337 (1984)
18. Heine, P., McGregor, J.A.: Trichomonas vaginalis: a reemerging pathogen. Clin. Obstet. Gynecol. **36**, 137–144 (1993)
19. Hobbs, M., Kazembe, P., Reed, A., et al.: *Trichomonas vaginalis* as a cause of urethritis in Malawian men. Sex. Transm. Dis. **26**, 381–387 (1999)

20. Jesus, J., Vannier-Santos, M., Britto, C., et al.: *Trichomonas vaginalis* virulence against epithelial cells and morphological variability: the comparison between a well-established strain and a fresh isolate. Parasitol. Res. **93**(5), 369–377 (2004)
21. Kigozi, G., Brahmbhatt, H., Wabwire-Mangen, F., et al.: Treatment of *Trichomonas* in pregnancy and adverse outcomes of pregnancy: a subanalysis of a randomized trial in Rakai, Uganda. Am. J. Obstet. Gynecol. **189**, 1398–1400 (2003)
22. Klebanoff, M., Carey, J., Hauth, J., et al.: Failure of metronidazole to prevent preterm delivery among pregnant women with asymptomatic Trichomonas vaginalis infection. N Engl J. Med. **345**, 487–493 (2001)
23. Koumans, E.H., Sternberg, M., Bruce, C., et al.: The prevalence of bacterial vaginosis in the United States, 2001–2004; associations with symptoms, sexual behaviors, and reproductive health. Sex. Transm. Dis. **34**(11), 864–869 (2007)
24. Kucknoor, A., Mundodi, V., Alderete, J.: The proteins secreted by *Trichomonas vaginalis* and vaginal epithelial cell response to secreted and episomally expressed AP65. J. Cell. Microbiol. **9**(11), 2586–2597 (2007)
25. Laga, M., Manoka, A., Kivuvu, M., et al.: Non-ulcerative sexually transmitted diseases as risk factors for HIV-1 transmission in women: results from a cohort study. AIDS **7**, 95–102 (1993)
26. Leroy, V., De Clercq, A., Ladner, J., et al.: Should screening of genital infections be part of antenatal care in areas of high HIV prevalence? A prospective cohort study from Kigali, Rwanda, 1992–1993. Genitourin. Med. **71**, 207–211 (1995)
27. Levi, M.H., Torres, J., Pina, C., et al.: Comparison of the InPouch TV culture system and Diamond's modified medium for detection of *Trichomonas vaginalis*. J. Clin. Microbiol. **35**, 3308–3310 (1997)
28. Madico, G., Quinn, T.C., Rompalo, K.T., et al.: Diagnosis of Trichomonas vaginalis infection by PCR using vaginal swab samples. J. Clin. Microbiol. **36**, 3205–3210 (1998)
29. McClelland, R., Sangare, L., Hassan, W., et al.: Infection with *Trichomonas vaginalis* increases the risk of HIV-1 acquisition. J. Infect. Dis. **195**, 698–702 (2007)
30. Minkoff, H., Grunebaum, A.N., Schwarz, A.H., et al.: Risk factors for prematurity and premature rupture of membranes: a prospectivestudy of the vaginal flora in pregnancy. Am. J. Obstet. Gynecol. **150**, 965–972 (1984)
31. Mundodi, V., Kucknoor, A., Alderete, J.: Antisense RNA decreases AP33 gene expression and cytoadherence by *T. vaginalis*. BMC Microbiol. **7**, 647 (2007)
32. Nanda, N., Michel, R.G., Kurdgelashvili, G., et al.: Trichomoniasis and its treatment. Expert Rev. Anti Infect. Ther. **4**(1), 125–135 (2006)
33. Patel, S.R., Wiese, W., Patel, S.C., et al.: Systematic review of diagnostic tests for vaginal trichomoniasis. Infect. Dis. Obstet. Gynecol. **8**, 248–257 (2000)
34. Petrin, D., Delgaty, K., Bhatt, R., et al.: Clinical and microbiological aspects of *Trichomonas vaginalis*. Clin. Microbiol. Rev. **2**, 300–317 (1998)
35. Price, M., Zimba, D., Hoffman, I.F., et al.: Addition of treatment for trichomoniasis to syndromic management of urethritis in Malawi: a randomized clinical trial. Sex. Transm. Dis. **30**, 516–522 (2003)
36. Provenazo, D., Alderete, J.: Analysis of human immunoglobulin-degrading cysteine proteinases of *Trichomonas vaginalis*. Infect. Immun. **69**(9), 3388–3395 (1995)
37. Rein, M.F., Muller, M.: Trichomonas vaginalis and trichomoniasis. In Holmes K.K. (ed.), Sexually Transmitted Diseases. New York: McGraw Hill; pp.481–492 (1990)
38. Ryu, J., Chung, H., Min, Y., et al.: Diagnosis of trichomoniasis by polymerase chain reaction. Yonsei Med. J. **40**, 56–60 (1999)
39. Sanderson, B., White, E., Baldson, M.: Amine content of vaginal fluid from patients with trichomoniasis and gardnerella associated non-specific vaginitis. J.Vener. Dis. **59**, 302–305 (1983)
40. Saurina, G.R., McCormack, W.M.: Trichomoniasis in pregnancy. Sex. Transm. Dis. **24**, 361–362 (1997)
41. Schwebke, J., Burgess, D.: Trichomoniasis. Clin. Microbiol. Rev. **17**(4), 794–803 (2004)
42. Sena, A., Miller, W., Hobbs, M., et al.: *Trichomonas vaginalis* infection in male sexual partners: implications for diagnosis, treatment, and prevention. Clin. Infect. Dis. **44**, 13–22 (2007)
43. Shaio, M., Lin, P., Liu, J., et al.: Generation of interleukin-8 from human monocytes in response to *Trichomonas vaginalis* stimulation. Infect. Immun. **63**(10), 3864–3870 (1995)
44. Solano-Gonzalez, E., Burrola-Barraza, E., Leon-Sicairos, C., et al.: The trichomonad cysteine proteinase TVCP4 transcript contains an iron-reponsive element. J. FEBS Lett. **561**(16), 2919–2928 (2007)
45. Sutcliffe, S., Giovannucci, E., Alderete, J., et al.: Plasma antibodies against *Trichomonas vaginalis* and subsequent risk of prostate cancer. Cancer Epidemiol. Biomark. Prev. **15**, 939–945 (2006)
46. Torok, M., Miller, W., Hobbs, M., et al.: The association between *Trichomonas vaginalis* infection and level of vaginal lactobacilli in non-pregnant women. J. Infect. Dis. **196**, 1102–1107 (2007)
47. Upcroft, P., Upcroft, J.A.: Drug targets and mechanisms of resistance in the anaerobic protozoa. Clin. Microbiol. Rev. **14**(1), 150–164 (2001)
48. Vancini, R., Bechimol, M.: Entry and intracellular location of *Mycoplasma hominis* in *Trichomonas vaginalis*. Arch. Microbiol. **189**(1), 7–18 (2008)
49. Van der Pol, B., Williams, J., Orr, D., et al.: Prevalence, incidence, natural history and response to treatment of *Trichomonas vaginalis* infection among adolescent women. J. Infect. Dis. **192**, 2039–2044 (2005)
50. Van der Shee, C., Sluiters, H., Van der Maijden, W.I., et al.: Host and pathogen interaction during vaginal infection by *Trichomonas vaginalis and Mycoplasma hominis* or *Ureaplasma urealyticum*. J. Microbiol. Methods **45**(1), 61–67 (2001)
51. Viikki, M., Pukkala, E., Nieminen, P., et al.: Gynaecological infections as risk determinants of subsequent cervical neoplasia. Acta Oncol. **39**, 71–75 (2000)
52. World Health Organization (WHO). Global prevalence and incidence of selected curable sexually transmitted diseases: overview and estimates. WHO, Geneva (1999)
53. Wiese, W.J., Patel, S.R., Patel, S.C., et al.: A meta-analysis of the Papanicolaou smear and wet mount for the diagnosis of vaginal trichomoniasis. Am. J. Med. **108**, 301–308 (2000)
54. Zhang, Z.F., Begg, C.B.: Is Trichomonas vaginalis a cause of cervical neoplasia? Results from a combined analysis of 24 studies. Int. J. Epidemiol. **23**, 682–690 (1994)

Part VI

Fungal Infections

Genital Candidiasis

46

Jack D. Sobel

Core Messages

- Candidiasis continues to be an extremely common cause of vulvovaginal symptoms and is still most commonly due to *Candida albicans.*
- Major progress has been made in recognizing the role of host genetic factors in pathogenesis of sporadic and recurrent vulvovaginal candidiasis (VVC).
- Diagnostic problems continue to prevail with frequent over diagnosis, but also self and practitioner dependent. Practitioners all too often fail to obtain microbiologic confirmation. PCR-based diagnosis may have a role in the future but current status is unconfirmed and not validated.
- No new antifungal drugs have been introduced in the last decade. Effective therapy is nevertheless achievable by prudent use of topical and oral systemic regimens. Recurrent vulvovaginal candidiasis (RVVC) can be well-controlled by long term suppressive maintenance antifungal regimens however, cure is often evasive.

46.1 Epidemiology

Information on the incidence of vulvovaginal candidiasis (VVC) is incomplete because VVC is not a reportable entity, and data collection is hampered by inaccuracies of diagnosis and the use of nonrepresentative study populations.

VVC affects most females (70–75%) at least once during their lives, most frequently young women in the child-bearing age, of whom 40 to 50 percent will experience a recurrence [1]. A small subpopulation of 5-8 percent of adult women has recurrent episodes of VVC, defined as ≥4 episodes per annum [2]. Authors indicate that VVC is responsible for 15 to 30 percent of vulvovaginal symptoms [3, 4]. Availability of over-the-counter antimycotics has further limited the ability to measure asymptomatic *Candida* carriage and VVC. Diagnosis and therapy of VVC, together with lost productivity, result in an estimated cost of 1 billion dollars annually in the United States [5]. In the United States, VVC is the second most common cause of vaginal infections following bacterial vaginosis (BV) [6, 7].

Point-prevalence studies indicate that *Candida* species may be isolated from the vagina of approximately 20% (range 10–80%) of asymptomatic healthy women [8].

46.2 Microbiology

Between 85 and 95 percent of yeast strains isolated from the vagina belong to the species *Candida albicans* [9, 10]. The remainder are non-*albicans* species, the commonest of which is *Candida glabrata.* Non-*albicans* species can induce vaginitis, which is

J.D. Sobel
Department of Medicine, Wayne State University School of Medicine, Detroit, MI, USA
e-mail: jsobel@med.wayne.edu

G. Gross and S.K. Tyring (eds.), *Sexually Transmitted Infections and Sexually Transmitted Diseases*,
DOI: 10.1007/978-3-642-14663-3_46, © Springer-Verlag Berlin Heidelberg 2011

clinically indistinguishable from that caused by *C. albicans*; moreover, they are often more resistant to therapy [9, 11, 12]. In many parts of the world, non-*albicans* isolates, notably *C. glabrata*, affect 10–30% of women [13, 14].

It has been suggested that the incidence of VVC caused by non-*albicans* strains is rising [15], owing to single-dose therapy, low-dosage azole maintenance regimens, and use of over-the-counter antimycotics. Several multicenter studies in the USA failed to confirm any increase in the prevalence of VVC caused by non-*albicans* species [16, 17]. Type 2 diabetes mellitus is a risk factor for *C. glabrata* vaginitis. Infrequent causes of vaginitis include *C. parapsilosis*, *C. tropicalis*, and *C. krusei* although most species of *Candida* have been associated with vaginitis [18, 19].

Yeast blastospores (blastoconidia) represent the phenotypic form responsible for vaginal transmission and asymptomatic colonization of the vagina. Germinated yeast with production of mycelia (hyphae) are found most commonly in symptomatic vaginitis.

46.3 *Candida* Virulence Factors

Colonization of the vagina requires yeast adherence to vaginal epithelial cells. *C. albicans* adheres in significantly higher numbers to such cells than do *non-albicans species* [20]. All *C. albicans* strains appear to adhere equally well to both exfoliated vaginal epithelial cells [20]. In contrast, there is considerable person-to-person variation in in vitro vaginal epithelial cell receptivity to *Candida* organisms in adherence assays [20]. Although unproven, it is quite likely that genetic factors increase receptivity in women with recurrent infections. The yeast adhesin appears to reside with the surface mannoprotein, but multiple adhesions have been identified (Als, hyphal-specific adhesin Hwplp).

Germination of *Candida* cells enhances colonization and facilitates tissue invasion. Factors that enhance or facilitate germination promote symptomatic vaginitis, whereas inhibition of germination may prevent vaginitis in asymptomatic yeast carriers.

Proteolytic enzymes, toxins, and phospholipase elaborated by yeast enhance virulence [21]. Secreted aspartyl proteinases elaborated by pathogenic *Candida* species have been identified in vaginal secretions in women with symptomatic vaginitis but not in those with asymptomatic colonization [22]. These proteolytic enzymes, which have broad substrate specificity, destroy free and cell-bound proteins that impair fungal colonization and invasion. Several genes governing proteinase production (SAP1, SAP2, and SAP3) have been cloned, and a strong correlation exists in both in vitro and experimental vaginitis between gene expression, aspartyl proteinase secretion, and ability to cause disease [23, 24]. Mycotoxin, including a vaginal-identified gliotoxin – may act to inhibit phagocytic activity or suppress the local immune system. High-frequency heritable switching occurs in colony morphology of most *Candida* species grown on amino acid-rich agar in vitro at 24°C [25]. The variant phenotypes represent a varying capacity to form mycelia spontaneously and express other virulence factors, including drug resistance and adherence. There is insufficient evidence that phenotypic switching occurs in vivo; however, this is an attractive hypothesis to explain spontaneous in vivo transformation from asymptomatic colonization to symptomatic vaginitis. Fresh clinical vaginal isolates obtained during acute vaginitis have been found to be in a high-frequency mode of switching.

Iron-binding by *Candida* organisms facilitates yeast virulence.

46.4 Pathogenesis

Candida organisms gain access to the vaginal lumen and secretions predominantly from the adjacent perianal area. Effective vaginal anti-*Candida* defense mechanisms allow long-term persistence of *Candida* organisms as vaginal commensals (Table 46.1). Two concepts are critical in understanding the pathogenesis of VVC: The first is the transformation of asymptomatic vaginal colonization to symptomatic VVC, and the second is the mechanism whereby some women suffer from recurrent VVC (RVVC) (Fig. 46.1).

Most if not all women carry *Candida* in the vagina sometime, yet without symptoms or signs of vaginitis, usually with a low concentration of yeast organisms. *Candida* may be either a commensal or a pathogen in the vagina, and it is very likely that changes in the host vaginal environment are necessary before the organism can induce pathologic effects.

Although the gut may well be the initial source of vaginal colonization by *Candida* organisms, controversy

Table 46.1 Vaginal Defense Mechanisms Against *Candida* species

Defense	Mechanism	Comments
Innate		
Vaginal epithelial cells	Inhibit *Candida* growth in vitro, cell contact required. No endocytosis	Protective role in vivo unknown. ↓ anti-*Candida* activity in women with RVVC
Mannose-binding lectin (MBL)	Epithelial cell associated. Binds to *Candida* surface mannan. Activates complement. Inhibits *Candida* growth	MBL is genetically determined. May provide individual host susceptibility to vaginal colonization and VVC
Activated lactoferrin	Fungistatic and cidal activity	Natural peptides in cervico-vaginal secretions (role unproven)
Vaginal bacterial flora	*Lactobacillus* spp. favored. Competition for nutrients. Bacteriocins and H_2O_2 inhibits yeast growth/germination	Protective role controversial
Phagocytic systems/ PMNs	Phagocytosis and intracellular killing decreases fungal load and prevents mucosal invasion	Protective role controversial PMNs not prominent in vaginal secretions
Mononuclear cells, complement	Mainly found in lamina propria in experimental vaginitis. Nitric oxide has anti-*Candida* activity	
Adaptive		
Humoral-immunogloblulin (S-IgA, IgM, IgG)	Following VVC systemic (IgM, IgG) and local (IgA) response. Experimental *Candida* vaginitis some but not all investigators show protective role by active and passive local immunization	Protective role not proven. Women with RVVC have high titers of vaginal anti-*Candida* IgG, IgA Anti-*Candida* IgE may contribute to symptoms
Cell-mediated immunity (CMI) T-cell response	Compartmentalization of vaginal CMI response from systemic CMI. Experimental studies-minimal role of systemic CMI but protection induced with local immunization. Hypothesis-protective role of Th-1 cytokine profile and Th-2 profile contributes to RVVC	Role extremely controversial Failure to detect Th-2 cytokines in women with RVVC IL-4 (Th-2) inhibits anti-*Candida* activity of nitric oxide (NO) and protective pro-inflammatory Th-1 cytokines

continues regarding the role of the intestinal tract as a source of reinfection in women with RVVC.

Asymptomatic male genital colonization with *Candida* is four times more common in male sexual partners of infected women [9]. Penile *Candida* organisms are present in approximately 20 percent of partners of women with RVVC [9]. *Candida* organisms are more commonly found in uncircumcised males. Infected partners usually carry identical strains, however, the contribution of sexual transmission to the pathogenesis of infection appears limited [26].

Following antimycotic therapy of VVC, negative vaginal *Candida* cultures turn positive within 30 days in 20 to 25 percent of women, indicating persistence of some strains of yeast and hence a vaginal as opposed to intestinal reservoir. Strains isolated before and after therapy are of the identical type in more than two-thirds of recurrences [9]. Small numbers of the microorganisms persist within the vaginal lumen, generally in numbers too small to be detected by conventional vaginal cultures, only to reemerge some weeks or months later.

46.5 Predisposing Factors

Although VVC is monomicrobial, causation is multifactorial. RVVC may be idiopathic or caused by multiple different mechanisms (Fig. 46.1). Factors that predispose to vaginal colonization may differ from those that facilitate transformation from asymptomatic colonization to symptomatic vaginitis.

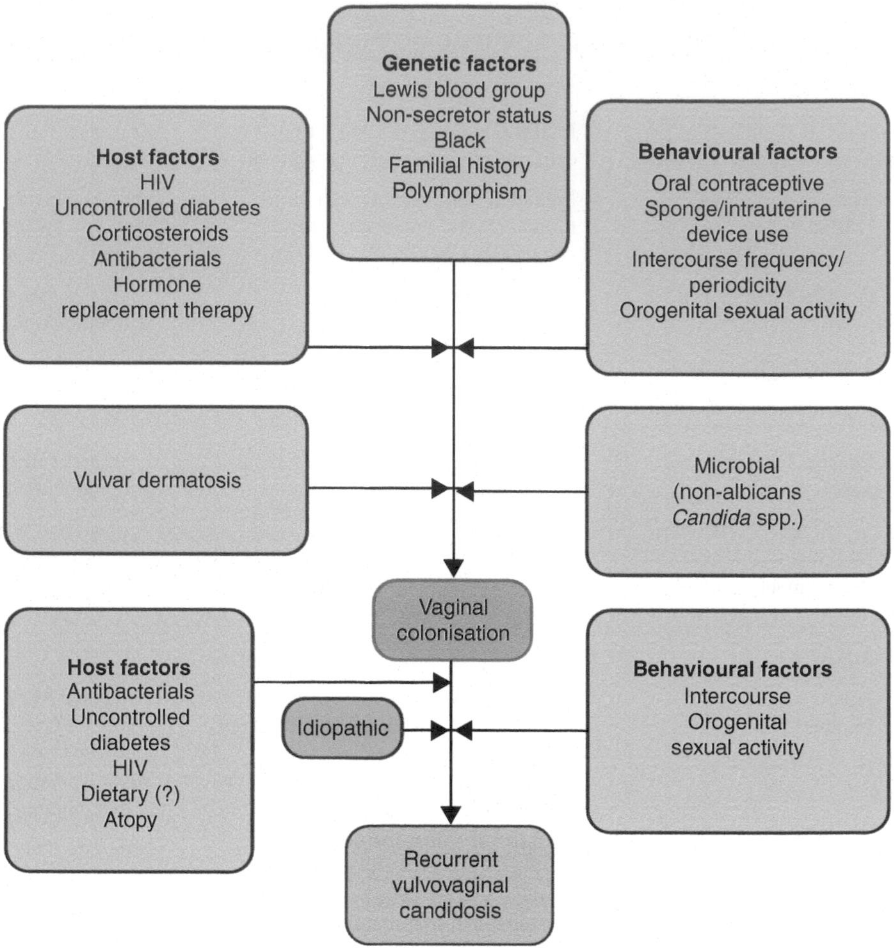

Fig. 46.1 Risk factors for recurrent vulvovaginal candidiasis (RVVC) (*OC* oral contraceptives, *IUD* intrauterine device, *NAC* non-albicans Candida species, *HIV* human immunodeficiency virus)

46.5.1 Genetic

Anecdotal reports of familial susceptibility to VVC, studies indicating increased VVC prevalence in African-American women, and ABO and Lewis blood group members all suggest a genetic basis [27]. Recently, in vivo polymorphism studies involving mannose-binding lectin (MBL) and experimental vaginitis in inbred and outbred mice, further support genetic susceptibility to *Candida* colonization or vaginitis [28].

46.5.2 Pregnancy

During pregnancy a higher prevalence of vaginal colonization and symptomatic vaginitis occurs [29]. Recurrences are more common and therapeutic response is reduced [30]. High levels of reproductive hormones, providing a higher glycogen content in the vaginal tissue, provide a carbon source for *Candida* organisms [31]. Estrogen also enhances the adherence of yeast to vaginal epithelial cells. A cytosol receptor or binding system, for female reproductive hormones has been documented in *C. albicans* resulting in enhanced mycelial formation.

46.5.3 Contraceptives

Many small, poorly controlled studies have produced conflicting data including increased vaginal colonization with *Candida* and symptomatic vaginitis following high estrogen-content oral contraceptive use [32]. Contradictory studies of women utilizing low-estrogen oral contraceptives are reported [33]. Increased carriage of yeast is reported in IUD, contraceptive sponge, diaphragm, and condom users, with or without use of spermicide [34]. Foxman, in an extensive study in college students, failed to identify increased risk of symptomatic VVC in users of oral contraceptives, diaphragms, condoms, or spermicides [32].

46.5.4 Diabetes Mellitus

Vaginal colonization with *Candida* is more frequent in diabetic women. Women with Type 2 diabetes are more prone to colonization with *C. glabrata* [35]. Although uncontrolled diabetes predisposes to symptomatic vaginitis, well controlled diabetics do not suffer from an increased prevalence of VVC. Although a glucose tolerance test is often recommended in women with RVVC, yield is extremely low; and testing is not justified in premenopausal women. Occasionally women with RVVC describe an association between "candy binges" and exacerbation of symptomatic VVC. Donders et al. performed glucose tolerance tests on women with RVVC [36]. An increased frequency of abnormal GTTs compatible with diabetes or prediabetes was not found. However, plasma glucose levels (within the normal range) were still significantly higher than in control subjects suggesting that a diet high in refined sugars may contribute to the risk of VVC [36].

On the other hand Ehrstrom & Rylander studied women with RVVC and found that vaginal concentrations of glucose were not increased compared to controls [37].

46.5.5 Antibiotics

Symptomatic VVC frequently follows vaginal or systemic antibiotics [38]. All antimicrobials appear responsible. Estimates of post-antibiotic VVC include a range of 28%–33% [39]. Vaginal colonization rates increase from approximately 10 percent to 30 percent (40]. Antibiotics, are thought to act by eliminating the protective vaginal bacterial flora that allows *Candida* overgrowth in the gastrointestinal tract, the vagina or both. In particular *Lactobacillus* species may provide colonization resistance and prevent germination, maintaining low numbers of yeast. Lactobacillus–yeast cell interaction include competition for nutrients, stearic interference by lactobacilli with *Candida* adherence, elaboration of H_2O_2 and inhibitory bacteriocins by lactobacilli, as well as a direct antibiotic-induced stimulatory effect on the growth of *Candida* species.

Not all studies confirm VVC occurrence following antibiotic regimens. Most women who receive antibiotics do not develop symptomatic VVC, in fact, the majority of women with acute VVC have not been recent recipients of antibiotics. Hence, only a subpopulation of women, already colonized with *Candida*, are at risk of vaginitis following antimicrobial therapy [41].

46.5.6 Behavioral Factors

The role of sexual behavior in causing symptomatic often recurrent VVC has been underestimated [26, 33]. Although non-sexually active females frequently develop VVC, the incidence of VVC increases dramatically in the second decade, corresponding to the onset of sexual activity [2]. Sexual transmission of *Candida* organisms may occur during vaginal intercourse [26]. Intercourse frequency has been questionably associated with acute vaginitis [26, 32]. In particular, receptive orogenital sex consistently emerges as a risk factor [42]. In spite of anecdotal evidence, Foxman found no evidence incriminating female hygiene habits as risk factors for VVC [32].

The use of well-ventilated clothing and cotton underwear may be of value in preventing infection. Foxman, however, found no increased risk for VVC among wearers of tight clothing or noncotton underwear [32]. There is no evidence confirming that iron deficiency predisposes to infection. Chemical contact, atopy, local allergy, or hypersensitivity reactions may alter the vaginal milieu and facilitate transformation from asymptomatic colonization to symptomatic vaginitis [43].

46.6 Transformation to Symptomatic Vaginitis

The mechanism whereby *Candida* organisms induce vulvovaginal inflammation is still obscure. Yeast cells are capable of producing extracellular proteases and phospholipase. The paucity of phagocytic cells in the vaginal discharge most likely reflects the lack of elaboration of chemotactic substances. Both blastoconidia and pseudohyphae are capable of destroying superficial cells by direct invasion.

During the symptomatic episode, there is the conspicuous appearance of pseudohyphae and hyphae. Hyphal elements enhance colonization and although representing the dominant invasive form, capable of penetrating intact epithelial cells, only the very superficial layers are involved [9]. Although symptoms are not always related to the yeast load, VVC is associated with greater numbers of *Candida* organisms and with hyphal elements.

It is likely that more than one pathogenic mechanism may exist. In the presence of pruritus, host hypersensitivity or immune mechanisms are likely to be involved. VVC is more common in women with atopy and allergic diseases [44]. Although clinical signs and symptoms are indistinguishable in infections caused by different *Candida* species, *C. glabrata* and *C. parapsilosis* tend to be associated with milder and often absent symptoms [18]. Occasionally, male partners of asymptomatic female carriers of *Candida* develop transient post-coital penile erythema and pruritus, suggesting that inflammation is due to hypersensitivity mechanisms. Much remains to be elucidated as to the role of the host versus microorganisms in inducing vulvovaginal inflammation.

46.7 Clinical Manifestations

Acute pruritus and vaginal discharge are the usual presenting complaints, but neither is specific to VVC [3, 6, 45]. Vaginal discharge is not invariably present and is frequently minimal. Although described as typically cottage-cheese-like, the discharge may vary from watery to homogeneously thick. Vaginal soreness, irritation, vulvar burning, dyspareunia, and external dysuria are common. Odor, if present, is minimal and inoffensive. Examination reveals erythema and swelling of the labia and vulva, often with fissures and pustulopapular peripheral lesions. The cervix is normal, and vaginal erythema is present together with adherent whitish discharge. Characteristically, symptoms are exacerbated in the week preceding menses. Several surveys indicate the unreliability of patient self-diagnosis.

46.8 Diagnosis

The lack of specificity of symptoms and signs precludes a diagnosis that is based on history and physical examination only [4, 6, 46]. The most specific symptom in VVC is pruritus, and even this criterion correctly predicted VVC in only 38 percent of patients [6].

Most patients with symptomatic vaginitis may be readily diagnosed by pH microscopic examination of vaginal secretions. A wet mount or saline preparation should routinely be done, not only to identify the presence of yeast cells and mycelia but also to exclude the presence of "clue cells" indicative of bacterial vaginosis, and motile trichomonads. A 10% potassium hydroxide (KOH) preparation is more sensitive in identifying yeast or hyphae (65 to 85 percent sensitivity) (Fig. 46.2). Vaginal pH is normal (4.0 to 4.5) in VVC, and pH in excess of 4.7 usually indicates bacterial vaginosis, trichomoniasis, or an uncommon mixed infection.

Unfortunately, up to 50 percent of patients with culture-positive symptomatic VVC will have negative microscopy [4]. Thus, although routine cultures are unnecessary if microscopy is positive, vaginal culture should be performed in symptomatic women with negative microscopy and a normal pH (Fig. 46.3) [4, 46]. The PAP smear, although specific, is insensitive, being positive in only about 25 percent of patients with culture-positive symptomatic VVC.

A positive culture alone does not necessarily indicate that yeast so identified are responsible for vaginal symptoms because 10–15% of asymptomatic women are colonized with *Candida* and hence are culture-positive. This is particularly the case for non-*albicans* *Candida* infection. Diagnosis of VVC requires a correlation of clinical findings, microscopic examination, and vaginal culture. There is no reliable serologic or commercial antigen detection technique available for the diagnosis of VVC.

Since the majority of clinicians are unable or unwilling to measure vaginal pH and perform microscopy, the majority of women with vulvovaginal symptoms remain incorrectly diagnosed and treated. PCR detection of *Candida* species in vaginal samples is possible but not available as a diagnostic test and may not prove a clinically useful test.

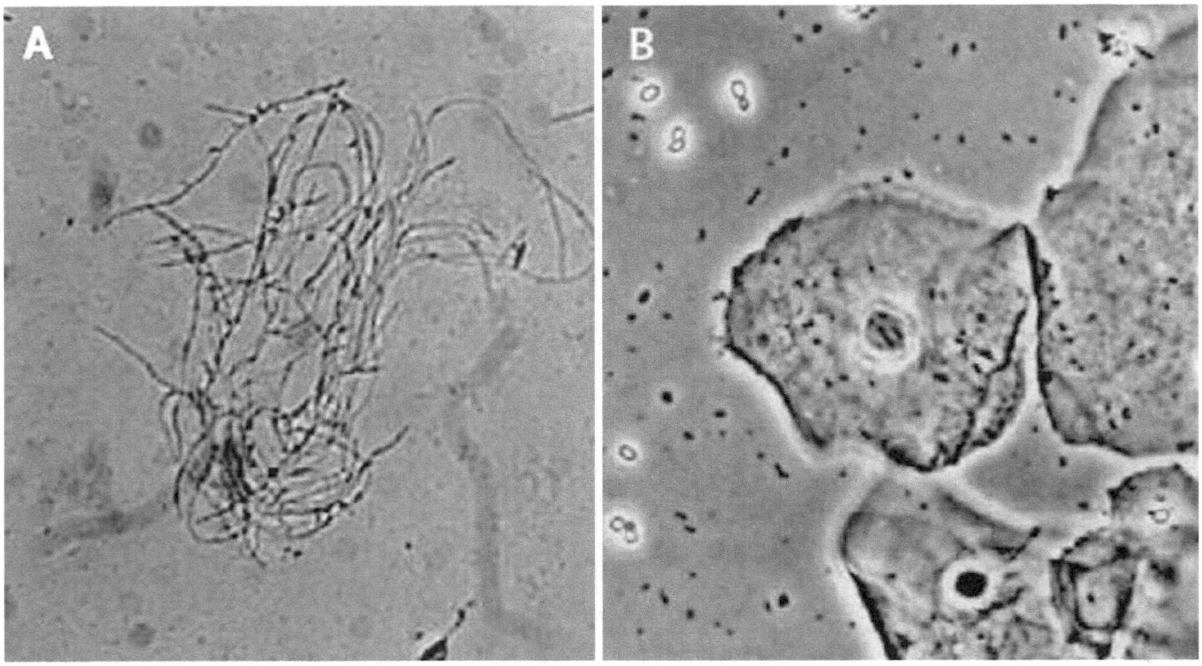

Fig. 46.2 Wet-mount examination of vaginal discharge from a woman with vulvovaginal candidiasis. (**a**) *C. albicans* hyphae 10× magnification; (**b**) Budding yeast *C. glabrata* 40× magnification

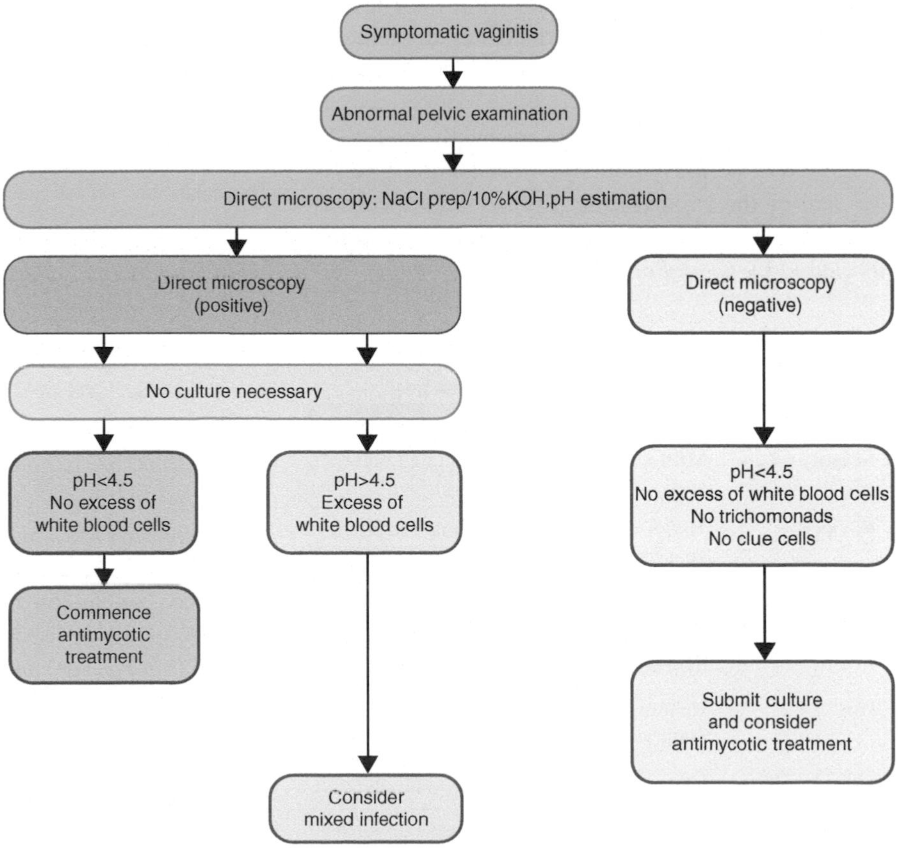

Fig. 46.3 Algorithm for diagnosis and treatment of vulvovaginal candidiasis

46.9 Treatment

46.9.1 *Acute Symptomatic Vaginitis*

Treatment of acute VVC requires individualization and a classification of VVC is available, which determines the selection and duration of antifungal therapy (Table 46.2). According to this classification, women with severe VVC do not respond adequately to single-dose and short-course therapy and require more prolonged therapy for 5–7 days [47]. Several effective topical azole agents are available in a variety of formulations (Table 46.3) [48]. Topical azoles are remarkably safe and well tolerated although not infrequent burning may be experienced. No evidence exists that any one formulation results in superior cure rates, nor evidence of the superiority of any specific azole [49]. Overall cure rates for topical azoles range from 80 to 90 percent. Oral azole agents achieve comparable or questionable marginally higher cure rates, although most patients prefer the convenience of oral administration, which eliminates local side-effects and messiness. Oral azoles suffer the drawback of potential systemic toxicity, which has dramatically limited the use of ketoconazole. In a meta-analysis of 17 trials published between 1989 and 1995 involving 2919 antifungal treatments for uncomplicated VVC, therapy was similarly effective when administered by the oral or the vaginal route [49]. Among the shortcomings of azoles is relatively poor efficacy in vaginitis caused by *C. glabrata*.

Table 46.2 Classification for vulvovaginal candidiasis

	Uncomplicated	Complicated
Severity	Mild to moderate and	Moderate to severe OR
Frequency	<4 episodes per year and	≥4 episodes per year OR
Microscopy	Pseudohyphae/ hyphae and	Budding yeast only OR
Host	Healthy, nongravid	Adverse factors (Pregnancy, diabetes, immunocompromised)
Treatment	Any short-course antimycotic therapy	Intensive regimens (avoid short-course)

Table 46.3 Azole therapy of vaginal candidiasis

Drug	Formulation	Dosage
Butoconazole	2% cream	5 gm × 3 days
	2% cream	Single dose
Clotrimazole	1% cream	5 gm × 7–14 days
	10% cream	5 gm single application
	100 mg vaginal tab	1 tab × 7 days
	100 mg vaginal tab	2 tab × 3 days
	500 mg vaginal tab	1 tab once
Miconazole	2% cream	5 gm × 7 days
	100 mg vaginal supp	1 supp × 7 days
	200 mg vaginal supp	1 supp × 3 days
	1,200 mg vaginal supp	1 supp once
Econazole	150 mg vaginal tab	1 tab × 3 days
	150 mg vaginal supp	Single dose
Fenticonazole	2% cream	5 gm × 7 days
Sertaconazole	300 mg supp	Single dose
Ticonazole	2% cream	5 gm × 3 days
	6.5% cream	5 gm single application
Teraconazole	0.4% cream	5 gm × 7 days
	0.8% cream	5 gm × 3 days
	80 mg vaginal supp	1 supp × 3 days
Fluconazole	150 mg tab	Single dose
Ketoconazole	200 mg tab	2 tab × 5 days
Itraconazole	100 mg tab	2 tab × 3 days

There has been a growing tendency to use shorter courses of topical (e.g., miconazole 1200 mg ovule) and oral agents [48]. Single-dose therapy by any route is effective in mild to moderate diseases. Vaginal clotrimazole (500-mg suppository), butoconazole as bioadhesive, and oral fluconazole (150 mg) possess pharmacokinetic properties that achieve therapeutic concentrations in the vagina for up to 5 days following single-dose administration. During pregnancy, topical azoles are more effective than nystatin and achieve acceptable cure rates; however, treatment for seven days may be necessary [30].

46.9.2 Management of Recurrent Vulvovaginal Candidiasis (RVVC)

Every effort should be made to eliminate factors that predispose one to VVC. In the majority of women, no correctable causal factors are apparent; moreover, RVVC is multifactorial in etiology. A small subgroup of women appear to benefit from restricting refined dietary sugar. Prior to therapy, mycological culture should be obtained to confirm diagnosis and identify the *Candida* specific species involved.

Successful therapy requires an induction course of either oral or topical azole to be continued until the patient is asymptomatic and culture-negative (7–14 d). In RVVC, failure to initiate a maintenance regimen results in clinical relapse in 50 percent of patients within 3 months [9, 17]. Maintenance-suppressive regimens include itraconazole 100 mg daily and once-weekly regimens of either 500 mg clotrimazole suppositories or 150 mg fluconazole orally. All three regimens are highly effective in preventing breakthrough vaginitis while on suppressive prophylaxis [9, 17, 50]. However, regardless of the maintenance regimen, cessation of therapy is accompanied by symptomatic relapse in half the women within a short time of stopping therapy [9, 17].

No benefit was demonstrated in several studies of treatment of male sexual partners [51]. Dennerstein reported a reduced rate of recurrence in RVVC in 15 patients during a 3-month period of depo-medroxyprogesterone acetate therapy [52]. The role of yogurt or lactobacillus probiotic therapy in preventing *Candida* vaginitis remains questionable. Occasional women on fluconazole with persistent pruritus benefit from addition of antihistamines [44].

An infrequently used alternative approach to maintenance of antifungals, is the use of systemic *Candida* antigen hyposensitization via the cutaneous route. Two small studies achieved encouraging results [53, 54]. This approach might be useful in women who are unable to tolerate maintenance azole suppressive therapy.

46.9.3 Resistant and non-albicans Candida vaginitis

In contrast to oral candidiasis, vaginitis, including RVVC caused by azole-resistant strains of *C. albicans*, is rare [13, 55, 56]. Vaginal isolation of *C. albicans* strains with higher MICs to fluconazole is, however, not rare and may be associated with breakthrough infections [57, 58]. In general, peak vaginal concentrations of fluconazole do not exceed 4 μg/gm, therefore, isolates with a fluconazole MIC > 8 μg/ml should be clinically resistant to conventional doses of fluconazole. In vitro susceptibility testing has not been validated or reliable in predicting clinical response in vaginitis. This is in sharp contrast to systemic and oral candidiasis. A partial explanation may relate to in vivo synergy between fluconazole and organic acids, e.g., acetic acid normally found in the vagina [59]. Adding acetic acid to the yeast-fluconazole mixture in vitro converts fungistatic fluconazole to fungicidal [59].

RVVC is not infrequently due to non-*albicans* species. *C. glabrata* is particularly common, and approximately half the strains show reduced sensitivity to fluconazole [60]. When *C. glabrata* is isolated from a symptomatic patient, it is essential to establish that this relatively virulent pathogen is in fact the cause of symptoms and is not serving as an innocent bystander. Vaginal boric acid 600 mg daily in a gelatin capsule for 14 days or amphotericin B suppositories are effective (70%) for refractory infection [60, 61]. When a history suggests RVVC, a maintenance regimen of alternate day and then twice-weekly boric acid should be considered. The long-term safety of intravaginal boric acid has not been confirmed, and boric acid should not be used in pregnancy. In patients who failed boric acid, a success rate of >90% was achieved with a two week course of topical 17% flucytosine alone or in combination with amphotericin B [60]. *C. krusei* vaginitis is resistant to fluconazole and flucytosine but usually responds to boric acid or other azoles [19].

46.10 Vulvovaginal Candidiasis In HIV-Positive Women

From the onset of the AIDS epidemic, the prevalence and significance of oral and esophageal candidiasis were recognized. As the numbers of women with HIV grew in the 1980s, vaginal candidiasis was increasingly reported; however, the attack rate of symptomatic *Candida* vaginitis in HIV-positive women remains undetermined.

Several studies have shown that *Candida* vaginal colonization is increased in HIV-positive women [8, 62]. Utilizing epidemiologic definitions of asymptomatic VVC, but including women with both *Candida* microscopy and culture-positive women, cross-sectional and cohort studies have documented a moderate increase of VVC in HIV-positive women not receiving antiretroviral therapy [63, 64]. The increased incidence of VVC in HIV-positive women was modest when compared with the occurrence of oropharyngeal candidiasis [64]. Higher HIV loads were significantly associated with increased odds of incident or persistent vaginal colonization and candidiasis. Duerr, who reported a different definition for VVC, did find an association between lower CD4 count and VVC [63]. VVC in HIV-infected women is not more severe or less likely to respond to therapy [65].

The microbiology of VVC in HIV-positive women appears identical to that of matched high-risk HIV-negative women, although with time and possible, but unmeasured, azole exposure, there is a tendency to isolate non-albicans Candida species, notably *C. glabrata [*66] and *Candida* isolates with fluconazole-reduced sensitivity. As with other forms of lower genital ulceration and inflammation, VVC has been associated with enhanced vaginal HIV shedding with increased genital-tract HIV RNA level [67]; whether VVC facilitate HIV transmission is still unknown.

Most women who experience a single episode of VVC today are obviously not HIV-infected and do not require testing. In women with RVVC, the issue is anything but clear as the overwhelming majority of women with RVVC are HIV-negative. Only women with RVVC who have risk factors for HIV infection should be tested.

Treatment of symptomatic VVC including RVVC in HIV-positive women is identical to that of HIV-negative persons.

46.10.1 Prevention of Vulvovaginal Candidiasis

Post-antibiotic VVC is a common problem, and women frequently resort to probiotic *Lactobacillus* spp. to prevent post-antibiotic VVC. Pirotta et al [41]. reported that neither oral nor vaginal lactobacillus administration prevented postantibiotic VVC. Many practitioners recommend prophylactic oral fluconazole 150 mg with onset and completion of antibiotics. Aimed at susceptible women only, fluconazole prophylaxis is effective in idiopathic recurrent VVC, and other categories of secondary RVVC, e.g., lichen sclerosus, and topical estrogen application.

Take-Home Pearls

- *C. albicans* continues to be the most frequent cause of vulvovaginal candidiasis.
- Non-albicans Candida species although less virulent than *C. albicans* also causes vulvovaginal signs and symptoms although disease manifestations tend to be less severe.
- When non-albicans Candida species are recovered on culture from symptomatic women, also search for and exclude other concomitant causes of vulvovaginal symptoms as these species especially *C. glabrata* are frequently innocent bystanders.
- Diagnosis of vulvovaginal candidiasis should always be confirmed by laboratory methods due to non-specificity of clinical findings.
- The only infectious agent causing normal pH vulvovaginal symptoms is *Candida.*
- Normal pH vulvovaginal symptoms are frequently caused by non-infectious causes e.g., eczema, contact dermatitis.
- Antibiotic use both local intravaginal or systemic is the commonest secondary cause of acute *Candida* vaginitis (VVC).
- One can prevent development of antibiotic induced VVC with prophylactic antifungals especially oral fluconazole.
- Role of PCR-based diagnosis remains problematic and is not without potential for overdiagnosis.
- Culture remains the most reliable current diagnostic test but requires 48–72 h.
- Oral and topical antimycotic therapy equally efficacious.
- Before prescribing antifungal therapy for *C. glabrata* presence, ensure no other cause for symptoms exist.
- Boric acid vaginal capsules one initial therapy for *C. glabrata* and resistant *Candida* vulvovaginitis.
- Oral fluconazole 150 mg once weekly remains highly effective maintenance therapy for recurrent *Candida* vaginitis given for at least 6 months.
- Probiotics have not been shown to be useful in prevention or treatment of VVC.

References

1. Hurley, R., De Louvois, J.: Candida vaginitis. Postgrad. Med. J. **55**, 645–647 (1979)
2. Foxman, B., Marsh, J.V., Gillespie, B., Sobel, J.D.: Frequency and response to vaginal symptoms among white and African American women: results of a random digit dialing survey. J. Womens Health **7**, 1167–1174 (1998)
3. Berg, A.O., Heidrich, F.E., Fihn, S.D., et al.: Establishing the cause of genitourinary symptoms in women in a family practice. Comparison of clinical examination and comprehensive microbiology. JAMA **251**, 620–625 (1984)
4. Eckert, L.O., Hawes, S.E., Stevens, C.E., Koutsky, L.A., Eschenbach, D.A., Holmes, K.K.: Vulvovaginal candidiasis: clinical manifestations, risk factors, management algorithm. Obstet. Gynecol. **92**, 757–765 (1998)
5. Foxman, B., Barlow, R., D'Arcy, H., Gillespie, B., Sobel, J.D.: Candida vaginitis: self-reported incidence and associated costs. Sex. Transm. Dis. **27**, 230–235 (2000)
6. Anderson, M.R., Klink, K., Cohrssen, A.: Evaluation of vaginal complaints. JAMA **291**, 1368–1379 (2004)
7. Goldacre, M.J., Watt, B., Loudon, N., Milne, L.J., Loudon, J.D., Vessey, M.P.: Vaginal microbial flora in normal young women. Br. Med. J. **1**, 1450–1455 (1979)
8. Carpenter, C.C., Mayer, K.H., Fisher, A., Desai, M.B., Durand, L.: Natural history of acquired immunodeficiency syndrome in women in Rhode Island. Am. J. Med. **86**, 771–775 (1989)
9. Sobel, J.D.: Epidemiology and pathogenesis of recurrent vulvovaginal candidiasis. Am. J. Obstet. Gynecol. **152**, 924–935 (1985)
10. Sobel, J.D.: Recurrent vulvovaginal candidiasis. A prospective study of the efficacy of maintenance ketoconazole therapy. N. Engl. J. Med. **315**, 1455–1458 (1986)
11. Erdem, H., Cetin, M., Timuroglu, T., Cetin, A., Yanar, O., Pahsa, A.: Identification of yeasts in public hospital primary care patients with or without clinical vaginitis. Aust. NZ. J. Obstet. Gynaecol. **43**, 312–316 (2003)
12. Holland, J., Young, M.L., Lee, O., C-A Chen, S.: Vulvovaginal carriage of yeasts other than *Candida albicans*. Sex. Transm. Infect. **79**, 249–250 (2003)
13. Bauters, T.G., Dhont, M.A., Temmerman, M.I., Nelis, H.J.: Prevalence of vulvovaginal candidiasis and susceptibility to fluconazole in women. Am. J. Obstet. Gynecol. **187**, 569–574 (2002)
14. Corsello, S., Spinillo, A., Osnengo, G., et al.: An epidemiological survey of vulvovaginal candidiasis in Italy. Eur. J. Obstet. Gynecol. Reprod. Biol. **110**, 66–72 (2003)
15. Cauwenbergh, G.: Vaginal candidiasis: Evolving trends in the incidence and treatment of non-*Candida albicans* infection. Curr. Probl. Obstet. Gynecol. Fertil. **8**, 241 (1990)
16. Sobel, J.D., Brooker, D., Stein, G.E., et al.: Single oral dose fluconazole compared with conventional clotrimazole topical therapy of Candida vaginitis. Fluconazole Vaginitis Study Group. Am. J. Obstet. Gynecol. **172**, 1263–1268 (1995)
17. Sobel, J.D., Wiesenfeld, H.C., Martens, M., et al.: Maintenance fluconazole therapy for recurrent vulvovaginal candidiasis. N. Engl. J. Med. **351**, 876–883 (2004)
18. Nyirjesy, P., Alexander, A.B., Weitz, M.V.: Vaginal Candida parapsilosis: pathogen or bystander? Infect. Dis. Obstet. Gynecol. **13**, 37–41 (2005)
19. Singh, S., Sobel, J.D., Bhargava, P., Boikov, D., Vazquez, J.A.: Vaginitis due to *Candida krusei*: epidemiology, clinical aspects, and therapy. Clin. Infect. Dis. **35**, 1066–1070 (2002)
20. Sobel, J.D., Myers, P.G., Kaye, D., Levison, M.E.: Adherence of *Candida albicans* to human vaginal and buccal epithelial cells. J. Infect. Dis. **143**, 76–82 (1981)
21. Macura, A.B., Voss, A., Melchers, W.J., Meis, J.F., Syslo, J., Heczko, P.B.: Characterization of pathogenetic determinants of *Candida albicans* strains. Zentralbl. Bakteriol. **287**, 501–508 (1998)
22. Taylor, B.N., Staib, P., Binder, A., et al.: Profile of *Candida albicans* – secreted aspartic proteinase elicited during vaginal infection. Infect. Immun. **73**, 1828–1835 (2005)
23. Naglik, J.R., Rodgers, C.A., Shirlaw, P.J., et al.: Differential expression of *Candida albicans* secreted aspartyl proteinase and phospholipase B genes in humans correlates with active oral and vaginal infections. J. Infect. Dis. **188**, 469–479 (2003)
24. Schaller, M., Bein, M., Korting, H.C., et al.: The secreted aspartyl proteinases Sap1 and Sap2 cause tissue damage in an in vitro model of vaginal candidiasis based on reconstituted human vaginal epithelium. Infect. Immun. **71**, 3227–3234 (2003)
25. Soll, D.R.: High-frequency switching in *Candida albicans* and its relations to vaginal candidiasis. Am. J. Obstet. Gynecol. **158**, 997–1001 (1988)
26. Reed, B.D., Zazove, P., Pierson, C.L., Gorenflo, D.W., Horrocks, J.: Candida transmission and sexual behaviors as risks for a repeat episode of Candida vulvovaginitis. J. Womens Health (Larchmt) **12**, 979–989 (2003)
27. Chaim, W., Foxman, B., Sobel, J.D.: Association of recurrent vaginal candidiasis and secretory ABO and Lewis phenotype. J. Infect. Dis. **176**, 828–830 (1997)
28. Babula, O., Lazdane, G., Kroica, J., Linhares, I.M., Ledger, W.J., Witkin, S.S.: Frequency of interleukin-4 (IL-4) -589 gene polymorphism and vaginal concentrations of IL-4, nitric oxide, and mannose-binding lectin in women with recurrent vulvovaginal candidiasis. Clin. Infect. Dis. **40**, 1258–1262 (2005)
29. Cotch, M.F.: Vaginal carriage of *Candida* spp in pregnancy. In: Interscience Conference on Antimicrobial Agents and Chemotherapy, Chicago, IL, 1991, p. 307.
30. Young, G.L., Jewell, D.: Topical treatment for vaginal candidiasis (thrush) in pregnancy. Cochrane Database Syst. Rev. 2006, 2.
31. Tarry, W., Fisher, M., Shen, S., Mawhinney, M.: *Candida albicans*: the estrogen target for vaginal colonization. J. Surg. Res. **129**, 278–282 (2005)
32. Foxman, B.: The epidemiology of vulvovaginal candidiasis: risk factors. Am. J. Public Health **80**, 329–331 (1990)
33. Barbone, F., Austin, H., Louv, W.C., Alexander, W.J.: A follow-up study of methods of contraception, sexual activity, and rates of trichomoniasis, candidiasis, and bacterial vaginosis. Am. J. Obstet. Gynecol. **163**, 510–514 (1990)
34. Demirezen, S., Dirlik, O.O., Beksac, M.S.: The association of Candida infection with intrauterine contraceptive device. Cent. Eur. J. Public Health **13**, 32–34 (2005)
35. de Leon, E.M., Jacober, S.J., Sobel, J.D., Foxman, B.: Prevalence and risk factors for vaginal Candida colonization in women with type 1 and type 2 diabetes. BMC Infect. Dis. **2**, 1–4 (2002)

36. Donders, G.G., Prenen, H., Verbeke, G., Reybrouck, R.: Impaired tolerance for glucose in women with recurrent vaginal candidiasis. Am. J. Obstet. Gynecol. **187**, 989–993 (2002)
37. Ehrström, S., Yu, A., Rylander, E.: Glucose in vaginal secretions before and after oral glucose tolerance testing in women with and without recurrent vulvovaginal candidiasis. Obstet. Gynecol. **108**(6), 1432–1437 (2006)
38. Spinillo, A., Capuzzo, E., Acciano, S., De Santolo, A., Zara, F.: Effect of antibiotic use on the prevalence of symptomatic vulvovaginal candidiasis. Am. J. Obstet. Gynecol. **180**, 14–17 (1999)
39. Pirotta, M.V., Gunn, J.M., Chondros, P.: "Not thrush again!" Women's experience of post-antibiotic vulvovaginitis. Med. J. Aust. **179**, 43–46 (2003)
40. Oriel, J.D., Waterworth, P.M.: Effects of minocycline and tetracycline on the vaginal yeast flora. J. Clin. Pathol. **28**, 403–406 (1975)
41. Pirotta, M.V., Garland, S.M.: Genital *Candida* species detected in samples from women in Melbourne, Australia, before and after treatment with antibiotics. J. Clin. Microbiol. **44**, 3213–3217 (2006)
42. Bradshaw, C.S., Morton, A.N., Garland, S.M., Morris, M.B., Moss, L.M., Fairley, C.K.: Higher-risk behavioral practices associated with bacterial vaginosis compared with vaginal candidiasis. Obstet. Gynecol. **106**, 105–114 (2005)
43. Neves, N.A., Carvalho, L.P., De Oliveira, M.A., et al.: Association between atopy and recurrent vaginal candidiasis. Clin. Exp. Immunol. **142**, 167–171 (2005)
44. Carvalho, L.P., Bacellar, O., Neves, N., de Jesus, A.R., Carvalho, E.M.: Downregulation of IFN-gamma production in patients with recurrent vaginal candidiasis. J. Allergy Clin. Immunol. **109**, 102–105 (2002)
45. Schaaf, V.M., Perez-Stable, E.J., Borchardt, K.: The limited value of symptoms and signs in the diagnosis of vaginal infections. Arch. Intern. Med. **150**, 1929–1933 (1990)
46. Bergman, J.J., Berg, A.O., Schneeweiss, R., Heidrich, F.E.: Clinical comparison of microscopic and culture techniques in the diagnosis of *Candida vaginitis*. J. Fam. Pract. **18**, 549–552 (1984)
47. Sobel, J.D., Kapernick, P.S., Zervos, M., et al.: Treatment of complicated Candida vaginitis: comparison of single and sequential doses of fluconazole. Am. J. Obstet. Gynecol. **185**, 363–369 (2001)
48. Reef, S.E., Levine, W.C., McNeil, M.M., et al.: Treatment options for vulvovaginal candidiasis, 1993. Clin. Infect. Dis. **20**(Suppl 1), S80–S90 (1995)
49. Watson, M.C., Grimshaw, J.M., Bond, C.M., Mollison, J., Ludbrook, A.: Oral versus intra-vaginal imidazole and triazole anti-fungal agents for the treatment of uncomplicated vulvovaginal candidiasis (thrush): a systematic review. BJOG **109**, 85–95 (2002)
50. Davidson, F., Mould, R.F.: Recurrent genital candidosis in women and the effect of intermittent prophylactic treatment. Br. J. Vener. Dis. **54**, 176–183 (1978)
51. Fong, I.W.: The value of treating the sexual partners of women with recurrent vaginal candidiasis with ketoconazole. Genitourin. Med. **68**, 174–176 (1992)
52. Dennerstein, G.J.: Depo-Provera in the treatment of recurrent vulvovaginal candidiasis. J. Reprod. Med. **31**, 801–803 (1986)
53. Rigg, D., Miller, M.M., Metzger, W.J.: Recurrent allergic vulvovaginitis: treatment with *Candida albicans* allergen immunotherapy. Am. J. Obstet. Gynecol. **162**, 332–336 (1990)
54. Rosedale, N., Browne, K.: Hyposensitisation in the management of recurring vaginal candidiasis. Ann. Allergy **43**, 250–253 (1979)
55. Mathema, B., Cross, E., Dun, E., et al.: Prevalence of vaginal colonization by drug-resistant *Candida* species in college-age women with previous exposure to over-the-counter azole antifungals. Clin. Infect. Dis. **33**, E23–E27 (2001)
56. Sobel, J.D., Vazquez, J.A.: Symptomatic vulvovaginitis due to fluconazole-resistant *Candida albicans* in a female who was not infected with human immunodeficiency virus. Clin. Infect. Dis. **22**, 726–727 (1996)
57. Richter, S.S., Galask, R.P., Messer, S.A., Hollis, R.J., Diekema, D.J., Pfaller, M.A.: Antifungal susceptibilities of *Candida* species causing vulvovaginitis and epidemiology of recurrent cases. J. Clin. Microbiol. **43**, 2155–2162 (2005)
58. Sobel, J.D., Zervos, M., Reed, B.D., et al.: Fluconazole susceptibility of vaginal isolates obtained from women with complicated Candida vaginitis: clinical implications. Antimicrob. Agents Chemother. **47**, 34–38 (2003)
59. Moosa, M.Y., Sobel, J.D., Elhalis, H., Du, W., Akins, R.A.: Fungicidal activity of fluconazole against *Candida albicans* in a synthetic vagina-simulative medium. Antimicrob. Agents Chemother. **48**, 161–167 (2004)
60. Sobel, J.D., Chaim, W., Nagappan, V., Leaman, D.: Treatment of vaginitis caused by *Candida glabrata*: use of topical boric acid and flucytosine. Am. J. Obstet. Gynecol. **189**, 1297–1300 (2003)
61. Phillips, A.J.: Treatment of non-albicans Candida vaginitis with amphotericin B vaginal suppositories. Am. J. Obstet. Gynecol. **192**, 2009–2012 (2005)
62. Rhoads, J.L., Wright, D.C., Redfield, R.R., Burke, D.S.: Chronic vaginal candidiasis in women with human immunodeficiency virus infection. JAMA **257**, 3105–3107 (1987)
63. Duerr, A., Heilig, C.M., Meikle, S.F., et al.: Incident and persistent vulvovaginal candidiasis among human immunodeficiency virus-infected women: Risk factors and severity. Obstet. Gynecol. **101**, 548–556 (2003)
64. Sobel, J.D., Ohmit, S.E., Schuman, P., et al.: The evolution of *Candida* species and fluconazole susceptibility among oral and vaginal isolates recovered from human immunodeficiency virus (HIV)-seropositive and at-risk HIV-seronegative women. J. Infect. Dis. **183**, 286–293 (2001)
65. Schuman, P., Capps, L., Peng, G., et al.: Weekly fluconazole for the prevention of mucosal candidiasis in women with HIV infection. A randomized, double-blind, placebo-controlled trial. Terry Beirn Community Programs for Clinical Research on AIDS. Ann. Intern. Med. **126**, 689–696 (1997)
66. Vazquez, J.A., Peng, G., Sobel, J.D., et al.: Evolution of antifungal susceptibility among *Candida* species isolates recovered from human immunodeficiency virus-infected women receiving fluconazole prophylaxis. Clin. Infect. Dis. **33**, 1069–1075 (2001)
67. Mostad, S.B., Overbaugh, J., DeVange, D.M., et al.: Hormonal contraception, vitamin A deficiency, and other risk factors for shedding of HIV-1 infected cells from the cervix and vagina. Lancet **350**, 922–927 (1997)

Part VII

STD and Travel Medicine

STDs and Travel Medicine

47

Rosella Creed, Anita K. Shetty, Parisa Ravanfar, and Stephen K. Tyring

Core Messages

- International travel contributes to the global spread of sexually transmitted diseases and resistant strains of infections.
- High-risk groups of travelers include truckers, seamen, sex tourists, and long-term visitors.
- A feeling of sexual freedom and lack of social constraints often contribute to casual sex encounters.
- Use of alcohol and other drugs is associated with decreased condom usage and leads to increased rates of STDs during travel.
- Patients often do not recognize the risk of acquiring STDs at a personal level, so pretravel advice should focus on educating patients on the risks abroad and emphasizing proper condom use in all sexual encounters.
- The physician must consider a patient's travel history as this may indicate that the patient has a strain of infection that may have a different susceptibility profile.

47.1 Introduction

Travel between regions of the world has played an important role in the spread of sexually transmitted diseases (STDs) between populations for centuries. After Columbus returned from the New World, an epidemic of a new disease, syphilis, emerged in Europe leading some to theorize that contact between the sailors and New World inhabitants was responsible for the introduction of syphilis to Europe. In recent years, phylogenetic evaluation of the various subspecies of *Treponema pallidum* and the evaluation of skeletal evidence of syphilis have proven that such a theory is plausible [1, 2]. Sailors traveling with James Cook during his expeditions led to the introduction of several STDs to Pacific Islanders [3].

In more recent times, international travel has contributed to the spread of HIV. The ability to fly across the world in hours has allowed people to transmit HIV and other STDs during the incubation period before there are any symptoms [4]. With traditional enzyme immunoassay testing, it may take 2–6 weeks to detect HIV, and with newer nucleic acid amplification tests, it still takes at least 9 days after infection for results to become positive [5]. If serologic testing is not done, it may take years for symptoms to develop that suggest HIV infection and in the meantime, the unaware person spreads the infection to others [6]

The World Tourism Organization estimates that there were 903 million international tourist arrivals in 2007, which includes people traveling for the purpose of leisure, business, or visiting friends and family [7]. As people travel, they may take infections from home to their destination and may bring back new infections from their destination. Often these people are traveling between a developed country, where STD rates are low, and a developing country, where STD rates are

R. Creed (✉)
Center for Clinical Studies, 451 N. Texas Avenue, Webster, TX 77598, USA
e-mail: rcreed@ccstexas.com, rosellacreed@gmail.com

A.K. Shetty and P. Ravanfar
Center for Clinical Studies, University of Texas, Health Science Center, 6655 Travis Street, Suite 100 Houston, TX 77030, USA
e-mail: pravanfar@ccstexas.com; anitaks@gmail.com

S.K. Tyring
Center for Clinical Studies, Houston TX, USA and Department of Dermatology, The University of Texas Health Science Center, Houston, TX, USA

G. Gross and S.K. Tyring (eds.), *Sexually Transmitted Infections and Sexually Transmitted Diseases*, DOI: 10.1007/978-3-642-14663-3_47, © Springer-Verlag Berlin Heidelberg 2011

high. This leads to the global spread of STDs and introduces new diseases or resistant strains to areas previously unaffected.

For the physician who encounters patients planning to travel or returning from travel, it is important to be aware of those at most risk for acquiring STDs abroad and understand the attitudes and behavior of travelers with respect to foreign sexual encounters. Prior to travel, physicians should assess the patient's level of risk and sex education and be able to advise patients on prevention of STDs. If a physician encounters someone who has a travel history, the physician must recognize that a familiar infection may have a different susceptibility profile or the infection may be unfamiliar to him/her altogether.

47.2 High-Risk Travelers

Travelers are a broad category. Short-term travelers are often defined as those who visit another place for 3 months or less [8]; long-term visitors to another country include Peace Corp volunteers, expatriates, missionaries, and those on extended business [4]. The general categories of travelers include tourists, businessmen, seafarers, airline workers, military personnel, truck drivers, immigrant workers, expatriate workers, and, though less easily defined, sex tourists [4]. Each category of traveler represents different attitudes, education levels, and sexual activity abroad [8]. Identification of those groups with the highest risk for acquiring STDs abroad is important in targeting education about preventive measures.

One theory regarding the epidemiology of STDs is that there is a "core group" of persons in whom an STD is most common and that this "core group" can spread the STD to the general population. Commercial sex workers (CSWs) in Africa and their patrons represent a core group in which there are many men having sex with a relatively small population of women, while long-distance truckers and seamen having sex with women along their routes represent a small population of men and a large population of women [8]. Truck drivers have made a significant contribution to the spread of HIV in many areas of the world that currently have high rates of infection, such as Africa and India [9, 10]. Seamen have been shown to have a rate of HIV infection that is much higher than the general population. In both truckers and seamen, knowledge about the risks of unprotected sex and AIDS is low [8, 9].

Long-term travelers also may engage in casual sexual encounters. A survey of 1,080 American Peace Corps volunteers showed that 39% engaged in sex with a partner from the host country but only 32% of unmarried volunteers admitted to using condoms every time they had sex. Male volunteers used condoms more often when they were drinking less alcohol and when they felt they were in a country with a high prevalence of HIV infection [11].

People who are traveling with the primary intention to visit friends or family may be comfortable in the country and in close contact with the local population. They are also more willing to purchase local condoms of poor quality, putting them at high risk for STDs [3].

Sex tourism has become a well-known lucrative business in Thailand and Eastern Europe [4]. The sex tourist is likely to engage in sex with a CSW, who is more likely to have an STD than someone in the general population of the country the tourist is visiting, so it would be most beneficial to target education on STD prevention at this group. Identifying the "sex tourist" is difficult though. Most people will not blatantly announce that their primary intention for traveling abroad is to engage in sex. It is also difficult to discern between those who are traveling primarily for sexual purposes and those who would be willing to engage in sex during their trip abroad if given the opportunity. Many sex tourists will travel as "individual tourists" [8]. A cross-sectional survey of Australians traveling to Thailand revealed that only 34% definitely planned to not have sex while traveling, and only 82% of the participants said that they would use a condom all the time [12]. In studies of those who are traveling for the purpose of sex, men, who make up approximately 90% of sex tourists, show preference for Thailand, the Philippines, Sri Lanka, the Caribbean islands, and Latin America. Women have some preference for Kenya and Haiti [8].

The goal of the physician during a pretravel visit is to identify these high-risk groups that need to be educated the most. This requires some amount of "profiling" of the high-risk traveler. Studies have shown that people with a higher likelihood of engaging in sex while traveling are male, single, traveling alone [13–15], less than 20 years old, users of illegal drugs, and alcohol abusers. Women with an early coitarche, history of alcohol abuse, history of extramarital affairs [14], and a history of many sexual partners are more likely to engage in sex abroad [14, 16]. There is also a second peak of people in their late 30s to mid-50s who are likely to engage in casual sex abroad [3]. The physician must also keep in mind the patient's education level, how that patient behaved on previous travels, if known, and what his or her sexual behavior is like in the home country. Someone who is promiscuous or inconsistently uses condoms at home is quite likely to behave similarly in another country. A study of Chinese businessmen who engaged in casual sex abroad showed that they had frequent changes of partners and had unprotected sex both at home and abroad [15]. A study of Japanese visitors to Hawaii reported that 86% of those surveyed had sex on their trip under the influence of alcohol, which was similar to their behavior in Japan. Rates of condom use during casual sex encounters were also similar regardless of whether the participants were in their home country or in Hawaii [17].

47.3 Sexual Attitudes and Behaviors

Identifying those who are at risk and counseling patients on responsible behavior abroad requires an understanding of their attitude toward casual sex abroad. Travelling abroad is freedom. People feel a sense of escape from their ordinary lives and express that in different ways during their travels. For some, this expression of freedom is in a sexual form. The sense of the exotic propels people to believe that what happens abroad remains a secret to everyone at home and that casual sexual encounters abroad have no personal consequences. During travel, people have more frequent casual sex encounters with less frequent condom use. These sexual encounters are often with someone who has had a high number of sexual partners. Men often have sex with CSWs, who have a high prevalence of STDs. Women are more likely to have sex with a fellow traveler, but that fellow traveler may also have had sex with local CSWs, so women may be indirectly affected, although they may not be wholly aware of this possibility [15].

Surveys assessing HIV and AIDS awareness in travel clinic patients have demonstrated that travelers often do not feel personally at risk for acquiring HIV even though they are aware that HIV is an STD [8]. A study of 757 patients at a London clinic found that 18.6% admitted to new sex partners during their last trip abroad, but only one third had used condoms 100% of the time [18]. Another study of Japanese men showed that 71% engaged in sex with a CSW in Bangkok, and although 76% admitted that this was risky, only 51% used condoms all the time [8]. Since this denial of risk and lack of prevention reflects the behavior at home frequently, the physician is faced with conveying to patients not only knowledge of STDs, but the importance of putting the knowledge into practice both at home and abroad.

47.4 Risk Education

The physician must remind the patient of the vast difference in the prevalence of STDs in developing countries when compared with developed countries. Even within a country, STDs are hyperendemic among certain groups, such as casual sex workers, so sexual encounters with members of those groups must include proper use of a condom [14]. In a study of street soliciting CSWs in Bangladesh, 56.7% of the women surveyed had 2 or more STDs [19]. Many CSWs in Sub-Saharan Africa and Southeast Asia are also seropositive for HIV (see Table 47.1). Recognizing casual sex workers is not always easy. In some countries, payment for sex may be in the form of food or the dream of emigration to a better place. These are still high-risk relationships [3]. Some variations do exist, e.g., the prevalence of gonorrhea in CSWs who solicit from hotels was 20% when compared with a 63% prevalence in CSWs who solicited on the streets [20].

It is difficult to estimate the amount of STDs that are transmitted during travel. A study of posttravel patients in a London clinic showed that 11.6% of the STDs diagnosed could have been contracted abroad [13]. Another survey of London clinic patients estimated that 5.7% contracted an STD on their last trip abroad [18]. In a study of HIV infection in travelers from the UK, the rate of infection in heterosexual patients who had traveled was 5.4%, compared with 1.8% for UK citizens and 33.2% for people originating from outside the UK [21]. Studies of gonococcal infection, which is easier to track owing to its acute nature, have estimated that 25–89% of gonorrhea cases were contracted abroad [8].

Table 47.1 Percentages of HIV seropositive female sex workers in selected countries

Country	Percentage of HIV seropositive female sex workers (%)
Zimbabwe	86
Malawi	70
Cote d'Ivoire	69
Kenya	55
India	50
Cambodia	39
Nigeria	29
Cameroon	18
Thailand	13
Argentina	8
Brazil	6
Vietnam	3
Mexico	3
France	2
Italy	2
Netherlands	2

Source: Wang and Celum [20]

Certain areas of the world have particularly high rates of STDs, such as Sub-Saharan Africa and Southeast Asia (See Fig. 47.1). Patients traveling to high-risk areas should be educated regarding this risk and on the proper precautions to take on their trip. Table 47.2 reviews the estimated prevalence of the most common STDs in the world. For the most common STDs in the world, gonorrhea, chlamydia, trichomonas, syphilis, herpes genitalis, hepatitis B, and HIV, the most affected areas are Sub-Saharan African and Southeast Asia.

47.5 Prevention and Pretravel Advice

Pretravel advice for those traveling to foreign countries should include a discussion of STDs and preventive measures. Patients may be more concerned with avoiding traveler's diarrhea, but it is important to also educate them on the risks of STDs in the area to which they are traveling. The only certain way to prevent the transmission of STDs is abstinence or a monogamous relationship between two uninfected individuals. If that is not possible or unlikely for the patient, the physician must emphasize that the proper use of high-quality condoms in 100% of sexual encounters is the next more important mode of prevention. Spermicides, such as nonoxynol-9, are unlikely to have a significant microbicidal effect on STDs and should not be recommended as a means of protection against STDs [22]. There is also the possibility that the irritating properties of nonoyxnol-9 can increase the frequency of genital lesions and could actually increase the transmission

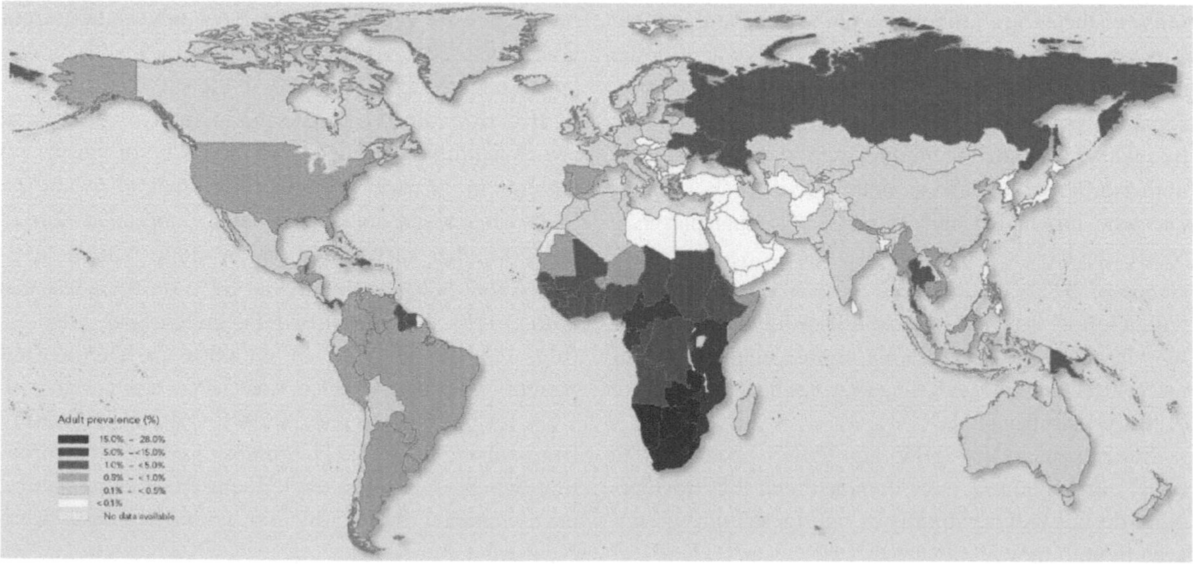

Fig. 47.1 HIV Infection in 2007 (World Health Organization [29])

Table 47.2 Prevalence of curable sexually transmitted diseases by region

Region	New cases among adults in 1999			
	Gonorrhea	Chlamydia	Syphilis	Trichomonas
North America	1.5 million	4 million	100,000	8 million
Latin American/Caribbean	7.5 million	9.5 million	3 million	18.5 million
North Africa/Middle East	1.5 million	3 million	370,000	5 million
Sub-Saharan Africa	17 million	16 million	4 million	32 million
Western Europe	1 million	5 million	140,000	11 million
Easter Europe/Central Asia	3.5 million	6 million	100,000	13 million
Eastern Asia	3 million	5.3 million	240,000	10 million
South Asia/Southeast Asia	27 million	43 million	4 million	76.5 million
Australia/New Zealand	120,000	340,000	10,000	610,000
Total	62 million	92 million	12 million	174 million

Source: World Health Organization [30]

rate of HIV [23]. Prior to travel, patients are often instructed on certain important items to incorporate into their travel kits. Physicians must remind patients that latex condoms need to be a part of every travel kit and should be used. Even if the traveler does not anticipate having sex on their trip, condoms should be carried. Purchasing condoms in the foreign country should be discouraged, since the manufacturing standards may not be equivalent to those of developed countries [3].

Travelers should be advised of certain general risks regarding STD transmission. STDs are more easily transmitted from males to females. Sex with anyone who has dermatological evidence of an STD should be avoided since this increases the risk of transmission of that STD as well as HIV and hepatitis. Travelers should be wary of engaging in sex under the influence of drugs and alcohol. Condom use is dramatically lower when people are under the influence of such substances. Bleeding during sex will increase the transmission rate of hepatitis and HIV [3]. The risk of transmitting HIV also increases if one or both parties have another STD. Genital ulcers in the seropositive individual can have HIV in the exudate. Genital ulcers in the seronegative partner can reduce the mucosal barrier and attract HIV susceptible cells to the surface, allowing for easier contraction of HIV. Nonulcerative STDs, such as gonorrhea and chlamydia, increase viral shedding in the genital tract and also lead to an elevated rate of HIV transmission [24].

There are very few other preventive measures that physicians can recommend to patients who may engage in sex while traveling. Patients who are members of the military, may be long-term or frequent travelers, or may be sex tourists should be particularly encouraged to receive the hepatitis B vaccine [14]. Many people are already vaccinated against HBV, but it is important to remember that the ACIP started to routinely recommend vaccination of infants in 1991, and vaccination of adolescents was recommended in 1996. Older generations are less likely to have been vaccinated and remain at risk [25]. The vaccine schedule typically requires a three-dose series over a 6-month period, but there are data to show that an accelerated schedule (0, 7, and 14 or 21-days, followed by a 1-year booster) can protect travelers as well, which is beneficial as travelers frequently present to their doctors too late to complete the typical (0, 1, and 6-month) series [26]. Though not usually considered a sexually transmitted disease, travelers to developing countries should also be encouraged to receive the hepatitis A vaccine; the recommended dosing scheduling is two injections 6–12 months apart. A combination vaccine protects against both HAV and HBV, which can be of benefit to travelers at risk for both types of hepatitis [23]. The typical dosing schedule is 0, 1, and 6 months, and both the initial and the 1-month doses must be given prior to travel for reliable protection against HAV. An accelerated schedule is also available for the combination vaccine. The HPV vaccine is also approved for females 9–26 years old and should be recommended to women in this age group who are sexually active. Like the HBV vaccine, the HPV vaccine three-shot series is administered over 6 months, which may limit its pretravel utilization [27].

Prophylactic use of antibiotics for certain common STDs, such as gonorrhea and chlamydia, is not advised. Chemoprophylaxis may lead to a false sense of security, placing patients at higher risk of contracting other STDs unaffected by the chemoprophylactic agents, such as HIV, hepatitis, and other viral STDs [14].

Patients should also be educated before their trip on the signs and symptoms of STDs so that they can seek early treatment and avoid complications if they do contract a disease. Patients should seek medical attention at the first sign of any vaginal or urethral discharge, any genital rash or sores, or pelvic pain [4]. Although many STDs can cause temporary symptoms, patients must be reminded that many of the consequences can be life-changing. Nontreatment of gonorrhea and chlamydia can lead to pelvic inflammatory disease and subsequent infertility or ectopic pregnancies in women. Hepatitis, HIV, herpes, and HPV have no cure and can be spread to future partners. Hepatitis can lead to chronic liver disease; HIV leads to AIDS and will shorten the patient's life considerably; HPV can lead to cervical cancer in women [3].

47.6 Posttravel Diagnosis and Treatment

Treating patients who have contracted an STD abroad can be a challenge to the physician because the susceptibility profile may be different for bacterial infections endemic to another country. The emergence of pencillinase-producing *Neisseria gonorrhoeae* in the 1970s and then tetracycline-resistant strains in the 1980s in many areas of the world prompted the CDC to change treatment recommendations. More recently, fluoroquinolone-resistance has emerged in many countries causing the CDC to warn against the use of fluoroquinolones in those who may have acquired gonorrhea abroad. In the USA, the overall prevalence of resistant strains is 6.8%, but areas of Southeast Asia have prevalence rates of well over 90%. Even in Germany and Austria, prevalence rates are estimated to be close to 50% and 60% , respectively [28].

Certain diseases, such as chancroid, granuloma inguinale, and lymphogranuloma venereum, are rare in the USA and may be misdiagnosed or inappropriately treated [3]. The physician must consider these diagnoses in those with a travel history to developing countries where these diseases are endemic.

47.7 Conclusions

International travel plays a large role in the global spread of sexually transmitted diseases. With more people than ever crossing borders and encountering new diseases and new strains of infections, it is important for the physician to initiate a pretravel discussion regarding the proper precautions that the patient should take to avoid acquiring an STD abroad. Physicians must also be prepared to recognize and treat STDs in patients returning from abroad to prevent further spread of the infection in the home country.

Take-Home Pearls

- International travel spreads known STDs and new, resistant strains.
- Travelers from developed countries to developing countries should be made aware of the vast difference in the incidence and prevalence of most STDs between their home country and their country of visit.
- High-risk travelers are often young, single males traveling alone. Long-term travelers are also at an elevated risk.
- To minimize the risk of acquiring STDs, patients should properly use condoms in every sexual encounter.
- Prior to travel, hepatitis B vaccination should be recommended for high-risk patients. Chemoprophylactic antibiotic treatment is not advised.
- The physician must be aware of the travel history of patients and consider that a resistant strain of common STDs or a rare STD may be present.

Acknowledgments We thank Charles D. Ericsson, University of Texas Health Science Center, Houston, Texas, USA.

References

1. Rothschild, B.M.: History of syphilis. Clin. Infect. Dis. **40**, 1454–1463 (2005)
2. Harper, K.N., Ocampo, P.S., Steiner, B.M., et al.: On the origin of the treponematoses: A phylogenetic approach. PLoS Negl. Trop. Dis. **2**, e148 (2008)
3. Ward, B.J., Plourde, P.: Travel and sexually transmitted infections. J. Travel Med. **13**, 300–317 (2006)
4. Memish, Z.A., Osoba, A.O.: Sexually transmitted diseases and travel. Int. J. Antimicrob. Agents **21**, 131–134 (2003)
5. Branson, B.M.: State of the art for diagnosis of HIV infection. Clin. Infect. Dis. **45**(Suppl 4), S221–S225 (2007)
6. Vergis, E.N., Mellors, J.W.: Natural history of HIV-1 infection. Infect. Dis. Clin. North Am. **14**, 809–825 (2000). v-vi
7. Organization WT. UNWTO World Tourism Barometer. http://www.unwto.org/facts/eng/pdf/barometer/UNWTO_Barom08_2_en_LR.pdf (2008). Accessed 20 Dec 2008;6.
8. Mulhall, B.P.: Sex and travel: studies of sexual behaviour, disease and health promotion in international travellers – a global review. Int. J. STD AIDS **7**, 455–465 (1996)
9. Sunmola, A.M.: Sexual practices, barriers to condom use and its consistent use among long distance truck drivers in Nigeria. AIDS Care **17**, 208–221 (2005)
10. Singh, Y.N., Malaviya, A.N.: Long distance truck drivers in India: HIV infection and their possible role in disseminating HIV into rural areas. Int. J. STD AIDS **5**, 137–138 (1994)
11. Moore, J., Beeker, C., Harrison, J.S., Eng, T.R., Doll, L.S.: HIV risk behavior among Peace Corps Volunteers. AIDS **9**, 795–799 (1995)
12. Mulhall, B.P., Hu, M., Thompson, M., et al.: Planned sexual behaviour of young Australian visitors to Thailand. Med. J. Aust. **158**, 530–535 (1993)
13. Hawkes, S., Hart, G.J., Bletsoe, E., Shergold, C., Johnson, A.M.: Risk behaviour and STD acquisition in genitourinary clinic attenders who have travelled. Genitourin. Med. **71**, 351–354 (1995)
14. Matteelli, A., Carosi, G.: Sexually transmitted diseases in travelers. Clin. Infect. Dis. **32**, 1063–1067 (2001)
15. Abdullah, A.S., Ebrahim, S.H., Fielding, R., Morisky, D.E.: Sexually transmitted infections in travelers: implications for prevention and control. Clin. Infect. Dis. **39**, 533–538 (2004)
16. Arvidson, M., Hellberg, D., Mardh, P.A.: Sexual risk behavior and history of sexually transmitted diseases in relation to casual travel sex during different types of journeys. Acta Obstet. Gynecol. Scand. **75**, 490–494 (1996)
17. Nemoto, T., Iwamoto, M., Morris, A., Yokota, F., Wada, K.: Substance use and sexual behaviors among Japanese tourists, students, and temporary workers in Honolulu, Hawaii. AIDS Educ. Prev. **19**, 68–81 (2007)
18. Hawkes, S., Hart, G.J., Johnson, A.M., et al.: Risk behaviour and HIV prevalence in international travellers. AIDS **8**, 247–252 (1994)
19. Mondal, N.I., Hossain, K., Islam, R., Mian, A.B.: Sexual behavior and sexually transmitted diseases in street-based female sex workers in Rajshahi City, Bangladesh. Braz. J. Infect. Dis. **12**, 287–292 (2008)
20. Wang, C.C., Celum, C.L.: Global risk of sexually transmitted diseases. Med. Clin. North Am. **83**, 975–995 (1999). vi
21. Hawkes, S., Malin, A., Araru, T., Mabey, D.: HIV infection among heterosexual travellers attending the Hospital for Tropical Diseases, London. Genitourin. Med. **68**, 309–311 (1992)
22. Roddy, R.E., Zekeng, L., Ryan, K.A., Tamoufe, U., Weir, S.S., Wong, E.L.: A controlled trial of nonoxynol 9 film to reduce male-to-female transmission of sexually transmitted diseases. N. Engl. J. Med. **339**, 504–510 (1998)
23. Wilkinson, D., Tholandi, M., Ramjee, G., Rutherford, G.W.: Nonoxynol-9 spermicide for prevention of vaginally acquired HIV and other sexually transmitted infections: systematic review and meta-analysis of randomised controlled trials including more than 5000 women. Lancet Infect. Dis. **2**, 613–617 (2002)
24. Fleming, D.T., Wasserheit, J.N.: From epidemiological synergy to public health policy and practice: The contribution of other sexually transmitted diseases to sexual transmission of HIV infection. Sex. Transm. Infect. **75**, 3–17 (1999)
25. Davis, J.P.: Experience with hepatitis A and B vaccines. Am. J. Med. **118**(Suppl 10A), 7S–15S (2005)
26. Keystone, J.S.: Travel-related hepatitis B: Risk factors and prevention using an accelerated vaccination schedule. Am. J. Med. **118**(Suppl 10A), 63S–68S (2005)
27. Markowitz, L.E., Dunne, E.F., Saraiya, M., Lawson, H.W., Chesson, H., Unger, E.R.: Quadrivalent human papillomavirus vaccine: Recommendations of the Advisory Committee on Immunization Practices (ACIP). MMWR Recomm. Rep. **56**, 1–24 (2007)
28. Newman, L.M., Moran, J.S., Workowski, K.A.: Update on the management of gonorrhea in adults in the United States. Clin. Infect. Dis. **44**(Suppl 3), S84–S101 (2007)
29. World Health Organization. http://www.who.int/hiv/facts/hiv2007/en/ (2009). Accessed Jan 3 2009.
30. World Health Organization. Global prevalence and incidence of selected curable sexually transmitted infections: Overview and estimates. http://www.who.int/hiv/pub/sti/who_hiv_aids_2001.02.pdf (2008). Accessed Dec 30 2008.

Part VIII

Therapeutic Challenges

Therapy-New Drugs

48

Anita K. Shetty, Devak G. Desai, Janice Wilson, and Stephen K. Tyring

Core Messages

- New medications for treatment of human immunodeficiency virus (HIV) are under investigation in the existing classes of nucleoside/nucleotide reverse transcriptase inhibitors, nonnucleoside reverse transcriptase inhibitors, and protease inhibitors.
- Emerging classes of medications for treatment of HIV include entry inhibitors, fusion inhibitors, CCR5 antagonists, CXCR4 antagonists, integration inhibitors, and maturation inhibitors.
- Photodynamic therapy and cidofovir are being studied as therapies for molluscum contagiosum.
- Emerging classes of medications for treatment of herpes simplex include nonnucleoside DNA polymerase inhibitors, helicase-primase complex inhibitors, portal protein inhibitors, topoisomerase II inhibitors, ribonucleotide reductase inhibitors, immune response inhibitors, and cyclin-dependent kinase inhibitors.
- Emerging therapies for human papillomavirus infection include photodynamic therapy, a nucleotide analog, and a catechin-based compound.
- New targets for antiviral drugs include cyclin-dependent kinases, helicase inhibitors, SF1 helicase-primase inhibitors, and SF3 helicase inhibitors.
- New antibiotics are available for treatment of *Neisseria gonorrhoeae, Chlamydia trachomatis.*

A.K. Shetty (✉), D.G. Desai, J. Wilson, and S.K. Tyring
Center for Clinical Studies, Houston, TX, USA
e-mail: anitaks@gmail.com

As the prevalence of sexually transmitted disease and resistance to current therapies increases, so does the necessity for new therapies. Current therapies for each disease have been covered in the corresponding chapter. This chapter will outline new and emerging therapies in the field of sexually transmitted disease. As a multitude of new medications are still in the early stages of development and clinical testing, only those with published results will be discussed here. While some medications are specific to one virus, others have targets that give them potential as treatments for multiple diseases.

48.1 Human Immunodeficiency Virus (HIV)

Antiretroviral therapy is the mainstay of treatment for HIV and acquired immunodeficiency syndrome (AIDS). The prevalence of resistance to the existing antiretrovirals is increasing, necessitating the formulation of new drugs within the existing drug classes as well as entirely new classes of drugs with novel mechanisms of action.

48.1.1 Nucleoside/Nucleotide Reverse Transcriptase Inhibitors (NRTIs)

Racivir [(±)-β-2′,3′-dideoxy-5-fluoro-3′-thiacytidine, (±)-FTC, or RCV] is a novel NRTI, which is currently in phase II development [1, 2]. It is a 50:50 mixture of the two β enantiomers of fluorocytosine (FTC) and has shown more potency in reducing HIV titers in the

G. Gross and S.K. Tyring (eds.), *Sexually Transmitted Infections and Sexually Transmitted Diseases*,
DOI: 10.1007/978-3-642-14663-3_48,

blood than either lamivudine (3TC) or (–)-FTC [3]. When used in combination with efavirenz and stavudine at doses of 200–600 mg once daily, a 2.1–2.6 $\log_{10}$ copies/mL reduction in viral load from baseline was seen at 14 days, with a continued >1 $\log_{10}$ copies/mL reduction from baseline at 35 days [4]. The drug's efficacy is currently being tested in patients with 3TC-resistant virus [2].

Apricitabine [(–)-2′-deoxy-3′-oxa-4′-thiocytidine, (–)dOTC, SPD754] is a cytosine analog of NRTI. In a phase I clinical study, apricitabine at doses of at 200–1,200 mg once daily versus placebo showed dose-dependent decreases in viral load in the treatment groups, ranging from a 1.16 to 1.44 $\log_{10}$ copies/mL reduction from baseline [5]. Intracellular levels of apricitabine are significantly reduced when taken in combination with 3TC, so this medication should not be dosed with 3TC or other cytidine analogs [1, 6].

Amdoxovir (diaminopurine dioxolane, DAPD) is a guanosine analog NRTI, which is deaminated intracellularly by adenosine deaminase to form dioxolane guanine (DXG). The active form of the drug is DXG-triphosphase [1, 7–9]. Both DAPD and DXG have activity against HIV virus resistant to zidovudine (AZT) and/or 3TC, as well as against multi-NRTI-resistant strains with the codon 69 insertion mutation [10–13]. In a Phase I/II study of treatment-experienced HIV-infected patients, 300–500 mg of amdoxovir given twice daily resulted in a decrease in viral load of 0.75–1.5 $\log_{10}$ copies/mL reduction in viral load from baseline [14]. Another series of patients with multi-drug-resistant HIV, treated for 2 weeks with amdoxovir 500 mg twice daily, with or without the addition of mycophenolate mofetil, showed an average decrease of 0.29 $\log_{10}$ copies/mL in viral load [7]. One other study showed that the use of amdoxovir 500 mg twice daily in treatment-experienced patients resulted in a mean 0.7 $\log_{10}$ copies/mL decrease in viral load after 15 days of therapy. The effect in treatment-naïve patients was a decrease of 1.5 $\log_{10}$ copies/mL in viral load [15]. Possible toxicities include lens opacification and obstructive nephropathy due to crystallization of the drug in the renal tubules [14].

Elvucitabine (β-2′,3′-didehydro-2′,3′-dideoxy-5-fluorocytidine, ACH-126 443, L-d4FC) is a L-cytidine analog that exhibits activity against HIV resistant to other nucleoside analogs, including AZT and 3TC. A Phase Ib study dosing treatment-experienced, HIV-infected patients with 50–100 mg/day of elvucitabine resulted in a 0.67–0.78 $\log_{10}$ copies/mL decrease in viral load from baseline by day 28. As several patients in this study developed bone marrow suppression, dosing was halted and current studies are examining the efficacy of lower doses of the drug [16]. One pharmacokinetic study suggests that co-administration with ritonavir may decrease bioavailability of elvucitabine [17].

GS-9148 ((5-(6-amino-purin-9-yl)-4-fluoro-2,5-dihydro-furan-2-yloxymethyl)phosphonic acid), a ribose-modified nucleoside phosphonate analog, is a novel HIV-1 nucleotide reverse transcriptase inhibitor. GS-9131 is the orally available phosphonoamidate prodrug of GS-9418, which has been shown to increase the intracellular metabolites of GS-9148 in peripheral blood mononuclear cells (PBMCs) of canine models. Although there is no available clinical data, GS-9131 and GS-9148 have shown promising activity against multiple subtypes of HIV-1 clinical isolates in PBMCs, synergy with multiple antiretrovirals in MT-2 cells infected with HIV-1, and inhibition of reverse transcriptase via GS-9148-DP, the diphosphate metabolite of GS-9148 [18]. Also, in a recent study with a canine model, GS-9148 was found to be inefficiently transported by the kidneys, indicating low potential for nephrotoxicity [19].

48.1.2 Nonnucleoside Reverse Transcriptase Inhibitors (NNRTIs)

Rilpivirine (TMC-278) is a novel NNRTI in development [20]. It is a diarylpyrimidine derivative, which potently inhibits wild-type and NNRTI-resistant HIV-1 in vitro and which also has an increased genetic barrier to resistance when compared with efavirenz (EFV) or nevirapine (NVP). Efficacy of dosing of 25–150 mg once daily was confirmed in a 48-week phase IIb study versus EFV in treatment-naïve individuals ($n=368$), showing viral load reduction of 2.63 $\log_{10}$ copies/mL in all dose groups, with viral load reduction to <50 copies/mL in at least 77% of patients at all doses, sustained over 48 weeks. Rilpivirine is tolerated well and has a lower incidence of neurologic and lipid abnormalities, as well as rash, when compared to efavirenz [21].

Calanolide A is a naturally occurring NNRTI isolated from the Malaysian tree *Calophyllum lanigerum*. In vitro, it has demonstrated activity against HIV-1, and has exhibited unique sensitivity to HIV-1 strains that are resistant to other drugs. A Phase I study of healthy individuals ($n=47$) showed that calanolide A is bioavailable at high twice-daily dosages (600–800 mg), exhibits a long half life, and is well-tolerated [22].

48.1.3 Protease Inhibitors (PIs)

Brecanavir (BCV, 640385) is a novel protease inhibitor (PI) in development. The drug has displayed great potency, with inhibitory concentrations achieved at subnanomolar doses against even HIV-1 viruses that are resistant to multiple other PIs [23–25]. In an efficacy study, which dosed HIV-positive individuals with 100 mg twice daily of brecanavir in addition to 300 mg twice daily of ritonavir, the observed analysis showed that 93% of participants had HIV-1 viral load <400 copies/mL, and 89% of participants had a viral load <50 copies/mL. The median CD4+ cell count increase was 84 cells/mm^3, and the regimen was generally well tolerated [24].

48.1.4 Entry Inhibitors (EIs)

This new class of antiretrovirals was developed based on the observation that HIV-1 requires a chemokine coreceptor (CCR5 or CXCR4), in addition to the CD4+ receptor, for viral entry into host cells [26].

Ibalizumab (previously known as TNX-355) is a humanized monoclonal antibody that binds CD4 and thus inhibits viral entry. A study involving 22 HIV-positive patients dosed intravenously with ibalizumab at 10 mg/kg weekly, 10 mg/kg loading dose followed by 6 mg/kg every 2 weeks, or 25 mg/kg every 2 weeks for a total of 9 weeks for all treatment arms resulted in 0.5–1.7 log_{10} decrease in viral load in 91% of the subjects [27].

PRO 140 is a humanized monoclonal antibody targeted against the CCR5 receptor. In vitro, it was shown to effectively inhibit HIV-1 at concentrations that do not interfere with CCR5 normal function. In a Phase Ib study of HIV-infected patients ($n=39$), administration of 0.5–5 mg/kg single intravenous doses of PRO 140 resulted in significant dose-dependent nadir reductions in viral load versus placebo (0.58–1.83 log_{10} copies/mL). The duration of response also correlated with dose; all groups returned to baseline viral loads by day 29 of the study. The treatment was well tolerated [28].

DCM205 is a novel small-molecule HIV-1 inhibitor that binds to gp120, the HIV envelope glycoprotein, thereby directly inhibiting the entry ability of the virus even in the absence of a cellular target [29]. DCM205 is therefore the first member of a class of potential new agents to prevent HIV infection.

48.1.4.1 Fusion Inhibitors

Currently, the only approved member of this new class is enfuvirtude [30–32].

48.1.4.2 CCR5 Antagonists

Maraviroc (UK-427,857) interferes with binding of HIV1 viral glycoprotein 120 (gp120) to the CCR5 coreceptor, which is the coreceptor utilized by the majority (>80%) of HIV-1 strains [33–35].

Vicriviroc (SCH 417690, SCH-D) is a CCR5 antagonist in Phase III clinical trials [36]. In a Phase II study of treatment-experienced HIV-infected patients ($n=116$), HAART therapy was supplemented by 20–30 mg vicriviroc once daily versus placebo. Patients receiving vicriviroc experienced significantly higher reduction in viral loads (1.75–1.77 log_{10} copies/mL compared to less than 1 log_{10} copies/mL for HAART-only patients). In addition, 53–56% of vicriviroc patients experienced viral loads below 50 copies/mL (compared to 14% for HAART-only patients) [37]. Thus, vicriviroc seems to be a promising agent for R5 HIV. However, an increased occurrence of malignancies demonstrated in an earlier Phase II trial has slowed progress [38].

48.1.4.3 CXCR4 Antagonists

AMD070 (AMD11070) is a CXCR4 antagonist similar to plerixafor (AMD3100). In two previous 10-day Phase II studies of HIV-infected patients, 200 mg doses of AMD070 administered twice daily demonstrated antiviral effects. In a recent Phase I study, AMD070 was administered to healthy patients ($n=23$) with a concomitant low dose of ritonavir, which was shown to increase the bioavailability of the experimental drug in comparison to an earlier Phase I study with mixed pharmacokinetic results [39]. AMD070 was well tolerated in all studies [39, 40].

KRH-3955 is a new CXCR4 antagonist that inhibits binding of anti-CXCR4 antibodies to the first, second, and third extracellular loops of CXCR4. In vitro data show that KRH-3955 has potent activity against X4 HIV-1, including strains resistant to enfuvirtide. In vivo data from a murine model demonstrated that KRH-3955 is bioavailable after oral administration, and an efficacy study in the human peripheral blood lymphocyte-severe combined immunodeficiency mouse model resulted in inhibition of HIV-1 infection, suggesting study of KRH-3955 as a prophylaxis against HIV infection [41].

48.1.5 Integrase Inhibitors (IIs)

Integrase, the target for this new drug class, is an enzyme required for stable replication of the HIV virus DNA and its incorporation into the host cell genome [42]. Raltegravir (MK-0518) is the first HIV integrase inhibitor to be approved for use.

Elvitegravir (GS 9137, JTK-303) is an integrase inhibitor currently in Phase III testing [43]. In a study of treatment-naïve and treatment-experienced HIV-infected individuals ($n=40$), 50 mg of ritonavir-boosted elvitegravir administered once daily, 200–800 mg of elvitegravir administered twice daily, and 800 mg of elvitegravir administered once daily resulted in greater than 1 $\log_{10}$ copies/mL reduction in viral load for all dosages, compared to 0.21 $\log_{10}$ copies/mL reduction for placebo. In addition, 50% of nonplacebo patients exhibited greater than 2 $\log_{10}$ copies/mL reduction in viral load [44]. The study also indicated that ritonavir greatly increased the bioavailability and half-life of elvitegravir [43, 44]. Other studies combining elvitegravir and ritonavir with PIs tipranavir and darunavir, the NNRTI etravirine, and the NRTIs zidovudine, didanosine, stavudine, abacavir, and emtricitabine/tenofovir show that elvitegravir can be co-administered with these drugs without any significant interactions [45–48]. Elvitegravir was well tolerated in all studies, but there are some concerns that resistance to other integrase inhibitors such as raltegravir seems to confer resistance to elvitegravir as well [43–48].

L-870812 is a type of integrase inhibitor known as an integrase strand transfer inhibitor (InSTI) that works by preventing the strand transfer step of HIV cDNA integration into the host genome, in which the 3′ OH ends of the cDNA are covalently linked to the cellular DNA. L-870812 has been shown to inhibit both cell-free and cell-associated HIV infection in a coculture model of autologous monocyte-derived dendritic cell cultures and CD4+ T-cells that represent mucosal cells that are normally the target of sexual HIV transmission. Therefore, L-870812 is a potential new candidate for the development of microbicidal prevention of HIV transmission [49].

48.1.6 Maturation Inhibitors (MIs)

Maturation inhibitors are a novel class of anti-HIV agents that focus on a previously untargeted step of the HIV life cycle: the assembly or release of mature, infective virion particles.

Bevirimat (PA-457, 3-*O*-(3′,3′-dimethylsuccinyl) betulinic acid) is the first maturation inhibitor to reach Phase II clinical trials. Bevirimat interferes with the late processing of gag polyprotein, a structural protein involved in assembly and budding of mature HIV particles, ultimately resulting in the release of noninfectious virions. In a Phase I/II study of treatment-experienced and treatment-naïve HIV-infected patients ($n=24$), single 75–250 mg doses of bevirimat were administered, resulting in 0.46–0.47 $\log_{10}$ copies/mL reduction in viral load for the 150 and 250 mg dosages [50]. A Phase I multiple-dose trial to determine optimal dosing was also completed, as well as a Phase I bioavailability study that determined the small bowel to be the site of optimal absorption [51, 52]. Bevirimat was well tolerated in all studies; it is currently in Phase IIb testing [53].

UK-201844 is a compound that seems to act as maturation inhibitor; it has displayed antiviral activity against HIV-1 in cell culture. In vitro studies have shown that UK-201844 interferes with normal processing of gp160 (Env gene) that results in noninfectious virions due to defective Env glycoproteins [54].

48.2 Molluscum Contagiosum

Because of the self-limiting nature of the disease, there have not been very many recent advances in the treatment of molluscum contagiosum. However, in immunocompromised patients (HIV+, etc.), molluscum contagiosum can become quite severe and difficult to treat, necessitating further study into novel treatments for the disease [55].

Photodynamic therapy with 20% 5-aminolevulinic acid (ALA-PDT) is FDA-approved for the treatment of actinic keratoses of the face and scalp. ALA-PDT involves applying a photosensitizing agent to the affected area of skin and then administering light to the region. No randomized controlled clinical trials have yet been performed regarding the use of ALA-PDT for the treatment of molluscum contagiosum, but numerous case reports describe successful treatments, and a case study performed on HIV-infected patients ($n=6$) reported a 75–80% reduction in lesion count after three to five treatments of 14 to 24 h of incubation with ALA and 16 min 40 s of blue light application. The treatment often causes a phototoxic reaction involving erythema, edema, pain, and/or itching, among other symptoms [56].

Cidofovir is an antiviral medication that is FDA-approved for the treatment of cytomegalovirus retinitis in immunocompromised hosts [57]. In vitro studies indicate that cidofovir competitively inhibits molluscum contagiosum DNA polymerase [58]. No randomized controlled clinical trials have been performed, but case reports have described success, and a small case study demonstrated the clearance of molluscum contagiosum lesions in AIDS patients ($n=4$) after one to three 2-week cycles of twice-daily cidofovir 1% cream application. Side-effects include dermatitis, erosion, itching, and postinflammatory hyperpigmentation [57].

48.3 Herpes Simplex Virus

Current classes of medications for herpesvirus infections can be divided into three groups: nucleoside analogs such as acyclovir, ganciclovir, penciclovir, and brivudin (approved only in Germany) and their prodrugs valacyclovir, valganciclovir, and famciclovir; nucleoside phosphonate (nucleotide) analogs such as cidofovir; and pyrophosphate analogs such as foscarnet. All these antiviral medications target the same active sites on viral kinases and viral DNA polymerases, so a virus resistant to one drug is often cross-resistant to other drugs [59, 60]. New medications are under development that target different enzymes or new binding sites.

48.3.1 Nonnucleoside Herpesvirus DNA Polymerase Inhibitors

Nonnucleoside DNA polymerase inhibitors target DNA polymerase in a novel fashion. Examples of this class of medications include PNU-26370, or naphthalene carboxamide, a representative of the novel class of these inhibitors known as 4-hydroxyquinoline-3-carboxamides. After additional chemical modification, this class yields 4-oxo-dihydroquinolines such as PNU-182171 and PNU-183792. In cell culture assays as well as in vitro studies, these compounds have been shown to inhibit the DNA polymerases of both HSV-1 and -2, as well as cytomegalovirus (CMV), varicella-zoster virus (VZV), and human herpesvirus 8 (HHV-8), but not those of HHV-6 [61–64].

48.3.2 Helicase–Primase Complex Inhibitors

Helicase–primase inhibitors are discussed at length in Sect. 48.5.2.1.

48.3.3 Portal Protein Inhibitors [60]

Portal protein inhibitors are a new class of anti-HSV drugs that target the HSV-1 portal complex, a 12-subunit homomer of U_L6 proteins, through which viral DNA enters the capsid to form a mature virion particle.

WAY-150138 is a small-molecule HSV-1 inhibitor that prevents the association of the portal complex with $U_L26.5$, a scaffolding protein that is involved in the incorporation of the portal complex into the capsid [65]. In vitro and cell culture studies have shown that WAY-150138 inhibits HSV-1 replication and, to a lesser extent, that of HSV-2, HCV, and VZV [66–68].

48.3.4 Cellular Topoisomerase II Inhibitor [60]

Many studies suggest that cellular topoisomerase II is required for DNA replication of HSV-1 [69–71]. Some new drugs are in development that inhibit HSV by blocking the action of topoisomerase II.

ICRF-193 is a specific inhibitor of topoisomerase II [71]. In cell-culture experiments, ICRF-193 prevented efficient HSV replication, and other topoisomerase II inhibitors, such as amsacrine, are being evaluated and developed for use against HSV [71–73].

48.3.5 Peptidomimetic Ribonucleotide Reductase Inhibitors

HSV uses its own ribonucleotides reductase (RNR) enzymes for DNA replication. BILD 1263 is a peptidomimetic HSV RNR inhibitor that was shown to inhibit HSV-1 and HSV-2 replication in cell culture, as well as inhibiting acyclovir-resistant HSV [74]. In a murine model in vivo, BILD 1263 was shown to reduce the severity of HSV-1 ocular disease [74, 75]. These results indicate that peptidomimetic RNR inhibitors are a potential new class of antiherpetic drugs. BILD 1263 derivatives BILD 1351, BILD 1357, and BILD 1633 have also been derived and studied, and they also exhibit anti-HSV activity [76–78].

48.3.6 Immune Response Modifiers

Immune response modifiers are agents that influence the immune response of an individual, favoring either the Th1 or Th2 branch and subsequent cytokine production. Immune response modifiers like imiquimod and resiquimod have shown anti-HSV activity in vivo.

Resiquimod in particular was selected for further development as an antiherpetic drug. Resiquimod is a toll-like receptor 7 and 8 agonist, and favors the Th1 branch of immune response (innate immunity). Resiquimod demonstrated marked efficacy in reducing outbreaks of genital herpes following its topical application [79]. More recent studies have further shown the potential of resiquimod as a genital herpes therapy. In a Phase II trial involving HSV-2-infected individuals ($n=75$), resiquimod 0.01% gel applied topically to lesions twice weekly for 3 weeks resulted in reduced rates of viral shedding and reduced lesion rates when compared with vehicle [80].

48.3.7 Cellular Cyclin-Dependent Kinase Inhibitors

Cellular cyclin-dependent kinases (CDK) are required for the replication and transcription of many viruses, including HSV [81]. CDK inhibitors such as roscovitine have demonstrated anti-HSV activity [82]; roscovitine is discussed in section 48.5.1.

48.4 Human Papilloma Virus

Since the FDA approval of the HPV quadrivalent vaccine, prevention via vaccination has been the hallmark of HPV therapy. However, HPV infection is extremely common and there are over 100 strains that infect humans [83]. Therefore, treatment options and the development of new therapies are important. Current treatments for skin and genital warts and most other manifestations of HPV infection include antiproliferative therapies such as podophyllotoxin and 5-fluorouracil, surgical and destructive therapies such as cryotherapy or curettage, antivirals like cidofovir, and immune response modulators like imiquimod [84]. Treatments of premalignant and malignant manifestations of HPV are not covered.

As for molluscum contagiosum, photodynamic therapy has been used off-label for treatment of verrucae vulgares and condylomata acuminata [56]. Case reports describe success with PDT; in addition, a pilot study treating periungual warts resulted in complete clearance in 90% of patients and low recurrence rates [56, 85]. Another pilot study treating periungual warts combined PDT with ablative CO_2 laser treatment, again achieving complete clearance in 90% of lesions and no recurrence [86]. However, results of a Phase III randomized control trial showed that combining CO_2 laser ablation with PDT to treat condyloma acuminata had no effect on recurrence rate of lesions [87].

The experimental agent GS-9191 is the prodrug of 9-(2-phosphonylmethoxyethyl) guanine (PMEG), a nucleotide analog. It is designed for use topically to treat lesions caused by HPV. PMEG-DP, the active metabolite of GS-9191, was shown to inhibit DNA polymerase α and β and only weakly inhibit mitochondrial DNA polymerase γ. In cell-culture assays, GS-9191 showed antiproliferative activity selectively against HPV-infected cells, and in a rabbit model, topical GS-9191 reduced the size of papilloma lesions in a dose-dependent manner [88]. GS-9191 is in clinical trials (Phase II completed at this time) for treatment of genital warts [89].

Polyphenon E is a catechin-based compound extracted from *Camellia sinesis*, a green tea plant, which has demonstrated immunomodulatory and antitumor activity [90]. In a Phase III study on the effects of Polyphenon E on anogenital warts, patients ($n=411$) were administered either 10% or 15% Polyphenon E ointment or placebo. Patients receiving Polyphenon E experienced significantly higher rates of complete clearance (51–53%) than patients receiving placebo (37%) [91]. An earlier Phase II/III study that tested the 10% cream formulation as well as the 15% ointment resulted in significant increased clearing only for the 15% ointment, suggesting that an ointment vector is more efficacious in delivery of Polyphenon E than a cream [90]. Polyphenon E caused mild to moderate local skin reactions in both studies, but was otherwise well tolerated [90, 91].

48.5 New Targets for Antiviral Drugs

48.5.1 Cyclin-dependent Kinases

Pharmacological cyclin-dependent kinase (CDK) inhibitors, which inhibit host-cell CDKs that are often utilized by viruses for replication of their genome, have been shown to inhibit replication of wild-type and multidrug-resistant strains of HIV, HSV-1, HSV-2, HCMV, EBV, and VZV. Since the action of the drug is on the host cell proteins, not on the viral proteins, mutations in viral genes may not overcome inhibition as easily. Roscovitine, a CDK inhibitor, was shown to inhibit replication of HSV-1, HSV-2, and HIV-1, including strains of HSV-1 and HIV-1 that were resistant to standard antiviral medications [82].

48.5.2 Helicase Inhibitors

The activity of viral helicases is essential for viral genome replication, transcription, and translation; they have thus been identified as targets for new antiviral medications. Inhibitors of viral helicases have the potential to treat the STIs HSV and HPV as well as other viral infections, such as hepatitis C and arboviruses. Helicases are motor proteins that use ATP hydrolysis to fuel the separation of nucleic acid strands. They are used in multiple steps of the viral life cycle, including separation of double-stranded DNA to initiate replication, separating duplexes of nucleic acid that occur after replication in single-stranded DNA viruses, as well as transcription of viral mRNAs, translation, and packaging nucleic acids into virions. Both large DNA viruses that invade the nucleus and viruses that replicate outside the nucleus almost always encode a helicase; retroviruses and negative sense single-stranded RNA viruses have not been reported to encode synthesis of helicases [92]. Helicase inhibitors have the potential for host-cell toxicity, since the helicase ATP-bending site is conserved in not only all classes of helicases but also in motor proteins, GTPases, kinases, ATPases, and mitochrondrial ATP synthase [92].

Viral helicases are generally grouped into one of the three superfamilies: superfamily 1 (SF1), superfamily 2 (SF2), superfamily 3 (SF3), and the DnaB family. The families are distinguished by specific conserved signature sequences, which may be conserved across all families, slightly different between families, or unique to a particular family. HSV UL5 protein, a 5′–3′ DNA helicase, is a member of SF1, while its UL9 protein, a 3′–5′ DNA helicase, is a member of SF2. The NS3 3′–5′ RNA/DNA helicase of hepatitis C virus is a member of SF2, while HPV's E1 DNA helicase is a member of SF3. Recent developments in assays now make it possible to identify new potent helicase inhibitors using high-throughput screening [93].

48.5.2.1 SF1 Helicase–Primase Inhibitors

The UL5 HSV helicase complexes tightly with the virus' primase (UL52), and this formation is required for their mutual function. This complex of helicase and primase is the target of new anti-HSV medications such as the aminothiazolylphenyl compound BILS 179 BS and the thiazole amide BAY 57-1293 [92, 94–96]. The mechanism of action of BILS 179 BS against HSV helicase–primase activity is likely through prevention of DNA release during translocation [95]. Several derivatives of the compound exist, including BILS 45 BS and BILS 22 BS (known as the Boehringer Ingelheim series) [95]. Murine studies show a dose-dependent reduction in HSV viral studies following administration of the BILS compounds [95, 97]. Incidence of mutations conferring resistance to BILS compounds is significantly less than those conferring resistance to acyclovir [98].

BAY 57–1293 is 50 times more potent in its anti-HSV activity than acyclovir and is also active against acyclovir-resistant HSV [99]. Resistance to BAY 57–1293 is approximately 10 times less frequent than acyclovir resistance [99]. The mechanism of action of BAY 57–1293 against HSV helicase–primase is through inhibition of DNA-stimulated ATPase activity, in a dose-dependent manner. The compound has shown activity against both HSV-1 and -2; it shortens healing time in HSV infection and is effective even when initiation of treatment is delayed, in contrast to the nucleoside analogs, which require early initiation for efficacy [99, 100].

48.5.2.2 SF3 Helicase Inhibitors

The E1 helicase of HPV is the current target of anti-HPV medications in development. Two major classes of molecules are under investigation: inhibitors that disrupt the interaction of HPV E1 helicase with its co-activator, HPV E2 protein, and inhibitors that specifically target HPV E1 helicase DNA unwinding [92]. HPV E1-E2 inhibitors 1–3 have been identified, of which inhibitor 3 is the most potent; these molecules target the E2 protein and inhibit HPV DNA replication in a dose-dependent manner. These molecules are active against the low-risk HPV types 6 and 11, but not against the high-risk HPV types [101]. E1 helicase-specific inhibitors are also under development, but initial efforts have yielded unstable molecules with poor cell permeability that have limited use in vivo [102].

48.6 New Antibiotics

48.6.1 *Neisseria Gonorrhoeae*

Emergence of quinolone-resistance strains worldwide has led to reliance on third-generation cephalosporins and the macrolide, azithromycin, as first-line treatment options. A new fluoroquinolone, zabofloxacin, has been shown in intro to have activity four- to eightfold greater (MIC_{90} 0.016 μg/mL) than ciprofloxacin against clinical isolates of *Neisseria gonorrhoeae* [103, 104]. Furthermore, zabofloxacin was tested against known ciprofloxacin-resistant strains of *N. gonorrhoeae* and shown to be highly effective (MIC_{90} 0.03–0.06 μg/mL). Further clinical trials are needed to determine proper dosing; however, single-dose regimens or short-course regimens may be able to treat uncomplicated gonococcal infections.

48.6.2 *Chlamydia Trachomatis*

Several new antimicrobials for *Chlamydia trachomatis* are being developed. Rifamycins, including rifampin, have been known for over 30 years to have excellent activity against *C. trachomatis.* The discovery of rapid one-step resistance to rifampin in *C. trachomatis* has limited the drug's therapeutic use [105]. A new rifamycin derivative, rifalazil, is currently being studied for persistent Chlamydia infections [106]. Rifalazil has many favorable characteristics that can be exploited to treat *C. trachomatis*: a relatively long half life (~60 h), high intracellular levels and tissue penetration, and low MIC_{90} (0.0025 μg/mL) [107]. Furthermore, recent studies show that some strains of rifampin-resistant strains of *C. trachomatis* remain susceptible to rifalazil [108]. Further studies are needed to confirm that rapid resistance is not acquired by *C. trachomatis*. However, initial studies of rifalazil are promising for the treatment of difficult-to-treat, persistent urogenital chlamydia infections. In addition, other rifamycin derivatives have shown promising activity against *C. trachomatis* infections. In vitro, compounds ABI-1662, ABI-1131, ABI-0046, and ABI-0204 show more favorable minimum inhibitory concentrations for wild-type and (except ABI-0204) rifampin-resistant *C. trachomatis* when compared with rifalazil [107].

48.6.3 Microbicides

Topical microbicides are a new focus of research designed to prevent transmission of sexually transmitted infections, including HIV, when applied vaginally [109]. In developing countries, heterosexual transmission remains the primary route of HIV infection. Furthermore, a concurrent STD infection such as gonorrhea, chlamydia, and herpes simplex virus can increase the risk of infection with HIV [110]. A topically vaginal compound may provide women an alternate, female-controlled, prophylaxis method. The ideal compound would prevent transmission of HIV and other STDs as well. There are four major classes of compounds being tested: (1) vaginal acid-buffering agents that maintain a protective vaginal pH and flora; (2) polymers that block the entry/fusion of virus to target cells; (3) detergents or surfactants that inactivate viral particles; (4) antiretroviral drugs specific for HIV. To date, several candidate compounds have advanced to clinical trials.

48.6.4 Drugs with Multiple Antibacterial Targets

One polyherbal cream, BASANT, is in Phase II clinical trials. BASANT, which is a combination of circumen, amla, reetha saponins, aloe vera, and rose water, has been shown to be effective against a number of different sexually transmitted pathogens in vitro, including *C. trachomatis*, *N. gonorrhea* (including clinical isolates resistant to several antibiotics), *Candida* spp., HIV, and HPV [111, 112].

48.7 Conclusion

A number of new therapies are being developed against viral and bacterial STIs. The search for such new agents is being driven by the development of resistance to current antimicrobial agents. Management of STIs, however, should not be totally dependent on new therapies, but should emphasize public health measures and new vaccines.

Take-Home Pearls

> Due to emerging resistance of sexually transmitted infections to current therapies, the necessity for new therapies has increased. Many of the drugs discussed in this chapter are still under investigation; regardless of whether they become available after testing, their use in elucidating new targets for treatment is invaluable.

> New medications under investigation in the existing classes for treatment of HIV include:
  Nucleoside/nucleotide reverse transcriptase inhibitors – racivir, apricitabine, amdoxovir, elvucitabine, and GS–9148.
  Nonnucleoside reverse transcriptase inhibitors – rilpivirine, calanolide A.
  Protease inhibitors – brecanavir.

> Emerging classes of medications for treatment of HIV include:
  Entry inhibitors – ibalizumab, PRO 140, DCM205.
  Fusion inhibitors – enfuvirtide.
  CCR5 antagonists – maraviroc, vicriviroc.
  CXCR4 antagonists – AMD070, KRH-3995.
  Integration inhibitors – elvitegravir, L-870812.
  Maturation inhibitors – bevirimat, UK-201844.

References

1. Otto, M.: New nucleoside reverse transcriptase inhibitors for the treatment of HIV infections. Curr. Opin. Pharmacol. **4**(5), 431–436 (2004)
2. Waters, L., Nelson, M.: New drugs. HIV Med. **6**(4), 225–231 (2005)
3. Otto, M., et al.: Single and multiple dose pharmacokinetics and safety of the nucleoside Racivir in male volunteers. In: Frontiers in Drug Development for Antiretroviral Therapies, Naples, FL, 2002
4. Herzmann, C., et al.: Safety, Pharmacokinetics, and Efficacy of (+/–)-{beta}-2', 3'-Dideoxy-5-Fluoro-3'-Thiacytidine with Efavirenz and Stavudine in Antiretroviral-Naive Human Immunodeficiency Virus-Infected Patients. Antimicrob. Agents Chemother. **49**(7), 2828 (2005)
5. Collins, P., et al.: Analysis of the genotypes of viruses isolated from patients after 10 days monotherapy with SPD754. In: 11th Conference on Retroviruses and Opportunistic Infections, San Francisco, CA, 2004
6. Bethell, R., et al.: Pharmacological evaluation of a dual deoxycytidine analogue combination: 3TC and SPD754.

In: Program and abstracts of the 11th Conference on Retroviruses and Opportunistic Infections, San Francisco, CA, 2004
7. Margolis, D., et al.: The use of [beta]-D-2, 6-diaminopurine dioxolane with or without mycophenolate mofetil in drug-resistant HIV infection. AIDS **21**(15), 2025 (2007)
8. Hernandez-Santiago, B., et al.: Short communication cellular pharmacology of 9-(beta-D-1, 3-dioxolan-4-yl) guanine and its lack of drug interactions with zidovudine in primary human lymphocytes. Antivir. Chem. Chemother. **18**(6), 343 (2007)
9. Gripshover, B., et al.: Amdoxovir versus placebo with enfuvirtide plus optimized background therapy for HIV-1-infected subjects failing current therapy (AACTG A5118) (Short communication). Antivir. Ther. **11**, 619–623 (2006)
10. Bazmi, H., et al.: In vitro selection of mutations in the human immunodeficiency virus type 1 reverse transcriptase that decrease susceptibility to (–)-ß-D-dioxolane-guanosine and suppress resistance to 3'-azido-3'-deoxythymidine. Antimicrob. Agents Chemother. **44**(7), 1783–1788 (2000)
11. Gu, Z., et al.: Mechanism of action and in vitro activity of 1', 3'-dioxolanylpurine nucleoside analogues against sensitive and drug-resistant human immunodeficiency virus type 1 variants. Antimicrob. Agents Chemother. **43**(10), 2376–2382 (1999)
12. Chong, Y., et al.: Molecular mechanism of DAPD/DXG against zidovudine-and lamivudine-drug resistant mutants: a molecular modelling approach. Antivir. Chem. Chemother. **13**, 115–128 (2002)
13. Mewshaw, J., et al.: Dioxolane guanosine, the active form of the prodrug diaminopurine dioxolane, is a potent inhibitor of drug-resistant HIV-1 isolates from patients for whom standard nucleoside therapy fails. J. Acquir. Immune Defic. Syndr. **29**(1), 11 (2002)
14. Thompson, M., et al. Preliminary results of dosing of amdoxovir in treatment-experienced patients. In: 10th Conference on Retroviruses and Opportunistic Infections, Boston, MA, 2003
15. Thompson, M., et al.: Short-term safety and pharmacodynamics of amdoxovir in HIV-infected patients. AIDS **19**(15), 1607 (2005)
16. Dunkle, L., et al.: Elvucitabine: potent antiviral activity demonstrated in multidrug-resistant HIV infection. Antivir. Ther. **8**(3), 2–12 (2003)
17. Colucci, P., Pottage, J.C., Robison, H., Turgeon, J., Schürmann, D., Hoepelman, I.M., Ducharme, M.P.: Multiple-dose pharmacokinetic behavior of elvucitabine, a nucleoside transcriptase inhibitor, administered over 21 days with lopinavir-ritonavir in human immunodeficiency virus type 1-infected subjects. Antimicrob. Agents Chemother. **53**(2), 662–669 (2009)
18. Cihlar, T., Ray, A.S., Boojamra, C.G., Hui, H., Laflamme, G., Vela, J.E., Grant, D., Chen, J., Myrick, F., White, K.L., Gao, Y., Lin, K.Y., Douglas, J.L., Parkin, N.T., Carey, A., Pakdaman, R., Mackman, R.L.: Design and profiling of GS-9148, a novel nucleotide analog active against nucleoside-resistant variants of human immunodeficiency virus type 1, and its orally bioavailable phosphonoamidate prodrug, GS-9131. Antimicrob. Agents Chemother. **52**(2), 655–665 (2008)
19. Cihlar, T., LaFlamme, G., Fisher, R., Carey, A.C., Vela, J.E., Mackman, R., Ray, A.S.: Novel nucleotide human immunodeficiency virus reverse transcriptase inhibitor GS-9148 with a low nephrotoxic potential: characterization of renal transport and accumulation. Antimicrob. Agents Chemother. **53**(1), 150–156 (2009)
20. Goebel, F., et al.: Short-term antiviral activity of TMC278-a novel NNRTI-in treatment-naive HIV-1-infected subjects. AIDS **20**(13), 1721 (2006)
21. Pozniak, A., et al. 48-week primary analysis of trial TMC278-C204: TMC278 demonstrates potent and sustained efficacy in ART-naive patients. In: Programs and Abstracts: 14th Conference on Retroviruses and Opportunistic Infections, Los Angeles, CA, 2007.
22. Eiznhamer, D.A., Creagh, T., Ruckle, J.L., Tolbert, D.T., Giltner, J., Dutta, B., Flavin, M.T., Jenta, T., Xu, Z.Q.: Safety and pharmacokinetic profile of multiple escalating doses of (+)-calanolide A, a naturally occurring nonnucleoside reverse transcriptase inhibitor, in healthy HIV-negative volunteers. HIV Clin. Trials **3**(6), 435–450 (2002)
23. Ford, S., et al.: Single-dose safety and pharmacokinetics of brecanavir, a novel human immunodeficiency virus protease inhibitor. Antimicrob. Agents Chemother. **50**(6), 2201–2206 (2006)
24. Lalezari, J., et al.: Preliminary safety and efficacy data of brecanavir, a novel HIV-1 protease inhibitor: 24 week data from study HPR10006. J. Antimicrob. Chemother. **60**(1), 170 (2007)
25. Reddy, Y., et al.: Safety and pharmacokinetics of brecanavir, a novel human immunodeficiency virus type 1 protease inhibitor, following repeat administration with and without ritonavir in healthy adult subjects? Antimicrob. Agents Chemother. **51**(4), 1202–1208 (2007)
26. Scarlatti, G., et al.: In vivo evolution of HIV-1 co-receptor usage and sensitivity to chemokine-mediated suppression. Nat. Med. **3**(11), 1259–1265 (1997)
27. Jacobson, J.M., Kuritzkes, D.R., Godofsky, E., DeJesus, E., Larson, J.A., Weinheimer, S.P., Lewis, S.T.: Safety, pharmacokinetics, and antiretroviral activity of multiple doses of ibalizumab (formerly TNX-355), and anti-CD4 monoclonal antibody, in human immunodeficiency virus type 1-infected adults. Antimicrob. Agents Chemother. **53**(2), 450–457 (2009)
28. Jacobson, J.M., Saag, M.S., Thompson, M.A., Fischl, M.A., Liporace, R., Reichman, R.C., Redfield, R.R., Fichtenbaum, C.J., Zingman, B.S., Patel, M.C., Murga, J.D., Pemrick, S.M., D'Ambrosio, P., Michael, M., Kroger, H., Ly, H., Rotshteyn, Y., Buice, R., Morris, S.A., Stavola, J.J., Maddon, P.J., Kremer, A.B., Olson, W.C.: Antiviral activity of single-dose PRO 140, a CCR5 monoclonal antibody, in HIV-infected adults. J. Infect. Dis. **198**(9), 1345–1352 (2008)
29. Duong, Y.T., Meadows, D.C., Srivastava, I.K., Gervay-Hague, J., North, T.W.: Direct inactivation of human immunodeficiency virus type 1 by a novel small-molecule entry inhibitor, DCM205. Antimicrob. Agents Chemother. **51**(5), 1780–1786 (2007)
30. Perno, C., et al.: Overcoming resistance to existing therapies in HIV-infected patients: The role of new antiretroviral drugs. J. Med. Virol. **80**(4), 565 (2008)
31. Kitchen, C., et al.: Fuvirtide antiretroviral therapy in HIV-1 infection. Ther. Clin. Risk Manag. **4**(2), 433–439 (2008)

32. Matthews, T., et al.: Case history: Enfuvirtide: the first therapy to inhibit the entry of HIV-1 into host CD4 lymphocytes. Nat. Rev. Drug Discov. **3**, 215–225 (2004)
33. Moyle, G., et al.: Epidemiology and predictive factors for chemokine receptor use in HIV-1 infection. J. Infect. Dis. **191**(6), 866–872 (2005)
34. Brumme, Z., et al.: Molecular and clinical epidemiology of CXCR4-using HIV-1 in a large population of antiretroviral-naive individuals. J. Infect. Dis. **192**(3), 466–474 (2005)
35. Ray, N.: Maraviroc in the treatment of HIV infection **2**, 151–161 (2008)
36. Klibanov, O.: Vicriviroc, a CCR5 receptor antagonist for the potential treatment of HIV infection. Curr. Opin. Investig. Drugs **10**(8), 845–859 (2009)
37. Hosein, S.: Anti-HIV agents. Vicriviroc. TreatmentUpdate **20**(2), 9–10 (2008)
38. Gulick, R.M., Su, Z., Flexner, C., Hughes, M.D., Skolnik, P.R., Wilkin, T.J., Gross, R., Krambrink, A., Coakley, E., Greaves, W.L., Zolopa, A., Reichment, R., Godfrey, C., Hirsch, M., Kuritzkes, D.R.: AIDS Clinical Trials Group 5211 Team, Phase 2 study of the safety and efficacy of vicriviroc, a CCR5 inhibitor, in HIV-1-infected, treatment-experienced patients: AIDS clinical trials group 5211. J. Infect. Dis. **196**(2), 304–312 (2007)
39. Cao, Y.J., Flexner, C., Dunaway, S., Park, J.G., Klingman, K., Wiggins, I., Conley, J., Radebaugh, C., Kashuba, A.D., MacFarland, R., Becker, S., Hendrix, C.W.: Effect of low-dose ritonavir on the pharmacokinetics of the CXCR4 anatagonist AMD070 in healthy volunteers. Antimicrob. Agents Chemother. **52**(5), 1630–1634 (2008)
40. Stone, N.D., Dunaway, S., Flexner, C., Tierney, C., Calandra, G.B., Becker, S., Cao, Y.J., Wiggins, I.P., Conley, J., MacFarland, R.T., Park, J.K., Lalama, C., Snyder, S., Kallungal, B., Klingman, K.L., Hendrix, C.W.: Multiple-dose escalation study of the safety, pharmacokinetics, and biologic activity of oral AMD070, a selective CXCR4 receptor inhibitor, in human subjects. Antimicrob. Agents Chemother. **51**(7), 2351–2358 (2007)
41. Murakami, T., Kumakura, S., Yamazaki, T., Tanaka, R., Hamatake, M., Okuma, K., Huang, W., Toma, J., Komano, J., Yanaka, M., Tanaka, Y., Yamamoto, N.: The novel CXCR4 antagonist KRH-3955 is an orally bioavailable and extremely potent inhibitor of human immunodeficiency virus type 1 infection: comparative studies with AMD3100. Antimicrob. Agents Chemother. **53**(7), 2940–2948 (2009)
42. Lataillade, M., Kozal, M.: The hunt for HIV-1 integrase inhibitors. AIDS Patient Care STDs **20**(7), 489–501 (2006)
43. Klibanov, O.: Elvitegravir, an oral HIV integrase inhibitor, for the potential treatment of HIV infection. Curr. Opin. Investig. Drugs **10**(2), 190–200 (2009)
44. DeJesus, E., Berger, D., Markowitz, M., Cohen, C., Hawkins, T., Ruane, P., Elion, R., Farthing, C., Zhong, L., Cheng, A.K., McColl, D., Kearney, B.P., for the 183-0101 Study Team: Antiviral activity, pharmacokinetics, and dose response of the HIV-1 integrase inhibitor GS-9137 (JTK-303) in treatment-naive and treatment-experienced patients. J. Acquir. Immune Defic. Syndr. **43**(1), 1–5 (2006)
45. Mathias, A.A., Hinkle, J., Shen, G., Enejosa, J., Piliero, P.J., Sekar, V., Mack, R., Tomaka, F., Kearney, B.P.: Effect of ritonaivr-boosted tipranavir or darunavir on the steady-state pharmacokinetics of elvitegravir. J. Acquir. Immune Defic. Syndr. **49**(2), 156–162 (2008)
46. Ramanathan, S., Kakuda, T., Mack, R., West, S., Kearney, B.P.: Pharmacokinetics of elvitegravir and etravirine following coadministration of ritonavir-boosted elvitegravir and etravirine. Antivir. Ther. **13**(8), 1011–1017 (2008)
47. Ramanathan, S., Shen, G., Cheng, A., Kearney, B.P.: Pharmacokinetics of emtricitabine, tenofovir, and GS-9137 following coadministration of emtricitabine/tenofovir disoproxil fumarate and ritonavir-boosted GS-9137. J. Acquir. Immune Defic. Syndr. **45**(3), 274–279 (2007)
48. Ramanathan, S., Shen, G., Hinkle, J., Enejosa, J., Kearney, B.P.: Pharmacokinetics of coadministered ritonavir-boosted elvitegravir and zidovudine, didanosine, stavudine or abacavir. J. Acquir. Immune Defic. Syndr. **46**(2), 160–166 (2007)
49. Terrazas-Aranda, K., Van Herrewege, Y., Hazuda, D., Lewi, P., Costi, R., Di Santo, R., Cara, A., Vanham, G.: Human immunodeficiency virus type 1 (HIV-1) integration: a potential target for microbicides to prevent cell-free or cell-associated HIV-1 infection. Antimicrob. Agents Chemother. **52**(7), 2544–2554 (2008)
50. Smith, P.F., Ogundele, A., Forrest, A., Wilton, J., Salzwedel, K., Doto, J., Allaway, G.P., Martin, D.E.: Phase I and II study of the safety, virologic effect, and pharmacokinetics/pharmacodynamics of single-dose 3-O-(3', 3'-dimethylsuccinyl)betulinic acid (bevirimat) against human immunodeficiency virus infection. Antimicrob. Agents Chemother. **51**(10), 3574–3581 (2007)
51. Connor, A., Evans, P., Doto, J., Ellis, C., Martin, D.E.: An oral human drug absorption study to assess the impact of site of delivery on the bioavailability of bevirimat. J. Clin. Pharmacol. **49**(5), 606–612 (2009)
52. Martin, D.E., Blum, R., Doto, J., Galbraith, H., Ballow, C.: Multiple-dose pharmacokinetics and safety of bevirimat, a novel inhibitor of HIV maturation, in healthy volunteers. Clin. Pharmacokinet. **46**(7), 589–598 (2007)
53. Qian, K., Yu, D., Chen, C.H., Huang, L., Morris-Natschke, S.L., Nitz, T.J., Salzwedel, K., Reddick, M., Allaway, G.P., Lee, K.H.: Anti-AIDS agents. 78. Design, synthesis, metabolic stability assessment, and antiviral evaluation of novel betulinic acid derivatives as potent anti-human immunodeficiency virus (HIV) agents. J. Med. Chem. **52**(10), 3248–3258 (2009)
54. Blair, W.S., Cao, J., Jackson, L., Jimenez, J., Peng, Q., Wu, H., Isaacson, J., Butler, S.L., Chu, A., Graham, J., Malfait, A.M., Tortorella, M., Patick, A.K.: Identification and characterization of UK-201844, a novel inhibitor that interferes with human immunodeficiency virus type 1 gp160 processing. Antimicrob. Agents Chemother. **51**(10), 3554–3561 (2007)
55. Bikowski Jr., J.: Molluscum contagiosum: the need for physician intervention and new treatment options. Cutis **73**(3), 202–206 (2004)
56. Gold, M.H., Moiin, A.: Treatment of verrucae vulgares and molluscum contagiosum with photodynamic therapy. Dermatol. Clin. **25**(1), 75–80 (2007)
57. Calista, D.: Topical cidofovir for severe cutaneous human papillomavirus and molluscum contagiosum infections in patients with HIV/AIDS. A pilot study. J. Eur. Acad. Dermatol. Venereol. **14**(6), 484–488 (2000)

58. Watanabe, T., Tamaki, K.: Cidofovir diphosphate inhibits molluscum contagiosum virus DNA polymerase activity. J. Investig. Dermatol. **128**(5), 1327–1329 (2008)
59. Visalli, R., van Zeijl, M.: DNA encapsidation as a target for anti-herpesvirus drug therapy. Antiviral Res. **59**(2), 73–87 (2003)
60. Eizuru, Y.: Development of new antivirals for herpesviruses. Antivir. Chem. Chemother. **14**, 299–308 (2003)
61. Brideau, R., et al.: Broad-spectrum antiviral activity of PNU-183792, a 4-oxo-dihydroquinoline, against human and animal herpesviruses. Antivir. Res. **54**(1), 19–28 (2002)
62. Knechtel, M., et al.: Inhibition of clinical isolates of human cytomegalovirus and varicella zoster virus by PNU-183792, a 4-oxo-dihydroquinoline. J. Med. Virol. **68**(2), 234–236 (2002)
63. Wathen, M.: Non-nucleoside inhibitors of herpesviruses. Rev. Med. Virol. **12**(3), 167–178 (2002)
64. Thomsen, D., et al.: Amino acid changes within conserved region III of the herpes simplex virus and human cytomegalovirus DNA polymerases confer resistance to 4-oxo-dihydroquinolines, a novel class of herpesvirus antiviral agents. J. Virol. **77**(3), 1868–1876 (2003)
65. Newcomb, W.W., Thomsen, D.R., Homa, F.L., Brown, J.C.: Assembly of the herpes simplex virus capsid: Identification of soluble scaffold-portal complexes and their role in formation of portal-containing capsids. J. Virol. **77**(18), 9862–9871 (2003)
66. Newcomb, W.W., Brown, J.C.: Inhibition of herpes simplex virus replication by WAY-150138: Assembly of capsids depleted of the portal and terminase proteins involved in DNA encapsidation. J. Virol. **76**(19), 10084–10088 (2002)
67. Pesola, J.M., Zhu, J., Knipe, D.M., Coen, D.M.: Herpes simplex virus 1 immediate-early and early gene expression during reactivation from latency under conditions that prevent infectious virus production. J. Virol. **79**(23), 14516–14525 (2005)
68. van Zeijl, M., Fairhurst, J., Jones, T.R., Vernon, S.K., Morin, J., LaRocque, J., Feld, B., O'Hara, B., Bloom, J.D., Johann, S.V.: Novel class of thiourea compounds that inhibit herpes simplex virus type 1 DNA cleavage and encapsidation: resistance maps to the UL6 gene. J. Virol. **74**(19), 9054–9061 (2000)
69. Boehmer, P.E., Lehman, I.R.: Herpes simplex virus DNA replication. Annu. Rev. Biochem. **66**, 347–384 (1997)
70. Ebert, S.N., Shtrom, S.S., Muller, M.T.: Topoisomerase II cleavage of herpes simplex virus type 1 DNA in vivo is replication dependent. J. Virol. **64**(9), 4059–4066 (1990)
71. Hammarsten, O., Yao, X., Elias, P.: Inhibition of topoisomerase II by ICRF-193 prevents efficient replication of herpes simplex virus type 1. J. Virol. **70**(7), 4523–4529 (1996)
72. Akanitapichat, P., Lowden, C., Bastow, K.F.: 1, 3-Dihydroxyacridone derivates as inhibitors of herpes virus replication. Antivir. Res. **45**(2), 123–134 (2000)
73. Goodell, J.R., Madhok, A.A., Hiasa, H., Ferguson, D.M.: Synthesis and evaluation of acridine- and acridone-based anti-herpes agents with topoisomerase activity. Bioorg. Med. Chem. **14**(16), 5467–5480 (2006)
74. Liuzzi, M., Deziel, R., Moss, N., Beauieu, P., Bonneau, A.M., Bousquet, C., Chafouleas, J.G., Garneau, M., Jaramillo, J., Krogsrud, R.L., et al.: A potent peptidomimetic inhibitor of HSV ribonucleotide reductase with antiviral activity in vivo. Nature **372**(6507), 695–698 (1994)
75. Brandt, C.R., Spencer, B., Imesch, P., Garneau, M., Déziel, R.: Evaluation of a peptidomimetic ribonucleotide reductase inhibitor with a murine model of herpes simplex virus type 1 ocular disease. Antimicrob. Agents Chemother. **40**(5), 1078–1084 (1996)
76. Duan, J., Liuzzi, M., Paris, W., Lambert, M., Lawetz, C., Moss, N., Jaramillo, J., Gauthier, J., Déziel, R., Cordingley, M.G.: Antiviral activity of a selective ribonucleotide reductase inhibitor against acyclovir-resistant herpes simplex virus type 1 in vivo. Antimicrob. Agents Chemother. **42**(7), 1629–1635 (1998)
77. Lawetz, C., Liuzzi, M.: The antiviral activity of the ribonucleotide reductase inhibitor BILD 1351 SE in combination with acyclovir against HSV type-1 in cell culture. Antivir. Res. **39**(1), 35–46 (1998)
78. Moss, N., Beaulieu, P., Duceppe, J.S., Ferland, J.M., Garneau, M., Gauthier, J., Ghiro, E., Goulet, S., Guse, I., Jaramillo, J., Llinas-Brunet, M., Malenfant, E., Plante, R., Poirer, M., Soucy, F., Wernic, D., Yoakim, C., Déziel, R.: Peptidomimetic inhibitors of herpes simplex virus ribonucleotide reductase with improved in vivo antiviral activity. J. Med. Chem. **39**(21), 4173–4180 (1996)
79. Spruance, S.L., Tyring, S.K., Smith, M.H., Meng, T.C.: Application of a topical immune response modifier, resiquimod gel, to modify the recurrence rate of recurrent genital herpes: a pilot study. J. Infect. Dis. **184**(2), 196–200 (2001)
80. Mark, K.E., Corey, L., Meng, T.C., Magaret, A.S., Huang, M.L., Selke, S., Slade, H.B., Tyring, S.K., Warren, T., Sacks, S.L., Leone, P., Bergland, V.A., Wald, A.: Topical resiquimod 0.01% gel decreases herpes simplex virus type 2 genital shedding: A randomized controlled trial. J. Infect. Dis. **195**(9), 1324–1331 (2007)
81. Schang, L.M., Phillips, J., Schaffer, P.A.: Requirement for cellular cyclin-dependent kinases in herpes simplex virus replication and transcription. J. Virol. **72**(7), 5626–5637 (1998)
82. Schang, L., et al.: Pharmacological cyclin-dependent kinase inhibitors inhibit replication of wild-type and drug-resistant strains of herpes simplex virus and human immunodeficiency virus type 1 by targeting cellular, not viral, proteins. J. Virol. **76**(15), 7874–7882 (2002)
83. Diaz, M.: Human papilloma virus: prevention and treatment. Obstet. Gynecol. Clin. North Am. **35**(2), 199–217 (2008). vii–viii
84. Ahmed, A.M., Madkan, V., Tyring, S.K.: Human papillomaviruses and genital disease. Dermatol. Clin. **24**(2), 157–165 (2006)
85. Schroeter, C.A., Kaas, L., Waterval, J.J., Bos, P.M., Neumann, H.A.: Successful treatment of periungual warts using photodynamic therapy: a pilot study. J. Eur. Acad. Dermatol. Venereol. **21**(9), 1170–1174 (2007)
86. Yoo, K.H., Kim, B., Kim, M.N.: Enhanced efficacy of photodynamic therapy with methyl 5-aminolevulinic acid in recalcitrant periungual warts after ablative carbon dioxide fractional laser: A pilot study. Dermatol. Surg. **35**(12), 1927–1932 (2009)

87. Szeimies, R.M., Schleyer, V., Moll, I., Stocker, M., Landthaler, M., Karrer, S.: Adjuvant photodynamic therapy does not prevent recurrence of condylomata acuminata after carbon dioxide laser ablation – A phase III, prospective, randomized, bicentric, double-blind study. Dermatol. Surg. **35**(5), 757–764 (2009)
88. Wolfgang, G.H., Shibata, R., Wang, J., Ray, A.S., Wu, S., Doerrfler, E., Reiser, H., Lee, W.A., Birkus, G., Christensen, N.D., Andrei, G., Snoeck, R.: GS-9191 is a novel topical prodrug of the nucleotide analog 9-(2-phosphonylmethoxyethyl) guanine with antiproliferative activity and possible utility in the treatment of human papillomavirus lesions. Antimicrob. Agents Chemother. **53**(7), 2777–2784 (2009)
89. Safety and Effectiveness Study of an Experimental Topical Ointment (GS-9191) for the Treatment of Genital Warts. [Electronic] 2007; 2009 Apr 7, cited 2009 Aug 21; GS-9191 Clinical Trial Record. Available from: http://www.clinicaltrials.gov/ct2/show/NCT00499967?term=gs+9191&rank=1.
90. Gross, G., Meyer, K.G., Pres, H., Thielert, C., Tawfik, H., Mescheder, A.: A randomized, double-blind, four-arm parallel-group, placebo-controlled Phase II/III study to investigate the clinical efficacy of two galenic formulations of Polyphenon E in the treatment of external genital warts. J. Eur. Acad. Dermatol. Venereol. **21**(10), 1404–1412 (2007)
91. Stockfleth, E., Beti, H., Orasan, R., Grigorian, F., Mescheder, A., Tawfik, H., Thielert, C.: Topical Polyphenon E in the treatment of external genital and perianal warts: a randomized controlled trial. Br. J. Dermatol. **158**(6), 1329–1338 (2008)
92. Frick, D., Lam, A.: Understanding helicases as a means of virus control. Curr. Pharm. Des. **12**(11), 1315–1338 (2006)
93. Frick, D.: Helicases as antiviral drug targets. Drug News Perspect. **16**(6), 355–362 (2003)
94. Crumpacker, C., Schaffer, P.: New anti-HSV therapeutics target the helicase-primase complex. Nat. Med. **8**(4), 386–391 (2002)
95. Crute, J., et al.: Herpes simplex virus helicase-primase inhibitors are active in animal models of human disease. Nat. Med. **8**(4), 386–391 (2002)
96. Kleymann, G.: Helicase primase: targeting the Achilles heel of herpes simplex viruses. Antivir. Chem. Chemother. **15**(3), 135–140 (2004)
97. Duan, J., et al.: Oral bioavailability and in vivo efficacy of the helicase-primase inhibitor BILS 45 BS against acyclovir-resistant herpes simplex virus type 1. Antimicrob. Agents Chemother. **47**(6), 1798–1804 (2003)
98. Liuzzi, M., et al.: Isolation and characterization of herpes simplex virus type 1 resistant to aminothiazolylphenyl-based inhibitors of the viral helicase-primase. Antivir. Res. **64**(3), 161–170 (2004)
99. Kleymann, G., et al.: New helicase-primase inhibitors as drug candidates for the treatment of herpes simplex disease. Nat. Med. **8**(4), 392–398 (2002)
100. Betz, U.A., Fischer, R., Kleymann, G., Hendrix, M., Rubsamen-Waigmann, H.: Potent In Vivo Antiviral Activity of the Herpes Simplex Virus Primase-Helicase Inhibitor BAY 57-1293. Antimicrob. Agents Chemother. **46**(6), 1766–1772 (2002)
101. White, P., et al.: Inhibition of human papillomavirus DNA replication by small molecule antagonists of the E1-E2 protein interaction*. J. Biol. Chem. **278**(29), 26765–26772 (2003)
102. Faucher, A., et al.: Discovery of small-molecule inhibitors of the ATPase activity of human papillomavirus E1 helicase. J. Med. Chem. **47**(1), 18–21 (2004)
103. Jones, R.N., Biedenbach, D., Ambrose, P.G., Wikler, M.A.: Zabofloxacin (DW-224a) activity against Neisseria gonorrhoeae including quinolone-resistant strains. Diagn. Microbiol. Infect. Dis. **62**(1), 110–112 (2008)
104. Park, H.S., Kim, H., Seol, M.J., Choi, D.R., Choi, E.C., Kwak, J.H.: In vitro and in vivo antibacterial activities of DW-224a, a new fluoronaphthyridone. Antimicrob. Agents Chemother. **50**(6), 2261–2264 (2006)
105. Keshishyan, H., Hanna, L., Jawetz, E.: Emergence of rifampin-resistance in *Chlamydia trachomatis*. Nature **244**(5412), 173–174 (1973)
106. Rothstein, D.M., van Duzer, J., Sternlicht, A., Gilman, S.C.: Rifalazil and other benzoxazinorifamycins in the treatment of chlamydia-based persistent infections. Arch. Pharm. **340**(10), 517–529 (2007)
107. Roblin, P.M., Reznik, T., Kutlin, A., Hammerschlag, M.R.: In vitro activities of rifamycin derivatives ABI-1648 (Rifalazil, KRM-1648), ABI-1657, and ABI-1131 against Chlamydia trachomatis and recent clinical isolates of Chlamydia pneumoniae. Antimicrob. Agents Chemother. **47**(3), 1135–1136 (2003)
108. Suchland, R.J., Bourillon, A., Denamur, E., Stamm, W.E., Rothstein, D.M.: Rifampin-resistant RNA polymerase mutants of Chlamydia trachomatis remain susceptible to the ansamycin rifalazil. Antimicrob. Agents Chemother. **49**(3), 1120–1126 (2005)
109. Madan, R.P., Keller, M., Herold, B.C.: Prioritizing prevention of HIV and sexually transmitted infections: first-generation vaginal microbicides. Curr. Opin. Infect. Dis. **19**(1), 49–54 (2006)
110. Galvin, S.R., Cohen, M.: The role of sexually transmitted disease in HIV transmission. Nat. Rev. Microbiol. **2**(1), 33–42 (2004)
111. Bhengraj, A.R., Dar, S., Talwar, G.P., Mittal, A.: Potential of a novel polyherbal formulation BASANT for prevention of *Chlamydia trachomatis* infection. Int. J. Antimicrob. Agents **32**(1), 84–88 (2008)
112. Talwar, G.P., Dar, S., Rai, M.K., Reddy, K.V., Mitra, D., Kulkarni, S.V., Doncel, G.F., Buck, C.B., Schiller, J.T., Muralidhar, S., Bala, M., Agrawal, S.S., Bansal, K., Verma, J.K.: A novel polyherbal microbicide with inhibitory effect on bacterial, fungal and viral genital pathogens. Int. J. Antimicrob. Agents **32**(2), 180–185 (2008)

Resistance of Sexually Transmitted Pathogens to Antibiotics and Antivirals

49

German A. Contreras and Cesar A. Arias

Core Messages

- Sexually transmitted diseases (STD) are a major health problem in both developed and developing countries and constitute one of the commonest acute illnesses in the world.
- Antibiotic resistance among the common STD pathogens is a worrisome phenomenon, especially among *Neisseria gonorrhoae* and the Human Immunodeficiency Virus (HIV).
- One of the most useful strategies to identify and control the emergence of resistance is the developing of structured surveillance programs that monitor and guide the use of antimicrobials in particular clinical settings.
- For an adequate management of any STD, it is crucial that the clinician and the public health authorities provide adequate information about adherence to medications and proper counseling to sexual partners, in order to avoid the steady increase in the rates of antimicrobial resistance.

G.A. Contreras
Molecular Genetics and Antimicrobial Resistance Unit, and Division of Pediatrics Infections Diseasas, Department of Pediatrics, University of Texas Medical School of Houston, Universidad El Bosque, Carrera 7 B Bis No 132 – 11, Houston, Texas, Bogotá, Colombia
e-mail: german.contreras@uth.tmc.edu

C.A. Arias (✉)
Molecular Genetics and Antimicrobial Resistance Unit
Carrera 7 B Bis No 132 – 11, Bogotá, Colombia and Division of Infectious Diseases, University of Texas Medical School at Houston Director, Molecular Genetics and Antimicrobial Resistance Unit,
6431 Fannin St, MSM 2.112 Houston, Texas, USA
e-mail: caa22@cantab.net

Sexually transmitted diseases (STD) are a major health problem in both developed and developing countries and constitute one of the commonest acute illnesses in the world.

The World Health Organization (WHO) has estimated a total of 340 million new cases of curable sexually transmitted diseases in adults per year [126]. Although these infections are preventable and easily treatable, many infections remain undiagnosed and untreated. Furthermore, the lack of adherence with the treatment and appropriate counseling cause a substantial social and economic impact worldwide. Additionally, the emergence of antibiotic resistance among the common STD pathogens is a worrisome phenomenon. For example, quinolone resistance in *Neisseria gonorrhoae* seems to be spreading at high rates. Similarly, the reports of azithromycin failure among syphilitic individuals and the emergence of antiretroviral resistance in HIV in numerous countries have made the management of such infections a difficult task. This chapter has for its objective the description of the epidemiological behavior of antimicrobial and antiviral resistance among the most common sexually transmitted pathogens; it also aims to describe the most important molecular mechanisms associated with antimicrobial resistance in each pathogen (Table 49.1).

49.1 Antimicrobial Resistance in *Neisseria Gonorrhoae*

Neisseria gonorrhoae is a gram-negative bacterial microorganism, which is transmitted mainly through sexual or perinatal contact. It is one of the most

G. Gross and S.K. Tyring (eds.), *Sexually Transmitted Infections and Sexually Transmitted Diseases*,
DOI: 10.1007/978-3-642-14663-3_49, © Springer-Verlag Berlin Heidelberg 2011

Table 49.1 Antimicrobial agents used in the treatment of sexually transmitted diseases

Etiologic agent	Drug of choice	Mechanism of resistance
Neisseria gonorrhoae[a]	Ceftriaxone	ND
	Cefixime	ND
	Spectinomycin	Enzyme inactivation
	Ciprofloxacin	Structural changes in DNA gyrase and topoisomerase IV Increase in the expression of efflux pumps Decreased porin expression
Treponema pallidum	Penicillin	Possible membrane protein with β-lactamase-like activity [16]
	Azithromycin	Point mutations in the 23 S rRNA
	Doxycycline	ND
	Ceftriaxone	ND
Chlamydia trachomatis	Azithromycin	Point mutations in the 23 S rRNA. *In vitro* analysis
	Doxycycline	ND
	Ofloxacin	Structural changes in DNA gyrase. *In vitro* analysis
	Levofloxacin	
Haemophilus ducreyi [b]	Azithromycin	ND
	Ceftriaxone	ND
	Ciprofloxacin	ND
	Erythromycin	ND
Human Immunodeficiency Virus	Nucleoside reverse transcriptase inhibitors	Mutations within the reverse transcriptase gene, leading to a failure to incorporate an analogue to the nascent DNA chain Thymidine analogue mutations help to increase the excision of nucleoside or nucleotide analogues from viral DNA
	Nonnucleoside reverse transcriptase inhibitors	Mutations within the active site of reverse transcriptase, reducing the affinity of the drugs
	Protease inhibitors	Mutations in the protease gene reduce affinity of the inhibitors for the enzyme
	Fusion inhibitors	Mutations in a crucial sequence of 10 amino acids within the *N*-terminal heptad repeat region of gp41
	Co-receptor antagonist	Point mutations in the V3 region of gp120 HIV viral strains with dual tropism (CCR5/CXCR4)
	Integrase inhibitors	Point mutations within the integrase gene
Herpes simplex virus	Acyclovir	Structural changes in the viral thymidine kinase enzyme
	Famciclovir (The prodrug of penciclovir)	
	Valacyclovir	Structural changes in the viral DNA polymerase
	Foscarnet	Structural changes in the viral DNA polymerase

[a]Reduced susceptibility to ceftriaxone and cefixime has been reported

[b]Reduced susceptibility to erythromycin and ciprofloxacin has been reported

ND not reported

common causes of STDs in both developed and developing countries. It affects neonates, adolescents, and adult populations, and the most common consequences found among infected individuals are infertility, ectopic pregnancy, blindness, and facilitation of human immunodeficiency virus (HIV) infection [110].

Numerous descriptions of STDs consistent with gonorrhea are present in old Chinese and Greek writings. Although several therapies were used, the actual treatment of gonococcal infections was only possible with the advent of antimicrobial therapy. The sulfonamides were used for this purpose in 1930 and since 1943 the use of penicillin was preferred.

The Centers for Disease Control and Prevention (CDC) currently recommend the use of third-generation cephalosporins (ceftriaxone and cefixime) as the first choice for the treatment of uncomplicated urogenital and anorectal gonorrheal infections [12]. For patients who cannot tolerate β-lactam drugs, spectinomycin (if available) is recommended as an alternative regimen [12]. If spectinomycin is not available and β-lactam desensitization is not an option, azithromycin may be considered for the treatment of uncomplicated gonococcal infections [12]. However, the use of macrolides should be restricted to prevent the emergence of antimicrobial resistance to this group of compounds. On the other hand, quinolones are no longer recommended for the management of such infections given the gradual increase in the prevalence of quinolone resistance in the USA and other countries [12]. Nevertheless, such antibiotics may be an alternative treatment option if antimicrobial susceptibility can be documented by culture and adherence to the treatment can be ensured.

In spite of available drug therapy, gonorrhea continues to be a public health problem in both developed and developing countries. This trend can be explained in part by the poor adherence to medications, the lack of proper counseling to sexual partners, and the gradual increase in the prevalence of antimicrobial resistance to the most common drugs, which limits their availability for the management of *N. gonorrhoae* infections. With this scenario, surveillance programs that monitor the trends of antimicrobial resistance in gonococci are of paramount importance worldwide.

49.2 Mechanisms of Resistance

49.2.1 *β-Lactam Antibiotics*

The bacterial cell wall is a vital structure and consists of a cross-linked polymer of polysaccharides and pentapeptides that mainly protects against the high osmotic pressures caused by the bacterial metabolism [104]. The β-lactam antibiotics are bactericidal inhibitors of the cell wall synthesis. They interact with membrane-bound proteins responsible for the polymerization of bacterial peptidoglycan (designated PBPs, for penicillin-binding proteins) resulting in the inhibition of the reactions of transpeptidation and transglycosylation that are necessary for the synthesis of the cell wall.

Resistance to this group of antibiotics in *N. gonorrhoeae* is mediated by several mechanisms: (1) the production of specific enzymes denominated β-lactamases, which disrupt the β-lactam ring; (2) alteration of the structure of the PBPs, leading to a decrease in the affinity of the antibiotic to its target; (3) reduction in the penetration of the antibiotic across the outer membrane by mutating specific porins, and (4) expulsion of the drug from the periplasmic space by the use of efflux pumps, which usually span the outer membrane.

The first reports of β-lactamase in *N. gonorrhoeae* were in 1976 from patients in Africa and the Far East [34, 92]. Later, the enzyme was also documented in the Americas and Europe [31, 57]. This β-lactamase (designated TEM-1) is found within a plasmid, which can be transferred to other strains of *N. gonorrhoeae* or other bacterial species [34, 65]. The enzyme has the ability to hydrolyze the amide bond of the β-lactam molecule and is able to inactivate benzylpenicillin, amino-penicillins (such as ampicillin), carboxypenicillins, ureidopenicillins, and narrow spectrum cephalosporins although it can be inhibited by clavulanic acid [58, 98, 103].

Additional to the β-lactamase enzyme, *N. gonorrhoeae* is capable of synthesizing PBPs with lower affinity for penicillins. Four specific genes that are involved in β-lactam resistance have been described and include the *penA* and *ponA* genes that encode altered forms of PBP2 and PBP1, respectively [40]. The *mtrR* locus encodes an efflux pump, which is part of the MtrC-MtrD-MtrE system. The operon encoding this efflux pump is highly regulated by a repressor protein, and mutations in the promoter region could lead to overexpression of the pump [40]

As indicated above, decreased cell permeability to β-lactam drugs can also influence the activity of these drugs. As an example, the *penB* gene encodes an outer membrane porin-denominated P1B, and mutations within the coding region of this gene have been associated with decreased production of this porin, which results in a reduction of the diffusion of penicillin across the outer membrane [50, 51, 88, 90, 100, 105].

49.2.2 Quinolones

The quinolones are inhibitors of the bacterial DNA synthesis, which results in bacterial cell death. This group of antibiotics interact with two members of the topoisomerase class of enzymes, DNA gyrase and topoisomerase IV, which are key enzymes involved in the synthesis of bacterial DNA [42]. The gyrase is a tetrameric enzyme composed of four subunits (two A and two B), encoded by the *gyrA* and *gyrB* genes, respectively. The action of the DNA gyrase results in relaxation of the supercoiled DNA, which is important for successful replication. The topoisomerase IV enzyme is also tetrameric, and it is composed of two subunits encoded by the *parC* and *parE* genes. This enzyme is responsible for separation of DNA strands during cell division [42].

Quinolone resistance in *N. gonorrhoae* is mediated by three mechanisms. The first (and most common) involves point mutations within the *gyrA* and *parC* genes resulting in conformational changes in the DNA gyrase and DNA topoisomerase IV enzymes. The amino acid changes reduce the affinity of quinolones to their target and prevent the binding of the drugs [47]. The most common *gyrA* mutations observed in *N. gonorrhoeae* are Ser91 and Asp95, which, alone or combined, can lead to an increase in the ciprofloxacin minimal inhibitory concentration (MIC) by 34- to 100-fold [72]. Mutations in the *parC* gene alone have not been associated with high level of resistance, but the presence of such mutations may contribute to increased MIC values [47].

The second mechanism of resistance to quinolones is characterized by a decrease in antibiotic uptake, which is usually due to overexpression of efflux pumps or to a decrease in the bacterial permeability. Overexpression of three types of efflux pumps has been associated with resistance to quinolones in *N. gonorrhoeae*, including the Mtr, FarA-FarB, and NorM systems [101, 102]. As occurs with β-lactams, the expression of these pumps is tightly regulated and specific mutations can change the level of expression dramatically [101].

49.3 Trends in Antimicrobial Resistance

Gonorrhea is one of the most common STD seen worldwide. It is estimated that 200 million cases occur every year. Furthermore, the numbers of cases of gonorrhea due to strains resistant to the most common antibiotics have sharply increased during the last years [42, 64]. Given the rise of this new threat and the necessity to improve and guide the empirical treatment, many countries have developed antimicrobial surveillance systems. Examples include the Gonococcal Antimicrobial Surveillance Program (GASP) in the Western Pacific region, the Gonococcal Isolate Surveillance Project in the USA, the Australian Gonococcal Surveillance Program (AGSP), and the Gonococcal Resistance to Antimicrobials Program (GRASP).

After its introduction, penicillin became one of the most effective therapies against *N. gonorrhoae*. However, during the mid-1980s, numerous outbreaks of high-level resistance to penicillin were reported in many areas of the USA and other countries [9, 97, 122]. Currently, the majority of the antimicrobial surveillance systems have reported a prevalence of resistance to penicillin of more than 90% in different regions of the world (the highest prevalence of resistance is found in the Western Pacific and Caribbean regions) [14, 30, 75, 125].

In this epidemiological context, antibiotics such as quinolones and cephalosporins emerged as new therapeutic options. Quinolones are oral antimicrobials, which used to have excellent activity against *N. gonorrhoae*. In 1993, the CDC recommended single dose of a fluoroquinolone for the treatment of gonococcal infections [15]. Unfortunately, the prevalence of fluoroquinolone resistance in *N. gonorrhoae* rapidly increased in many parts of Asia and the Pacific region [71, 110]. This phenomenon led the CDC in 2000 to not recommend the use of quinolones for the treatment of gonorrhea in patients who acquired these organisms in the Western Pacific region or Asia. After 2000, the trend of increased quinolone resistance continued. Resistance was initially documented among men who have sex with men (MSM) and among heterosexual males throughout the USA and other locations different from the Asia and Pacific regions. As a consequence, the CDC (2006) do not currently endorse the use of quinolones for the treatment of gonococcal infections and associated conditions such as pelvic inflammatory disease in any population [2, 11, 12, 30, 35, 64].

The increase in quinolone resistance has decreased dramatically the available therapeutic options. As stated above, broad spectrum cephalosporins are now recommended as the drugs of choice for the management of uncomplicated urogenital and anorectal gonorrhea [12]. True resistance to ceftriaxone or cefixime has not been reported yet in any surveillance system. However, a number of isolates with decreased susceptibility to ceftriaxone and cefixime have been described from the Pacific region and the United States [14, 21, 22, 30, 71, 120, 125]. Thus, local health departments must remain vigilant for the emergence of cephalosporin resistance in gonococci.

Spectinomycin is a safe alternative for the treatment of uncomplicated *N. gonorrhoae* infections with cure rates above 98% in the majority of series reported. The limitation is that the compound is not widely available. Resistance is limited, and has been occasionally reported in the Western pacific region and in some countries of South America [14, 30, 44].

49.4 Antimicrobial Resistance in *Treponema pallidum*

Syphilis is one of the oldest STD described in human history and continues to be a global health problem. Several strategies and compounds have been used through history for the treatment of syphilis, including hot baths, mercury, spartan diet, and salvarsan. The arsphenamine compound (salvarsan) was the most effective treatment since it reduced the severity of the disease and became the drug of choice until 1943 [49]. Penicillin was later discovered and the effectiveness against syphilis demonstrated and since then, penicillin became the drug of choice for the treatment of syphilis. According to the latest CDC STD guidelines [12], penicillin continues to be the first line of therapy for the management of any state of syphilis. Alternative regimens are considered only for allergic patients (except pregnant women, who should be desensitized and treated with penicillin) and include doxycycline, tetracycline, ceftriaxone, and azithromycin [12].

49.4.1 Penicillin Resistance

Possible treatment failures of syphilis after courses of penicillin have been reported since 1960, but no mechanism has been characterized [45, 48, 54, 112, 114]. Recently, a novel *T. pallidum* membrane-bound protein (designated Tp47) with the ability to bind and hydrolyze penicillin was characterized [16]. The protein does not share any homology at the amino acid level with previously described PBPs or β-lactamases [28] and its activity is restricted to the hydrolysis of penicillins, sparing the cephalosporins [16]. The level of β-lactamase activity is high and is regulated by feedback inhibition of the reaction product, which is likely to prevent the development of a fully penicillin-resistant phenotype [16]. The characterization of this mechanism indicated that the selection of mutants that may overcome product inhibition and therefore become fully resistant to penicillin is theoretically possible [16]. Adequate antimicrobial surveillance programs to evaluate *T. pallidum* susceptibility and treatment failures should be implemented to characterize the cases and determine the mechanism of resistance.

49.4.2 Macrolide Resistance

Macrolides such as erythromycin and azithromycin have been used for the treatment of syphilitic patients who are allergic to penicillin. In 1973, the first report of erythromycin failure in a pregnant woman who was treated with this antibiotic for 12 days was documented [38]. Despite serologic evidence of a response, she delivered an infant with congenital syphilis [38]. Subsequently, several reports of treatment failure appeared in the literature occurring among patients in different stages of syphilis [55, 108]. In 2002, several groups of patients who experienced azithromycin failure from both the United States and Ireland [10, 62, 73, 79, 128] were characterized. These individuals had a clinical picture suggestive of primary syphilis, indicating that they had acquired strains that were already resistant.

Macrolides are antibiotics that produce inhibition of bacterial protein synthesis. The 50 S subunit of the bacterial ribosome is the target of macrolides. This group of antibiotics inhibit the peptidyl-transferase moiety of the ribosome (composed of 23 S rRNA and proteins), thus blocking translation [23]. The mechanisms of resistance to macrolides in bacteria involve drug efflux, drug inactivation (usually by production of specific methyltransferases encoded by the *erm* genes), or alterations in the drug target site. In the case of *T. pallidum*, the resistance has been linked to spontaneous point mutations in specific nucleotides of the 23 S rRNA gene [107]. This structural change confers resistance to erythromycin and precludes the use of other types of macrolides such as azithromycin.

49.5 Antimicrobial Resistance in *Chlamydia trachomatis*

Chlamydia trachomatis is also an important and costly (more than 1 billion in medical cost) cause of STD. Although the clinical impact of *C. trachomatis* is widely recognized, information related to antimicrobial susceptibility and mechanism of resistance is limited, mainly due to the lack of appropriate and standardized methods for testing and reporting antimicrobial resistance [117]. Thus, the true incidence and prevalence of drug resistance and its clinical impact is not well known. The treatment of *C. trachomatis* is really affordable and the recommended regimen could include either of the following antibiotics: azithromycin, doxycycline, erythromycin, ofloxacin, or levofloxacin [12].

49.6 Mechanisms of Resistance

The majority of mechanisms of antibiotic resistance described in *C. trachomatis* have been characterized using *in vitro* models, although *in vivo* failures have been documented [7, 33, 66, 70, 84, 106]. In the case of quinolones, emergence of resistance has been observed after serial exposures to subinhibitory concentrations of these compounds [29, 82, 102]. A Ser83→Ile substitution in the *gyrA* gene with intact *gyrB, parC,* and *parE* genes has been observed in the quinolone-resistant strains studied [29, 82, 102].

Clinical isolates exhibiting resistance to macrolides have also been characterized [78]. The organisms were resistant *in vitro* to erythromycin, azithromycin, and josamycin. The mechanism of resistance involved mutations in the 23 S rRNA gene, which alters the binding site of the drugs [78].

49.7 Antimicrobial Resistance in *Haemophilus ducreyi*

H. ducreyi is the etiologic agent of chancroid, which is a clinical condition characterized by genital ulcers and regional lymphadenopathy. It is one of the most common etiologic agents of genital ulcers in developing countries. The presence of genital ulcers of any etiology is associated with increased risk of transmission of HIV [35]. The current recommended regimens for the treatment of chancroid include azithromycin ceftriaxone, ciprofloxacin, or erythromycin [12]. Structured antibiotic resistance surveillance programs for *H. ducreyi* are not available due to difficulties of organism isolation, identification, and problems related to the standardization of inoculum size for susceptibility testing [113]. It is therefore difficult to estimate the true incidence of resistance in *H. ducreyi*.

49.8 Mechanisms of Resistance

The first cases of penicillin resistance in *H. ducreyi* were reported in Canada [53]. The isolates exhibited an MIC of ≥ 128 μg/ml for penicillin and ampicillin, and the presence of the β-lactamase TEM-1 was documented [53]. Similar to the enzyme described in *N. gonorrhoae* (see above), the β-lactamase has the ability to hydrolyze benzylpenicillin, aminopenicillins, carboxypenicillins, ureidopenicillins, and narrow-spectrum cephalosporins [53]. Broad spectrum cephalosporins (such as ceftriaxone) remain stable and resistance to these compounds has not been yet documented.

Trimethoprim-sulfamethoxazole (TMS) was also used in the past for the treatment of chancroid. However, resistance to this antibiotic emerged mainly due to inappropriate and indiscriminate use. The antibacterial activity of TMS is due to the inhibition of bacterial folic acid synthesis. The first reaction of folic acid synthesis is characterized by the formation of dihydrofolic acid from *p*-aminobenzoic acid (PABA) and dihydropteroate diphosphate. This reaction is catalyzed by the dihydropteroate synthetase enzyme. Dihydrofolic acid is subsequently converted to tetrahydrofolate, which is the active form of folic acid, by the action of the dihydrofolate reductase enzyme. TMS inhibits both enzymes of the folic acid pathway. Resistance to this combination is due mainly to the presence of altered dihydropteroate synthetase and dihydrofolate reductase enzymes with reduced affinity for the antibiotics due to specific structural changes [41].

49.9 Antiretroviral Resistance in Human Immunodeficiency Virus (HIV)

HIV infection is one of the most important pandemic diseases of the 21st century. It is estimated that 40.3 million people live with HIV and more than 25 million deaths have occurred due to HIV since its emergence in the early 1980s [114]. Currently, there are 6 groups of antiretrovirals (ARV) approved for the treatment of HIV. Each group targets a specific step of the HIV life cycle (Fig. 49.1). The introduction of highly active antiretroviral therapy (HAART) (which includes the combination of three ARVs) has substantially reduced the severity of acute HIV infection and disease progression [89].

One of the main problems related to the treatment of HIV is the rapid emergence of resistance to several compounds. Resistance is constantly promoted due to: (1) suboptimal use of HAART regimens; (2) difficulties on patients' adherence and tolerability; (3) presence of high degree of polymorphism in circulating HIV strains and, (4) lack of an appropriate system for monitoring HAART failure. These factors have led to a gradual increase in the prevalence of ARV resistance in both developed and developing countries [5, 25, 43, 58, 59, 67, 87, 91, 99, 104].

Owing to this worrisome trend, the pipeline for new groups of ARVs runs full. The latest groups of approved compounds include integrase inhibitors, fusion inhibitors, and chemokine antagonists (Fig. 49.1) [27, 37, 39, 68, 93]. Therefore, HIV resistance is an expansive field, which changes rapidly and a comprehensive review of this topic is beyond the scope of this chapter. We focus on the main mechanisms of resistance associated with each ARV approved for HIV treatment and the reader is referred to other publications [13, 46, 111] for a more detailed review of this topic [11, 126, 127].

49.9.1 Resistance to Nucleoside and Nucleotide Analogues Reverse Transcriptase Inhibitors (NRTIs)

These groups of ARVs are competitive inhibitors of the natural deoxynucleotide triphosphates, and act by blocking the DNA polymerase function of the viral reverse transcriptase (RT) enzyme. Usually, the NRTIs are phosphorylated by cellular kinases from the host cell (the triphosphate forms of these drugs have high affinity for the HIV-1 RT), and compete with the natural enzymatic substrates. Subsequently, these compounds are incorporated into the growing DNA chain, promoting termination of replication due to the fact that they lack a 3′ hydroxyl group, which allows the formation of a phosphodiester bond with the incoming nucleotide [20].

The mechanism of resistance to this group of drugs is due to the presence of several mutations inside the RT (Table 49.2) that leads to an inability of the enzyme to incorporate the compounds to the nascent DNA chain, or to an increase in the excision of the nucleoside or nucleotide analogues from the viral nascent DNA [20]. The excision mechanism is characterized by an attack to the phosphodiester bond with ATP or pyrophosphate, resulting in a removal of the nucleoside/nucleotide analogue from the DNA, permitting the RT to progress with the incorporation of other nucleotides in the normal fashion [52, 118].

49.9.2 Resistance to Nonnucleoside Reverse Transcriptase Inhibitors (NNRTIs)

These types of drugs are noncompetitive inhibitors of RT. They bind to a site located near the catalytic site of the RT but different from the binding site of NRTIs. By interacting with the RT, they produce alterations in the catalytic activity of the enzyme, which eventually results in its inhibition. Conversely to NTRI, they do not need a phosphorylation step or intracellular processing to be activated and, therefore, they are very active against HIV-1 (but lack activity against HIV-2).

The mechanism of resistance is due to the presence of mutations located in the site of the interaction with RT (Table 49.2) [6, 36]. Usually, the presence of resistance to one NNRTI confers resistance to several other drugs from the same group. On the other hand, cross-resistance does not occur between NRTI and NNRTI. Additionally, it has been observed that strains of HIV, which harbor numerous NRTI mutations (e.g., M41L, L210W, and T215Y), may have increased susceptibility

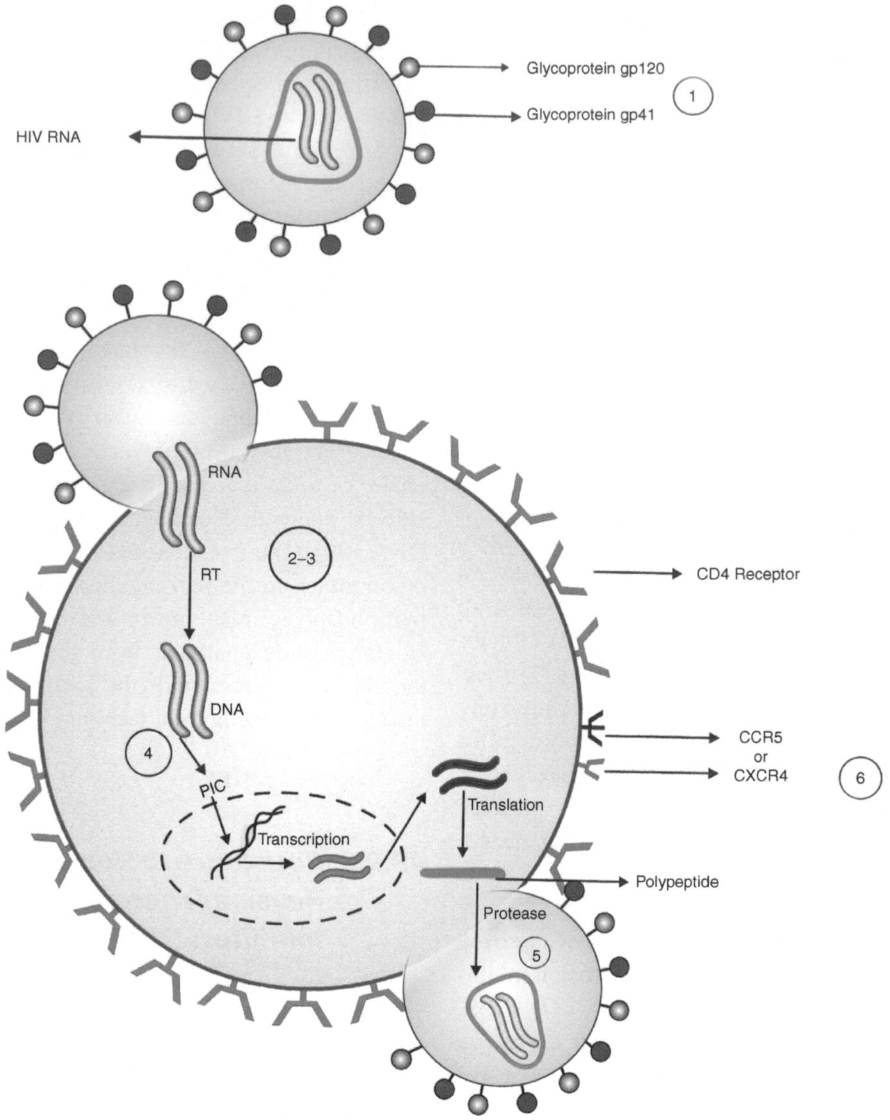

Fig. 49.1 *Schematic Representation of the HIV Cycle Infecting a Cell.* Circled numbers indicate steps inhibited by antiretroviral drugs. *1*, Fusion inhibitors block the entry of the HIV by altering the interaction of gp120 and gp41 with the CD4 receptor; *2* and *3*, nucleoside and nucleotide reverse transcriptase inhibitors (NRTIs) and nonnucleoside reverse transcriptase inhibitors (NNRTIs) interact with the reverse transcriptase enzyme; *4*, integrase inhibitors block the incorporation of viral cDNA into the host DNA; *5*, protease inhibitors alter the processing of new virions; *6*, Co-receptor antagonists block the entry of the HIV by interacting with the chemokine receptors CCR5 and CXCR4 on the surface of the eukaryotic cell (*PIC* Pre-integration complex, *RT* Reverse Transcriptase)

to the NNRTI, which could be useful in selected therapeutic situations [121].

Etravirine is a new NNRTI, which has high in vitro activity against wild-type and several NNRTI-resistant strains of HIV [1, 115]. Experienced patients treated with etravirine showed high rates of virological suppression and increased CD4 counts at week 24 of treatment [69, 95]. Resistance to this new ART drug is due to the presence of specific mutations within the RT. Mutations such as E138K, V197F, and Y181CIV are associated with high levels of resistance or with reduced clinical virology response [116, 118–120].

Table 49.2 Most common mutations involved in resistance of HIV among the different types of antiretroviral drugs

Mutations	Antiretroviral drug
Mutations conferring resistance to NRTIs[a]	
Thymidine analogue mutations (TAM)	
M41L, D67N, L210W, T215FY	Confers resistance to abacavir, didanosine, tenofovir, stavudine, and zidovudine
K70R, K219QE	Confers resistance to stavudine and zidovudine
Multi-NRTI mutations	
T69INS, Q151M, A62V	Confers resistance to abacavir, didanosine, tenofovir, stavudine, zidovudine, lamivudine, and emtricitabine
NRTI discriminatory mutation	
M184V	Confers resistance to lamivudine, emtricitabine, abacavir, and didanosine
Mutations conferring resistance to NNRTIs[b]	
A986G, L100I, K101EP, E138K, V179DEF,V181CIV, Y188LHC, M230L, F227C, G190E	Confers resistance to nevirapine, delavirdine, efavirenz, and etravirine
K103NS, V106AM, V1081, K238NT	Confers resistance to nevirapine, delavirdine, efavirenz
G190AS	Confers resistance to nevirapine, efavirenz, etravirine
P225H	Resistance to efavirenz
F227L	Confers resistance nevirapine
P236L	Confers resistance to delavirdine
E138K, V179F, Y181CIV, Y188L, G190SE, F227C	Confers high levels of resistance and/or clinical evidence of reduced virological response to etravirine
Mutations conferring resistance to protease inhibitors	
L90M, I84VAC	Confers resistance to atazanavir, darunavir, fosamprenavir, indinavir, lopinavir, nelfinavir, saquinavir, tipranavir
V82ATFS	Confers resistance to atazanavir, fosamprenavir, indinavir, lopinavir, and nelfinavir
I54VTALM	Confers resistance to atazanavir, fosamprenavir, indinavir, lopinavir, nelfinavir, saquinavir
G73ST	Confers resistance to atazanavir, darunavir, fosamprenavir, indinavir, nelfinavir, saquinavir
G48VM	Confers resistance to atazanavir, lopinavir, nelfinavir, saquinavir
M46L	Confers resistance to atazanavir, fosamprenavir, indinavir, lopinavir, nelfinavir, tipranavir
Mutations conferring resistance to fusion inhibitors	
G36DEVS, I37V, V38EAMG, Q40H, N42T, N43DKS, L44M, L45M	Confers resistance to enfuvirtide
Mutations conferring resistance to integrase inhibitors	
E92Q, F121Y, E138AK, G140AS, Q148HRK, N155H	Confers resistance to raltegravir
T66I, E92Q, F121Y, E138AK, G140AS, S147G, Q148HRK, S153Y, N155H, R263K	Confers resistance to elvitegravir

[a]*NRTIs* nucleoside and nucleotide analogues reverse transcriptase inhibitors
[b]*NNTRIs* nonnucleoside reverse transcriptase inhibitors

49.9.3 Resistance to Protease Inhibitors (PIs)

The HIV protease is a key enzyme involved in the posttranslational cleavage of viral structural proteins such as the Gag and Gag-Pol polyproteins, which encode the protein components of the viral core, the protease itself, the RT, and the integrase enzyme. The protease is important in the assembly of mature viral particles during the late stages of the HIV cycle (Fig. 49.1).

Resistance to PIs is mediated by the presence of different amino acid substitutions in the catalytic domain of the enzyme or in distant sites from the active site of the protease (Table 49.2) [24, 80]. These mutations produce changes in the quantity and nature of the points of contact between the enzyme and the PI, leading to a reduced affinity of the drug for the target enzyme [20].

49.9.4 Resistance to Fusion Inhibitors

HIV entry into the host cell is a crucial step in HIV infection and progression. This process is characterized by the interaction of a number of viral and host proteins. HIV harbors a glycoprotein complex designated gp160, which is formed by the gp120 (external glycoprotein) and gp41 (transmembrane glycoprotein) components. The entry process starts with the binding of gp120 to the cell surface via the CD4 receptor of the host cell (Fig. 49.1). The interaction with CD4 subsequently leads to conformational changes inside the gp120 protein. The structural change uncovers hidden contact sites that are capable of binding to additional receptors, which belong to the family of chemokine receptors (CCR5 or CXCR4). The gp120 protein has a high degree of genetic variability. Currently, five variable (V1–V5) and four constant (C1–C4) regions have been identified in gp120 [37]. The binding to either CCR5 or CXR4 is determined by the amino acid composition of the variable regions (particularly V1–V2 and V3 loops). Additionally, the HIV cell tropism is determined by the utilization of a specific chemokine receptor. Once the binding to the chemokine receptor has occurred, further conformational changes in gp120 are evidenced. The latter process is characterized by exposure of gp41, which eventually leads to fusion of the viral envelope to the host cell membrane and then, entry of the viral core into the cellular cytoplasm [37].

Enfuvirtide was the first HIV fusion inhibitor approved for use in the treatment-experienced patients [39, 83]. This antiviral is a synthetic peptide that mimics amino acids 127–162 of the protein. Enfuvirtide binds to and blocks the entry and infectivity of HIV [76]. The mechanism of resistance to this drug results from mutations in a crucial sequence of 10 amino acids within the *N*-terminal heptad repeat region of gp41 (Table 49.2) [60, 61].

49.9.5 Co-receptor Antagonist Resistance

As mentioned previously, the chemokine receptors (CCR5 and CXCR4) are crucial molecules that mediate HIV entry into the host cell and initiate the viral cycle (Fig. 49.1). During the first stages of the immune response against HIV, normal T cells secrete inhibitory chemokines such as MIP 1α (macrophage inflammatory protein 1α), MIP 1β (macrophage inflammatory protein 1 β), and RANTES (regulated on activation, normal T-cell expressed, and secreted) in order to control viral replication. However, when HIV has established a chronic infection process, the production of such chemokines partially arrests the HIV replication. Furthermore, it has documented that defects in CCR5 expression severely decrease acute HIV infection [37]. All these observations have led to the development of maraviroc, which is an antagonist of the CCR5 chemokine receptor and thus inhibits the entry of HIV into the host cell [37]. Other CCR5 inhibitors are currently under development (e.g., vicriviroc, aplaviroc, INCB9471, and PRO140) [37]. Antagonists of the CXCR4 receptor and inhibitors of other steps in the process of viral entry are also undergoing clinical development [37].

Resistance to this group of ARVs is mainly due to the presence of viral strains that have the ability to switch chemokine receptor preference. Normally, CCR5 tropism is commonly found during the early stages of the infection and persist during the course of the infection. In later stages of the disease, the HIV might evolve dual tropism (CCR5 and CXCR4 co-receptor tropism) or exclusive CXCR4 tropism [85, 123]. In naïve patients, ca. 12–19% have viral populations exhibiting dual tropism, and less than 1% of the patients are infected with CXCR4-tropic viruses [85, 125]. In contrast, 22–48% of treatment-experienced patients have dual viral populations, and 2–4% are infected with CXCR4-tropic viruses [8, 85, 125]. Thus, it is quite likely that during maraviroc treatment, selection of viral populations with the ability to use either dual or exclusive CXCR4 tropism may occur. Another less common mechanism includes the presence of mutations within the V3 region of gp120, which increases the affinity of gp120 for CCR5, a mechanism that is independent of drug binding to CCR5 [37, 96].

49.9.6 *Resistance to Integrase Inhibitors*

Integrase is also one of the key enzymes involved in the life cycle of HIV (Fig. 49.1). The main function of the integrase enzyme is to catalyze the insertion of the viral cDNA into the genome of infected cells. The integration of viral DNA to the host chromosome is divided into two sequential reactions. The first one is designated 3′-processing and is characterized by the cytosolic cleavage of a conserved di-nucleotide motif. This reaction produces 3′-hydroxyl DNA ends of the newly reverse-transcribed proviral cDNA and takes place in the cytoplasm of the CD4+ T cell [93]. The integrase enzyme remains linked to the viral cDNA and joins both ends of the viral DNA within an intracellular particle denominated pre-integration complex (PIC), which translocates to the nucleus (Fig. 49.1). During the second reaction, the integrase catalyzes the insertion of the viral genome into the host chromosome, linking the 3′-hydroxyl DNA ends to the 5′-DNA phosphate of a host chromosome [27, 93].

When the PIC structure is formed in the host cell, the integrase inhibitors bind to the catalytic site of the enzyme. The complex of drugs bound to the viral PIC particle enters the nucleus of the infected cell. However, the drugs actually inhibit the catalytic site of the enzyme and the integrase–viral DNA complex cannot be joined to the cellular DNA, blocking effectively the viral cycle [68].

A number of integrase inhibitors have been synthesized and studied in preclinical and clinical settings. Raltegravir and elvitegravir are two compounds that have progressed to full development. Raltegravir has recently been FDA approved for the treatment of multiresistant HIV infections [27]. However, there are a number of reports that highlight the emergence of resistance to this class of medications, which usually involves mutations in the integrase gene (Table 49.2) [56, 77].

49.10 Herpes Simplex Virus Resistance to Antiviral Drugs

Herpes simplex virus (HSV) infections are among the most common chronic viral infections. These viruses cause marked morbidity and mortality, including fatal disseminated infections in immunosuppressed patients [19, 32, 94]. The introduction of viral medications active against the HSVs has substantially improved the clinical management of these infections. The current CDC STD guidelines recommend the use of acyclovir, valacyclovir, and famciclovir (the prodrug of penciclovir) as the drugs of choice for the management of HSV infections [12]. As an alternative, foscarnet is available and it has been approved for the treatment of acyclovir-resistant mucocutaneous HSV infections [3, 81].

The extensive use of acyclovir has led to the emergence of viral strains resistant to this compound. Nonetheless, the prevalence of resistant strains does not seem to have increased dramatically since the first cases were reported in 1982 [2]. The highest rates of acyclovir resistance are found among immunocompromised individuals [3], including patients with hematological malignancies, bone marrow graft recipients, and patients with HIV [18, 26, 74, 86].

49.11 Mechanisms of Resistance

Acyclovir and penciclovir are nucleoside analogues of guanosine. In order to be active, the compounds undergo three sequential phosphorylation steps to yield the triphosphate form. The first phosphorylation step is completed by the viral thymidine kinase (TK) and is carried out within the infected cells. Subsequently, phosphorylations are completed by the host enzyme kinases. The final product competes with the natural nucleotide dGTP, leading to selective inhibition of the viral DNA polymerase, which results in an impaired ability to incorporate additional nucleotides. Foscarnet is a pyrophosphate analogue that directly inhibits herpes virus DNA polymerase without undergoing phosphorylation.

The mechanism of resistance to acyclovir is usually mediated by mutations in the viral TK, which may lead to two situations: (1) inability of the enzyme to recognize acyclovir as a substrate or, (2) complete elimination of TK activity (the most common mechanism reported) [81]. Alternatively, mutations in the DNA polymerase, (which alter the affinity of acyclovir triphosphate for the enzyme), can also lead to (1) alterations in the rate of incorporation of acyclovir-triphosphate and deoxyguanosine-triphosphate; (2) decreased incorporation of acyclovir-triphosphate into the growing DNA chain, and (3) polymerase instability, which results in decreased enzyme inactivation following incorporation of the acyclovir triphosphate [63, 81]. Mutations in the TK produce cross-resistance with other compounds including penciclovir, whereas mutations in the DNA polymerase are also associated with cross-resistance to foscarnet [4].

There is a biological cost for the virus when emergence of resistance occurs [3]. For instance, HSV strains that have complete elimination of TK activity are less neurovirulent and are also unable to undergo full reactivation from latency. Nonetheless, they can be responsible for extensive mucocutaneous disease among immunodeficient hosts [17].

49.12 Concluding Remarks

Antimicrobial resistance in STD pathogens is a widely disseminated phenomenon in the hospital and the community affecting dramatically the clinical outcome of a great number of individuals. One of the most dramatic examples of this trend is the continuous emergence of resistance in *N. gonorrhoae*. One of the most useful strategies to identify and control the emergence of resistance is the developing of structured surveillance programs that monitor and guide the use of antimicrobials in particular clinical settings. For instance, surveillance systems for *N. gonorrhoae* have immensely contributed in the control of the emergence of quinolone resistance and the management of such infections. Similarly, the creation and construction of antiretroviral databases for HIV has led to the development of better therapeutic combinations for naïve and experienced patients. However, surveillance programs are not available for all STD pathogens. Thus, the creation of these programs should be encouraged in both the developing and developed worlds.

Education and prevention programs for STD are also crucial to curtail and control the emergence and dissemination of multidrug-resistant strains. Thus, continuous interaction with patients and sexual partners (when feasible) is of paramount importance so as to improve treatment adherence, provide the most suitable management for each STD, and explain the long-term complications for such infections.

Microorganisms evolve continuously, and the clinician will always face important therapeutic challenges due to the molecular adaptation that STD pathogens undergo in a hostile environment such as the human body. It is important that all healthcare workers dealing with STD recognize that microbial evolution cannot be stopped, and all available resources should be directed toward delaying this process.

Take-Home Pearls

- One of the key factors in the decision-making process for the treatment of any STD is the understanding of the factors that influence the local epidemiology of sexually transmitted pathogens and the rates of resistance to common antimicrobial agents.
- *Neisseria gonorrhoae* isolates with decreased susceptibility to ceftriaxone and cefixime have been described in several areas of the world. Thus, clinicians and local health departments must remain vigilant for the emergence of cephalosporin resistance in gonococci.
- Quinolones should not be used for the treatment of gonococcal infections and associated conditions such as pelvic inflammatory disease, due to the high prevalence of resistance.
- Penicillin continues to be the first line of therapy for the management of any state of syphilis.
- Antiretroviral resistance in HIV continues to evolve and is mainly related to the lack of adherence to antiretroviral regimens. Clinicians treating HIV patients should make drug adherence a top priority among their patients.

> The extensive use of acyclovir has led to the emergence of HSV strains resistant to this compound and the highest rates of acyclovir resistance are found among immunocompromised individuals.
> Education and prevention programs for STDs that include continuous communication with patients and sexual partners are crucial in the management of these infections in order to prevent and control the emergence and dissemination of multidrug-resistant strains and avoid the long-term complications of STDs worldwide.

References

1. Andries, K., Azijn, H., Thielemans, T.: TMC125, a novel next-generation nonnucleoside reverse transcriptase inhibitor active against nonnucleoside reverse transcriptase inhibitor-resistant human immunodeficiency virus type 1. Antimicrob. Agents Chemother. **48**, 4680–4686 (2004)
2. Australian Gonococcal Surveillance Program: Annual report of the Australian Gonococcal Surveillance Programme, 2006. Commun. Dis. Intell. **31**, 180–184 (2007)
3. Bacon, T.H., Levin, M.J., Leary, J.J., et al.: Herpes simplex virus resistance to acyclovir and penciclovir after two decades of antiviral therapy. Clin. Microbiol. Rev. **16**, 114–128 (2003)
4. Blot, N., Schneider, P., Young, P., et al.: Treatment of acyclovir and foscarnet-resistant herpes simplex virus infection with cidofovir in a child after an unrelated bone marrow transplant. Bone Marrow Transplant. **26**, 903–905 (2000)
5. Booth, C.L., Garcia-Diaz, A.M., Youle, M.S., et al.: Prevalence and predictors of antiretroviral drug resistance in newly diagnosed HIV-1 infection. J. Antimicrob. Chemother. **59**, 517–524 (2007)
6. Boyer, P.L., Currens, M.J., McMahon, J.B., et al.: Analysis of nonnucleoside drug-resistant variants of human immunodeficiency virus type 1 reverse transcriptase. J. Virol. **67**, 2412–2420 (1993)
7. Bragina, E.Y., Gomberg, M.A., Dmitriev, G.A.: Electronmicroscopic evidence of persistent chlamydial infection following treatment. J. Eur. Acad. Dermatol. Venereol. **15**, 405–409 (2001)
8. Brumme, Z.L., Goodrich, J., Mayer, H.B., et al.: Molecular and clinical epidemiology of CXCR4-using HIV-1 in a large population of antiretroviral-naive individuals. J. Infect. Dis. **192**, 466–474 (2005)
9. Centers for Disease Control (CDC): Chromosomally mediated resistant *Neisseria gonorrhoae* – United States. MMWR Morb. Mortal Wkly. Rep. **33**, 408–410 (1984)
10. Centers for Disease Control and Prevention: Azithromycin treatment failures in syphilis infections – San Francisco, California, 2002–2003. MMWR Morb. Mortal Wkly. Rep. **53**, 197–198 (2004)
11. Centers for Disease Control and Prevention: Increases in fluoroquinolone-resistant Neisseria gonorrhoae among men who have sex with men–United States, 2003, and revised recommendations for gonorrhea treatment, 2004. MMWR Morb. Mortal Wkly. Rep. **53**, 335–338 (2004)
12. Centers for Disease Control and Prevention: Sexually transmitted diseases treatment guidelines, 2006. MMWR Morb. Mortal Wkly. Rep. **55**, 1–94 (2006)
13. Centers for Disease Control and Prevention: Investigation of a new diagnosis of multidrugresistant, dual-tropic HIV-1 infection – New York City, 2005. MMWR Morb. Mortal Wkly. Rep. **55**, 793–796 (2006)
14. Centers for Disease Control and Prevention. Sexually Transmitted Disease Surveillance 2005 Supplement, Gonococcal Isolate Surveillance Project (GISP) Annual Report 2005. Atlanta, GA: U.S. Department of Health and Human Services, Centers for Disease Control and Prevention, January 2007.
15. Centers for Disease Control and Prevention (1993) Sexually transmitted diseases treatment guidelines. MMWR 42 (No. RR-14).
16. Cha, J.Y., Ishiwata, A., Mobashery, S.: A novel beta-lactamase activity from a penicillin-binding protein of *Treponema pallidum* and why syphilis is still treatable with penicillin. J. Biol. Chem. **279**, 14917–14921 (2004)
17. Chatis, P.A., Crumpacker, C.S.: Resistance of herpesviruses to antiviral drugs. Antimicrob. Agents Chemother. **36**, 1589–1595 (1992)
18. Chen, Y., Scieux, C., Garrait, V., et al.: Resistant herpes simplex virus type 1 infection: an emerging concern after allogeneic stem cell transplantation. Clin. Infect. Dis. **31**, 927–935 (2000)
19. Christophers, J., Clayton, J., Craske, J., et al.: Survey of resistance of herpes simplex virus to acyclovir in northwest England. Antimicrob. Agents Chemother. **42**, 868–872 (1998)
20. Clavel, F., Hance, A.J.: HIV drug resistance. N Engl J. Med. **350**, 1023–1035 (2004)
21. Clendennen, T.E., Echeverria, P., Saengeur, S., et al.: Antibiotic susceptibility survey of *Neisseria gonorrhoae* in Thailand. Antimicrob. Agents Chemother. **36**, 1682–1688 (1992)
22. Clendennen, T.E., Hames, C.S., Kees, E.S., et al.: In vitro antibiotic susceptibility of *Neisseria gonorrhoae* isolates in the Philippines. Antimicrob. Agents Chemother. **36**, 277–281 (1992)
23. Cocito, C., Di Giambattista, M., Nyssen, E., Vannuffel, P.: Inhibition of protein synthesis by streptogramins and related antibiotics. J. Antimicrob. Chemother. **39**(Suppl A), 7–13 (1997)
24. Condra, J.H., Schleif, W.A., Blahy, O.M., et al.: In vivo emergence of HIV-1 variants resistant to multiple protease inhibitors. Nature **374**, 569–571 (1995)
25. Corvasce, S., Violin, M., Romano, L., et al.: Evidence of differential selection of HIV-1 variants carrying drug-resistant mutations in seroconverters. Antivir. Ther. **11**, 329–334 (2006)
26. Danve-Szatanek, C., Aymard, M., Thouvenot, D., et al.: Surveillance network for herpes simplex virus resistance to

antiviral drugs: 3-year follow-up. J. Clin. Microbiol. **42**, 242–249 (2004)
27. Dayam, R., Al-Mawsawi, L.Q., Neamati, N.: HIV-1 integrase inhibitors: an emerging clinical reality. Drugs R&D **8**, 155–168 (2007)
28. Deka, R.K., Machius, M., Norgard, M.V., Tomchick, D.R.: Crystal structure of the 47-kDa lipoprotein of *Treponema pallidum* reveals a novel penicillin-binding protein. J. Biol. Chem. **277**, 41857–41864 (2002)
29. Dessus-Babus, S., Bébéar, C.M., Charron, A., et al.: Sequencing of gyrase and topoisomerase IV quinolone-resistance-determining regions of *Chlamydia trachomatis* and characterization of quinolone-resistant mutants obtained in vitro. Antimicrob. Agents Chemother. **42**, 2474–2481 (2474)
30. Dillon, J.A., Ruben, M., Li, H., et al.: Challenges in the control of gonorrhea in South America and the Caribbean: monitoring the development of resistance to antibiotics. Sex. Transm. Dis. **33**, 87–95 (2006)
31. Dillon, J.R., Duck, P., Thomas, D.Y.: Molecular and phenotypic characterization of penicillinase-producing Neisseria gonorrhoae from Canadian sources. Antimicrob. Agents Chemother. **19**, 952–957 (1981)
32. Domingo Gordo, B., Luezas Morcuende, J.J., Vidal Fernández, P., et al.: Bilateral acute retinal necrosis due to herpes simplex virus in inmunocompetent people and acyclovir resistance. Arch. Soc. Esp. Oftalmol. **77**, 327–330 (2002)
33. Dreses-Werringloer, U., Padubrin, I., Köhler, L., et al.: Detection of nucleotide variability in rpoB in both rifampin-sensitive and rifampin-resistant strains of *Chlamydia trachomatis*. Antimicrob. Agents Chemother. **47**, 2316–2318 (2003)
34. Elwell, L.P., Roberts, M., Mayer, L.W., et al.: Plasmid-mediated beta-lactamase production in *Neisseria gonorrhoae*. Antimicrob. Agents Chemother. **11**, 528–533 (1977)
35. Erbelding, E., Quinn, T.C.: The impact of antimicrobial resistance on the treatment of sexually transmitted diseases. Infect. Dis. Clin. North Am. **11**, 889–903 (1997)
36. Esnouf, R.M., Ren, J., Hopkins, A.L., et al.: Unique features in the structure of the complex between HIV-1 reverse transcriptase and the bis(heteroaryl)piperazine (BHAP) U-90152 explain resistance mutations for this nonnucleoside inhibitor. Proc. Natl Acad. Sci. USA **94**, 3984–3989 (1997)
37. Esté, J.A., Telenti, A.: HIV entry inhibitors. Lancet **370**, 81–88 (2007)
38. Fenton, L.J., Light, I.J.: Congenital syphilis after maternal treatment with erythromycin. Obstet. Gynecol. **47**, 492–494 (1976)
39. Fletcher, C.V.: Enfuvirtide, a new drug for HIV infection. Lancet **361**, 1577–1578 (2003)
40. Folster, J.P., Shafer, W.M.: Regulation of mtrF expression in *Neisseria gonorrhoae* and its role in high-level antimicrobial resistance. J. Bacteriol. **187**, 3713–3720 (2005)
41. Foster, T.J.: Plasmid-determined resistance to antimicrobial drugs and toxic metal ions in bacteria. Microbiol. Rev. **47**, 361–409 (1983)
42. Forterre, P., Gribaldo, S., Gadelle, D., Serre, M.C.: Origin and evolution of DNA topoisomerases. Biochimie **89**, 427–446 (2007)
43. Fox, J.M., Fidler, S., Weber, J.: Resistance to HIV drugs in UK may be lower in some areas. BMJ **332**, 179–180 (2006)
44. Fox, K.K., Knapp, J.S.: Antimicrobial resistance in *Neisseria gonorrhoae*. Curr. Opin. Urol. **9**, 65–70 (1999)
45. Gager, W.E., Israel, C.W., Smith, J.L.: Presence of spirochaetes in paresis despite penicillin therapy. Br. J. Vener. Dis. **44**, 277–282 (1968)
46. Geretti, A.M.: Epidemiology of antiretroviral drug resistance in drug-naïve persons. Curr. Opin. Infect. Dis. **20**, 22–32 (2007)
47. Ghanem, K.G., Giles, J.A., Zenilman, J.M.: Fluoroquinolone-resistant *Neisseria gonorrhoae*: the inevitable epidemic. Infect. Dis. Clin. North Am. **19**, 351–365 (2005)
48. Giles, J.A., Falconio, J., Yuenger, J.D., et al.: Quinolone resistance-determining region mutations and por type of Neisseria gonorrhoae isolates: resistance surveillance and typing by molecular methodologies. J. Infect. Dis. **189**, 2085–2093 (2004)
49. Giles, A.J., Lawrence, A.G.: Treatment failure with penicillin in early syphilis. Br. J. Vener. Dis. **55**, 62–64 (1979)
50. Gill, M.J., Simjee, S., Al-Hattawi, K., et al.: Gonococcal resistance to beta-lactams and tetracycline involves mutation in loop 3 of the porin encoded at the penB locus. Antimicrob. Agents Chemother. **42**, 2799–2803 (1998)
51. Hagman, K.E., Pan, W., Spratt, B.G., et al.: Resistance of *Neisseria gonorrhoae* to antimicrobial hydrophobic agents is modulated by the mtrRCDE efflux system. Microbiology **141**, 611–622 (1995)
52. Hammer, S.M.: Nucleoside analogue reverse transcriptase inhibitor options: a re-examination of the class. Top. HIV Med. **14**, 140–143 (2006)
53. Hammond, G.W., Lian, C.J., Wilt, J.C., et al.: Antimicrobial susceptibility of *Haemophilus ducreyi*. Antimicrob. Agents Chemother. **13**, 608–612 (1978)
54. Hardy, J.B., Hardy, P.H., Oppenheimer, E.H., et al.: Failure of penicillin in a newborn with congenital syphilis. JAMA **212**, 1345–1349 (1970)
55. Hashisaki, P., Wertzberger, G.G., Conrad, G.L., et al.: Erythromycin failure in the treatment of syphilis in a pregnant woman. Sex. Transm. Dis. **10**, 36–38 (1983)
56. Hazuda, D.J., Miller, M.D., Nguyen, B.Y., et al.: Resistance to the HIV-integrase inhibitor raltegravir: analysis of protocol 005, a phase 2 study in patients with triple-class resistant HIV-1 infection. XVI International Drug Resistance Workshop. Antivir. Ther. **12**, S10 (2007)
57. Hermida, M., Roy, C., Baró, M.T., Reig, R., Tirado, M.: Characterization of penicillinase-producing strains of *Neisseria gonorrhoae*. Eur. J. Clin. Microbiol. Infect. Dis. **12**, 45–48 (1993)
58. Jacoby, G.A., Munoz-Price, L.S.: The new beta-lactamases. N Engl J. Med. **352**, 380–391 (2005)
59. Jayaraman, G.C., Archibald, C.P., Kim, J., et al.: A population-based approach to determine the prevalence of transmitted drug-resistant HIV among recent versus established HIV infections: results from the Canadian HIV strain and drug resistance surveillance program. J. Acquir. Immune Defic. Syndr. **42**, 86–90 (2006)
60. Johnson, V.A., Brun-Vezinet, F., Clotet, B., et al.: Update of the drug resistance mutations in HIV-1: Fall 2006. Top. HIV Med. **14**, 125–130 (2006)

61. Johnson, V.A., Brun-Vézinet, F., Clotet, B., et al.: Update of the drug resistance mutations in HIV-1: 2007. Top. HIV Med. **15**, 119–125 (2007)
62. Katz, K.A., Klausner, J.D.: Azithromycin resistance in *Treponema pallidum*. Curr. Opin. Infect. Dis. **21**, 83–91 (2008)
63. Kimberlin, D.W., Whitley, R.J.: Antiviral resistance: mechanisms, clinical significance, and future implications. J. Antimicrob. Chemother. **37**, 403–421 (1996)
64. Knapp, J.S., Ohye, R., Neal, S.W., et al.: Emerging in vitro resistance to quinolones in penicillinase-producing *Neisseria gonorrhoae* strains in Hawaii. Antimicrob. Agents Chemother. **38**, 2200–2203 (1994)
65. Knapp, J.S., Zenilman, J.M., Biddle, J.W., et al.: Frequency and distribution in the United States of strains of *Neisseria gonorrhoae* with plasmid-mediated, high-level resistance to tetracycline. J. Infect. Dis. **155**, 819–822 (1987)
66. Kutlin, A., Kohlhoff, S., Roblin, P., et al.: Emergence of resistance to rifampin and rifalazil in *Chlamydophila pneumoniae* and *Chlamydia trachomatis*. Antimicrob. Agents Chemother. **49**, 903–907 (2005)
67. Lapadula, G., Izzo, I., Gargiulo, F., et al.: Updated prevalence of genotypic resistance among HIV-1 positive patients naïve to antiretroviral therapy: a single center analysis. J. Med. Virol. **80**, 747–753 (2006)
68. Lataillade, M., Kozal, M.J.: The hunt for HIV-1 integrase inhibitors. AIDS Patient Care STDs **20**, 489–501 (2006)
69. Lazzarin, A., Campbell, T., Clotet, B., et al.: DUET-2 study group. Efficacy and safety of TMC125 (etravirine) in treatment-experienced HIV-1-infected patients in DUET-2: 24-week results from a randomised, double-blind, placebo-controlled trial. Lancet **370**, 39–48 (2007)
70. Lefèvre, J.C., Lépargneur, J.P.: Comparative in vitro susceptibility of a tetracycline-resistant Chlamydia trachomatis strain isolated in Toulouse (France). Sex. Transm. Dis. **25**, 350–352 (1998)
71. Guoming, L., Chen, Q., Wang, S.: Resistance of Neisseria gonorrhoae epidemic strains to antibiotics: report of resistant isolates and surveillance in Zhanjiang, China: 1998–1999. Sex. Transm. Dis. **27**, 115–118 (2000)
72. Lindback, E., Rahman, M., Jalal, S., et al.: Mutations in gyrA, gyrB, parC, and parE in quinolone-resistant strains of *Neisseria gonorrhoae*. APMIS **110**, 651–657 (2002)
73. Lukehart, S.A., Godornes, C., Molini, B.J., et al.: Macrolide resistance in *Treponema pallidum* in the United States and Ireland. N Engl J. Med. **351**, 154–158 (2004)
74. Malvy, D., Treilhaud, M., Bouée, S., et al.: A retrospective, case-control study of acyclovir resistance in herpes simplex virus. Clin. Infect. Dis. **41**, 320–326 (2005)
75. Martin, I.M., Hoffmann, S., Ison, C.A.: ESSTI Network. European Surveillance of Sexually Transmitted Infections (ESSTI): the first combined antimicrobial susceptibility data for *Neisseria gonorrhoae* in Western Europe. J. Antimicrob. Chemother. **58**, 587–593 (2006)
76. Matthews, T., Salgo, M., Greenberg, M., et al.: Enfuvirtide: the first therapy to inhibit the entry of HIV-1 into host CD4 lymphocytes. Nat. Rev. Drug Discovery **3**, 215–225 (2004)
77. McColl, D.J., Fransen, S., Gupta, S., et al.: Resistance and cross-resistance to first generation integrase inhibitors: insights from a phase 2 study of elvitegravir (GS-9137). XVI International Drug Resistance Workshop. Antivir. Ther. **538**(12), S11 (2007)
78. Misyurina, O.Y., Chipitsyna, E.V., Finashutina, Y.P., et al.: Mutations in a 23 S rRNA gene of *Chlamydia trachomatis* associated with resistance to macrolides. Antimicrob. Agents Chemother. **48**, 1347–1349 (2004)
79. Mitchell, S.J., Engelman, J., Kent, C.K., et al.: Azithromycin-resistant syphilis infection: San Francisco, California, 2000–2004. Clin. Infect. Dis. **42**, 337–345 (2006)
80. Molla, A., Korneyeva, M., Gao, Q., et al.: Ordered accumulation of mutations in HIV protease confers resistance to ritonavir. Nat. Med. **2**, 760–766 (1996)
81. Morfin, F., Thouvenot, D.: Herpes simplex virus resistance to antiviral drugs. J. Clin. Virol. **26**, 29–37 (2003)
82. Morrissey, I., Salman, H., Bakker, S., et al.: Serial passage of *Chlamydia* spp. in sub-inhibitory fluoroquinolone concentrations. J. Antimicrob. Chemother. **49**, 757–761 (2002)
83. Morse, C., Maldarelli, F.: Enfuvirtide antiviral activity despite rebound viremia and resistance mutations: fitness tampering or a case of persistent braking on entering? J. Infect. Dis. **195**, 318–321 (2007)
84. Mourad, A., Sweet, R.L., Sugg, N., et al.: Relative resistance to erythromycin in *Chlamydia trachomatis*. Antimicrob. Agents Chemother. **18**, 696–698 (1980)
85. Moyle, G.J., Wildfire, A., Mandalia, S., et al.: Epidemiology and predictive factors for chemokine receptor use in HIV-1 infection. J. Infect. Dis. **191**, 866–872 (2005)
86. Nugier, F., Colin, J.N., Aymard, M., et al.: Occurrence and characterization of acyclovir-resistant herpes simplex virus isolates: report on a two-year sensitivity screening survey. J. Med. Virol. **36**, 1–12 (1992)
87. Oette, M., Kaiser, R., Daumer, M., et al.: (2006) Primary HIV drug resistance and efficacy of first-line antiretroviral therapy guided by resistance testing. J. Acquir. Immune Defic. Syndr. **41**, 573–581 (2006)
88. Olesky, M., Hobbs, M., Nicholas, R.A.: Identification and analysis of amino acid mutations in porin IB that mediate intermediate-level resistance to penicillin and tetracycline in *Neisseria gonorrhoae*. Antimicrob. Agents Chemother. **46**, 2811–2820 (2002)
89. Panel on Antiretroviral Guidelines for Adult and Adolescents. Guidelines for the use of antiretroviral agents in HIV-1-infected adults and adolescents. Department of Health and Human Services. January 29, 2008; pp. 1–128.
90. Pan, W., Spratt, B.G.: Regulation of the permeability of the gonococcal cell envelope by the mtr system. Mol. Microbiol. **11**, 769–775 (1994)
91. Petroni, A., Deluchi, G., Pryluka, D., et al.: Update on primary HIV-1 resistance in Argentina: emergence of mutations conferring high-level resistance to nonnucleoside reverse transcriptase inhibitors in drug-naive patients. J. Acquir. Immune Defic. Syndr. **42**, 506–510 (2006)
92. Phillips, I.: Beta-lactamase-producing, penicillin-resistant gonococcus. Lancet **2**, 656–657 (1976)
93. Pommier, Y., Johnson, A.A., Marchand, C.: Integrase inhibitors to treat HIV/AIDS. Nat. Rev. Drug Discov. **4**, 236–248 (2005)
94. Pottage, J.C., Kessler, H.A.: Herpes simplex virus resistance to acyclovir: clinical relevance. Infect. Agents Dis. **4**, 115–124 (1995)

95. Poveda, E., Garrido, C., de Mendoza, C., et al.: Prevalence of etravirine (TMC-125) resistance mutations in HIV-infected patients with prior experience of non-nucleoside reverse transcriptase inhibitors. J. Antimicrob. Chemother. **60**, 1409–1410 (2007)
96. Pugach, P., Marozsan, A.J., Ketas, T.J., Landes, E.L., Moore, J.P., Kuhmann, S.E.: HIV-1 clones resistant to a small molecule CCR5 inhibitor use the inhibitor-bound form of CCR5 for entry. Virology **361**, 212–228 (2007)
97. Rice, R.J., Biddle, J.W., JeanLouis, Y.A., DeWitt, W.E., Blount, J.H., Morse, S.A.: Chromosomally mediated resistance in *Neisseria gonorrhoae* in the United States: results of surveillance and reporting, 1983–1984. J. Infect. Dis. **153**, 340–345 (1986)
98. Roberts, M.C.: Plasmids of *Neisseria gonorrhoae* and other *Neisseria* species. Clin. Microbiol. Rev. **2**(Suppl), S18–S23 (1989)
99. Rodrigues, R., Scherer, L.C., Oliveira, C.M., et al.: Low prevalence of primary antiretroviral resistance mutations and predominance of HIV-1 clade C at polymerase gene in newly diagnosed individuals from south Brazil. Virus Res. **116**, 201–207 (2006)
100. Ropp, P.A., Hu, M., Olesky, M., et al.: Mutations in ponA, the gene encoding penicillin-binding protein 1, and a novel locus, penC, are required for high-level chromosomally mediated penicillin resistance in *Neisseria gonorrhoae*. Antimicrob. Agents Chemother. **46**, 769–777 (2002)
101. Rouquette-Loughlin, C., Dunham, S.A., Kuhn, M., Balthazar, J.T., Shafer, W.M.: The NorM efflux pump of *Neisseria gonorrhoae* and *Neisseria meningitidis* recognizes antimicrobial cationic compounds. J. Bacteriol. **185**, 1101–1106 (2003)
102. Rupp, J., Solbach, W., Gieffers, J.: Variation in the mutation frequency determining quinolone resistance in *Chlamydia trachomatis* serovars L2 and D. J. Antimicrob. Chemother. **61**, 91–94 (2008)
103. Samaha-Kfoury, J.N., Araj, G.F.: Recent developments in beta lactamases and extended spectrum beta lactamases. BMJ **327**, 1209–1213 (2003)
104. Scheffers, D.J., Pinho, M.G.: Bacterial cell wall synthesis: new insights from localization studies. Microbiol. Mol. Biol. Rev. **69**, 585–607 (2005)
105. Shet, A., Berry, L., Mohri, H., et al.: Tracking the prevalence of transmitted antiretroviral drug-resistant HIV-1: a decade of experience. J. Acquir. Immune Defic. Syndr. **41**, 439–446 (2006)
106. Somani, J., Bhullar, V.B., Workowski, K.A., et al.: Multiple drug-resistant *Chlamydia trachomatis* associated with clinical treatment failure. J. Infect. Dis. **181**, 1421–1427 (2000)
107. Stamm, L.V., Bergen, H.L.: A point mutation associated with bacterial macrolide resistance is present in both 23 S rRNA genes of an erythromycin-resistant *Treponema pallidum* clinical isolate. Antimicrob. Agents Chemother. **44**, 806–807 (2000)
108. Stürmer, M., Staszewski, S., Doerr, H.W.: Quadruple nucleoside therapy with zidovudine, lamivudine, abacavir and tenofovir in the treatment of HIV. Antivir. Ther. **12**, 695–703 (2007)
109. Sukasem, C., Churdboonchart, V., Sukeepaisarncharoen, W., Piroj, W., Inwisai, T., Tiensuwan, M., Chantratita, W.: Genotypic resistance profiles in antiretroviral-naive HIV-1 infections before and after initiation of first-line HAART: impact of polymorphism on resistance to therapy. Int. J. Antimicrob. Agents **1**, 277–281 (2008)
110. Tapsall, J.W.: Antibiotic resistance in *Neisseria gonorrhoae*. Clin. Infect. Dis. Suppl. **4**, S263–S268 (2005)
111. Taylor, B.S., Sobieszczyk, M.E., McCutchan, F.E., Hammer, S.M.: The challenge of HIV-1 subtype diversity. N Engl J. Med. **358**, 1590–1602 (2008)
112. Tramont, E.C.: Persistence of Treponema pallidum following penicillin G therapy. Report of two cases. JAMA **236**, 2206–2207 (1976)
113. Trees, D.L., Morse, S.A.: Chancroid and Haemophilus ducreyi: an update. Clin. Microbiol. Rev. **8**, 357–375 (1995)
114. UNAIDS. Global overview. In: UNAIDS (2007) AIDS Epidemic Update December 2007. WHO Library Cataloguing-in-Publication Data.
115. Vingerhoets, J., Azijn, H., Fransen, E., et al.: TMC125 displays a high genetic barrier to the development of resistance: evidence from in vitro selection experiments. J. Virol. **79**, 12773–12782 (2005)
116. Vingerhoets, J., Buelens, A., Peeters, M., et al.: Impact of baseline mutations on the virological response to TMC125 in the phase III clinical trials DUET-1 and DUET-2 [abstract]. HIVDRW (2007)
117. Vingerhoets, J., Janssen, K., Welkenhuysen-Gybels, J., et al.: Impact of baseline K103N or Y181C on the virological response to the NNRTI TMC125: analysis of study TMC125-C223 [abstract]. HIVDRW (2006)
118. Vivet-Boudou, V., Didierjean, J., Isel, C., et al.: Nucleoside and nucleotide inhibitors of HIV-1 replication. Cell. Mol. Life Sci. **63**, 163–186 (2006)
119. Wang, S.A., Lee, M.V., O'Connor, N., et al.: Multidrug-resistant *Neisseria gonorrhoae* with decreased susceptibility to cefixime – Hawaii, 2001. Clin. Infect. Dis. **37**, 849–852 (2003)
120. Wang, S.A., Papp, J.R., Stamm, W.E., et al.: Evaluation of antimicrobial resistance and treatment failures for *Chlamydia trachomatis*: a meeting report. J. Infect. Dis. **191**, 917–923 (2005)
121. Whitcomb, J.M., Huang, W., Limoli, K., et al.: Hypersusceptibility to non-nucleoside reverse transcriptase inhibitors in HIV-1: Clinical, phenotypic and genotypic correlates. AIDS **16**, F41–F47 (2002)
122. Whittington, W.L., Knapp, J.S.: Trends in resistance of *Neisseria gonorrhoae* to antimicrobial agents in the United States. Sex. Transm. Dis. **15**, 202–210 (1988)
123. Wilkin, T.J., Su, Z., Kuritzkes, D.R., et al.: HIV type 1 chemokine coreceptor use among antiretroviral-experienced patients screened for a clinical trial of a CCR5 inhibitor: AIDS Clinical Trial Group A5211. Clin. Infect. Dis. **44**, 591–595 (2007)
124. Wittek, M., Stürmer, M., Doerr, H.W., Berger, A.: Molecular assays for monitoring HIV infection and antiretroviral therapy. Expert Rev. Mol. Diagn. **7**, 237–246 (2007)
125. WHO Western Pacific Gonococcal Antimicrobial Surveillance Programme: Surveillance of antibiotic resistance in

Neisseria gonorrhoae in the WHO Western Pacific Region, 2005. Commun. Dis. Intell. **30**, 430–433 (2006)
126. World Health Organization: Global prevalence and incidence of selected curable sexually transmitted infections; overview and estimates. World Health Organization, Geneva (2001)
127. Yerly, S., von Wyl, V., Ledergerber, B., et al.: Transmission of HIV-1 drug resistance in Switzerland: a 10-year molecular epidemiology survey. AIDS **21**, 2223–2229 (2007)
128. Zhou, P., Qian, Y., Xu, J., et al.: Occurrence of congenital syphilis after maternal treatment with azithromycin during pregnancy. Sex. Transm. Dis. **34**, 472–474 (2007)

Part IX

Prevention and Vaccines

50 Viral Hepatitis Vaccines

Melissa L. Diamantis and Stephen K. Tyring

Core Messages

- HAV and HBV are prevalent worldwide, cause significant morbidity and mortality, and are vaccine-preventable.
- Current recommendations advocate vaccination of non-immune adults at risk of exposure, including travelers to HAV or HBV endemic areas, individuals with high risk of contracting a sexually-transmitted infection, illegal drug users, and healthcare workers.
- All infants at birth should receive a HBV vaccine, and all children at age 1 year should receive a HAV vaccine.
- HAV is transmitted via the fecal-oral route and causes acute hepatitis that generally resolves in 4-6 weeks.
- HBV is bloodborne pathogen and is a major cause of liver failure, liver cancer, and cirrhosis, with 367 million chronic carriers of HBV worldwide; the most common exposures include sexual risk factors and IV drug use.
- HCV is a blood-borne pathogen. Sexual transmission of HCV is possible but inefficient.
- No vaccine or immunoglobulin is currently available against HCV. Potential HCV vaccine candidates include recombinant proteins, recombinant viruses, DNA constructs, synthetic peptides, and virus like particles; in particular, HCV envelope glycoprotein E1.
- In phase II clinical trials, a recombinant hepatitis E virus vaccine has proven safe and highly efficacious in prevention of HEV infection in a high-risk population in Nepal.

50.1 Hepatitis A

50.1.1 Epidemiology and Transmission

Hepatitis A virus (HAV) is the most common cause of viral hepatitis worldwide, with approximately 30% of acute viral hepatitis in the USA caused by HAV. HAV is transmitted by the fecal–oral route, by person-to-person contact, and through contamination of food and water. Blood-borne transmission is uncommon, and transmission through saliva has not been demonstrated. The fecal–oral route is the primary means of HAV infection in the USA, with the majority of cases among men who have sex with men (MSM), persons who use illegal drugs, and international travelers [1]. Vaccination for hepatitis A is the most effective means of preventing HAV transmission among persons at risk for infection.

Since the hepatitis A vaccine became available in 1995, hepatitis A became a disease that is vaccine-preventable. Since implementation of recommendations for routine HAV vaccination in 1999, HAV infection has declined sharply to the lowest rate ever recorded [2]. During 1995–2006, hepatitis A incidence declined 90% to a rate of 1.2 cases per 100,000 [3]. HAV mortality rates have also declined over the past decade [4]. Hospitalizations, ambulatory visits, and their associated expenditures due to hepatitis A disease have declined substantially across the USA, with greater

M.L. Diamantis (✉) and S.K. Tyring
Department of Dermatology,
The University of Texas Medical School at Houston,
6655 Travis, Suite 120, Houston, TX 77030-1312, USA
e-mail: melissa.l.diamantis@uth.tmc.edu;
stephen.k.tyring@uth.tmc.edu

G. Gross and S.K. Tyring (eds.), *Sexually Transmitted Infections and Sexually Transmitted Diseases*,
DOI: 10.1007/978-3-642-14663-3_50,

declines seen in the 17 states that followed vaccination recommendations for HAV [5]. The expansion in 2006 of recommendations for routine HAV vaccination to include all children in the USA aged 12–23 months is expected to reduce hepatitis A rates further [6].

50.1.2 Clinical Course

Greatest infectivity is 2 weeks before onset of clinical illness with fecal shedding that continues for 2 to 3 weeks after onset of symptoms. HAV has an incubation period of about 28 days with a 15–50 day range. Symptoms vary from mild illness to fulminant hepatic failure and are largely dependent on age. Children and young adults typically have subclinical infection, whereas older children and adults are typically symptomatic, with jaundice occurring in >70% of patients [7]. HAV infection typically has an abrupt onset and common symptoms include malaise, fatigue, myalgias, arthralgias, headache, abdominal discomfort, nausea, vomiting, anorexia, fever, dark urine, and pruritus. Physical examination reveals jaundice, hepatomegaly, and, in rare cases, lymphadenopathy, splenomegaly, or rash.

50.1.3 Diagnosis

The diagnosis of an acute HAV infection is made by the identification of IgM anti-HAV antibodies. During the recovery or immunity phase, patients have IgG anti-HAV antibodies. Infection with HAV does not result in chronic hepatitis: the illness duration is usually less than 2 months with almost all cases of acute HAV hepatitis resolving in 4–6 weeks. Acute liver failure is relatively rare with an overall case-fatality rate of 0.3%; however, the rate is 1.8% among adults older than 50 years of age [6].

50.1.4 Prevention

Both a HAV vaccine and immunoglobulin (Ig) can be administered for prevention of HAV infection. The HAV vaccine was initially approved for persons aged ≥2 years, but in 2005, the vaccine became approved for children aged ≥12 months. All children should receive a hepatitis A vaccine at age 1 year [6]. Three inactivated vaccines are available for the prevention of HAV. Two single antigen HAV vaccines include HAVRIX (GlaxoSmithKline Biologicals) and VAQTA (Merck & Co., Inc.). A combination vaccine, TWINRIX (GlaxoSmithKline Biologicals), contains both HAV and hepatitis B virus (HBV) antigens. The vaccine should be administered intramuscularly (IM) into the deltoid muscle with a two-dose schedule for the single antigen vaccines and a three-dose schedule for the combined vaccine. Table 50.1 lists the dosing regimen for the three vaccines.

The HAV vaccine should be given to all high-risk groups that include travelers to endemic areas, MSM, users of injection (IV) and noninjection drugs, persons with clotting-factor disorders, persons with chronic liver disease, and persons with high occupational risk for infection (research personnel working with HAV or HAV-infected primates). In the USA, vaccination for HAV should occur in children residing in areas where the incidence of hepatitis A is twice the national average and people living in communities with local outbreaks of HAV [6].

Table 50.1 Hepatitis A single antigen and combined vaccine dosing and schedule [6]

Vaccine	Age (years)	Dose	Volume (mL)	Dose schedule (months)[a]
HAVRIX	1–18	720 (EL.U.[b])	0.5	0, 6–12
	≥18	1,440 (EL.U.)	1.0	
VAQTA	1–18	25 Units	0.5	0, 6–18
	≥18	50 Units	1.0	
TWINRIX	≥18	720 (EL.U.)/20 mcg	1.0	0, 1, 6

[a]0 months represents timing of initial dose; subsequent numbers represent months after initial dose

[b]Enzyme-linked immunosorbent assay units

Persons with liver transplants or awaiting liver transplants should be vaccinated. The safety of the HAV vaccine has not been determined in pregnancy; however, because the vaccine is formalin-inactivated, the theoretic risk to the developing fetus is expected to be low [6]. Simultaneous administration with other vaccines does not decrease the immune response or increase the frequency of adverse effects [8–10]. No major adverse side effects exist, and the most commonly reported local reaction was tenderness at the injection site [11].

Antibody production in response to HAV infection results in lifelong immunity to HAV. A recent review concluded that protective levels of anti-HAV antibodies could be present for at least 25 years in adults and for at least 14–20 years in children, according to estimates of antibody persistence derived from mathematical models. A hepatitis A booster vaccination is, therefore, not necessary in fully vaccinated individuals [12, 13].

Vaccination should be initiated at least 4 weeks before travel to an endemic area. A single-antigen hepatitis A vaccine will often have detectable anti-HAV antibodies by 2 weeks after the first vaccine dose. By 1 month after the first dose, 94–100% of adults have protective antibody levels, and 100% of adults develop protective antibody levels after the second dose [6]. There is no data regarding risk of HAV among persons vaccinated 2–4 weeks before departure; therefore, persons traveling to an endemic area in less than 4 weeks may require immediate protection with immunoglobulin 0.02 mL/kg IM as well as the first dose of HAV vaccine. These injections should be given at different anatomic sites. Travelers who are allergic to a vaccine component or who elect not to undergo vaccination should receive a single dose of Ig 0.02 mL/kg IM if the desired duration of protection is up to 3 months or 0.06 mL/kg IM if the desired duration is 2–5 months. The dose should be repeated if travel exceeds 5 months [6].

50.1.5 Postexposure Prophylaxis and Treatment

Immunoglobulin (0.02 mL/kg IM) should be given as soon as possible (i.e., within 2 weeks of last exposure) to unvaccinated individuals. Efficacy when administered greater than 2 weeks after exposure has not been established. Persons who have been administered 1 dose of HAV vaccine ≥1 month before exposure to HAV do not need Ig. Household and sexual contacts and persons who have shared illegal drugs with a person who has serologically confirmed HAV by IgM anti-HAV testing should receive Ig and the first dose of vaccine at different anatomic sites. The hepatitis A vaccine is not licensed to be used as postexposure prophylaxis; more studies need to be completed before the vaccine can be recommended in this setting. If a food handler receives a diagnosis of HAV, Ig should be given to other food handlers in the same establishment and to patrons who can be identified ≤2 weeks after the exposure. Ig should be administered to all previously unvaccinated staff and attendees of daycare centers if one or more cases of HAV are recognized in children or cases are recognized in two or more households of center attendees [6].

50.2 Hepatitis B

50.2.1 Epidemiology

Hepatitis B virus infections are a major cause of liver failure, liver cancer, and cirrhosis. Worldwide, there are 367 million chronic carriers of HBV and an estimated 620,000 to 1 million deaths per year from both chronic infection-related cirrhosis and acute hepatitis B infection [13–15]. In Western countries, the disease is relatively rare and acquired primarily in adulthood, whereas in Asia and most of Africa, chronic HBV infection is common and usually acquired perinatally or in childhood [16]. In 2006, a total of 4,713 acute cases of hepatitis B were reported nationwide with an overall incidence of 1.6 cases per 100,000 population, which was the lowest ever recorded and represents a decline of 81% since 1990 [3]. There continues to be higher rates of hepatitis B among adults, particularly males aged 25–44 years, reflecting the need to vaccinate adults at risk for HBV infection, e.g., MSM, IV drug users, persons with multiple sexual partners, and persons whose sex partners are infected with HBV [3].

High risk groups for HBV infection include individuals with history of multiple blood transfusions, patients on hemodialysis, healthcare workers, IV drug users, household and heterosexual contacts of HBV carriers, MSM, residents and employees of residential care facilities, travelers to hyperendemic regions, and natives of Alaska, Asia, and the Pacific Islands. Since 2001, the proportion of persons who reported either sexual or IV drug use as sources of HBV infection has increased gradually, whereas other sources of transmission have declined, including hemodialysis (0.2%), blood transfusion (0.6%), and occupational exposure to blood (0.5%) [3]. When information regarding exposures during the incubation period was available, approximately one third reported at least one sexual risk factor: 8%, sexual contact with a person known to have hepatitis B; 34%, multiple sexual partners; and 15%, MSM. Injection drug use was reported for 16% of persons [3]. One study found that a national program for routine HBV vaccination of adults at STD clinics would be cost-saving to society, with a net economic savings of approximately $526 million [17].

50.2.2 Mode of Transmission

HBV is transmitted through perinatal transmission, sexual contact, and parenteral exposure to blood via needlestick injury, IV drug use, or transfusion. Person-to-person transmission of HBV can also occur in the setting of nonsexual interpersonal contacts over an extended period, such as household contacts. The highest concentrations of virus are found in the blood; however, semen and saliva also have been demonstrated to be infectious [14]. HBV is transmitted efficiently by sexual contact among heterosexuals and MSM. Risk factors associated with sexual transmission among adolescents and young adults are unprotected sex with an infected partner, unprotected sex with multiple partners, MSM, history of another STD, anal intercourse, and illegal IV drug use [3, 18–20]. Approximately 79% of newly acquired cases of hepatitis B are associated with high-risk sexual activity or IV drug use [3].

50.2.3 Diagnosis

Serologic testing is required for the diagnosis of acute or chronic HBV infection. The presence of IgM antibody to hepatitis B core antigen (IgM anti-HBc antibody) is diagnostic of acute or recently acquired HBV infection. Anti-HBsAg is produced after a resolved infection and is the only antibody marker present after immunization. Chronic HBV infection is indicated by the persistence of HBsAg or HBV DNA for at least 6 months and anti-HBc with a negative test for IgM anti-HBc antibody. Serologic testing for HBsAg is the primary way to identify persons with chronic HBV infection.

Routine testing for HBsAg is recommended for pregnant women, infants born to HBsAg-positive mothers, household contacts and sexual partners of HBV-infected persons, persons born in countries with HBsAg prevalence ≥8%, HIV-infected individuals, and persons exposed to blood that warrant postexposure prophylaxis (i.e., needlestick injury and sexual assault). In 2008, the CDC expanded its recommendations to include routine HBsAg testing for populations with HBsAg prevalence of ≥2%, persons born in geographic regions with HBsAg prevalence of ≥2%, MSM, injection drug users, persons receiving immunosuppressive therapy, and persons with liver disease of unknown etiology [21].

50.2.4 Clinical Course

Acute hepatitis B infection can be self-limited with elimination of the virus or can result in chronic infection. Incubation period for HBV infection ranges from 6 weeks to 6 months, with illness that typically manifests 2–3 months after HBV exposure. Acute infection may be asymptomatic, especially in infants, young children, and immunosuppressed patients. Approximately 30–50% of persons aged >5 years have clinical symptoms of acute illness. Acute illness typically lasts 2–4 months and symptoms include malaise, fatigue, headache, abdominal pain, nausea, vomiting, anorexia, fever, jaundice, dark urine, and pruritus. Clinical signs include jaundice, liver tenderness, and possibly hepatosplenomegaly [21]. The case-fatality rate of acute hepatitis B infection is approximately 1%.

Chronic HBV infection encompasses a spectrum of disease ranging from asymptomatic to chronic hepatitis to cirrhosis to liver cancer. The risk of progression to chronic infection is related inversely to age at the time of infection. HBV infection becomes chronic in 90% of infants, up to 50% of children aged 1–5 years, and <5%

of older children and adults [22]. HIV-infected patients and patients on hemodialysis are at an increased risk for chronic infection [23, 24]. Chronic HBV infection runs an indolent course until the onset of cirrhosis or end-stage liver disease later in life [21]. In patients with chronic HBV, 30% progress to cirrhosis and 5–10% progress to hepatocellular carcinoma with or without preceding cirrhosis. Persons with histologic evidence of hepatic inflammation or fibrosis are at higher risk for hepatocellular carcinoma than HBV-infected persons without such evidence [25]. Potential extra-hepatic manifestations of HBV include palpable purpura, arthritis, glomerulonephritis, polyarteritis nodosa, cryoglobulinemia, papular acrodermatitis, serum-sickness like "arthritis-dermatitis," idiopathic thrombocytopenic purpura, lichen planus, Mooren's corneal ulcer, Sjogren's syndrome, porphyria cutanea tarda, and necrotizing cutaneous vasculitis [26, 27]. Approximately 0.5% of patients with chronic HBV infection have spontaneous resolution of infection annually [22].

50.2.5 Prevention

Two single-antigen HBV vaccines are available: Recombivax HB (Merck & Co., Inc.) and Engerix-B (GlaxoSmithKline Biologicals). Three combination vaccines are available: Twinrix (GlaxoSmithKline Biologicals), Comvax (Merck & Co., Inc.), and Pediarix (GlaxoSmithKline Biologicals). The latter two are used for vaccination of infants and young children. Twinrix contains recombinant HBsAg and inactivated hepatitis A virus. Comvax contains recombinant HBsAg and *Haemophilus influenzae* type b polyribosylribitol phosphate conjugated to *Neisseria meningitidis* outer membrane protein complex. Pediarix contains recombinant HBsAg, DTaP (diphtheria and tetanus toxoids and acellular pertussis adsorbed), and inactivated poliovirus [28]. The recommended HBV dose varies by product and age of recipient as seen in Tables 50.2 and 50.3.

HBV vaccine should be considered for everyone, particularly individuals with a history of multiple blood transfusions, patients on hemodialysis, patients with chronic liver disease, healthcare workers, household and heterosexual contacts of HBV carriers, IV drug users, MSM, HIV-infected individuals, persons seeking treatment in STD clinics, residents and employees of residential care facilities, international travelers to hyperendemic regions, and natives of Alaska, Asia, and the Pacific Islands.

Vaccination consists of at least 3 intramuscular doses of HBV vaccine administered at 0, 1, and 6 months. See Tables 50.2 and 50.3 for recommended doses. The HBV vaccine produces a protective antibody response in 30–55% of healthy adults aged ≤40 years after the first dose, 75% after the second dose, and >90% after the third dose [29, 30]. Vaccine-induced immune memory has been demonstrated to persist for at least 15 20 years. Even when anti-HBs concentrations decline to < 10 mIU/mL, nearly all vaccinated individuals remain protected against HBV infection due to the preservation of immune memory through selective expansion and differentiation of clones of HBsAg-specific memory B and T lymphocytes [31, 32]. Long-term protection has been demonstrated by rapid development of anamnestic antibody response in 5–7 days among vaccines who no longer have detectable anti-HBs. Accumulated data from a large number of studies indicate that, despite antibody decline or loss, immune memory exhibits long-term persistence [13]. Based on current data, in general, there is no necessity for booster doses for fully vaccinated immunocompetent individuals [13]. Booster doses, higher doses, or revaccination can be considered when anti-HBs levels decline to <10 mIU/mL on annual testing to elicit

Table 50.2 HBV vaccines for adults: recommended doses and schedule

Vaccine	Group	Dose (mcg)	Volume (mL)	Dose schedule (months)
Recombivax HB	≥20 years	10	1.0	0, 1, 6 or 0, 1, 4 or 0, 2, 4
	HD & IC ≥20 years	40	1.0	0, 1, 6
Engerix-B	≥20 years	20	1.0	0, 1, 6 or 0, 1, 4 or 0, 2, 4
	HD & IC ≥20 years	40	2.0	0, 1, 2, 6
Twinrix	≥18 years	20	1.0	0, 1, 6

HD hemodialysis patients, *IC* immunocompromised patients

Table 50.3 HBV vaccines for children: recommended doses and schedule

Vaccine	Group	Dose (mcg)	Volume (mL)	Dose schedule (months)
Recombivax HB	<1 year	5	0.5	0, 1, 6
	1–10 years	5	0.5	0, 1, 6
	11–15 years	10	1.0	0, 4–6 (two-dose adult schedule)
	11–19 years	5	0.5	0, 1, 6
Engerix-B	<1 year	10	0.5	0, 1, 6 or 0, 1, 2, 12
	1–10 years	10	0.5	0, 1, 6 or 0, 1, 2, 12
	11–19 years	10	0.5	0, 1, 6 or 0, 1, 2, 12
Comvax[a]	6 weeks–71 months	5	0.5	2, 4, 12–15
Pediarix[b]	6 weeks – 6 years	10	0.5	2, 4, 6

[a]Combined hepatitis B-*Haemophilus influenzae* type b conjugate vaccine. This vaccine cannot be administered before age 6 weeks or after age 71 months

[b]Combined hepatitis B-diphtheria, tetanus, pertussis-inactivated poliovirus vaccine. This vaccine cannot be administered at birth, before age 6 weeks, or after age 7 years

protective levels of immunity in persons with an ongoing risk for exposure, hyporesponders, and immunocompromised individuals [28].

The CDC recommends a universal vaccination program for all infants and sexually active adolescents in the USA. Prevaccination screening for previous exposure or infection is recommended in high-risk groups to avoid vaccinating recovered individuals or those with chronic infection. For patients who require rapid immunity such as last minute travelers and short-term correctional inmates, the dosage schedule can be escalated to 0, 1, and 2 months or even 0, 7, and 14 days, but a follow-up booster at 6 months is required for long-lasting immunity [28]. Administering three doses over 3 weeks and a fourth dose at 12 months provides rapid initial protection for most individuals for whom the standard 6-month vaccination schedule would not be suitable [33].

Infants born to HBsAg-positive mothers should receive HBV vaccine and hepatitis B Ig (HBIg) 0.5 mL within 12 h of birth. Hepatitis B vaccine is 70–95% effective as postexposure prophylaxis in preventing mother-to-infant HBV transmission when the first dose is administered within 24 h after birth [34]. Infants who become HBV-infected have approximately 90% risk for developing chronic HBV infection and, when chronically infected, have a 25% risk for dying prematurely from cirrhosis or liver cancer [35]. Immunized infants should be tested at approximately 12 months of age for HBsAg, anti-HBs, and anti-HBc. The presence of HBsAg indicates the infant is actively infected. The presence of both anti-HBs and anti-HBc suggests that the infection had occurred but was probably modified by immunoprophylaxis and that immunity is likely to be prolonged. The presence of anti-HBs alone is indicative of vaccine-induced immunity.

50.2.6 Postexposure Prophylaxis

The standard dose of HBIg (0.06 mL/kg) provides passively acquired anti-HBs and temporary protection for 3–6 months. Susceptible sexual partners of individuals with HBV and victims of needlestick injury with HBV contamination should receive HBIg and the first dose of HBV vaccine at different sites of the body preferably within 48 h but no more than 7 days after exposure. A second dose of HBIg can be administered 30 days after exposure, and the vaccination schedule should be completed. Postexposure prophylaxis with HBIg and lamivudine or adefovir should be used after liver transplantation for end-stage liver disease that results from HBV.

50.3 Other Hepatitis Virus Vaccines

Several preclinical, phase I, and phase II clinical trials are in existence for the development of a hepatitis C virus (HCV) vaccine for both prophylactic and therapeutic purposes. No vaccine is currently available against HCV, and immunoglobulin does not provide protection. Potential HCV vaccine candidates include recombinant proteins, recombinant viruses, DNA constructs, synthetic peptides, and virus-like particles [36–38]. In particular, the HCV envelope glycoprotein E1 has been widely employed as a potential vaccine antigen in clinical research [39]. Many vaccine trials for both prophylaxis and immunotherapy are in progress and use diverse delivery methods and formulations, but little information is available about their efficacy at present.

A recombinant hepatitis E virus (rHEV) vaccine was evaluated for safety and efficacy in a phase II, randomized, double-blind, placebo-controlled trial. Healthy adults susceptible to hepatitis E virus (HEV) infection in Nepal were randomly assigned to receive three doses of rHEV vaccine (898 subjects) or placebo (896 subjects). After three vaccine doses, the rHEV vaccine was 95.5% effective in prevention of clinically overt hepatitis E. The rHEv vaccine was proven safe and highly efficacious in preventing clinically overt hepatitis in a high-risk population [40].

50.4 Summary

Hepatitis A virus (HAV) and hepatitis B virus (HBV) are prevalent worldwide, cause significant morbidity and mortality, and are vaccine-preventable. Since the implementation of routine HAV and HBV vaccination in the USA, the overall incidence, morbidity, and mortality of both viruses have declined in the past decade to the lowest ever recorded in the USA. Current recommendations advocate vaccination of nonimmune adults at risk of exposure, including travelers to HAV or HBV endemic areas, individuals with high risk of contracting a sexually transmitted infection, illegal drug users, and healthcare workers. Hepatitis A and hepatitis B immunoglobulins are also available for postexposure prophylaxis in unvaccinated individuals.

Hepatitis A is the most common cause of viral hepatitis worldwide and is transmitted primarily via the fecal–oral route. Hepatitis A causes acute hepatitis, is detected by IgM anti-HAV antibodies, and generally resolves in 4–6 weeks. All children at age 1 year should receive a HAV vaccine, which provides lifelong immunity and requires no booster. Three HAV inactivated vaccines exist: two single antigen vaccines (Havrix and Vaqta) and one combination vaccine containing HBV and HAV antigens (Twinrix).

Hepatitis B virus is a blood-borne pathogen and is a major cause of liver failure, liver cancer, and cirrhosis, with 367 million chronic carriers of HBV worldwide. The most common exposures include sexual risk factors (i.e., multiple sexual partners, MSM) and injection drug use. HBV vaccination should be considered for everyone, particularly individuals at high risk. Five HBV vaccines exist: two single antigen vaccines (Recombivax and Energix-B) and three combination vaccines (Twinrix, Comvax, and Pediarix). Vaccine-induced immune memory lasts 15–20 years and requires no booster.

Vaccines for prophylaxis of hepatitis E virus (HEV) and hepatitis C virus (HCV) as well as immunotherapy for HCV are not available yet but are currently being developed in clinical trials. In a phase II clinical trial, a recombinant HEV vaccine was 95.5% effective in prevention of clinically overt hepatitis E in a high-risk population. Potential HCV vaccine candidates include recombinant proteins, recombinant viruses, DNA constructs, synthetic peptides, and virus-like particles.

Take-Home Pearls

- All children should receive a HAV vaccine at age 1 year.
- HAV vaccination provides lifelong immunity and requires no booster.
- Three HAV vaccines exist: 2 single antigen vaccines (Havrix and Vaqta) and 1 combination vaccine containing HBV and HAV antigens (Twinrix).
- HAV vaccination generally requires a 2-dose schedule (although the combination vaccine requires a 3-dose schedule).
- HAV vaccination should occur at least 4 weeks prior to travel to an endemic area.
- HAV vaccination and immunoglobulin should be given to persons traveling to an endemic area in less than 4 weeks.
- Immunoglobulin (and HAV vaccine) should be given within 2 weeks of last exposure to unvaccinated individuals.
- Vaccinated individuals with 1 dose of HAV vaccine $\geq$ 1 month before exposure to HAV do not need immunoglobulin.

> All infants should receive a HBV vaccine at birth.
> No boosters are necessary for fully vaccinated immunocompetent individuals.
> Booster doses or revaccination can be considered when anti-HBs levels decline in annual testing in persons with an ongoing risk for exposure, hypo-responders, and immunocompromised individuals.
> Five HBV vaccines exist: 2 single antigen vaccines (Recombivax and Energix-B) and 3 combination vaccines (Twinrix, Comvax, and Pediarix).
> HBV vaccination generally requires a 3-dose schedule (although there is an accelerated 2-dose schedule for adolescents).
> Chronic HBV infection: 90% of infants, up to 50% of children aged 1-5 years, and <5% of older children and adults.
> Chronic HBV infection: 30% progress to cirrhosis; 5-10% progress to hepatocellular carcinoma (with or without preceding cirrhosis).
> HBV vaccination and immunoglobulin should be given to infants born to HBsAg-positive mothers within 12 hours of birth.
> HBV Immunoglobulin provides passively acquired anti-HBs and temporary protection for 3-6 months.

References

1. Diamond, C., et al.: Viral hepatitis among young men who have sex with men: prevalence of infection, risk behaviors, and vaccination. Sex. Transm. Dis. **30**(5), 425–432 (2003)
2. Wasley, A., Samandari, T., Bell, B.P.: Incidence of hepatitis A in the United States in the era of vaccination. JAMA **294**(2), 194–201 (2005)
3. Wasley, A., Grytdal, S., Gallagher, K.: Surveillance for acute viral hepatitis – United States, 2006. MMWR Surveill. Summ. **57**(2), 1–24 (2008)
4. Vogt, T.M., et al.: Declining hepatitis A mortality in the United States during the era of hepatitis A vaccination. J. Infect. Dis. **197**(9), 1282–1288 (2008)
5. Zhou, F., et al.: Impact of hepatitis A vaccination on health care utilization in the United States, 1996–2004. Vaccine **25**(18), 3581–3587 (2007)
6. Fiore, A.E., Wasley, A., Bell, B.P.: Prevention of hepatitis A through active or passive immunization: recommendations of the Advisory Committee on Immunization Practices (ACIP). MMWR Recomm. Rep. **55**(RR-7), 1–23 (2006)
7. Lednar, W.M., et al.: Frequency of illness associated with epidemic hepatitis A virus infections in adults. Am. J. Epidemiol. **122**(2), 226–233 (1985)
8. Bienzle, U., et al.: Immunogenicity of an inactivated hepatitis A vaccine administered according to two different schedules and the interference of other "travellers" vaccines with the immune response. Vaccine **14**(6), 501–505 (1996)
9. Jong, E.C., et al.: An open randomized study of inactivated hepatitis A vaccine administered concomitantly with typhoid fever and yellow fever vaccines. J. Travel Med. **9**(2), 66–70 (2002)
10. Gil, A., et al.: Interference assessment of yellow fever vaccine with the immune response to a single-dose inactivated hepatitis A vaccine (1440 EL.U.). A controlled study in adults. Vaccine **14**(11), 1028–1030 (1996)
11. CDC, Prevention of hepatitis A through active or passive immunization. In: Recommendations of the Advisory Committee on Immunization Practices (ACIP). 2006.
12. Van Damme, P., et al.: Hepatitis A booster vaccination: is there a need? Lancet **362**(9389), 1065–1071 (2003)
13. Van Damme, P., Van Herck, K.: A review of the long-term protection after hepatitis A and B vaccination. Travel Med. Infect. Dis. **5**(2), 79–84 (2007)
14. Bond, W.W., Petersen, N.J., Favero, M.S.: Viral hepatitis B: aspects of environmental control. Health Lab. Sci. **14**(4), 235–252 (1977)
15. Goldstein, S.T., et al.: A mathematical model to estimate global hepatitis B disease burden and vaccination impact. Int. J. Epidemiol. **34**(6), 1329–1339 (2005)
16. Lavanchy, D.: Hepatitis B virus epidemiology, disease burden, treatment, and current and emerging prevention and control measures. J. Viral Hepat. **11**(2), 97–107 (2004)
17. Miriti, M.K., et al.: Economic benefits of hepatitis B vaccination at sexually transmitted disease clinics in the U.S. Public Health Rep. **123**(4), 504–513 (2008)
18. Workowski, K.A., Berman, S.M.: Sexually transmitted diseases treatment guidelines. MMWR Recomm. Rep. **55** (RR-11), 1–94 (2006)
19. Silverman, A.L., et al.: Tattoo application is not associated with an increased risk for chronic viral hepatitis. Am. J. Gastroenterol. **95**(5), 1312–1315 (2000)
20. Hwang, L.Y., et al.: Relationship of cosmetic procedures and drug use to hepatitis C and hepatitis B virus infections in a low-risk population. Hepatology **44**(2), 341–351 (2006)
21. Weinbaum, C.M., et al.: Recommendations for identification and public health management of persons with chronic hepatitis B virus infection. MMWR Recomm. Rep. **57**(RR-8), 1–20 (2008)
22. Lok, A.S., McMahon, B.J.: Chronic hepatitis B. Hepatology **45**(2), 507–539 (2007)
23. Tsouchnikas, I., et al.: Loss of hepatitis B immunity in hemodialysis patients acquired either naturally or after vaccination. Clin. Nephrol. **68**(4), 228–234 (2007)
24. Hyams, K.C.: Risks of chronicity following acute hepatitis B virus infection: a review. Clin. Infect. Dis. **20**(4), 992–1000 (1995)
25. Weissberg, J.I., et al.: Survival in chronic hepatitis B. An analysis of 379 patients. Ann. Intern. Med. **101**(5), 613–616 (1984)
26. Baig, S., Alamgir, M.: The extrahepatic manifestations of hepatitis B virus. J. Coll. Physicians Surg. Pak. **18**(7), 451–457 (2008)

27. Pyrsopoulos, N.T., Reddy, K.R.: Extrahepatic manifestations of chronic viral hepatitis. Curr. Gastroenterol. Rep. **3**(1), 71–78 (2001)
28. Mast, E.E., et al.: A comprehensive immunization strategy to eliminate transmission of hepatitis B virus infection in the United States: recommendations of the Advisory Committee on Immunization Practices (ACIP) Part II: immunization of adults. MMWR Recomm. Rep. **55**(RR-16), 1–33 (2006). quiz CE1-4
29. Andre, F.E.: Summary of safety and efficacy data on a yeast-derived hepatitis B vaccine. Am. J. Med. **87**(3A), 14S–20S (1989)
30. Zajac, B.A., et al.: Overview of clinical studies with hepatitis B vaccine made by recombinant DNA. J. Infect. **13**(Suppl A), 39–45 (1986)
31. Banatvala, J.E., Van Damme, P.: Hepatitis B vaccine – do we need boosters? J. Viral Hepat. **10**(1), 1–6 (2003)
32. Bauer, T., Jilg, W.: Hepatitis B surface antigen-specific T and B cell memory in individuals who had lost protective antibodies after hepatitis B vaccination. Vaccine **24**(5), 572–577 (2006)
33. Keystone, J.S., Hershey, J.H.: The underestimated risk of hepatitis A and hepatitis B: benefits of an accelerated vaccination schedule. Int. J. Infect. Dis. **12**(1), 3–11 (2008)
34. Mast, E.E., et al.: A comprehensive immunization strategy to eliminate transmission of hepatitis B virus infection in the United States: recommendations of the Advisory Committee on Immunization Practices (ACIP) part 1: immunization of infants, children, and adolescents. MMWR Recomm. Rep. **54**(RR-16), 1–31 (2005)
35. Dumolard, L., Gacic-Dobo, M., Shapiro, C.N., Wiersma, S., Wang, S.A.: Implementation of Newborn Hepatitis B Vaccination – Worldwide, 2006. Morb. Mortal Wkly. Rep. **57**(46), 1249–1252 (2008)
36. Bukh, J., et al.: Studies of hepatitis C virus in chimpanzees and their importance for vaccine development. Intervirology **44**(2–3), 132–142 (2001)
37. Youn, J.W., et al.: Sustained E2 antibody response correlates with reduced peak viremia after hepatitis C virus infection in the chimpanzee. Hepatology **42**(6), 1429–1436 (2005)
38. Elmowalid, G.A., et al.: Immunization with hepatitis C virus-like particles results in control of hepatitis C virus infection in chimpanzees. Proc. Natl. Acad. Sci. USA **104**(20), 8427–8432 (2007)
39. Nevens, F., et al.: A pilot study of therapeutic vaccination with envelope protein E1 in 35 patients with chronic hepatitis C. Hepatology **38**(5), 1289–1296 (2003)
40. Shrestha, M.P., et al.: Safety and efficacy of a recombinant hepatitis E vaccine. N. Engl. J. Med. **356**(9), 895–903 (2007)

Prophylactic HPV Vaccines

51

Lutz Gissmann

Core Messages

> › Antibodies directed against conformational epitopes of papillomavirus virus capsids have been demonstrated to convey protection against viral infections. HPV vaccines are based on virus-like particles (VLP) that assemble after expression of the major structural protein L1 and are able to induce neutralizing antibodies. The currently available vaccines (Cervarix® and Gardasil®) differ in their composition (bivalent: HPV 16,18; quadrivalent: HPV 6,11,16,18) as well as in the added adjuvant. Large placebo-controlled double-blind, randomized clinical trials in women demonstrated an excellent safety profile and close to 100% protection against persistent infection and disease induced by the vaccine types (lesions at the outer genitals and precursors of cervical cancer). Several questions (e.g. sustainability of protection) still remain and are being addressed in population-based studies with many years of follow-up.

51.1 The Principle of Vaccination

Microbial infections are controlled by the different arms of the immune system. The first line of defense is the so-called innate immunity, which consequently reacts fast but at the expense of low specificity. Specialized molecules (toll-like receptors: TLR) at the cell surface or in the cytoplasm of certain immune cells recognize incoming agents or damaged/dead cells either through their surface structure or specific nucleic acid sequences when they have been released within a cell. Interaction with the specific ligands activates the TLRs, leading to a signal cascade *via* other molecules (e.g. MyD88 and NFkB) into the nucleus, thus activating several families of genes that code for inflammatory cytokines (e.g., TNF-α, IL-6, and IL-12), costimulatory molecules on antigen-presenting cells (APC) or type I interferons [1]. These molecules by themselves trigger T- or B-cells, the specificity of which is achieved by presentation of microbial peptides in association with MHC molecules at the surface of APCs or by binding of the antigen to B cell-associated immunoglobulins.

Vaccination against infectious agents is typically based on induction of neutralizing antibodies that will bind to the microbe and thus label it for inactivation by macrophages or, mostly in case of viruses, prevent its entry into the cell. Classical vaccines are being made by chemical inactivation of the infectious agents or by adaptation through several passages in cell culture [2]. Gene technology methods now permit the production of the immunogenic molecules of the agent (subunit vaccine) (for review see [3]). To further improve the safety and efficacy of individual vaccines, modern research aims to identify such molecules and to understand the specific immune mechanisms against the particular pathogen.

L. Gissmann
Program Infections and Cancer, German Cancer Research Center (DKFZ), Im Neuenheimer Feld 242,
69120 Heidelberg, Germany
e-mail: l.gissmann@dkfz.de

G. Gross and S.K. Tyring (eds.), *Sexually Transmitted Infections and Sexually Transmitted Diseases*,
DOI: 10.1007/978-3-642-14663-3_51, © Springer-Verlag Berlin Heidelberg 2011

51.2 Immune Biology of HPV Infections

Papillomavirus infections are mostly undetected by the immune system as they remain restricted to the affected epithelium. There is no viremic phase, and the viral proteins are fully expressed only in the superficial, differentiated cells. The escape from immune surveillance is required to establish a persistent infection as part of the survival strategy of some papillomaviruses (particularly the high-risk HPV types) that produce very low virus progeny. In addition, such HPV types seem to be able to actively suppress the antiviral effect of the immune system, most effectively already at the level of the innate response. This was suggested by the results of a clinical study that demonstrated the inverse correlation between the expression of the E7 gene within a cervical lesion and its response to interferon [4]. Experimental data corroborated this observation by demonstrating the interference of the E6 and E7 proteins of HPV 16 and 18 with the expression of TLR 9 [5] and of type I interferons as well as with downstream events within the interferon-induced pathways (for review see [6]). Another immune-inhibitory effect of the viral oncoproteins is the inhibition of migration of APCs from the epithelium as required to exert their function within the lymph nodes [7, 8] and the strong reduction of the amount of surface MHC I molecules that are necessary for specific recognition by cytotoxic T cells [9].

The immunosuppressive properties of papillomaviruses notwithstanding, the immune system does participate in the control of HPV infections. There are several lines of evidence in favour of this statement. For instance, there is an increased risk of HPV infections and associated lesions in immunosuppressed patients. HIV-positive women with reduced $CD4^+$ cell count are up to eightfold more likely to develop a persistent genital HPV infection and a cervical dysplasia [10]. Further, in some of the HPV-infected individuals, virus-specific T helper and/or cytotoxic T cells can be detected that are typically directed against the early proteins E2, E6, and E7 (for summary see [11–13]) and are often associated with the regression of the lesion. In regressing warts infiltrating macrophages, NK cells and/or $CD4^+$ lymphocytes have been detected [14, 15]. Successful treatment of anal lesions with interferon goes along with infiltration by Thelper 1 cells that are characteristic for a delayed-type hypersensitivity reaction. When treatment fails, the patients show a depletion of Langerhans cells, reduction of MHC II expression in keratinocytes and of the cytokines IL-1a, -1b, and GM-CSF [16]. The inverse expression pattern has been noted in patients after successful treatment of genital warts with an immune modulator (imiquimod) that stimulates the innate immune system via TLR 7 [17, 18]. Antibodies that develop in about 50% of the infected individuals don't seem to play a role in controlling an existing HPV infection. During the natural course of an infection humoral immune response against early HPV proteins can only occasionally be detected and occurs typically only in patients with HPV-related malignant diseases [19–21]. Measurable antibodies directed against the viral structural proteins occur in about half of the infected subjects and are considered a marker for virus persistence.

As discussed earlier, protection against viral infections is mostly conferred by neutralizing antibodies. There are several arguments that this is also true in case of papillomaviruses: (1) Antibodies against mucosal papillomaviruses in some cases protect against reinfection by the same type, the depending on the antibody titer [22, 23]. (2) The original definition of HPV types made on the basis of the nucleotide sequence of their DNA ("genotypes") seems to correlate with the antigenic properties of the respective virus particles ("serotypes"). Sera from naturally infected individuals or from vaccinated women show no or only a limited response to other HPV types [24]. This immunologic signature permits the assumption that during evolution different HPV types have developed as consequence of the selection pressure by the humoral immune system. (3) Direct proof for a protective role of antibodies stems from experiments with animal papillomaviruses in their natural host, i.e. in cattle, dogs, or rabbits. The lesions induced by these viruses that closely resemble the HPV-related diseases were shown to be preventable by previous immunization with virus particles [25–27].

51.3 Design of Prophylactic HPV Vaccines

The concept of the currently available prophylactic HPV vaccines for prevention of anogenital infections and associated diseases is based on the data obtained with the earlier-mentioned animal models. Although early studies with L1 protein expressed in *Escherichia coli* had provided promising results [28], virus-like particles proved to be the most suitable vaccine candidates as they induced efficient protection against the cognate papillomavirus. It was demonstrated that protection was conferred by high titers of neutralizing antibodies induced by the immunization since naïve animals transfused with IgG from vaccinated ones became protected against viral challenge [25]. Neutralizing antibodies are directed against conformational epitopes on the surface of the virions; therefore, only complete particles are able to induce an efficient immune protection. As of today, papillomaviruses cannot be propagated to high titers in cell culture systems. Therefore, the option for generating a "classical" vaccine, namely inactivated particles derived from live stocks, was per se excluded. Instead, methods for the development of a subunit vaccine needed to be established.

Early studies with bacteriophages and later on with viruses from plants and animals had revealed their capacity to form particles, given a high concentration of the respective structural proteins [29]. This ability proved to hold true for the papillomaviruses as well [29, 30]. Production of the major structural protein (L1) by the aid of recombinant expression systems (L1-recombinant yeast or insect cells infected by L1-recombinant baculoviruses) leads to assembly of pentameric capsomeres, 72 of which form a virus-like particle (VLP). VLPs appear to be indistinguishable from authentic virus particles to the immune system. In animal experiments as well as in clinical trials, high levels of antibodies were induced, which efficiently neutralize the cognate HPV with a high degree of specificity, although cross-reactivity against other HPV types have also been reported [31, 32]. VLPs are completely apathogenic since they lack the HPV genome. Contamination with viral DNA, if it occurs at all, is restricted to the L1 gene, the only sequence that is present during the manufacturing process.

Initial clinical trials demonstrated a very good safety profile in humans and the efficient induction of antibodies even in the absence of an adjuvant [33, 34]. The good immunogenicity is in contrast to the situation after natural infection that leads only in 50–70% of the infected individuals to detectable antibodies of low titers [35]. Even in the presence of measurable antibodies, women proved to be only incompletely protected against reinfection by the same HPV type [36]. The difference in antibody response after infection and vaccination may be explained by the much higher antigen dose that is administered during vaccination. More importantly, it is based on the exposure of the virus particles to the immune system in the non-natural compartment as it happens after intramuscular immunization. Studies on isolated immune cells have revealed that VLPs very efficiently activate circulating APCs (dendritic cells) that are responsible for initiating an immune response but fail to do so in case of the epithelium-based Langerhans cells with the equivalent function [7]. The biological reason behind this observation is the earlier mentioned ability of papillomaviruses to suppress the local immune response, securing the virus persistence. Yet this suppression does not work (as it is not necessary) in the artificial environment where papillomaviruses normally never meet. The circulating antibodies induced by the vaccination reach the mucosal surface, most likely by diffusion ("transudation") into the cervical mucus, thus preventing the infection [37]. In addition, direct exposure of the incoming virus to the serum-derived antibodies may occur since a small wounding of the epithelium seems to be required as initial step of HPV infection [38]. During the early phases of vaccine development, the local route of administration had also been considered for immunization. In fact, in mouse experiments and in a clinical study, intranasal or intrabroncheal immunization induced local IgA antibodies [39]. However, such antibodies are of lower titers and shorter sustainability when compared with a systemic immune response.

At present, two vaccines have been licensed in several countries, i.e. Cervarix® manufactured by GlaxoSmithKline (GSK) and Gardasil® by Merck Sharp Dome (MSD), in certain countries marketed by Sanofi Pasteur MSD (SPMSD). They consist of VLPs, generated by assembly of the major structural protein L1. Both products contain VLPs of HPV 16 and 18, the two most important cancer-related virus types. Gardasil® has also VLPs of the HPV types 6 and 11 that cause the majority of genital warts ("quadrivalent vaccine"). The amount of protein and the recommended three times immunization scheme are similar. Production is by generation of the individual VLPs (produced in yeast or in insect cells by the aid of recombinant baculovirus) that are subsequently mixed together. A notable difference is the used adjuvant: both products contain the classical aluminium hydroxide as standard of most vaccines that are in use today and that have been injected into many millions of people. As required for the formation of antibodies, aluminum salts induce a Th2 response that has been reported in Gardasil®-immunized women [40]. The mode of action is based not only on a slow release of the antigen but also on the induction of an inflammatory response via the intracellular innate immune response system (Nalp 3) that is only recently being unravelled in more detail (for review see [41]). Cervarix® has in addition monophosphoryl Lipid A (MPL), a detoxified lipopolysaccharide prepared from *Salmonella minnesota* that activates the system via TLR4 (for review see [42]) and leads to a balanced Th1/Th2 response [43]. One cannot compare the published antibody titers following immunization with Gardasil® or Cervarix® since they have been measured by different analytical methods, namely by a competition assay using type-specific monoclonal antibodies followed by detection by Luminex-based fluorescence (MSD) [44] or by an IgG specific ELISA (GSK). A study aiming at the direct comparison of the immunogenicity of both vaccines has recently been conducted [45]. Women (n=1,106) were stratified by age (18–26, 27–35, and 36–45 years) and randomized 1:1 to receive either Gardasil® or Cervarix®. Neutralizing antibodies were measured by a newly developed assay based on HPV 16 and 18 pseudovirions that are generated in genetically modified mammalian cells in culture and contain the gene of alkaline phosphatase whose activity can be easily measured on "infection" of 393TT cells [46]. Preincubation of the pseudovirions with sera may lead to a reduction in enzymatic activity, thus indicating the presence of neutralizing activity. Analysis of the sera from the head-to-head comparative trial revealed superior immunogenicity of Cervarix, i.e. two- to fourfold (seven- to ninefold) higher serum antibody titers against HPV 16 (HPV 18) in the different age groups, along with higher antibody levels in the cervicovaginal secretions and more HPV 16- and 18-specific circulating memory B-cells [45]. This study did not address efficacy; hence, it is unknown whether the observed differences correlate with the capacity to protect against infection and disease.

As reported for the comparative trial [45] as well as for the clinical studies of the individual vaccines (see below), immunization induced seroconversion in almost all recipients. Average titers were 10- to 100-fold higher when compared with naturally developing antibodies [47, 48]. Antibody titers were similar after immunization with the quadrivalent and with an HPV 16 monovalent vaccine as well as in combination of Gardasil® with a hepatitis B vaccine arguing against the exhaustion of the immune system [49, 50]. Comparison of the immunogenicity in individuals of different age groups revealed a decrease with age and an elevated response in case of a preexisting antibodies as the consequence of an earlier infection [51, 52]. The maximal antibody level was reached after the third immunization, followed by a decrease to a stable plateau up to 14-fold above the level of natural titers, as shown in a follow up of up to 75 months after the first immunization [52–54]. From a Cervarix® recipient cohort, 8.4 years of sustained antibody titers were reported in oral presentations. HPV-specific immunization activates immune memory as demonstrated by a further immunization with Gardasil® 5 years after completion of the first series leading to a rapid increase of antibodies up to the initial maximal titer [55]. It is unclear, however, whether a natural exposure to HPV induces a booster effect or whether a repeated vaccination will become necessary in later years to come. This information will not be available before many years of follow-up of a vaccinated population when we will have learned what antibody levels are required to protect against the infection and associated disease [56].

51.4 Clinical Studies

The first data on the efficacy of prophylactic HPV vaccination came from a randomized controlled trial (sponsored by Merck) with about 2,400 women (16–23 years) that received a monovalent HPV 16 vaccine or placebo. Follow up at 48 months revealed 100% efficacy against HPV 16 induced CIN 2/3 (12 vs. 0 cases) and 94% efficacy against persistent HPV 16 infections (111 vs. 7 cases) [57, 58]. In an extended follow up of 8.5 years, encompassing 270 women, there was 100% efficacy against HPV 16 infection (0 vs. 6) and HPV 16 related cervical lesions (0 vs. 3 cases, 95% CI < 0–100%; not significant) [59].

Results from two phase II and three phase III double-blind, randomized, placebo-controlled clinical trials with >40,000 women have been published [47, 48, 53, 54, 60, 61]; another population-based study in

Costa Rica is ongoing [62]. Participants of the published trials were between 15 and 26 years of age with less than five or seven sex partners, respectively. Follow up was for at least 4 years. The placebo consisted either of the adjuvant used in the vaccine, of aluminium hydroxide, or a licensed Hepatitis A vaccine. In one study, NaCl in a physiologic concentration was given to the women in the control arm [63]. HPV positivity (defined by DNA and/or antibody positivity) was in most studies not an exclusion criterion. Yet in the final analysis, HPV positive women were stratified into the intention-to treat (ITT) group as opposed to the according-to-protocol (ATP) group comprising women who had no measurable marker for previous infection with the vaccine types, received all three immunizations, and delivered all samples as defined in the study protocol. Data from the phase II studies (for review see [64–66]) were confirmed by the larger phase III trials (n>32,000) that were pivotal for licensing of the vaccines [54, 60]. For a detailed review of these trials named FUTURE I and FUTURE II (Gardasil®) and PATRICIA (Cervarix®), see [67].

As expected from a protein-based vaccine, both products were well tolerated. Very few participants left the study because of adverse effects. The most frequently reported minor symptoms, i.e. pain, local swelling, and reddening at the injection site, and fever were slightly elevated in the vaccine group (e.g. fever 12.4% vs. 10.9%) [60, 68]. There was no increase in severity of symptoms with the second or third vaccination or in those women who had been infected by HPV before vaccination [60]. The number of women with severe adverse effects was statistically not different in the placebo- and vaccine groups (for meta-analysis of the data see [66]). There were no negative effects in women who became pregnant during the study yet the immunization during pregnancy is not recommended.

The ATP analyses revealed an efficacy of 96–98% for the HPV vaccination type-specific end points, i.e. incident or persistent infection of HPV (6 or 11 in case of Gardasil®) 16 or 18, CIN or lesions at the outer genitals induced by the vaccine types. Within the ITT analyses, efficacy was much lower (17–44% for CIN 2 or worse) due to the inclusion of lesions caused by nonvaccine types, of participants who received less than the three recommended immunizations as well as of women positive for HPV antibody and/or DNA at baseline whose infections were not influenced in their course by the vaccination. It needs to be mentioned, however, that these values refer to the difference between placebo- and vaccine group after 30 months but were increasing during follow up. Thus, it is to be expected that the benefit from vaccination will increase with time.

Combined analyses of the three Gardasil® studies and an MSD-sponsored study with HPV 16 VLPs in the ATP group revealed efficacy against vaccine-type lesions of 98% for CIN3, 100% for VIN2/3 or Va2/3, and 100% for adenocarcinoma in situ (AIS). The respective values from the ITT analysis were 44% (CIN3) and 71% (VIN2/3, VaIN2/3) and 18% for CIN 2/3 or AIS induced by any HPV type [68, 69]. Women with proven infection by at least one of the vaccine types were still completely protected against CIN2+ or AIS caused by another vaccine type.

Confirming the previous results from the Cervarix® phase II study, the PATRICIA trial reported protection against persistent infections by the nonvaccine types 31/33/45/52/58 (30%) or against CIN2+ induced by these types (53%) [54]. The respective numbers of the Gardasil® trials are 25% and 33% (not significant) [70]. The immunologic basis for this cross-protection is not yet known as neutralization assays with pseudovirions of the nonvaccine types did not show higher titers in the Cervarix® vaccinated women compared with the Gardasil® recipients [45, 9]. Yet, from the clinical data, one can calculate that theoretically Cervarix® (Gardasil®) could prevent 79% (72%) of squamous cell carcinomas and 87% (77%) of adenocarcinomas [67].

The first success of the vaccination in a real-life situation was reported from Australia where Gardasil® was given to young women in a mass vaccination program. Analysis of the proportion of patients in an STD clinic diagnosed with genital warts revealed a 48% drop in 2008 compared with the years 2004–2007 within the vaccinated cohort (aged 12–26 years). Reduction in the nonvaccinated cohort (>27 years) was 9% (not significant). Interestingly, there was also a decrease of male wart patients (17%), suggesting a herd effect due to the reduction of the virus load in this population [71].

In addition to the phase II and III studies discussed earlier, safety and immunogenicity of Gardasil® and Cervarix® was also evaluated in girls and boys between 9 and 15 years in comparison to young women (15–26 years) [63, 72, 73]. For both products, more than 99% of the participants developed antibodies. The titers in the younger individuals were up to 2.7-fold higher. The reported side effects were not significantly different from earlier trials. A similar safety profile was recorded in women up to 55 years [45]. We expect relevant information from further follow up of the phase III trials and from other studies initiated by either company, such as efficacy after only two vaccine doses, protection against genital warts in males (Gardasil®), as well as safety and immunogenicity in HIV positive patients bearing an extremely high risk for HPV-related anogenital disease.

Other important questions need to be addressed in large population-based studies. They include the role of vaccinating young boys to efficiently build herd immunity, the minimal antibody titer necessary for immune protection or the risk to shift the prevalence of different HPV types in case the vaccine types can be eliminated [56]. Also, the issue of prevention of cervical cancer can only be evaluated in such large studies (comparing the incidence before and several years after introduction of the vaccine) because, for ethical reasons, follow up in placebo-controlled trials cannot exceed the endpoint of a high-grade lesion that needs immediate treatment. Data from cancer registries may also ultimately prove the role of HPV infection in squamous cancer of the head and neck and provide information about a putative association to other cancers that at present is still only speculative (e.g. cancer of the lung or esophagus).

51.5 Future Development of HPV Vaccines

Because of the multiplicity of the high-risk HPV types, the incidence of cervical cancer can – even under optimal use of the currently available vaccines – only be reduced by 70–80% (see above). The obvious strategy to reach a closer to 100% protection is the addition of VLPs of other HPV types into a future vaccine. In fact, Merck is currently exploring this option with a nonvalent vaccine. A caveat is a putative exhaustion of the immune system by overloading with too many antigens at the same time. Also, in case of the more rare HPV types the evaluation of efficacy against disease is not feasible except in very large and expensive studies. Here the authorities responsible for the licensing process must agree to a softer endpoint, i.e. persistent infection. A possible alternative to the "add-on" approach is the "heterogenization" of VLPs by including L1 genes of different types into the expression system or by engineering type-specific neutralizing epitopes into an L1 backbone. The structure of the resulting materials is expected to be extremely complex; hence, standardizing of the manufacturing process of such a product might be difficult. In addition, the multiplicity of the epitopes per HPV type will decrease, and it will most likely need to be compensated by higher protein concentration.

A promising approach to bypass the immunologic identity of the individual HPV types is the use of the minor structural protein L2 that can be present in up to 72 copies per particle [74]. Immunization with L2 or with highly conserved immunogenic peptides derived thereof induces cross-neutralizing antibodies but at relatively low titers. However, they can be improved by applying the epitope in an oligomerized form [24, 75–77]. Future developments to improve the immune response will include the use of a very potent novel adjuvant as proven effective in non-human primates that had been immunized with poorly immunogenic HPV 16 capsomeres [78].

For theoretical reasons, which have also been confirmed in the clinical trials that have been discussed earlier, the available bivalent or quadrivalent vaccines do not exhibit any therapeutic activity, i.e. women with a persisting infection are not protected against the development of the resulting lesion but may only benefit on the long run from protection of a possible novel infection with the same or one of the other vaccine types [54]. Therefore, the development of a therapeutic vaccine is of high priority. The basis for the development of HPV-specific therapeutic vaccines is the fact that, in persistently infected cells, the early viral genes E6 and E7 are expressed, and that, these proteins are required to maintain the proliferative state of HPV transformed cells and prevent their apoptosis [79, 80]. Therefore, they are the prime target for an immune therapeutic strategy of HPV-related neoplasia although other early proteins (E1, E2) may be conceivable (for review see [81]).

Several therapeutic vaccination trials (phase I or II) that use a variety of different antigen formulations with cervical cancer patients, individuals affected by intraepithelial neoplasias (CIN, VIN, VAIN, and AIN) and healthy volunteers have been published [82–86]. The older literature has been reviewed before [64]. Immunizations were generally well tolerated and major side effects, if any, were not attributable to the vaccine. Immune responses were detected in most of the study participants (antibodies, CTL, Th1, DTH, production of cytokines), and there were some promising clinical responses in patients with intraepithelial lesions, i.e. precursors to cervical, vulval, or perianal cancer (CIN, VIN, and AIN). With the exception of two recent trials that used peptides to target VIN III lesions [87, 88] all studies demonstrated a poor correlation between clinical response and immune response within the individual patients. This implies that we need more information about the immune effector functions to improve HPV-specific immunotherapy.

Another line of development is the generation of vaccines that combine prophylactic and therapeutic properties. The rationale behind this strategy is the fact that young women that had cleared their persistent infections (with or without clinical signs thereof) are still at risk for reinfection [89]. A current development comprises chimeric VLPs that consist of L1 molecules fused to the nonstructural protein E6 and/or E7. Studies in animal models and a clinical trial have demonstrated immunogenicity and safety; efficacy was so far only shown in the animal experiments [84, 90]. The concept of combinatory HPV vaccines appears particularly attractive for countries with less developed infrastructure where it might be difficult to reach young women before they become sexually active.

Low-resource countries bear the highest burden of cervical cancer (about 80% of the cases occurring worldwide). In the absence of any kind of Pap screening, vaccination is the only realistic option to reduce the incidence of this disease. Obviously, it is hard to imagine that the current vaccines will be widely used in such areas as they are by far too expensive and require refrigeration for storing. Here the manufacturers are asked to work on their pricing policy; governments and NGOs must cooperate to organize the distribution. The situation might change once the patent protection has been expired and generic products become available that are made by providers that do not have to include the high costs for the initial clinical development into their calculation. As this will not happen before at least 10 more years, other options need to be explored, i.e. the production in cheaper expression systems such as *E. coli* or other suitable bacteria. Unfortunately, HPV L1 proteins are mostly insoluble; thus, VLPs can only be recovered after long and again costly processes. Recently, it has been demonstrated that L1 can be kept in solution when expressed as glutathione S- transferase (GST)-fusion protein. Because of the high affinity of GST to glutathione, the fusion protein can easily be purified by affinity chromatography. Enzymatic removal of GST leads to generation of large amounts of pentameric capsomers [13]. They were shown to be of similar immunogenicity when compared with VLPs, most likely because they are able to assemble to larger particles under physiologic conditions during the process of immunization. In contrast, capsomeres obtained from L1 molecules carrying point mutations that preclude assembly are of low immunogenicity that, however, can be compensated for by the addition of a potent adjuvant [79, 91]. Another system for cost-effective production of HPV vaccines may be recombinant plants that, so far, express VLPs only in relative small amounts [92, 93]. Yet, the extremely low cost of production of plants and the ease of purification of proteins therefrom, along with the expected improvement in protein yield, may render this technology attractive in the near future. A further challenge, particularly, for settings with low hygiene standards is the design of a vaccine suited for noninvasive ("needle-less") application, such as by direct exposure to mucosal surfaces. Studies in mice and with human volunteers have demonstrated immunogenicity of HPV 16 VLPs after intranasal or intrabroncheal application, but the titers were lower and short living when compared with i.m. immunization [94, 95]. Hope for improvements comes from novel adjuvants and by the aid of recombinant viral and bacterial vectors such as Salmonella or Adeno-Associated Viruses (AAV) that can be applied locally and may persist within the immunized organism, thus facilitating a long antigen stimulus [96, 97].

Take-Home Pearls

- HPV vaccines are based on virus-like particles (VLP) that are able to induce neutralizing antibodies. The currently available vaccines (Cervarix® and Gardasil®) differ in their composition (HPV 16 and 18 with or without HPV 6 and 11) and in the added adjuvant. Pivotal clinical trials demonstrated an excellent safety profile and close to 100% protection against persistent infection and disease induced by the vaccine types. Open questions still remain that are being addressed in population-based studies.

References

1. Kawai, T., Akira, S.: TLR signaling. Semin. Immunol. **19**, 24–32 (2007)
2. Jenson, H.B.: Pocket Guide to Vaccination and Prophylaxis. W.B. Saunders, Philadelphia (1999)
3. Ellis, R.W.: Technologies for making new vaccines. In: Plotkin, S.A., Orenstein, W.A., Offit, P.A. (eds.) Vaccines, pp. 1177–1197. Philadelphia, Saunders (2004)
4. Schneider, A., Papendick, U., Gissmann, L., De Villiers, E.M.: Interferon treatment of human genital papillomavirus infection: importance of viral type. Int. J. Cancer **40**, 610–614 (1987)
5. Hasan, U.A., Bates, E., Takeshita, F., Biliato, A., Accardi, R., Bouvard, V., Mansour, M., Vincent, I., Gissmann, L., Iftner, T., et al.: TLR9 expression and function is abolished by the cervical cancer-associated human papillomavirus type 16. J. Immunol. **178**, 3186–3197 (2007)
6. Koromilas, A.E., Li, S., Matlashewski, G.: Control of interferon signaling in human papillomavirus infection. Cytokine Growth Factor Rev. **12**, 157–170 (2001)
7. Fausch, S.C., Da Silva, D.M., Rudolf, M.P., Kast, W.M.: Human papillomavirus virus-like particles do not activate Langerhans cells: a possible immune escape mechanism used by human papillomaviruses. J. Immunol. **169**, 3242–3249 (2002)
8. Matthews, K., Leong, C.M., Baxter, L., Inglis, E., Yun, K., Backstrom, B.T., Doorbar, J., Hibma, M.: Depletion of Langerhans cells in human papillomavirus type 16-infected skin is associated with E6-mediated down regulation of E-cadherin. J. Virol. **77**, 8378–8385 (2003)
9. Gruener, M., Bravo, I.G., Momburg, F., Alonso, A., Tomakidi, P.: The E5 protein of the human papillomavirus type 16 down-regulates HLA-I surface expression in calnexin-expressing but not in calnexin-deficient cells. Virol. J. **4**, 116 (2007). GSK (2009)
10. Strickler, H.D., Burk, R.D., Fazzari, M., Anastos, K., Minkoff, H., Massad, L.S., Hall, C., Bacon, M., Levine, A.M., Watts, D.H., et al.: Natural history and possible reactivation of human papillomavirus in human immunodeficiency virus-positive women. J. Natl. Cancer Inst. **97**, 577–586 (2005)
11. Konya, J., Dillner, J.: Immunity to oncogenic human papillomaviruses. Adv. Cancer Res. **82**, 205–238 (2001)
12. Scott, M., Nakagawa, M., Moscicki, A.B.: Cell-mediated immune response to human papillomavirus infection. Clin. Diagn. Lab. Immunol. **8**, 209–220 (2001)
13. Stern, P.L., Brown, M., Stacey, S.N., Kitchener, H.C., Hampson, I., Abdel-Hady, E.S., Moore, J.V.: Natural HPV immunity and vaccination strategies. J. Clin. Virol. **19**, 57–66 (2000)
14. Aiba, S., Rokugo, M., Tagami, H.: Immunohistologic analysis of the phenomenon of spontaneous regression of numerous flat warts. Cancer **58**, 1246–1251 (1986)
15. Coleman, N., Birley, H.D., Renton, A.M., Hanna, N.F., Ryait, B.K., Byrne, M., Taylor-Robinson, D., Stanley, M.A.: Immunological events in regressing genital warts. Am. J. Clin. Pathol. **102**, 768–774 (1994)
16. Arany, I., Muldrow, M., Tyring, S.K.: Correlation between mRNA levels of IL-6 and TNF alpha and progression rate in anal squamous epithelial lesions from HIV-positive men. Anticancer Res. **21**, 425–428 (2001)
17. Arany, I., Tyring, S.K., Stanley, M.A., Tomai, M.A., Miller, R.L., Smith, M.H., McDermott, D.J., Slade, H.B.: Enhancement of the innate and cellular immune response in patients with genital warts treated with topical imiquimod cream 5%. Antivir. Res. **43**, 55–63 (1999)
18. Hemmi, H., Kaisho, T., Takeuchi, O., Sato, S., Sanjo, H., Hoshino, K., Horiuchi, T., Tomizawa, H., Takeda, K., Akira, S.: Small anti-viral compounds activate immune cells via the TLR7 MyD88-dependent signaling pathway. Nat. Immunol. **3**, 196–200 (2002)
19. Galloway, D.A.: Serological assays for the detection of HPV antibodies. In: Munoz, N., Bosch, F.X., Shah, K.V., Meheus, A. (eds.) The Epidemiology of Human Papillomavirus and Cervical Cancer, pp. 147–161. Lyon, IARC Scientific Publications (1992)
20. Jochmus-Kudielka, I., Schneider, A., Braun, R., Kimmig, R., Koldovsky, U., Schneweis, K.E., Seedorf, K., Gissmann, L.: Antibodies against the human papillomavirus type 16 early proteins in human sera: correlation of anti-E7 reactivity with cervical cancer. J. Natl. Cancer Inst. **81**, 1698–1704 (1989)
21. Meschede, W., Zumbach, K., Braspenning, J., Scheffner, M., Benitez-Bribiesca, L., Luande, J., Gissmann, L., Pawlita, M.: Antibodies against early proteins of human papillomaviruses as diagnostic markers for invasive cervical cancer. J. Clin. Microbiol. **36**, 475–480 (1998)
22. Ho, G.Y., Studentsov, Y., Hall, C.B., Bierman, R., Beardsley, L., Lempa, M., Burk, R.D.: Risk factors for subsequent cervicovaginal human papillomavirus (HPV) infection and the protective role of antibodies to HPV-16 virus-like particles. J. Infect. Dis. **186**, 737–742 (2002)
23. Viscidi, R.P., Ahdieh-Grant, L., Clayman, B., Fox, K., Massad, L.S., Cu-Uvin, S., Shah, K.V., Anastos, K.M., Squires, K.E., Duerr, A., et al.: Serum immunoglobulin G response to human papillomavirus type 16 virus-like particles in human immunodeficiency virus (HIV)-positive and risk-matched HIV-negative women. J. Infect. Dis. **187**, 194–205 (2003)
24. Pastrana, D.V., Gambhira, R., Buck, C.B., Pang, Y.-Y.S., Thompson, C.D., Culp, T.D., Christensen, N.D., Lowy, D.R., Schiller, J.T., Roden, R.B.S.: Cross-neutralization of cutaneous and mucosal Papillomavirus types with anti-sera to the amino terminus of L2. Virology **337**, 365–372 (2005)
25. Breitburd, F., Kirnbauer, R., Hubbert, N.L., Nonnenmacher, B., Trin-Dinh-Desmarquet, C., Orth, G., Schiller, J.T., Lowy, D.R.: Immunization with viruslike particles from cottontail rabbit papillomavirus (CRPV) can protect against experimental CRPV infection. J. Virol. **69**, 3959–3963 (1995)
26. Kirnbauer, R., Chandrachud, L.M., O'Neil, B.W., Wagner, E.R., Grindlay, G.J., Armstrong, A., McGarvie, G.M., Schiller, J.T., Lowy, D.R., Campo, M.S.: Virus-like particles of bovine papillomavirus type 4 in prophylactic and therapeutic immunization. Virology **219**, 37–44 (1996)
27. Suzich, J.A., Ghim, S.J., Palmer-Hill, F.J., White, W.I., Tamura, J.K., Bell, J.A., Newsome, J.A., Jenson, A.B., Schlegel, R.: Systemic immunization with papillomavirus L1 protein completely prevents the development of viral mucosal papillomas. Proc. Natl. Acad. Sci. USA **92**, 11553–11557 (1995)

28. Pilacinski, W.P., Glassman, D.L., Glassman, K.F., Reed, D.E., Lum, M.A., Marshall, R.F., Muscoplat, C.C., Faras, A.J.: Immunization against bovine papillomavirus infection. Ciba Found. Symp. **120**, 136–156 (1986)
29. Salunke, D.M., Caspar, D.L., Garcea, R.L.: Self-assembly of purified polyomavirus capsid protein VP1. Cell **46**, 895–904 (1986)
30. Kirnbauer, R., Taub, J., Greenstone, H., Roden, R., Durst, M., Gissmann, L., Lowy, D.R., Schiller, J.T.: Efficient self-assembly of human papillomavirus type 16 L1 and L1-L2 into virus-like particles. J. Virol. **67**, 6929–6936 (1993)
31. Alba-Lucia Combita, M.-M.B.A.T.O.O.P.C.: Serologic response to human oncogenic papillomavirus types 16, 18, 31, 33, 39, 58 and 59 virus-like particles in colombian women with invasive cervical cancer. Int. J. Cancer **97**, 796–803 (2002)
32. Pastrana, D.V., Buck, C.B., Pang, Y.-Y.S., Thompson, C.D., Castle, P.E., FitzGerald, P.C., Kruger Kjaer, S., Lowy, D.R., Schiller, J.T.: Reactivity of human sera in a sensitive, high-throughput pseudovirus-based papillomavirus neutralization assay for HPV16 and HPV18. Virology **321**, 205–216 (2004)
33. Brown, D.R., Fife, K.H., Wheeler, C.M., Koutsky, L.A., Lupinacci, L.M., Railkar, R., Suhr, G., Barr, E., Dicello, A., Li, W., et al.: Early assessment of the efficacy of a human papillomavirus type 16 L1 virus-like particle vaccine. Vaccine **22**, 2936–2942 (2004)
34. Harro, C.D., Pang, Y.Y., Roden, R.B., Hildesheim, A., Wang, Z., Reynolds, M.J., Mast, T.C., Robinson, R., Murphy, B.R., Karron, R.A., et al.: Safety and immunogenicity trial in adult volunteers of a human papillomavirus 16 L1 virus-like particle vaccine. J. Natl. Cancer Inst. **93**, 284–292 (2001)
35. Carter, J.J., Koutsky, L.A., Hughes, J.P., Lee, S.K., Kuypers, J., Kiviat, N., Galloway, D.A.: Comparison of human papillomavirus types 16, 18, and 6 capsid antibody responses following incident infection. J. Infect. Dis. **181**, 1911–1919 (2000)
36. Viscidi, R.P., Schiffman, M., Hildesheim, A., Herrero, R., Castle, P.E., Bratti, M.C., Rodriguez, A.C., Sherman, M.E., Wang, S., Clayman, B., et al.: Seroreactivity to human papillomavirus (HPV) types 16, 18, or 31 and risk of subsequent HPV infection: results from a population-based study in Costa Rica. Cancer Epidemiol. Biomarkers Prev. **13**, 324–327 (2004)
37. Nardelli-Haefliger, D., Wirthner, D., Schiller, J.T., Lowy, D.R., Hildesheim, A., Ponci, F., De Grandi, P.: Specific antibody levels at the cervix during the menstrual cycle of women vaccinated with human papillomavirus 16 virus-like particles. J. Natl. Cancer Inst. **95**, 1128–1137 (2003)
38. Kines, R.C., Thompson, C.D., Lowy, D.R., Schiller, J.T., Day, P.M.: The initial steps leading to papillomavirus infection occur on the basement membrane prior to cell surface binding. Proc. Natl. Acad. Sci. USA **106**, 20458–20463 (2009)
39. Balmelli, C., Roden, R., Potts, A., Schiller, J., De Grandi, P., Nardelli-Haefliger, D.: Nasal immunization of mice with human papillomavirus type 16 virus-like particles elicits neutralizing antibodies in mucosal secretions. J. Virol. **72**, 8220–8229 (1998)
40. Ruiz, W., McClements, W.L., Jansen, K.U., Esser, M.T.: Kinetics and isotype profile of antibody responses in rhesus macaques induced following vaccination with HPV 6, 11, 16 and 18 L1-virus-like particles formulated with or without Merck aluminum adjuvant. J. Immune Based Ther. Vaccines **3**, 2 (2005)
41. De Gregorio, E., Tritto, E., Rappuoli, R.: Alum adjuvanticity: unraveling a century old mystery. Eur. J. Immunol. **38**, 2068–2071 (2008)
42. Baldridge, J.R., McGowan, P., Evans, J.T., Cluff, C., Mossman, S., Johnson, D., Persing, D.: Taking a toll on human disease: toll-like receptor 4 agonists as vaccine adjuvants and monotherapeutic agents. Expert Opin. Biol. Ther. **4**, 1129–1138 (2004)
43. Ismaili, J., Rennesson, J., Aksoy, E., Vekemans, J., Vincart, B., Amraoui, Z., Van Laethem, F., Goldman, M., Dubois, P.M.: Monophosphoryl lipid A activates both human dendritic cells and T cells. J. Immunol. **168**, 926–932 (2002)
44. Opalka, D., Lachman, C.E., MacMullen, S.A., Jansen, K.U., Smith, J.F., Chirmule, N., Esser, M.T.: Simultaneous quantitation of antibodies to neutralizing epitopes on virus-like particles for human papillomavirus types 6, 11, 16, and 18 by a multiplexed luminex assay. Clin. Diagn. Lab. Immunol. **10**, 108–115 (2003)
45. Einstein, M.H., Baron, M., Levin, M.J., Chatterjee, A., Edwards, R.P., Zepp, F., Carletti, I., Dessy, F.J., Trofa, A.F., Schuind, A., et al.: Comparison of the immunogenicity and safety of Cervarix() and Gardasil((R)) human papillomavirus (HPV) cervical cancer vaccines in healthy women aged 18–45 years. Hum. Vaccin. **5**, 705–719 (2009)
46. Buck, C.B., Pastrana, D.V., Lowy, D.R., Schiller, J.T.: Generation of HPV pseudovirions using transfection and their use in neutralization assays. Methods Mol. Med. **119**, 445–462 (2005)
47. Harper, D.M., Franco, E.L., Wheeler, C., Ferris, D.G., Jenkins, D., Schuind, A., Zahaf, T., Innis, B., Naud, P., De Carvalho, N.S., et al.: Efficacy of a bivalent L1 virus-like particle vaccine in prevention of infection with human papillomavirus types 16 and 18 in young women: a randomised controlled trial. Lancet **364**, 1757–1765 (2004)
48. Villa, L.L., Costa, R.L., Petta, C.A., Andrade, R.P., Paavonen, J., Iversen, O.E., Olsson, S.E., Hoye, J., Steinwall, M., Riis Johannessen, G., et al.: High sustained efficacy of a prophylactic quadrivalent human papillomavirus types 6/11/16/18 L1 virus-like particle vaccine through 5 years of follow-up. Br. J. Cancer **95**, 1459–1466 (2006)
49. Garland, S.M., Steben, M., Hernandez-Avila, M., Koutsky, L.A., Wheeler, C.M., Perez, G., Harper, D.M., Leodolter, S., Tang, G.W., Ferris, D.G., et al.: Noninferiority of antibody response to human papillomavirus type 16 in subjects vaccinated with monovalent and quadrivalent L1 virus-like particle vaccines. Clin. Vaccine Immunol. **14**, 792–795 (2007)
50. Wheeler, C.M., Bautista, O.M., Tomassini, J.E., Nelson, M., Sattler, C.A., Barr, E.: Safety and immunogenicity of co-administered quadrivalent human papillomavirus (HPV)-6/11/16/18 L1 virus-like particle (VLP) and hepatitis B (HBV) vaccines. Vaccine **26**, 686–696 (2008)
51. Giuliano, A.R., Lazcano-Ponce, E., Villa, L., Nolan, T., Marchant, C., Radley, D., Golm, G., McCarroll, K., Yu, J., Esser, M.T., et al.: Impact of baseline covariates on the immunogenicity of a quadrivalent (types 6, 11, 16, and 18) human papillomavirus virus-like-particle vaccine. J. Infect. Dis. **196**, 1153–1162 (2007)

52. Villa, L.L., Ault, K.A., Giuliano, A.R., Costa, R.L., Petta, C.A., Andrade, R.P., Brown, D.R., Ferenczy, A., Harper, D.M., Koutsky, L.A., et al.: Immunologic responses following administration of a vaccine targeting human papillomavirus types 6, 11, 16, and 18. Vaccine **24**, 5571–5583 (2006)
53. Harper, D.M., Franco, E.L., Wheeler, C.M., Moscicki, A.B., Romanowski, B., Roteli-Martins, C.M., Jenkins, D., Schuind, A., Costa Clemens, S.A., Dubin, G.: Sustained efficacy up to 4.5 years of a bivalent L1 virus-like particle vaccine against human papillomavirus types 16 and 18: follow-up from a randomised control trial. Lancet **367**, 1247–1255 (2006)
54. Paavonen, J., Naud, P., Salmeron, J., Wheeler, C.M., Chow, S.N., Apter, D., Kitchener, H., Castellsague, X., Teixeira, J.C., Skinner, S.R., et al.: Efficacy of human papillomavirus (HPV)-16/18 AS04-adjuvanted vaccine against cervical infection and precancer caused by oncogenic HPV types (PATRICIA): final analysis of a double-blind, randomised study in young women. Lancet **374**, 301–314 (2009)
55. Olsson, S.E., Villa, L.L., Costa, R.L., Petta, C.A., Andrade, R.P., Malm, C., Iversen, O.E., Hoye, J., Steinwall, M., Riis-Johannessen, G., et al.: Induction of immune memory following administration of a prophylactic quadrivalent human papillomavirus (HPV) types 6/11/16/18 L1 virus-like particle (VLP) vaccine. Vaccine **25**, 4931–4939 (2007)
56. Lehtinen, M., Apter, D., Dubin, G., Kosunen, E., Isaksson, R., Korpivaara, E.L., Kyha-Osterlund, L., Lunnas, T., Luostarinen, T., Niemi, L., et al.: Enrolment of 22, 000 adolescent women to cancer registry follow-up for long-term human papillomavirus vaccine efficacy: guarding against guessing. Int. J. STD AIDS **17**, 517–521 (2006)
57. Koutsky, L.A., Ault, K.A., Wheeler, C.M., Brown, D.R., Barr, E., Alvarez, F.B., Chiacchierini, L.M., Jansen, K.U.: A controlled trial of a human papillomavirus type 16 vaccine. N. Engl. J. Med. **347**, 1645–1651 (2002)
58. Mao, C., Koutsky, L.A., Ault, K.A., Wheeler, C.M., Brown, D.R., Wiley, D.J., Alvarez, F.B., Bautista, O.M., Jansen, K.U., Barr, E.: Efficacy of human papillomavirus-16 vaccine to prevent cervical intraepithelial neoplasia: a randomized controlled trial. Obstet. Gynecol. **107**, 18–27 (2006)
59. Rowhani-Rahbar, A., Mao, C., Hughes, J.P., Alvarez, F.B., Bryan, J.T., Hawes, S.E., Weiss, N.S., Koutsky, L.A.: Longer term efficacy of a prophylactic monovalent human papillomavirus type 16 vaccine. Vaccine **27**, 5612–5619 (2009)
60. Garland, S.M., Hernandez-Avila, M., Wheeler, C.M., Perez, G., Harper, D.M., Leodolter, S., Tang, G.W., Ferris, D.G., Steben, M., Bryan, J., et al.: Quadrivalent vaccine against human papillomavirus to prevent anogenital diseases. N. Engl. J. Med. **356**, 1928–1943 (2007)
61. Villa, L.L., Costa, R.L., Petta, C.A., Andrade, R.P., Ault, K.A., Giuliano, A.R., Wheeler, C.M., Koutsky, L.A., Malm, C., Lehtinen, M., et al.: Prophylactic quadrivalent human papillomavirus (types 6, 11, 16, and 18) L1 virus-like particle vaccine in young women: a randomised double-blind placebo-controlled multicentre phase II efficacy trial. Lancet Oncol. **6**, 271–278 (2005)
62. Herrero, R., Hildesheim, A., Rodriguez, A.C., Wacholder, S., Bratti, C., Solomon, D., Gonzalez, P., Porras, C., Jimenez, S., Guillen, D., et al.: Rationale and design of a community-based double-blind randomized clinical trial of an HPV 16 and 18 vaccine in Guanacaste, Costa Rica. Vaccine **26**, 4795–4808 (2008)
63. Reisinger, K.S., Block, S.L., Lazcano-Ponce, E., Samakoses, R., Esser, M.T., Erick, J., Puchalski, D., Giacoletti, K.E., Sings, H.L., Lukac, S., et al.: Safety and persistent immunogenicity of a quadrivalent human papillomavirus types 6, 11, 16, 18 L1 virus-like particle vaccine in preadolescents and adolescents: a randomized controlled trial. Pediatr. Infect. Dis. J. **26**, 201–209 (2007)
64. Gissmann, L.: Human papillomavirus vaccines. In: Meisels, A., Morin, C. (eds.) Modern Uterine cytopathology, pp. 169–200. Chicago, ASCP Press (2007)
65. Koutsky, L.A., Harper, D.M.: Chapter 13: Current findings from prophylactic HPV vaccine trials. Vaccine **24**(suppl 3), S114–S121 (2006)
66. Rambout, L., Hopkins, L., Hutton, B., Fergusson, D.: Prophylactic vaccination against human papillomavirus infection and disease in women: a systematic review of randomized controlled trials. CMAJ **177**, 469–479 (2007)
67. Harper, D.M.: Currently approved prophylactic HPV vaccines. Expert Rev. Vaccines **8**, 1663–1679 (2009)
68. Joura, E.A., Leodolter, S., Hernandez-Avila, M., Wheeler, C.M., Perez, G., Koutsky, L.A., Garland, S.M., Harper, D.M., Tang, G.W., Ferris, D.G., et al.: Efficacy of a quadrivalent prophylactic human papillomavirus (types 6, 11, 16, and 18) L1 virus-like-particle vaccine against high-grade vulval and vaginal lesions: a combined analysis of three randomised clinical trials. Lancet **369**, 1693–1702 (2007)
69. Ault, K.A.: Effect of prophylactic human papillomavirus L1 virus-like-particle vaccine on risk of cervical intraepithelial neoplasia grade 2, grade 3, and adenocarcinoma in situ: a combined analysis of four randomised clinical trials. Lancet **369**, 1861–1868 (2007)
70. Brown, D.R., Kjaer, S.K., Sigurdsson, K., Iversen, O.E., Hernandez-Avila, M., Wheeler, C.M., Perez, G., Koutsky, L.A., Tay, E.H., Garcia, P., et al.: The impact of quadrivalent human papillomavirus (HPV; types 6, 11, 16, and 18) L1 virus-like particle vaccine on infection and disease due to oncogenic nonvaccine HPV types in generally HPV-naive women aged 16–26 years. J. Infect. Dis. **199**, 926–935 (2009)
71. Fairley, C.K., Hocking, J.S., Gurrin, L.C., Chen, M.Y., Donovan, B., Bradshaw, C.S.: Rapid decline in presentations of genital warts after the implementation of a national quadrivalent human papillomavirus vaccination programme for young women. Sex. Transm. Infect. **85**, 499–502 (2009)
72. Block, S.L., Nolan, T., Sattler, C., Barr, E., Giacoletti, K.E., Marchant, C.D., Castellsague, X., Rusche, S.A., Lukac, S., Bryan, J.T., et al.: Comparison of the immunogenicity and reactogenicity of a prophylactic quadrivalent human papillomavirus (types 6, 11, 16, and 18) L1 virus-like particle vaccine in male and female adolescents and young adult women. Pediatrics **118**, 2135–2145 (2006)
73. Pedersen, C., Petaja, T., Strauss, G., Rumke, H.C., Poder, A., Richardus, J.H., Spiessens, B., Descamps, D., Hardt, K., Lehtinen, M., et al.: Immunization of early adolescent females with human papillomavirus type 16 and 18 L1 virus-like particle vaccine containing AS04 adjuvant. J. Adolesc. Health **40**, 564–571 (2007)

74. Buck, C.B., Cheng, N., Thompson, C.D., Lowy, D.R., Steven, A.C., Schiller, J.T., Trus, B.L.: Arrangement of L2 within the papillomavirus capsid. J. Virol. **82**, 5190–5197 (2008)
75. Alphs, H.H., Gambhira, R., Karanam, B., Roberts, J.N., Jagu, S., Schiller, J.T., Zeng, W., Jackson, D.C., Roden, R.B.: Protection against heterologous human papillomavirus challenge by a synthetic lipopeptide vaccine containing a broadly cross-neutralizing epitope of L2. Proc. Natl. Acad. Sci. USA **105**, 5850–5855 (2008)
76. Jagu, S., Karanam, B., Gambhira, R., Chivukula, S.V., Chaganti, R.J., Lowy, D.R., Schiller, J.T., Roden, R.B.: Concatenated multitype L2 fusion proteins as candidate prophylactic pan-human papillomavirus vaccines. J. Natl. Cancer Inst. **101**, 782–792 (2009)
77. Rubio, I., Bolchi, A., Moretto, N., Canali, E., Gissmann, L., Tommasino, M., Muller, M., Ottonello, S.: Potent anti-HPV immune responses induced by tandem repeats of the HPV16 L2 (20–38) peptide displayed on bacterial thioredoxin. Vaccine **27**, 1949–1956 (2009)
78. Stahl-Hennig, C., Eisenblatter, M., Jasny, E., Rzehak, T., Tenner-Racz, K., Trumpfheller, C., Salazar, A.M., Uberla, K., Nieto, K., Kleinschmidt, J., et al.: Synthetic double-stranded RNAs are adjuvants for the induction of T helper 1 and humoral immune responses to human papillomavirus in rhesus macaques. PLoS Pathog. **5**, e1000373 (2009)
79. Butz, K., Ristriani, T., Hengstermann, A., Denk, C., Scheffner, M., Hoppe-Seyler, F.: siRNA targeting of the viral E6 oncogene efficiently kills human papillomavirus-positive cancer cells. Oncogene **22**, 5938–5945 (2003)
80. DeFilippis, R.A., Goodwin, E.C., Wu, L., DiMaio, D.: Endogenous human papillomavirus E6 and E7 proteins differentially regulate proliferation, senescence, and apoptosis in HeLa cervical carcinoma cells. J. Virol. **77**, 1551–1563 (2003)
81. Nieto, K., Gissmann, L., Schädlich, L.: Human papillomavirus (HPV)-specific immune therapy: failure and hope. Antivir. Ther. **15**, 951–957 (2010)
82. Hallez, S., Simon, P., Maudoux, F., Doyen, J., Noel, J.C., Beliard, A., Capelle, X., Buxant, F., Fayt, I., Lagrost, A.C., et al.: Phase I/II trial of immunogenicity of a human papillomavirus (HPV) type 16 E7 protein-based vaccine in women with oncogenic HPV-positive cervical intraepithelial neoplasia. Cancer Immunol. Immunother. **53**, 642–650 (2004)
83. Kaufmann, A.M., Nieland, J.D., Jochmus, I., Baur, S., Friese, K., Gabelsberger, J., Gieseking, F., Gissmann, L., Glasschroder, B., Grubert, T., et al.: Vaccination trial with HPV16 L1E7 chimeric virus-like particles in women suffering from high grade cervical intraepithelial neoplasia (CIN 2/3). Int. J. Cancer **121**, 2794–2800 (2007)
84. Kenter, G.G., Welters, M.J., Valentijn, A.R., Lowik, M.J., Berends-van der Meer, D.M., Vloon, A.P., Drijfhout, J.W., Wafelman, A.R., Oostendorp, J., Fleuren, G.J., et al.: Phase I immunotherapeutic trial with long peptides spanning the E6 and E7 sequences of high-risk human papillomavirus 16 in end-stage cervical cancer patients shows low toxicity and robust immunogenicity. Clin. Cancer Res. **14**, 169–177 (2008)
85. Santin, A.D., Bellone, S., Palmieri, M., Zanolini, A., Ravaggi, A., Siegel, E.R., Roman, J.J., Pecorelli, S., Cannon, M.J.: Human papillomavirus type 16 and 18 E7-pulsed dendritic cell vaccination of stage IB or IIA cervical cancer patients: a phase I escalating-dose trial. J. Virol. **82**, 1968–1979 (2008)
86. Welters, M.J., Kenter, G.G., Piersma, S.J., Vloon, A.P., Lowik, M.J., Berends-van der Meer, D.M., Drijfhout, J.W., Valentijn, A.R., Wafelman, A.R., Oostendorp, J., et al.: Induction of tumor-specific CD4+ and CD8+ T-cell immunity in cervical cancer patients by a human papillomavirus type 16 E6 and E7 long peptides vaccine. Clin. Cancer Res. **14**, 178–187 (2008)
87. Kenter, G.G., Welters, M.J., Valentijn, A.R., Lowik, M.J., Berends-van der Meer, D.M., Vloon, A.P., Essahsah, F., Fathers, L.M., Offringa, R., Drijfhout, J.W., et al.: Vaccination against HPV-16 oncoproteins for vulvar intraepithelial neoplasia. N. Engl. J. Med. **361**, 1838–1847 (2009)
88. Viscidi, R.P., Snyder, B., Cu-Uvin, S., Hogan, J.W., Clayman, B., Klein, R.S., Sobel, J., Shah, K.V.: Human papillomavirus capsid antibody response to natural infection and risk of subsequent HPV infection in HIV-positive and HIV-negative women. Cancer Epidemiol. Biomarkers Prev. **14**, 283–288 (2005)
89. Schafer, K., Muller, M., Faath, S., Henn, A., Osen, W., Zentgraf, H., Benner, A., Gissmann, L., Jochmus, I.: Immune response to human papillomavirus 16 L1E7 chimeric virus-like particles: induction of cytotoxic T cells and specific tumor protection. Int. J. Cancer **81**, 881–888 (1999)
90. Schadlich, L., Senger, T., Gerlach, B., Mucke, N., Klein, C., Bravo, I.G., Muller, M., Gissmann, L.: Analysis of modified human papillomavirus type 16 L1 capsomeres: the ability to assemble into larger particles correlates with higher immunogenicity. J. Virol. **83**, 7690–7705 (2009)
91. Biemelt, S., Sonnewald, U., Galmbacher, P., Willmitzer, L., Muller, M.: Production of human papillomavirus type 16 virus-like particles in transgenic plants. J. Virol. **77**, 9211–9220 (2003)
92. Maclean, J., Koekemoer, M., Olivier, A.J., Stewart, D., Hitzeroth, I.I., Rademacher, T., Fischer, R., Williamson, A.L., Rybicki, E.P.: Optimization of human papillomavirus type 16 (HPV-16) L1 expression in plants: comparison of the suitability of different HPV-16 L1 gene variants and different cell-compartment localization. J. Gen. Virol. **88**, 1460–1469 (2007)
93. Nardelli-Haefliger, D., Lurati, F., Wirthner, D., Spertini, F., Schiller, J.T., Lowy, D.R., Ponci, F., De Grandi, P.: Immune responses induced by lower airway mucosal immunisation with a human papillomavirus type 16 virus-like particle vaccine. Vaccine **23**, 3634–3641 (2005)
94. Schiller, J.T., Lowy, D.R.: Prospects for cervical cancer prevention by human papillomavirus vaccination. Cancer Res. **66**, 10229–10232 (2006)
95. Kuck, D., Lau, T., Leuchs, B., Kern, A., Muller, M., Gissmann, L., Kleinschmidt, J.A.: Intranasal vaccination with recombinant adeno-associated virus type 5 against human papillomavirus type 16 L1. J. Virol. **80**, 2621–2630 (2006)
96. Revaz, V., Zurbriggen, R., Moser, C., Schiller, J.T., Ponci, F., Bobst, M., Nardelli-Haefliger, D.: Humoral and cellular immune responses to airway immunization of mice with human papillomavirus type 16 virus-like particles and mucosal adjuvants. Antivir. Res. **76**, 75–85 (2007)
97. Daayana, S., Elkord, E., Winters, U., Pawlita, M., Roden, R., Stern, P.L., Kitchener, H.C.: Phase II trial of imiquimod and HPV therapeutic vaccination in patients with vulval intraepithelial neoplasia. Br. J. Cancer **102**, 1129–1136 (2010)

HSV Prevention

52

Parisa Ravanfar, Natalia Mendoza, Anita K. Shetty, Rosella Creed, and Stephen K. Tyring

Core Messages

- Herpes simplex virus is the most common ulcerating disease of the genital mucosa.
- Almost 90% of the world population is HSV-1 positive and approximately 50 million people in the US have genital herpes.
- A prophylactic vaccine should ideally induce sterilizing immunity, which must be broad, durable, and effective at all sites of potential HSV entry.
- The objective of a therapeutic vaccine is to prevent herpes recurrences or at least minimize their rate, duration, and severity while decreasing transmissibility.

52.1 Introduction

Genital herpes is caused by the herpes simplex virus type 1 (HSV-1) or herpes simplex virus type 2 (HSV-2). The majority of genital herpes cases are due to HSV-2 infection. Genital herpes is the most common ulcerating disease of the genital mucosa; 45–90% of the world population is HSV-1 positive and 40–60% of the United States population is HSV-1 positive. Approximately 50 million people in the United States have genital herpes (i.e., are HSV-2 seropositive) and a million new genital herpes cases occur annually. There is also evidence indicating that HSV-2 infection is a significant cofactor for HIV infection. Owing to the significant morbidity that HSV infection may cause, an HSV vaccine could create a significant public health impact. There are prophylactic and therapeutic herpes simplex virus vaccines currently under investigation. Benefits of an HSV vaccine may include reduction in risk of HSV acquisition, reduction in severity of disease, reduction in neonatal herpes, reduction in transmission of herpes, and reduction in transmission of HIV.

52.2 Virology

Both HSV-1 and HSV-2 belong to the family Herpesviridae, subfamily Alphaherpesvirinae. They are large, complex enveloped viruses composed of an outer lipid envelope covered with viral glycoproteins, an intermediate tegument layer, and an icosahedral nucleocapsid containing the viral DNA genome (Fig. 52.1). The viral genome is a double-stranded DNA consisting of two covalently linked components: a 126-kb long region and a 26-kb short region that are flanked by inverted repeat sequences, which allow for isomerization and recombination of the long and short regions [2]. Both HSV-2 and HSV-1 encode over 80 different polypeptides.

Infection is initiated when HSV attaches to cell surface receptors of the host and fuses its envelope to the plasma membrane, thus releasing the capsid that is transported to the nuclear pores where the viral DNA enters the nucleus of the host cell. While in the host cell, transcription, DNA synthesis, capsid assembly, DNA packaging, and envelopment occur for viral

P. Ravanfar (✉), N. Mendoza, A.K. Shetty, and R. Creed
Center for Clinical Studies, Houston, TX 77030, USA
e-mail: pravanfar@ccstexas.com

S.K. Tyring
Department of Dermatology, Center for Clinical Studies,
University of Texas Health Science Center, Houston, TX, USA

G. Gross and S.K. Tyring (eds.), *Sexually Transmitted Infections and Sexually Transmitted Diseases*,
DOI: 10.1007/978-3-642-14663-3_52, © Springer-Verlag Berlin Heidelberg 2011

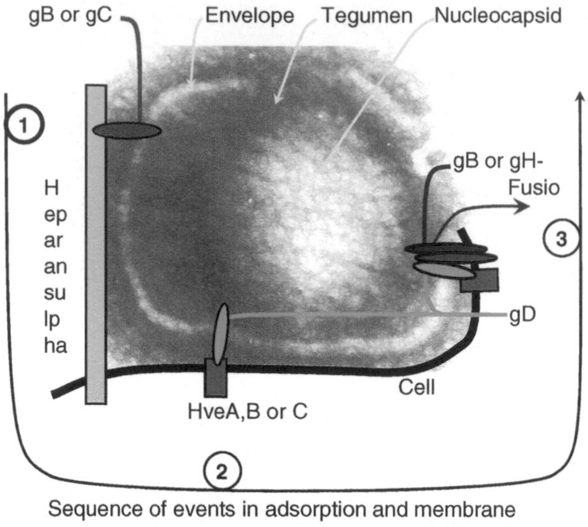

Fig. 52.1 HSV composition and entry. Electron micrograph of negatively stained HSV particle with indications of major structural elements. Important mediators of adsorption to cells (1) receptor binding (2) and fusion of membranes (3) during the process of infection are drawn stylistically ([1]. Permission pending)

replication, the viral surface glycoproteins allow for attachment and penetration of the virus into the host cells. There are at least 11 of these glycoproteins that are currently known [2]. The glycoproteins are the main targets in mediating protective humoral responses and some glycoproteins have been tested in subunit vaccines, which are discussed later.

The viral proteins and RNA are produced in three stages: the α, or immediate early proteins, the β, or early proteins, and the γ, or late gene products. The α proteins control the reproductive cycle of the virus and block antigenic peptide presentation on the infected cell surfaces [3]. Next, the β proteins regulate viral nucleic acid metabolism, including viral thymidine kinase and viral DNA polymerase, and are the main targets for antiviral chemotherapy. Last, the γ products are the structural proteins of the virion [3].

HSV has two unique infectious characteristics that affect human disease. First, the virus is capable of invading and infecting the central nervous system (CNS). The deletion of almost any gene that is not required for replication decreases the ability of the virus to invade and replicate in the CNS [2]. The capability to invade the CNS has been mapped to viral glycoprotein genes [2].

Another prime characteristic of HSV infection is the capability to establish latent infection. Once the virus enters and infects the nerve endings, it undergoes retrograde transportation into the nuclei of the sensory ganglia where it multiplies in a few sensory neurons. The viral genome remains in an episomal state in most infected neurons for the life of the human host. However, reactivation can occur and may be induced by factors such as physical or emotional stress, ultraviolet light exposure, tissue damage, fever, menstruation, and especially immune suppression. The latent virus can be recovered from the trigeminal, sacral, and vaginal ganglia either unilaterally or bilaterally [4].

52.3 Clinical Pathophysiology

HSV-1 infections are spread via respiratory droplets or direct exposure to infected saliva. HSV-2 is typically transmitted by genital contact involving mucous membranes or open or damaged skin.

Herpes viruses cause cytolytic infections, thus causing pathologic change s due to cell necrosis and inflammatory changes. Vesicles are formed from fluid accumulation between the dermis and the epidermal skin layers. The fluid is later absorbed and the vesicles dry to form scabs. Lesions often begin as clusters of small papules, which progress to vesicles on an erythematous base. The vesicles rupture on mucous membranes and form shallow painful ulcers. Lesions coalesce and usually heal over several weeks.

The average incubation period from exposure to development of symptoms in true primary herpes is 4 days; however, incubation time can range from 1 to 26 days. Prodromal symptoms are common and include local pain, tingling, itching, and burning. Constitutional symptoms of fever, fatigue, myalgias, and headache often occur during the primary HSV infection.

Local pain is a common symptom and patients with genital herpes may also have pain in the groin area secondary to local adenopathy. Women often present with complaints of genital swelling, discharge, and dysuria.

Many primary infections are asymptomatic. Up to 80% of women with HSV-2 antibodies have no clinical history of infection. Symptomatic primary infections are often more severe than recurrent infections, and recurrent lesions are common.

52.4 Epidemiology

It is estimated that approximately 40–60 million people in the United States are infected with HSV-2, with an estimated incidence of 1–2 million infections and 600,000–800,000 clinical cases/year [5]. Twenty to twenty-five percent of US adults test seropositive for HSV-2 antibodies by 40 years of age. The prevalence of HSV-2 in 30–40-year-olds is approximately 30%. Prevalence is higher in women compared to men, especially in younger populations. Approximately one out of every four women, compared to almost one out of every eight men, is infected with HSV-2 in the United States. The higher prevalence in women is most likely due to the higher male-to-female rate of transmission compared to female-to-male transmission. Prevalence rates as high as 40% have been reported in women aged 15–19 years, living in countries such as Costa Rica, Kenya, and Mexico [5].

Risk factors associated with genital HSV infection include older age, female gender, African-American race, low socioeconomic status, low education level, a prior sexually transmitted infection, and high number of total lifetime sexual partners [6].

52.5 HSV Prevention

HSV prevention can be difficult because of the widespread nature of the disease. More than two-thirds of adults are infected with HSV-1 and/or HSV-2 [7]. Furthermore, the majority of individuals who are infected with HSV are unaware of their infection as the majority of HSV infections are asymptomatic. To complicate matters further, most HSV seropositive individuals, whether or not they are aware of their infection, experience asymptomatic viral shedding, which leads to high rates of transmission. Although the only method of guaranteeing prevention of genital herpes is through abstinence from any genital–genital or oral–genital contact, this is rarely possible in the adult population. Therefore, there are other ways to reduce the risk of HSV transmission. For example, patients should avoid mucosal contact with herpetic lesions. Prodromal symptoms and herpetic outbreaks increase the risk of HSV transmission and mucosal contact should be avoided at these stages.

The consistent use of condoms between outbreaks has also been demonstrated to decrease the risk of HSV infection during times of asymptomatic shedding. One study found that condom use during more than 25% of sex acts was associated with protection against HSV-2 acquisition for women (adjusted HR, 0.085; 95% CI, 0.01–0.67) [8]. However, consistent condom use did not provide statistically significant prevention against HSV-2 for men [8]. One possible explanation for this gender difference may be due to the difference in HSV shedding. For example, penile skin is the most common site of HSV shedding in heterosexual men and male condom use would consequently reduce transmission from penile skin [9]. However, the vulvar and perianal areas are the most common sites of HSV shedding in women and men are likely to be exposed to these areas during sexual contact despite condom use [9].

Antiviral drug therapy in patients known to have genital herpes has also been proven to significantly decrease the risk of HSV transmission. Valacyclovir 500 mg to 1 g taken daily has been shown to decrease the risk of HSV transmission by 50%, as well as decrease the risk of development of genital herpes lesions by 77% [7,10]. One study demonstrated that valacyclovir 500 mg taken daily (by the HSV-2 seropositive patient) in immunocompetent, heterosexual, HSV-2 serodiscordant couples significantly reduced HSV transmission, significantly prolonged the time to development of a symptomatic first episode of genital herpes among the partners of valacyclovir recipients, and significantly reduced the number of days of asymptomatic viral shedding [10] (Fig. 52.2). Acyclovir may also be used for chronic suppressive therapy, dosed as 400 mg twice daily or 200 mg three to five times daily (Fig. 52.3). One study found acyclovir 400 mg twice daily to be just as effective as valacyclovir 500 mg twice daily in reducing HSV recurrences and viral shedding [11]. Chronic suppressive therapy with famciclovir 250 mg twice daily may also be administered, but studies indicate that valacyclovir may be slightly superior to famciclovir in the prevention of HSV shedding and genital herpes recurrence [12].

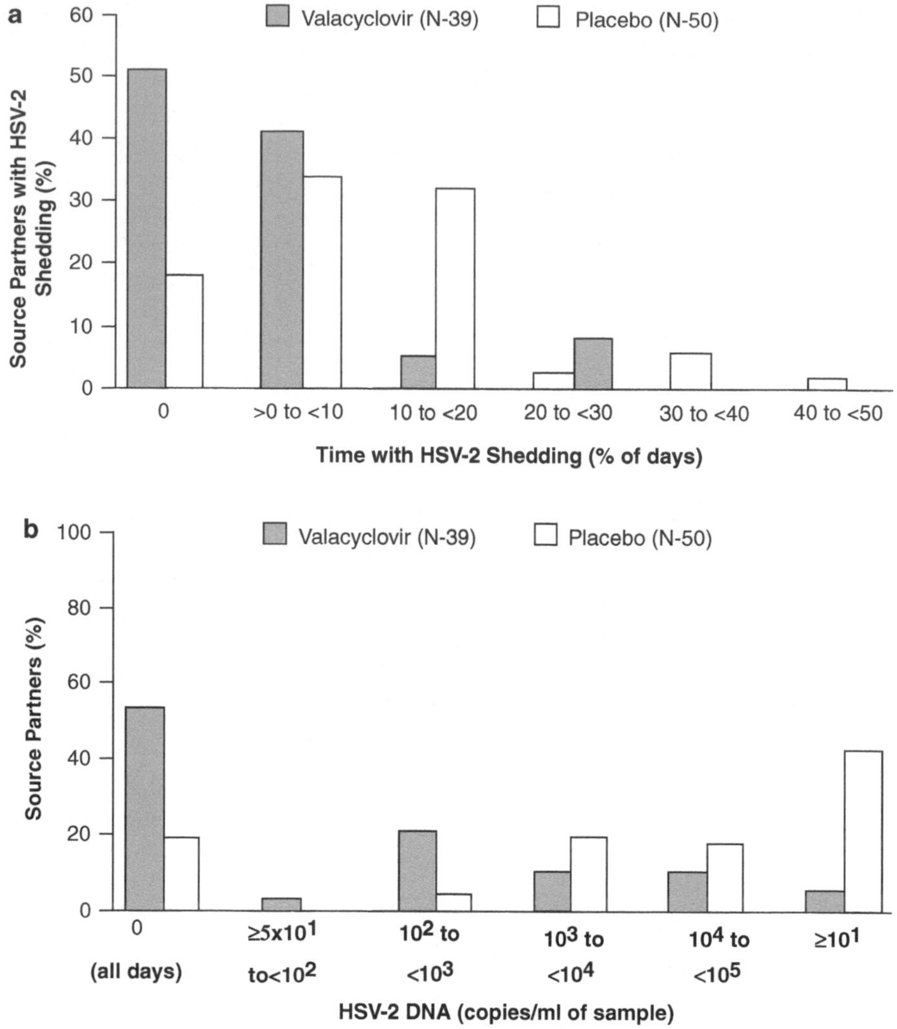

Fig. 52.2 Frequency and titer of HSV-2 shedding among Valacyclovir-treated when compared with Placebo-treated source partners ([10]. Permission pending)

52.5.1 Microbicides

The use of vaginal microbicides in the prevention of HSV is a recent area of investigation. Small interfering RNAs (siRNAs) are about 20 bp long and associate with a silencing complex, leading to sequence-specific hybridization with cytoplasmic mRNAs and selective degradation or inactivation of the mRNAs by arresting translation (Fig. 52.4). Palliser et al. administered anti-HSV-2 siRNA lipoplexes (siRNAs combined with catatonic lipids) to the vaginal epithelia of mice and demonstrated prevention of viral infection and shedding, as well as protection against HSV-2 challenge [13]. It was shown that the use of two siRNAs administered even hours after exposure to the virus reduced infection [13]. Furthermore, the antiviral response was demonstrated to last 9 or more days [13]. Further studies utilizing cholesterol-conjugated (chol)-siRNAs have demonstrated prevention in the transmission of HSV-2 for a week in mice by targeting and "silencing" the HSV-2 receptor, nectin-1. The cholesterol combination is also proposed to cause less vaginal irritation than the lipoplexes [14]. However, prevention is delayed for a few days until the receptor is downmodulated, and thus attacking a second gene, UL29, found in the virus would provide additional immediate protection [14]. Vaginal microbicides against HSV-2 appear to have great potential in prevention of HSV-2 transmission.

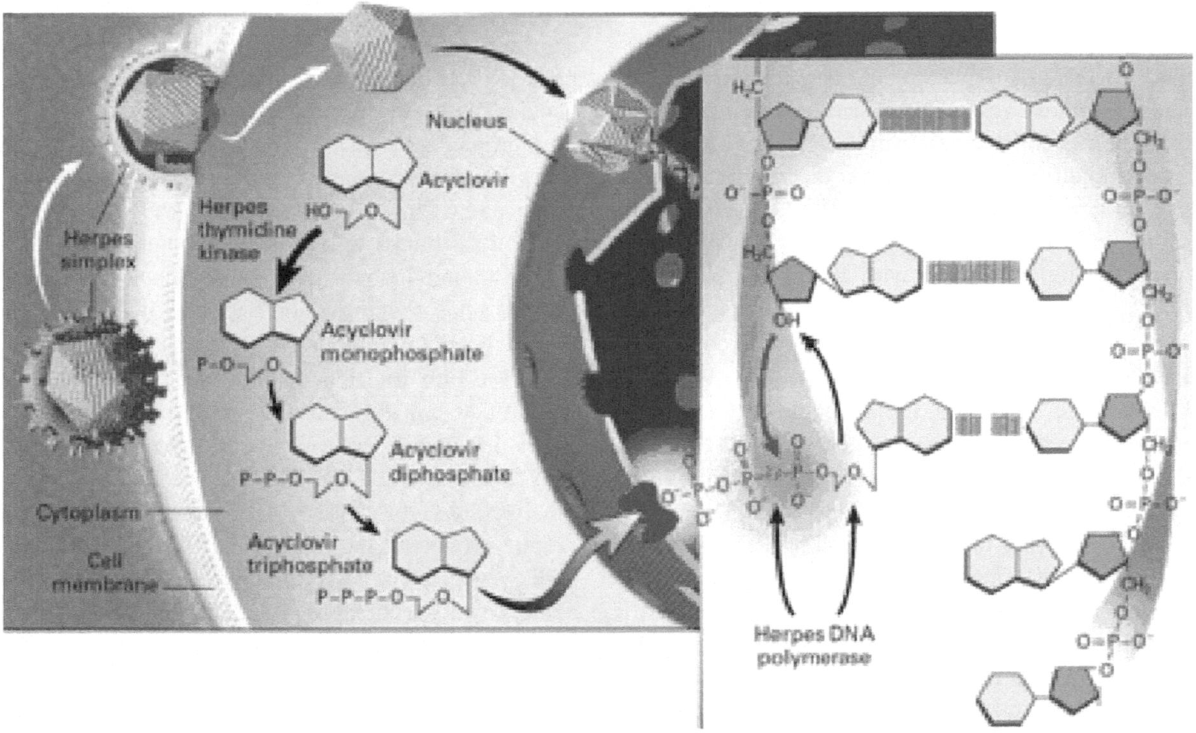

Fig. 52.3 Mechanism of action of acyclovir in cells infected by herpes simplex virus (N. Engl. J. Med. **340**(16), 1255–1268 (22 Apr 1999). Permission pending)

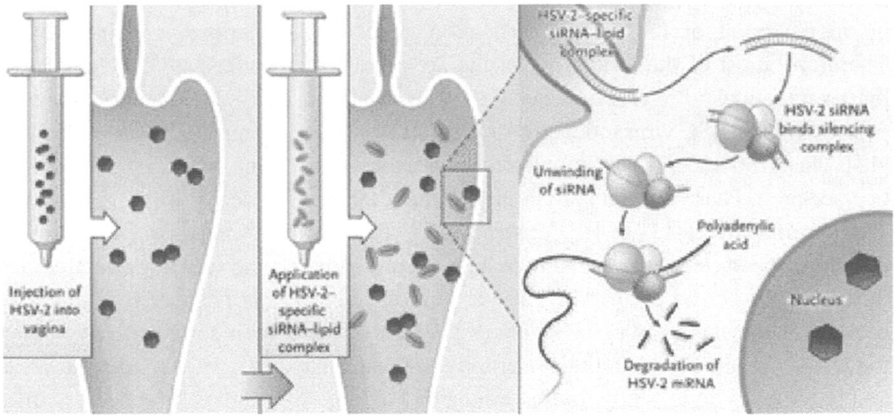

Fig. 52.4 Assaulting herpes simplex virus 2 (HSV-2) in mice (N. Engl. J. Med. **354**(9), 970 (2 Mar 2006). Permission pending)

52.5.2 Potential Vaccines

52.5.2.1 Prophylactic HSV-2 Vaccines

A prophylactic vaccine should ideally induce sterilizing immunity, which must be broad, durable, and effective at all sites of potential HSV entry [15]. A vaccine must induce an immune response that is stronger than the response induced from a natural infection. The types of vaccines that have undergone clinical evaluation for HSV prophylaxis include: attenuated live virus vaccines, subunit vaccines, and DNA vaccines.

Attenuated Live Virus Vaccines

The objective of a live attenuated vaccine is to stimulate an immune response by causing a primary infection, then establishing latency in the ganglia. However, there should not be reactivation of the virus, even in immunocompromised patients. The key factor is the stability of attenuation since genetic recombination could theoretically occur with a wild-type virus [15]. R7020 was a live attenuated HSV vaccine tested in clinical trials [16]. The vaccine was derived from an HSV-1 strain with a deleted portion of the thymidine kinase gene and with replacement of the interval inverted repeats and adjacent genes with a portion of the HSV-2 genome encoding for glycoproteins (g) G, D, I, and a portion of E [16]. Although the vaccine displayed promising results in animal models by providing protection against wild-type virus challenges, the vaccine was poorly immunogenic in clinical trials. It was also poorly tolerated at high doses and the clinical trial was brought to a halt due to adverse events [17].

A novel, live attenuated HSV-2 vaccine candidate has been created by Xenova/GlaxoSmithKline®, which uses a replication-impaired virus with an essential gene deletion. The virus mutant lacks the essential glycoprotein gH (ICP8 gene mutation) and is referred to as a disabled infectious single cycle (DISC) virus vaccine [18]. When the DISC virus infects a human cell, the virus replicates up to the point of the deleted replication gene [19]. Therefore, most of the viral components are produced, but no infectious virions are created [19]. The structural proteins of the DISC virus induce a host immune response [15]. The DISC vaccine was initially tested as a therapeutic vaccine in Phase II clinical trials in the United States. The vaccine was tested in HSV-2 seropositive patients. Although the vaccine was found to be safe, there was no difference in herpes recurrence rate or viral shedding between the vaccine and placebo groups [20]. However, the DISC vaccine has potential as a prophylactic vaccine and is currently under study for this indication [15].

Other live, genetically attenuated vaccines are also in clinical studies; these include replication-impaired virus vaccines and those that are impaired in both replication and establishment of latency.

Subunit Vaccines

HSV subunit vaccines use recombinant DNA technology to produce large quantities of one or two glycoproteins, free of whole virus or DNA, which are administered with adjuvants. There are 11 HSV envelope glycoproteins; unlike RNA viruses, there is only minor strain differentiation in the major surface proteins of HSV [15].

A prophylactic vaccine consisting of truncated gD2 and gB2 glycoproteins with the adjuvant MF59 was produced by Chiron®. The vaccine was studied in two randomized double-blind, placebo-controlled studies [21]. Although in the first 5 months of both studies the vaccine appeared promising, with a 50% reduction rate of HSV-2 acquisition in the vaccine group, the effect was only transient and the vaccine was found to be ineffective at the end of 1 year [21]. Also, it was found that male vaccinees were not protected against HSV-2 acquisition [21]. The vaccine did not reduce the likelihood or severity of symptomatic disease, despite producing high titers of HSV-2-specific antibodies, which suggests that neutralizing antibodies alone are not sufficient to protect against HSV-2 infection [22].

GlaxoSmithKline® developed a single component gD2 vaccine with AS04 adjuvant (alum plus monophosphoryl lipid A) that appears to be very promising. The vaccine produced a strong immune response and provided protection from HSV-2 challenge in animal models. The vaccine was then tested in clinical trials with administration at 0 month, 1 month, and 6 months. It was demonstrated in Phase I studies to be safe, well-tolerated, and induced gD-specific neutralizing antibodies and T helper 1 cell-mediated immune response [23, 24]. The vaccine went into two large, double-blind controlled multicenter phase III clinical trials. The vaccine was 73% efficacious against genital herpes disease in women who were both HSV-1 and HSV-2 seronegative [23]. However, it was found that the vaccine was not effective in women who were previously seropositive for HSV-1 and also in men regardless of their seropositivity status (Fig. 52.5) [23]. The difference in sex-specific efficacy is not fully understood, but may be related to differences in mucosal immunity between men and women. A large phase III efficacy trial with NIH collaboration is being conducted to assess the prophylactic efficacy and safety of the vaccine in the prevention of genital herpes in 7,550 women aged 18–30 years who are both HSV-1 and HSV-2 seronegative (The Herpevac Trial for Women). The vaccine trial is double-blinded, randomized, and uses the hepatitis A vaccine as control, with approximately 20 month follow-up after administration at 0, 1, and 6 months.

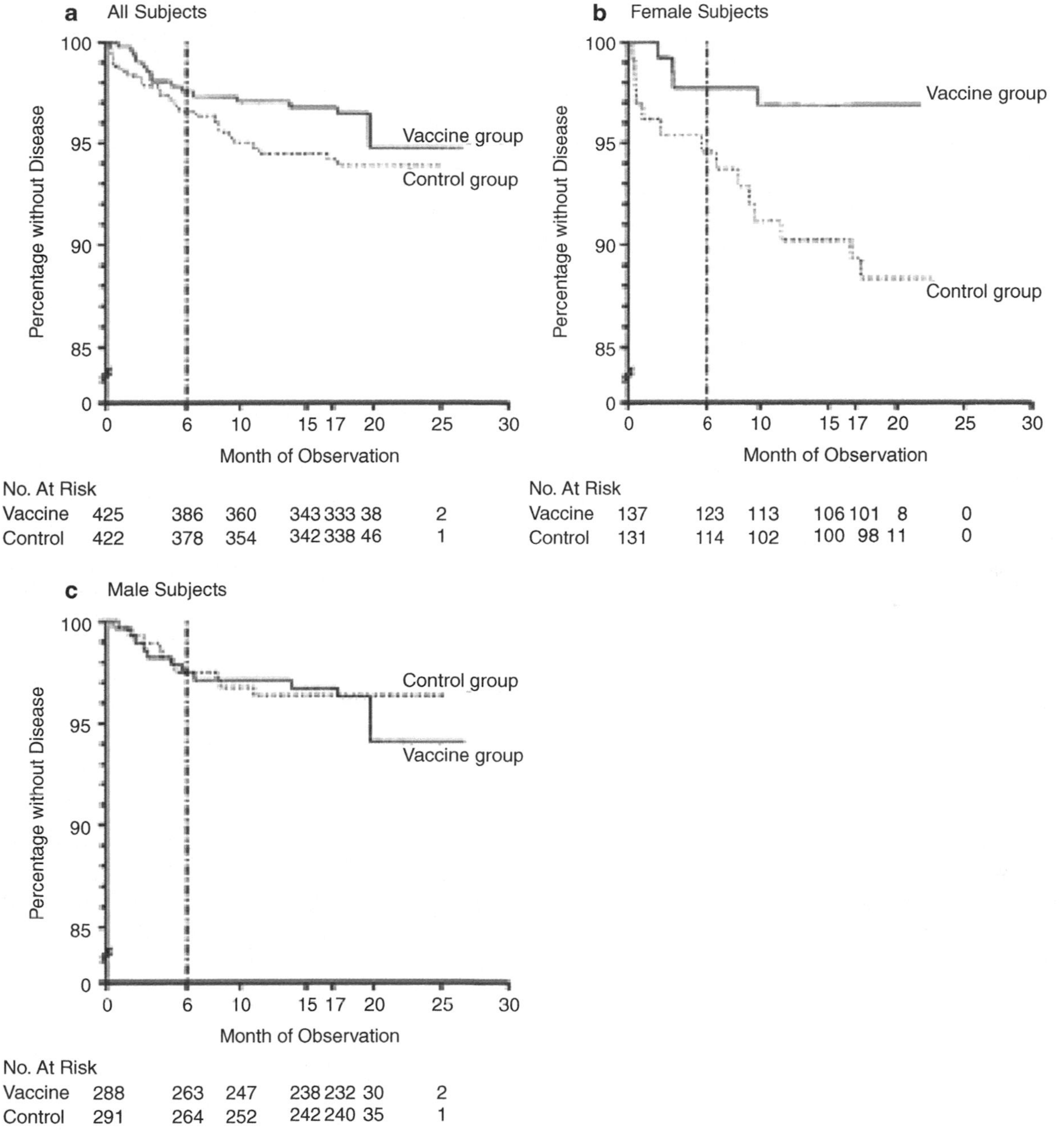

Fig. 52.5 Kaplan–Meier plots for study 1, showing time to occurrence of genital herpes disease in subjects who were seronegative for herpes simplex virus type 1 (HSV-1) and herpes simplex virus type 2 (HSV-2) at base line ([23]. Permission pending)

52.5.2.2 Therapeutic HSV-2 Vaccines

The objective of a therapeutic vaccine is to prevent herpes recurrences or at least minimize their rate, duration, and severity while decreasing transmissibility through preventing or limiting viral reactivation in the ganglion or by minimizing virus replication after egression from the nerve, prior to transport to the mucosal surface [15]. There are currently no therapeutic vaccines available and many previous trials with potential therapeutic vaccines demonstrated disappointing results. Therapeutic vaccine candidates that have been shown to be ineffective include: non-specific live vaccines such as the vaccinia vaccine that did not show any of the theorized cross-protection; autoinoculation of live HSV, which not only did not prevent HSV reactivation episodes, but lesions often occurred at the injection site as well [25, 26]; and whole, inactivated virion vaccines including heat-killed whole virus vaccines from HSV-2 (Lupidon G) and HSV-1 (Lupidon H) [27, 28]. Inactivated subunit vaccines have also not proven effective, to date. These include the NFU.Ac.HSV-1(S)MRC (Skinner) vaccine, which is composed of HSV-1 glycoproteins prepared by formalin inactivation and detergent extractions. Clinical trials of the Skinner vaccine against placebo did not demonstrate clear efficacy or immunogenicity [15, 29]. Clinical trials of recombinant glycoprotein vaccines have been conducted using a gD2-alum vaccine and a gD2gB2-MF59 vaccine, but therapeutic potential was not seen [30]. The gD2gB2-MF59 vaccine has not demonstrated significant reduction in HSV recurrence by either culture or clinical assessment and has not been shown to affect viral shedding [15, 30].

52.6 Conclusion

There is still much that is not known about cellular and mucosal responses to HSV infection. Further research should be conducted to gauge immune responses to HSV and to identify HSV-2 antigens that will generate effective immunity. The Herpevac trial for women appears to have great prophylactic potential. A vaccine that protects women against HSV could decrease the rate of neonatal HSV infection, as well as drastically decrease the spread of genital herpes infections. However, the fact that many adults are HSV-1 seropositive may limit the utility of this vaccine [5]. Furthermore, needle-free mucosal vaccines are being investigated in animal models and appear to have potential as vaccine candidates. Regardless of potential vaccines, behavioral measures must still be emphasized to patients in order to prevent genital herpes transmission.

Take-Home Pearls

- There are currently no preventive or therapeutic vaccines available for HSV infections.
- The Herpevac trial for women appears to have great prophylactic potential.
- The only method of guaranteeing prevention of genital herpes is through. abstinence from any genital-genital or oral-genital contact.
- Further HSV vaccine studies are needed.

References

1. Ellermann-Eriksen, S.: Macrophages and cytokines in the early defense. Virol. J. **2**, 59 (2005). doi:10.1186/1743-422X-2-59
2. Whitley, R.J., Roizman, B.: Herpes simplex viruses: is a vaccine tenable? J. Clin. Invest. **110**(2), 145–151 (July 2002)
3. Roizman, B., Pellett, P.E.: Herpesviridae. In: Knipe, D.M., Howley, R.M. (eds.) Fields Virology, 4th edn, pp. 2381–2397. Lippincott Williams & Wilkins, Philadelphia (2001)
4. Whitley, R.J.: Herpes simplex vaccines. In: Levine, M.M., Kaper, J.B., Rappuoli, R., Liu, M., Good, M. (eds.) New Generation Vaccines. Marcel Dekker, New York (2002)
5. World Health Organization. http://www.who.int/vaccine_research/diseases/soa_std/en/index3.html (2009). Accessed 2 May 2009
6. Fatahzadeh, M., Schwartz, R.A.: Human herpes simplex virus infections: epidemiology, pathogenesis, symptomatology, diagnosis, and management. J. Am. Acad. Dermatol. **57**(5), 737–763 (Nov 2007)
7. Herpevac Trial for Women. http://www.niaid.nih.gov/dmid/stds/herpevac/about_herpes.html (2009). Accessed 2 May 2009
8. Wald, A., Langenberg, A.G., Link, K., Izu, A.E., Ashley, R., Warren, T., Tyring, S., Douglas Jr., J.M., Corey, L.: Effect of condoms on reducing the transmission of herpes simplex virus type 2 from men to women. JAMA **285**(24), 3100–3106 (27 June 2001)
9. Wald, A., Zeh, J., Selke, S., et al.: Reactivation of genital herpes simplex virus type 2 infection in asymptomatic HSV-2 seropositive persons. N. Engl. J. Med. **342**, 844–850 (2000)
10. Corey, L., Wald, A., Patel, R., Sacks, S.L., Tyring, S.K., Warren, T., et al.: Once-daily valacyclovir to reduce the risk of transmission of genital herpes. N. Engl. J. Med. **350**(1), 11–20 (1 Jan 2004)
11. Gupta, R., Wald, A., Krantz, E., Selke, S., Warren, T., Vargas-Cortes, M., et al.: Valacyclovir and acyclovir for suppression of shedding of herpes simplex virus in the genital

tract. J. Infect. Dis. **190**(8), 1374–1381 (15 Oct 2004) [Epub; 20 Sept 2004]

12. Wald, A., Selke, S., Warren, T., Aoki, F.Y., Sacks, S., Diaz-Mitoma, F., Corey, L.: Comparative efficacy of famciclovir and valacyclovir for suppression of recurrent genital herpes and viral shedding. Sex. Transm. Dis. **33**(9), 529–533 (Sept 2006)
13. Palliser, D., Chowdhury, D., Wang, Q.-Y., et al.: An siRNA-based microbicide protects mice from lethal herpes simplex virus 2 infection. Nature **439**, 89–94 (2006)
14. Wu, Y., Navarro, F., Lal, A., Basar, E., Pandey, R.K., Manoharan, M., Feng, Y., Lee, S.J., Lieberman, J., Palliser, D.: Durable protection from herpes simplex virus-2 transmission following intravaginal application of siRNAs targeting both a viral and host gene. Cell Host Microbe **5**(1), 84–94 (22 Jan 2009)
15. Stanberry, L.R.: Clinical trials of prophylactic and therapeutic herpes simplex virus vaccines. Herpes **11**(suppl 3), 161A–169A (Aug 2004)
16. Meignier, B., Longnecker, R., Roizman, B.: In vivo behavior of genetically engineered herpes simplex viruses R7017 and R7020: construction and evaluation in rodents. J. Infect. Dis. **158**(3), 602–614 (Sept 1988)
17. Whitley, R.J.: Prospects for vaccination against herpes simplex virus. Pediatr Ann. **22**(12), 726, 729–732 (Dec 1993)
18. McLean, C.S., Erturk, M., Jennings, R., Challanain, D.N., Minson, A.C., Duncan, I., et al.: Protective vaccination against primary and recurrent disease caused by herpes simplex virus (HSV) type 2 using a genetically disabled HSV-1. J. Infect. Dis. **170**, 1100–1109 (1994)
19. Forrester, A., Farrell, H., Wilkinson, G., Kaye, J., Davis-Poynter, N., Minson, T.: Constuction and properties of a mutant of herpes simplex virus type 1 with glycoprotein H coding sequences deleted. J. Virol. **66**, 341–348 (1992)
20. de Bruyn, G., Vargas-Cortez, M., Warren, T., Tyring, S.K., Fife, K.H., Lalezari, J., et al.: A randomized controlled trial of a replication defective (gH deletion) herpes simplex virus vaccine for the treatment of recurrent genital herpes among immunocompetent subjects. Vaccine **24**(7), 914–920 (13 Feb 2006) [Epub; 21 Sept 2005]
21. Corey, L., Langenberg, A.G., Ashley, R., Sekulovich, R.E., Izu, A.E., Douglas Jr., J.M., et al.: Recombinant glycoprotein vaccine for the prevention of genital HSV-2 infection: two randomized controlled trials. Chirion HSV Vaccine Study Group. JAMA **282**, 331–340 (1999)
22. Brown, Z.A., Vontver, L.A., Benedetti, J., Critchlow, C.W., Sells, C.J., Berry, S., Corey, L.: Effects on infants of a first episode of genital herpes during pregnancy. N. Engl. J. Med. **317**(20), 1246–1251 (12 Nov 1987)
23. Stanberry, L.R., Spruance, S.L., Cunningham, A.L., Bernstein, D.I., Mindel, A., Sacks, S., Tyring, S., et al.: Glycoprotein-D-adjuvant vaccine to prevent genital herpes. GlaxoSmithKline Herpes Vaccine Efficacy Study Group. N. Engl. J. Med. **347**(21), 1652–1661 (21 Nov 2002)
24. Bernstein, D.I., Aoki, F.Y., Tyring, S.K., Stanberry, L.R., St-Pierre, C., Shafran, S.D., Leroux-Roels, G., Van Herck, K., Bollaerts, A., Dubin, G.: GlaxoSmithKline Herpes Vaccine Study Group. Safety and immunogenicity of glycoprotein D-adjuvant genital herpes vaccine. Clin. Infect. Dis. **40**(9), 1271–1281 (1 May 2005)
25. Blank, H., Haines, H.G.: Experimental human reinfection with herpes simplex. J. Invest. Dermatol. **61**(4), 223–225 (Oct 1973). virus
26. Lazar, M.P.: Vaccination for recurrent herpes simplex infection; initiation of a new disease site following the use of unmodified material containing the live virus. AMA Arch. Derm. **73**(1), 70–71 (Jan 1956)
27. Mastrolorenzo, A., Tiradritti, L., Salimbeni, L., Zuccati, G.: Multicentre clinical trial with herpes simplex virus vaccine in recurrent herpes infection. Int. J. STD AIDS **6**(6), 431–435 (Nov–Dec 1995)
28. Weitgasser, H.: Controlled clinical study of the herpes antigens LUPIDON H and LUPIDON G. Z. Hautkr. **52**(11), 625–628 (1 June 1977)
29. Skinner, G.R., Turyk, M.E., Benson, C.A., Wilbanks, G.D., Heseltine, P., Galpin, J., Kaufman, R., Goldberg, L., Hartley, C.E., Buchan, A.: The efficacy and safety of Skinner herpes simplex vaccine towards modulation of herpes genitalis; report of a prospective double-blind placebo-controlled trial. Med. Microbiol. Immunol. **186**(1), 31–36 (June 1997)
30. Straus, S.E., Wald, A., Kost, R.G., McKenzie, R., Langenberg, A.G., Hohman, P., Lekstrom, J., et al.: Immunotherapy of recurrent genital herpes with recombinant herpes simplex virus type 2 glycoproteins D and B: results of a placebo-controlled vaccine trial. J. Infect. Dis. **176**(5), 1129–1134 (Nov 1997)

HIV Prevention

53

Parisa Ravanfar, Natalia Mendoza, Anita K. Shetty, Rosella Creed, and Stephen K. Tyring

Core Messages

- The number of people living with HIV has risen from approximately 8 million in 1990 to 42 million in 2007.
- A successful vaccine must either prevent infection in HIV-negative individuals, or at least reduce the viral load in those already infected.
- There are multiple classes of HIV vaccines: fowlpox vector, canarypox vectors, DNA plasmid, lipopeptides, live-attenuated vesicular stomatitis virus vectors, modified vaccinia Ankara (MVA) vector, nonreplicating adenoviral vector, peptides, proteins, and VEE vectors.
- HIV research is also focused on the development of vaginal and rectal microbicides for the prevention of HIV transmission.

53.1 HIV Epidemiology

Acquired immune deficiency syndrome (AIDS) was first recognized in the United States in 1981. Human immunodeficiency virus (HIV) was identified in 1983 and was clearly demonstrated to be the causative agent of AIDS in 1984. The number of people living with HIV has risen from approximately 8 million in 1990 to 42 million in 2007, with 74% of these individuals living in Sub-Saharan Africa [1]. In 2007, there were 2.7 million new HIV infections and 2 million HIV-related deaths [1]. The estimated number of adults and children living with HIV in the United States was 1.2 million in 2007, of which 24–27% were undiagnosed and unaware of being HIV-positive [2]. Over 25 million people have died from AIDS. The prevalence of HIV among 15–24 year olds in the United States is estimated to be 0.7 among US males and 0.3 among US females [1]. About 14,000 individuals become newly infected everyday, 95% of whom live in developing countries [1]. The United Nations (UN) estimates that there are currently >14 million AIDS orphans and that number is estimated to be 25 million by 2010.

P. Ravanfar (✉), N. Mendoza, A.K. Shetty, and R. Creed
Center for Clinical Studies, Houston, TX 77030, USA
e-mail: pravanfar@ccstexas.com

S.K. Tyring
Department of Dermatology, Center for Clinical Studies, University of Texas Health Science Center, Houston, TX, USA

53.2 HIV Virology

HIV is a human retrovirus and belongs to the family Retroviridae; subfamily Lentivirus. HIV-1 and HIV-2 are cytopathic viruses. HIV-1 causes the majority of HIV disease worldwide.

The mature HIV virion has a spherical morphology of 100–120 nm in diameter consisting of a dense nucleocapsid core that is composed of the genomic RNA molecules, the viral protease (PR), reverse transcriptase (RT), integrase (IN), Vpu, Vif, Vpr, and Nef, and cellular factors. The nucleocapsid core is surrounded by a lipid bilayer membrane [3]. The HIV-1 genome consists of two identical 9.2 kb single-stranded RNA molecules while within the virion. However, the

G. Gross and S.K. Tyring (eds.), *Sexually Transmitted Infections and Sexually Transmitted Diseases*,
DOI: 10.1007/978-3-642-14663-3_53,

persistent form of the HIV-1 genome is double-stranded DNA when it is within infected cells [4].

HIV infection is initiated by the attachment of the virion to the cell surface through high-affinity binding between the extracellular domain of HIV-1, namely the gp120 protein, and host cell receptors [4, 5]. HIV has a high affinity for CD4+ T lymphocytes and monocytes. CD4 is the major host cell receptor for HIV-1 and HIV-2, and the chemokine receptors, CCR5 and CXCR4, are the main HIV-1 coreceptors [6]. After binding, viral and cellular membranes fuse, thus releasing the virus into the host cell cytoplasm. Viral uncoating involves cellular factors and the viral proteins MA, Nef, and Vif. The viral RNA genome is then retrotranscribed into a double-stranded DNA by the viral RT [4]. Reverse transcription is achieved through the presence of the cellular protein APOBEC3G (or CEM15). The DNA translocates into the host nucleus where it becomes integrated into the host cell chromosomes by the viral enzyme, integrase.

53.2.1 HIV Clades

HIV clades are taxonomic subgroups of HIV that are categorized by geographical region and each clade has genetic similarities and markers. The ability of HIV to rapidly mutate its envelope proteins and evade the host's immune system makes the development of an HIV vaccine very challenging. There are two major HIV clades. These are: clade M, or Main, and clade O, or Outgroup. The main (M) clade is responsible for the majority of HIV infections, and the outgroup (O) HIV clade is less common. The M clade has eight different subtypes, lettered A–H. Certain geographic areas are associated with a particular clade. For example, clades A and D are the most common in East Africa, clade B is the most common in Europe and the Americas, and clade C is the most common in East Africa.

53.3 HIV Pathophysiology

HIV is transmitted through contact with blood and blood-related products, as well as semen, vaginal fluid, pre-ejaculate, and breast milk. Thus, HIV is transmitted both parenterally and sexually. HIV disease is characterized by an acquired immunodeficiency resulting from a progressive quantitative and qualitative deficiency in the subset CD4+ T lymphocytes. The host's risk of becoming infected with opportunistic diseases increases as their number of CD4+ T cells fall.

During initial HIV infection, the virus undergoes significant replication in the CD4 T cells prior to the initiation of an HIV-specific immune response, resulting in an explosion of viremia and spread of the virus to various organ tissues [7]. A clinically latent phase ranging from weeks to years is followed by a chronic and progressive phase of viral replication. The destruction of CD4 cells results in decreased immunity, resulting in opportunistic infections as well as increased risk of malignancy. The HIV epidemic has created a surge of opportunistic diseases that were previously uncommon in medicine.

53.4 HIV Vaccines

Once HIV was discovered to be the causative agent of AIDS, considerable scientific energy was devoted to the development of a vaccine. A successful vaccine must either prevent infection in HIV-negative individuals, or at least reduce the viral load in those already infected. There are multiple HIV vaccine classes currently under study. These classes include: fowlpox vector vaccines, canarypox vectors, DNA plasmid vaccines, lipopeptides, live-attenuated vesicular stomatitis virus vectors, modified vaccinia Ankara (MVA) vector vaccines, nonreplicating adenoviral vector vaccines, peptides, proteins, and VEE Vectors (see Table 53.1).

Table 53.1 List of HIV vaccine classes under study

HIV Vaccine Classes Under Study
Fowlpox vector vaccines
Nonreplicating adenoviral vector vaccines
DNA plasmid vaccines
Canarypox vectors
Lipopeptides
Live-attenuated vesicular stomatitis virus vectors
Modified vaccinia ankara (MVA) vector vaccines
Nonreplicating adenoviral vector vaccines
Peptides
Proteins
VEE vectors

53.4.1 Fowlpox Vector Vaccines

Poxviruses such as canarypox, vaccinia, and fowlpox are the most commonly used live-vectors for HIV vaccines under investigation [8]. This is because poxviruses can both accommodate large amounts of foreign DNA and infect mammalian cells. This allows for the expression of a significant amount of foreign proteins [8].

The fowlpox virus (FPV) belongs to the *Poxviridae* family, genus *Avipoxvirus*. Although the fowlpox virus can only infect avian cells [8], avipox-based recombinants have demonstrated expression of foreign genes and the induction of protective immunity [9, 10].

Various studies suggest that mammalian species immunized by recombinant fowlpox virus can result in both humoral and cell-mediated immunity to the expressed transgene product without any resulting local or systemic adverse effects [8, 11–15].

53.4.1.1 Safety

The concern for potential systemic infection is minimal as fowlpox cannot replicate in nonavian species.

53.4.1.2 Immunogenicity

FPV vaccines have been utilized in various animal models for prevention of various infectious agents [9, 10, 12, 15, 16]. Protective immunogenicity from infectious agents, including immunodeficiency viruses and plasmodium parasites, has been demonstrated in various animal models.

An immunization series that consists of a DNA vaccine primer followed by a booster recombinant fowlpox-based vaccine has demonstrated some protection in animal primates after challenging them with an immunodeficiency virus [8].

53.4.2 Nonreplicating Adenoviral Vector Vaccines

Nonreplicating viral vector vaccines are created through deletion of one or more genes from a virus capable of entering human cells [17]. The deleted genes are then replaced by transgenes, which are inserted segments of DNA encoding HIV proteins. The result is a viral vector that is incapable of replication. The vector enables the HIV transgenes to enter the cells, resulting in expression of the HIV peptides or proteins [17].

Therefore, nonreplicating viral vector vaccines can carry HIV antigens into the cytoplasm of antigen-presenting cells without the risk of the host being infected with HIV. The viral antigens are processed with MHC class I and presented on the cell surface to CD8 cells, which creates an HIV-specific cytotoxic T-cell response [17].

Viral vectors composed of adenoviruses with gene deletions, referred to as adenovectors, are under study as potential HIV vaccines. Adenovectors were originally created to be used as gene therapy delivery vehicles [17]. The adenovirus type 5 (Ad5) vectors have been studied in animal and early clinical trials as possible HIV vaccines. The Ad5 vector is incapable of replication due to inactivation of the E1 gene. Adenovector HIV vaccines have significant prophylactic potential in that they have produced both high-titer antibody and high-frequency cytotoxic T cell (CTL) responses in animal models [18]. They have also shown protection in primates challenged with an immunodeficiency virus [18]. Some phase I studies that administered an adenoviral vector vaccine containing the HIV gag gene as a series of injections or as a booster following a primer DNA vaccine elicited significant Gag-specific CD8 responses in humans [17, 19].

53.4.2.1 Safety

Adenovectors have been evaluated as potential gene therapy agents for various human diseases, including cancer, cystic fibrosis, and cardiovascular disease. The majority of these have employed vectors based on Ad5. The adenovectors have also been administered via various routes such as aerosol, intradermal, intramyocardial, intrapleural, and intratumoral [17, 20–28]. Gene therapy studies with Ad5 have shown side effects to be mild, local, or absent in the majority of cases when the agents were administered intradermally or intramuscularly, and no significant toxicities due to the vector were reported [17, 20–28]. A dose-escalation trial of an HIV-1 Gag-Ad5 vaccine in humans demonstrated self-limited adverse events that were more common at higher doses of the vaccine as well as in subjects lacking pre-existing neutralizing antibody to Ad5. Such adverse events consisted of moderate reactions at the injection site, malaise, and myalgias [17].

The adenovectors under investigation in HIV vaccine studies have deletions in the E1 region and some in the E3 and/or E4 regions, which allow for the production of a vector that is incapable of replication. Nevertheless, all adenovectors are initially tested for cytopathic effects in tissue culture prior to use in human trials [17]. However, there is always the theoretical possibility that an adenovector vaccine could undergo recombination with a wild-type adenovirus that is concurrently infecting a vaccine recipient, leading to possible replication [17].

53.4.2.2 Immunogenicity

Studies in primates have illustrated the ability of adenovectors to induce strong CD8 T-cell responses to encoded HIV antigens as well as strong antibody responses [17, 18].

Ad5 is endemic in many areas. Neutralizing antibodies to Ad5 have been detected in 30–70% of vaccine trial participants in the United States and the seroprevalence of neutralizing antibodies to Ad5 is almost 90% in Sub-Saharan Africa [17]. A prior immunity to the Ad5 vector may lower the host's immune response to an Ad5 vaccine [17].

Theories in resolving this attenuation include increasing the vaccine dosage, using a heterologous prime-boost approach, or both [17, 18]. Boosters with adenovectors based on alterative serotypes, such as Ad24 or canarypox vector, have been associated with an improvement in cellular immune responses after administration of an Ad5-adenovector primer [17].

53.4.3 DNA Plasmid Vaccines

DNA vaccines often consist of plasmids with a gene encoding the target antigen that is transcriptionally controlled by a promoter region active in human cells. They are typically administered intramuscularly. DNA vaccines were first tested in persons who were already HIV-positive, and later studied as preventative vaccines in HIV-negative individuals [29, 30]. Humans have typically demonstrated weak immune responses to DNA alone; however, combination vaccines with adjuvants or with recombinant viral vectors in prime-boost approaches have demonstrated considerable HIV-specific CD8 responses and produced protective responses in primate models [30].

53.4.3.1 Safety

Studies indicate that DNA vaccines rarely integrate into cellular DNA. However, the risk of integration could potentially increase as vectors are modified or adjuvanted to increase immunogenicity. There is concern that an integrated vaccine could cause insertional mutagenesis through activation of oncogenes or inactivation of tumor suppressor genes [30]. There is also the theoretical possibility of an integrated plasmid DNA vaccine resulting in chromosomal instability by induction of chromosomal breaks or rearrangements [30].

Vaccine-associated autoimmunity is also another safety concern, but there are currently no definitive data supporting this possibility [30].

The production of DNA plasmids involves the selection of bacterial cells carrying the plasmid. Selection is obtained by culturing the cells in the presence of an antibiotic to which resistance is enabled by a gene in the plasmid. This leads to the concern that resistance to the same antibiotic might be acquired by vaccinees who receive the selected plasmid [30]. However, this concern is subdued by the fact that the antibiotic resistance genes contained in vaccine plasmids replicate through a bacterial origin of replication sequence rather than a mammalian one and are therefore unable to be expressed outside of bacterial cells [30]. In addition, the antibiotic that is selected is often not an antibiotic typically used to treat human infections [30].

53.4.3.2 Immunogenicity

The immune response to DNA vaccines is achieved through the uptake of plasmids into cells, such as dendritic and muscle cells, resulting in expression of the target antigen gene. Proteins are then produced and processed as intracytoplasmic antigens and subsequently as peptides that bind to Class I MHC molecules. The presentation of these peptides on the cell surface produces a CD8 T-lymphocyte response. The plasmid-encoded proteins also have been shown to stimulate an antibody response, signifying B lymphocyte stimulation. DNA vaccines thus mimic viral infection by stimulating both cellular and humoral immune responses [30].

DNA vaccine studies with primates that are later challenged with an immunodeficiency virus have shown that DNA vaccines provide a level of protection from HIV infection. These studies include vaccines such as a DNA plasmid primer with recombinant modified vaccinia Ankara (MVA) boost [31], DNA plasmid with cytokine (interleukin-2) adjuvant [32], DNA plasmid with nonionic blocked copolymer adjuvant, with or without recombinant adenovirus booster [18], DNA plasmid primer with recombinant fowlpox virus booster [15, 33, 34], and DNA plasmid primer with cytokine (interleukin-12) adjuvant plus recombinant gp140 protein boost [35].

Many other studies have failed to demonstrate protection in primates challenged with SIV or SHIV viruses after vaccination with DNA vaccine-containing regimens [36, 37].

53.4.4 Modified Vaccinia Ankara (MVA) Vector Vaccines

Modified Vaccinia Ankara (MVA) is a highly attenuated strain of vaccinia virus that was produced at the end of the smallpox eradication [38]. MVA lacks about 10% of the vaccinia genome and is incapable of efficiently replicating in primate cells [39], but is still able to provide similar levels of recombinant gene expression to vaccinia viruses in human cells [40].

53.4.4.1 Safety

MVA has been administered to various mammalian species [38, 41] without any reported serious adverse events. The use of MVA as a recombinant HIV vaccine is under clinical investigation in humans [38].

The vaccinia vaccine has some rare reported serious adverse events, such as myocarditis, pericarditis, and myopericarditis [38, 42]. Although MVA is an attenuated vaccinia virus and does not replicate in the human body as efficiently as vaccinia, it is not known if MVA can induce the same side-effects as vaccinia.

53.4.4.2 Immunogenicity

MVA vaccines have shown immunogenic and protective properties against infectious agents such as immunodeficiency viruses, influenza, parainfluenza, measles virus, flaviviruses, plasmodium parasites, and smallpox [38].

Viral vector vaccine combination studies have been conducted and have demonstrated significant prophylactic potential in mice models. For example, fowlpox-based and MVA-based vaccines in combination induce immunity and protection against challenge with Plasmodium parasites [43]. As previously mentioned, DNA-based HIV vaccines administered with recombinant MVA-based vaccine boosters expressing HIV antigen have some potential [31]. The immunization regimen combining a DNA-primer vaccine with a recombinant MVA-based vaccine booster has been shown to provide some protection in primates after challenging with an immunodeficiency virus. Unfortunately, vaccination did not prevent infection in these studies, but rather, resulted in lower viral loads, increased CD4 counts, and reduced rates of morbidity and mortality in vaccinated animals versus controls [31, 38, 44–46].

53.5 Potential HIV Microbicides

Since the introduction of an HIV vaccine is still years away, there is also HIV research focused on the production of vaginal and rectal microbicides for the prevention of HIV transmission. There are five classes of HIV microbicides that are divided according to where they disrupt the pathway of sexual transmission of HIV: surfactants/membrane disruptors, vaginal milieu protectors, viral entry inhibitors, reverse transcriptase inhibitors, and those of unknown mechanism [47].

53.5.1 Surfactants/Membrane Disruptors

Surfactants were the earliest agents investigated as topical HIV microbicides. They provide contraception and offer protection against many possible sexually transmitted diseases, including HIV. The first of these microbicides formally studied for HIV prevention was nonoxynol (N-9). N-9 is an effective over-the-counter spermicide and disrupts the HIV envelope [48–50]. However, clinical trials failed to reveal efficacy in HIV prevention and were associated with a higher incidence of genital ulcers [49].

Another studied agent is C31G (Savvy, Cellegy Pharmaceuticals, Quakertown, PA, USA), which is composed of cetyl betaine and myristamine oxide. It was demonstrated as safe and effective against bacteria such as *C. trachomatis*, as well as viruses such as HSV and HIV [51–53]. However, clinical trials did not reveal any statistically significant results due to the low HIV seroprevalence rate in the studies [47].

The "Invisible Condom"® consisting of sodium lauryl sulfate is a surfactant that has been demonstrated to disrupt both enveloped and nonenveloped viruses [54]. This compound covers the vaginal wall as a liquid at room temperature and then transforms into a gel at body temperature. The "invisible condom" is still under investigation.

53.5.2 Vaginal Milieu Protectors

Vaginal milieu protectors work by maintaining or enhancing the natural protective mechanisms of the vaginal canal provided by lactobacilli allowing for the acidic pH. A pH of 4–5.8 has been demonstrated to inactivate HIV [55–57]. Compounds currently under clinical investigation in this class include carbopol (BufferGel, ReProtect, Baltimore, MD, USA), which is a polyacrylic acid that buffers twice its volume of semen to a pH of 5 or less [58]. Animal and/or in vitro trials have shown BufferGel to be spermicidal as well as virucidal against HIV, HSV, and HPV [56, 59]. Another gel is Acidform®, which is already approved as a sexual lubricant, but is currently under study as a microbicide because of its acid-buffering and bioadhesive properties [47].

The use of exogenous lactobacilli for vaginal colonization is another strategy under investigation [60–63]. Bioengineered lactobacilli created to express proteins that bind to HIV and block viral fusion or host entry are also being developed [47].

53.5.3 Entry Inhibitors

Viral entry inhibitors can prevent HIV infection by blocking either the attachment of HIV to host cells, the fusion of HIV to the host cell, or the entry of HIV into host cells.

Anion polymers function as viral entry inhibitors by using their negative charge to interrelate with the HIV envelope proteins and impede the attachment of HIV to CD4+ cells [64, 65]. There are multiple anionic polymers under investigation as possible HIV microbicides.

CCR5 inhibitors also work as potential HIV entry inhibitors. Macrophage-tropic HIV strains can predominate in the early stages of viral transmission and require CCR5 as a co-receptor [66]. PSC-RANTES is a formulated inhibitor of the CCR5 coreceptor and has been demonstrated in vitro as having antiviral activity against all HIV clades as well as providing protection from SHIV SF126 in macaques [67–69]. CMPD167, consisting of cyclopentane, is another receptor antagonist that has provided promising results in animal model studies [70].

Compounds under development and/or testing as viral fusion inhibitors include C52-L, which inhibits gp41-mediated viral-cell fusion, and cyanovirin-N, a lectin agent extracted from cyanobacterium that prevents fusion by binding high mannose residues in the HIV envelope [70–72].

53.5.4 Reverse Transcriptase Inhibitors

The use of antiretrovirals, namely reverse transcriptase inhibitors, for HIV prevention is under investigation. The nucleoside reverse transcriptase inhibitor, tenofovir, is active as a diphosphate and has a prolonged intracellular half-life of 5–50 h, depending on the cell type [73, 74]. Tenofovir was shown to be successful as pre-exposure prophylaxis in macaques [75, 76]. The use of vaginal tenofovir gel is being studied in clinical trials. There are also two nonnucleoside reverse transcriptase inhibitors (NNRTIs), TMC120 and UC781, that are in clinical trials as potential topical microbicides. Both TMC120 and UC781 appear to have low systemic absorption, good safety profiles and unlike first generation NNRTs, they usually require at least two mutations for viral resistance to occur, rather than one [77–81]. TMC120 is also in clinical trials as a slow release vaginal ring, allowing for monthly dosing [47].

53.5.5 Microbicide Agents with Unknown Mechanism

There are several agents under study as potential microbicides whose mechanisms of action are not fully understood yet. One such agent is Praneem (Panacea Biotech Ltd, New Delhi, India), which is developed from a mixture of extracts from the Indian neem tree (*Azadirachta indica*), saponins from *Sapindus mukorossi* trees, and menthe citrate oil [82]. Praneem was originally created as a spermicide, but appears to have antimicrobial and antiviral properties and is currently in clinical trials [82–85].

53.6 HIV Prevention: Behavioral and Social Aspects

53.6.1 Education

Access to education alone promotes HIV prevention. There is a strong correlation between higher levels of education and safer sex practices, as well as delayed sexual debut [86]. Moreover, school attendance allows students to have access to sexual education and HIV prevention programs. There is a preconceived notion that sexual education programs would encourage earlier sexual activity; however, data support that sex education delays the onset of sexual intercourse and is associated with safer sex practices in those educated [86]. For those who do not have access to formal schooling, peer education and community education activities allow for all socioeconomic classes to be educated in HIV-preventative issues (see Table 53.2).

53.6.2 Prevention of Mother-to-Child Transmission

In addition to preventing HIV infection in females, as well as preventing unintended pregnancies in women who are already HIV-positive, there is also the important aspect of preventing vertical transmission of HIV from mother to child. First, HIV testing should be available to all pregnant women. This allows for early initiation of antiretroviral agents to HIV-positive pregnant women in addition to proper healthcare and support. Antiretroviral therapy administered in a timely manner causes a significantly decreased rate of vertical HIV transmission [87, 88].

53.6.3 Safe Sex Practices

The male latex condom is the most cost-effective and most easily available method of reducing the risk of

Table 53.2 HIV prevention methods

HIV Prevention Methods	Supportive Strategies
Education	Access to education, sex education
Prevention of mother-to-child transmission	HIV testing for pregnant women, early initiation of antiretroviral therapy for HIV-positive women
Safe sex practices	Male and female condoms
Male circumcision	Education
Universal precautions and blood safety	Providing clean needles to IV drug users, use of gloves and protective equipment
HIV postexposure prophylaxis	Initiate prior to 48 h from exposure as a 28-day course
Microbicides	Surfactants/membrane disruptors, vaginal milieu protectors, entry inhibitors, reverse transcriptase inhibitors
Pre-exposure prophylaxis	For use in high-risk individuals. Under investigation

HIV transmission, in addition to other sexually transmitted diseases [89]. The female condom is also just as effective as the male condom in reducing HIV transmission and is progressively becoming more available [89]. The advantages of using condoms should be incorporated in sexual education programs and should take into account cultural beliefs of the target population. The general population should have the knowledge to use them properly and should have male and female condoms available in order to maximize the effectiveness of safe sex practices and sexual/HIV education [89].

53.6.4 HIV Prevention Among Key Populations

It is important to recognize the patient populations that are at most risk for HIV infection so that preventative resources may be allocated appropriately. For example, sex workers, men who have sex with men, IV drug users, and prisoners are at higher risk for HIV infection than the general population. According to UNAIDS (Joint United Nations Programme on HIV/AIDS), to ensure the most effective use of resources, HIV prevention programs should place priority on high-risk populations and should be guided by epidemiological surveillance [90]. In addition, it is critical that people who are already HIV infected be incorporated into HIV prevention strategies [90].

53.6.5 Male Circumcision

Male circumcision has proven to significantly reduce the risk of heterosexual HIV transmission [91]. Based on clinical evidence and need to reduce the rate of HIV transmission, the World Health Organization (WHO) and the UNAIDS recommended that male circumcision be recognized as an important aspect of aiding in HIV prevention in heterosexual men [91]. (For further reading see chapter 54, page 715–739).

53.6.6 Universal Precautions and Blood Safety

Direct exposure to HIV in blood is the most effective mode of HIV transmission, although not the most frequent cause of transmission. Preventing unsafe injections and providing clean needles can aid in HIV prevention. In the healthcare setting, adherence to universal precautions such as routine use of gloves, use of protective equipment, safe disposal of needles and other sharp objects, and timely administration of a 4-week prophylactic course of antiretroviral medication when indicated are paramount to HIV prevention in the healthcare setting [92]. Proper training of workers who may potentially be exposed to body fluids is another effective prevention strategy. HIV transmission through blood transfusions is relatively uncommon, especially in developed countries. However, the incidence is higher in areas with weak healthcare systems, as well as when blood supplies are scarce such as during wars, disasters, or epidemics [92].

53.6.7 Postexposure Prophylaxis

Postexposure HIV prophylaxis (HIV-PEP) is the immediate administration of antiretroviral medications after exposure to HIV-infected blood or bodily fluids in order to prevent HIV seroconversion. HIV-PEP is most effective when initiated prior to 48 h postexposure and is not effective when initiated after 72 h from exposure [93–95]. It is also most effective when administered as a 28-day course of drug therapy, rather than a 3 or 10 days course [93–95]. Since HIV-PEP is not 100% effective, primary HIV prevention must also be stressed [93]. Many developed countries utilize HIV-PEP after possible occupational exposures in healthcare settings. HIV-PEP is also being progressively used and/or studied in other situations such as sexual assault survivors, rape survivors in refugee camps, and persons in high-risk communities [93]. There is no evidence linking risk behavior with HIV-PEP use or in communities in which HIV-PEP is available [96]. Both the International Labour Organization and the WHO concluded in 2005 that HIV-PEP must be part of comprehensive HIV prevention, occupational health, and postrape care service policies [93, 94].

53.7 Pre-exposure Prophylaxis

There is significant evidence suggesting the use of antiretroviral drugs in reducing the risk of HIV infection. The CDC, the National Institutes of Health

(NIH), and Family Health International (FHI) are among the organizations that are sponsoring clinical trials of pre-exposure prophylaxis (PrEP). The use of an antiretroviral drug taken as a daily oral preventative is the same rational as the use of prophylactic antimalarial medication taken prior to traveling to malaria-endemic areas. An effective daily preventative treatment could provide a female-controlled prevention method and therefore reduce HIV infections in high-risk individuals [97].

The concept behind this form of prevention is that if HIV replication could be inhibited when the virus first enters the body, then it may not be able to establish a permanent infection [97]. Other proven preventive measures such as postexposure prophylaxis and antiretroviral treatment to prevent mother-to-child transmission support PrEP. Primate studies have demonstrated that tenofovir can reduce the transmission of an immunodeficiency virus when administered before and immediately after a single retroviral exposure [98–100]. Furthermore, pre-exposure tenofovir plus emtricitabine has shown to provide significant protection to primates that were repeatedly exposed to an immunodeficiency virus [98, 100]. Both tenofovir and tenofovir plus emtricitabine have favorable resistance and safety profiles. Also, the fact that the drugs are taken orally once daily with or without food make them convenient for patients and thus encourages medication compliance [97]. The use of PrEP is promising as an effective HIV-prevention strategy, but clinical trial results must first be obtained to verify this possibility.

53.8 Conclusion

With the HIV-epidemic still ongoing worldwide, it is critical that HIV-prevention methods continue to be implemented and evaluated, see Table 53.2. The preventative measures discussed within this chapter are not to be used solely, but would provide the highest yield when used in combination and effectively. It is critical that a strong healthcare infrastructure be in place in order to provide appropriate HIV-preventive measures.

Take-Home Pearls

- Sex education delays the onset of sexual intercourse and is associated with safer sex practices.
- Antiretroviral therapy administered in a timely manner causes a significantly decreased rate of vertical HIV transmission.
- The male latex condom is the most cost-effective and most easily available method of reducing the risk of HIV transmission.
- Male circumcision has proven to significantly reduce the risk of heterosexual HIV transmission.
- Universal precautions such as routine use of gloves, use of protective equipment, safe disposal of needles and other sharp objects, and timely administration of a four-week prophylactic course of antiretroviral medication when indicated are paramount to HIV prevention in the healthcare setting.
- Multiple HIV vaccines and microbicides are currently under study.

References

1. UNAIDS: 2008 Report on the global AIDS epidemic. http://www.unaids.org/en/KnowledgeCentre/HIVData/GlobalReport/2008/2008_Global_report.asp). Accessed 3 Jan 2009
2. Cases of HIV Infection and AIDS in the United States and Dependent Areas: Centers for Disease Control and Prevention, Atlanta (2006)
3. Hirsch, M.S., Curran, J.: Human immunodeficiency viruses. In: Fields, B.N. (ed.) Virology, 4th edn, pp. 1953–1975. Lipincott-Raven, Philadelphia (1990)
4. Sierra, S., Kupfer, B., Kaiser, R.: Basics of the virology of HIV-1 and its replication. J. Clin. Virol. **34**(4), 233–244 (2005)
5. Moore, J.P., Jameson, B.A., Weiss, R.A., Sattentau, Q.J. (eds.): The HIV-Cell Fusion Reaction. CRC, Boca Raton (1993)
6. Clapham, P.R., McKnight, A.: Cell surface receptors, virus entry and tropism of primate lentiviruses. J. Gen. Virol. **83**(Pt 8), 1809–1829 (2002)
7. Dennis, L., Kasper, E.B., Fauci, A., Hauser, S., Longo, D., Jameson, J.L. (eds.): Harrison's Principles of Internal Medicine, 16th edn. McGraw-Hill Professional, New York (2004)
8. Philippon, V.: Class: fowlpox vector vaccines. http://chi.ucsf.edu/vaccines/vaccines?page=vc-01-03 (2008). Accessed 15 Dec 2008

9. Taylor, J., Weinberg, R., Kawaoka, Y., Webster, R.G., Paoletti, E.: Protective immunity against avian influenza induced by a fowlpox virus recombinant. Vaccine **6**(6), 504–508 (1988)
10. Taylor, J., Weinberg, R., Languet, B., Desmettre, P., Paoletti, E.: Recombinant fowlpox virus inducing protective immunity in non-avian species. Vaccine **6**(6), 497–503 (1988)
11. Kent, S.J., Stallard, V., Corey, L., et al.: Analysis of cytotoxic T lymphocyte responses to SIV proteins in SIV-infected macaques using antigen-specific stimulation with recombinant vaccinia and fowl poxviruses. AIDS Res. Hum. Retroviruses **10**(5), 551–560 (1994)
12. Kent, S.J., Zhao, A., Best, S.J., Chandler, J.D., Boyle, D.B., Ramshaw, I.A.: Enhanced T-cell immunogenicity and protective efficacy of a human immunodeficiency virus type 1 vaccine regimen consisting of consecutive priming with DNA and boosting with recombinant fowlpox virus. J. Virol. **72**(12), 10180–10188 (1998)
13. Nacsa, J., Radaelli, A., Edghill-Smith, Y., et al.: Avipox-based simian immunodeficiency virus (SIV) vaccines elicit a high frequency of SIV-specific CD4+ and CD8+ T-cell responses in vaccinia-experienced SIVmac251-infected macaques. Vaccine **22**(5–6), 597–606 (2004)
14. Radaelli, A., Zanotto, C., Perletti, G., et al.: Comparative analysis of immune responses and cytokine profiles elicited in rabbits by the combined use of recombinant fowlpox viruses, plasmids and virus-like particles in prime-boost vaccination protocols against SHIV. Vaccine **21**(17–18), 2052–2064 (2003)
15. Robinson, H.L., Montefiori, D.C., Johnson, R.P., et al.: Neutralizing antibody-independent containment of immunodeficiency virus challenges by DNA priming and recombinant pox virus booster immunizations. Nat. Med. **5**(5), 526–534 (1999)
16. Kent, S.J., Zhao, A., Dale, C.J., Land, S., Boyle, D.B., Ramshaw, I.A.: A recombinant avipoxvirus HIV-1 vaccine expressing interferon-gamma is safe and immunogenic in macaques. Vaccine **18**(21), 2250–2256 (2000)
17. Peiperl, L.: Class: nonreplicating adenoviral vector vaccines. http://chi.ucsf.edu/vaccines/vaccines?page=vc-01-02 (2008). Accessed 14 Dec 2008
18. Shiver, J.W., Fu, T.M., Chen, L., et al.: Replication-incompetent adenoviral vaccine vector elicits effective anti-immunodeficiency-virus immunity. Nature **415**(6869), 331–335 (2002)
19. Harvey, B.G., Leopold, P.L., Hackett, N.R., et al.: Airway epithelial CFTR mRNA expression in cystic fibrosis patients after repetitive administration of a recombinant adenovirus. J. Clin. Invest. **104**(9), 1245–1255 (1999)
20. Hay, J.G., McElvaney, N.G., Herena, J., Crystal, R.G.: Modification of nasal epithelial potential differences of individuals with cystic fibrosis consequent to local administration of a normal CFTR cDNA adenovirus gene transfer vector. Hum. Gene Ther. **6**(11), 1487–1496 (1995)
21. Harvey, B.G., Worgall, S., Ely, S., Leopold, P.L., Crystal, R.G.: Cellular immune responses of healthy individuals to intradermal administration of an E1-E3- adenovirus gene transfer vector. Hum. Gene Ther. **10**(17), 2823–2837 (1999)
22. Rosengart, T.K., Lee, L.Y., Patel, S.R., et al.: Six-month assessment of a phase I trial of angiogenic gene therapy for the treatment of coronary artery disease using direct intramyocardial administration of an adenovirus vector expressing the VEGF121 cDNA. Ann. Surg. **230**(4), 466–470 (1999); discussion 70–72
23. Rosengart, T.K., Lee, L.Y., Patel, S.R., et al.: Angiogenesis gene therapy: phase I assessment of direct intramyocardial administration of an adenovirus vector expressing VEGF121 cDNA to individuals with clinically significant severe coronary artery disease. Circulation **100**(5), 468–474 (1999)
24. Sterman, D.H., Treat, J., Litzky, L.A., et al.: Adenovirus-mediated herpes simplex virus thymidine kinase/ganciclovir gene therapy in patients with localized malignancy: results of a phase I clinical trial in malignant mesothelioma. Hum. Gene Ther. **9**(7), 1083–1092 (1998)
25. Clayman, G.L., Frank, D.K., Bruso, P.A., Goepfert, H.: Adenovirus-mediated wild-type p53 gene transfer as a surgical adjuvant in advanced head and neck cancers. Clin. Cancer Res. **5**(7), 1715–1722 (1999)
26. Swisher, S.G., Roth, J.A., Nemunaitis, J., et al.: Adenovirus-mediated p53 gene transfer in advanced non-small-cell lung cancer. J. Natl. Cancer Inst. **91**(9), 763–771 (1999)
27. Gahery-Segard, H., Molinier-Frenkel, V., Le Boulaire, C., et al.: Phase I trial of recombinant adenovirus gene transfer in lung cancer. Longitudinal study of the immune responses to transgene and viral products. J. Clin. Invest. **100**(9), 2218–2226 (1997)
28. Tursz, T., Cesne, A.L., Baldeyrou, P., et al.: Phase I study of a recombinant adenovirus-mediated gene transfer in lung cancer patients. J. Natl. Cancer Inst. **88**(24), 1857–1863 (1996)
29. Boyer, J.D., Cohen, A.D., Vogt, S., et al.: Vaccination of seronegative volunteers with a human immunodeficiency virus type 1 env/rev DNA vaccine induces antigen-specific proliferation and lymphocyte production of beta-chemokines. J. Infect. Dis. **181**(2), 476–483 (2000)
30. Peiperl. L.: DNA plasmid vaccines. http://chi.ucsf.edu/vaccines/vaccines?page=vc-01-01 (2008). Accessed 15 Dec 2008
31. Amara, R.R., Villinger, F., Altman, J.D., et al.: Control of a mucosal challenge and prevention of AIDS by a multiprotein DNA/MVA vaccine. Science (New York, NY) **292**(5514), 69–74 (2001)
32. Barouch, D.H., Santra, S., Schmitz, J.E., et al.: Control of viremia and prevention of clinical AIDS in rhesus monkeys by cytokine-augmented DNA vaccination. Science (New York, NY) **290**(5491), 486–492 (2000)
33. Amara, R.R., Villinger, F., Staprans, S.I., et al.: Different patterns of immune responses but similar control of a simian-human immunodeficiency virus 89.6P mucosal challenge by modified vaccinia virus Ankara (MVA) and DNA/MVA vaccines. J. Virol. **76**(15), 7625–7631 (2002)
34. Wee, E.G., Patel, S., McMichael, A.J., Hanke, T.: A DNA/MVA-based candidate human immunodeficiency virus vaccine for Kenya induces multi-specific T cell responses in rhesus macaques. J. Gen. Virol. **83**(Pt 1), 75–80 (2002)
35. Habel, A., Chanel, C., Le Grand, R., et al.: DNA vaccine protection against challenge with simian/human immunodeficiency virus 89.6 in rhesus macaques. Dev. Biol. **104**, 101–105 (2000)
36. Hanke, T., Samuel, R.V., Blanchard, T.J., et al.: Effective induction of simian immunodeficiency virus-specific cytotoxic T lymphocytes in macaques by using a multiepitope gene and DNA prime-modified vaccinia virus Ankara boost vaccination regimen. J. Virol. **73**(9), 7524–7532 (1999)

37. Horton, H., Vogel, T.U., Carter, D.K., et al.: Immunization of rhesus macaques with a DNA prime/modified vaccinia virus Ankara boost regimen induces broad simian immunodeficiency virus (SIV)-specific T-cell responses and reduces initial viral replication but does not prevent disease progression following challenge with pathogenic SIVmac239. J. Virol. **76**(14), 7187–7202 (2002)
38. Philippon, V.: Class: modified vaccinia ankara (MVA) vectorvaccines.http://chi.ucsf.edu/vaccines/vaccines?page=vc-01-04 (2008). Accessed 14 Dec 2008
39. Meyer, H., Sutter, G., Mayr, A.: Mapping of deletions in the genome of the highly attenuated vaccinia virus MVA and their influence on virulence. J. Gen. Virol. **72**(Pt 5), 1031–1038 (1991)
40. Sutter, G., Moss, B.: Nonreplicating vaccinia vector efficiently expresses recombinant genes. Proc. Natl. Acad. Sci. USA **89**(22), 10847–10851 (1992)
41. Stittelaar, K.J., Kuiken, T., de Swart, R.L., et al.: Safety of modified vaccinia virus Ankara (MVA) in immune-suppressed macaques. Vaccine **19**(27), 3700–3709 (2001)
42. Centers for Disease Control and Prevention: Smallpox vaccination. http:www.bt.cdc.gov/agent/smallpox/vaccination). Accessed 14 Dec 2008
43. Anderson, R.J., Hannan, C.M., Gilbert, S.C., et al.: Enhanced CD8+ T cell immune responses and protection elicited against Plasmodium berghei malaria by prime boost immunization regimens using a novel attenuated fowlpox virus. J. Immunol. **172**(5), 3094–3100 (2004)
44. Verrier, B., Le Grand, R., Ataman-Onal, Y., et al.: Evaluation in rhesus macaques of Tat and rev-targeted immunization as a preventive vaccine against mucosal challenge with SHIV-BX08. DNA Cell Biol. **21**(9), 653–658 (2002)
45. Barouch, D.H., Santra, S., Kuroda, M.J., et al.: Reduction of simian-human immunodeficiency virus 89.6P viremia in rhesus monkeys by recombinant modified vaccinia virus Ankara vaccination. J. Virol. **75**(11), 5151–5158 (2001)
46. Muthumani, K., Bagarazzi, M., Conway, D., et al.: A Gag-Pol/Env-Rev SIV239 DNA vaccine improves CD4 counts, and reduce viral loads after pathogenic intrarectal SIV(mac)251 challenge in rhesus Macaques. Vaccine **21**(7–8), 629–637 (2003)
47. Cutler, B., Justman, J.: Vaginal microbicides and the prevention of HIV transmission. Lancet Infect. Dis. **8**(11), 685–697 (2008 Nov)
48. Van Damme, L., Ramjee, G., Alary, M., et al.: Effectiveness of COL-1492, a nonoxynol-9 vaginal gel, on HIV-1 transmission in female sex workers: a randomized controlled trial. Lancet **360**, 971–977 (2002)
49. Roddy, R.E., Zekeng, L., Ryan, K.A., Tamoufe, U., Weir, S.S., Wong, E.L.: A controlled trial of nonoxynol-9 film to reduce male-to-female transmission of sexually transmitted diseases. N. Engl. J. Med. **339**, 504–510 (1998)
50. Bourinbaiar, A.S., Lee-Huang, S.: The efficacy of nonoxynol-9 from an in vitro point of view. AIDS **10**, 558–559 (1996)
51. Bax, R., Douville, K., McCormick, D., Rosenberg, M., Higgins, J., Bowden, M.: Microbicides—evaluating multiple formulations of C31G. Contraception **66**, 365–368 (2002)
52. Ballagh, S.A., Baker, J.M., Henry, D.M., Archer, D.F.: Safety of single daily use for one week of C31G HEC gel in women. Contraception **66**, 369–375 (2002)
53. Mauck, C.K., Weiner, D.H., Creinin, M.D., Barnhart, K.T., Callahan, M.M., Bax, R.: A randomized phase I vaginal safety study of three concentrations of C31G vs extra strength gynol II. Contraception **70**, 233–240 (2004)
54. Piret, J., Desormeaux, A., Bergeron, M.G.: Sodium lauryl sulfate, a microbicide effective against enveloped and non-enveloped viruses. Curr. Drug Targets **3**, 17–30 (2002)
55. Martin, L.S., McDougal, J.S., Loskoski, S.L.: Disinfection and inactivation of the human T lymphotropic virus type III/lymphadenopathy-associated virus. J. Infect. Dis. **152**(2), 400–403 (1985)
56. Ongradi, J., Ceccherini-Nelli, L., Pistello, M., Specter, S., Bendinelli, M.: Acid sensitivity of cell-free and cell-associated HIV-1: clinical implications. AIDS Res. Hum. Retroviruses **6**, 1433–1436 (1990)
57. O'Connor, T.J., Kinchington, D., Kangro, H.O., Jeffries, D.J.: The activity of candidate virucidal agents, low pH and genital secretions against HIV-1 in vitro. Int. J. STD AIDS **6**, 267–272 (1995)
58. Olmsted, S.S., Dubin, N.H., Cone, R.A., Moench, T.R.: The rate at which human sperms are immobilized and killed by mild acidity. Fertil. Steril. **73**, 687–693 (2000)
59. Zeitlin, L., Hoen, T.E., Achilles, S.L., et al.: Tests of Buffergel for contraception and prevention of sexually transmitted diseases in animal models. Sex. Transm. Dis. **28**, 417–423 (2001)
60. Klebanoff, S.J., Coombs, R.W.: Viricidal effect of Lactobacillus acidophilus on human immunodeficiency virus type 1: possible role in heterosexual transmission. J. Exp. Med. **174**, 289–292 (1991)
61. Martin, H.L., Richardson, B.A., Nyange, P.M., et al.: Vaginal lactobacilli, microbial flora, and risk of human immunodeficiency virus type 1 and sexually transmitted disease acquisition. J. Infect. Dis. **180**, 1863–1868 (1999)
62. Patton, D.L., Sweeney YT, Cosgrove, Antonio, M.A., Rabe, L.K., Hillier, S.L.: Lactobacillus crispatus capsules: single-use safety study in the Macaca nemestrina model. Sex. Transm. Dis. **30**, 568–570 (2003)
63. Antonio, M.A., Hillier, S.L.: DNA fingerprinting of Lactobacillus crispatus strain CTV-05 by repetitive element sequence-based PCR analysis in a pilot study of vaginal colonization. J. Clin. Microbiol. **41**, 1881–1887 (2003)
64. Schols, D., Pauwels, R., Desmyter, J., De, C.E.: Dextran sulfate and other polyanionic anti-HIV compounds specifically interact with the viral gp120 glycoprotein expressed by T-cells persistently infected with HIV-1. Virology **175**, 556–561 (1990)
65. Mitsuya, H., Looney, D.J., Kuno, S., Ueno, R., Wong-Staal, F., Broder, S.: Dextran sulfate suppression of viruses in the HIV family: inhibition of virion binding to CD4+ cells. Science **240**, 646–649 (1988)
66. Maeda, K., Nakata, H., Ogata, H., Koh, Y., Miyakawa, T., Mitsuya, H.: The current status of, and challenges in, the development of CCR5 inhibitors as therapeutics for HIV-1 infection. Curr. Opin. Pharmacol. **4**, 447–452 (2004)
67. Lederman, M.M., Veazey, R.S., Offord, R., et al.: Prevention of vaginal SHIV transmission in rhesus macaques through inhibition of CCR5. Science **306**, 485–487 (2004)
68. Torre, V.S., Marozsan, A.J., Albright, J.L., et al.: Variable sensitivity of CCR5-tropic human immunodeficiency virus type 1 isolates to inhibition by RANTES analogs. J. Virol. **74**, 4868–4876 (2000)
69. Kawamura, T., Gulden, F.O., Sugaya, M., et al.: R5 HIV productively infects Langerhans cells, and infection levels

are regulated by compound CCR5 polymorphisms. Proc. Natl Acad. Sci. USA **100**, 8401–8406 (2003)
70. Veazey, R.S., Klasse, P.J., Schader, S.M., et al.: Protection of macaques from vaginal SHIV challenge by vaginally delivered inhibitors of virus-cell fusion. Nature **438**, 99–102 (2005)
71. Lu, M.: Stabilizing peptides and their use in the preparation of stabilized HIV inhibitors. World Intellectual Property Organization Patent WO-04/106364A1 (2004)
72. Bewley, C.A., Otero-Quintero, S.: The potent anti-HIV protein cyanovirin-N contains two novel carbohydrate binding sites that selectively bind to Man(8) D1D3 and Man(9) with nanomolar affinity: implications for binding to the HIV envelope protein gp120. J. Am. Chem. Soc. **123**, 3892–3902 (2001)
73. Balzarini, J., Zhang, H., Herdewijn, P., Johns, D., De Clercq, E.: Intracellular metabolism and mechanism of antiretrovirus action of 9-(2-phosphony lmethoxyethyl) adenine, a potent anti-human immunodeficiency virus compound. Proc. Natl Acad. Sci. USA **88**, 1499–1503 (1991)
74. Aquaro, S., Caliò, R., Balzarini, J., Bellocchi, M.C., Garaci, E., Perno, C.F.: Macrophages and HIV infection: therapeutical approaches toward this strategic virus reservoir. Antiviral Res. **55**, 209–225 (2002)
75. Tsai, C.C., Follis, K.E., Sabo, A., et al.: Prevention of SIV infection in macaques by (R)-9-(2-phosphonylmethoxypropyl)adenine. Science **270**, 1197–1199 (1995)
76. Otten, R.A., Smith, D.K., Adams, D.R., et al.: Efficacy of post exposure prophylaxis after intravaginal exposure of pig-tailed macaques to a human-derived retrovirus (human immunodeficiency virus type 2). J. Virol. **74**, 9771–9775 (2000)
77. Balzarini, J., Pelemans, H., Aquaro, S., et al.: Highly favorable antiviral activity and resistance profile of the novel thiocarboxanilide pentenyloxy ether derivatives UC-781 and UC-82 as inhibitors of human immunodeficiency virus type 1 replication. Mol. Pharmacol. **50**, 394–401 (1996)
78. Borkow, G., Barnard, J., Nguyen, T.M., Belmonte, A., Wainberg, M.A., Parniak, M.A.: Chemical barriers to human immunodeficiency virus type 1 (HIV-1) infection: retrovirucidal activity of UC781, a thiocarboxanilide nonnucleoside inhibitor of HIV-1 reverse transcriptase. J. Virol. **71**, 3023–3030 (1997)
79. Buckheit, R.W., Snow, M.J., Fliakas-Boltz, V., et al.: Highly potent oxathiin carboxanilide derivatives with efficacy against nonnucleoside reverse transcriptase inhibitor-resistant human immunodeficiency virus isolates. Antimicrob. Agents Chemother. **41**, 831–837 (1997)
80. Balzarini, J., Naesens, L., Verbeken, E., et al.: Preclinical studies on thiocarboxanilide UC-781 as a virucidal agent. AIDS **12**, 1129–1138 (1998)
81. Di Fabio, S., Van, R.J., Giannini, G., et al.: Inhibition of vaginal transmission of HIV-1 in hu-SCID mice by the nonnucleoside reverse transcriptase inhibitor TMC120 in a gel formulation. AIDS **17**, 1597–1604 (2003)
82. Talwar, G.P., Raghuvanshi, P., Mishra, R., et al.: Polyherbal formulations with wide spectrum antimicrobial activity against reproductive tract infections and sexually transmitted pathogens. Am. J. Reprod. Immunol. **43**, 144–151 (2000)
83. Joshi, S.N., Katti, U., Godbole, S., et al.: Phase I safety study of Praneem polyherbal vaginal tablet use among HIV-uninfected women in Pune, India. Trans. R. Soc. Trop. Med. Hyg. **99**, 769–774 (2005)
84. Joglekar, N.S., Joshi, S.N., Navlakha, S.N., Katti, U.R., Mehendale, S.M.: Acceptability of Praneem polyherbal vaginal tablet among HIV uninfected women and their male partners in Pune India—phase I study. Indian J. Med. Res. **123**, 547–552 (2006)
85. Josh, S.N., Dutta, S., Kumar, B.K., et al.: Expanded safety study of Praneem polyherbal vaginal tablet among HIV-uninfected women in Pune, India: a phase II clinical trial report. Sex. Transm. Infect. **84**, 343–37 (2008)
86. UNAIDS: Education: in and out of school settings. http://www.unaids.org/en/PolicyAndPractice/Prevention/Education/. . Accessed 29 Dec 2008
87. UNAIDS: Prevention of mother-to-child transmission of HIV. http://www.unaids.org/en/PolicyAndPractice/Prevention/PMTCT/. Accessed 29 Dec 2008
88. WHO: Guidance on global scale-up of the prevention of mother-to-child transmission of HIV. http://www.who.int/hiv/pub/guidelines/pmtct_scaleup2007/en/index.html. Accessed 29 Dec 2009
89. UNAIDS: Condoms. http://www.unaids.org/en/PolicyAndPractice/Prevention/Condoms/. Accessed 29 Dec 2008
90. UNAIDS: HIV prevention among key populations. http://www.unaids.org/en/PolicyAndPractice/Prevention/HIVprevKeyPopulations/. Accessed 29 Dec 2008
91. UNAIDS. Male circumcision: http://www.unaids.org/en/PolicyAndPractice/Prevention/MaleCircumcision/. Accessed 29 Dec 2008
92. UNAIDS: Universal precautions and blood safety. http://www.unaids.org/en/PolicyAndPractice/Prevention/UnivPrecaution/). Accessed 29 Dec 2008
93. UNAIDS: HIV post-exposure prophylaxis. http://www.unaids.org/en/PolicyAndPractice/Prevention/HIVPEP/. Accessed 29 Dec 2008
94. WHO. Post-exposure prophylaxis to prevent HIV transmission. http://www.who.int/hiv/pub/prophylaxis/pep_guidelines/en/index.html. Accessed 28 Dec 2008
95. Young, T., Arens, F., Kennedy, G., Laurie, J., Rutherford, G.: Antiretroviral post-exposure prophylaxis (PEP) for occupational HIV exposure. Cochrane Database Syst. Rev. **2007**, CD002835 (2007)
96. Martin, J.N., Roland, M.E., Neilands, T.B., Krone, M.R., Bamberger, J.D., et al.: Use of postexposure prophylaxis against HIV infection following sexual exposure does not lead to increases in high-risk behavior. AIDS **18**, 787–792 (2004)
97. CDC: CDC trials of pre-exposure prophylaxis for hiv prevention. http://www.cdc.gov/HIV/resources/factsheets/prep.htm. Accessed 2 Feb 2009
98. Tsai, C.C., Follis, K.E., Sabo, A., Beck, T.W., Grant, R.F., et al.: Prevention of SIV infection in macaques by (R)-9-(2-phosphonylmethoxypropyl)adenine. Science **270**, 1197–1199 (1995)
99. Van Rompay, K.K., Miller, M.D., Marthas, M.L., Margot, N.A., Dailey, P.J., et al.: Prophylactic and therapeutic benefits of short-term 9-[2-(R)-(phosphonomethoxy)propyl]adenine (PMPA) administration to newborn macaques following oral inoculation with simian immunodeficiency virus with reduced susceptibility to PMPA. J. Virol. **74**, 1767–1774 (2000)
100. Subbarao, S., Otten, R.A., Ramos, A., Kim, C., Jackson, E., et al.: Chemoprophylaxis with tenofovir disoproxil fumarate provided partial protection against infection with simian human immunodeficiency virus in macaques given multiple virus challenges. J. Infect. Dis. **194**, 904–911 (2006)

The Role of Circumcision in Preventing STIs

54

Brian J. Morris and Xavier Castellsague

Core Messages

- Male circumcision affords substantial protection against genital ulcer disease (GUD), human immunodeficiency virus (HIV), high-risk types of human papillomavirus (HPV), herpes simplex virus type 2 (HSV-2), *Treponema pallidum* (syphilis), *Haemophilus ducreyi* (chancroid), *Trichomonas vaginalis*, and *Candida albicans* (thrush).
- It offers little or no protection against *Neisseria gonorrhea*, *Chlamydia trachomatis*, and nonspecific urethritis.
- In the female sexual partner, circumcision of the male partner is associated with greatly reduced HPV, chlamydia, HSV-2, Trichomonas, and bacterial vaginosis.
- At the population level, increased rate of male circumcision should reduce heterosexually acquired HIV/AIDS, as well as genital HPV, penile and cervical cancer, prostate cancer, genital herpes, infertility in each sex, pelvic inflammatory disease, and ectopic pregnancy.
- Male circumcision is an important component of strategies to reduce the global burden of many STIs.

B.J. Morris (✉)
School of Medical Sciences and Bosch Institute, Sydney Medical School, The University of Sydney, Bldg F13, New South Wales, 2006, Australia
e-mail: brian.morris@sydney.edu.au

X. Castellsague
Cancer Epidemiology Research Program (CERP), Istitut Català d'Oncologia (ICO), Hospitalet de Llobregat, Av Gran Via s/n, Km. 2.7, Barcelona 08907, Spain
e-mail: xcastellsague@ico.scs.es

54.1 Introduction

This chapter describes the effect of male circumcision on incidence of various sexually transmitted infections (STIs). Protection against STIs is just one of the many benefits that circumcision confers [1, 2].

54.2 Ulcerative and Nonulcerative STIs Other Than HPV and HIV

The first medical link between circumcision and protection against STIs concerned syphilis in 1855 [3]. This was confirmed in 1891, when protection against genital herpes (HSV-2) and urethritis was also noted [4]. Subsequent reports showed protection against syphilis and chancroid, but for nonulcerative STIs and HSV-2, both protection (1.3- to 3-fold) or no protection have been reported [5–18].

The reports of protection against nonulcerative STIs tend to be in earlier studies and those in developing nations, whereas more recent studies have tended to show little or no difference. However, it is important to note that some of these data are based on studies of men attending STI clinics. Such data should be viewed with caution, since any protective effect afforded by circumcision against a particular STI will mean lower presentation of circumcised men to a STI clinic. For this reason, reports in the literature that involve STI clinic attendees are likely to be biased away from detection of association with lack of circumcision. Studies involving general populations are therefore more likely to yield reliable data.

A review in 1998 of 11 studies [19] noted only 2 of 6 studies that showed an association of HSV-2 with

G. Gross and S.K. Tyring (eds.), *Sexually Transmitted Infections and Sexually Transmitted Diseases*,
DOI: 10.1007/978-3-642-14663-3_54, © Springer-Verlag Berlin Heidelberg 2011

lack of circumcision [15, 17]. For gonorrhea, it was 5 of 7 [16, 20] and with chlamydial, nongonococcal, or other types of urethritis, 2 of 8 [6, 9, 16].

A meta-analysis of ulcerative STIs examined 26 research articles (from the United States, United Kingdom, Australia, Africa, India, and Peru) and found circumcision protected against chancroid and syphilis, but for HSV-2, it was only 12% lower [21] (Table 54.1).

Consistent with this, a study by the US Centers for Disease Control and Prevention found 12% lower HSV-2 seroprevalence (13.7% vs. 11.6%) in circumcised men [22]. HSV-2 infection per sex act was 0.013 in uncircumcised men, compared with 0.0074 in circumcised men (RR 0.56; $P = 0.005$) [23]. Two small longitudinal studies of STIs common in New Zealand produced conflicting results. One found a 3.2-fold higher rate of STIs, including 2.5 times more chlamydia, to age 25 in the uncircumcised men [24]. The other saw no difference [25]. This included similar HSV-2 seroprevalence [7].

In two randomized controlled trials (RCTs), lower HSV-2 seroprevalence was seen in the men who had been circumcised. HSV-2 was 45% lower in the trial in Orange Farm, South Africa [26], and was 30% lower in the trial in Rakai, Uganda [27]. Interestingly, although HSV-2 seroincidence has been found not to differ between circumcised and uncircumcised men [7, 28], the incidence of genital ulcer disease (GUD), including herpetic lesions, has been reported to be twice as high in uncircumcised men [29]. This might suggest that circumcision reduces the recurrence of genital lesions arising from HSV-2 infection. Such a possibility is supported by a small Indian study that found recurrence to be 20 times lower in men who underwent circumcision compared to men who remained uncircumcised, and interval between bouts was longer in the circumcised men [30]. A study of Black heterosexual 18–25-year-old men attending an STI clinic in the United States found that, although HSV-2 did not differ, the seroprevalence of HSV-1 was 2.8 times higher in those who were not circumcised [28].

Table 54.1 Meta-analysis, showing protection by circumcision against ulcerative STIs

STI	Studies	Relative Risk (Confidence Interval)
Syphilis	14 of 14 studies	0.61 (0.54–0.83) 0.53 (0.34–0.83)[a]
Chancroid	6 of 7 studies	0.12–1.11[b]
HSV-2	6 of 10 studies	0.88 (0.77–1.01)

[a]When circumcision was done prior to first sexual intercourse
[b]Individual study RR, since meta-analysis was not possible

The data emanating from Rakai, Uganda, was from two RCTs in that locality. One of these (RCT-2) involved men with a higher sexual-risk profile. An initial report, focused primarily on HIV prevention, found that circumcision afforded 48% protection against GUD [31]. In a subsequent report, GUD was 39% lower in circumcised men in RCT-2 but did not differ in RCT-1 [32]. Later, GUD was found to be present in 1.9% of uncircumcised men and 0.8% of those who had undergone circumcision, and period prevalence of GUD was reported as being 46% lower in the circumcised [33]. Circumcision was associated with a reduction in GUD of 49% in those who were HSV-2 seronegative. No difference in syphilis seroprevalence was found [32], but only 2% of men were infected with this STI. Although it was suggested at the time that the RCT might have been insufficiently powered to reach a valid conclusion [34], positive syphilis serology was, however, found in 7% of men in each group in a later report, which also tested for *T. pallidum* DNA and found positive results for this organism in 7/56 swabs from genital ulcers in uncircumcised men, but none of the ulcers in 25 circumcised men [33]. In this report, HSV-2 seroprevalence was 27% and 28% in each respective group, and in men with genital ulcers, HSV-2 DNA was found in 48% and 39% of swabs ($P = 0.62$) [33]. None of the ulcers in either group contained DNA for *Haemophilus ducreyi* or HSV-1. A large proportion of those whose test was STI negative had a non-STI as a cause of the ulceration. It was suggested that most of the ulcers were a result of infection by non-STI pathogens of tears in the foreskin and its attached frenulum, pointing out that tearing occurs commonly in uncircumcised men during intercourse [33].

Incident syphilis was 2.9 times lower in a study in Sydney, Australia, of circumcised, as opposed to uncircumcised, men who had sex with men (MSM), and was ten times lower in those who only engaged in insertive anal intercourse [35]. Similarly, a study of MSM in Seattle, USA, found syphilis to be twofold lower in those who were circumcised and was completely absent from the 11% who said they were insertive-only [36]. In the US study, seroprevalence of HSV-2 was 34% lower, although in this and the Australian study, the differences in HSV-2 and HSV-1 seroprevalence as a function of circumcision status were not statistically significant.

A meta-analysis by Van Howe that reported higher sexually acquired urethritis in circumcised men [37] has been shown to be erroneous, since, astonishingly, much of the data he used bore little resemblance to that in the source publications cited, leading to a published critique [38] and an erratum by the journal that effectively invalidates his conclusions [39].

For nonspecific urethritis (NSU), a meta-analysis of the 10 studies sourced in Van Howe's report shows that NSU was in fact slightly but not significantly lower (not higher) in circumcised men: summary OR = 0.92 (95% CI 0.64–1.3) [38].

Similar findings were obtained in the RCT in South Africa, the prevalence of gonorrhea being lower in circumcised men but not significantly so: adjusted odds ratio (AOR) = 0.91 [40]. In this trial, *Chlamydia trachomatis* was 42% lower, and *T. vaginalis* was 46% lower, the latter showing a statistically significant 51% reduction in an as-treated analysis, with AOR being 0.47 [41]. An RCT in Kenya, however, observed similar prevalence of *N. gonorrhea*, *C. trachomatis*, and *T. vaginalis* in circumcised and uncircumcised men [42].

In an Australian survey, circumcised men had less penile candidiasis (OR 0.40) [43], where yeast infection can follow female sexual contact.

Why does the prepuce increase risk? The warm moist environment under the prepuce favors bacterial replication. It traps microorganisms in a pool of smegma, so facilitating transmission. The inner preputial lining, being mucosal, is delicate, so it and the frenulum can tear during intercourse (Fig. 54.1). The prepuce presents a larger area for infection. As such, it is more prone to Chancroid, although syphilis and HSV-2 infect the genitalia more widely.

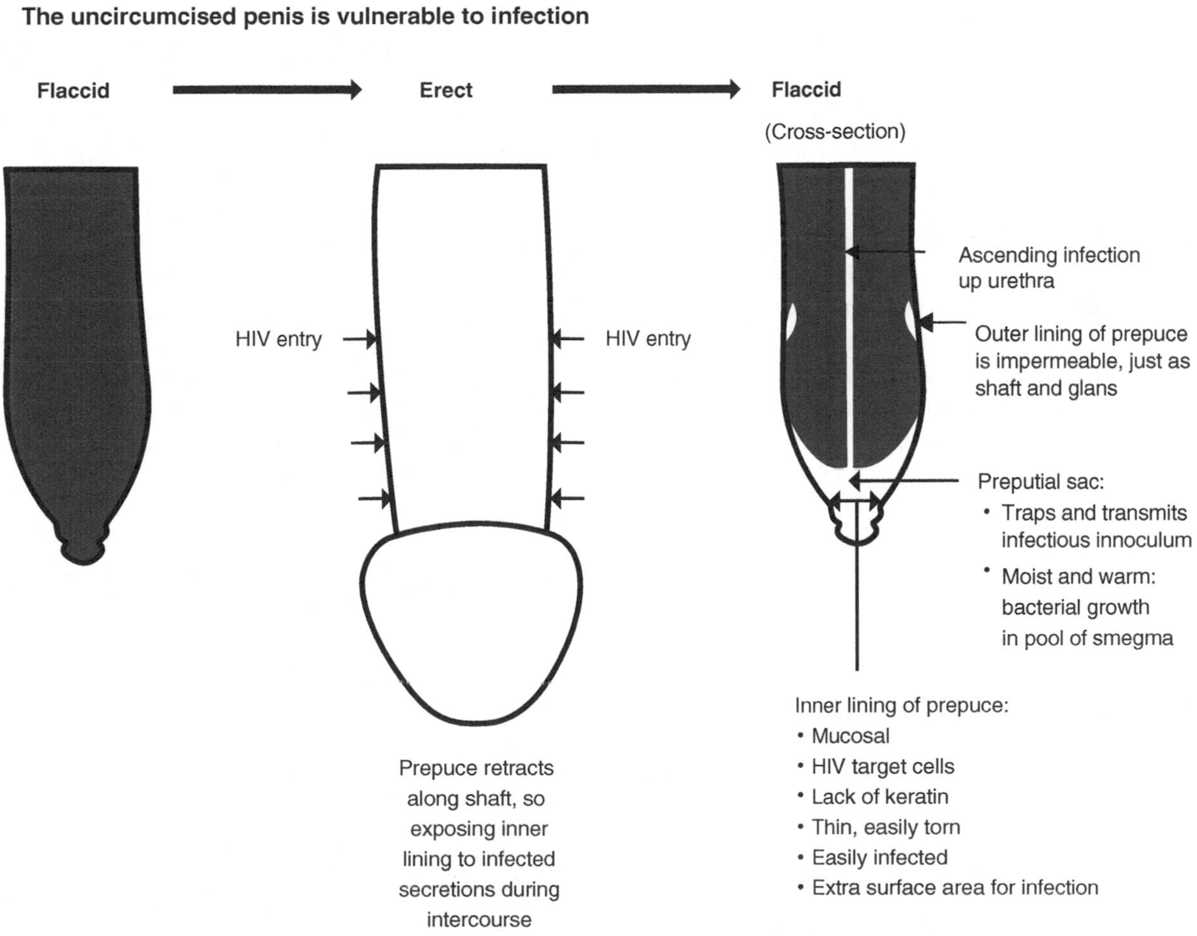

Fig. 54.1 Aspects of the uncircumcised penis that increase its risk for infection during and after intercourse

54.3 HPV and Penile Cancer

54.3.1 Incidence

Lifetime penile cancer risk in an uncircumcised man is 1 in 600–900 (US and Danish data) [44], whereas in circumcised men, it is only 1 in 50,000–12,000,000 [45, 46]. Of the 50,000 penile cancer cases in the United States from 1930 to 1990 (10,000 being fatal), only 10 were in circumcised men [47], and these had been circumcised later in life. Thus, neonatal circumcision virtually abolishes the risk [48]. In five major series in the United States, starting in 1932 [49], not one man with invasive penile cancer had been circumcised neonatally [50]. Two other US studies found it was 22 times higher [51–53].

The overall annual incidence of malignant penile cancer (mostly squamous cell carcinoma) in the United States from 1973 to 2002 was 0.69/100,000 [54]. For 1993–2002, it was 0.58/100,000 overall, but was 1.01/100,000 in Hispanics (lower circumcision) compared with 0.51/100,000 in other Whites (higher circumcision) [54]. In the United States, the difference in rate according to race has been attributed to differences in circumcision prevalence [55]. The total lifetime cost of new HPV16 and -18 related cases of penile cancer in the United States in 2003 (25% of total cases) has been estimated as US$ 4.4 million [56].

When circumcision is performed later in life, protection is not as great [57], particularly if "vigorous" ritual circumcision is involved [58]. For carcinoma in situ (rarely fatal), the protective effect is lower [50, 52, 53].

Penile cancer is seen as an "emerging problem" in which "public health measures, such as prophylactic use of circumcision, have proven successful" [59], and "circumcision should be performed in childhood [as a] prophylactic [to penile cancer]" [60]. The rising incidence of penile cancer has, moreover, been linked to decreases in neonatal circumcision in certain countries [61, 62].

In underdeveloped countries, penile cancer incidence is much higher: three to ten cases per 100,000 per year [44]. Where circumcision is uncommon, it can represent 10–22% of all male cancers [63–65]. In Uganda, it is the most common malignancy in males, leading to calls for greater circumcision [66]. The low rate in Nigeria where men are circumcised contrasts with high rates in Uganda [67] and other noncircumcising locations such as Puerto Rico and Brazil [68, 69].

In Israel, where almost all males are circumcised, the rate of penile cancer is only 0.1/100,000 [67].

54.3.2 Cause

High-risk HPVs have been implicated in cancer of the penis. High-risk (oncogenic) HPVs are less common in circumcised men [70–77]. A large, multination study in 2002 involving Spain, Thailand, the Philippines, Columbia, and Brazil found HPV in 19.6% of 847 uncircumcised men, but only 5.5% of 292 circumcised men (AOR = 0.37) [71]. A meta-analysis in 2009 of data from 14 studies (5 United States, 2 Mexican, 2 Australian, and one each from England, Denmark, South Korea, Kenya, and a multinational study referred to above, and involving 5,880 circumcised and 4,257 uncircumcised men) found that the protective effect had an OR of 0.52 (95% CI = 0.33–0.82) [78] (Fig. 54.2). Low-risk HPV types that manifest as visible warts tend to occur more commonly on the shaft of the penis, a site of infection unlikely to be affected by circumcision, and the meta-analysis found that circumcision afforded only a slight reduction in these (OR 0.89; 95% CI 0.59–1.33) [78]. An earlier meta-analysis by Van Howe [79] has been criticized severely [80] and should be disregarded.

The protection afforded by circumcision against HPV is supported by two RCTs (reviewed in: [81]). In Uganda, among men aged 15–49 years, one can see a decrease in prevalence of high-risk HPV on swabs from the coronal sulcus from a prevalence of 38% at enrolment down to 18% at 24 months after having been circumcised, compared with a decrease from 37% to 28% in the men who remained uncircumcised, indicating a 35% efficacy of the circumcision [32]. Circumcised men were, moreover, 65% less likely to be infected by multiple high-risk HPV types. In the other RCT, in South Africa involving men aged 18–24 years, high-risk HPV in urethral swabs was 16% in urethral swabs 21 months after circumcision, compared with 25% in the men who were not randomized to the circumcision arm of the trial, pointing to a 35% efficacy [40]. It was further found that circumcision reduced the incidence of new high-risk HPV infection by 42% [81]. Protection against nonhigh-risk types was 34% [32].

The distribution of HPV types on the penis appears to be important, with much higher prevalence of

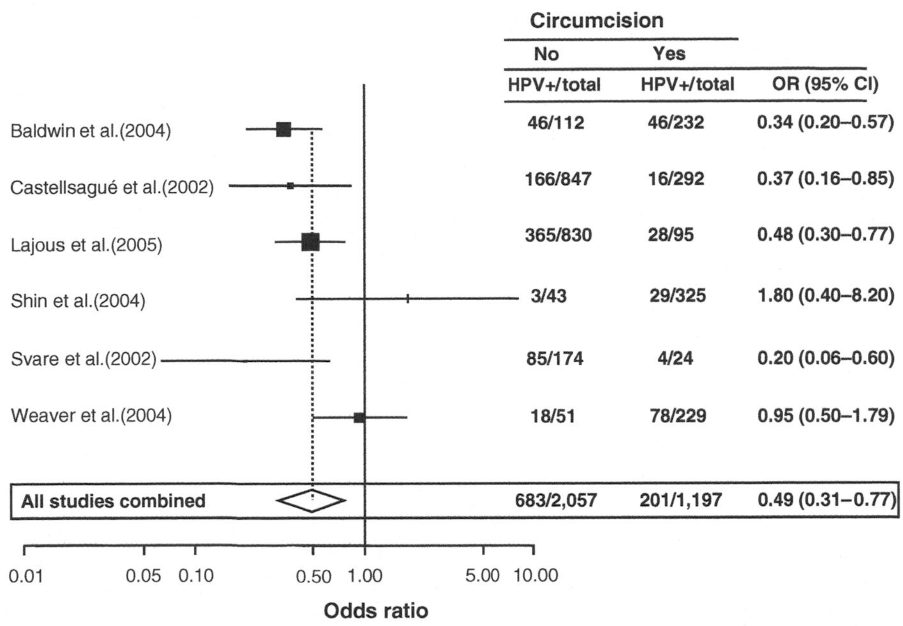
Circumcision
No
Yes
HPV+/total
HPV+/total
OR (95% CI)
Baldwin et al.(2004) 46/112 46/232 0.34 (0.20–0.57)
Castellsagué et al.(2002) 166/847 16/292 0.37 (0.16–0.85)
Lajous et al.(2005) 365/830 28/95 0.48 (0.30–0.77)
Shin et al.(2004) 3/43 29/325 1.80 (0.40–8.20)
Svare et al.(2002) 85/174 4/24 0.20 (0.06–0.60)
Weaver et al.(2004) 18/51 78/229 0.95 (0.50–1.79)
All studies combined 683/2,057 201/1,197 0.49 (0.31–0.77)
0.01
0.05
0.10
0.50
1.00
5.00
10.00
Odds ratio

Fig. 54.2 Meta-analysis of studies exploring the association between being circumcised and penile HPV (Adapted from data in [78, 80])

high- risk types with proximity to the tip of the penis. In one study, the distribution was 28% prepuce, 24% shaft, 17% scrotum, 16% glans, and 6% urine [82]. In another, involving uncircumcised men, high-risk HPV was 31% on the glans/coronal sulcus and 12% on the shaft [83]. The HIM study, involving men in the United States, Mexico, and Brazil, found both high-risk (OR 0.70) and low-risk (OR 0.63) HPV types to be lower in circumcised men [84], HPV prevalence ranging from 41% on the shaft to 4.7% in semen [85]. In this study, the strength of the association between circumcision and reduced HPV decreased with distance from the prepuce/urethra, AOR being 0.17 for the urethra, 0.44 for the glans/corona, 0.53 for the shaft, and no difference for scrotum, perianal area, anal canal, and semen [85]. A study in Hawaii found HPV infection of the glans/coronal sulcus was much higher in uncircumcised men (46% vs. 29%) [72].

Despite similar HPV seroprevalence [86], circumcised men clear penile oncogenic HPV infections six times faster than uncircumcised men [87]. This would further explain their lower risk of penile cancer, and of cervical cancer in their female partner(s). Indeed, in a study of healthy Mexican military men, OR for persistent HPV infection was ten times higher in those who were not circumcised [74].

High-risk HPVs are not easily seen and most infections are subclinical. Prevalence is higher in uncircumcised men with balanoposthitis [73]. Easily seen genital warts, however, are caused by low-risk HPV types [88]. The low-risk HPVs that cause these more commonly infect the shaft, as well as the penis generally, so, not surprisingly, circumcision has been reported to have less of a protective effect against low-risk types (OR 0.89; 95% CI = 0.59–1.33) [78]. RCT data showed protection against nonhigh-risk HPV of 34% (RR 0.65; 95% CI 0.49–0.91; $P = 0.01$).

Most (93%) men whose female partner had squamous intraepithelial lesions (SIL) had penile intraepithelial neoplasia (PIN) [89], consistent with the sexually transmission of HPV. Oncogenic HPV was found in 75% of patients with PIN grade I, 93% with PIN grade II, and 100% of PIN grade III (one step short of penile cancer), and PIN was more common in the uncircumcised [89]. Condom use may lower HPV infection [70].

Phimosis is associated strongly with invasive penile carcinoma (adjusted OR 16) [57] and 11 [90]), and phimosis is seen in 45–85% of patients [57, 91]. A notable feature is dysplastic changes in skin of the preputial sac [92]. The length of the prepuce is probably not a factor, however [93].

Smegma under the prepuce may be carcinogenic [94–97]. It causes chronic inflammation and recurrent infections leading to preputial adhesions and phimosis [57, 92]. Male horses produce large amounts of smegma and have a high penile cancer incidence (23% of cancers) [98]. Geldings do not get erections that would normally help eliminate smegma and have ten times more penile cancer than stallions [98]. A study in Sweden found that despite affected men reporting a history of smegma, smegma was not, however, associated with invasive squamous cell carcinoma or carcinoma in situ [99].

Chronic-relapsing balanitis of bacterial, mycotic, or viral origin may increase risk of invasive penile cancer [100, 101]. It occurred in 45% of penile cancer patients, but only 8% of controls [52, 91]. Penile lichen sclerosis (balanitis xerotica obliterans [BXO]), an inflammatory disorder that can lead to meatal stenosis or phimosis, is associated with penile carcinoma (reviewed in [59]). Incidence in such patients is 28% [102]. Of these, 77% had squamous cell carcinoma and 23% carcinoma in situ. The rate of HPV infection is 2.6 times higher in BXO [103]. Although oncogenic HPVs were seen in 17% of BXO cases cf. 9% of controls, lichen sclerosis was considered a preneoplastic condition unrelated to HPV infection (reviewed in [59]). Recurrent HSV-2 balanitis may be cocarcinogenic [104, 105].

Of all factors, lack of circumcision is the primary prerequisite for penile cancer [50, 90, 106]. There is, moreover, no evidence that improved penile hygiene reduces penile cancer risk in an uncircumcised man [19, 57]. Circumcision in early childhood, by eliminating phimosis, helps prevent penile cancer [90]. Furthermore, the cause can be sexual transmission of oncogenic HPV in young men or, in older men, a mode unrelated to HPV (reviewed in [59]).

In view of the low 5-year survival [107, 108], and adverse physical, emotional, and psychosexual consequences [109], it is surprising that "despite overwhelming evidence from urological surgeons that neoplasm of the penis is a lethal disease that can be prevented by removal of the prepuce, some physicians continue to argue against routine newborn circumcision in a highly emotional and aggressive fashion" [61].

54.4 Prostate Cancer

Risk of prostate cancer correlates with a history of STIs [110–119]. If there is a role for a STI, the nature of this is unclear. There is no consistent evidence for HPV being involved, however. Human polyoma virus BKV [120] or xenotropic murine leukemia virus-related virus (XMVR) [121] could play a role. The common STI *T. vaginalis* has been implicated, especially for risk of extraprostatic prostate cancer (OR 2.2) and clinically relevant, potentially lethal prostate cancer (OR 2.7) [122]. Prostate cancer incidence is 1.6- to 2-fold higher in uncircumcised men [118, 123–125] and is low among Jews [126]. However, more research is needed to confirm the link with lack of circumcision, but if true, would account for 24–40% (45–67,000) extra prostate cancer cases in the United States (where 40% of 70-year-olds are not circumcised), and US$0.8–1.6B in extra costs for treatment and terminal care each year [127].

54.5 HPV and Cervical Cancer

There is now overwhelming evidence for a link between lack of male circumcision and increased risk of cervical cancer (see reviews [1, 2]). UNAIDS and IARC data from 117 developing countries noted a cervical cancer incidence of 35/100,000 women/year in 51 countries with a low (<20%) circumcision prevalence, but 20/100,000 women/year in 52 countries with a high (>80%), circumcision prevalence ($P < 0.001$) [128]. Of all factors, the strongest association was with lack of male circumcision.

In 2002, a large, well-designed study of 1,913 couples in five global locations in Europe, Asia, and South America found monogamous women whose male partner was "high-risk" (i.e., had had six or more sexual partners as well as early sexual debut) were 5.6 times more likely to have cervical cancer if the partner was uncircumcised (adjusted OR 0.42) [71]. Circumcision was also protective in women whose partner had an intermediate sexual behavior risk index (OR 0.50). Genital HPV types are highly infectious, meaning any skin-to-skin contact, such as during foreplay, could lead to infection. This study found no significant difference in HPV infection between condom users (OR 0.83) and nonusers (OR 0.67). The higher HPV infection in uncircumcised men could be because the more delicate, easily infected, mucosal lining of the prepuce, when retracted during intercourse, becomes wholly exposed to vaginal secretions of an infected woman (Fig. 54.1). Women with cervical cancer are, not surprisingly, more likely to have partners with PIN [129], this being 93% in one study [89].

HPV can be transmitted to the mouth during oral sex and is an independent risk factor for some oral cancers [130]. In the past decade, breast tumors have also been found to contain high-risk HPVs [131, 132]. These were the same type(s) as present in the cervix of each patient [133, 134], so supporting a STI contribution to at least some breast cancers [135]. Consistent with this, women with HPV-positive breast cancer were significantly younger than those with HPV-negative breast cancer [136]. HPV-associated koilocytes have, moreover, been found in breast skin and lobules from normal and ductal carcinoma in situ and invasive ductal carcinoma [137, 138]. HPV can, moreover, be found in the bloodstream of cervical cancer patients [139] as well as male blood donors, attached to blood cells [140]. A viral etiology might include mouse mammary tumor virus (MMTV) and Epstein-Barr virus (EBV) [131]. A role for uncircumcised male partner(s) in sexual transmission of an STI responsible for mouth or breast cancer will require further research.

A vaccine against the two types of HPV seen in approx. 70% of cervical cancers is starting to be used in countries that can afford it. It offers only limited protection against the numerous other high-risk HPV types [141], is best given before commencement of sexual activity, was approved for girls only, and uptake has not been universal. A randomized, placebo-controlled, double-blind trial involving 5,455 women aged 16–24 found, however, that vaccination (with Gardasil) reduced the rate of cervical lesions by only 20% over the 3 years of the study [142]. In one analysis, HPV vaccination was found to not be cost effective, even under favorable assumptions for vaccination programs [143]. A review of cost-effectiveness studies by others, however, suggested that vaccination of girls against HPV might be cost effective [144]. For uptake of 80% in 12-year-old girls, the HPV vaccine could reduce cervical cancer by 38–82% after 60 years of an ongoing vaccination program should vaccine protection last 20 years [145]. Vaccination of boys, however, was not cost effective [144, 145]. Male circumcision thus offers a valuable adjunct to the vaccine. Male circumcision also offers protection against acquisition of several other common STIs by women.

54.6 Other STIs in Female Partners

54.6.1 HSV-2 in Women

History of sexual intercourse (ever) with an uncircumcised man increased risk of HSV-2 infection (OR 2.2; 95% CI 1.4–3.6, after multivariate logistic regression analysis) in 1,207 Pittsburgh women aged 18–30 years (HSV-2 seroprevalence 25%) [146]. A RCT saw two-fold higher HSV-2 infection over 12 months in 800 wives of uncircumcised men [147]. These women also had higher symptomatic GUD (increased 30%). However, a study in Africa showed no difference, although most represented reactivation of existing HSV-2 in this high prevalence setting [148]. Overall, it would seem that circumcision could help counter the worldwide epidemic of HSV-2.

54.6.2 Chlamydia in Women

A 5.6-fold higher seropositivity for *Chlamydia trachomatis* has been noted in women with an uncircumcised partner [149]. This study involved 305 couples in five countries. The finding also applied to women who had only ever had one sexual partner. *C. pneumoniae*, which is not transmitted sexually, did not differ. In uncircumcised men, infected cervicovaginal secretions may be trapped under the prepuce for longer, so increasing risk of penile urethral infection and transmission to the vagina during sex [149]. An African study was, however, negative [150].

54.6.3 Bacterial Vaginosis and Trichomonas in Women

Bacterial vaginosis (BV) is associated with a range of adverse health outcomes, including premature labor, postpartum endometriosis, pelvic inflammatory disease, and increased risk of STIs. A study in Pittsburgh, where incidence was 36 cases/100 woman-years, found that women who had had an uncircumcised male partner(s) in the preceding 4 months were 1.9 times more likely to have BV [151]. In a large RCT, circumcision of the male partner reduced the risk of any BV in their wives by 40% and severe BV by 61% [152]. *T. vaginalis* (TV) was reduced by 48% [152]. This contrasts with a prospective study that found no difference in trichomonal, chlamydial, or gonococcal infection in women in two African countries and Thailand [150].

54.7 Sexually Transmitted HIV

54.7.1 How the Prepuce Increases Infection Risk

Vaginal intercourse accounts for more than 80% [153] of the 30 million HIV infections in men worldwide [73]. A link with lack of circumcision was first proposed in 1986 [154] and now at least 50 epidemiological studies have confirmed higher HIV in heterosexual men who are uncircumcised [155–158].

During an erection, the prepuce is pulled half-way up the shaft of the penis (Fig. 54.1), so causing its thin keratin lining to become even thinner [159] and exposing its inner surface to vaginal secretions during intercourse [160]. These become trapped physically in the preputial sac, which provides a hospitable environment for pathogenic organisms in a pool of smegma [161]. The prepuce's high surface area, risk of tearing during intercourse, and inflammation (balanitis) were also invoked. Unlike the inner prepuce, the glans of each type of penis has a similar amount of protective keratin [160, 162]. Infected cells in vaginal fluids or semen can adhere to mucosal surfaces and migrate through lesions [163]. Preputial wetness, an indicator of poor hygiene, conveys a 40% increase in infection risk, possibly because virions attach for longer, healing after trauma is lower, and microulcerations caused by balanitis are more common [164]. Penile wetness is more common in men with a long prepuce [165]. Lesions, created by GUD (more common in the uncircumcised) also facilitate HIV entry [166].

HIV, applied to fresh preputial tissue in vitro, was taken up rapidly by the inner lining but not by the outer epithelium [167]. Simian immunodeficiency virus does the same to infect monkeys [168]. Surprisingly, however, in one study, glans, prepuce, meatus, and urethra in explant culture were reported to be equally susceptible to HIV infection [169].

The mucosal inner prepuce is rich in immune-system cells [167]. The urethra, although mucosal, lacks these, and it is not considered a site of HIV infection. Interestingly, circumcised men with high sexual activity have lower HIV, leading to a suggestion that repeated contact of the urethral meatus (that contains a small number of HIV receptors) [159] with subinfectious inoculums might induce an immune response [170]. The small area exposed would lessen the likelihood of the immune system being overwhelmed, as compared with the prepuce [170]. Mucosal alloimmunization may indeed protect against HIV [171].

Immune system cells in the inner lining of the prepuce act as a "Trojan horse" in uptake of HIV, which binds to receptors CD1a, CD4, CCR5, CXCR4, HLA-DR, and DC-SIGN, particularly on Langerhans cells, which are closer to the surface [172] and send dendritic projections up between keratinocytes [159].

Langerhans cells contain Langerin, which helps internalize and transport HIV to regional lymph nodes [173]. Direct HIV infection of T cells is at least as important, however [174, 175]. Success in establishing a systemic infection might, nevertheless, depend on early interaction of HIV with Langerhans cells [174]. At low viral loads Langerin is able to clear HIV, shunting it to intracellular granules for degradation, but this mechanism becomes overwhelmed at higher viral loads [176, 177].

Finally, larger foreskin surface area is associated with higher HIV prevalence [178].

54.7.2 Epidemiological Research – Heterosexual

In developing countries other than in Sub-Saharan Africa, adult HIV prevalence in 2004 was 0.76% for 11 with low (<20%) and 0.09% for 17 with high (>80%) rates of circumcision [128] – i.e., was eight-fold higher where circumcision was less common. In Sub-Saharan African countries, these figures were 16% for 8 countries with low and 3% for 22 with high circumcision rates [128], independent of Muslim and Christian religion. The current data implicating male circumcision in the prevention of HIV infection satisfies six of Hill's nine criteria of causality (strength of association, consistency, temporality, biological plausibility, coherence, and experiment) [179]. After considering all factors, lack of circumcision has emerged as the major driving force behind the AIDS epidemic [180].

In a meta-regression analysis of 27 studies, lack of circumcision in susceptible men was associated with an infectivity difference versus circumcised men of 8.1 transmissions per 1,000 exposures (range 0.4–16) [181]. Infectivity was, moreover, only weakly associated with geographical region (Africa versus United States/Europe) [181]. In high-risk contexts, such as when the male is uncircumcised, heterosexual infectivity can exceed 0.1, i.e., one transmission per ten contacts, which exceeds by two orders of magnitude the value of 0.001 that is cited commonly [181]. This was later extended to a meta-analysis of 43 publications based on 25 different study populations [182]. It showed female-to-male infectivity, during the asymptomatic phase, of 0.04% per sex act for high income countries and 0.38% for low income countries.

54.7.2.1 United States

DNA sequencing of archival specimens suggested that HIV moved out of Africa to Haiti around 1966 and from there migrated to the United States around 1969, circulating cryptically in the latter for approx. 12 years before AIDS was first recognized in 1981 [183].

A report in 1993 of heterosexual men attending a STI clinic in New York City found HIV to be 2.1% in 405 who were uncircumcised, but only 0.6% in 308 who were circumcised (risk ratio = 4.1) [184].

Heterosexual contact accounted for 15% of HIV infections men in the United States in 2005, this route having grown by 42% over the years [185]. High-risk heterosexual contact accounted for 31–33% of HIV/AIDS cases diagnosed in 2006 [186, 187]. Men comprised 36% and women 64% of heterosexually acquired infections in 2007 [186]. In 2009, it was reported that, among African American men in Baltimore with known heterosexual exposure to infected partner(s), HIV was 51% lower in those who were circumcised [188]. The various findings have led to calls for greater circumcision in the United States [189].

54.7.2.2 United Kingdom, Europe, Russia, and Central Asia

The low circumcision rate in these regions has been accompanied by a rise in heterosexual transmission, provoking calls in the United Kingdom for a change in circumcision guidelines [190]. The proportion of infections due to female to male transmission in Europe is much higher than in the United States, consistent with the influence of the much lower rate of circumcision in Europe [191–193].

54.7.2.3 Asia

Adult HIV incidence in countries with high circumcision rates (Philippines, Bangladesh, and Indonesia) is 0.03–0.06%, compared with 1.8–2.4% for those with low circumcision rates (Thailand, India, and Cambodia) [192], being 3–6% in Thai military conscripts [194]. A prospective study in India of 2,298 men initially not infected saw a 6.7-fold higher HIV infection in the uncircumcised (adjusted RR 0.14) [195]. Another study found HIV incidence in Muslim men (circumcised) was 1% compared with 4.4% in Hindu men (uncircumcised) (OR 0.42), despite Muslim men having more sex partners and visits to commercial sex workers [196]. This finding was not influenced by concurrent infection with other STIs. A later study of 4,800 men noted 2.5 times higher HIV infection in those who were uncircumcised, with circumcision stated as being the factor having the highest impact on reducing HIV rate [197]. In another Indian study, of 1,925 men, HIV prevalence was 1.1% in the 90% who were uncircumcised but zero in the circumcised [198]. The clear benefits of circumcision have led to calls in India for physicians to inform patients in the interests of ethical responsibility [199]. Similarly, in China, there has been a call to establish surgical standards and training protocols for the promotion of circumcision for STI reduction [200].

54.7.2.4 South America

In Rio de Janeiro 13% of 799 men aged <30 years were circumcised, and HIV prevalence in these was 70% lower than in those who were not circumcised [201].

54.7.2.5 Middle East

Muslim men are circumcised and Middle Eastern countries have a very low prevalence of HIV [202]. HIV and syphilis were not seen at all in STI patients in Kuwait [203].

54.7.2.6 Sub-Saharan Africa

Observational Studies

Striking differences in HIV incidences in Sub-Saharan Africa correlate with circumcision practice [204]. Rates in Botswana, Swaziland, and South Africa are 40%, 33%, and 25%, respectively, with most infections from heterosexual intercourse [205]. Risk from a single act of unprotected vaginal sex in a study of Kenyan truck drivers was 1 in 78 in an uncircumcised man and 1 in 200 in a circumcised man [206]. When 422 HIV-negative men in Nairobi were followed for a year a tenfold higher infection occurred in the uncircumcised (RR 8.2 by logistic regression analysis) [161]. Risk during a single exposure was one in six in this study.

Couples in Uganda, in whom one partner was HIV-positive, were followed prospectively for 30 months, and 17 seroconversions/100 person-years were observed in the uncircumcised men, but none in the circumcised, despite them having regular unprotected sex [207, 208]. Behaviors in Muslim men have been excluded [207]. Viral load is a factor, with no HIV transmission being seen for <1,500 copies of HIV-1 RNA/ml serum, but above this a dose-response increase in infection was noted [208]. For men with a viral load of less than 50,000 copies/mL, there was no transmission of HIV to the female partner if the man was circumcised, but if the man was not circumcised, transmission was 9.6/100 person-years [207]. Postcoital washing did not reduce HIV acquisition [209].

Fastidious matching of circumcised and uncircumcised Luo groups, each from nine Christian churches in Kenya, again noted higher HIV in the uncircumcised [210]. Frequency of sexual intercourse and higher rate of other risk factors did not contribute in a Ugandan study [211]. Muslims had a lower risk profile for all factors, except condom use (OR 0.3). Biological factors – circumcision and STIs – were more important than behavior; those who considered themselves at low risk being more likely to get a HIV infection [212]. Age at circumcision may [207, 213], or may not [210], be important.

A large systematic meta-analysis in 2000 of 27 studies, 21 of which had found lower HIV in circumcised men, showed, after adjusting 15 for potential confounding factors, 2.4-fold higher HIV in those not circumcised [157]. In men at high risk, HIV incidence was 3.7 times higher in the uncircumcised. Only one of these studies had verified circumcision status by physical examination [214]. Since self-report of circumcision status is often inaccurate (67–81% in African studies [215, 216] and 69–84% in studies in the United States [217, 218]), and some men have only a partial circumcision, the protective effect of circumcision could be even greater.

Randomized Controlled Trials

Three RCTs were begun in the early 2000s. The first involved 3,274 uncircumcised men aged 18–24 in a semiurban region of South Africa [219]. It was to run for 21 months, but so striking was the benefit of circumcision (60%) that at 18 months it was stopped so the control group could be offered circumcision. Protection was 61% after controlling for behavioral factors such as higher sexual activity in the intervention group. A per-protocol analysis to correct for the dilutional effect of cross-overs, so treating men who were actually circumcised as circumcised and vice-versa showed the protective effect was 76%. It concluded that "circumcision provides a degree of protection against acquiring HIV infection equivalent to what a vaccine of high efficacy would have achieved" and that circumcision "could be incorporated rapidly into the national plans of countries where most males are not circumcised," just as in South Korea, where circumcision has risen from virtually zero 50 years ago to 85% today [220]. Furthermore, circumcision "is an inexpensive means of prevention, performed only once, and ... over a wide age range, from childhood to adulthood" and "the number of HIV infections that could be avoided ... is high."

RCTs in Kenya [221] and Uganda [31] were similarly stopped early by the monitoring committees due to the marked preventative effect. These studies involved, respectively, 2,784 and 4,996 uncircumcised men aged 18–24 and 15–40 [31, 221]. In each, the as-treated protective effect of circumcision was 60%. Extensive analyses of the data dismissed a contribution from other, potentially confounding factors. After excluding four invalid subjects in the Kenyan trial, 2-year HIV incidence was 1.6% in the circumcised group and 4.2% in the control group, i.e., the true protective effect was 68% [221]. The reduction in HIV infection after circumcision occurred irrespective of number of partners. Moreover, unlike the South African trial, the Kenyan and Ugandan RCTs saw no risk compensation. Only 1.5% [221] and 3.6% [31] of subjects had adverse events from the circumcision itself, and these resolved quickly. None reported moderate or severe pain, and almost all were "very," and none "not," satisfied with their circumcision [221]. At the time, just 10–20% of the HIV infections prevented by circumcision were considered to be due to reduction in STIs (primarily GUD) [222].

A random-effects meta-analysis of the RCT data and of 15 observational studies that adjusted for potential confounders found a RR of 0.42 for each [158] (Fig. 54.3). A meta-analysis by others of the RCT data obtained similar findings [223]. Meta-analysis of data for "as-treated" subjects yielded a summary RR of 0.35 (95% CI 0.24–0.54) [158]. Thus, circumcision reduced HIV infection by 65%. An extensive Cochrane review in 2009, incorporating the RCT results, concluded that "inclusion of male circumcision into current HIV prevention measures guidelines [sic] is warranted" [224]. Follow-up data from men in the Rakai trial in Kenyan showed that by 3.5 years, not only was the protective effect sustained, but it was

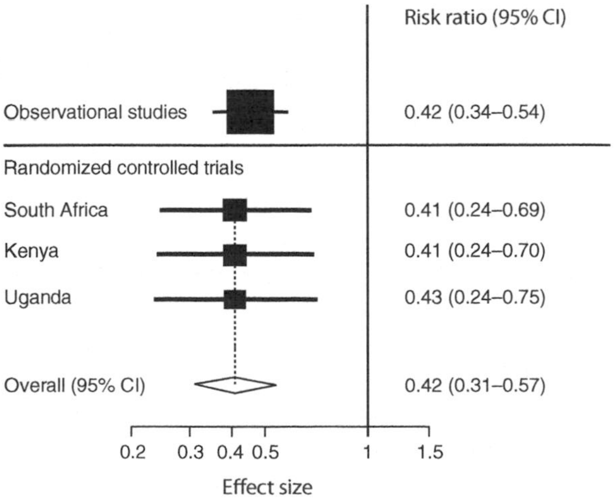

Fig. 54.3 Effect of circumcision on HIV prevention. Shown is risk ratio for 15 observational studies that adjusted for potential confounding factors, and below this, a random effects meta-analysis of the RCTs intention-to-treat findings (Modified from [158], with correction)

increased [225], consistent with an earlier suggestion that "early stopping may have underestimated the effect [of circumcision]" [158].

54.7.3 Synergy with GUD?

Although the prepuce seems to be the weak point for HIV infection of uncircumcised men, a man with GUD or lesions anywhere on the penis will be at increased risk irrespective of circumcision status [226]. Indeed, men with HSV-2 appeared to have a two [227] or three to five times [228] higher risk of acquiring HIV, and men with both viruses seemed more likely to transmit HIV [227]. It has been suggested that HIV and HSV-2 may be in a vicious cycle of infection, each exacerbating infection by the other [29]. Such a synergy between each was seen in the South African RCT described earlier [23, 41].

In the Ugandan RCT, HSV-2 was not significantly higher, however, in HIV positive men, and it was suggested that HIV and syphilis are most likely markers of increased sexual activity [27]. An analysis of RCT data found that protection against STIs contributed little to the overall protective effect that circumcision has against HIV infection [229]. In the South African RCT, the protective effect of circumcision against HIV infection appeared, moreover, to be independent of HSV-2 serostatus [26, 41, 165]. Similarly, in the Kenyan RCT, only 8.6% of the reduction in HIV associated with circumcision was mediated by reduction in HSV-2, and for GUD was only 11% [33]. The Rakai data suggested that most of the reduction in HIV was from nonherpetic ulceration [33]. It was suggested that the ulcers responsible for HIV infection were likely caused by traumatic lesions of the foreskin, and attached frenulum in particular [33]. Such tearing occurs commonly when uncircumcised men have sexual intercourse [160]. Inflammation of the foreskin is more common in men who have HIV, HSV-2, or smegma [230]. HSV-2 suppressive therapy has, however, failed to decrease HIV acquisition in men, as seen in two RCTs [226]. A RCT in women similarly found HSV-2 suppressive therapy had no effect on them becoming infected with HIV [231]. HIV positive inflammatory cells are enriched in lesions caused by HSV-2 and persist for months after healing, so this might explain why anti-HSV-2 therapy has failed to reduce acquisition of HIV [232].

In men infected with high-risk (but not low-risk) HPV, prevalence of HIV is 3.8-fold higher [233].

Whether HPV facilitates HIV acquisition remains to be determined.

54.7.4 Implications, Lives Saved, and Costs

Other prevention measures "have often been unsuccessful in restricting the spread of HIV" [221]. In the case of antiretroviral therapy, the pace of new HIV infections is outstripping supply. And as far as a vaccine is concerned, "there is little promise that an effective vaccine will be available within the next 15 years" [221]. Prevention is preferable, and circumcision is cheaper than antivirals.

Condom use in the RCTs was low, despite free supply. Circumcision is once only, does not have to be "applied," is not inconvenient, apart for abstinence from sex for a few weeks, and reduces numerous other problems [1, 2]. Moreover, "neonatal circumcision or circumcision of younger boys will provide a simpler, safer, and cheaper option" [31].

Analysis of the dynamics of the epidemic suggests that heterosexual transmission of HIV probably peaked during the 1990s [234]. For a circumcision efficacy of 50%, when HIV incidence is 1.3/100 person-years (as in Uganda), 35 surgeries would prevent one HIV infection over 10 years if all underwent circumcision [31]. For South Africa (HIV 3.8/100 person-years), fewer circumcisions would achieve this. Targeting any age group in this country was shown to be cost effective, leading to a suggestion that the UNAIDS target age group range (12–30) should be widened to include older men [235]. The cumulative net cost for rolling out medical adult male circumcision in South Africa has been estimated as US$ 919 million for the first 5 years and would be US$672M over the first 10 years; over 20 years the net savings would be US$ 2.3 billion [236]. In Zambia, increasing circumcision to 100% (from 10%) would reduce adult HIV prevalence from 27% down to 7% [237]. WHO/ANAIDS estimates show circumcision could avert 2 million new infections and 0.3 million deaths over the next 10 years in Sub-Saharan Africa, and a further 4 million new infections and 3 million deaths in the 10 years after that, a quarter being in South Africa [238]. They equated circumcision with condom use or a vaccine. In South Africa, each 1,000 circumcisions would prevent 308 HIV infections over 10 years, at a cost of US$ 181 per HIV infection averted, a net saving of US$ 2.4 million [239]. For an 80% uptake of circumcision, HIV prevalence would be reduced by 45–67% in both men and women within a decade in countries with high HIV [240]. If uptake was 50%, HIV would be reduced 25–41% [240]. Other modeling predicted that, for a 60% efficacy, 19 surgeries would prevent one HIV infection in both sexes at a cost per infection averted of US$ 1,269 [241]. In Botswana scale-up of adult and neonatal circumcision to 80% by 2012 would avert 70,000 new HIV infections through 2025 at a cost per HIV infection averted of US$ 689 [242]. The reduction achieved could be sufficient to "abort the epidemic" [241]. By 2020, complete male circumcision in an average country could reduce HIV prevalence from 12% to 6% [243]. In Zimbabwe, the 25% HIV rate predicted for no circumcision would be just 13%. Circumcision cost (in Kenya) is US$ 20 for supplies, obtained locally, and US$ 13 for the procedure itself in a government hospital and US$ 77 in a private hospital [244]. To 1999, circumcision had likely prevented 10 million HIV infections in Africa and Asia [155]. For 14 Sub-Saharan countries in which circumcision is <20% and HIV >5%, and assuming >85% of men get circumcised, initial 5-year cost will be US$922M (private)/US$397M (public) [245]. This would require 1,912 circumcisers (0.23/10,000 adults). In years 6–10 the number needed would reduce to 504 and cost to US$ 208 million/US$ 84 million. This analysis found five to eight circumcisions would be needed to prevent one HIV infection. Although expensive, the roll-out of circumcision would be cost effective, sustainable, and have important other benefits to public health.

"Circumcision must now be deemed to be a proven intervention for reducing the risk of heterosexually acquired HIV infection in adult men" [31]. In March 2007, in endorsing circumcision, the WHO and UNAIDS stated "the efficacy of male circumcision in reducing female to male HIV transmission has now been proven beyond reasonable doubt. This is an important landmark in the history of HIV prevention" [246]. It went on to recommend circumcision for men and boys, as well as infants, since in infants circumcision is "less complicated and risky." The RCTs were an "extraordinary development" and circumcision a "potent intervention in HIV prevention." "Global expansion of male circumcision programs [is a] vital tool for control of HIV infection" [247].

54.7.5 Epidemiological Research – Men Who Have Sex with Men (MSM)

In New York City, the epicenter of the HIV epidemic, HIV prevalence in MSM is 8.4% [248], which is higher than in Uganda (7%) and Kenya (7.4%) [249]. However, unlike heterosexual transmission, the data for the effectiveness of circumcision in HIV prevention among MSM is not as consistent as it is for the former [248]. This can be attributed to the mixture of sexual practices – receptive anal intercourse is unlikely to relate to circumcision status, whereas insertive might.

Among the 15% who were uncircumcised in a Seattle study of MSM, HIV was 2.2 times higher [250]. A later study in Seattle of 4,749 men attending a STI clinic found no difference, however [36]. Findings in STIs clinics should, however, be viewed with caution because any protective effect that circumcision may have against STIs means a selective bias against attendance of circumcised men at STI clinics, meaning the population studied is not representative of the general population of men. In six US cities, a study of 3,257 mostly white MSM from 1995–1997 showed lack of circumcision doubled the risk of acquiring HIV [251]. A meta-analysis that excluded studies that did not meet rigid inclusion criteria found incidence of HIV was 51% lower in circumcised MSM [252]. Another study in the United States of 1,154 Black and 1,091 Latino MSM was negative, however [253]. A meta-analysis performed in the United States found HIV was 53% lower in circumcised men for studies conducted before the introduction of antiretroviral therapy [254]. These authors found that a protective effect of circumcision was more likely to be seen in higher quality studies. For MSM who were primarily insertive, those who were circumcised had 29% lower HIV infection [254].

In Lima, Peru, 4% of circumcised and 21% of uncircumcised MSM had HIV [255].

Logically, circumcision should be protective during insertive, but not receptive, anal intercourse. Indeed, in a study of MSM in Sydney, Australia, MSM who engaged only in insertive anal intercourse had an 89% lower HIV prevalence if they were circumcised [256]. Similarly, in Africa, men who were insertive-only were 80% less likely to have HIV [257]. In an STI clinic population in Seattle, men who were insertive-only had a 45% lower risk [36]. Nevertheless, a RCT should be helpful. Owing to the high rate of circumcision in the US population of MSM (70–80%), such a trial could be considered in countries such as in Peru and Ecuador (circumcision rate 10%) where there is strong support for doing so [258]. Modeling in a resource-rich setting (Sydney, Australia) showed that circumcision of MSM, especially those who were insertive only, would be cost effective for HIV prevention, with one infection prevented for every 118 circumcisions for men in the insertive-only category [259].

It has been suggested that anal intercourse may present a higher viral load than vaginal intercourse, higher load being known to increase infection risk [208].

A lesser-known high-risk activity of MSM – "docking" [260] – involves insertion of the penis under the prepuce of the partner. The ejaculate then makes direct contact with the inner preputial lining.

54.7.6 Epidemiological Research – The Female Partners

One would think that if a man is HIV-positive, whether he is circumcised or not should make little difference to whether a woman he has sex with will become infected [261]. Based on data from Africa, an exception might exist in the case of women from high-risk settings (hazards ratio = 0.16) [261]. A meta-analysis of all relevant studies found that male circumcision reduced the risk to women by 20%, which was not significant [262]. A later report noted a reduction in risk of 38% for seven sites in eastern Africa [263]. Of course, a reduction in HIV prevalence in men will lower the HIV prevalence and thus lower the risk to women indirectly [264].

54.7.7 Risk Compensation

The protection circumcision affords could lead men to increase risky sexual behavior ("risk compensation") [265]. But this did not happen in two of the three RCTs [31, 221, 266]. In the South African trial, all five sexual behavior factors increased, but HIV infections were lower [219]. In the Kenyan trial, men in the circumcised arm were less likely to use condoms in the first 6 months after circumcision, but thereafter all risk behaviors did not differ [31], as seen by others [267]. Most men delayed sex after their circumcision, but early sex was not associated with HIV risk [268].

54.7.8 Acceptability and Satisfaction

Most population groups are willing to accept circumcision to reduce HIV. This includes those in Tanzania [216], Kenya [269], Botswana [270], and South Africa [271, 272]. Among cultures that normally did not circumcise, circumcision rate has increased to 23% overall, and to 57% among those with ≥8 years of education [216]. Mean age of getting it done was 17 years. Health was the main reason given.

A review of 13 studies from nine countries found 65% of men (range 29–87%) were willing to get circumcised, and 69% of women (range 47–79%) preferred circumcision for their partner [273]. Furthermore, 79% (50–90%) of men and 81% (70–90%) of women wanted to get their sons circumcised.

A follow-up survey in Kenya 30 days after circumcision showed 99% of the men were very satisfied, as were 92% of their partners, and 96% had resumed general activities within the first week [244, 274]. None of the men and only 0.3% of partners were very dissatisfied with the outcome. By 3 days, 83% of those with regular employment had resumed working, rising to 93% by 1 week and 99% by 1 month [274]. Resumption of sex occurred in 10% by 1 month and by 65% by 3 months [274]. Much the same was seen in Zimbabwe [275]. At 3 months 98.5% of men were "very satisfied" in the South African RCT [219], as were 99.5% in the Kenyan RCT [221].

54.7.9 Ethical and Other Challenges

Obstacles that could impede the full roll-out of circumcision include cost, supply of sufficient competent circumcisers, circumcision training, adequacy of clinics and resources, best age, risk compensation, conflict between individuals within families, societal objections, prioritization of individuals in the face of limited resources, education to ensure circumcision is not seen as a panacea, and ethical issues such as obstacles to changing the culture, and the need make circumcision safer in cultures that do circumcise [276]. Increased uptake might lead to stigmatization of uncircumcised men as being less "safe" [277]. Ensuring safe circumcisions will require all stakeholders to work together [278].

The challenges seem minor, however, when compared with the perceived benefit. Many concerns have little validity. Most cultures are neutral on circumcision [279]. Those generally opposed include Indians of Hindu or Sikh faiths. But even here, a study in India of mostly Hindu mothers with male children found that after being informed about the risks and benefits of circumcision 81% said they would definitely have their sons circumcised if it was provided in a safe hospital setting free of charge, and 7% said they would probably have it done [280].

As stated by Stemple "At this nexus of health and rights, it is important not to pit one set of rights against another artificially. …." To move unnecessarily incrementally [sic!] as a result of violations concerns risks reinforcing too simplistic a conceptualise of right – thwarting efforts to realize the highest attainable standard of health for populations in urgent need of HIV preventions strategies. A violations-only approach to human rights is unduly limiting; indeed it overlooks the duty of states affirmatively to create conditions necessary for the fulfilment of rights. Symbolically, a non-violative, rights-respecting rollout [of circumcision] is indispensable to encouraging men to elect 'the procedure [281]' and, to quote from Clark and coworkers from the Institute of Catholic Bioethics, "Mandating neonatal male circumcision is an effective therapy that has minimal risks, is cost efficient and will save human lives. To deny individuals access to this effective therapy is to deny them the dignity and respect all persons deserve. Neonatal male circumcision is medically necessary and ethically imperative" [282].

The speed of the roll-out of circumcision will be increased by enlisting and training paramedical as well as traditional and religious figures [283]. A voucher system has been suggested [283]. More funding and doctors are needed. Had a "parachute approach" to evidence-based medicine been applied in the early 1990s millions of lives would have been saved [284].

54.7.10 Condoms

Condoms, when always used, reduce HIV infection by 80–90% [285]. Condom use remains low, however [286], with 45% of the sexually active population of western countries not using them [287]. In Zimbabwe, 78% had never used condoms [288]. In US studies, 38% of US adults [289] and 16% of men and 24% of women [290] never used condoms during heterosexual sex with a nonprimary partner. Of female STI clinic attendees in Baltimore, 25% stated consistent use and 48% had not used them in the previous 2 weeks [291]. Male DNA was, however, detected in the vagina in all, albeit at higher levels in nonusers [291]. Among American college students, 40% had not used condoms in the previous 6 months and <50% intended to use them in the next month [292]. Only 25% of younger Australians always used condoms, 25% never having done so [293]. In Mexico 51% of young men and 23% of young women reported using condoms, consistent use being 30% [294]. Of 13,293 Mexican public school students, among the 37% with high HIV/AIDS knowledge, condom use was higher in males (OR 1.4), but lower in females (OR 0.7) [295].

Condoms can, moreover, be applied incorrectly, may break, and certain cultures may object to their use. Even when the female partner was known to be infected and condoms were made available continuously, 89% did not use them [208].

Interestingly, it has been found that condom use did not influence rate of HIV transmission, only circumcision status did [160]. A review of ten studies from Africa found no association between condom use and reduction in HIV infection, one finding it increased infection [296]. Similarly, in a large Indian study, odds of having HIV were significantly higher for those who said they had used condoms always or often in the past 6 months [197]. Condom use ever was associated with a 2.7-fold higher HIV prevalence in another study from India, and it was suggested that this may be because those with high-risk behavior start using condoms after they learn that they have become infected [198]. Alternatively, the apparent ineffectiveness of condoms may be because men assess their risk and use condoms accordingly. For example, in the Kenyan RCT, men used condoms 70% of the time with sex workers, 40% of the time with casual partners, and 18% of the time with their usual partner. Moreover, unless a condom is used during all sex play then the risk remains of contact between the inner lining of the prepuce and HIV-laden secretions, sperm (in the case of homosexual sex), and cells or tissues of an infected sex partner. Diaphragms have been found to provide no protection against HIV [297].

Circumcision should be promoted as part of a package that includes safe-sex (condoms) and fidelity. There are now two "ABC's: 'abstinence, behavior and condoms', and 'antivirals, barriers and circumcision'. Consistent condom use has not reached a sufficiently high level, even after many years of widespread and often aggressive promotion, to produce a measurable slowing of new infections" [298]. Unlike most other approaches, circumcision is a practical, once-off preventative strategy whose effectiveness has been proven. Funding and resources have, however, been allocated disproportionately to each measure, and increased focus is needed for male circumcision programs [298].

54.7.11 Misinformation from Opponents of Circumcision

There has been a concerted attempt by individuals and organizations opposed to male circumcision to distort and otherwise misrepresent the findings that have emanated from good research studies that have attested to the benefits of circumcision. In the case of HIV, a meta-analysis by Van Howe [299] has been criticized by some leading figures in the field for its incorrect use of statistical methods and other transgressions [300, 301]. More recently, an opinion piece by others countering the evidence that circumcision can prevent HIV infection has led to a detailed rebuttal by 48 authors that included academic experts worldwide, as well as representatives of WHO, UNAIDS, and the World Bank [193]. The latter publication documents the reasons for scale-up of circumcision in the fight against HIV/AIDS.

54.8 Conclusion

Male circumcision is a very effective component of STI-prevention messages, especially as condoms are not a panacea, even when used consistently [302]. Indeed, when coupled with the enormous evidence for other extensive benefits of this low risk procedure over the lifetime of males, the current evidence leads to a conclusion that circumcision should be regarded as "a biomedical imperative for the twenty-first century" [1]. So strong is the evidence that male circumcision is now regarded as a "surgical vaccine" for STI prevention. Moreover, to quote a UNAIDS document, "access to accurate information about male circumcision is a human right" [303]. Globally, 30% of males aged 15 years or more are circumcised [279], a high number for an intervention such as this. Although males can be circumcised at any age, the neonatal period appears best, since at this age the procedure is cheaper, simpler, more convenient, safer, does not involve stitches, need involve only a local anesthetic, means no anxiety by the male or others later about whether to have it done, can be pain-free, and is most likely to result in an optimum outcome. Efforts aimed at further increasing the rate of circumcision internationally should help in lowering the burden of STIs around the world.

Take-Home Pearls

- Circumcision prevents several types of common STIs.
- Risk to men of HIV infection acquired heterosexually is reduced at least threefold.
- Risk of syphilis is halved.
- Risk of HPV infection is reduced two- to fourfold.
- Risk of invasive penile cancer is reduced more than 20-fold.
- Risk of HSV-2, thrush, and trichomonas in men is reduced by up to half.
- Risk of cervical cancer (caused by high-risk HPV) in the female partner is reduced by two- to sixfold.
- Risk of Chlamydia in the female partner may be reduced by up to sixfold.
- Risk of HSV-2 in the female partner is halved.
- Risk of bacterial vaginosis and trichomonas in the female partner is reduced by half.
- There are many other benefits of circumcision besides STI prevention, including a marked reduction in urinary tract infections over the lifetime, elimination of phimosis and paraphimosis, lowering of balanitis and other inflammatory skin conditions, and improved genital hygiene.
- Good research, including data from two RCTs, has shown there is no adverse effect of male circumcision on sexual function, satisfaction, or sensitivity of the penis.
- While circumcision can be performed at any age, the neonatal period is the best time.

References

1. Morris, B.J.: Why circumcision is a biomedical imperative for the 21st century. BioEssays **29**, 1147–1158 (2007)
2. Morris, B.J.: Circumcision: an evidence-based appraisal - medical, health and sexual (Review). http://www.circinfo.net (>1,000 refs) (2010)
3. Hutchinson, J.: On the influence of circumcision in preventing syphilis. Medical Times and Gazette II:542-543. www.historyofcircumcision.net (1855)
4. Remondino, P.C.: 1891 History of circumcision: from the earliest times to the present: moral and physical reasons for its performance, with a history of eunuchism, hermaphrodism, etc. and of the different operations practiced upon the prepuce. Physicians' and students' ready reference series; No. 11 (Republished 1990). FA Davis, Philadelphia
5. Asin, J.: Chancroid; a report of 1, 402 cases. Am. J. Syph. Gonorrhea Vener. Dis. **36**, 483–487 (1952)
6. Cook, L.S., Koutsky, L.A., Holmes, K.K.: Circumcision and sexually transmitted diseases. Am. J. Public Health **84**, 197–201 (1994)
7. Dickson, N., van Roode, T., Paul, C.: Herpes simplex virus type 2 status at age 26 is not related to early circumcision in a birth cohort. Sex. Transm. Dis. **32**, 517–519 (2005)
8. Diseker, R.A., Peterman, T.A., Kamb, M.L., et al.: Circumcision and STD in the United States: cross sectional and cohort analysis. Sex. Transm. Infect. **76**, 474–479 (2000)
9. Donovan, B., Basset, I., Bodsworth, N.J.: Male circumcision and common sexually transmissible diseases in a developed nation setting. Genitourin. Med. **70**, 317–320 (1994)
10. Hammond, G.W., Slutchuk, M., Scatliff, J., et al.: Epidemiologic, clinical, laboratory, and therapeutic features of an urban outbreak of chancroid in North America. Rev. Infect. Dis. **2**, 867–879 (1980)
11. Hand, E.A.: Circumcision and venereal disease. Arch. Dermatol. Syphilol. **60**, 341–346 (1949)
12. Hart, G.: Factors associated with genital chlamydial and gonoccocal infection in males. Genitourin. Med. **69**, 393–396 (1993)

13. Latif, A.S., Katzenstein, D.A., Bassett, M.T., et al.: Genital ulcers and transmission of HIV among couples in Zimbabwe. AIDS **3**, 519–523 (1989)
14. Parker, J.D., Banatvala, J.E.: Herpes genitalis; clinical and virological studies. Br. J. Vener. Dis. **43**, 212–216 (1967)
15. Parker, S.W., Stewart, A.J., Wren, M.N., et al.: Circumcision and sexually transmissible diseases. Med. J. Aust. **2**, 288–290 (1983)
16. Smith, G., Greenup, R., Takafuji, E.: Circumcision as a risk factor for urethritis in racial groups. Am. J. Publ. Health **77**, 452–454 (1987)
17. Taylor, P.K., Rodin, P.: Herpes genitalis and circumcision. Br. J. Ven. Dis. **51**, 274–277 (1975)
18. Wilson, R.A.: Circumcision and venereal disease. Can. Med. Assoc. J. **56**, 54–56 (1947)
19. Moses, S., Bailey, R.C., Ronald, A.R.: Male circumcision: assessment of health benefits and risks. Sex Transm. Inf. **74**, 368–373 (1998)
20. Laumann, E.O., Maal, C.M., Zuckerman, E.W.: Circumcision in the United States. Prevalence, prophyactic effects, and sexual practice. J. Am. Med. Assoc. **277**, 1052–1057 (1997)
21. Weiss, H.A., Thomas, S.L., Munabi, S.K., et al.: Male circumcision and risk of syphilis, chancroid, and genital herpes: a systematic review and meta-analysis. Sex. Transm. Infect. **82**, 101–109 (2006)
22. Xu, F., Markowitz, L.E., Sternberg, M.R., et al.: Prevalence of circumcision and herpes simplex virus type 2 infection in men in the United States: the National Health and Nutrition Examination Survey (NHANES), 1999-2004. Sex. Transm. Dis. **34**, 479–484 (2007)
23. Mahiane, S.G., Legeai, C., Taljaard, D., et al.: Transmission probabilities of HIV and herpes simplex virus type 2, effect of male circumcision and interaction: a longitudinal study in a township of South Africa. AIDS **23**, 377–383 (2009)
24. Fergusson, D.M., Boden, J.M., Horwood, L.J.: Circumcision status and risk of sexually transmitted infection in young adult males: an analysis of a longitudinal birth cohort. Pediatrics **118**, 1971–1977 (2006)
25. Dickson, N.P., van Roode, T., Herbison, P., et al.: Circumcision and risk of sexually transmitted infections in a birth cohort. J. Pediatr. **152**, 383–387 (2008)
26. Sobngwi-Tambekou, J., Taljaard, D., Lissouba, P., et al.: Effect of HSV-2 serostatus on acquisition of HIV by young men: results of a longitudinal study in Orange Farm, South Africa. J. Infect. Dis. **199**, 958–964 (2009)
27. Tobian, A.A.R., Charvat, B., Ssempijja, V., et al.: Factors associated with the prevalence and incidence of herpes simplex virus type 2 infection among men in Rakai, Uganda. J. Infect. Dis. **199**, 945–949 (2009)
28. Van Wagoner, N.J., Geisler, W.M., Sizemore, J.M., Jr., et al.: Herpes simplex virus in African American heterosexual males: the roles of age and male circumcision. Sex Transm. Dis. **37**, 217–222 (2010)
29. Bailey, R.C., Mehta, S.D.: Circumcision's place in the vicious cycle involving herpes simplex virus type 2 and HIV. J. Infect. Dis. **199**, 923–925 (2009)
30. Jerath, V.P., Mahajan, V.K.: Does circumcision influence recurrences in herpes genitalis? Indian J. Dermatol. Venereol. Leprol. **75**, 575–578 (2009)
31. Gray, R.H., Kigozi, G., Serwadda, D., et al.: Male circumcision for HIV prevention in men in Rakai, Uganda: a randomised trial. Lancet **369**, 657–666 (2007)
32. Tobian, A.A.R., Serwadda, D., Quinn, T.C., et al.: Male circumcision for the prevention of HSV-2 and HPV infections and syphilis. N. Engl. J. Med. **360**, 1298–1309 (2009)
33. Gray, R.H., Serwadda, D., Tobian, A.A.R., et al.: Effects of genital ulcer disease and herpes simplex virus type 2 on the efficacy of male circumcision for HIV prevention: analyses from the Rakai trials. PLoS Med **6**, e1000187 (8 pp.) (2009)
34. Golden, M.R., Wasserheit, J.N.: Prevention of viral sexually transmitted infections–foreskin at the forefront. N. Engl. J. Med. **360**, 1349–1351 (2009)
35. Templeton, D.J., Jin, F., Prestage, G.P., et al.: Circumcision and risk of sexually transmissible infections in a community-based cohort of HIV-negative homosexual men in Sydney, Australia. J. Infect. Dis. **200**, 1813–1819 (2009)
36. Jameson, D.R., Celum, C.L., Manhart, L., et al.: The association between lack of circumcision and HIV, HSV-2, and other sexually transmitted infections among men who have sex with men. Sex Transm. Dis. **37**, 147–152 (2010)
37. Van Howe, R.S.: Genital ulcerative disease and sexually transmitted urethritis and circumcision: a meta-analysis. Int. J. STD AIDS **18**, 799–809 (2007)
38. Waskett, J.H., Morris, B.J., Weiss, H.A.: Errors in meta-analysis by Van Howe. Int. J. STD AIDS **20**, 216–218 (2009)
39. Anonymous: Erratum for Van Howe, Int. J. STD AIDS **18**(12), 799–809. Int. J. STD AIDS **20**, 592 (2009)
40. Auvert, B., Sobngwi-Tambekou, J., Cutler, E., et al.: Effect of male circumcision on the prevalence of high-risk human papillomavirus in young men: results of a randomized controlled trial conducted in orange farm, South Africa. J. Infect. Dis. **199**, 14–19 (2009)
41. Sobngwi-Tambekou, J., Taljaard, D., Nieuwoudt, M., et al.: Male circumcision and *Neisseria gonorrhoeae*, *Chlamydia trachomatis*, and *Trichomonas vaginalis*: observations in the aftermath of a randomised controlled trial for HIV prevention. Sex. Transm. Infect. **85**, 116–120 (2009)
42. Mehta, S.D., Moses, S., Agot, K., et al.: Adult male circumcision does not reduce the risk of incident *Neisseria gonorrhoeae*, *Chlamydia trachomatis*, or *Trichomonas vaginalis* infection: results from a randomized, controlled trial in Kenya. J. Infect. Dis. **200**, 370–378 (2009)
43. Richters, J., Smith, A.M., de Visser, R.O., et al.: Circumcision in Australia: prevalence and effects on sexual health. Int. J. STD AIDS **17**, 547–554 (2006)
44. Kochen, M., McCurdy, S.: Circumcision and risk of cancer of the penis. A life-table analysis. Am. J. Dis. Child. **134**, 484–486 (1980)
45. Wiswell, T.E.: Neonatal circumcision: a current appraisal. Focus Opin. Pediat. **1**, 93–99 (1995)
46. Wiswell, T.E.: Circumcision circumspection. N. Engl. J. Med. **36**, 1244–1245 (1997)
47. Schoen, E.J.: The relationship between circumcision and cancer of the penis. CA Cancer J. Clin. **41**, 306–309 (1991)
48. Schoen, E.J.: Neonatal circumcision and penile cancer. Evidence that circumcision is protective is overwhelming. Br. Med. J. **46**, 313 (1996)
49. Wolbarst, A.L.: Circumcision and penile cancer. Lancet **i**, 150–153 (1932)

50. Maden, C., Sherman, K.J., Beckmann, A.M., et al.: History of circumcision, medical conditions, and sexual activity and risk of penile cancer. J. Nat. Cancer Inst. **85**, 19–24 (1993)
51. Carver, B.S., Venable, D.D., et al.: Squamous cell carcinoma of the penis: a retrospective review of forty-five patients in northwest Louisiana. South Med. J. **95**, 822–825 (2002)
52. Schoen, E.J., Oehrli, M., Colby, C.J., et al.: The highly protective effect of newborn circumcision against invasive penile cancer. Pediatrics **105**, e36 (4 pp.) (2000)
53. Schoen, E.J., Wiswell, T.E., Moses, S.: New policy on circumcision – cause for concern. Pediatrics **105**, 620–623 (2000)
54. Barnholtz-Sloan, J.S., Maldonado, J.L., Pow-sang, J., et al.: Incidence trends in primary malignant penile cancer. Urol. Oncol. **25**, 361–367 (2007)
55. Goodman, M.T., Hernandez, B.Y., Shvetsov, Y.: Demographic and pathologic differences in the incidence of invasive penile cancer in the United States, 1995–2003. Cancer Epidemiol. Biomarkers Prev. **16**, 1833–1839 (2007)
56. Hu, D., Goldie, S.: The economic burden of noncervical human papillomavirus disease in the United States. Am. J. Obstet. Gynecol. **198**, 500.e1–500.e7 (2008)
57. Tsen, H.F., Morgenstern, H., Mack, T., et al.: Risk factors for penile cancer: results of a population-based case-control study in Los Angeles County (United States). Cancer Causes Control **12**, 267–277 (2001)
58. Seyam, R.M., Bissada, N.K., Mokhtar, A.A., et al.: Outcome of penile cancer in circumcised men. J. Urol. **175**, 557–561 (2006)
59. Micali, G., Nasca, M.R., Innocenzi, D., et al.: Penile cancer. J. Am. Acad. Dermatol. **54**, 369–391 (2006)
60. Sanchez Merino, J.M., Parra Muntaner, L., Jiminez Rodriguez, M., et al.: Epidoid carcinoma of the penis. Arch. Esp. Urol. **53**, 799–808 (2000)
61. Dagher, R., Selzer, M.L., Lapides, J.: Carcinoma of the penis and the anti-circumcision crusade. J. Urol. **110**, 79–80 (1973)
62. Sandeman, T.F.: Carcinoma of the penis. Australasian Radiol. **34**, 12–16 (1990)
63. American Cancer Society: Cancer statistics. http://www.cancer.org/docroot/CRI/content/CRI_2_4_1X_What_are_the_key_statistics_for_penile_cancer_35.asp?rnav=cri (2005)
64. Gross, G., Pfister, H.: Role of human papillomavirus in penile cancer, penile intraepithelial squamous cell neoplasias and in genital warts. Med. Microbiol. Immunol. **193**, 35–44 (2004)
65. Narayana, A.S., Olney, L.E., Loening, S.A.: Carcinoma of the penis: analysis of 219 cases. Cancer **49**, 2185–2191 (1982)
66. Dodge, O.G., Linsell, C.A.: Carcinoma of the penis in Uganda and Kenya Africans. Cancer **18**, 1255–1263 (1963)
67. World Health Organization: International Agency for Research on Cancer 1966–1997: Cancer Incidence in Five Countries, vol. 1–7 (1997)
68. Favorito, L.A., Nardi, A.C., Ronalsa, M., et al.: Epidemiologic study on penile cancer in Brazil. Int. Braz. J. Urol. **34**, 587–591 (2008)
69. Villa, L.L., Lopez, A.: Human papillomavirus sequence in penile carcinomas in Brazil. Int. J. Cancer **37**, 853–855 (1986)
70. Baldwin, S.B., Wallace, D.R., Papenfuss, M.R., et al.: Condom use and other factors affecting penile human papillomavirus detection in men attending a sexually transmitted disease clinic. Sex. Transm. Dis. **31**, 601–607 (2004)
71. Castellsague, X., Bosch, F.X., Munoz, N., et al.: Male circumcision, penile human papillomavirus infection, and cervical cancer in female partners. N. Engl. J. Med. **346**, 1105–1112 (2002)
72. Hernandez, B.Y., Wilkens, L.R., Zhu, X., et al.: Circumcision and human papillomavirus infection in men: a site-specific comparison. J. Infect. Dis. **197**, 787–794 (2008)
73. Kohn, F.-M., Pflieger-Bruss, S., Schill, W.-B.: Penile skin diseases. Andrologia **31**(suppl 1), 3–11 (1999)
74. Lajous, M., Mueller, N., Cruz-Valdez, A., et al.: Determinants of prevalence, acquisition, and persistence of human papillomavirus in healthy Mexican military men. Cancer Epidemiol. Biomarkers Prev. **14**, 1710–1716 (2005)
75. Niku, S.D., Stock, J.A., Kaplan, G.W.: Neonatal circumcision (Review). Urol. Clin. N. Am. **22**, 57–65 (1995)
76. Shin, H.R., Franceschi, S., Vaccarella, S., et al.: Prevalence and determinants of genital infection with papillomavirus, in female and male university students in Busan, South Korea. J. Infect. Dis. **190**, 468–478 (2004)
77. Svare, E.I., Kjaer, S.K., Worm, A.M., et al.: Risk factors for genital HPV DNA in men resemble those found in women: a study of male attendees at a Danish STD clinic. Sex. Transm. Infect. **78**, 215–218 (2002)
78. Bosch, F.X., Albero, G., Castellsagué, X.: Male circumcision, human papillomavirus and cervical cancer: from evidence to intervention. J. Fam. Plann. Reprod. Health Care **35**, 5–7 (2009)
79. Van Howe, R.S.: Human papillomavirus and circumcision: a meta-analysis. J. Infect. **54**, 490–496 (2007)
80. Castellsague, X., Albero, G., Cleries, R., et al.: HPV and circumcision: a biased, inaccurate and misleading meta-analysis. J. Infect. **55**, 91–93 (2007)
81. Gray, R.H.: Infectious disease: Male circumcision for preventing HPV infection. Nat. Rev. Urol. **6**, 298–299 (2009)
82. Weaver, B.A., Feng, Q., Holmes, K.K., et al.: Evaluation of genital sites and sampling techniques for detection of human papillomavirus DNA in men. J. Infect. Dis. **189**, 677–685 (2004)
83. Smith, J.S., Backes, D.M., Hudgens, M.G., et al.: Prevalence and risk factors of human papillomavirus infection by penile site in uncircumcised Kenyan men. Int. J. Cancer **126**, 572–577 (2009)
84. Giuliano, A.R., Lazcano, E., Villa, L.L., et al.: Circumcision and sexual behavior: factors independently associated with human papillomavirus detection among men in the HIM study. Int. J. Cancer **124**, 1251–1257 (2009)
85. Nielson, C.M., Schiaffino, M.K., Dunne, E.F., et al.: Associations between male anogenital human papillomavirus infection and circumcision by anatomic site sampled and lifetime number of female sex partners. J. Infect. Dis. **199**, 7–13 (2009)
86. Dickson, N.P., Ryding, J., van Roode, T., et al.: Male circumcision and serologically determined human papillomavirus infection in a birth cohort. Cancer Epidemiol. Biomarkers Prev. **18**, 177–183 (2009)
87. Lu, B., Wu, Y., Nielson, C.M., et al.: Factors associated with acquisition and clearance of human papillomavirus

infection in a cohort of US men: a prospective study. J. Infect. Dis. **199**, 362–371 (2009)
88. Katelaris, P.M., Cossart, Y.E., Rose, B.R., et al.: Human papillomavirus: the untreated male reservoir. J. Urol. **140**, 300–305 (1988)
89. Aynaud, O., Ionesco, M., Barrasso, R.: Penile intraepithelial neoplasia – specific clinical features correlate with histologic and virologic findings. Cancer **74**, 1762–1767 (1994)
90. Daling, J.R., Madeleine, M.M., Johnson, L.G., et al.: Penile cancer: importance of circumcision, human papillomavirus and smoking in in situ and invasive disease. Int. J. Cancer **116**, 606–616 (2005)
91. Dillner, J., von Krogh, G., Horenblas, S., et al.: Etiology of squamous cell carcinoma of the penis. Scand. J. Urol. Nephrol. **205**(Suppl), 189–193 (2000)
92. Reddy, C.R., Devendranath, V., Pratap, S.: Carcinoma of penis: role of phimosis. Urology **24**, 85–88 (1984)
93. Velazquez, E.F., Bock, A., Soskin, A., et al.: Preputial variability and preferential association of long phimotic foreskins with penile cancer: an anatomic comparative study of types of foreskin in a general population and cancer patients. Am. J. Surg. Pathol. **27**, 994–998 (2003)
94. Dennis, E.J., Heins, H.C., Latham, E., et al.: The carcinogenic effect of human smegma: an experimental study. I. Preliminary report. Cancer Epidemiol. Biomarkers Prev. **9**, 671–680 (1956)
95. Heins Jr., H.C., Dennis, E.J.: The possible role of smegma in carcinoma of the cervix. Am. J. Obstet. Gynecol. **76**, 726–733 (1958)
96. Pratt-Thomas, H.R., Heins, H.C., Latham, E., et al.: Carcinogenic effect of human smegma: an experimental study. Cancer **9**, 671–680 (1956)
97. Reddy, D.G., Baruah, I.K.: Carcinogenic action of human smegma. Arch. Pathol. **75**, 414 (1963)
98. Schoeberlein, W.: Bedeutung und Haeufigkeit von Phimose und Smegma (Significance and frequency ofr phimosis and smegma) (Translated by Kasper, J.P., 1997; edited by Bailis, S.A., 1997). Muench Med. Wschr. **7**, 373–377 (1966)
99. Madsen, B.S., van den Brule, A.J., Jensen, H.L., et al.: Risk factors for squamous cell carcinoma of the penis–population-based case-control study in Denmark. Cancer Epidemiol. Biomarkers Prev. **17**, 2683–2691 (2008)
100. Haneke, E.: Skin diseases and tumors of the penis. Urol. Int. **37**, 172–182 (1982)
101. Sayed, E.I., Viraben, R., Bazex, J., et al.: Carcinome verruqueux du penis. Nouv. Dermatol. **12**, 112–113 (1993)
102. Pietrzak, P., Hadway, P., Corbishley, C.M., et al.: Is the association between balanitis xerotica obliterans and penile carcinoma underestimated? BJU Int. **98**, 74–76 (2006)
103. Nasca, M.R., Innocenzi, D., Micali, G.: Association of penile lichen sclerosus and oncogenic human papillomavirus infection. Int. J. Dermatol. **45**, 681–683 (2006)
104. Fernando, J.J., Wanas, T.M.: Squamous carcinoma of the penis and previous recurrent balanitis: a case report. Genitourin. Med. **67**, 153–155 (1991)
105. zur Hausen, H.: Herpes simplex virus in human genital cancer. Int. Rev. Exp. Pathol. **25**, 307–326 (1983)
106. Bailis, S.A.: Circumcision – The debate goes on. Pediatrics **105**, 682 (2000)
107. Ozsahin, M., Jichlinski, P., Weber, D.C., et al.: Treatment of penile carcinoma: to cut or not to cut? Int. J. Radiat. Oncol. Biol. Phys. **66**, 674–679 (2006)
108. Zouhair, A., Coucke, P.A., Jeanneret, W., et al.: Radiation therapy alone or combined surgery and radiation therapy in squamous-cell carcinoma of the penis? Eur. J. Cancer **37**, 198–203 (2001)
109. Opjordsmoen, S., Waehre, H., Aass, N., et al.: Sexuality in patients treated for penile cancer; patient's experience and doctor's judgement. Br. J. Urol. **73**, 554–560 (1994)
110. Adami, H.O., Kuper, H., Andersson, S.O., et al.: Prostate cancer risk and serologic evidence of human papilloma virus infection: a population-based case-control study. Cancer Epidemiol Biomarkers Prev **12**, 872–875 (2003)
111. Correa, P.: Is prostate cancer an infectious disease? Int. J. Epidemiol. **34**, 197–198 (2005)
112. Dennis, L.K., Dawson, D.V.: Meta-analysis of measures of sexual activity and prostate cancer. Epidemiology **13**, 72–79 (2002)
113. Dillner, J., Knekt, P., Boman, J., et al.: Sero-epidemiological association between human-papillomavirus infection and risk of prostate cancer. Int. J. Cancer **75**, 564–567 (1998)
114. Fernandez, L., Galan, Y., Jimenez, R., et al.: Sexual behaviour, history of sexually transmitted diseases, and the risk of prostate cancer: a case-control study in Cuba. Int. J. Epidemiol. **34**, 193–197 (2005)
115. Hayes, R.B., Pottern, L.M., Strickler, H., et al.: Sexual behaviour, STDs and risks for prostate cancer. Br. J. Cancer **82**, 718–725 (2000)
116. Oliver, J.C., Oliver, R.T., Ballard, R.C.: Influence of circumcision and sexual behaviour on PSA levels in patients attending a sexually transmitted disease (STD) clinic. Prostate Cancer Prostatic Dis. **4**, 228–231 (2001)
117. Radhakrishnan, S., Lee, A., Oliver, T., et al.: An infectious cause for prostate cancer. BJU Int. **99**, 239–240 (2007)
118. Ross, R.K., Shimizu, H., Paganini-Hill, A., et al.: Case-control studies of prostate cancer in blacks and whites in southern California. J. Natl. Cancer Inst. **78**, 869–874 (1987)
119. Taylor, M.L., Mainous 3rd, A.G., Wells, B.J.: Prostate cancer and sexually transmitted diseases: a meta-analysis. Fam. Med. **37**, 506–512 (2005)
120. Balis, V., Sourvinos, G., Soulitzis, N., et al.: Prevalence of BK virus and human papillomavirus in human prostate cancer. Int. J. Biol. Markers **22**, 245–251 (2007)
121. Schlaberg, R., Choe, D.J., Brown, K.R., et al.: XMRV is present in malignant prostatic epithelium and is associated with prostate cancer, especially high-grade tumors. Proc. Natl. Acad. Sci. USA **106**, 16351–16356 (2009)
122. Stark, J.R., Judson, G., Alderete, J.F., et al.: Prospective study of *Trichomonas vaginalis* infection and prostate cancer incidence and mortality: Physicians' Health Study. J. Natl. Cancer Inst. **101**, 1406–1411 (2009)
123. Apt, A.: Circumcision and prostatic cancer. Acta Med. Scand. **178**, 493–504 (1965)
124. Ewings, P., Bowie, C.: A case-control study of cancer of the prostate in Somerset and east Devon. Br. J. Cancer **74**, 661–666 (1996)
125. Ravich, A., Ravich, R.A.: Prophylaxis of cancer of the prostate, penis, and cervix by circumcision. N Y State J. Med. **51**, 1519–1520 (1951)

126. Alderson, M.: Occupational Cancer. Butterworths, London (1986)
127. Morris, B.J., Waskett, J., Bailis, S.A.: Case number and the financial impact of circumcision in reducing prostate cancer. BJU Int. **100**, 5–6 (2007)
128. Drain, P.K., Halperin, D.T., Hughes, J.P., et al.: Male circumcision, religion, and infectious diseases: an ecologic analysis of 118 developing countries. BMC Infect. Dis. **6**, 172 (110 pp.) (2006)
129. Barrasso, R., De Brux, J., Croissant, O., et al.: High prevalence of papillomavirus associated penile intraepithelial neoplasia in sexual partners of women with cervical intraepithelial neoplasia. N. Engl. J. Med. **317**, 916–923 (1987)
130. Zelkowitz, R.: Cancer. HPV casts a wider shadow. Science **323**, 580–581 (2009)
131. Amarante, M.K., Watanabe, M.A.: The possible involvement of virus in breast cancer. J. Cancer Res. Clin. Oncol. **135**, 329–337 (2009)
132. Lawson, J.S., Gunzburg, W.H., Whitaker, N.J.: Viruses and human breast cancer. Future Microbiol. **1**, 33–51 (2006)
133. Hennig, E.M., Suo, Z., Thoresen, S., et al.: Human papillomavirus 16 in breast cancer of women treated for high grade cervical intraepithelial neoplasia (CIN III). Breast Cancer Res. Treat. **53**, 121–135 (1999)
134. Widschwendter, A., Brunhuber, T., Wiedemair, A., et al.: Detection of human papillomavirus DNA in breast cancer of patients with cervical cancer history. J. Clin. Virol. **31**, 292–297 (2004)
135. Kan, C.Y., Iacopetta, B.J., Lawson, J.S., et al.: Identification of human papillomavirus DNA gene sequences in human breast cancer. Br. J. Cancer **93**, 946–948 (2005)
136. Lawson, J.S., Kan, C.Y., Iacopetta, B.J., et al.: Are some breast cancers sexually transmitted? Br. J. Cancer **95**, 1708 (2006)
137. Heng, B., Glenn, W.K., Ye, Y., et al.: Human papilloma virus is associated with breast cancer. Br. J. Cancer **101**, 1345–1350 (2009)
138. Lawson, J.S., Glenn, W.K., Heng, B., et al.: Koilocytes indicate a role for human papilloma virus in breast cancer. Br. J. Cancer **101**, 1351–1356 (2009)
139. Tseng, C.J., Pao, C.C., Lin, J.D., et al.: Detection of human papillomavirus types 16 and 18 mRNA in peripheral blood of advanced cervical cancer patients and its association with prognosis. J. Clin. Oncol. **17**, 1391–1396 (1999)
140. Chen, A.C., Keleher, A., Kedda, M.A., et al.: Human papillomavirus DNA detected in peripheral blood samples from healthy Australian male blood donors. J. Med. Virol. **81**, 1792–1796 (2009)
141. Herrero, R.: Human papillomavirus (HPV) vaccines: limited cross-protection against additional HPV types. J. Infect. Dis. **199**, 919–922 (2009)
142. Garland, S.M., Hernandez-Avila, M., Wheeler, C.M., et al.: Quadrivalent vaccine against human papillomavirus to prevent anogenital diseases. N. Engl. J. Med. **356**, 1928–1943 (2007)
143. de Kok, I.M.C.M., van Ballegooijen, M., Habbem, J.D.F.: Cost-effectiveness analysis of human papillomavirus vaccination in the Netherlands. J. Natl. Cancer Inst. **101**, 1083–1092 (2009)
144. Brisson, M., Van de Velde, N., Boily, M.C.: Economic evaluation of human papillomavirus vaccination in developed countries. Public Health Genom. **12**, 343–351 (2009)
145. Choi, Y.H., Jit, M., Gay, N., et al.: Transmission dynamic modelling of the impact of human papillomavirus vaccination in the United Kingdom. Vaccine **28**, 4091–4102 (2010)
146. Cherpes, T.L., Meyne, L.A., Krohn, M.A., et al.: Risk factors for infection with herpes simplex virus type 2: role of smoking, douching, uncircumcised males, and vaginal flora. Sex. Transm. Dis. **30**, 405–410 (2003)
147. Tobian, A., Serwadda, D., Quinn, T., et al.: Trial of male circumcision: prevention of HSV-2 in men and vaginal infections in female partners, Rakai, Uganda. 15th Conference on Retroviruses and Opportunistic Infections, Boston, abstract 28LB (2008)
148. Brankin, A.E., Tobian, A.A., Laeyendecker, O., et al.: Aetiology of genital ulcer disease in female partners of male participants in a circumcision trial in Uganda. Int. J. STD AIDS **20**, 650–651 (2009)
149. Castellsague, X., Peeling, R.W., Franceschi, S., et al.: *Chlamydia trachomatis* infection in female partners of circumcised and uncircumcised adult men. Am. J. Epidemiol. **162**, 907–916 (2005)
150. Turner, A.N., Morrison, C.S., Padian, N.S., et al.: Male circumcision and women's risk of Incident chlamydial, gonococcal, and trichomonal Infections. Sex. Transm. Dis. **35**, 689–695 (2008)
151. Cherpes, T.L., Hillier, S.L., Meyn, L.A., et al.: A delicate balance: risk factors for acquisition of bacterial vaginosis include sexual activity, absence of hydrogen peroxide-producing lactobacilli, black race, and positive herpes simplex virus type 2 serology. Sex. Transm. Dis. **35**, 78–83 (2008)
152. Gray, R.H., Kigozi, G., Serwadda, D., et al.: The effects of male circumcision on female partners' genital tract symptoms and vaginal infections in a randomized trial in Rakai, Uganda. Am. J. Obstet. Gynecol. **200**, e1–e7 (2009)
153. Joint United Nations Programme on HIV/AIDS. The HIV/AIDS Situation in Mid 1996: Global and Regional Highlights. United Nations, Geneva (UNAIDS fact sheet) (1996)
154. Fink, A.J.: A possible explanation for heterosexual male infection with AIDS. N. Engl. J. Med. **314**, 1167 (1986)
155. Fischbacher, C.M.: Circumcision of newborn boys. Lancet **353**, 669–670 (1999)
156. Siegfried, N., Muller, M., Volmink, J., et al.: Male circumcision for prevention of heterosexual acquisition of HIV in men. Cochrane Database Syst. Rev. CD003362 (2003)
157. Weiss, H.A., Quigley, M.A., Hayes, R.J.: Male circumcision and risk of HIV infection in sub-Saharan Africa: a systematic review and meta-analysis. AIDS **14**, 2361–2370 (2000)
158. Weiss, H.A., Halperin, D., Bailey, R.C., et al.: Male circumcision for HIV prevention: from evidence to action? (Review). AIDS **22**, 567–574 (2008)
159. McCoombe, S.G., Short, R.V.: Potential HIV-1 target cells in the human penis. AIDS **20**, 1491–1495 (2006)
160. Szabo, R., Short, R.V.: How does male circumcision protect against HIV infection? Br. Med. J. **320**, 1592–1594 (2000)

161. Cameron, B.E., Simonsen, J.N., D'Costa, L.J., et al.: Female to male transmission of human immunodeficiency virus type 1: risk factors for seroconversion in men. Lancet **ii**, 403–407 (1989)
162. Bailey, R.C.: Male circumcision as an effective HIV prevention strategy: current evidence. 8th Conference on Retroviruses and Opportunistic Infections, Chicago, S22, 2001. http://www.retroconference.org//requested_lectures.cfm?ID=383& mode =send
163. Kaizu, M., Weiler, A.M., Weisgrau, K.L., et al.: Repeated intravaginal inoculation with cell-associated simian immunodeficiency virus results in persistent infection of nonhuman primates. J. Infect. Dis. **194**, 912–916 (2006)
164. O'Farrell, N., Morison, L., Moodley, P., et al.: Association between HIV and subpreputial penile wetness in uncircumcised men in South Africa. J. Acquir. Immune Defic. Syndr. **43**, 69–77 (2006)
165. O'Farrell, N., Chung, C.K., Weiss, H.A.: Foreskin length in uncircumcised men is associated with subpreputial wetness. Int. J. STD AIDS **19**, 821–823 (2008)
166. Alanis, M.C., Lucidi, R.S.: Neonatal circumcision: A review of the world's oldest and most controversial operation. Obstet. Gynecol. Surv. **59**, 379–395 (2004)
167. Patterson, B.K., Landy, A., Siegel, J.N., et al.: Susceptibility to human immunodeficiency virus-1 infection of human foreskin and cervical tissue grown in explant culture. Am. J. Pathol. **161**, 867–873 (2002)
168. Miller, C.: Localization of simian immunodeficiency virus-infected cells in the genital tract of male and female rhesus macaques. J. Reprod. Immunol. **4**, 331–339 (1998)
169. Fischetti, L., Barry, S.M., Hope, T.J., et al.: HIV-1 infection of human penile explant tissue and protection by candidate microbicides. AIDS **23**, 319–328 (2009)
170. Wawer, M.J., Reynolds, S.J., Serwadda, D., et al.: Might male circumcision be more protective against HIV in the highly exposed? An immunological hypothesis. AIDS **19**, 2181–2182 (2005)
171. Peters, B., Whittall, T., Babaahmady, K., et al.: Effect of heterosexual intercourse on mucosal alloimmunisation and resistance to HIV-1 infection. Lancet **363**, 518–524 (2004)
172. Donoval, B.A., Landay, A.L., Moses, S., et al.: HIV-1 target cells in foreskins of African men with varying histories of sexually transmitted infections. Am. J. Clin. Pathol. **125**, 386–391 (2006)
173. Turville, S.G., Cameron, P.U., Handley, A., et al.: Diversity of receptors binding HIV on dendritic cell subsets. Nat. Immunol. **3**, 975–983 (2002)
174. Boggiano, C., Littman, D.R.: HIV's vagina travelogue. Immunity **26**, 145–147 (2007)
175. Hladik, F., Sakchalathorn, P., Ballweber, L., et al.: Initial events in establishing vaginal entry and infection by human immunodeficiency virus type-1. Immunity **26**, 257–270 (2007)
176. de Witte, L., Nabatov, A., Pion, M., et al.: Langerin is a natural barrier to HIV-1 transmission by Langerhans cells. Nat. Med. **13**, 367–371 (2007)
177. Schwartz, O.: Langerhans cells lap up HIV-1. Nat. Med. **13**, 245–246 (2007)
178. Kigozi, G., Wawer, M., Ssettuba, A., et al.: Foreskin surface area and HIV acquisition in Rakai, Uganda (size matters). AIDS **23**, 2209–2213 (2009)
179. Byakika-Tusiime, J.: Circumcision and HIV infection: assessment of causality. AIDS Behav. **12**, 835–841 (2008)
180. O'Farrell, N.: Enhanced efficiency of female-to-male HIV transmission in core groups in developing countries. Sex. Transm. Dis. **28**, 84–91 (2001)
181. Powers, K.A., Poole, C., Pettifor, A.E., et al.: Rethinking the heterosexual infectivity of HIV-1: a systematic review and meta-analysis. Lancet **8**, 553–563 (2008)
182. Boily, M.C., Baggaley, R.F., Wang, L., et al.: Heterosexual risk of HIV-1 infection per sexual act: systematic review and meta-analysis of observational studies. Lancet Infect. Dis. **9**, 118–129 (2009)
183. Gilbert, M.T., Rambaut, A., Wlasiuk, G., et al.: The emergence of HIV/AIDS in the Americas and beyond. Proc. Natl. Acad. Sci. USA **104**, 18566–18570 (2007)
184. Telzak, E.E., Chiasson, M.A., Bevier, P.J., et al.: HIV-1 seroconversion in patients with and without genital ulcer disease. Ann. Intern. Med. **119**, 1181–1186 (1993)
185. US Centers for Disease Control and Prevention: HIV/AIDS surveillance report: cases of HIV infection and AIDS in the United States and dependent areas, 2005, vol. 17. Revised edition [cited]. http://www.cdc.gov/hiv/topics/surveillance/resources/reports/2005report/default.htm (2007)
186. Centers for Disease Control and Prevention, HIV/AIDS Surveillance Reports [cited]. http://www.cdc.gov/hiv/topics/surveillance/resources/reports/
187. Xu, X., Patel, D.A., Dalton, V.K., et al.: Can routine neonatal circumcision help prevent human immunodeficiency virus transmission in the United States? (Review). Am. J. Mens Health **3**, 79–84 (2009)
188. Warner, L., Ghanem, K.G., Newman, D.R., et al.: Male circumcision and risk of HIV infection among heterosexual African American men attending Baltimore sexually transmitted disease clinics. J. Infect. Dis. **199**, 59–65 (2009)
189. Sullivan, P.S., Kilmarx, P.H., Peterman, T.A., et al.: Male circumcision for prevention of HIV transmission: what the new data mean for HIV prevention in the United States. PLoS Med. **4**(e223), 1162–1166 (2007)
190. Macdonald, A., Humphreys, J., Jaffe, H.W.: Prevention of HIV transmission in the United Kingdom: what is the role of male circumcision? Sex. Transm. Infect. **84**, 158–160 (2008)
191. Gray, R.H., Quinn, T.C., Serwadda, D., et al.: The ethics of research in developing countries. N. Engl. J. Med. **343**, 361–362 (2000)
192. Halperin, D., Bailey, R.: Male circumcision and HIV infection: 10 years and counting. Lancet **354**, 1813–1815 (1999)
193. Wamai, R.G., Weiss, H.A., Hankins, C., et al.: Male circumcision is an efficacious, lasting and cost-effective strategy for combating HIV in high-prevalence AIDS epidemics: Time to move beyond debating the science. Future HIV Ther. **2**, 399–405 (2008)
194. Mastro, T., Satten, G., Nopkesorn, T., et al.: Probability of female-to-male transmission of HIV-1 in Thailand. Lancet **343**, 204–207 (1994)
195. Reynolds, S.J., Shepherd, M.E., Risbud, A.R., et al.: Male circumcision and risk of HIV-1 and other sexually transmitted infections in India. Lancet **363**, 1039–1040 (2004)
196. Talukdar, A., Khandokar, M.R., Bandopadhyay, S.K., et al.: Risk of HIV infection but not other sexually transmitted

diseases is lower among homeless Muslim men in Kolkata. AIDS **21**, 2231–2235 (2007)

197. Dandona, L., Dandona, R., Kumar, G.A., et al.: Risk factors associated with HIV in a population-based study in Andhra Pradesh state of India. Int. J. Epidemiol. **37**, 1274–1286 (2008)
198. Munro, H.L., Pradeep, B.S., Jayachandran, A.A., et al.: Prevalence and determinants of HIV and sexually transmitted infections in a general population-based sample in Mysore district, Karnataka state, southern India. AIDS **22**(suppl 5), S117–S125 (2008)
199. Madhivanan, P., Krupp, K.: Doesn't the public have the right to know that male circumcision protects against HIV? Indian J. Med. Ethics **6**, 5–6 (2009)
200. Li, P.S., Lü, N.Q., Cheng, Y., et al.: The need for high-quality training and surgical standards for adult male circumcision in China (Article in Chinese). Zhonghua Nan Ke Xue **15**, 390–394 (2009)
201. Périssé, A.R., Schechter, M., Blattner, W.: Association between male circumcision and prevalent HIV infections in Rio de Janeiro, Brazil. J. Acquir. Immune Defic. Syndr. **50**, 435–437 (2009)
202. Short, R.V.: New ways of preventing HIV infection: thinking simply, simply thinking. (Review). Philos. Trans. R. Soc. Lond. B Biol. Sci. **361**, 811–820 (2006)
203. Al-Mutairi, N., Joshi, A., Nour-Eldin, O., et al.: Clinical patterns of sexually transmitted diseases, associated sociodemographic characteristics, and sexual practices in the Farwaniya region of Kuwait. Int. J. Dermatol. **46**, 594–599 (2007)
204. Orroth, K.K., Freeman, E.E., Bakker, R., et al.: Understanding the differences between contrasting HIV epidemics in east and west Africa: results from a simulation model of the Four Cities Study. Sex. Transm. Infect. **83**(suppl 1), i5–i16 (2007)
205. Schmid, G.P., Buve, A., Mugyeny, P., et al.: Transmission of HIV-1 infection in sub-Saharan Africa and effect of elimination of unsafe injections. Lancet **363**, 482–488 (2004)
206. Baeten, J.M., Richardson, B.A., Lavreys, L., et al.: Female-to-male infectivity of HIV-1 among circumcised and uncircumcised Kenyan men. J. Infect. Dis. **191**, 546–553 (2005)
207. Gray, R.H., Kiwanuka, N., Quinn, T., et al.: Male circumcision and HIV aquisition and transmission: cohort studies in Raiki, Uganda. AIDS **14**, 42371–42381 (2000)
208. Quinn, T.C., Wawer, M.J., Sewankambo, N., et al.: Viral load and heterosexual transmission of human immunodeficiency virus type 1. N. Engl. J. Med. **342**, 921–929 (2000)
209. Makumbi, F.E., Gray, R.H., Wawer, M., et al.: Male post-coital penile cleansing and the risk of HIV-acquisition in rural Rakai district, Uganda. 4th International AIDS Society Conference, Sydney (2007) (late-breaker abstract)
210. Agot, K.E., Ndinya-Achola, J.O., Kreiss, J.L., et al.: Risk of HIV-1 in Kenya. A comparison of circumcised and uncircumcised men. Epidemiology **15**, 157–163 (2004)
211. Bailey, R.C., Neema, S., Othieno, R.: Sexual behaviors and other HIV risk factors in circumcised and uncircumcised men in Uganda. J. Acquir. Immune Defic. Syndr. **22**, 294–301 (1999)
212. Johnson, K., Way, A.: Risk factors for HIV infection in a national adult population: evidence from the 2003 Kenya Demographic and Health Survey. J. Acquir. Immune Defic. Syndr. **42**, 627–636 (2006)
213. Kelly, R., Kiwanuka, N., Wawer, M.J., et al.: Age of male circumcision and risk of HIV infection in rural Uganda. AIDS **13**, 399–405 (1999)
214. Urassa, M., Todd, J., Boerma, J.T., et al.: Male circumcision and susceptibility to HIV infection among men in Tanzania. AIDS **11**, 73–80 (1997)
215. Brown, J.E., Micheni, K.D., Grant, E.M., et al.: Varieties of male circumcision: a study from Kenya. Sex. Transm. Dis. **28**, 608–612 (2001)
216. Nnko, S., Washija, R., Urassa, M., et al.: Dynamics of male circumcision practices in Northwest Tanzania. Sex. Transm. Dis. **28**, 214–218 (2001)
217. Diseker, R.A., Lin, L.S., Kamb, M.L., et al.: Fleeting foreskins: the misclassification of male circumcision status. Sex. Transm. Dis. **28**, 330–335 (2001)
218. Risser, J.M., Risser, W.L., Eissa, M.A., et al.: Self-assessment of circumcision status by adolescents. Am. J. Epidemiol. **159**, 1095–1097 (2004)
219. Auvert, B., Taljaard, D., Lagarde, E., et al.: Randomized, controlled intervention trial of male circumcision for reduction of HIV infection risk: the ANRS 1265 trial. PLoS Med. **2**(e298), 1112–1122 (2005)
220. Kim, D.S., Lee, J.Y., Pang, M.G.: Male circumcision: a South Korean perspective. BJU Int. **83**(suppl 1), 28–33 (1999)
221. Bailey, R.C., Moses, S., Parker, C.B., et al.: Male circumcision for HIV prevention in young men in Kisumu, Kenya: a randomised controlled trial. Lancet **369**, 643–656 (2007)
222. Desai, K., Boily, M.C., Garnett, G.P., et al.: The role of sexually transmitted infections in male circumcision effectiveness against HIV-insights from clinical trial simulation. Emerg. Themes Epidemiol. **3**, 19 (16 pp.) (2006)
223. Mills, E., Cooper, C., Anema, A., et al.: Male circumcision for the prevention of heterosexually acquired HIV infection: a meta-analysis of randomized trials involving 11, 050 men. HIV Med. **9**, 332–335 (2008)
224. Siegfried, N., Muller, M., Deeks, J.J., et al.: Male circumcision for prevention of heterosexual acquisition of HIV in men. Cochrane Database Syst. Rev. CD003362 (38 pp.) (2009)
225. Bailey, R.C., Moses, S., Parker, C.B., et al.: The protective effect of male circumcision is sustained for at least 42 months: results from the Kisumu, Kenya Trial. In: XVII International AIDS Conference, Mexico City, 2008
226. Tobian, A.A., Quinn, T.C.: Herpes simplex virus type 2 and syphilis infections with HIV: an evolving synergy in transmission and prevention. Curr. Opin. HIV AIDS **4**, 294–299 (2009)
227. Stephenson, J.: New HIV prevention strategies urged: averting new infections key to controlling pandemic. J. Am. Med. Assoc. **292**, 1163–1164 (2004)
228. Todd, J., Grosskurth, H., Changalucha, J., et al.: Risk factors influencing HIV infection incidence in a rural African population: a nested case-control study. J. Infect. Dis. **193**, 458–466 (2006)
229. Boily, M.C., Desai, K., Masse, B., et al.: Incremental role of male circumcision on a generalised HIV epidemic through its protective effect against other sexually transmitted infections: from efficacy to effectiveness to population-level impact. Sex. Transm. Infect. **84**(Suppl 2), i28–i34 (2008)

230. Johnson, K.E., Sherman, M.E., Ssempiija, V., et al.: Foreskin inflammation is associated with HIV and herpes simplex virus type-2 infections in Rakai, Uganda. AIDS **23**, 1807–1815 (2009)
231. Watson-Jones, D., Weiss, H.A., Rusizoka, M., et al.: Effect of herpes simplex suppression on incidence of HIV among women in Tanzania. N. Engl. J. Med. **358**, 1560–1571 (2008)
232. Zhu, J., Hladik, F., Woodward, A., et al.: Persistence of HIV-1 receptor-positive cells after HSV-2 reactivation is a potential mechanism for increased HIV-1 acquisition. Nat. Med. **15**, 886–892 (2009)
233. Auvert, B., Lissouba, P., Cutler, E., et al.: Association of oncogenic and nononcogenic human papillomavirus with HIV incidence. J. Acquir. Immune Defic. Syndr. **53**, 111–116 (2010)
234. Shelton, J.D., Halperin, D.T., Wilson, D.: Has global HIV incidence peaked? Lancet **367**, 1120–1122 (2006)
235. White, R.G., Glynn, J.R., Orroth, K.K., et al.: Male circumcision for HIV prevention in sub-Saharan Africa: who, what and when? AIDS **22**, 1841–1850 (2008)
236. Auvert, B., Marseille, E., Korenromp, E.L., et al.: Estimating the resources needed and savings anticipated from roll-out of adult male circumcision in Sub-Saharan Africa. PLoS ONE **3**, e2679 (8 pp.) (2008)
237. Cohen, J.: HIV/AIDS. Prevention cocktails: combining tools to stop HIV's spread. Science **309**, 1002–1005 (2005)
238. Williams, B.G., Lloyd-Smith, J.O., Gouws, E., et al.: The potential impact of male circumcision on HIV in Sub-Saharan Africa. PLoS Med **3**(e262), 1032–1040 (2006)
239. Kahn, J.G., Marseille, E., Auvert, B.: Cost-effectiveness of male circumcision for HIV prevention in a South African setting. PLoS Med. **3**(e517), 2349–2358 (2006)
240. Nagelkerke, N.J., Moses, S., de Vlas, S.J., et al.: Modelling the public health impact of male circumcision for HIV prevention in high prevalence areas in Africa. BMC Infect. Dis. **7**, 16 (15 pp.) (2007)
241. Gray, R.H., Li, X., Kigozi, G., et al.: The impact of male circumcision on HIV incidence and cost per infection prevented: a stochastic simulation model from Rakai, Uganda. AIDS **21**, 845–850 (2007)
242. Bollinger, L.A., Stover, J., Musuka, G., et al.: The cost and impact of male circumcision on HIV/AIDS in Botswana. J. Int. AIDS Soc. **12**, 7 (2009)
243. Londish, G.J., Murray, J.M.: Significant reduction in HIV prevalence according to male circumcision intervention in sub-Saharan Africa. Int. J. Epidemiol. **37**, 1246–1253 (2008)
244. Krieger, J.N., Bailey, R.C., Opeya, J., et al.: Adult male circumcision: results of a standardized procedure in Kisumu District, Kenya. BJU Int. **96**, 1109–1113 (2005)
245. Auvert, B., Kahn, J.G., Korenromp, E., et al.: Cost of the roll-out of male circumcision in sub-Saharan Africa. 7th International AIDS Society Conference, WEAC105 (2007)
246. World Health Organization and UNAIDS: New data on male circumcision and HIV prevention: policy and programme implications [cited]. http://who.int/hiv/mediacentre/MCrecommendations_en.pdf (2007)
247. Sahasrabuddhe, V.V., Vermund, S.H.: The future of HIV prevention: control of sexually transmitted infections and circumcision interventions. Infect. Dis. Clin. N. Am. **21**, 241–257 (2007)
248. Manning, S.E., Thorpe, L.E., Ramaswamy, C., et al.: Estimation of HIV prevalence, risk factors, and testing frequency among sexually active men who have sex with men, aged 18–64 years–New York City, 2002. J. Urban Health **84**, 212–215 (2007)
249. McKinney, C.M., Klingler, E.J., Paneth-Pollak, R., et al.: Prevalence of adult male circumcision in the general population and a population at increased risk for HIV/AIDS in New York City. Sex. Transm. Dis. **35**, 814–817 (2008)
250. Kreiss, J.K., Hopkins, S.G.: The association between circumcision status and human immunodeficiency virus infection among homosexual men. J. Infect. Dis. **168**, 1404–1408 (1993)
251. Buchbinder, S.P., Vittinghoff, E., Heagerty, P.J., et al.: Sexual risk, nitrite inhalant use, and lack of circumcision associated with HIV seroconversion in men who have sex with men in the United States. J. Acquir. Immune Defic. Syndr. **39**, 82–89 (2005)
252. Fankem, S.L., Wiysonge, C.S., Hankins, C.A.: Male circumcision and the risk of HIV infection in men who have sex with men. Int. J. Epidemiol. **37**, 353–355 (2008)
253. Millett, G.A., Ding, H., Lauby, J., et al.: Circumcision status and HIV infection among Black and Latino men who have sex with men in 3 US cities. J. Acquir. Immune Defic. Syndr. **46**, 643–650 (2007)
254. Millett, G.A., Flores, S.A., Marks, G., et al.: Circumcision status and risk of HIV and sexually transmitted infections among men who have sex with men: a meta-analysis. JAMA **300**, 1674–1684 (2008)
255. Sanchez, J., Lama, J.R., Peinado, J., et al.: High HIV and ulcerative sexually transmitted infection incidence estimates among men who have sex with men in Peru: awaiting for an effective preventive intervention. J. Acquir. Immune Defic. Syndr. **51**(Suppl 1), S47–S51 (2009)
256. Templeton, D.J., Jin, F., Mao, L., et al.: Circumcision and risk of HIV infection in Australian homosexual men. AIDS **23**, 2347–2351 (2009)
257. Lane, T., Raymond, H.F., Dladla, S., et al.: High HIV prevalence among men who have sex with men in Soweto, South Africa: results from the Soweto Men's Study. AIDS Behav. **13**, 7 Aug (9 pp.) (2009)
258. Guanira, J., Lama, J., Goicochea, P., et al.: How willing are gay men to "cut off" the epidemic? Circumcision among MSM in the Andrean region. 4th International AIDS Society Conference on HIV Pathogenesis, Treatment and Prevention, Sydney, Australia, WEAC102 (2007)
259. Anderson, J., Wilson, D., Templeton, D.J., et al.: Cost-effectiveness of adult circumcision in a resource-rich setting for HIV prevention among men who have sex with men. J. Infect. Dis. **200**, 1803–1812 (2009)
260. Short, R.V.: The HIV/AIDS pandemic: New ways of preventing infection in men. Reprod. Fert. Dev. **16**, 555–559 (2004)
261. Turner, A.N., Morrison, C.S., Padian, N.S., et al.: Men's circumcision status and women's risk of HIV acquisition in Zimbabwe and Uganda. AIDS **21**, 1779–1789 (2007)
262. Weiss, H.A., Hankins, C.A., Dickson, K.: Male circumcision and risk of HIV infection in women: a systematic review and meta-analysis. Lancet Infect. Dis. **9**, 669–677 (2009)

263. Baeten, J.M., Donnell, D., Inambo, M., et al.: Male circumcision and risk of male-to-female HIV-1 transmission: a multinational prospective study. 5th International AIDS Society Conference, Cape Town, South Africa, LBPEC06
264. Chersich, M.F., Rees, H.V.: Vulnerability of women in southern Africa to infection with HIV: biological determinants and priority health sector interventions. AIDS **22**(suppl 4), S27–S40 (2008)
265. Cassell, M.M., Halperin, D.T., Shelton, J.D., et al.: Risk compensation: the Achilles' heel of innovations in HIV prevention? Br. Med. J. **332**, 605–607 (2006)
266. Mattson, C.L., Campbell, R.T., Bailey, R.C., et al.: Risk compensation is not associated with male circumcision in Kisumu, Kenya: a multi-faceted assessment of men enrolled in a randomized controlled trial. PLoS ONE **3**, e2443 (9 pp.) (2008)
267. Agot, K.E., Kiarie, J.N., Nguyen, H.Q., et al.: Male circumcision in Siaya and Bondo Districts, Kenya: prospective cohort study to assess behavioral disinhibition following circumcision. J. Acquir. Immune Defic. Syndr. **44**, 66–70 (2007)
268. Mehta, S.D., Gray, R.H., Auvert, B., et al.: Does sex in the early period after circumcision increase HIV-seroconversion risk? Pooled analysis of adult male circumcision clinical trials. AIDS **23**, 1557–1564 (2009)
269. Bailey, R.C., Muga, R., Poulussen, R., et al.: The acceptability of male circumcision to reduce HIV infections in Nyanza Province, Kenya. AIDS Care **14**, 27–40 (2002)
270. Kebaabetswe, P., Lockman, S., Mogwe, S., et al.: Male circumcision: an acceptable strategy for HIV prevention in Botswana. Sex. Transm. Infect. **79**, 214–219 (2003)
271. Lagarde, E., Dirk, T., Puren, A., et al.: Acceptability of male circumcision as a tool for preventing HIV infection in a highly infected community in South Africa. AIDS **17**, 89–95 (2003)
272. Rain-Taljaard, R.C., Lagarde, E., Taljaard, D.J., et al.: Potential for an intervention based on male circumcision in a South African town with high levels of HIV infection. AIDS Care **15**, 315–327 (2003)
273. Westercamp, N., Bailey, R.C.: Acceptability of male circumcision for prevention of HIV/AIDS in sub-Saharan Africa: a review. AIDS Behav. **11**, 341–355 (2007)
274. Krieger, J.N., Bailey, R.C., Opeya, J.C., et al.: Adult male circumcision outcomes: experience in a developing country setting. Urol. Int. **78**, 235–240 (2007)
275. Halperin, D.T., Fritz, K., McFarland, W., et al.: Acceptability of adult male circumcision for sexually transmitted disease and HIV prevention in Zimbabwe. Sex. Transm. Dis. **32**, 238–239 (2005)
276. Rennie, S., Muula, A.S., Westreich, D.: Male circumcision and HIV prevention: ethical, medical and public health tradeoffs in low-income countries. J. Med. Ethics **33**, 357–361 (2007)
277. Karim, Q.A.: Prevention of HIV by male circumcision. Effective but integration with existing sexual health services remains the biggest challenge. Br. Med. J. **335**, 4–5 (2007)
278. Meissner, O., Buso, D.L.: Traditional male circumcision in the Eastern Cape–scourge or blessing? S. Afr. Med. J. **97**, 371–373 (2007)
279. World Health Organization/UNAIDS: Male circumcision: global trends and determinants of prevalance, safety and acceptability. http://whqlibdoc.who.int/publications/2007/9789241596169_eng.pdf. World Health Organization, Geneva (42 pp.) (2008)
280. Madhivanan, P., Krupp, K., Chandrasekaran, V., et al.: Acceptability of male circumcision among mothers with male children in Mysore, India. AIDS **22**, 983–988 (2008)
281. Stemple, L.: Health and human rights in today's fight against HIV/AIDS. AIDS **22**(suppl 2), S113–S121 (2008)
282. Clark, P.A., Eisenman, J., Szapor, S.: Mandatory neonatal male circumcision in Sub-Saharan Africa: medical and ethical analysis. Med. Sci. Monit. **12**, RA205–RA213 (2007)
283. Griffith, D., Bellows, B., Potts, M.: Cut to the chase: quickly achieving high coverage male circumcision. J. Epidemiol. Community Health **61**, 612 (2007)
284. Potts, M., Prata, N., Walsh, J., et al.: Parachute approach to evidence based medicine. Br. Med. J. **333**, 701–703 (2006)
285. Halperin, D.T., Steiner, M.J., Cassell, M.M., et al.: The time has come for common ground on preventing sexual transmission of HIV. Lancet **364**, 1913–1915 (2004)
286. Ferrante, P., Delbue, S., Mancuso, R.: The manifestation of AIDS in Africa: an epidemiological overview. J. Neurovirol. **11**(suppl 1), 50–57 (2005)
287. Donovan, B., Ross, M.W.: Preventing HIV: determinants of sexual behaviour (review). Lancet **355**, 1897–1901 (2000)
288. Yahya-Malima, K.I., Matee, M.I., Evjen-Olsen, B., et al.: High potential of escalating HIV transmission in a low prevalence setting in rural Tanzania. BMC Publ. Health **7**, 103 (10 pp.) (2007)
289. Anderson, J.E., Wilson, R., Doll, L., et al.: Condom use and HIV risk behaviors among US adults: data from a national survey. Fam. Plann. Perspect. **31**, 24–28 (1999)
290. Sanchez, T., Finlayson, T., Drake, A., et al.: Human immunodeficiency virus (HIV) risk, prevention, and testing behaviors–United States, National HIV Behavioral Surveillance System: men who have sex with men, November 2003-April 2005. MMWR Surveill. Summ. **55**, 1–16 (2006)
291. Jadack, R.A., Yuenger, J., Ghanem, K.G., et al.: Polymerase chain reaction detection of Y-chromosome sequences in vaginal fluid of women accessing a sexually transmitted disease clinic. Sex. Transm. Dis. **33**, 22–25 (2006)
292. Beckman, L.J., Harvey, S.M., Tiersky, L.A.: Attitudes about condoms and condom use among college students. J. Am. Coll. Health **44**, 243–249 (1996)
293. Kang, M., Rochford, A., Johnston, V., et al.: Prevalence of *Chlamydia trachomatis* infection among 'high risk' young people in New South Wales. Sex. Health **3**, 253–254 (2006)
294. Caballero-Hoyos, R., Villasenor-Sierra, A.: [Socioeconomic strata as a predictor factor for constant condom use among adolescents] (Spanish). Rev. Saúde Pública **35**, 531–538 (2001)
295. Tapia-Aguirre, V., Arillo-Santillan, E., Allen, B., et al.: Associations among condom use, sexual behavior, and knowledge about HIV/AIDS. A study of 13,293 public school students. Arch. Med. Res. **35**, 334–343 (2004)
296. Slaymaker, E.: A critique of international indicators of sexual risk behaviour. Sex. Transm. Infect. **80**(Suppl 2), ii13–ii21 (2004)
297. Padian, N.S., van der Straten, A., Ramjee, G., et al.: Diaphragm and lubricant gel for prevention of HIV acquisition in

southern African women: a randomised controlled trial. Lancet **370**, 251–261 (2007)
298. Potts, M., Halperin, D.T., Kirby, D., et al.: Public health. Reassessing HIV prevention. Science **320**, 749–750 (2008)
299. Van Howe, R.: Circumcision and HIV infection: review of the literature and meta-analysis. Int. J. STD AIDS **10**, 8–16 (1999)
300. Moses, S., Nagelkerke, N.J.D., Blanchard, J.F.: Commentary: analysis of the scientific literature on male circumcision and risk for HIV infection. Int. J. STD AIDS **10**, 626–628 (1999)
301. O'Farrell, N., Egger, M.: Commentary: circumcision in men and the prevention of HIV infection: a 'meta-analysis' revisited. Int. J. STD AIDS **11**, 137–142 (2000)
302. Low, N., Broutet, N., Adu-Sarkodie, Y., et al.: Global control of sexually transmitted infections. Lancet **368**, 2001–2016 (2006)
303. UNAIDS: Safe, voluntary, informed male circumcision and comprehensive hiv prevention programming: guidance for decision-makers on human rights, ethical & legal considerations. http://data.unaids.org/pub/Manual/2007/070613_humanrightsethicallegalguidance_en.pdf (2007)

Physical Barrier Methods and Microbicides

55

Kelly B. Conner, Aron J. Gewirtzman, and Stephen K. Tyring

Core Messages

- STIs represent a significant source of morbidity and mortality and cause significant financial strain worldwide.
- Prevention is the first and most cost-effective step in controlling the spread of STIs.
- The mainstay of prevention is abstinence which is 100% effective but impractical for obvious social reasons.
- When abstinence fails, various forms of physical barrier methods and potentially microbicides may aid in the prevention of STIs.

55.1 Introduction

Sexually transmitted infections (STIs) are an extremely important cause of morbidity and mortality that cause significant strain on health-care costs and resources. It is estimated by the Center of Disease Control that 19 million new cases of STIs occur annually in the United States, generating 14.7 billion dollars in health-care costs [1]. Many of those infected are unaware and therefore are undiagnosed and untreated. The sequelae of being untreated can be devastating.

Fortunately, STIs are largely preventable along with their inherent complications. Prevention is complicated and involves physical, chemical, behavioral, and social factors. The mainstays of prevention of STIs are abstinence, barrier methods, and sexual discretion within a monogamous relationship. Barrier methods include the male and female condom and cervical diaphragms. Vaccines have been created for Hepatitis B and for two of the carcinogenic strains of HPV and two nononcogenic strains, but most STIs are not preventable by this method [2]. A new method with many promising formulas in clinical trials is to use microbicides, which are liquids or gels that prevent STI transmission using physical, biological, and biochemical barriers.

55.2 The Male Condom

55.2.1 History

The first published description of the condom occurred in 1564 when Gabriel Fallopius advised the use of "a small linen cloth made to fit the glans" to prevent the spread of syphilis. Fallopius conducted an experiment in which 1,100 men were "protected" from contracting syphilis by using the linen sheaths. The name condom is ascribed to many sources, such as the city of Condom in Gascony and a doctor Qundom, the physician of King Charles II. The famous lover Casanova was said to have used the condom frequently to avoid sexually transmitted disease and many other references to

K.B. Conner
University of Texas Health Science Center, Houston, TX, USA

A.J. Gewirtzman
Center for Clinical Studies, Houston, TX, USA

S.K. Tyring (✉)
Center for Clinical Studies, Houston, TX and
Department of Dermatology, University of Texas Health Science Center, 6655 Travis Street, Suite 100, Houston, TX 77030, USA
e-mail: styring@ccstexas.com

G. Gross and S.K. Tyring (eds.), *Sexually Transmitted Infections and Sexually Transmitted Diseases*,
DOI: 10.1007/978-3-642-14663-3_55,

condoms appear in early eighteenth century literature. Early condoms were commonly composed of fish bladders or the dried intestines of cattle and sheep. During the eighteenth century and beyond, using condoms became more prominent, especially in wealthier classes and slowly spread to the lower classes towards the beginning of the 1800s. Affordable condoms became conceivable after the vulcanization of rubber in 1843, but it was many years before society, as well as the medical community, would strongly support condom use for prevention of venereal disease. During World War I, condoms were considered a last resort measure because of fears that they would promote sexual activity and indiscretion among recruits. The U.S. Army learned a difficult lesson when almost 7 million days of active duty were lost to venereal disease. They took a completely different approach in World War II by promoting condom use, now more efficient by the introduction of latex in the 1930s. The campaign was a success and condoms have since been the foundation of modern sexually transmitted disease prevention [3].

55.2.2 Mechanism of Action

Male condoms are intended to cover the penis and urethra, preventing the passage of ejaculate and secretions from entering the female genital tract as well as protect the male urethra from cervical and vaginal secretions that may contain infectious agents. Most modern condoms are made of thin latex rubber that forms a protective, impermeable barrier to fluids. Alternatively, they can be made of polyurethane or lambskin. Today, condoms are manufactured to be affordable, easy to obtain, simple to use, and exceptionally effective in preventing STIs.

55.2.3 Efficacy in Preventing STIs

While condoms are widely known to be effective at blocking the passage of spermatazoa to prevent pregnancy, bacteria such as *Neisseria gonorrhoea* and viruses such as the human immunodeficiency virus (HIV) are considerably smaller than sperm. Manufacturers test condom integrity using a "Water Leak Test" in which water added to the condom under pressure is used to detect the presence of defects, but researchers have developed more sensitive tests. In a study by Lytle et al., a bacteriophage approximately 27 nm in size was used to assess for virus passage through condoms after a simulation of normal intercourse [4–6]. To put it into perspective, HIV is approximately 110 nm in size and hepatitis B virus, the smallest sexually transmitted virus, is approximately 40 nm in size. It was determined that 2.6% of latex condoms allowed some virus penetration, the median level being 7×10^{-4} ml of fluid. This compares favorably to the average ejaculate of approximately 3 mL of fluid. Therefore, even the few condoms that do allow virus penetration only allowed volumes several orders of magnitude lower than if no condom was used at all [6, 7]. This study along with several others that reproduced similar results proved that latex condoms were very effective in preventing the passage of tiny infectious particles when used correctly. A formal meta-analysis of 25 studies documenting the seroconversion rate of serodiscordant heterosexual couples showed that the use of condoms resulted in a proportionate reduction in HIV acquisition by 80% [8]. The study did not indicate whether the participants used the condoms properly with each and every sexual act; therefore, the results estimate effectiveness with user variability rather than efficacy. Wald et al. found that condom use during more than 25% of sex acts was associated with protection against Herpes Simplex Virus type 2 (adjusted hazard ratio, 0.085) for women but not for men (adjusted hazard ratio, 2.02) [9]. One possible explanation for the apparent lack of protection in men is that virus is shed from perianal and vulvar areas, which are left exposed. Suprapubic skin and the scrotum are not covered by the male condom. Another study found that the incidence of genital human papillomavirus infection was 37.8/100 patient-years-at-risk among women whose partners used condoms for all instances of intercourse during 8 months before testing. Comparatively, the incidence of genital human papillomavirus in women whose partners used condoms less than 5% of the time was 89.3/100 patient-years-at-risk [10].

A condom reaches its highest efficacy only when it is applied correctly, remains intact, and is secure on the penis. In a study involving 892 women over 6 months who used over 21,000 male condoms and kept a journal documenting condom failures, 2.3% of condoms broke while 1.3% slipped. The study also found that such failure rates decreased with increased condom use, increased coital frequency, and in conjunction with spermicides, indicating that social factors and experience with condoms play an important role in their efficacy [11]. Although not a perfect means of prevention, the male latex condom effectively reduces the rate of transmission of STIs and, apart from abstinence, is the best preventative method available today.

55.3 The Female Controlled Barrier Methods

55.3.1 The Female Condom

The FDA approved the use of the female condom in the early 1990s. Its development grew out of the need for female-controlled contraception and STI protection. Although male condoms are the most commonly used type of condom, some relationships, especially in countries with a gender-based power differential, put women in a vulnerable state with little control over their own protection. Their partners might dislike the feel of a male condom and refuse to use it or they may have no control over their sexual encounters at all [12].

The female condom is made of latex or polyurethane and is a pouch-like device designed to fit loosely inside of the vagina, protecting the cervical and vaginal epithelium as well as the surrounding perineum from ejaculate and secretions. The device consists of two rings: a closed interior ring and an open exterior ring. The closed interior ring is to be placed near the cervix while the external ring lies outside of the vagina. The inner sheath that connects the rings serves as a barrier and reservoir for ejaculate. Because the device does not have to be fit tightly around the penis it can be made with thicker rubber and therefore potentially offer greater protection by reducing the incidence of tears. Acceptability studies for the female condom demonstrated that women are amenable to using this form of contraception with proper education and training on its correct use [13].

Studies have demonstrated that female condoms offer protection against STIs that is comparable to that of male condoms. French et al. developed a randomized controlled trial in which 1,442 women were divided into male-condom and female-condom groups and found no statistically significant difference in STI acquisition between users of either barrier method [14]. A similar study was performed in Kenya in which 1,752 women with significant STI risk were separated into male and female condom groups, and STI prevalence did not vary between the two groups over 1 year [15]. While more studies are required to fully understand the efficacy of the female condom, it remains a valuable and empowering tool for women to prevent STIs.

55.3.2 Cervical Barriers

Cervical barrier devices such as the diaphragm are a discrete, female-controlled method of contraception, but there is also evidence to suggest that protection of the cervix may help prevent transmission of STIs. Chlamydia and gonorrhea replicate in cervical epithelium and cause cervicitis. These organisms are incapable of replicating adequately in the vaginal epithelium; therefore, if the cervix is protected from invasion the incidence of transmission decreases. The endocervical epithelium is more fragile and thin than vaginal epithelium and can be compromised by other STIs [16]. It has been shown that the expression of CD4 cells and CCR5 chemokine receptors is higher in the cervix than in the vagina, indicating more risk for HIV transmission at the cervix [17]. There is also a significant reduction in the transmission of HIV when other STIs have been properly prevented or treated in which diaphragms may play a role [18]. While there are few experimental studies to evaluate the effectiveness of diaphragms in protecting against STIs, there have been numerous observational studies indicating there is some protection in using these devices. Three studies observed a decrease in the prevalence of gonorrhea in diaphragm users versus nonusers [19–21]. Another study observed a lower incidence of Cervical Intraepithelial Neoplasia among users of the diaphragm [22]. A recent study in which South African women were taught to use diaphragms with a spermicide in an effort to prevent HIV acquisition illustrated that while the device did not increase the risk of HIV, it unfortunately added no benefit to preventing disease transmission [23]. Although it seems that evidence for the direct prevention of HIV by cervical barrier methods is lacking, there does seem to be evidence that it helps prevent other STIs and by doing so indirectly decreases the risk of HIV acquisition.

55.4 Microbicides

55.4.1 What Is a Microbicide?

A microbicide is a biological or chemical agent that can kill microbes and may potentially be used to prevent the transmission of sexually transmitted infectious agents. Topical microbicides that may safely be in contact with vaginal or rectal mucosa have been proposed to prevent the transmission of STIs by forming a chemical, physical, and biological barrier against infectious agents. It is postulated that with the development of an effective topical microbicide, STI protection could be delivered as inexpensively as condoms, would serve as an effective resource in lower socioeconomic environments and would provide an additional discrete female-controlled method for STI prevention [24].Although such a microbicide is not yet approved for this use, many formulas are in Phase II and III trials and researchers are hopeful that an effective topical microbicide will be on the market soon.

55.4.2 History of Microbicides

The original concept of microbicides began from the widespread availability of over-the-counter spermicides used for contraception. The active ingredient of most spermicides is nonoxyl-9 (N-9), a neutral surfactant and detergent that has structural affinity for membrane lipids. At cytotoxic doses it functions by damaging the phospholipid cell membranes of sperm, resulting in increased permeability, leakage of cellular contents, and cell death [25]. Unfortunately, the doses required to induce this spermicidal activity are also damaging to vaginal epithelial cells and normal vaginal flora and therefore frequent use can increase the risk of vaginal irritation and ulceration [26]. Researchers in the early 1980s began to question the possibility that it could also destroy the envelopes of viral particles and potentially be effective in preventing STI transmission. With the onset of the AIDS epidemic came a national feeling of urgency to develop effective methods to prevent HIV transmission. After much debate and numerous studies, N-9 was considered inappropriate for STI protection and potentially increases the risk of HIV transmission due to the induction of ulcerations [27–30].

55.4.3 Potential Microbicidal Strategies

Despite the failure of N-9 as a potential microbicidal formula, many other compounds and formulas are currently undergoing clinical trials. An ideal microbicide may be on the horizon that may provide a safe and effective alternative to condoms in the prevention of STIs. The Alliance for Microbicide Development publishes a list of the most up-to-date ongoing clinical trials www.microbicide.com.

Several mechanisms of action have been targeted for the clinical development of topical microbicides. The first method is to augment the innate antimicrobial factors of the vagina by restoring or maintaining vaginal pH. For example, BufferGel, now in Phase II/IIB clinical trials, is proposed to prevent the alkalization of the vagina after intercourse and therefore maintain the vagina's protective acidic environment that is thought to inhibit the overgrowth of harmful organisms [31]. It has been shown that a low pH inhibits transmission of HIV [32]. Viral entry and fusion inhibitors are being studied as another mechanism under development. They are meant to inhibit the entry and fusion of HIV to host cells. Currently, in Phase III trials, PRO 2000, a large sulfated polymer, competes against HIV for the entry into host cells by binding to CD4 and blocking gp120 [33, 34]. Another method is to interfere with the viral replication cycle by using classic antiretroviral mechanisms that target the reverse transcriptase enzyme of HIV. In the oral form, nucleoside and non-nucleoside reverse transcriptase inhibitors with protease inhibitors are the mainstay of current HIV therapy. Drawing upon the success of these pharmaceuticals, researchers hope to develop a gel based delivery system. An example is tenofovir gel, now in phase IIB trials, and TMC 120, a formula containing dapivirine that entered Phase 3 trials in mid 2008 [24]. Other methods of delivery such as a vaginal ring, which may facilitate the continuous release of antiretroviral agents, are also being investigated [35].

Despite these promising microbicidal strategies, the development of microbicides has been met with many roadblocks and failures. A study involving the cotton-based microbicide, Ushercell, was halted in 2007 when results suggested that it might actually increase the risk of infection. In February 2008, Carraguard, a product developed from seaweed extract, proved to be ineffective in preventing HIV in a large study involving 6,000 women in South Africa [36].

55.5 Conclusion

STIs are a largely avoidable cause of morbidity and mortality, but prevention is complex and involves physical, chemical, behavioral, and social factors. The mainstays of prevention of STIs are abstinence, barrier methods, and sexual discretion within a monogamous relationship. The prevention of STIs remains an important area of research and study. Newer methods of protection such as female-controlled barrier methods and the development of topical microbicides represent a new hope for patients at risk for contracting sexually transmitted infections.

Take-Home Pearls

- The male latex condom effectively reduces the rate of transmission of STIs and, apart from abstinence, is the best preventative method available today.
- Female-controlled barrier methods include the female condom, cervical diaphragm, and potentially in the future, microbicides.
- Studies have demonstrated that female condoms offer protection against STIs that is comparable to that of male condoms.
- Cervical diaphragms, while obviously useful for contraception, are also somewhat protective from STIs as the cervix is more vulnerable to infection than the vaginal epithelium.
- There are many promising formulas of microbicides, which are liquids or gels that prevent STI transmission using physical, biological, and biochemical barriers. Phase II and III trials are underway to develop a safe and effective microbicide. Examples include BufferGel, PRO 2000, tenofovir gel, and TMC 120.

References

1. Centers for Disease Control and Prevention: Sexually Transmitted Disease Surveillance, 2006. U.S Department of Health and Human Services, Atlanta (Nov 2007)
2. Speck, L.M., Tyring, S.K.: Vaccines for the prevention of human papillomavirus infections. Skin. Ther. Lett. **11**(6), 1–3 (2006)
3. Valdiserri, R.O.: Cum hastis sic clypeatis: the turbulent history of the condom. Bull. N. Y. Acad. Med. **64**(3), 237–245 (1988)
4. Carey, R.F., Lytle, C.D., Cyr, W.H.: Implications of laboratory tests of condom integrity. Sex. Transm. Dis. **26**(4), 216–220 (1999)
5. Lytle, C.D., et al.: A sensitive method for evaluating condoms as virus barriers. J. AOAC Int. **80**(2), 319–324 (1997)
6. Lytle, C.D., et al.: An in vitro evaluation of condoms as barriers to a small virus. Sex. Transm. Dis. **24**(3), 161–164 (1997)
7. Cayley Jr., W.E.: Effectiveness of condoms in reducing heterosexual transmission of HIV. Am. Fam. Physician **70**(7), 1268–1269 (2004)
8. Davis, K.R., Weller, S.C.: The effectiveness of condoms in reducing heterosexual transmission of HIV. Fam. Plann. Perspect. **31**(6), 272–279 (1999)
9. Wald, A., et al.: Effect of condoms on reducing the transmission of herpes simplex virus type 2 from men to women. JAMA **285**(24), 3100–3106 (2001)
10. Winer, R.L., et al.: Condom use and the risk of genital human papillomavirus infection in young women. N. Engl. J. Med. **354**(25), 2645–2654 (2006)
11. Macaluso, M., et al.: Mechanical failure of the latex condom in a cohort of women at high STD risk. Sex. Transm. Dis. **26**(8), 450–458 (1999)
12. Amaro, H.: Love, sex, and power. Considering women's realities in HIV prevention. Am. Psychol. **50**(6), 437–447 (1995)
13. Elias, C., Coggins, C.: Acceptability research on female-controlled barrier methods to prevent heterosexual transmission of HIV: where have we been? where are we going? J. Womens Health Gend. Based Med. **10**(2), 163–173 (2001)
14. French, P.P., et al.: Use-effectiveness of the female versus male condom in preventing sexually transmitted disease in women. Sex. Transm. Dis. **30**(5), 433–439 (2003)
15. Feldblum, P.J., et al.: Female condom introduction and sexually transmitted infection prevalence: results of a community intervention trial in Kenya. AIDS **15**(8), 1037–1044 (2001)
16. Moench, T.R., Chipato, T., Padian, N.S.: Preventing disease by protecting the cervix: the unexplored promise of internal vaginal barrier devices. AIDS **15**(13), 1595–1602 (2001)
17. Patterson, B.K., et al.: Repertoire of chemokine receptor expression in the female genital tract: implications for human immunodeficiency virus transmission. Am. J. Pathol. **153**(2), 481–490 (1998)
18. Grosskurth, H., et al.: Impact of improved treatment of sexually transmitted diseases on HIV infection in rural Tanzania: randomised controlled trial. Lancet **346**(8974), 530–536 (1995)
19. Magder, L.S., et al.: Factors related to genital Chlamydia trachomatis and its diagnosis by culture in a sexually transmitted disease clinic. Am. J. Epidemiol. **128**(2), 298–308 (1988)

20. Rosenberg, M.J., et al.: Barrier contraceptives and sexually transmitted diseases in women: a comparison of female-dependent methods and condoms. Am. J. Publ. Health **82**(5), 669–674 (1992)
21. Austin, H., Louv, W.C., Alexander, W.J.: A case-control study of spermicides and gonorrhea. JAMA **251**(21), 2822–2824 (1984)
22. Becker, T.M., et al.: Contraceptive and reproductive risks for cervical dysplasia in southwestern Hispanic and non-Hispanic white women. Int. J. Epidemiol. **23**(5), 913–922 (1994)
23. Padian, N.S., et al.: Diaphragm and lubricant gel for prevention of HIV acquisition in southern African women: a randomised controlled trial. Lancet **370**(9583), 251–261 (2007)
24. Howett, M.K., Kuhl, J.P.: Microbicides for prevention of transmission of sexually transmitted diseases. Curr. Pharm. Des. **11**(29), 3731–3746 (2005)
25. Schill, W.B., Wolff, H.H.: Ultrastructure of human spermatozoa in the presence of the spermicide nonoxinol-9 and a vaginal contraceptive containing nonoxinol-9. Andrologia **13**(1), 42–49 (1981)
26. Weir, S.S., et al.: Nonoxynol-9 use, genital ulcers, and HIV infection in a cohort of sex workers. Genitourin. Med. **71**(2), 78–81 (1995)
27. Fleming, D.T., Wasserheit, J.N.: From epidemiological synergy to public health policy and practice: the contribution of other sexually transmitted diseases to sexual transmission of HIV infection. Sex. Transm. Infect. **75**(1), 3–17 (1999)
28. Dayal, M.B., et al.: Disruption of the upper female reproductive tract epithelium by nonoxynol-9. Contraception **68**(4), 273–279 (2003)
29. Kreiss, J., et al.: Efficacy of nonoxynol 9 contraceptive sponge use in preventing heterosexual acquisition of HIV in Nairobi prostitutes. JAMA **268**(4), 477–482 (1992)
30. Gollub, E.L.: The female condom: STD protection in the hands of women. Am. J. Gynecol. Health **7**(4), 91–92 (1993)
31. Ballagh, S.A., et al.: A Phase I study of the functional performance, safety and acceptability of the BufferGel Duet. Contraception **77**(2), 130–137 (2008)
32. Olmsted, S.S., et al.: Low pH immobilizes and kills human leukocytes and prevents transmission of cell-associated HIV in a mouse model. BMC Infect. Dis. **5**, 79 (2005)
33. Keller, M.J., et al.: PRO 2000 gel inhibits HIV and herpes simplex virus infection following vaginal application: a double-blind placebo-controlled trial. J. Infect. Dis. **193**(1), 27–35 (2006)
34. Rusconi, S., et al.: Naphthalene sulfonate polymers with CD4-blocking and anti-human immunodeficiency virus type 1 activities. Antimicrob. Agents Chemother. **40**(1), 234–236 (1996)
35. Woolfson, A.D., et al.: Intravaginal ring delivery of the reverse transcriptase inhibitor TMC 120 as an HIV microbicide. Int. J. Pharm. **325**(1–2), 82–89 (2006)
36. Albrecht, H.: Report from the 4th IAS conference on HIV pathogenesis, treatment and prevention. Disappointing data from anti-HIV microbicide trials. AIDS Clin. Care **19**(10), 85 (2007)

Part X

Laboratorial Diagnosis

Novel Diagnostic Methods

56

Thomas Meyer

Core Messages

› Novel diagnostic tests based on molecular techniques are increasingly used in routine testing of sexually transmitted infections, but classical methods like serology and culture are still important and remain the mainstay to diagnose certain diseases, e.g. syphilis and gonorrhoea.

› Apart from detection of sexually transmitted infections molecular tests are also used to characterize pathogens and course of disease by quantification and molecular typing of pathogens, susceptibility testing as well as characterization of factors associated with virulence and disease progression.

› Sophisticated molecular methods like ultra deep sequencing, and DNA-arrays will improve identification of infections with multiple pathogens, as well as pathogen subtypes or variants, even when present in low frequency (for instance: minor viral quasispecies carrying resistance associated mutations).

56.1 Introduction

Sexually transmitted infections and diseases (STI, STD) are caused by a number of different pathogens including bacteria, viruses, fungi, and parasites. The WHO has stated more than 20 different infectious agents transmitted by sexual contacts. Yet, there is no clear definition of STI. Infections of *T. pallidum*, *N. gonorrhea*, or *H. ducreyi* are almost always acquired by sexual contacts and cause typical venereal diseases, like lues, gonorrhea, or chancroid, while others although transmitted by sexual contacts, primarily affect organs outside the genital tract and do not result in venereal disease (HIV, HBV, CMV). Furthermore, some reports indicate sexual transmission of pathogens, which in most cases were transmitted by other routes, e.g., EBV and adenovirus [1,2]. Thus, some authors prefer the term sexually transmissible infection.

According to WHO-estimates, the incidence of curable STIs has increased from 250 million in 1990 to 340 million in 1999 [3]. Increased frequency of STIs and STDs during last years was also reported for many countries [4–6]. Various reasons may account for the increase in STI-incidence, including changes of sexual behavior, lack of education, lack of prevention, traveling, increase of predisposing conditions (like HIV-infection and other STDs), increased testing (for instance through screening programs), and improved reporting of positive cases. In addition, improvement of diagnostic tests did also significantly contribute to more frequent detection of STIs.

56.2 Historical Review

In 1906, von Wassermann, Neisser, and Bruck developed the first serologic test to detect STI/STD, the Wassermann-test, which was used to diagnose syphilis [7]. Extracts of *T. pallidum* containing fetal liver tissues were used in a complement fixation test to detect syphilitic antibodies. The assay later also proved to be

T. Meyer
Institute of Medical Microbiology, Virology and Hygiene, University Hospital Hamburg-Eppendorf, University of Hamburg, Martinistr. 52, 20246 Hamburg, Germany
e-mail: th.meyer@uke.de

G. Gross and S.K. Tyring (eds.), *Sexually Transmitted Infections and Sexually Transmitted Diseases*,
DOI: 10.1007/978-3-642-14663-3_56,

effective using tissues without treponemes and the molecule binding syphilitic antibodies was identified as cardiolipin, a lipoid compound liberated through treponema-mediated tissue destruction. Testing for lipoid antibody is still an important tool for both detecting active *T. pallidum* infection and treatment monitoring. Even today, no culture system for *T. pallidum* has been established for laboratory diagnosis, which is in contrast to many other bacterial and viral STI pathogens.

Antibody detection by serological assays can also be used to diagnose other STIs, in particular in case of disseminating pathogens causing systemic immune responses, like HIV and HBV. Antibody testing, however, is less important for STIs confined to the genital tract epithelium. For instance, in HPV infections and Chlamydia trachomatis (CT) infections of the lower genital tract, antibody production is weak and delayed usually, and sometimes not all detectable in peripheral blood. In contrast, CT infections ascending to upper genital tract or invasive CT infections, like LGV, are associated with strong antibody responses, which can be exploited for diagnostic purposes.

The next generation of diagnostic assays was represented by antigen tests and nucleic acid hybridization tests, which have been developed for detection of CT, Neisseria gonorrhoeae (NG), HSV, HBV, HIV, and others. As an important advantage to culture, these tests do not depend on viable pathogens and are generally faster to perform and to produce results.

Some of these tests were designed to detect pathogens like CT, NG, and HSV in anogenital swabs. In general, analytical and clinical sensitivity was not improved compared to culture [8]. In addition, specificity of these tests is limited, owing to antigenic similarities or nucleotide sequence homologies to other microbial agents, including nonpathogenic strains. Antigen assays are also used to detect viral antigens in blood (HBs-antigen, CMV pp65 antigen, HIV-1 p24 antigen). These assays are sensitive and specific and still represent widely distributed primary tests to analyze viremia of HBV, HIV, and CMV infections.

A major technical improvement in laboratory diagnostics was represented by the development of methods for nucleic acid amplification and application to detection of infectious disease pathogens, which started in the early 1990s. Nucleic acids amplification tests (NAATs) are the most sensitive assays, which in principle are able to detect single infectious agents. PCR was the first NAAT, developed in 1985 [9], followed by several other amplification techniques, summarized in Table 56.1. Basically, signal amplification and target amplification techniques are distinguished. Most of the amplification technologies are used in commercial tests available for detection of various pathogens.

The high sensitivity of NAATs also relates to an important problem associated with the introduction of NAATs to routine diagnostic testing, since it represents a potential risk of minimal contaminations to cause false-positive results. A number of preventive measures have been shown to be indispensable requirements, which need to be strictly followed in order to produce reliable results of NAATs [10]. These prerequisites are also subject to guidelines of quality control [11,12]. In addition, carry-over contamination by amplified products can be prevented by selective destruction of PCR products using UTP instead of TTP for amplification and uracil-N-glycosylase-treatment prior to new amplification reactions, which is used in commercial assays of Roche (AmpErase). The development of closed systems for real-time amplification, which allow

Table 56.1 Nucleic acid amplification technologies

Method	Nucleic Acid Template	Enzymes	Temperature Profile	Quantification
bDNA	DNA/RNA	None	Isothermal	Yes
Qβ-Replicase	DNA	Qβ-replicase	Isothermal	No
PCR	DNA/RNA	DNA-polymerase	Cyclic	Yes
LCR	DNA/RNA	DNA-ligase	Cyclic	Yes
NASBA	RNA (DNA)	Reverse transcriptase RNA polymerase	Isothermal	Yes
SDA	DNA (RNA)	DNA-polymerase restriction-endonuclease	Isothermal	Yes

detection and measurement of amplification products during amplification reactions without opening test tubes, also prevents carry-over contamination efficiently.

In the following, novel diagnostic tests will be described for selective pathogens of STI. In addition to detection of these pathogens, molecular tests are also used for molecular typing, resistance testing, and characterization of pathogenic properties.

56.3 Chlamydia trachomatis

C. trachomatis (CT) infections can be detected by a number of different methods, as shown in Table 56.2. Culture of chlamydia on cell monolayers has been the gold standard of CT diagnostics for a long time because typical intracellular inclusion bodies provide high specificity [12]. On the other hand, dependence on vital bacteria limits sensitivity of culture. By comparing, different methods for CT detection culture were shown to have a sensitivity of at best 70–85% [8,12–15]. Sensitivity of CT antigen tests and hybridization assays is similar to cell culture or even worse, while the highest sensitivity was demonstrated for NAATs (Fig. 56.1, Table 56.2). Thus, cell culture does not represent an appropriate reference method. Instead of culture, NAATs are now considered as gold standard for CT testing [16]. According to CDC recommendations, NAATs are the test of choice for CT detection, while antigen tests (EIA, DFA, and rapid point-of-care tests) are no longer recommended owing to low sensitivity and low specificity [12, 17]. Although some technical modifications of novel CT antigens test have improved sensitivity [18, 19], detection rate in clinical specimens is still lower than for NAATs, even after using gray-zone

Table 56.2 Sensitivity and specificity of *Chlamydia trachomatis* detection tests

Method	Sensitivity	Specificity
Culture	70–85%	100%
Antigen test (EIA)	53–76%	95%
Antigen test (DFA)	70–90%	98–100%
Hybridization	65–96%	96–100%
Amplification (NAAT)	90–100%	99–100%

Based on data from [8, 12, 13, 15, 17, 21, 24, 30]

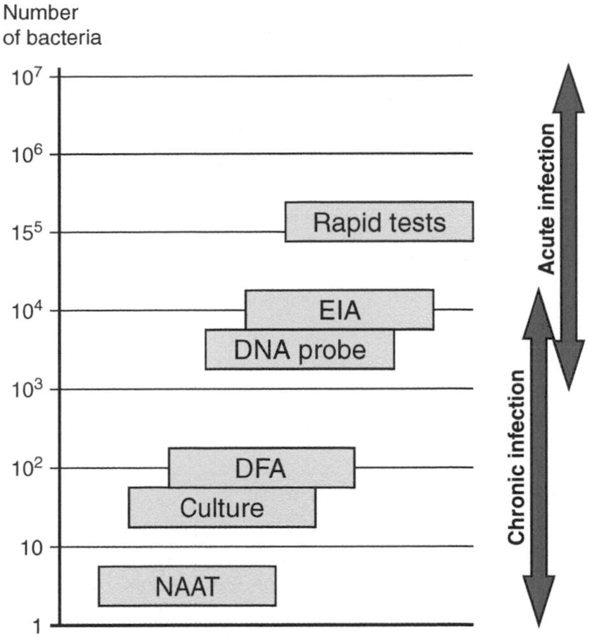

Fig. 56.1 Detection limits of tests for diagnosis of C. trachomatis infections

testing [20]. Moreover, specificity of antigen tests of 95% on an average will result in low positive predictive values (PPV) in most clinical settings, since predictive values depend on prevalence of infection. Considering a prevalence of 5%, the PPV of antigen tests with a sensitivity of 70% and a specificity of 95% is only 42.2%, in contrast to 90.6% for NAATs with a sensitivity of 95% and specificity of 99.5%. However, with lower prevalence, the PPV of NAATs will also be less than 90%. According to CDC recommendations, positive results of NAATs should be confirmed when PPV is <90% [12]. Thus, for CT testing of low-prevalence populations (e.g. screening programs), retesting of positive samples using the same test or another NAAT would be required. A negative confirmatory test may indicate not only a false-positive result of the first test but also a false-negative result of confirmatory test. As shown recently, using one NAAT to confirm the test result of another NAAT is not suitable, owing to different sensitivities of NAATs and low amount of target in specimens, which may result in inhomogeneous distribution in aliquots [21].

Several commercial NAATs for CT-detection using different amplification techniques are available (Table 56.3). In general, good agreement of results obtained by NAAT was reported. By comparing SDA (Becton

Table 56.3 Amplification tests for *Chlamydia trachomatis* and *Neisseria gonorrhoeae*

Method	Company/Assay	Target	
		C. trachomatis	*N. gonorrhoeae*
PCR	Roche, Cobas Amplicor; TaqMan	pCCT1	Cytosine DNA methyltransferase
	Abbott, m2000	pCCT1	Opa
	Qiagen, Artus C. trachomatis Plus RG	Omp1	–
LCR	Abbott LCx[a]	pCCT1	Opa
TMA	GenProbe: AmpCT, APTIMA	16S-rRNA	16S-rRNA
SDA	Becton Dickinson: ProbeTec-ET	pCCT1	Pilin gene-inverting Protein homologue
Hybrid Capture	Digene/Qiagen HC-II CT/NG	pCCT1	Plasmid and genomic
		Genomic DNA	DNA

[a]Assay has been taken off the market

Dickinson), TMA (GenProbe), and LCR (Abbott) with the novel Abbott m2000 assay, concordant results were found in 96–100% of swabs and 94–100% in urine specimens [22]. The discrepant results, however, indicate that not all NAATs are identical, but some differences of sensitivity and specificity do exist, which depend on different analytical sensitivities, specimen type, method of DNA extraction, presence of inhibitors, and CT variants. The APTIMA Combo2 assay (AC2, GenProbe) appears to be the most sensitive NAAT [21, 23], with somewhat lower specificity [24, 25]. However, lower specificity might be artificial for a test with highest sensitivity when uniquely positive samples cannot be confirmed by less-sensitive assays.

In general, analytical sensitivity is higher for isothermal amplification techniques (TMA and SDA) compared to NAATs using cyclic amplification (PCR and LCR), as well as for NAATs detecting multicopy targets compared to single-copy targets. Most commercial NAATs detect sequences located in the cryptic plasmid of CT, present in about ten copies per bacteria. The AC2 assay amplifies RNA sequences of 16S-rRNA, present in even higher copy numbers. Using such targets decreases the limit of detection with respect to the number of bacteria. On the other hand, sensitivity of these tests may be impaired because rRNAs are present in replicating bacteria predominately, and CT-strains with variant plasmids or no plasmids at all have been reported [26, 27]. In 2006, a new variant of CT was identified in Sweden, characterized by a 322 bp deletion in the cryptic plasmid [28]. The variant was found to be responsible for up to 30% of CT infections in Sweden, but yet was detected very rarely outside Sweden [29]. Importantly, the variant was not detected by some commercial assays used at that time, since the deletion includes the target region of these tests.

Frequency of detected infections also depends on the clinical material analyzed. NAATs for CT can be used for different clinical specimens including swabs, urine, sperm, and tissues. So far, only first catch urine (FCU), cervical smears, and vaginal smears (the latter only for AC2) were FDA-cleared. According to an earlier study comparing CT detection by SDA in different specimen types, cervical smears were shown to be superior to urine for CT detection in women, while urethral smears and urine were equally suitable for testing men [30]. Subsequent studies showed no significant difference between smears and urine also for women. By comparing different NAATs (LCR, PCR, TMA) for detection of CT in urine, cervical, urethral, and vaginal smears (self-collected or taken by physician), the highest rate of CT-positive samples was found in self-collected vaginal smears [31]. Skidmore et al. recently conducted a study on paired FCU and vulvo-vaginal swabs and found 88% versus 92% of true positives in urine and swabs, respectively, thus confirming higher detection rate in vulvo-vaginal swabs [20]. According to the authors, a systematic review and meta-analysis of studies is required to conclusively decide whether vulvo-vaginal swabs or urine is the superior specimen for CT-testing.

Another factor influencing the detection rate is represented by substances inhibiting the amplification procedure. Inhibition is associated with the specimen

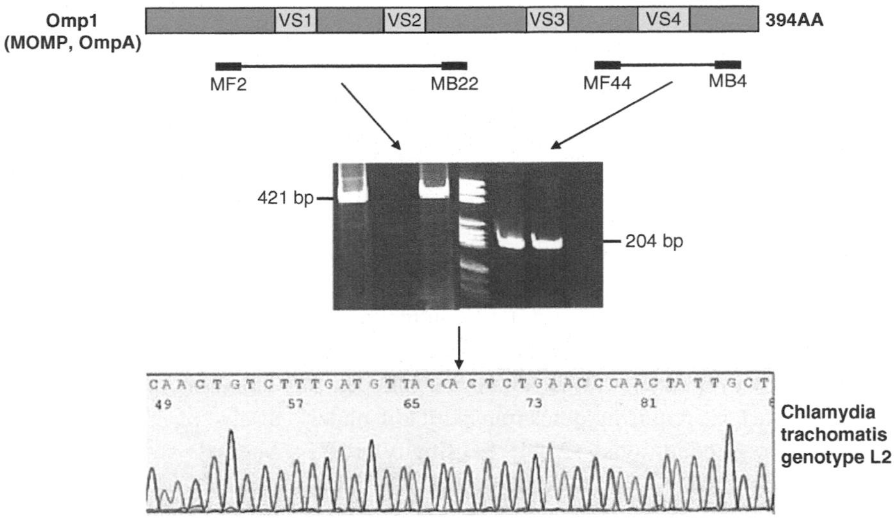

Fig. 56.2 Identification of LGV-strains by genotyping

type used, as in particular urine samples have been shown to frequently contain inhibitors [32]. The recent Health Technology Assessment (HTA) report from UK describes 13% of FCU samples inhibitory to PCR, and, moreover 16% of vulvo-vaginal swabs were also inhibitory to PCR. Using SDA technology, the number of inhibitory specimens was smaller (7% of FCU and <0.1% of vulvo-vaginal swabs), indicating that NAATs differ with respect to vulnerability to inhibitors, and the importance to control amplification efficacy [33]. As shown in Table 56.3, almost all currently available NAATs contain systems to control amplification/inhibition. GenProbe´s AC2 assay represents an exception; however, for this test very low rate of inhibition in both, urine (0.3%), cervical swabs (1.7%), and vaginal swabs (1.3%) have been reported [34].

56.4 Lymphogranuloma Venereum (LGV)

Chlamydia trachomatis (CT) causes different diseases correlating with particular CT serovars/genotypes. Serovars A–C are associated with ocular infections and may cause trachoma in persisting infections [35], serovars D–K cause anogenital infections and are also associated with conjunctivitis [36], while LGV is associated with serovars L1, L2, and L3. LGV is endemic in Africa, South-East Asia, South America, and the Caribbean, but represents a rare disease in Europe and North America [37]. Recently, however, an outbreak of LGV caused by L2 among MSM has been noticed in several European countries and North America. Confirmation of LGV requires presence of anorectal or inguinal symptoms, detection of *C. trachomatis* and identification of serovars L1, L2, or L3. CT-genotypes can be identified by sequence analysis of variable domains (VD) of Omp1 (Fig. 56.2) or by type-specific PCR tests [38, 136, 140]. Sequence analysis also provides information for epidemiology. In the Netherlands, the recent LGV outbreak was found to be caused by a variant of L2, named L2b. The same L2b variant was also shown to be present in San Francisco in the early 1980s [41]. In addition, some other variants of L2 were described in Vienna [42]. These variants show the same two mutations differing L2b from L2 and contain another one or two additional mutations. Probably, L2b has been imported to Europe some time ago and since then has acquired additional mutations resulting in sequence divergence.

56.5 Neisseria gonorrhea

As described for CT, NAATs were also increasingly used for detection of *N. gonorrhoeae* (gonococci NG). In contrast to CT, traditional assays like direct examination of smears and culture are still useful for NG diagnosis. Microscopic examination of smears for NG (intracellular Gram-negative diplococci) is much more sensitive than microscopy for CT. Sensitivity of Gram staining for NG was reported to be 90%

in symptomatic men, but is considerably lower in asymptomatic men (50–75%) and in women (30–50%) [17, 43]. Direct staining of smears for CT (Giemsa) is useful only for conjunctivitis of newborns (high bacterial loads) but not suitable for detection of urogenital CT infections [8].

Isolation of NG by culture is also easier than for CT. NG can be grown on several solid selective media (modified Thayer-Martin, Martin-Lewis). Sensitivity of NG culture is higher than for CT cell culture and is still considered the gold standard in diagnosis of gonorrhoea. However, as for CT, isolation of NG depends on viable bacteria requiring quick transportation under optimal storage conditions [12, 44]. Sensitivity of NG culture was shown to be impaired by specimen collection device, viability in transportation systems, and culture media used [45, 46] as well as by antibiotic (pre)treatment. Identification of NG in cultured bacteria requires confirmation by biochemical, serological, or coagulation tests. Therefore, time to results may take up to 3 days or longer.

Similar to CT, several tests that do not depend on viable organisms, but detect structural components of the bacteria have been developed to improve diagnosis of NG infection. Commercial antigen tests (Gonozyme, Abbott) and hybridization assays (Gen Probe Pace2, Digene/Qiagen HC-II) are faster than culture. Sensitivities and specificities of hybridization tests are similar to or less than culture [17, 44, 47, 48]. The antigen tests were taken off the market due to poor sensitivity [49].

Improved sensitivity of NG detection when compared with culture was reported for NAATs with specificities usually >98% [17, 49, 50]. Performances of commercial assays have been analyzed in many different studies with varying results depending on the patient population and reference standard used [49]. Next to commercial NAATs, a number of in-house assays have been published, for which performance data are limited, because most of them were investigated in single studies only [49]. Accuracy of all these NAATs may be affected by genetic variability and genome plasticity of NG. Horizontal transfer of genetic material within the genus Neisseria can cause false-positive results due to acquisition of gonococcal genes by commensal neisseria [51]. Loss of target regions has been shown to be responsible for reduced sensitivity [52, 53]. As described for CT, inhibitory substances may also cause false-negative results. Internal controls were required to indicate inhibition of NAATs [54], which are generally included in commercial assays but mostly not in in-house assays.

Four commercial NAATs are currently available for NG (Table 56.3). These tests can be used to detect NG with high sensitivity in urethral, cervical, and vaginal swabs [17, 43]. Considering urine specimens, higher sensitivity of PCR was found for males than for females and for symptomatic versus asymptomatic males [30,55]. Subsequently sensitivity of testing female urines for GC was improved to 85% and 91% using SDA and TMA, but did not reach sensitivities of testing cervical swabs of 97% and 99% in these studies [30, 56]. Vaginal swabs, another noninvasive, patient-taken material of women may be superior to urine. As has been shown for CT [57], it was also reported for NG detection that self-taken vaginal swabs performed better than clinician-obtained cervical swabs [58].

Testing anorectal and oropharyngeal swabs by NAATs has been shown to be more sensitive than culture to diagnose pharyngeal and rectal gonorrhea [59–61]. It is important to consider that cross-reactivity with commensal neisseria may potentially reduce specificity of testing these materials for NG [53, 62]. Commercial NAATs are not licensed for anorectal and pharyngeal swabs but only for material from urogenital sites where commensal neisseria are relatively uncommon [63]. Using these tests for testing rectal and pharyngeal swabs may lead to false-positive results and lower positive predictive values [61, 64]. Thus, NAAT-positive results obtained with extragenital specimens should be confirmed by culture or another NAAT using a different target in order to raise the PPV. Compared to CT, the prevalence of NG can be higher in particular groups, like MSM, but is generally lower in the general population. For the latter NG, confirmatory tests might also be considered, because even when using a test with 99% sensitivity and specificity, the PPV will be less than 50% when the prevalence is less than 1% [65].

In summary, NAATs provide a number of advantages over other diagnostic tests. Besides high sensitivity and specificity, NAATs offer high flexibility, as the same specimen can be used for detection of multiple STI pathogens. All commercial companies providing NAATs for CT offer test kits, which are able to detect CT and NG simultaneously at almost the same price as for CT test kits. Usually, NAATs need only 3–5 h for up to 92 specimens; therefore, final results were obtained within one day under routine conditions. In addition, NAATs can be used for noninvasive specimens and do not require viable organisms, requiring less stringent transport conditions. Compared to swabs transported in liquid medium, dry swabs, which can be sent by mail, have been shown to be as accurate for CT/NG testing [66].

In general, NAAT are more expensive than traditional tests like culture, which is usually mentioned as a major disadvantage of NAAT, but some commercial NAATs for CT/NG are now fully automated (Becton-Dickinson Viper; Gen-Probe TIGRIS). These systems allow high throughput with very low hands-on-time and thus minimize personal costs.

On the other hand, NAATs are not suitable as test of cure since DNA can be detected for several weeks after treatment but do not represent viable organisms [12,67]. Patients with persistent symptoms under antibiotic treatment may be infected with potentially resistant strains. In this case, identification by culture and resistance testing is advised, because use of commercial NAATs for NG detection does not provide information about antibiotic susceptibility. NG isolates have been shown to be resistant against many different antibiotics. Resistance against ampicillin, erythromycin, tetracyclines, and quinolones has been observed increasingly during the last years [68–70]. Culture and susceptibility testing still represents the gold standard but the sensitivity of culture being less 100% and the decreased use of culture for diagnostics in favor of NAATs requests culture-independent techniques to identify antibiotic resistance.

Resistance of NG to quinolones (QRNG) depends on mutations of the quinolone target enzymes gyrase and topoisomerase. Two regions of gyrA and parC were identified to be associated with QRNG and were thus termed QR-determining region [71, 72]. Several different point mutations and amino acid changes located in this region confer decreased susceptibility and resistance to quinolones [73]. GyrA mutations alone are sufficient for resistance [74, 75], but mutations in both gyrA and parC are associated with higher levels of resistance [76]. In a study from China, almost all QRNG could have been identified by analyzing S91P of gyrA [77].

Based on these data, several molecular methods for testing QRNG have been described. These include direct sequencing of PCR products spanning the QR determining region [39, 63, 112,], denaturing HPLC analysis of PCR products [72], PCR using primers with specific restriction sites [74], mismatch amplification using mutation-specific primers [78], and oligonucleotide biochips for gyrA and parC mutations [75, 79].

In addition, real-time fluorometric PCR systems using TaqMan probes or Light Cycler and FRET probes have been used to differentiate between wild-type and mutated gyrA and parC [80–82]. These tests have a high sensitivity and specificity for detection of QRNG compared to susceptibility testing of cultured bacteria and can also be used in urine specimens [82]. They clearly facilitate and accelerate detection of resistance to quinolones; however, current molecular tests are largely limited to quinolones. Reduced susceptibility to cefixime in clinical isolates of Neisseria gonorrhoeae was linked to amino acid changes in penicillin-binding protein 2 [83]. To introduce molecular testing for antibiotic resistance in routine diagnostics, it would be important to extend these tests to other relevant antibiotics with emerging resistance.

56.6 Treponema pallidum

Diagnosis of syphilis is based primarily on clinical symptoms, serology, and direct detection of pathogens. Serology is central to laboratory testing, usually performed by a combination of nontreponemal (Rapid plasma regain [RPR] test or Venereal Disease research Laboratory [VDRL] test) and treponemal tests (*Treponema pallidum* particle agglutination [TPPA], *Treponema pallidum* hemagglutination assay [TPHA], fluorescent treponema antibody absorption test [FTA-Abs test], enzyme immunoassay [EIA], Western blot). Serology follows a two-step diagnostic procedure using VDRL, TPPA, or EIA as a screening test and confirmation of reactive samples by another test (FTA-Abs, EIA, TPPA, or Western blot).

In the early phase of infection, serology is negative, since development of antibodies may take up to 4 weeks [84]. Seronegative cases of secondary syphilis have been reported in HIV-infected immunocompromised patients [85]. In addition, serology may lack sensitivity for diagnosis of neurosyphilis and congenital syphilis.

Definite diagnosis of syphilis in suspicious cases with negative or borderline serology requires demonstration of *T. pallidum* in clinical specimens either by dark-field (dark-ground) microscopy, direct fluorescent antibody test or silver stain (Warthin–Starry, Dieterle), or by detection of bacterial DNA in mucosal swabs or tissue samples. Dark-field microscopy has limited sensitivity and is not useful for oral and rectal swabs owing to nonpathogenic spirochetes, which may be present at these sites. Problems with background staining and limited sensitivity were also shown for silver staining [86, 87]. Both sensitivity and specificity was improved by immunohistochemistry [88].

There are also several PCR assays that have been described to successfully detect *T. pallidum* in fresh material and formalin-fixed paraffin-embedded biopsy specimens, though with sensitivities ranging from 40% to 100% [89–94]. Differences are likely to depend on the target regions (TP47kd protein, basic membrane protein (bmp), pol-1, tmpC), clinical material (swabs, biopsies, blood), and amplification technique used (gel-based standard/nested PCR, real-time PCR). Palmer et al. described a detection limit of 800 target gene copies using gel-based PCR test [93]. A threshold of 10 treponemes per PCR reaction was reported for nested PCR and gelelectrophoretic analysis of PCR products [90]. The detection limit was even lower for real-time PCR, which was shown to detect as few as two copies [95]. Also, in a comparative study of Koek et al., real-time PCR for *T. pallidum* was at least as sensitive as gel-based nested PCR, confirming the high analytical sensitivity of real-time PCR [96].

PCR testing of smears or biopsies from suspicious clinical lesions appears to be useful to confirm or exclude early syphilis. Palmer et al. reported sensitivity and specificity of 94.7% and 98.6% for primary syphilis, including two patients being PCR positive prior to seroconversion. In addition, PCR was more sensitive to detect primary lesions than dark-field microscopy [93]. These findings are confirmed by 95% agreement of serology and PCR in patients with early syphilis recently described by Leslie et al. using a more sensitive real-time PCR assay [95]. In contrast, detection rate in lesions from patients with secondary syphilis is lower, but was again shown to be more sensitive than dark-field microscopy or silver staining [89, 93, 97]. Kouznetsov et al. were able to detect *T. pallidum* DNA in blood (PBMC) of all six patients with secondary syphilis and also in PMBC from five out of seven patients with latent syphilis [90]. Detection of *T. pallidum* DNA in blood from patients with latent syphilis has also been reported in other studies [98, 99].

In conclusion, PCR appears useful to rapidly confirm or rule out early syphilis in cases of unclear serologic results, but is inferior for later disease stages. However, PCR may be used as an adjunctive test to confirm congenital syphilis and neurosyphilis [100, 101], as well as to demonstrate involvement of particular organs like lymph nodes, sternal bone, stomach, or vitreus in the pathogenic process [102–105].

Furthermore, in the light of increasing resistance of *Treponema pallidum* to macrolides [106, 107] and considering the lack of suitable in vitro system to culture *T. pallidum*, molecular analysis of resistance associated mutations have gained interest recently. As the genetic basis for macrolide resistance, the mutation A2058G of the 23S rRNA gene was identified, which alters the active site of macrolides on ribosomes [107, 108]. This mutation can be detected using a PCR assay spanning the corresponding 23S rRNA region and subsequent sequence analysis of the PCR product or by MboII digestion [107]. Recently, a real-time PCR assay was developed, which allows discrimination of azithromycin-resistant and -susceptible *T. pallidum* strains by melting-curve analysis of PCR products [109]. These assays provide an important diagnostic supplement for management of syphilis patients treated with azithromycin instead of penicillin G by reasons of penicillin allergy, discomfort of intramuscular administered penicillin, and lower rate of side-effects with azithromycin.

56.7 HPV

Papillomaviruses represent a large group of small DNA viruses within the family of Papovaviridae. About 100 types of human papillomaviruses (HPV) have been identified, with more than 40 of them infecting the anogenital mucosa [110]. HPV have been shown to be causally involved in development of cervical cancer and were also associated with other anogenital and extragenital cancers [111–113]. Anogential HPV types differ with respect to their oncogenic properties. Based on epidemiologic and molecular studies, HPV types 16, 18, and several others were characterized as high-risk (HR) HPV types with increased risk of malignant progression of dysplastic epithelial lesions (Fig. 56.3). In contrast, HPV types 6, 11, and others are classified as low-risk (LR) HPV types, which are frequently

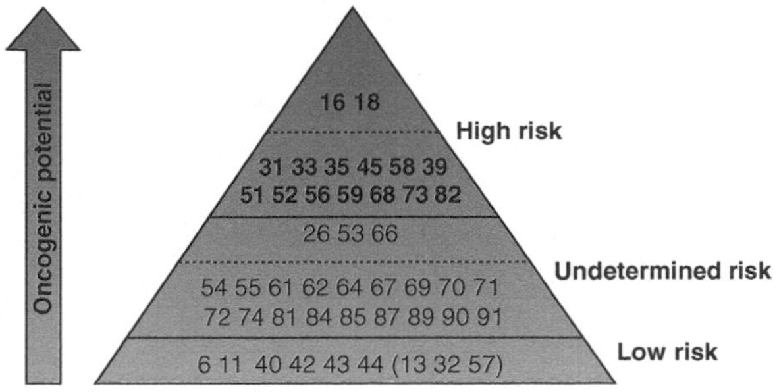

Fig. 56.3 Oncogenic potential of genital HPV Classification according to [144]

detected in benign lesions (e.g., condylomata acuminata). For a number of other genital HPV types, the oncogenic properties were not yet characterized, but current epidemiologic data indicate low oncogenicity of these HPV types.

Although being a prerequisite for cervical cancer, only a small number of HR-HPV infections lead to dysplastic and neoplastic lesions, indicating that additional factors are involved in carcinogenesis. HR HPV infections are detected more frequently in young individuals [114]. In women of age 15–25, the highest HPV prevalence of more than 20% was found. With increasing age, prevalence is decreasing below 5% of women aged 30 years and above. Most HPV infections acquired by young women resolve spontaneously within a period of 12 months [115–117]. Failure of immunologic elimination results in persistent infection, which may progress towards dysplasia and neoplasia in a small number of cases (Fig. 56.4) [116].

For women with normal cytology, the risk for development of high-grade squamous intraepithelial lesions (HSIL) within 5 years was shown to be >10-fold higher in HPV-positive compared to HPV-negative women [118]. The risk of progression depends on HPV type and viral load [119, 120]. HPV types 16 and 18 represent the highest risk for CIN3 and cervical cancer [119]. In addition, malignant progression is associated with certain cytogenetic and molecular changes (Fig. 56.4).

Based on the close association of HPV and cervical carcinogenesis, the viral infection has become a central target of prevention strategies including screening and vaccination. Testing for HPV is used for both primary screening and triage of women with abnormal cytology [121, 122].

Since replication of viral genomes, expression of capsid proteins, and assembly of viral particles occur in different cell layers of the epidermis, HPV cannot be grown in conventional cell cultures [123]. Although HPV induce humoral immune responses, detection of antibodies is not useful for detection of HPV infection, as antibodies detected may result from both present and past infection [124]. Most useful methods for

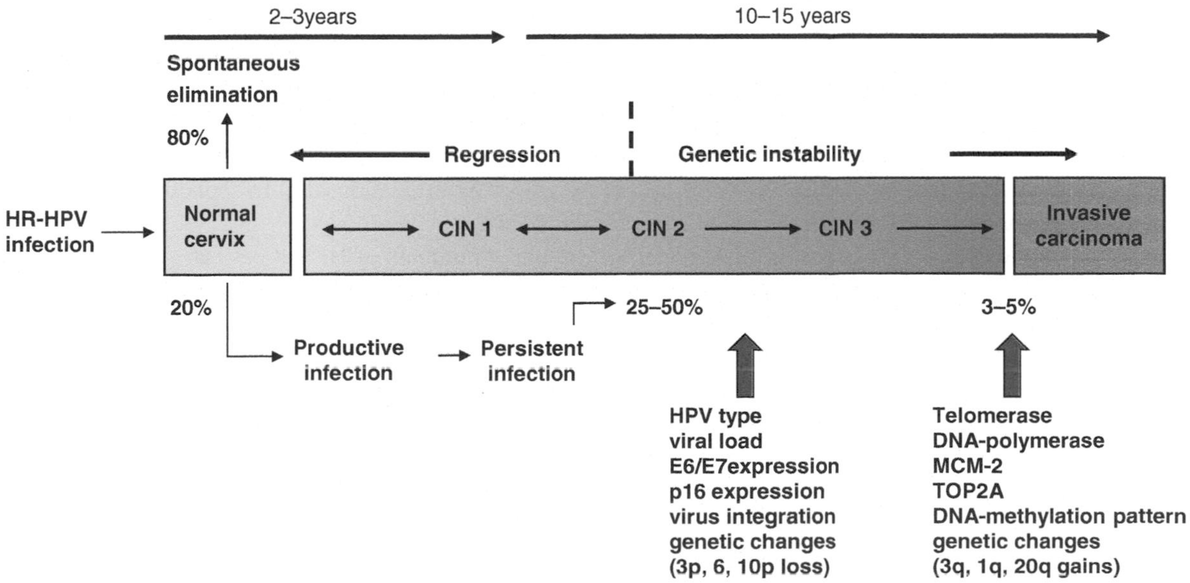

Fig. 56.4 HPV-induced carcinogenesis

detection of HPV infections are molecular techniques based on identification of viral nucleic acids [125]. Initially applied hybridization assays like Southern blot, Dot blot, and in situ hybridization are no longer used for routine HPV testing because they are labor-intensive and lack sensitivity and specificity. Current HPV testing is performed using signal and target amplification systems detecting HPV sequences in DNA isolated from swabs or biopsies.

The Hybrid Capture Test (HC-II, Digene/Qiagen) represents a signal amplification method, based on hybridization of RNA-probes with target DNA sequences. DNA–RNA hybrids are captured with immobilized monoclonal antibodies and detected with multiple anti-DNA/RNA antibodies conjugated with phosphatase and using chemiluminescent substrates [126]. The test is able to differentiate between LR and HR HPV using two different probe cocktails including 5 LR HPV types (6, 11, 42, 43, 44) and 13 HR HPV types (16, 18, 31, 33, 35, 39, 45, 51, 52, 56, 58, 59, 68), but does not permit identification of individual HPV types. HC-II is approved by the FDA and has been used in many clinical studies. The detection limit of 1,000 copies makes it less sensitive than most PCR assays [127], but was shown sufficient to detect HSIL with a high sensitivity (97%) [128]. Of importance, specificity of HC-II can be impaired due to cross-reactivity with HPV types of unknown oncogenic potential [129, 130]. Improvement of specificity was reported by using HPV-specific oligonucleotides instead of anti-DNA antibodies to capture RNA/DNA hybrids [131].

Another widely used method for HPV detection is PCR, which depends on target amplification. Using type-specific primers, individual HPV types can be detected with high sensitivity [132]. However, more attractive are consensus PCR assays detecting a broad spectrum of HPV types. Primers of consensus HPV PCRs bind to conserved regions, mainly located in the L1 gene [125]. The analytical sensitivity of most PCR assays is generally higher than for HC-II and ranges between 10 and 1,000 copies, depending on the HPV type and use of type-specific versus consensus primer [127, 133]. A commercial PCR test provided by Roche (HPV-Amplicor) includes all HR HPV types, though in contrast to HC-II, it is not FDA-approved.

HPV testing has been shown to be more sensitive than cytology (Pap smear) for identification of dysplasia in a number of studies [134], but the positive predictive value of HR-HPV testing for cervical dysplasia is relatively low, e.g., many HR-HPV infections are clinically unapparent and will not induce epithelial changes. Therefore, additional markers are required to evaluate the risk of progression. Some of these potential progression markers shown in Fig. 56.4 are now being used or considered to be used in novel diagnostic assays.

Importance of HPV typing relates to different oncogenic properties of individual HPV types. In addition, identification of persistent infection also requires HPV typing. Usually, HPV types are identified by analysis of consensus PCR products, for which a number of techniques have been developed, including RFLP [135], direct sequencing [136], microplate hybridization [137], reverse hybridization [138, 139], DNA microarray hybridization [140, 141], and luminex suspension array technology [142]. RFLP analysis is labor-intensive and has limited sensitivity to detect presence of multiple HPV types. Similarly, direct sequencing of PCR products will also not allow identification of minority genotypes. Reverse hybridization represents a more attractive technique for HPV typing. It depends on immobilization of HPV-type specific probes on a solid phase and hybridization of PCR products added in the liquid phase. The technique is suitable to identify multiple HPV types in one sample using only a small amount of PCR product. Several commercial assays are available including 27 (Inno-LiPA, Innogenetics) and 37 genital HPV types (Linear Array, Roche). The same principle of hybridization is applied in DNA chips. A commercial low-density array (Papillocheck, Greiner One Bio) contains oligonucleotides derived from the E1 region of 24 genital HPV types immobilized on a plastic device, which are used for hybridization of corresponding fluorophore-labelled E1-PCR products.

Large numbers of HPV types can also be analyzed simultaneously using Luminex xMAP suspension array technology, which depends on hybridization of PCR products to fluorescence-labeled polystyrene beads, conjugated with type-specific oligonucleotides. To distinguish beads with different oligonucleotides, various ratios of two spectrally different fluorophores are used to create up to 100 different bead sets with specific absorption spectra. The technique thus may include up to 100 different HPV types and was reported to be fast and easy to perform, making it a preferential technique for high throughput analyses [142]. In addition, use of biotinylated primers and streptavidin-phycoerythrin conjugate permits quantification of PCR products.

HPV viral load may be a valuable predictor of disease. To calculate copy numbers of individual HPV types, real-time PCR assays using TaqMan 5' exonuclease system or LightCycler technology can be used, which detect type-specific HPV DNA and human DNA in the same assay or in separate assays [120, 143–145]. In a retrospective case control study in Sweden, it was shown that patients with cervical cancer had higher HPV 16 viral loads in their preceding cervical smear with normal cytology than HPV 16 positive controls without cancer [145]. Relation of HPV 16 and HPV 18 viral copy numbers with severity of cervical lesions was also reported [143]. However, accuracy of single viral load measurements are limited, due to high variability of HPV DNA concentrations and the fact that both extensive CIN3 lesion with low replication and small CIN1 lesion with extensive replication may result in a similar overall copy number. By comparing viral loads of HPV 16, 18, 31, and 33 in cervical smears of women with normal cytology, CIN3 thresholds have been determined to rule out CIN3 [120], which may be used as a marker for less aggressive management of HPV 16 positive women with normal cytology.

As another potential marker to indicate disease progression, expression of HR-HPV oncogenes was suggested. By comparing DNA and RNA concentration of HPV 16 E6 and E7 in ASCUS, LSIL, and HSIL, an increase of both DNA and RNA copy numbers was observed with expanding severity of lesions [146]. Since higher RNA than DNA copy numbers were detected in HSIL, the authors hypothesized quantification of oncogene transcripts to be a more sensitive marker of early cellular changes indicating progression towards HSIL and invasive cancer, than DNA copy number. In this study, a real-time PCR and reverse transcription PCR for quantification of HPV 16 E6 and E7 DNA and RNA was used [146]. In addition, transcripts of cellular housekeeping genes were analyzed to control RNA integrity. This is of particular importance when analyzing mRNAs, which are rapidly degraded by intracellular RNAses. Expression of HPV oncogenes can also be analyzed with a commercial assay (PreTect HPV-Proofer, NorChip/BioMerieux), that depends on real-time multiplex NASBA to amplify E6/E7 transcript of HPV 16, 18, 31, 33, and 45 [147]. In a 2-year follow-up study of 77 women with ASCUS or LSIL, it was demonstrated that patients tested positive for RNA are much more likely to develop CIN2+ lesions than patients with positive consensus HPV DNA PCR result at enrolment [148]. While showing the same high sensitivity to identify patients with progressive disease, PreTect HPV-Proofer was much more specific than HPV DNA PCR and could improve triage of women with ASCUS and LSIL.

Transcription-mediated amplification (TMA), which is used in APTIMA assays of Gen-Probe, was recently applied to HPV transcripts. A prototype commercial assay (APTIMA-HPV) has been developed for detection of E6/E7 transcripts of 14 HR-HPV types including those of PreTect-HPV Proofer and evaluated in a preliminary cross-sectional study [149]. HPV E6/E7 mRNA was detected in 94% of CIN3 and all of five cervical cancers, but also in parts of CIN1, CIN2, LSIL, ASCUS, and even in specimens of normal cytology. Using a higher cutpoint resulted in lower frequency of HPVE6/E7 transcripts in lesions <CIN2, without affecting frequency in CIN3 and cancer. According to the authors, the optimal cutpoint needs to be evaluated in order to use the assay to identify precancer and to predict progression [149].

HPV oncogene transcript analysis can also be used to detect integration of HPV into the host cell genome. Transcripts of integrated viral oncogenes are characterized by human sequences at the 3' end, resulting in larger mRNA molecules compared to transcripts of episomal viruses. These transcripts were detected by a technique called APOT (amplification of papillomavirus oncogene transcripts) in 88% of cervical cancers, but in only 16% of CIN3 lesions, 5% of CIN2 lesions, and none of CIN1 lesions [150]. However, especially in HPV 16-associated cancers, the viral genome was not always found to be integrated [151].

As shown in Fig. 56.4, there are several other candidate markers that in case of HR-HPV positive results may increase specificity to detect cervical disease. They are based on molecular changes occurring in cervical carcinogenesis. More than 200 genes have been identified by gene expression profiling that were upregulated in cervical cancer compared to normal cervical epidermis [152, 153]. In particular, p16^{INK4a}, members of the MCM (minichromosome maintenance proteins) family, cyclin D1, and topoisomerase 2a (TOP2a) were shown to be strongly overexpressed in cervical cancer. Some of these factors may serve as surrogate markers of HPV oncogene activity [154]. Expression of p16^{INK4a}

was shown to be a specific marker of cervical dysplasia [155]. According to the combined data of studies analyzing p16^{INK4a} in cervical lesions, protein expression is found in 0–18% in normal cytology, 81–100% in HSIL, and 97–100% in cervical cancer [156]. Actually, p16^{INK4a} represents a tumor suppressor, functioning as inhibitor of cyclin-dependent kinases [157]. Overexpression of p16 in cervical dysplasia and neoplasia results from negative feedback loop of cell cycle progression induced by HPV E7-mediated pRB-activation and E2F-expression [157], hence reflecting HPV E7 activity. Based on p16^{INK4a} reactivity of HR-HPV-positive LSIL, detection of p16^{INK4a}, which is also available as commercial test (CINTec™, Dako) might be used to identify patients at risk to progress to HSIL and cervical cancer [158].

ProEx™C (Becton Dickinson) represents another biomarker reagent to detect aberrant S-phase induction based on immunocytochemical detection of MCM2 and TOP2a, two proteins associated with DNA replication and overexpressed in cervical neoplasia [159, 160]. In a preliminary study, MCM2/TOP2a expression was demonstrated in (10/10) HSIL, 5/10 LSIL, 2/10 ASCUS, and in none of the ten specimens with normal cytology [161]. Use of ProEx™C to indicate progressive cervical disease needs to be confirmed in larger trials. However, these biomarkers may potentially supplement conventional screening and HPV testing in the future by helping to more precisely define patients at risk for cancer development and thus reducing patient anxiety and also overall screening costs.

56.8 HIV

Diagnosis of HIV-infection is based primarily on serologic assays detecting HIV-1/HIV-2-specific antibodies, which will appear in virtually all infected patients. With the exception of acute infection and vertical infection, methods depending on direct detection of virus particles (culture) or structural components (p24 antigen viral RNA) are of minor importance for primary diagnosis. Serology is performed by a two-step testing procedure using first a sensitive screening test (EIA), which when reactive, must be confirmed by specific tests (Western blot). Latest screening tests (fourth-generation tests) detect both HIV antibodies and antigen (p24). In case of recently acquired HIV infection, these tests may produce reactive results, which cannot be confirmed by Western blot (detecting antibody only) and thus require verification by testing for viral antigen or RNA, which can be detected several weeks before seroconversion. In children of HIV-positive mothers, detection of viral RNA or proviral cDNA by NAATs permits identification or exclusion of HIV-infection much earlier than serology, since maternal antibodies can be detected for up to 18 months [162].

Quantification of viral load to monitor antiretroviral treatment is considered the most important application of NAATs. In addition, molecular assays are used to analyze disease progression, subtype identification, co-receptor use, and susceptibility testing. Currently used amplification techniques include both target (PCR, NASBA) and signal amplification (branched DNA). These methods allow quantitative analysis and are available in several commercial assays.

The first quantitative HIV-PCR test of Roche (Cobas Amplicor HIV-1 monitor) has been replaced recently by Cobas TaqMan HIV-1 test. Whereas the Amplicor assay used endpoint quantification by photometric measurement of enzyme-linked color reaction, the TaqMan system is based on real-time amplification. It allows more precise quantification, because PCR products are measured during the exponential phase of amplification, as accumulation of amplicons result in increasing reporter fluorescence emission of cleaved TaqMan probes [163]. The amount of target is related to a critical cycle when fluorescent signals exceed a threshold value. This threshold cycle is inversely related to the target concentration and can be used for quantification. Real-time PCR has decreased the limit of detection from 400 to 40 copies/mL and has extended the dynamic range from 400–750,000 to 40–10^7 (Table 56.4). The technique of real-time PCR is also used in tests of Abbott and Siemens (Abbott RealTime HIV1 and New VERSANT HIV-1 RNA 1.0 assay, kPCR), displaying almost the same sensitivity and dynamic range [164]. The assays differ with respect to the HIV-1 subtypes detected. As shown in Table 56.4, the Abbott assay detects HIV subgroups O and N in addition to group M subtypes A–H, probably due to the use of HIV 1 integrase as a target, which contains more conserved regions than the gag and pol region.

NASBA, which is based on isothermal amplification using reverse transcriptase, RNAse H, and T7 RNA polymerase, was also used for HIV-1 detection.

Table 56.4 Commercial quantitative HIV-1 assays

HIV Test/Company	Detection Limit	Range	Subtypes Detected
Cobas TaqMan (Roche)	40	40–107	Group M, subtypes A–H
RealTime HIV-1 (Abbott)	40	40–107	Group M, subtypes A–H Group O and N
NewVersant kPCR (Siemens)	34	34–107	Group M, subtypes A–G Group O
NucliSens HIV-1 (BioMerieux)	50	50.3 × 106	Group M, subtypes A–J
Versant HIV-RNA3.0 (Siemens)	50	50–5 × 105	Group M, subtypes A–G

Amplification products generated by T7 RNA polymerase are represented by ssRNA copies, which can be detected real time with molecular beacons [165]. A commercial version, NucliSens HIV-1, is provided by BioMerieux, detecting group M subtypes A–J with a detection limit and dynamic range similar to real-time PCR (see Table 56.4).

The technique of branched DNA represents a method of signal amplification. It is applied in Siemens HIV RNA quantification assay (Versant HIV-RNA 3.0) [166]. Genomic HIV RNA molecules were immobilized using plate-coated capture probes and then hybridized with a second series of target-specific probes (preamplifier), which provide binding of branched DNA molecules. These actually represent the amplification step as they carry multiple binding sites for AP-labeled probes, subsequently used to generate chemiluminescent signals, which are proportional to the amount of target sequences [167, 168]. Although target amplification has generally higher analytical sensitivity than signal amplification, the detection limit of the Versant assay (50 copies/mL) is not much different from real-time PCR and NASBA; the dynamic range of 50–500,000 copies/mL, however, is smaller. The Versant HIV RNA assay was shown to detect group M subtypes A–G.

Although good agreement of HIV-NAATs was shown in many comparative studies [169–173], it should be considered that accurate determination of viral load may be affected by diversity of HIV-1. In particular, HIV-1 non-B subtypes have been shown to be underestimated or were not detected at all by some tests [174, 175]. All commercial assays for HIV-1 quantification described above are equipped with automated sample preparation, but complete automation including transfer of isolated RNAs to the amplification unit is available for the Roche TaqMan system only (Cobas AmpliLink).

Molecular assays have also been developed to analyze patients' HIV strains with respect to subtype, coreceptor use, and susceptibility against antiretroviral drugs. Phenotypic resistance testing involves amplification of relevant pol-regions (containing mutations associated with resistance to protease and reverse transcriptase-inhibitors) incorporation into corresponding pol-deleted HIV-1 vectors to generate recombinant viruses and subsequent infection of cell lines used to analyze replication in the presence of various concentrations of antiretroviral drugs [176, 177]. The technique is offered by some companies (Antivirogram, Tibotec-VIRCO; PhenoSense ViroLogic/Monogram) but is tedious, lengthy, and expensive.

In routine diagnostics, phenotypic resistance testing is largely replaced by genotypic assays, which depend on direct sequencing of PCR products and identification of known resistance-associated mutations [178].

Genotypic resistance testing was first based on sequence analysis of reverse transcriptase (RT) and protease [179,180]. Currently, antiretroviral therapy also includes drugs directed against integrase, gp41, and gp120 in addition to protease and RT, resulting in extension of sequence analysis to corresponding HIV gene regions. Because of the complex pattern of mutations, several sequence analysis tools, like Stanford database (http://hivdb.stanford.edu), are used to predict resistance/susceptibility to antiretroviral drugs. At present, more than 20 interpretation systems are available, including those of two commercial assays for HIV-1 genotyping (TRUEGENE, Siemens; ViroSeq, Abbott). Some degree of discordance has been found by comparing interpretation algorithms [181], probably resulting from the fact that most of them depend on rule-based interpretation considering expert opinion and published data. Other systems, like geno-2-pheno and Vircotype provide virtual phenotypes [182, 183]. These systems are based on large databases of genotype–phenotype-pairs and use bioinformatics tools (decision trees, neuronal networks, support vector machines, etc.) to predict phenotype more accurately from sequence data.

The value of genotypic resistance testing was confirmed in several studies [179, 184] and HIV-1 genotyping has now been implemented in both national and international treatment guidelines. With the recent approval of CCR 5 antagonist Maraviroc for HIV-1 treatment, the analysis of co-receptor use has become important since the drug can be used only for CCR5 tropic viruses. Both phenotypic and genotypic assays based on the V3-loop of gp120 were used to identify tropism of HIV [60, 185]. Discrepancies between genotypic and phenotypic assays have been described, but even by comparing two phenotypic assays, only 85% concordance was found [186]. Discordant findings may relate to non-V3-sequences determining the tropism [176, 187] and presence of CXC4 minorities below the detection limit of phenotypic and genotypic assays, which represents 5% and 20%, respectively, of an individual sequence in the whole population [60, 188]. An additional limitation for molecular tropism assays and resistance tests is represented by the minimum number of viral copies required, which was reported to be around 1,000/mL for Trofile (Monogram), TRUEGENE, and ViroSeq.

Sensitivity may be improved by some modifications like nested PCR and more efficient nucleic acid extraction [189, 190]. Minor variants can be detected by PCR using specific primers for nucleic acid changes [191]. The method is suitable for detection of key mutations, but impractical to analyze all resistance-associated mutations, which would require a large number of PCR tests. Similarly, line probe assays (such as INNO-LiPA HIV-1 line probe assay, Innogenetics) can be used to identify some key mutations but are unable to consider the wide spectrum of polymorphisms associated with resistance and the high variability of HIV-1 strains [192]. In contrast, high-density DNA microarray chips may cope with the task of high-grade sequence variability. DNA chips potentially have the capacity to include all relevant mutations and HIV-1 subtypes, but may encounter problems to identify insertions and deletions as has been shown for a commercial test (Affymetrix HIV-1 Gene Chip) [193]. In addition, these tests need to be redesigned with any novel relevant polymorphism identified.

Recently, a novel genome sequencing technique [194] was applied to identify rare HIV-sequences [195, 196]. This technique, called ultradeep sequencing (or massively parallel sequencing), depends on clonal amplification of cDNA fragments and subsequent pyrosequencing on a pico-titer plate device using Genome Sequencer FLX system (454 Life Sciences/Roche). Basic modules of the technology are shown in Fig. 56.5. Based on the generation of 8–12,000 sequences per sample, the technique was shown to identify minorities representing as little as 0.2% of the whole population and thus significantly improves detection of minor variants in a population of HIV-1 quasispecies [195].

56.9 HBV

Similar to HIV, primary diagnosis of HBV infection depends on serology, usually by testing for HBs antigen and antibodies against HBs and HBc. In addition, molecular assays targeting viral DNA may be used in case of suspected infection with HBs antigen not detectable, e.g., acute infection, occult infection, and HBs antigen variants [197]. Detection and quantification of viral DNA, however, is used predominately to determine activity of viral replication to predict progression of chronic HBV-related liver disease, as well as initiation and monitoring of antiviral treatment [198–201]. Molecular assays are also used to identify HBV genotypes and to characterize individual strains with respect to mutations/polymorphisms associated with virulence, immune escape, and resistance against antiviral drugs [202, 203].

Active HBV infection is known to be associated with a wide range of viral DNA concentrations in blood, which may even exceed 10^{10} viral genome copies/mL [204]. Thus, quantitative HBV NAATs require a wide dynamic range, achieved best by using real-time amplification. In addition, high sensitivity is also important to identify early treatment failure, respectively, emergence of drug-resistant strains under antiviral therapy. A number of HBV PCR assays with high sensitivity have been developed in-house, but these tests usually lack standardization and validation [205–208].

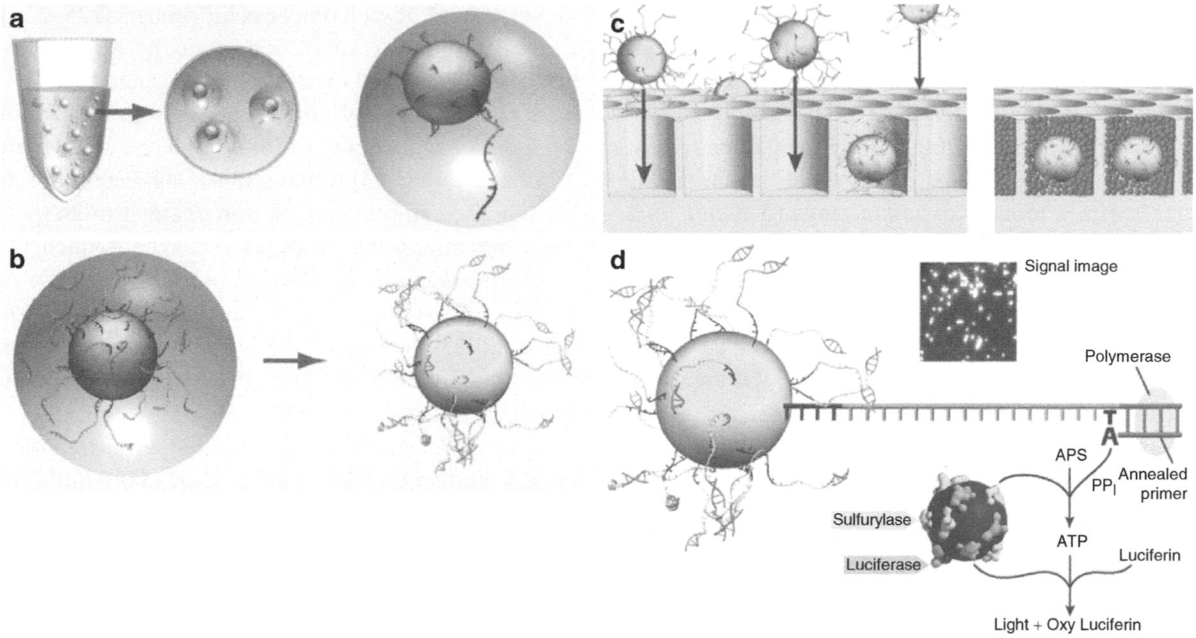

Fig. 56.5 Genome sequencer FLX system. (**a**) Single stranded template (sst) DNA with specific adaptors, generated by blunt end ligation of adaptors to fragmented genomic DNA or by using appropriate primers during PCR, is immobilized onto DNA capture beads. Beads were used in excess to achieve binding of only one DNA molecule per bead. (**b**) By adding PCR reagents in a water-in-oil mixture sst DNA is amplified on emulsified beads called micro-reactors, allowing clonal amplification (emulsion-based clonal amplification – emPCR). (**c**) After removal of the emulsion beads containing millions of copies of clonally amplified sst DNA molecules were transferred onto pico-titer plates containing wells small enough to contain single beads only. (**d**) Amplified sst DNAs are analyzed by pyro-sequencing (sequencing-by-synthesis) using the Genome Sequencer 20 instrument. Incorporation of nucleotides results in a chemiluminescent signal detected by the CCD camera of the instrument. All wells of the pico-titer plate were analyzed simultaneously, resulting in up to 200.000 reads in parallel. (photograph from Roche Diagnostics GmbH, Mannheim, Germany; with permission)

Commercial NAATs for quantification of HBV viral load are similar to those for HIV and are offered by the same companies. Both Roche and Abbott provide automated real-time PCR assays (Cobas TaqMan HBV Monitor, Abbott RealTime HBV), with similar detection limits of 12 and 10 IU/mL, respectively [199, 209–211]. The dynamic range of quantification was reported to be broader for the Abbott assay (10–10^9 IU/mL compared to 54–1.1 × 10^8 IU/mL for Cobas TaqMan) [199, 209–211]. The former Cobas Amplicor HBV Monitor test of Roche depended on endpoint quantification of PCR products with a lower sensitivity and smaller dynamic range [210, 211].

Siemens also offers the bDNA signal amplification system for HBV quantification (Versant HBV DNA 3.0) with a detection limit of 357 IU/ml and a dynamic range of 357–1.8 × 10^8 IU/mL [212]. Expression of HBV DNA concentrations in units is preferred to copy numbers, since calibration against the WHO HBV DNA standard has revealed test-dependent differences of copy numbers (one IU corresponds to 5.8 DNA copies for Cobas TaqMan and 5.6 DNA copies for bDNA). The HBV hybrid capture test 2 (Digene/Qiagen) represents another signal amplification system based on hybridization of a chemiluminescent probe [213]. The assay is less sensitive than real-time PCR and bDNA with a detection limit of approx. 3,500 IU/mL (8,000 copies/mL) for the ultrasensitive version. The dynamic range of quantification was reported 3,500 IU/mL to 5 x 10^8 IU/mL [203].

Currently, eight HBV genotypes with distinct geographic distribution are distinguished, designated A–H [214]. Accurate quantification of genotypes A–F has been demonstrated for Cobas TaqMan, Abbott RealTime HBV, HC-II, and bDNA [199, 209, 211, 212, 215]. Genotype G was also detected, but tested for in single samples only. Using a highly conserved region of HBV surface gene, genotype-independent quantification of HBV DNA by a real-time PCR assay was reported recently [207]. The assay correlated well with Cobas TaqMan assay and, moreover, was found to be more sensitive (limit of detection: 5 IU/mL) with a broader dynamic range (5 IU/mL to 2 × 10^9 IU/mL).

By comparing different HBV NAATs, concordant results were found especially for real-time PCR assays [211]. Less good agreement was described between real-time PCRs and bDNA [210, 216]. Of importance, several studies have shown nonspecific reactions for the bDNA assay in samples with values close to the positive cut off, reducing specificity of the test [210, 212, 216]. Significant deviation of quantitative results was also described. Ronsin et al. reported 18% of blood specimen with more than 0.5 log difference with higher values produced by bDNA [210]. The differences most likely relate to different amplification techniques, but may also depend on different extraction procedures.

In general, target amplification assays are more sensitive and more specific than signal amplification tests and display broader dynamic range, but on the other hand have higher intra- and interassay variability and may underestimate viral load. These differences must be considered when switching between different assays. It is generally recommended to use the same assay in longitudinal studies and during treatment monitoring.

Clinical outcome and response to antiviral treatment depends on both viral load and HBV genotype. Genotype C is associated with more aggressive liver disease than genotype B, probably because genotype B is associated with earlier HBe seroconversion [217, 218]. Moreover, since response to interferon alpha (IFNα) is lower for genotypes C and D, when compared with A and B [219–221], genotyping is recommended before initiation of antiviral treatment [197]. A number of techniques have been described to identify HBV genotypes, mainly based on analysis of preS and S region. Direct sequencing of PCR products is usually considered the most accurate method [222]. A commercial sequencing test for HBV genotyping is offered by Siemens (TRUEGENE). Other commercial HBV typing tests are based on reverse hybridization (INNO-LiPA, Innogenetics) [223] and chip hybridization of PCR products (BioMerieux/Affymetrix) [224]. In addition, melting curve analysis of real-time PCR products or PCR with type-specific primers [225–227], as well as analysis of PCR products by RFLP [228] have been described to identify HBV genotypes.

By comparing INNO-LiPA and chip-hybridization with direct sequencing of PCR products, concordant results of INNO-LiPA and sequencing were reported in 273/275 samples (99.3%), in contrast to 268/275 (97.5%) comparing chip-analysis with sequencing [222]. In addition, the INNO-LiPA HBV genotyping test is well suited to detect mixed genotype infections [222]; however, single nucleotide polymorphisms or deletions may produce indeterminate results [223].

Current guidelines indicate initiation of treatment of HBV infection when viral load >2,000 IU/mL and treatment monitoring by viral load controls after 6 weeks, 12 weeks, and then in intervals of 3–6 months. Sustained virologic response is assumed when viral load falls below 2,000 IU/mL, ideally below 60 IU/mL [197]. On the other hand, tenfold increase of viral load indicates treatment failure, which among other reasons may result from emergence of drug-resistant viruses.

Next to IFNα, a growing number of nucleoside inhibitors were used for HBV treatment, including lamivudine, adefovir, entecavir, tenofovir, telbivudine, emtricitabine, and clevudine. All these drugs target the viral polymerase/reverse transcriptase; hence, resistance is associated with specific mutations in the viral pol-gene, which can be analyzed by genotypic and phenotypic assays [229, 230].

Commercial genotypic tests depend on sequence analysis of PCR products (TRUEGENE, Siemens, Affygene, Sangtec) and reverse hybridization (INNO-LiPA DR2.0, Innogenetics). Concordance of 89–95% between INNO-LiPA and sequencing has been reported [231, 232]. High concordance of results was also reported in a study comparing INNO-LiPA and TRUEGENE [233]. False-negative results of the line assay may result from polymorphisms affecting hybridization [231]. In addition, testing with line assays allows identification of known mutations only. As described for HIV, the expanding number of drugs to treat chronic hepatitis B will result in more complex pattern of mutations (cross-resistance mutations and compensatory mutations), which will complicate interpretation. Some sequence analysis tools described for HIV are also available for characterization and quantification of HBV resistance (e.g., geno-2-pheno HBV, and HIV-GRADE, HBV tool) and will become increasingly useful considering the growing number of antiviral agents.

DNA microarrays have also been used to analyze drug-resistant HBV. Tran et al. reported 92.8% concordance with sequencing [234]. Sensitivity of chips might be reduced by unknown polymorphisms, which affect hybridization. In addition, regular updates of probes will be required to cover newly identified sequence variations of clinical relevance. Nevertheless, DNA chip technology bears great potential for future applications, as it provides the capacity to utilize large numbers of probes in high density, necessary to analyze all relevant mutations and polymorphisms in parallel. Recently, such an HBV chip has been designed, which allows identification of HBV genotype and testing for polymorphisms at about 150 sites, associated with drug-resistance (lamivudine, adefovir, entecavir), immune, vaccine and diagnostic escape (HBs antigen variation), as well as viral activity and disease progression (HBe antigen downregulating mutations) [234].

Take-Home Pearls

› NAATs have replaced culture as gold standard for Chlamydia trachomatis (CT) testing, because they are the most sensitive tests to detect genitourinary CT infections with specificity comparable to culture.

› For gonorrhoea NAATs are also more sensitive and faster than culture, but bacterial culture is still preferred over NAAT due to higher specificity and feasibility of subsequent susceptibility testing.

› Laboratory diagnosis of syphilis is primarily based on serology. Direct detection of treponema pallidum by NAAT is useful in early seronegative phase of infection and may be applied as an adjunctive test in neurosyphilis and congenital infection.

› Customary tests to detect and differentiate HPV are based on identification of viral nucleic acids by target or signal amplification. As high-risk HPV detection has low predictive value for cervical cancer development, additional molecular tests to analyze viral load, oncogene expression, integration and cell cycle markers can be used to define patients at risk for malignant progression.

› Primary diagnosis of HBV and HIV infection is based on serologic tests mainly. Management of patients with confirmed HBV and HIV infection, however, involves various molecular tests for virus quantification, subtype identification, as well as for identification of mutations/polymorphisms associated with pathogenicity, disease progression, and resistance against antiviral drugs.

References

1. Bradshaw, C.S., Denham, I.M., Fairley, C.K.: Characteristics of adenovirus associated urethritis. Sex. Transm. Infect. **78**, 445–447 (2002)
2. Crawford, D.H., Swerdlow, A.J., Higgins, C., et al.: Sexual history and Epstein-Barr virus infection. J. Infect. Dis. **186**, 731–736 (2002)
3. World Health Organization: Global prevalence and incidence of selected curable sexually transmitted infections: overview and estimates. WHO, Geneva (2001)
4. Centers for Disease Control and Prevention: Increases in gonorrhea – eight western states 2000-2005. MMWR **56**, 222–225 (2007)
5. Fenton, K.A., Lowndes, C.M., for the ESSTI-Network: Recent trends in the epidemiology of sexually transmitted infections in the European Union. Sex. Transm. Infect. **80**, 255–263 (2004)
6. McDonald, N., Dougan, S., McGarrigle, C.A., et al.: Recent trends in diagnosis of HIV and other sexually transmitted infections in England and Wales among men who have sex with men. Sex. Transm. Infect. **80**, 492–497 (2004)
7. Von Wassermann, A., Neisser, A., Bruck, C.: Eine serodiagnostische Reaktion bei Syphilis. Dtsch Med. Wochenschr. **32**, 745–746 (1906)
8. Black, C.M.: Current methods of laboratory diagnosis of Chlamydia trachomatis infections. Clin. Microbiol. Rev. **10**, 160–184 (1997)
9. Mullis, K.B., Faloona, F.: Specific synthesis of DNA in vitro via a polymerase catalyzed chain reaction. Meth. Enzymol. **155**, 335–350 (1987)
10. Kwok, S.: Procedures to minimize PCR product carry-over. In: Innis, M.A., et al. (eds.) PCR Protocols: A Guide to Methods and Applications, pp. 142–145. Academic, San Diego (1990)
11. Burkhardt, H.J.: Standardization and quality control of PCR analyses. Clin. Chem. Med. Lab **38**, 87–91 (2000)
12. Johnson, R.E., Newhall, W.J., Papp, J.R., et al.: Screening tests to detect *Chlamydia trachomatis* and *Neisseria gonorrhoeae* infections. MMWR **51**(RR-15), 1–38 (2002)
13. Howell, M.R., Quinn, T.C., Brathwaite, W., et al.: Screening women for Chlamydia trachomatis in family planning clinics. Sex. Transm. Dis. **25**, 108–117 (1998)
14. Schachter, J.: The more you look the more you find. How much is there? Sex. Transm. Dis. **25**, 229–231 (1998)

15. Watson, E.J., Templeton, A., Russell, I., et al.: The accuracy and efficacy of screening tests for *Chlamydia trachomatis*: a systematic review. J. Med. Microbiol. **51**, 1021–1031 (2002)
16. Jespersen, D.J., Flatten, K.S., Jones, M.F., et al.: Prospective comparison of cell cultures and nucleic acid amplification tests for laboratory diagnosis of *Chlamydia trachomatis* infections. J. Clin. Microbiol. **43**, 5324–5326 (2005)
17. Gaydos, C.A., Quinn, T.C.: Urine nucleic acid amplification tests for the diagnosis of sexually transmitted infections in clinical practice. Curr. Opin. Infect. Dis. **18**, 55–66 (2005)
18. Tanaka, M., Nakayama, H., Sagiyama, K., et al.: Evaluation of a new amplified enzyme immunoassay (EIA) for the detection of Chlamydia trachomatis in male urine, female endocervical swab, and patient obtained vaginal swab specimens. J. Clin. Pathol. **53**, 350–354 (2000)
19. Waites, K.B., Smith, K.R., Crum, M.A., et al.: Detection of *Chlamydia trachomatis* endocervical infections by ligase chain reaction versus ACCESS Chlamydia antigen assay. J. Clin. Microbiol. **37**, 3072–3073 (1999)
20. Skidmore, S., Horner, P., Herring, A., et al.: Vulvovaginal swab or first-catch urine specimen to detect *Chlamydia trachomatis* in women in a community setting? J. Clin. Microbiol. **44**, 4389–4394 (2006)
21. Schachter, J., Chow, J.M., Howard, H., et al.: Detection of *Chlamydia trachomatis* by nucleic acid amplification testing. Our evaluation suggests that CDC-recommended approaches for confirmatory testing are ill-advised. J. Clin. Microbiol. **44**, 2512–2517 (2006)
22. Marshall, R., Chernesky, M., Jang, D., et al.: Characteristics of the m2000 automated sample preparation and multiplex real-time PCR system for detection of *Chlamydia trachomatis* and *Neisseria gonorrhoeae*. J. Clin. Microbiol. **45**, 747–651 (2007)
23. Chernesky, M.A., Jang, D.A.: APTIMA transcription-mediated amplification assays for *Chlamydia trachomatis* and *Neisseria gonorrhoeae*. Expert Rev. Mol. Diagn. **6**, 519–525 (2006)
24. Gaydos, C.A., Theodore, M., Dalesio, N., et al.: Comparison of three nucleic acid amplification tests for detection of *Chlamydia trachomatis* in urine specimens. J. Clin. Microbiol. **42**, 3041–3045 (2004)
25. Lowe, P., O'Loughlin, P., Evans, K., et al.: Comparison of the Gen-Probe APTIMA Combo 2 assay to the AMPLICOR CT/NG assay for detection of *Chlamydia trachomatis* and *Neisseria gonorrhoeae* in urine samples from Australian men and women. J. Clin. Microbiol. **44**, 2619–2621 (2006)
26. An, Q., Radcliffe, G., Vassallo, R., et al.: Infection with a plasmid-free variant Chlamydia related to *Chlamydia trachomatis* identified by using multiple assays for nucleic acid detection. J. Clin. Microbiol. **30**, 2814–2821 (1992)
27. Magbanua, J.P., Goh, B.T., Michel, C.E., et al.: *Chlamydia trachomatis* variant not detected by plasmid-based nucleic acid amplification tests: molecular characterization and failure of single dose azithromycin. Sex. Transm. Infect. **83**, 339–343 (2007)
28. Ripa, T., Nilsson, P.A.: A *Chlamydia trachomatis* strain with a 377-bp deletion in the cryptic plasmid causing false negative nucleic acid amplification tests. Sex. Transm. Dis. **34**, 255–256 (2007)
29. Savage, E.J., Ison, C.A., van de Laar, M.J.W.: Results of a Europe-wide investigation to assess the presence of a new variant of *Chlamydia trachomatis*. Eurosurveillance **12**, E3–E4 (2007)
30. Van der Pol, B., Ferrero, D., Buck-Barrington, L., et al.: Multicenter evaluation of the BDProbeTec ET system for the detection of *Chlamydia trachomatis* and *Neisseria gonorrhoeae* in urine specimens, female endocervical swabs, and male urethral swabs. J. Clin. Microbiol. **39**, 1008–1016 (2001)
31. Schachter, J., McCormack, W.M., Chermensky, M.A., et al.: Vaginal swabs are appropriate specimens for diagnosis of genital tract infections with *Chlamydia trachomatis*. J. Clin. Microbiol. **41**, 3784–3789 (2003)
32. Mahony, J.B., Chong, S., Jang, D., et al.: Urine specimens from pregnant and non pregnant women inhibitory to amplification of *Chlamydia trachomatis* nucleic acid by PCR, ligase chain reaction, and transcription-mediated amplification: identification of urinary substances associated with inhibition and removal of inhibitory activity. J. Clin. Microbiol. **36**, 3122–3126 (1998)
33. Low, N., McCarthy, A., Macleod, J., et al.: Epidemiological, social, diagnostic and economic evaluation of population screening for genital chlamydial infection. Health Technol. Assess. **11**(8), 1–84 (2007)
34. Chernesky, M.A., Jang, D.A., Luinstra, K., et al.: High analytical sensitivity and low rates of inhibition may contribute to detection of Chlamydia trachomatis in significantly more women by the APTIMA Combo 2 assay. J. Clin. Microbiol. **44**, 400–405 (2006)
35. Mabey, D.C., Solomon, A.W., Foster, F.: Trachoma. Lancet **362**, 223–229 (2003)
36. Stamm, W.E.: Chlamydia trachomatis infections of the adult. In: Holmes, K.K., Mardh, P.A., Sparling, F.P., et al. (eds.) Sexually Transmitted Diseases, 3rd edn, pp. 407–422. McGraw-Hill, New York (1999)
37. Mabey, D., Peeling, R.W.: Lymphogranuloma venereum. Sex. Transm. Infect. **78**, 90–92 (2002)
38. Dean, D., Stephens, R.S.: Identification od individual genotypes of *Chlamydia trachomatis* from experimentally mixed serovars and mixed infections among trachoma patients. J. Clin. Microbiol. **32**, 1506–1510 (1994)
39. Meyer, T., Arndt, R., van Krosigk, A., et al.: Repeated detection of lymphogranuloma venereum caused by *Chlamydia trachomatis* L2 in homosexual men in Hamburg. Sex. Transm. Infect. **81**, 91–92 (2005)
40. Morre, S.A., Spaargaren, J., Fennema, J.S.A.: Real-time polymerase chain reaction to diagnose Lymphogranuloma venereum. Emerg. Infect. Dis. **11**, 1311–1312 (2005)
41. Spaargaren, J., Fennema, H.A.S., Morre, S.A., et al.: New lymphogranuloma venereum *Chlamydia trachomatis* variant, Amsterdam. Emerg. Infect. Dis. **11**, 1090–1092 (2005)
42. Stary, G., Meyer, T., Bangert, C., et al.: New *Chlamydia trachomatis* L2 strains identified in a recent outbreak of lymphogranuloma venereum in Vienna, Austria. Sex. Transm. Dis. **35**, 377–382 (2008)
43. Bignell, C., Ison, C.A., Jungmann, E.: Gonorrhoea. Sex. Transm. Infect. **82**(suppl IV), iv6–iv9 (2006)
44. Koumans, E.H., Johnson, R.E., Knapp, J.S., et al.: Laboratory testing for *Neisseria gonorrhoeae* by recently

introduced nonculture tests: a performance review with clinical and public health considerations. Clin. Infect. Dis. **27**, 1171–1180 (1998)
45. Lauer, B.A., Masters, H.B.: Toxic effects of calcium alginate swabs on *Neisseria gonorrhoeae*. J. Clin. Microbiol. **26**, 54–56 (1988)
46. Young, H., Moyes, A.: An evaluation of pre-poured selective media for the isolation of *Neisseria gonorrhoeae*. J. Med. Microbiol. **44**, 253–260 (1996)
47. Schachter, J., Hook, E.W.I.I.I., McCormack, W.M., et al.: Ability of the Digene hybrid capture II test to identify *Chlamydia trachomatis* and *Neisseria gonorrhoeae* in cervical specimens. J. Clin. Microbiol. **37**, 3668–3671 (1999)
48. Stary, A., Kopp, W., Zahel, B., et al.: Comparison of DNA-probe test and culture for the detection of *Neisseria gonorrhoeae* in genital samples. Sex. Transm. Dis. **20**, 243–247 (1993)
49. Whiley, D.M., Tapsall, J.W., Sloots, T.P.: Nucleic acid amplification testing for *Neisseria gonorrhoeae*: an ongoing challenge. J. Mol. Diagn. **8**, 3–15 (2006)
50. Hardwick, C., White, D., Osman, H.: An audit of the results of the Roche Amplicor gonorrhoea test on female genital samples: a cheaper and more sensitive method than culture in an urban English population. Int. J. STD AIDS **18**, 347–348 (2007)
51. Frosch, M., Meyer, T.F.: Transformation-mediated exchange of virulence determinants by co-cultivation of pathogenic Neisseriae. FEMS Microbiol. Lett. **79**, 345–349 (1992)
52. Bruisten, S.M., Noordhoek, G.T., van den Brule, A.J., et al.: Multi-center validation of the cppB gene as a PCR target for detection of *Neisseria gonorrhoeae*. J. Clin. Microbiol. **42**, 4332–4334 (2004)
53. Palmer, H.M., Mallinson, H., Wood, R.L., et al.: Evaluation of the specificities of five DNA amplification methods for the detection of *Neisseria gonorrhoeae*. J. Clin. Microbiol. **41**, 835–837 (2003)
54. Hoofar, J., Cook, N., Malorny, B., et al.: Making internal amplification control mandatory for diagnostic PCR. J. Clin. Microbiol. **41**, 5835 (2003)
55. Martin, D.H., Cammarata, C., van der Pol, B., et al.: Multicenter evaluation of AMPLICOR and automated COBAS AMOLICOR CT/NG tests for *N. gonorrhoeae*. J. Clin. Microbiol. **38**, 3544–3549 (2000)
56. Gaydos, C.A., Quinn, T.C., Wills, D., et al.: Performance of the APTIMA Combo 2 assay for the multiplex detection of *Chlamydia trachomatis* and *Neisseria gonorrhoeae* in female urine and endocervical swab specimens. J. Clin. Microbiol. **41**, 304–309 (2003)
57. Hook, E.W.I.I.I., Smith, K., Mullen, C., et al.: Diagnosis of genitourinary *Chlamydia trachomatis* infections by using the ligase chain reaction on patient-obtained vaginal swabs. J. Clin. Microbiol. **35**, 2133–2135 (1997)
58. Madico, G., Romplao, A.M., Gaydos, C.A., et al.: Evaluation of use of a single intravaginal swab to detect multiple sexually transmitted infections in active-duty military women. Clin. Infect. Dis. **33**, 1455–1461 (2001)
59. Stary, A., Ching, S.F., Teodorowicz, L., et al.: Comparison of ligase chain reaction and culture for detection of *Neisseria gonorrhoeae* in genital and extragenital specimens. J. Clin. Microbiol. **35**, 239–242 (1997)
60. Whitcomb, J.M., Huang, W., Fransen, S.: Development and characterization of a novel single-cycle recombinant-virus assay to determine human immunodeficiency virus type 1 coreceptor tropism. Antimicrob. Agents Chemother. **51**, 566–575 (2007)
61. Young, H., Manavi, K., McMillan, A.: Evaluation of ligase chain reaction for the non-cultural detection of rectal and pharyngeal gonorrhea in men who have sex with men. Sex. Transm. Infect. **79**, 484–486 (2003)
62. Farrell, D.J.: Evaluation of AMPLICOR *Neisseria gonorrhoeae* PCR using cppB nested PCR and 16S rRNA PCR. J. Clin. Microbiol. **37**, 386–390 (1999)
63. Knapp, J., Rice, R.J.: Neisseria and Bramhamella. In: Murray, P.R., Baron, E.J., Pfaller, M.A., Tenover, F.C., Yolken, R.H. (eds.) Manual of Clinical Microbiology, pp. 324–340. ASM Press, Washington (1995)
64. Leslie, D.E., Azzalo, F., Ryan, N., et al.: An assessment of the Roche Amplicor *Chlamydia trachomatis/Neisseria gonorrhoeae* multiplex PCR assay in routine diagnostic use of a variety of specimen types. Commun. Dis. Intell. **27**, 373–379 (2003)
65. Diemert, D.J., Libman, M.D., Lebel, P.: Confirmation by 16S rRNA PCR of the COBAS AMPLICOR CT/NG test for diagnosis of *Neisseria gonorrhoeae* infection in a low-prevalence population. J. Clin. Microbiol. **40**, 4056–4059 (2002)
66. Gaydos, C.A., Crotchfield, K.A., Shah, N., et al.: Evaluation of dry and wet transported intravaginal swabs in detection of *Chlamydia trachomatis* and *Neisseria gonorrhoeae* infections in female soldiers by PCR. J. Clin. Microbiol. **40**, 758–761 (2002)
67. Bachmann, L.H., Desmond, R.A., Stephens, J., et al.: Duration of persistence of gonococcal DNA detected by ligase chain reaction in men and women following recommended therapy for uncomplicated gonorrhea. J. Clin. Microbiol. **40**, 3596–3601 (2002)
68. Centers for Disease Control and Prevention: Update to CDC's sexually transmitted diseases treatment guidelines, 2006: fluorochinolones no longer recommended for treatment of gonococcal infections. MMWR **56**, 332–336 (2007)
69. Fenton, K.A., Ison, C., Johnson, A.P., et al.: GRASP collaboration: Ciprofloxacin resistance in *Neisseria gonorrhoeae* in England and Wales in 2002. Lancet **361**, 1867–1869 (2003)
70. World Health Organisation: Increases in fluorochinolone-resistant *Neisseria gonorrhoeae* among men who have sex with men – United States 2003, and revised recommendations for gonorrhea treatment. MMWR **53**, 335–338 (2004)
71. Belland, R.J., Morrison, S.G., Ison, C., et al.: *Neisseria gonorrhoeae* acquires mutations in analogous regions of gyrA and parC in fluorochinolone-resistant isolates. Mol Microbiol **14**, 371–380 (1994)
72. Shigemura, K., Shirakawa, T., Okada, H., et al.: Rapid detection of gyrA and parC mutations in fluorochinolone-resistant *Neisseria gonorrhoeae* by denaturing high-performance liquid chromatography. J. Microbiol. Meth. **59**, 425–421 (2004)
73. Giles, J.A., Falconio, J., Yuenger, J.D., et al.: Quinolone-resistance determining region mutations and por type of *Neisseria gonorrhoeae* isolates: resistance surveillance and

typing by molecular methodologies. J. Infect. Dis. **189**, 2085–2093 (2004)
74. Deguchi, T., Yasuda, M., Nakano, M., et al.: Quinolone-resistant *Neisseria gonorrhoeae*: correlation of alterations in the gyrA subunit of DNA gyrase and the ParC subunit of topoisomerase IV with antimicrobial susceptibility profiles. Antimicrob. Agents Chemother. **40**, 1020–1023 (1996)
75. Zhou, W., Du, W., Cao, H., et al.: Detection of gyra and parC mutations associated with ciprofloxacin resistance in *Neisseria gonorrhoeae* by use of oligonucleotide biochip technology. J. Clin. Microbiol. **42**, 5819–5824 (2004)
76. Lindback, E., Gharizadeh, B., Ataker, F., et al.: DNA gyrase gene in *Neisseria gonorrhoeae* as indicator for resistance to ciprofloxacin and species verification. Int. J. STD AIDS **16**, 142–147 (2005)
77. Yang, Y., Liao, M., Gu, W.M., et al.: Antimicrobial susceptibility and molecular determinants of quinolone resistance in *Neisseria gonorrhoeae* isolates from Shanghai. J. Antimicrob. Chemother. **58**, 868–872 (2006)
78. Sultan, Z., Nahar, S., Wretlind, B., et al.: Comparison of mismatch amplification mutation assay with DNA sequencing for characterization of fluorochinolone resistance in *Neisseria gonorrhoeae*. J. Clin. Microbiol. **42**, 591–594 (2004)
79. Booth, S.A., Drebot, M.A., Martin, I.E., et al.: Design of oligonucleotide arrays to detect point mutations: molecular typing of antibiotic resistant strains of *Neisseria gonorrhoeae* and hantavirus infected deer mice. Mol. Cell. Probes **17**, 77–84 (2003)
80. Giles, J., Hardick, J., Yuenger, J., et al.: Use of Applied Biosystems 7900HT sequence detection system and TaqMan assay for detection of quinolone-resistant *Neisseria gonorrhoeae*. J. Clin. Microbiol. **42**, 3281–3283 (2004)
81. Shigemura, K., Shirakawa, T., Tanaka, K., et al.: Rapid detection of the fluorochinolone resistance-associated ParC mutation in *Neisseria gonorrhoeae* using TaqMan probes. Int. J. Urol. **13**, 277–281 (2006)
82. Siedner, M.J., Pandori, M., Castro, L., et al.: Real-time PCR assay for detection of quinolone-resistant *Neisseria gonorrhoeae* in urine samples. J. Clin. Microbiol. **45**, 1250–1254 (2007)
83. Takahata, S., Senju, N., Osaki, Y., et al.: Amino acid substitutions in mosaic penicillin-binding protein 2 associated with reduced susceptibility to cefixime in clinical isolates of *Neisseria gonorrhoeae*. Antimicrob. Agents Chemother. **50**, 3638–3645 (2006)
84. Larsen, S.A., Steiner, B.M., Rudolph, A.H.: Laboratory diagnosis and interpretation of tests for syphilis. Clin. Microbiol. Rev. **8**, 1–21 (1995)
85. Johnson, P.D., Graves, S.R., Stewart, L., et al.: Specific syphilis serological tests may become negative in HIV infection. AIDS **5**, 419–423 (1991)
86. Cummings, M.C., Lukehart, S.A., Narra, C., et al.: Comparison of methods for the detection of *Treponema pallidum* in lesions of early syphilis. Sex Transm. Dis. **23**, 366–369 (1996)
87. Engelkens, H.J., ten Kate, F.J., Judanarso, J., et al.: The localization of treponemes and characterization of the inflammatory infiltrate in skin biopsies from patients with primary or secondary syphilis, or early infectious yaws. Genitourin. Med. **69**, 102–197 (1993)
88. Hoang, M.P., High, W.A., Molberg, K.H.: Secondary syphilis: a histologic and immunohistochemical evaluation. J. Cutan. Pathol. **31**, 595–599 (2004)
89. Berhof, W., Springer, E., Bräuninger, W., et al.: PCR testing for treponema pallidum in paraffin-embedded skin biopsy specimens: test design and impact on the diagnosis of syphilis. J. Clin. Pathol. **61**, 390–395 (2008)
90. Kouznetsov, A.V., Weisenseel, P., Trommler, P., et al.: Detection of the 47-kilodalton membrane immunogen gene of *Treponema pallidum* in various tissue sources of patients with syphilis. Diagn. Microbiol. Infect. Dis. **51**, 143–145 (2005)
91. Liu, H., Rodes, B., Chen, C.Y., et al.: New tests for syphilis: rational design of a PCR method for detection of *Treponema pallidum* in clinical specimens using unique regions of the DNA polymerase I gene. J. Clin. Microbiol. **39**, 1941–1946 (2001)
92. Orle, K.A., Gates, C.A., Martin, D.H., et al.: Simultaneous PCR detection of *Haemophilus ducreyi*, *Treponema pallidum* and herpes simplex virus types 1 and 2 from genital ulcers. J. Clin. Microbiol. **34**, 49–54 (1996)
93. Palmer, H.M., Higgins, S.P., Herring, A.J., et al.: Use of PCR in the diagnosis of early syphilis in the United Kingdom. Sex. Transm. Infect. **79**, 479–483 (2003)
94. Wenhai, L., Jianzhong, Z., Cao, Y.: Detection of *Treponema pallidum* in skin lesions of secondary syphilis and characterization of the inflammatory infiltrate. Dermatology **208**, 94–97 (2004)
95. Leslie, D.E., Azzato, F., Karapangiotidis, T., et al.: Development of a real-time PCR assay to detect *Treponema pallidum* in clinical specimens and assessment of the assay's performance by comparison with serological testing. J. Clin. Microbiol. **45**, 93–96 (2007)
96. Koek, A.G., Bruisten, S.M., Dierdorp, M., et al.: Specific and sensitive diagnosis of syphilis using a real-time PCR for *Treponema pallidum*. Clin. Microbiol. Infect. **12**, 1233–1236 (2006)
97. Buffet, M., Grange, P.A., Gerhardt, P., et al.: Diagnosing *Treponema pallidum* in secondary syphilis by PCR and immunohistochemistry. J. Invest. Dermatol. **127**, 2345–2350 (2007)
98. Castro, R., Prieto, E., Aguas, M.J., et al.: Detection of *Treponema pallidum* sp pallidum DNA in latent syphilis. Int. J. STD AIDS **18**, 842–845 (2007)
99. Pietravalle, M., Pimpinelli, F., Maini, A., et al.: Diagnostic relevance of polymerase chain reaction technology for *T. pallidum* in subjects with syphilis in different phase of infection. New Microbiol. **22**, 99–104 (1999)
100. Woznicova, V., Smajs, D., Wechsler, D., et al.: Detection of *Treponema pallidum* subsp pallidum from skin lesions, serum, and cerebrospinal fluid in an infant with congenital syphilis after clindamycin treatment of the mother during pregnancy. J. Clin. Microbiol. **45**, 659–661 (2007)
101. Wu, C.C., Tsai, C.N., Wong, W.R., et al.: Early congenital syphilis and erythema multiforme-like bullous targetoid lesions in a 1-day-old newborn: detection of *Treponema pallidum* genomic DNA from the targetoid plaque using nested polymerase chain reaction. J. Am. Acad. Dermatol. **55**, S11–S15 (2006)
102. Chen, Y.C., Chi, K.H., George, R.W., et al.: Diagnosis of gastric syphilis by direct immunofluorescence staining and

real-time PCR testing. J. Clin. Microbiol. **44**, 3452–3456 (2006)
103. Kandelaki, G., Kapila, R., Fernandes, H.: Destructive osteomyelitis associated with early secondary syphilis in an HIV-positive patient diagnosed by *Treponema pallidum* DNA polymerase chain reaction. AIDS Patient Care STDs **21**, 229–233 (2007)
104. Kouznetsov, A.V., Prinz, J.C.: Molecular diagnosis of syphilis: the Schaudinn-Hoffmann lymph-node biopsy. Lancet **360**, 388–389 (2002)
105. Rajan, M.S., Pantelidis, P., Tong, C.Y., et al.: Diagnosis of *Treponema pallidum* in vitreous samples using real-time polymerase chain reaction. Br. J. Ophthalmol. **90**, 647–648 (2006)
106. Katz, K.A., Klausner, J.D.: Azithromycin resistance in *Treponema pallidum*. Curr. Opin. Infect. Dis. **21**, 83–91 (2008)
107. Lukehart, S.A., Godornes, C., Molini, B.J., et al.: Macrolide resistance in *Treponema pallidum* in the United States and Ireland. N. Engl. J. Med. **351**, 154–158 (2004)
108. Stamm, L.V., Bergen, H.L.: A point mutation associated with bacterial macrolide resistance is present in both 23S rRNA genes of an erythromycin-resistant *Treponema pallidum* clinical isolate. Antimicrob. Agents Chemother. **44**, 806–807 (2000)
109. Pandori, M.W., Gordones, C., Castro, L., et al.: Detection of azithromycin resistance in *Treponema pallidum* by real-time PCR. Antimicrob. Agents Chemother. **51**, 3425–3430 (2007)
110. DeVilliers, E.M., Fauquet, C., Broker, T.R., et al.: Classification of papillomaviruses. Virology **324**, 17–27 (2004)
111. Munoz, N., Bosch, F.X., de Sanjose, S., et al.: Epidemiologic classification of human papillomavirus types associated with cervical cancer. N. Engl. J. Med. **348**, 518–527 (2003)
112. Walboomers, J.M., Jacobs, J.V., Manos, M.M., et al.: Human papillomavirus is a necessary cause of invasive cervical cancer worldwide. J. Pathol. **189**, 12–19 (1999)
113. Zur Hausen, H.: Papillomavirus causing cancer: evasion from host cell control in early events in carcinogenesis. J. Natl. Cancer Inst. **92**, 690–698 (2000)
114. DeRoda Husman, A.M., Walboomers, J.M., Hopman, E., et al.: HPV prevalence in cytomorphologically normal cervical scrapes of pregnant women as determined by PCR: the age-related pattern. J. Med. Virol. **46**, 97–102 (1995)
115. Moscicki, A.B., Shiboski, S., Broering, J., et al.: The natural history of human papillomavirus infection as measured by repeated DNA testing in adolescent and young women. J. Pediatr. **132**, 277–284 (1998)
116. Rodriguez, A.C., Schiffman, M., Herrero, R. et al.: Rapid clearance of human papillomavirus and implications for clinical focus on persistent infections. J. Natl. Cancer Inst. **100**, 513–517 (2008)
117. Woodman, C.B.J., Collins, S., Winter, H., et al.: Natural history of cervical human papillomavirus infection in young women: a longitudinal cohort study. Lancet **357**, 1831–1836 (2001)
118. Liaw, K.L., Glass, A.G., Manos, M.M., et al.: Detection of human papillomavirus in cytologically normal women and subsequent cervical squamous intraepithelial lesions. J. Natl. Cancer Inst. **91**, 954–960 (1999)
119. Khan, M.J., Castle, P.E., Lörincz, A.T., et al.: The elevated 10-year risk of cervical precancer and cancer in women with human papillomavirus (HPV) type 16 or 18 and the possible utility of type-specific HPV testing in clinical practice. J. Natl. Cancer Inst. **97**, 1072–1079 (2005)
120. Snijders, P.J.F., Hogewoning, C.J.A., Hesselink, A.T., et al.: Determination of viral load thresholds in cervical scrapings to rule out CIN3 in HPV 16, 18, 31, and 33-positive women with normal cytology. Int. J. Cancer **119**, 1102–1107 (2006)
121. Solomon, D., Schiffman, M., Tarone, R.: Comparison of three management strategies for patients with atypical squamous cells of undetermined significance: baseline results from a randomized trial. J. Natl. Cancer Inst. **93**, 293–299 (2001)
122. Wright, T.C., Schiffman, M., Solomon, D., et al.: Interim guidance for the use of human papillomavirus DNA testing as an adjunct to cervical cytology for screening. Obstet. Gynecol. **103**, 304–309 (2004)
123. Doorbar, J.: The papillomavirus life cycle. J. Clin. Virol. **32**(suppl 1), S7–S15 (2005)
124. Dillner, J., Meijer, C.J.L.M., van Krogh, G., et al.: Epidemiology of human papillomavirus infection. Scand. J. Urol. Nephrol. **205**(suppl), 194–200 (2000)
125. Moljin, A., Kleter, B., Quint, W., et al.: Molecular diagnosis of human papillomavirus (HPV) infections. J. Clin. Virol. **32**(suppl), S43–S51 (2005)
126. Lörincz, A.T.: Hybrid capture method for detection of human papillomavirus DNA in clinical specimens: a tool for clinical management of equivocal Pap smears and for population screening. J. Obstet. Gynecol. Res. **22**, 629–636 (1996)
127. Poljak, M., Brencic, A., Seme, K., et al.: Comparative evaluation of first and second generation Digene hybrid capture assays for detection of human papillomavirus associated with high or intermediate risk for cervical cancer. J. Clin. Microbiol. **37**, 796–797 (1999)
128. Clavel, C., Masure, M., Bory, J.P., et al.: Hybrid capture II based human papillomavirus detection: a sensitive test to detect in routine high grade cervical lesions: a preliminary study on 1518 women. Br. J. Cancer **80**, 1306–1311 (1999)
129. Schneede, P., Hillemanns, P., Ziller, F., et al.: Evaluation of HPV testing by Hybrid capture II for routine gynaecologic screening. Acta Obstet. Gynecol. Scand. **80**, 750–752 (2001)
130. Vernon, S.D., Unger, E.R., Williams, D.: Comparison of human papillomavirus detection and typing by cycle sequencing, line blotting and hybrid capture. J. Clin. Microbiol. **38**, 651–655 (2000)
131. Castle, P.E., Lörincz, A.T., Scott, D.R., et al.: Comparison between prototype Hybrid Capture 3 and Hybrid Capture 2 papillomavirus DNA assays for detection of high-grade cervical intraepithelial neoplasia and cancer. J. Clin. Microbiol. **41**, 4022–4030 (2003)
132. Van den Brule, A.J., Meijer, C.J.L.M., Bakels, V., et al.: Rapid detection of human papillomavirus in cervical scrapings by combined general primer-mediated and type-specific polymerase chain reaction. J. Clin. Microbiol. **28**, 2739–2743 (1990)
133. Cope, J.U., Hildesheim, A., Schiffman, M., et al.: Comparison of the hybrid capture tube test and PCR for detection of human papillomavirus DNA in cervical specimens. J. Clin. Microbiol. **35**, 2262–2265 (1997)

134. Cusick, J., Clavel, C., Petry, U., et al.: Overview of the European and North American studies on HPV testing in primary cervical cancer screening. Int. J. Cancer **119**, 1095–1101 (2006)
135. Meyer, T., Arndt, R., Stockfleth, E., et al.: Strategy for typing human papillomavirus by RFLP analysis of PCR products and subsequent hybridization with a generic probe. Biotechniques **19**, 632–639 (1995)
136. Van Doorn, L.J., Kleter, B., Quint, W.G.V.: Molecular detection and genotyping of human papillomavirus. Expert Rev. Mol. Diagn. **1**, 394–402 (2001)
137. Jacobs, M.V., Snijders, P.J.F., van den Brule, A.J., et al.: A general primer GP5+/GP6+ mediated PCR-enzyme immunoassay method for rapid detection of 14 high risk and 6 low risk human papillomavirus genotypes in cervical scrapings. J. Clin. Microbiol. **35**, 791–795 (1997)
138. Gravitt, P.E., Peyton, C.L., Apple, R.J., et al.: Genotyping of 27 human papillomavirus types by using L1 consensus PCR products by a single hybridization, reverse line blot detection method. J. Clin. Microbiol. **36**, 3020–3027 (1998)
139. Kleter, B., van Doorn, L.J., Schrauwen, L., et al.: Development and clincal evaluation of a highly sensitive PCR-reverse hybridization line probe assay for detection and identification of anogenital human papillomavirus. J. Clin. Microbiol. **37**, 2508–2517 (1999)
140. Klaasen, C.H., Prinsen, C.F., de Valk, H.A., et al.: DNA microarray format for detection and subtyping of human papillomavirus. J. Clin. Microbiol. **42**, 2152–2160 (2004)
141. Park, T.C., Kim, C.J., Koh, Y.M., et al.: Human papillomavirus genotyping by the DNA chip in the cervical neoplasia DNA. Cell Biol. **23**, 119–125 (2004)
142. Schmitt, M., Bravo, I.G., Snijders, P.J.F., et al.: Bead-based multiplex genotyping of human papillomavirus. J. Clin. Microbiol. **44**, 504–512 (2006)
143. Carcopino, X., Henry, M., Benmoura, D., et al.: Determination of HPV type 16 and 18 viral load in cervical smears of women referred to colposcopy. J. Med. Virol. **78**, 1131–1140 (2006)
144. Hesselink, A.T., van den Brule, A.J., Groothuismink, Z.M., et al.: Comparison of three different PCR methods for quantifying human papillomavirus type 16 DNA in cervical crape specimens. J. Clin. Microbiol. **43**, 4868–4871 (2005)
145. JosefsonAM, M.P.K.E., Ylitalo, N., et al.: Viral load of human papillomavirus 16 as a determinant for development of cervical carcinoma in situ: a nested case-control study. Lancet **355**, 2189–2193 (2000)
146. Wang-Johänning, F., Lu, D.W., Wang, Y., et al.: Quantitation of human papillomavirus 16 E6 and E7 DNA and RNA in residual material from ThinPrep Papanicolao tests using real-time polymerase chain reaction analysis. Cancer **94**, 2199–2210 (2002)
147. Molden, T., Kraus, I., Karlsen, F., et al.: Comparison of human papillomavirus messenger RNA and DNA detection: a cross-sectional study of 4136 women >30 years of age with a 2-year follow-up of high-grade squamous intraepithelial lesions. Cancer Epidemiol. Biomarkers Prev. **14**, 367–372 (2005)
148. Molden, T., Nygard, J.F., Kraus, I., et al.: Predicting CIN2+ when detecting HPV mRNA and DNA by PreTect HPV-Proofer and consensus PCR: a 2-year follow-up of women with ASCUS or LSIL Pap smear. Int. J. Cancer **114**, 973–976 (2005)
149. Castle, P.E., Dockter, J., Giachetti, C., et al.: A cross-sectional study of a prototype carcinogenic human papillomavirus E6/E7 messenger RNA assay for detection of cervical precancer and cancer. Clin. Cancer Res. **13**, 2599–2605 (2007)
150. Klaes, R., Woerner, S.M., Ridder, R., et al.: Detection of high-risk cervical intraepithelial neoplasia and cervical cancer by amplification of transcripts derived from integrated papillomavirus oncogenes. Cancer Res. **59**, 6132–6136 (1999)
151. Hudelist, G., Manavi, M., Pischinger, K.I.D., et al.: Physical state and expression of HPV DNA in benign and dysplastic cervical tissue: different levels of viral integration are correlated with lesion grade. Gynecol. Oncol. **92**, 873–880 (2004)
152. Chen, Y., Miller, C., Mosher, R., et al.: Identification of cervical cancer markers by cDNA and tissue microarrays. Cancer Res. **63**, 1927–1935 (2003)
153. Santin, A.D., Zhan, F., Bignotti, E., et al.: Gene expression profiles of primary HPV16- and HPV18-infected early stage cervical cancers and normal cervical epithelium: identification of novel candidate molecular markers for cervical cancer diagnosis and therapy. Virology **331**, 269–291 (2005)
154. Malinowski, D.P.: Molecular diagnostic assays for cervical neoplasia: emerging markers for the detection of high-grade cervical disease. Biotechniques **38**(Suppl), S17–S23 (2005)
155. Klaes, R., Friedrich, T., Spitkovsky, D., et al.: Overexpression of p16(INK4a) as a specific marker for dysplastic and neoplastic epithelial cells of the cervix uteri. Int. J. Cancer **92**, 276–284 (2001)
156. Dehn, D., Torkko, K.C., Shroyer, K.R.: Human papillomavirus testing and molecular markers of cervical dysplasia and carcinoma. Cancer **111**, 1–14 (2007)
157. Zhang, H.S., Postigo, A.A., Dean, D.C.: Active transcriptional repression by the Rb-E2F complex mediates G1 arrest triggered by p16INK4a, TGFbeta, and contact inhibition. Cell **97**, 53–61 (1999)
158. Murphy, N., Ring, M., Killalea, A.G., et al.: p16(INK4a) as a marker for cervical dyskaryosis: CIN and cGIN in cervical biopsies and ThinPrep smears. J. Clin. Pathol. **56**, 56–63 (2003)
159. Freeman, A., Morris, L.S., Mills, D., et al.: Minichromosome maintenance proteins as biological markers of dysplasia and malignancy. Clin. Cancer Res. **5**, 2121–2132 (1999)
160. Kastan, M., Bartek, J.: Cell-cycle checkpoints and cancer. Nature **432**, 316–323 (2004)
161. Shroyer, K.R., Homer, P., Heinz, D., et al.: Validation of a novel immunocytochemical assay for topoisomerase II alpha and minichromosome maintenance protein 2 expression in cervical cytology. Cancer Cytopthol. **108**, 324–330 (2006)
162. Rossi, A.: Early diagnosis of HIV infection in infants. Report of a consensus workshop, Siena, Italy January 17-18, 1992. JAIDS **5**, 1168–1178 (1992)
163. Heid, C.A., Stevens, J., Livak, K.J.: Real-time quantitative PCR. Genome Res. **6**, 986–994 (1996)
164. Wittek, M., Stürmer, M., Doerr, H.W., et al.: Molecular assays for monitoring HIV infection and antiretroviral therapy. Expert Rev. Mol. Diagn. **7**, 237–246 (2007)

165. Wuesten, J.J., Carpay, W.M., Oosterlaken, T.A., et al.: Principles of quantitation of viral loads using nucleic acid sequence-based amplification in combination with homogeneous detection using molecular beacons. Nucleic Acids Res. **30**, e26 (2002)
166. Collins, M.L., Irvine, B., Tyner, D., et al.: A branched DNA signal amplification assay for quantification of nucleic acid targets below 100 molecules/mL. Nucleic Acids Res. **25**, 2979–2984 (1997)
167. Tsongalis, G.J.: Branched DNA technology in molecular diagnostics. Am. J. Pathol. **126**, 448–453 (2006)
168. Urdea, M.S.: Branched DNA signal amplification. Biotechnology **12**, 926–928 (1994)
169. Berger, A., Scherzed, L., Stürmer, M., et al.: Comparative evaluation of the COBAS Amplicor HIV-1 Monitor ultrasensitive test, the new COBAS Ampliprep/COBAS Amplicor HIV-1 Monitor and the Versant HIV RNA 3.0 assay for quantification of HIV-1 RNA in plasma samples. J. Clin. Virol. **33**, 43–51 (2005)
170. Braun, P., Ehret, R., Wiesmann, F., et al.: Comparison of four commercial quantitative HIV-1 assays for viral load monitoring in clinical daily routine. Clin. Chem. Lab **45**, 93–99 (2007)
171. Gomes, P., Palma, A.C., Cabanas, J., et al.: Comparison of the COBAS TAQMAN HIV-1 HPS with VERSANT HIV-1 RNA 3.0 assay (bDNA) for plasma RNA quantitation in different HIV-1 subtypes. J. Virol. Meth. **135**, 223–228 (2006)
172. Lam, H.Y., Chen, J.H., Wong, K.H., et al.: Evaluation of NucliSense EasyQ HIV-1 assay for quantification of HIV-1 subtypes prevalent in South-East Asia. J. Clin. Virol. **38**, 39–43 (2007)
173. Swanson, P., Huang, S., Abravaya, K., et al.: Evaluation of performance across the dynamic range of the Abbott RealTime HIV-1 assay as compared to Versant HIV-1 RNA 3.0 and Amplicor HIV-1 Monitor v1.5 using serial dilutions of 39 group M and O viruses. J. Virol. Meth. **141**, 49–57 (2007)
174. Foulongne, V., Montes, B., Didelot-Rousseau, et al.: Comparison of the LCx human immunodeficiency virus (HIV) RNA quantitative, RealTime HIV, and COBAS AmpliPrep-COBAS TaqMan assays for quantitation of HIV type 1 RNA in plasma. J. Clin. Microbiol. **44**, 2963–2966 (2006)
175. Gueudin, M., Plantier, J.C., Lernee, V., et al.: Evaluation of the Roche Cobas TaqMan and Abbott RealTime extraction-quantification system for HIV-1 subtypes. AIDS **44**, 500–505 (2007)
176. Huang, W., Toma, J., Fransen, S.: Coreceptor tropism can be influenced by amino acid substitutions in the gp41 transmembrane subunit of human immunodeficiency virus type 1 envelope protein. J. Virol. (2008). doi:10.1128/JVI02676-07
177. Mracna, M., Becker-Pergola, G., Dileanis, J., et al.: Performance of applied biosystems ViroSeq HIV-1 genotyping system for sequence-based analysis of non-subtype B human immunodeficiency virus type 1 from Uganda. J. Clin. Microbiol. **39**, 4323–4327 (2001)
178. Shafer, R.W., Rhee, S.Y., Pillay, D., et al.: HIV-1 protease and reverse transcriptase mutations for drug resistance surveillance. AIDS **21**, 215–223 (2007)
179. Durant, J., Clevenbergh, P., Halfon, P., et al.: Drug-resistance genotyping in HIV-1 therapy: the VIRADAPT randomised controlled trial. Lancet **353**, 2195–2199 (1999)
180. Wilson, J.W.: Update on antiretroviral drug resistance testing: combining laboratory technology with patient care. AIDS Read. **13**, 25–30 (2003)
181. Stürmer, M., Berger, A., Preiser, W.: HIV-1 genotyping: comparison of two commercially available assays. Expert Rev. Mol. Diagn. **4**, 281–291 (2004)
182. Beerenwinkel, N., Däumer, M., Oette, M., et al.: Geno-2-pheno: estimating phenotypic drug resistance from genotypes. Nucleic Acids Res. **13**, 3850–3855 (2003)
183. Larder, B., Revell, A., Wang, D., et al.: The development of artificial neural networks to predict virological response to combination HIV therapy. Antivir. Ther. **12**, 15–24 (2007)
184. Tural, C., Ruiz, L., Holtzer, C., et al.: Clinical utility of HIV-1 genotyping and expert advice: the Havana trial. AIDS **16**, 209–218 (2002)
185. Petropoulous, C.J., Parkin, N.T., Limoli, K.L., et al.: A novel phenotypic drug susceptibility assay for human immunodeficiency virus type 1. Antimicrob. Agents Chemother. **44**, 920–928 (2000)
186. Skrabal, K., Low, A.J., Dong, W., et al.: Determining human immunodeficiency virus coreceptor use in a clinical setting: degree of correlation between two phenotypic assays and a bioinformatic model. J. Clin. Microbiol. **45**, 279–284 (2007)
187. Hoffman, N.G., Seillier-Moiseiwitsch, F., Ahn, J.H., et al.: Variability in the human immunodeficiency virus type 1 gp120 env protein linked to phenotype-associated changes in the V3 loop. J. Virol. **76**, 3852–3864 (2002)
188. D´Aquila, R.T.: Limits of resistance testing. Antivir. Ther. **5**, 71–76 (2000)
189. Elbeik, T., Hoo, B.S., Campodonico, M.E., et al.: In vivo emergence of drug-resistant mutations at less than 50 HIV-1 RNA copies/mL that are maintained at viral rebound in longitudinal plasma samples from human immunodeficiency virus type-1-infected patients on highly active antiretroviral therapy. J. Hum. Virol. **4**, 317–328 (2001)
190. McClernon, D.R., Ramsey, E., Clair, M.S.: Magnetic silica extraction for low-viremia human immunodeficiency type 1 genotyping. J. Clin. Microbiol. **45**, 572–574 (2007)
191. Metzner, K.J., Rauch, P., Walter, H.: Detection of minor populations of drug-resistant HIV-1 in acute seroconverters. AIDS **4**, 1819–1825 (2005)
192. Stuyver, L., Wyseur, A., Rombout, A., et al.: Line probe assay for rapid detection of drug-selected mutations in the human immunodeficiency virus type 1 reverse transcriptase gene. Antimicrob. Agents Chemother. **41**, 284–291 (1997)
193. Hanna, G.J., Johnson, V.A., Kuritzkes, D.R., et al.: Comparison of sequencing by hybridization and cycle sequencing for genotyping of human immunodeficiency virus type 1 reverse transcriptase. J. Clin. Microbiol. **38**, 2715–272 (2000)
194. Margulies, M., Egholm, M., Altman, W., et al.: Genome sequencing in microfabricated high-density picolitre reactors. Nature **437**, 376–380 (2005)
195. Hoffmann, C., Minkah, N., Leipzig, J., et al.: DNA bar coding and pyrosequencing to identify rare HIV drug resistance mutations. Nucleic Acid Res. **35**, e91 (2007). doi:10.1093/nar/gkm435
196. Wang, C., Mitsuya, Y., Gharizadeh, B., et al.: Characterization of mutation spectra with ultra-deep

pyrosequencing: application to HIV-1 drug resistance. Genome Res. **17**, 1195–1201 (2007)
197. Cornberg, M., Protzer, U., Dollinger, M.M., et al.: Prophylaxis, diagnostics and therapy of hepatitis B virus (HBV) infection: upgrade of the guideline, AWMF register 021/011. Z. Gastroenterol. **45**, 1–50 (2007)
198. Allice, T.F., Cerutti, F., Pittaluga, S., et al.: COBAS AmpliPrep-COBAS TaqMan hepatitis B virus (HBV) test: a novel automated real-time PCR assay for quantification of HBV DNA in plasma. J. Clin. Microbiol. **45**, 828–834 (2007)
199. Chevaliez, S., Bouvier-Alias, M., Laperche, S. et al.: Performance of the Cobas Ampliprep/Cobas TaqMan (CAP/CTM) real-time polymerase chain reaction assay for hepatitis B virus DNA quantification. J. Clin. Microbiol. 46: doi:10.1128/JCM.01248-07 (2008)
200. Lok, A.S., McMahon, B.J.: Chronic hepatitis. B. Hepatology **45**, 507–539 (2007)
201. Pawlotsky, J.M.: Hepatitis B virus (HBV) DNA assays (methods and practicle use) and viral kinetics. J. Hepatol. **39**(suppl 1), S31–S35 (2003)
202. Niesters, H.G., Pas, S.D., de Man, R.A.: Detection of hepatitis B virus genotypes and mutants: current status. J Clin Virol **34**(suppl 1), S4–S8 (2005)
203. Valsamakis, A.: Molecular testing in the diagnosis and management of chronic hepatitis B. Clin. Microbiol. Rev. **20**, 426–439 (2007)
204. Ter Borg, F., Jones, E.A.: Prediction of hepatic inflammatory activity in hepatitis B. Lancet **352**, 1555 (1998)
205. Abe, A., Inoue, K., Tanaka, T., et al.: Quantitation of hepatitis B virus genomic DNA by real-time detection PCR. J. Clin. Microbiol. **37**, 2899–2903 (1999)
206. Chen, R.W., Piiparinen, H., Seppanan, M., et al.: Real-time PCR for detection and quantitation of hepatitis B virus DNA. J. Med. Virol. **68**, 250–256 (2001)
207. Liu, Y., Hussain, M., Wong, S., et al.: A genotype-independent real-time PCR assay for quantification of hepatitis B virus DNA. J. Clin. Microbiol. **45**, 553–558 (2007)
208. Pas, S.D., Fries, E., de Man, R.A., et al.: Development of a quantitative real-time detection assay for hepatitis B virus DNA and comparison with two commercial assays. J. Clin. Microbiol. **38**, 2897–2901 (2000)
209. Hochberger, S., Althof, D., Gallegos de Schrott, R., et al.: Fully automated quantitation of hepatitis B virus (HBV) DNA in human plasma by the COBAS AmpliPrep/COBAS TaqMan system. J. Clin. Virol. **35**, 373–380 (2006)
210. Ronsin, C., Pillet, A., Bali, C., et al.: Evaluation of the COBAS AmpliPrep-Total nucleic acid isolation-COBAS TaqMan hepatitis B virus (HBV) quantitative test and comparison to the VERSANT HBV DNA 3.0 assay. J. Clin. Microbiol. **44**, 1390–1399 (2006)
211. Thibault, V., Pichoud, C., Mullen, C., et al.: Characterization of a new sensitive PCR assay for quantification of viral DNA isolated from patients with hepatitis B virus infection. J. Clin. Microbiol. **45**, 3948–3953 (2007)
212. Yao, J.D., Beld, M.G., Oon, L.L., et al.: Multicenter evaluation of the VERSANT hepatitis B virus DNA 3.0 assay. J. Clin. Microbiol. **42**, 800–806 (2004)
213. Konnick, E.Q., Erali, M., Ashwood, E.R., et al.: Evaluation of the COBAS Amplicor HBV Monitor assay and comparison with the ultrasensitive HBV Hybrid Capture II assay for quantification of hepatitis B virus DNA. J. Clin. Microbiol. **43**, 596–603 (2005)
214. Fung, S.K., Lok, A.S.: Hepatitis B virus genotypes: do they play a role in the outcome of HBV infection? Hepatology **40**, 790–792 (2004)
215. Niesters, H.G., Krajden, M., Cork, L., et al.: Multi-center evaluation of the Digene Hybrid Capture II signal amplification technique for the detection of hepatitis B virus DNA in serum samples and testing of EUROHEP standards. J. Clin. Microbiol. **38**, 2150–2155 (2000)
216. Garbuglia, A.R., Angeletti, C., Lauria, F.N., et al.: Comparison of Versant HBV DNA 3.0 and COBAS AmpliPrep-COBAS TaqMan assays for hepatitis B DNA quantitation: possible clinical implications. J. Virol. Meth. **146**, 274–280 (2007)
217. Chu, C., Hussain, M., Lok, A.S.: Hepatitis B virus genotype B is associated with earlier HBeAg seroconversion compared with hepatitis B virus genotype C. Gastroenterology **122**, 1756–1762 (2002)
218. Kobayashi, M., Arase, Y., Ikeda, K., et al.: Clinical characteristics of patients infected with hepatitis B virus genotypes A, B, and C. J. Gastroenterol. **37**, 35–39 (2002)
219. Janssen, H.L., van Zonneveld, M., Senturk, H., et al.: Pegylated interferon alpha 2b alone or in combination with lamivudine for HBeAg-positive chronic hepatitis B: a randomised trial. Lancet **365**, 123–129 (2005)
220. Kao, J.H., Chan, P.J., Lai, M.Y., et al.: Hepatitis B genotypes correlate with clinical outcomes in patients with chronic hepatitis B. Gastroenterology **118**, 554–559 (2000)
221. Kao, J., Chen, P., Lai, M., et al.: Genotypes and clinical phenotypes of hepatitis B virus in patients with chronic hepatitis B virus infection. J. Clin. Microbiol. **40**, 1207–1209 (2002)
222. Pas, S.D., Tran, N., de Man, R.A., et al.: Comparison of reverse hybridization, microarray and sequence analysis for genotyping hepatitis B virus. J. Clin. Microbiol. **46**, 1268–1273 (2008)
223. Osiowy, C., Giles, E.: Evaluation of the INNO-LiPA HBV genotyping assay for determination of hepatitis B virus genotype. J. Clin. Microbiol. **41**, 5473–5477 (2003)
224. Vernet, G., Tran, N.: The DNA-Chip technology as a new molecular tool for the detection of HBV mutants. J. Clin. Virol. **34**(Suppl.1), S49–S53 (2005)
225. Liu, W.C., Mizokami, M., Buti, M., et al.: Simultaneous quantification and genotyping of hepatitis B virus for genotypes A to G by real-time PCR and two-step melting curve analysis. J. Clin. Microbiol. **44**, 4491–4497 (2006)
226. Naito, H., Hayashi, S., Abe, K.: Rapid and specific genotyping system for hepatitis B virus corresponding to six major genotypes by PCR using type-specific primers. J. Clin. Microbiol. **39**, 362–364 (2001)
227. Yeh, S.H., Tsai, C.Y., Kao, J.H., et al.: Quantification and genotyping of hepatitis B virus in a single reaction by real-time PCR and melting curve analysis. J. Hepatol. **41**, 659–666 (2004)
228. Lindh, M., Gonzales, J.E., Norkrans, G., et al.: Genotyping of hepatitis B virus by restriction pattern analysis of a pre S amplicon. J. Virol. Meth. **72**, 163–174 (1998)
229. Durantel, D., Brunelle, M.N., Gros, E., et al.: Resistance of human hepatitis B virus to reverse transcriptase inhibitors:

from genotypic to phenotypic testing. J. Clin. Virol. **34**(suppl 1), S34–S43 (2005)
230. Shaw, T., Bartholomeusz, A., Locarnini, S.: HBV drug resistance: mechanisms, detection and interpretation. J. Hepatol. **44**, 593–606 (2006)
231. Lok, A.S., Zoulim, F., Locarnini, S., et al.: Monitoring drug-resistance in chronic hepatitis B virus (HBV)-infected patients during lamivudine therapy: evaluation of performance of INNO-LiPA DR assay. J. Clin. Microbiol. **40**, 3729–3734 (2002)
232. Osiowy, C., Villeneuve, J.P., Heathcote, E.J., et al.: Detection of rtN236T and rtA181V/T mutations associated with resistance to adefovir dipivoxil in samples from patients with chronic hepatitis B virus infection by the INNO-LiPA HBV DR line probe assay (version 2). J. Clin. Microbiol. **44**, 1994–1997 (2006)
233. Roque-Afonso, A.M., Ferey, M.P., Mackiewicz, V., et al.: Monitoring the emergence of hepatitis B virus polymerase gene variants during lamivudine therapy in human immunodeficiency virus coinfected patients: performance of CLIP sequencing and line probe assay. Antivir. Ther. **8**, 627–634 (2003)
234. Tran, N., Berne, R., Chann, R., et al.: European multicenter evaluation of high density DNA probe arrays for detection of hepatitis B virus resistance mutations and identification of genotypes. J. Clin. Microbiol. **44**, 2792–2800 (2006)
235. Hertogs, K., de Bethune, M.P., Miller, V., et al.: A rapid method for simultaneous detection of phenotypic resistance to inhibitors of protease and reverse transcriptase in recombinant human immunodeficiency virus type 1 isolates from patients treated with antiretroviral drugs. Antimicrob. Agents Chemother. **42**, 269–276 (1998)
236. Whiley, D.M., Buda, P.J., Freeman, K., et al.: A real-time PCR assay for the detection of *Neisseria gonorrhoeae* in genital and extragenital specimens. Diagn. Microbiol. Infect. Dis. **52**, 1–5 (2005)

Part XI

Special Aspects of STIs and STDs in Comparison to Other Conditions

57 Genitoanal Dermatoses

Gerd Gross

Core Messages

- A considerable amount of cutaneous genitoanal conditions are unrelated to sexually transmitted infections.
- Dermatoses are equally seen at genitoanal sites of both genders.
- A wide number of differential diagnoses exist. History taking, physical examination together with simple tests as takings swabs, urine and serum are necessary to exclude a sexually transmitted infection.
- Taking a biopsy is one of the most useful procedures to diagnose correctly.
- Immunofluorescence staining is particularly helpful to differentiate autoimmune disorders such as bullous dermatoses and others.
- Organization of the chapter is done by 8 subchapters:
  - Normal variations of the genitoanal skin
  - Infectious diseases
  - Bullous diseases
  - Genetic disorders
  - Genitoanal manifestations of systemic disease
  - Inflammatory dermatoses
  - Genitoanal tumors
  - Genitoanal pain
- At the beginning of each subchapter there is a list of relevant differential diagnoses.

G. Gross
Department of Dermatology and Venereology, University of Rostock, Strempelstraße 13, 18057 Rostock, Germany
e-mail: gerd.gross@med.uni-rostock.de

57.1 Introduction

A large number of genital and perianal diseases are caused by sexually transmitted infectious agents. However, a considerable amount of cutaneous conditions of this area are unrelated to such agents.

Dermatoses located on the vulva may equally be seen at the male external genitalia. The same applies to perineal and perianal sites. The majority of these require dermatologic expertise [3]. For this reason, this chapter deals with genitoanal skin conditions without making any difference to the gender affected. Genitoanal dermatoses may patients, since disconcert might be afraid of a sexually transmitted disease or a malignant condition. Exclusion of these conditions is therefore essential.

The morphology of lesions can offer useful clues to the underlying pathomechanism and the likely causing agent. There is no doubt that physical examination provides the most valuable preliminary information as to the possible etiology. It enhances the thinking about differential diagnosis by establishing the category of cutaneous and mucocutaneous lesions that should be considered. Thus at the beginning of each subchapter relevant differential diagnoses are mentioned. This is to ameliorate understanding differences between similarly appearing clinical conditions and to establish a correct diagnosis.

Simple diagnostic procedures may be helpful in the diagnosis. They may also be the basis for the management of genitoanal dermatoses in both genders. For instance, relief from pain and pruritus may be accelerated and problems in sexual partnership can be prevented [34].

G. Gross and S.K. Tyring (eds.), *Sexually Transmitted Infections and Sexually Transmitted Diseases*,
DOI: 10.1007/978-3-642-14663-3_57,

57.2 Diagnostic Procedures

Diagnosis comprises history taking, clinical examination, and standardized simple tests by taking swabs and serum as well as collecting urine to exclude sexually transmitted infections. Taking a biopsy is often necessary especially if diagnosis remains unclear.

Specimens for immunofluorescence snap-frozen by liquid nitrogen have to be taken in special cases to rule out pemphigus, bullous pemphigoid, lichen planus, and other cutaneous autoimmune disorders.

The patient's history is essential, particularly the description of local and systemic symptoms and of major complaints. It should include earlier cutaneous disorders, contact sensitivities, allergies, earlier genitoanal infections and venereal diseases, operations, hospitalization, current or past medications. Excessive use of hygiene products has to be considered. Taking the sexual history, it should be clarified whether there is a risk of sexual trauma.

Careful examination has to be done with gloved hands under good light and a magnification aid such as a hand lens or a colposcope/peniscope (magnification eight to ten times). When examining the outer genitalia, it is important to consider morphologic changes at different ages and at physiological states such as pregnancy.

Both surfaces of the labia minora and, in case of male patients, the outer and inner aspects of the prepuce, the coronal sulcus, and the glans have to be carefully inspected. The same is true for the urethra, the perianal and perineal skin, and the anus of both genders. The clitoris has to be inspected by retracting the clitoral prepuce.

Documentation of the conditions is necessary. If permission is obtained, a photograph should be taken to record the actual disorder.

Examination of the genitoanal area covers hairs, hair follicles, the surrounding mucocutaneous areas such as mons pubis, the upper thighs, and urethral orificium. Palpation of inguinal–femoral, cervical, and axillary areas for the presence of lymph nodes is in line with a complete examination. This also includes inspection of the oral mucosa. A number of genital dermatoses may affect both sites simultaneously or the oral mucosa only. Such dermatoses are pemphigus, bullous pemphigoid, herpes simplex virus infection, syphilis (particularly secondary syphilis), lichen planus, candidiasis, HPV infections and related lesions.

57.2.1 Biopsy

Skin biopsies are very useful procedures in the diagnosis of genitoanal dermatoses. As a rule, biopsies are performed under local anesthesia in the outpatient setting. Different techniques have been used to take a biopsy from lesions at the vulva, the perianal skin, and the penis.

The most common techniques used are punch biopsy and shave biopsy (scissor snip technique). The punch biopsy is preferably used in skin ulcers and inflammatory conditions. Disposable punch biopsy instruments range in size from 2 to 8 mm (Fig. 57.1).

The lesional tissue is anesthetized using lidocaine 1% or 2%. Infiltration anesthesia of perianal and vulvar areas is best performed with epinephrine as an adjuvant in order to achieve hemostasis. Epinephrine, however, should be avoided in penile biopsies to prevent necrosis. Local anesthesia with a cream, consisting in a mixture of prilocaine and lidocaine (EMLA cream) can be used to prevent

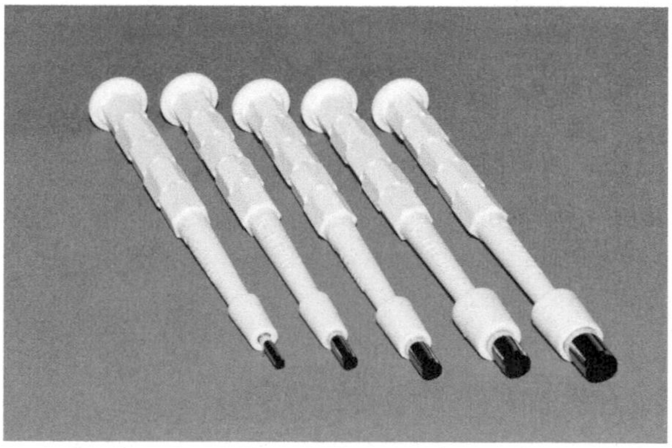

Fig. 57.1 Punch biopsy instruments at sizes ranging from 2 to 8 mm in diameter

pain if applied about 60 min before injection of anesthesia at mucous membranes or keratinized skin, respectively.

This method enables to produce a probe for microscopic examination. Bleeding can be stopped with pressure or chemical cautery (ferric chloride, or silver nitrate). Alternatively, one or two sutures are helpful to achieve hemostasis.

In case of shave biopsy or scissor-snip excision technique, a sample of superficial skin is removed by scissor with anesthesia.

57.2.2 Further Investigation

Histological examination of a tissue sample is regarded as the gold standard. If herpes simplex infection is in question, a Tzanck smear may be helpful. A more sensitive method, however, is the direct immunofluorescence test on exfoliated cells using HSV1, HSV2, and VZV-specific monoclonal antibodies (see Chapter 21 on pages 217 to 248).

Further investigations may comprise microbiological tests with swabs taken for bacterial, yeast, and viral cultures. Another option for detection of infectious agents may be the detection of nuclear acids. Patch tests are used in cases of suspected allergic contact dermatitis and an underlying delayed type hypersensitivity (type IV immune reaction). Prick testing is required to investigate urticarial (type I) reactions. In such conditions, radioimmunoabsorbent assays may also be helpful.

Genitoanal dermatoses may be asymptomatic. However, many patients present complaints such as itching or pruritus. There is a clear influence by psychological factors. Continuous itching will lead to scratching and thickening and lichenification of the skin.

Pain is a rare complaint of patients presenting with a genitoanal dermatosis.

Differential diagnosis is always done on a morphological basis. Dermatoses at flexural sites of the genitoanal areas are particularly difficult to diagnose. Both clinical examination and histology may be complicated by secondary overgrowth and also by irritant contacts from therapies. Furthermore, neoplastic disorders can be mistaken as simple dermatoses. This requires always taking a biopsy from any condition unresponsive to treatment.

57.3 Clinical Manifestations

57.3.1 Normal Variations on the Genitoanal Skin

57.3.1.1 Genital Papillomatosis

Differential Diagnosis

- Genital warts

Genital papillomatosis is a regular finding in both women and men. On the penis, this condition has been described as pearly penile papules or hirsutoid papillomas [1]. The lesions may simulate condylomata acuminata (Fig. 57.2). However, there are characteristic clinical findings for clear differentiation. Discrete acuminata structures are distributed in parallel rows circumferentially around the coronal sulcus (Fig. 57.2).

Histology shows hypertrophic papillae covered by a normal epithelium. At magnification, the papular lesions do not show the typical vascular pattern of mucosal condylomata and they do not coalesce. Vulvar papillomatosis, also described as micropapillomatosis labialis, is found on the inner surface of the labia minora in many women (Fig. 57.3). It consists in bilateral and commonly symmetric tiny finger-like projections that do not coalesce. Histologically, the epithelium contains glycogen-rich pale keratinocytes, which can be, in general, mistaken as koilocytes. Pearly penile papules and vulvar papillomatosis are definitely not associated with HPV [5, 31]. This and their regular surface and arrangement of the vessels help to differentiate these lesions from condylomata acuminata. Therapy is not indicated. Sometimes, papillomatosis is associated with vulvodynia (see page 835).

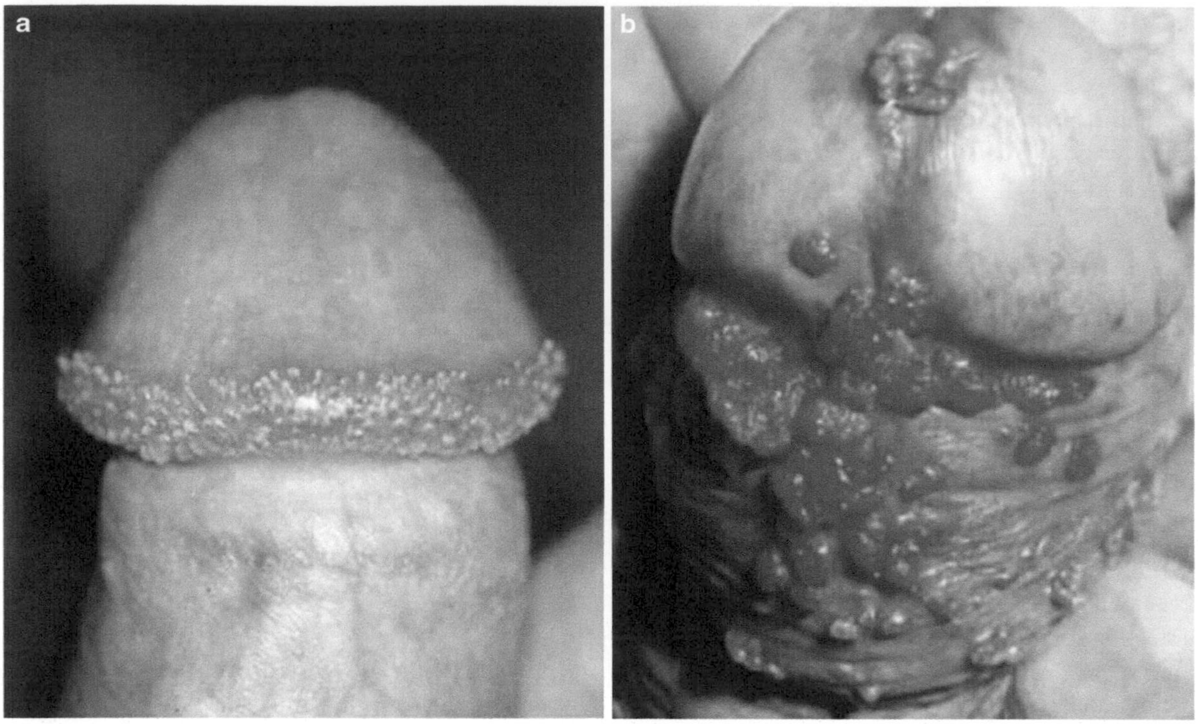

Fig. 57.2 (**a**) Pearly penile papules (syn.: hirsuties papillaris):digitate micropapular lesions located on the coronal sulcus. (**b**) Condylomata acuminata on the inner part of the prepuce and on the glans. The meatus urethra is involved

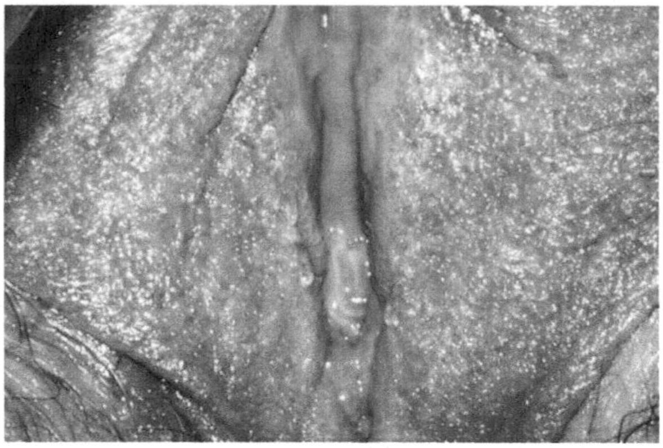

Fig. 57.3 Micropapillomatosis vulvae: Noncoalescent tiny monomorphous papillae on the labia minora and the vestibule

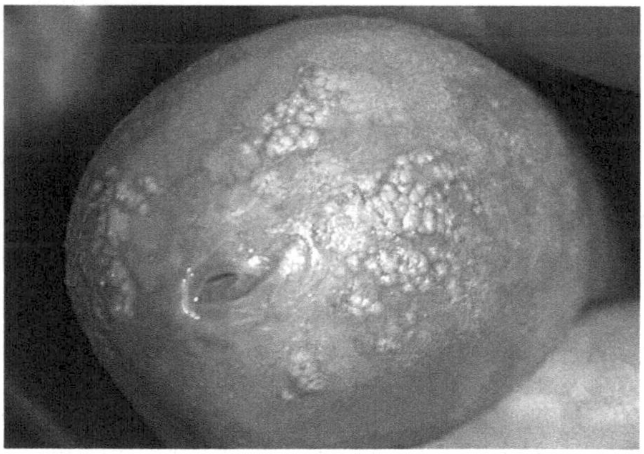

Fig. 57.4 Fordyce spots on the glans

57.3.1.2 Fordyce Spots

Differential Diagnoses

- Lichen nitidus
- Genital warts

These are yellowish papules which can be mistaken for genital warts. In women, they consist in simply ectopic sebaceous glands of the labial epithelium in different numbers. Similarly, such lesions are regular findings on the prepuce (Fig. 57.4). Sebaceous glands are also seen at the lips and oral mucosa (Fig. 57.5). Lichen nitidus is another differential diagnosis, which however is quite rarely found (Fig. 57.6).

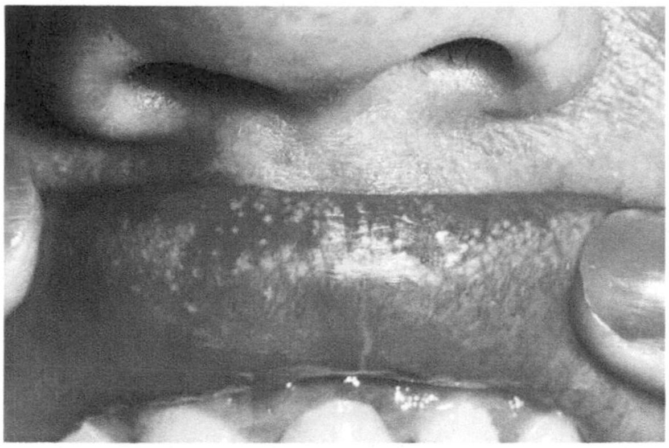

Fig. 57.5 Yellowish lesions (sebaceous glands) on the lips

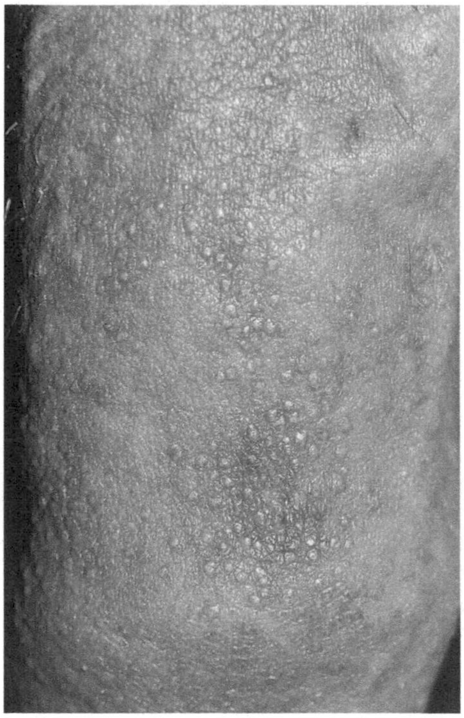

Fig. 57.6 Discrete shiny micropapular lesions of lichen nitidus on the penile shaft

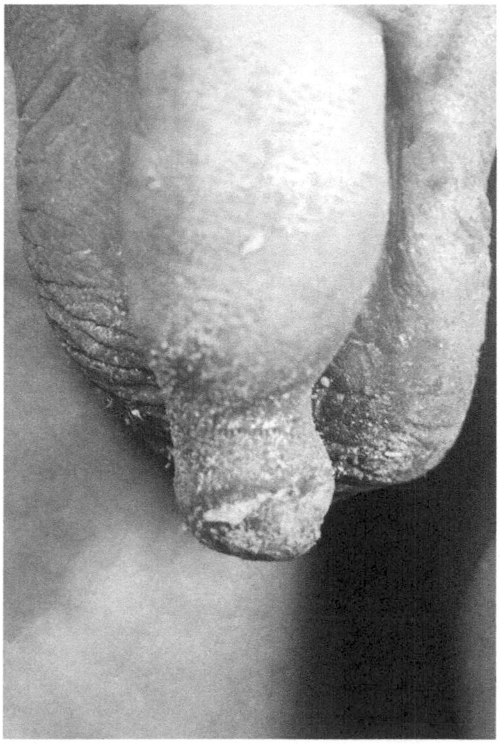

Fig. 57.7 Congenital phimosis

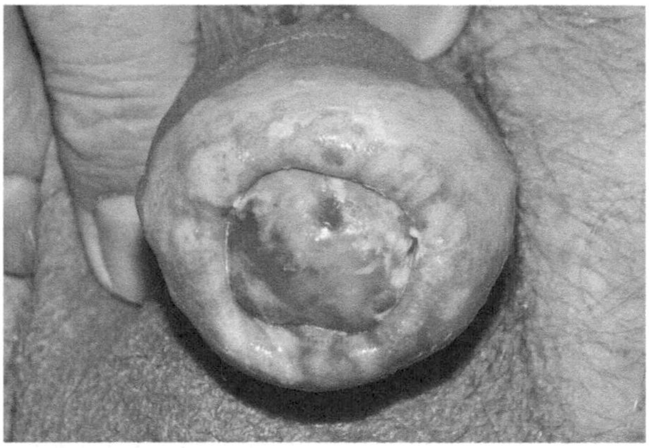

Fig. 57.8 Phimosis and lichen sclerosus: pallor, atrophy, and sclerosis contribute to balanitis xerotica obliterans (lichen sclerosus)

57.3.1.3 Phimosis

Phimosis is a normal condition in the male in the early years of life. This physiologic type of phimosis may lead to recurrent balanoposthitis. Medical or surgical treatment is rarely required for separating foreskin from the glans penis (Fig. 57.7) Later in life, phimosis can be caused by various infections and especially by lichen sclerosus (Fig. 57.8). Laser or cautery applied for treatment of genital warts may result in iatrogenic phimosis or paraphimosis. If phimosis is causing recurrent balanitis, circumcision is required (see Chap. 54). Phimosis is a risk factor for the development of penile cancer (see Chap. 37).

57.4 Infectious Diseases

57.4.1 Bacterial Infection

Bacterial infections with streptococci and staphylococci are promoted by the warm, moist, and occlude environment of the genitoanal and inguinal areas. Initially, a staphylococcal infection leads to folliculitis, which consists of perifollicular pustules (folliculitis) or nodules, which may then develop into an abscess and finally an ulcer. Typical predispositions are obesity and diabetes. In recurrent cases malignancy and immunodeficiency have to be occluded. Local washing with antiseptic solutions and treatment with topical antibiotics are often sufficient. Oral antibiotics such as dicloxacillin and others should be given according to cultural results.

57.4.1.1 Erysipelas (Syn. Cellulitis)

Differential Diagnoses

- Erythrasma
- Contact dermatitis
- Figurate erythema
- Erythema chronicum migrans
- Horpes zoster

Streptococci or less frequently staphylococci cause erysipelas by an infection of lymph vessels in the dermis. The most common cause is *Streptococcus pyogenes*. Clinical features of erysipelas consist in an edematous erythema growing centrifugally (Fig. 57.9). Sometimes vesicles, bullae, and skin necrosis may aggravate the course. Severe erysipelas is a well-known hazard of radical surgery in the genitoanal area and the lower abdominal skin. Irradiation is a further risk. Patients suffer from fever, chills, and malaise. Lymphedema may be complicated by erysipelas. In turn, erysipelas may lead to lymphedema and in chronic and recurrent disease elephantiasis may result. The golden standard of therapy is still systemic penicillin, clindamycin, or erythromycin accompanied by wet wrappings. Choice of antibiotics should depend on the result of cultures of probes taken from suspicious places of entry.

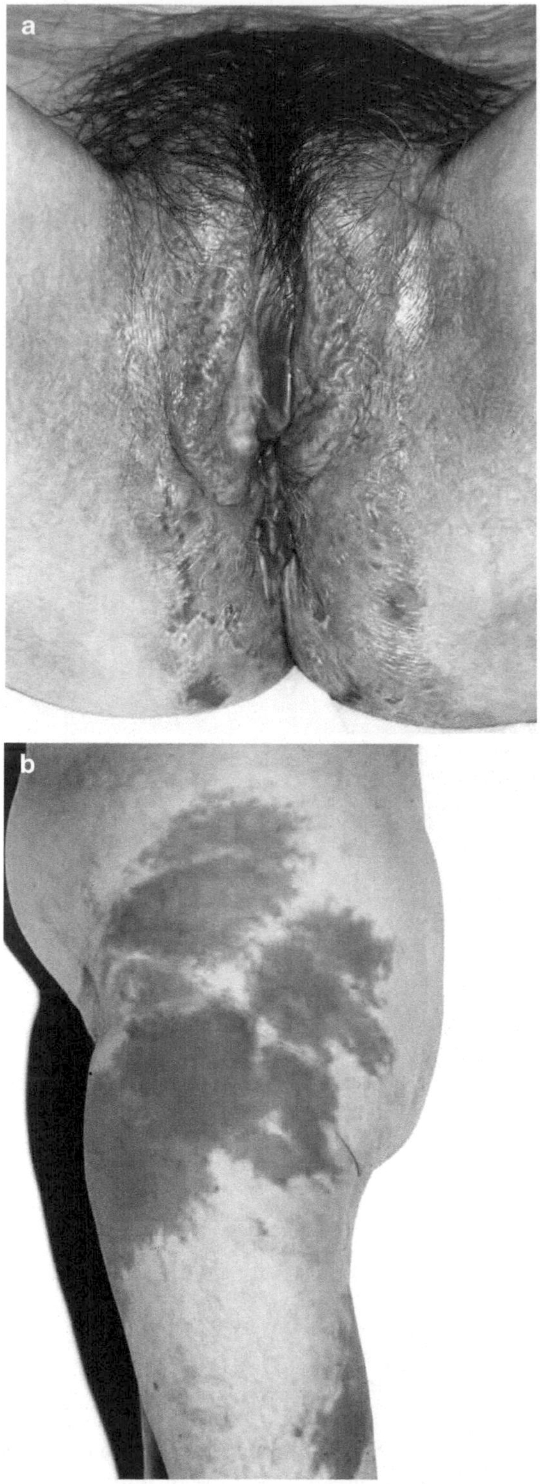

Fig. 57.9 (**a**) Erysipelas on the labia majora and the pubic skin. (**b**) Multicentric erysipelas: Spreading inflammation together with lymphatic damage due to previous x-ray irradiation

57.4.1.2 Perianal Streptococcal Dermatitis

Differential Diagnoses

- Contact Eczema

This condition is characterized by a painful erythema of the perianal skin and sometimes the buttocks. It is rarely seen in adults, but children are frequently affected [35]. It is caused by group A beta-hemolytic streptococci. Treatment is with penicillin [20].

57.4.1.3 Erythrasma

Differential Diagnoses

- Psoriasis inversa
- Seborrheic dermatitis
- Fungal infection
- Yeast
- Intertrigo

This mostly asymptomatic noninflammatory dermatosis is located at intertriginous areas such as the genitoanal and inguinal folds (Fig. 57.10) as well as the axillae (Fig. 57.12). It is caused by *Corynebacterium minutissimum*, which is a part of the normal skin flora. Typical features are erythematous patches leading to confluent large reddish to brownish areas. The borders of the lesions are sharp, which is in contrast to other similar lesions.

Diagnosis of erythrasma is often based solely on clinical grounds.

A simple diagnostic help is Wood's light examination (UVA 365 nm) which produces a coral-red fluorescence (due to a porphyrin in *C. minutissimum*) [27] (Fig. 57.11). Staining of scales with PAS or Gram may be helpful. Erythrasma of the groins has to be differentiated from psoriasis inversa, seborrheic dermatitis, fungal infections, and yeast infections. Treatment consists mainly in hygienic measures, topical and if necessary systemic antibiotic therapy, especially with erythromycin.

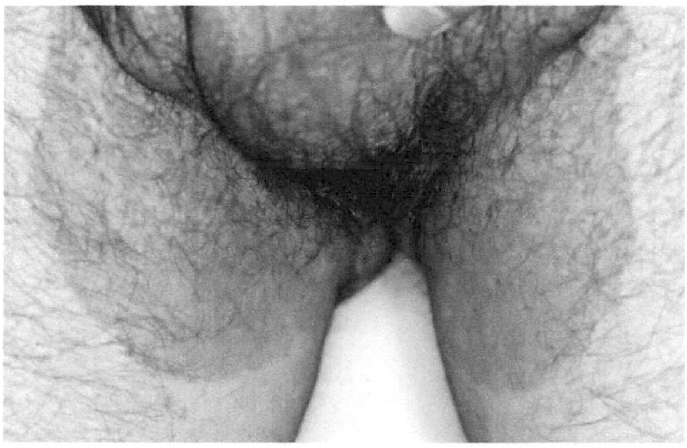

Fig. 57.10 Erythrasma on the groins in a patient suffering from diabetes

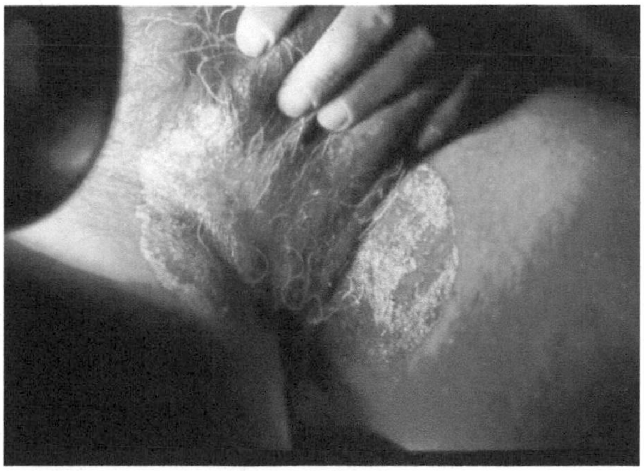

Fig. 57.11 Wood's light (ultraviolet rays, 365 nm) leads to coral-pink fluorescence

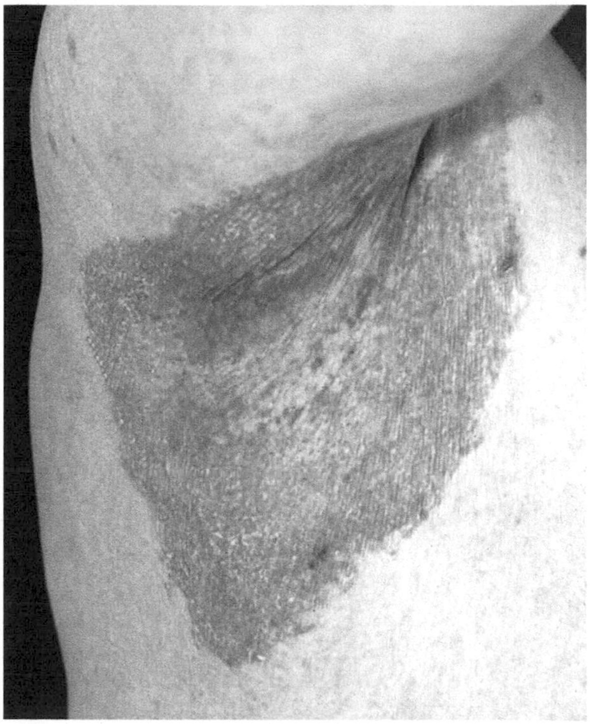

Fig. 57.12 Axillar involvement of erythrasma

57.4.2 Fungal Infections

57.4.2.1 Yeast Infection

Differential Diagnoses

- Psoriasis inversa
- Fungal infection
- Erythrasma

The most common cause of yeast infection is *Candida albicans* (see Chap. 46 page 613). Topical symptoms of yeast balanitis in the male are pruritus and rarely pain. Women may suffer from a milky discharge (Fig. 57.13). On inspection, confluent red spots with whitish patches are seen.

Small "satellite" lesions at the border are further typical findings. Fissuring and slight ulcerations may occur on the prepuce, the glans, the fourchette, and the vagina. The most common site of candida infection in males is the glans and prepuce (Fig. 57.14). Penile shaft, the inguinal and anal folds may also be affected.

Differential diagnosis should be based on clinical inspection and laboratory test results. Psoriasis inversa, other fungal infections, and erythrasma have to be considered. In painful cases, genital herpes should be

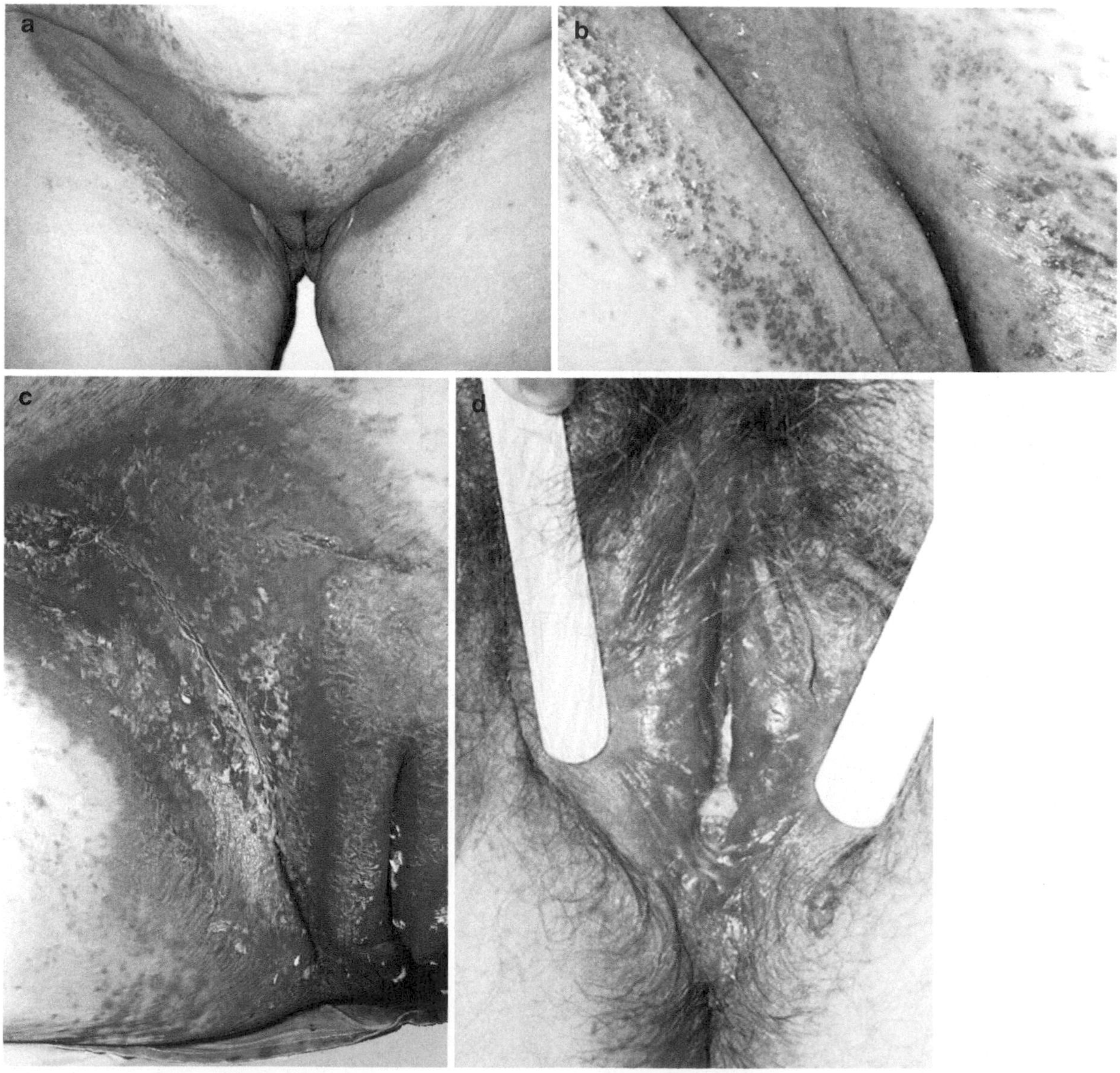

Fig. 57.13 Candidosis (female). (**a**) The groins are chiefly affected. (**b**) Peripheral "satellite lesions" are typical features. (**c**) Severe vulvitis due to *Candida albicans*. (**d**) Thick, curdish discharge. The vagina is erythematous. (**e**) Microscopic detection of hyphae in the corneal layer of the epidermis (PAS-staining)

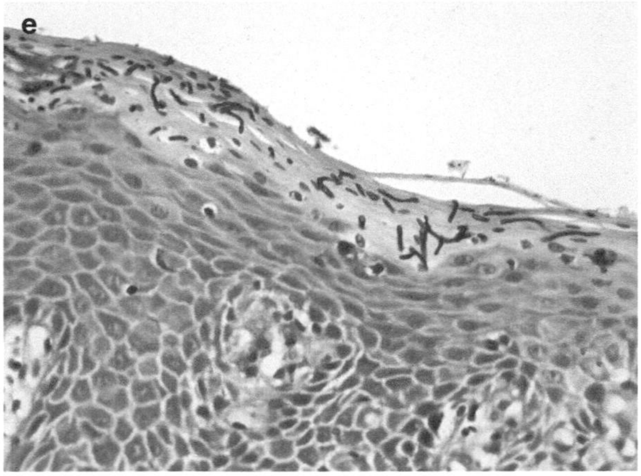

Fig. 57.13 (continued)

excluded by viral culture or immunofluorescence investigation. For further information please refer to the Chap. 21 on page 217.

57.4.2.2 Dermatophytic Infections

Differential Diagnoses

- Psoriasis
- Seborrheic dermatitis
- Erythrasma

Causes of dermatophytic infections of the groins are *Trichophyton rubrum*, *T. mentagrophytes*, and *Epidermophyton floccosum.*

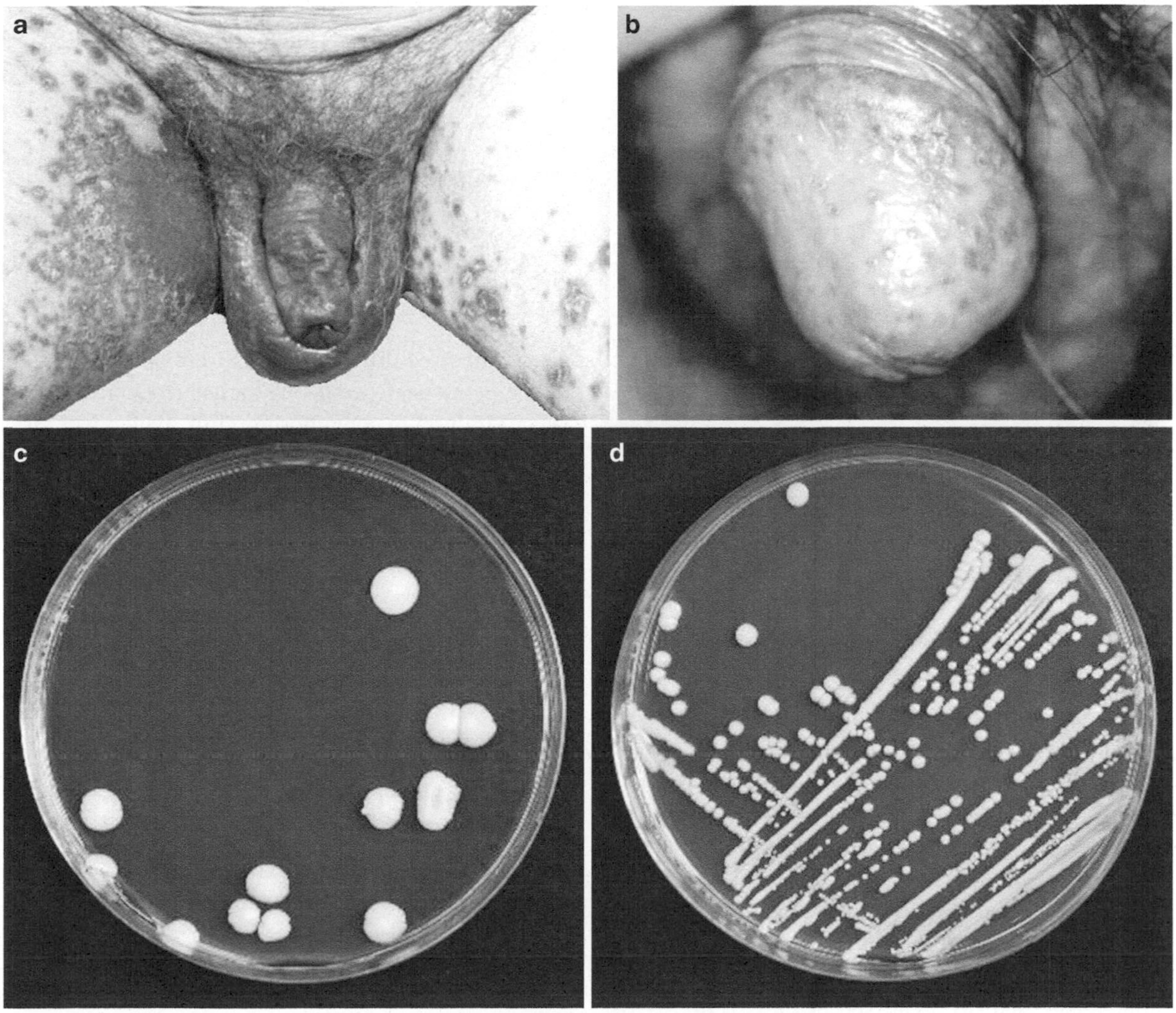

Fig. 57.14 Candidosis in the male. (**a**) Candidosis affecting the scrotum, penis, and the groins. (**b**) Balanitis candidomycetica with discrete erosive lesions on the glans. (**c**) Culture of *Candida albicans* on Sabouraud's medium, 24 h at 37°C. (**d**) Candida albicans in culture, 48 h at 37°C

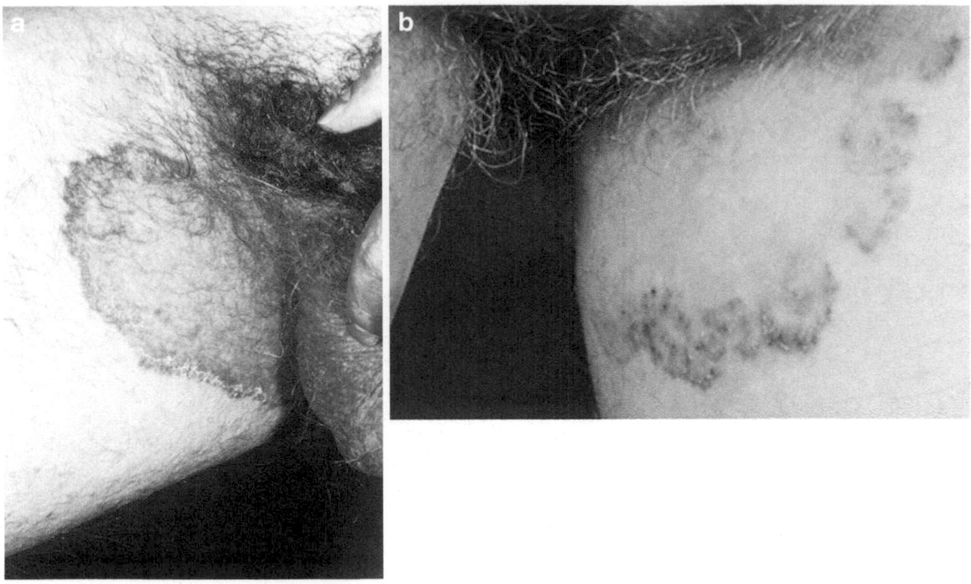

Fig. 57.15 (**a**) Tinea cruris. (**b**) Older lesion with central clearing

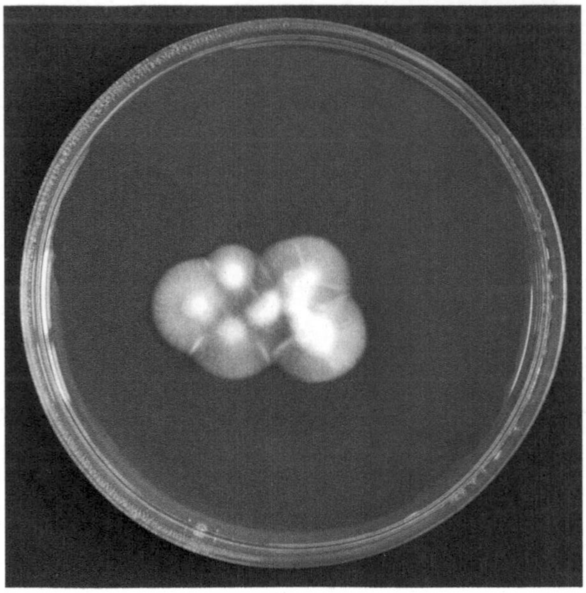

Fig. 57.16 Culture of *Trichophyton rubrum* with white cottony colony (Sabouraud's glucose agar, 3 weeks at 24°C)

In the male, tinea cruris can be accompanied by genital dermatophytic infection. The most characteristic findings of dermatophyte infections of the folds are their asymmetrical growth, their well-defined spreading border, and in chronic courses, itching (Figs. 57.15 and 57.16). The most important differential diagnoses are yeast infection, seborrheic dermatitis, and erythrasmas, (Fig. 57.10). Detection of the fungi by culture helps to differentiate and to treat successfully (Fig. 57.16). Treatment consists primarily in local antifungal therapy, such as imidazole cream. In recalcitrant disease, oral imidazole therapy is recommendable. It is the goal to continue local and/or systemic antifungal therapy until fungal infection is definitely no longer detectable. However, side effects have to be taken into account, when treatment is given for more than 1 month.

57.4.3 Viral Infections

There are three different DNA-viruses that may often infect genitoanal cutaneous and mucocutaneous tissues: Molluscum contagiosum virus, which is a virus of the poxvirus group, human papillomaviruses, and herpesviruses. Over the time, age of persons affected by viral infections has clearly changed. Nowadays, infections seem to occur more frequently in young adults. In earlier times, transfer of virus was mainly during childhood through close personal contact. Actually some associated diseases develop later in life due to close sexual contacts.

57.4.3.1 Genital Herpes

Differential Diagnoses

- Herpes zoster
- Behcet's disease
- Yeast

Herpes simplex virus (HSV2 > HSV1) infection can be sexually transmitted and lead to genital herpes. It is

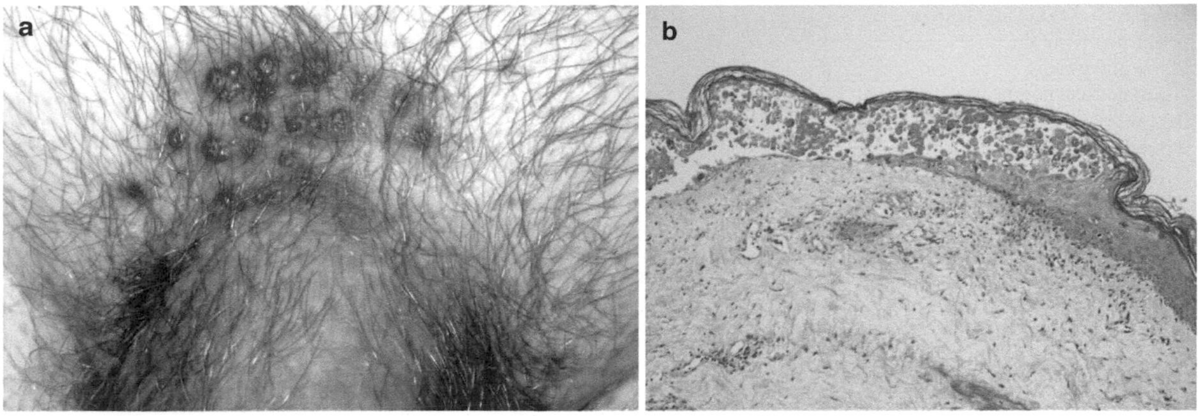

Fig. 57.17 (**a**) Grouped vesicles of genital herpes. (**b**) Histology: Subcorneal vesicle with multinuclear giant cells

characterized by painful, grouped, vesicular, and erosive lesions at the genitoanal skin, the buttocks, and the adjacent mucosa (Fig. 57.17). Sometimes, HSV-infection remains subclinical and unrecognized. Recurrences which are due to persistence of HSV-DNA in regional ganglia help to differentiate genital herpes from herpes zoster (see Chap. 20 and 21). Herpes is painful. In contrast yeast is itching.

57.4.3.2 Varicella and Herpes Zoster

Differential Diagnoses

- Genital herpes
- Behcet's disease
- Arthropod reaction
- Folliculitis

The primary infection with varicella-zoster virus (VZV) usually occurs in children. It results in varicella (chickenpox), which is a generalized rash of papules, vesicles, pustules, and crusts. Occasionally, the genitoanal area is affected including mucosal surfaces such as the vulva, the glans, and the anus. Healing of lesions takes up to 2 weeks with the potential of scar formation. Similar to HSV-DNA VZV-DNA persists in the sensory root ganglion cells and cranial ganglion cells. Herpes zoster (shingles) develops when VZV is reactivated. This is usually seen in elderly people >50 years of age and in persons with impaired cell-mediated immunity (immunosuppressive therapy, HIV-infection etc.).

Skin lesions in herpes zoster are unilateral and asymmetrical. Often, they are preceded by prodromal symptoms such as pain along a cutaneous dermatome. Further prodromi can be headache, fatigue, and fever, occurring about 7–10 days prior to the skin eruption. Red, partially urticaria-like papules and plaques develop along the involved dermatome, followed by grouped vesicles and bullae that may coalesce and become hemorrhagic (Fig. 57.18).

Regional lymphadenopathy is a frequent finding seen in about 15% of herpes zoster patients. If lumbosacral nerves and the S3-dermatome are involved in VZV reactivation, lesions develop unilaterally on the buttocks, the vulva, the penis, and the scrotum (Fig. 57.18).

Cutaneous complications of herpes zoster are postinflammatory hyperpigmentation and depigmentation as well as scar formation (Fig. 57.19). Sometimes, second-line lesions may develop within a previously affected dermatome. This may be psoriasis or lymphoma. Rarely zoster lesions become hemorrhagic and necrotic. Chronic pain persisting after healing of the skin is most common in patients older than 50 years of age. Rarely vulvodynia and penodynia may result. Another rare complication of shingles in immunodeficient patients is dissemination of lesions, resulting in a varicella-like clinical picture (Fig. 57.20). This is reminiscent of severe depression of the cellular immunity. There are rare cases of herpes zoster of the genitoanal region affecting urination and defecation [46].

Diagnosis of manifest VZV-infection is primarily clinical. Virus detection of blister fluid and swabs from the blister ground using immunofluorescence test or polymerase chain reaction technique is helpful to differentiate between shingles and herpes simplex in difficult cases.

Adults with varicella require a specific antiviral treatment because the course of disease is more severe and complicated than in children. Especially pneumonitis is an important complication. The drug of

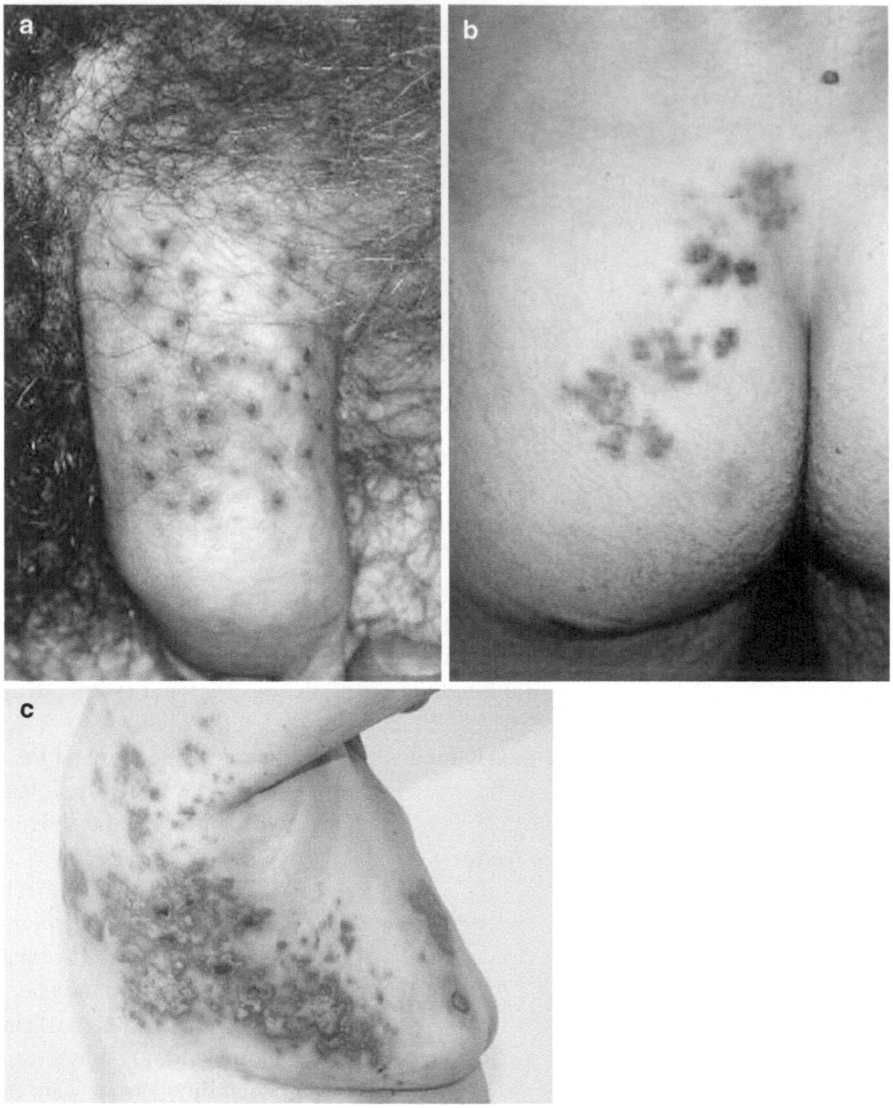

Fig. 57.18 (**a**) Genital herpes zoster involving the third sacral nerve root. Asymmetrical penile aspect. (**b**) Left gluteal aspect with grouped herpes vesicles (same patient as in **a**). (**c**) Thoracic zoster: grouped vesicles in the fourth thoracal dermatome

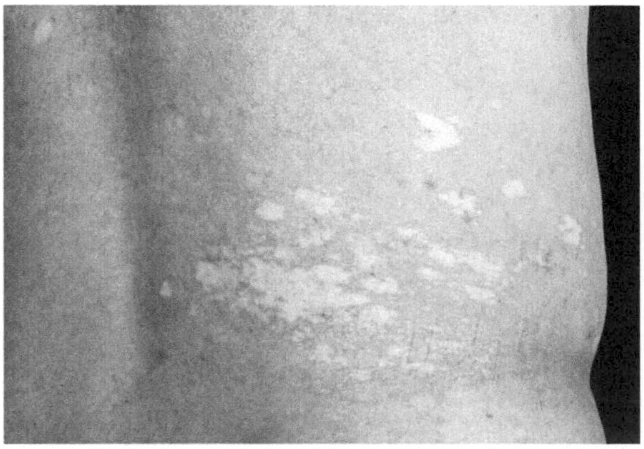

Fig. 57.19 Depigmented scarring after herpes zoster

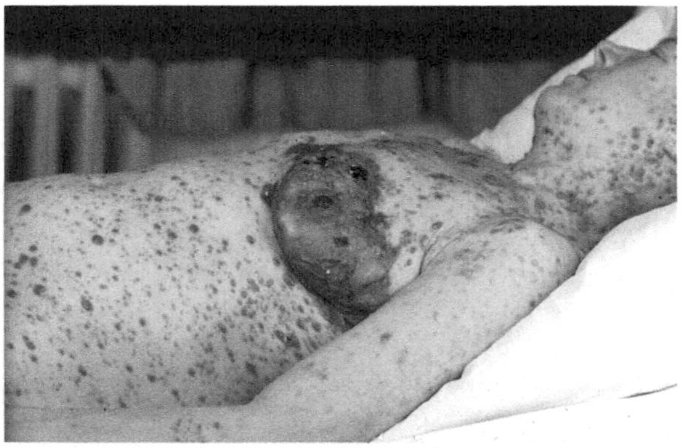

Fig. 57.20 Disseminated thoracal herpes zoster

choice for adult varicella is peroral acyclovir 800 mg, five times a day. In severe cases, intravenous aciclovir (8 mg/kg body-weight per day, for 7–10 days) must be considered.

The goal of herpes zoster management is accelerated healing of skin lesions, control of pain, and prevention of long-term complications, mainly postherpetic neuralgia and ophthalmic sequelae. Most recently, a report has shown the elevated risk of stroke in patients suffering from shingles, mainly of the ophthalmic nerve [23].

In patients with herpes zoster, antiviral therapy with oral aciclovir 800 mg five times a day for 7 days is the therapy of choice. An alternative for severe cases particularly in older patients and those with zoster in one of the three branches of the trigeminal nerve is intravenous acyclovir (8 mg/kg body-weight, three times a day, for 7 days). Other options of antiviral therapy are valacyclovir 1 g or famciclovir 500–750 mg three times a day for 7 days, respectively. Consequent oral administration of amitriptyline, carbamazepine, gabapentin, or pregabalin is essential, since it may contribute to prevent or reduce postherpetic pain. Local therapy of genitoanal herpes zoster consists in desiccating and antiseptic lotions.

57.4.4 Parasitic Infections

Infestations by scabies or pubic lice have been an ever increasing problem. These diseases cause pruritus in almost everyone who acquires them.

Infections with scabies and pubic lice result from close personal and sexual contact. In men, a common manifestation of scabies is papulonodular lesions on the scrotum and the penile shaft (Fig. 57.21 scabies). (Further reading Chap. 43 and 44). In general, symptoms at the genitoanal area of women are less severe than in men.

57.5 Bullous Diseases

A number of different blistering conditions affect the genitoanal skin and mucosal surfaces. Benign familial chronic pemphigus (Hailey-Hailey's disease) and Darier's disease are discussed in the chapter on genetic disorders (Chapter 57 page 792).

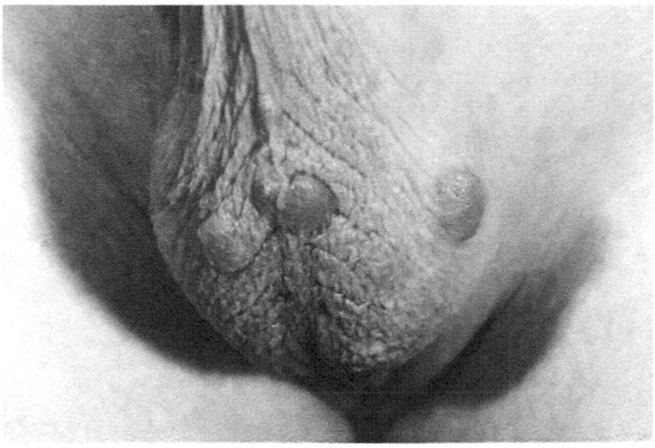

Fig. 57.21 Nodular scabies on the scrotal skin

Anogenital involvement is a regular finding of pemphigus vulgaris and pemphigoid. The pathogenesis of immunobullous disorders is based on the presence of antibodies directed against epidermal and basement membrane zone tissues.

Diagnosis consists in direct immunofluorescence of nonlesional skin to detect antigen material and in indirect immunofluorescence to investigate circulating antibodies in the blood (Fig. 57.22).

57.5.1 Bullous Pemphigoid

Differential Diagnoses

- Erythrasma
- Lichen ruber
- Genital herpes
- Pemphigus
- Epidermolysis bullosa acquisita

Bullous pemphigoid equally affects men and women at any age including children. However, it occurs mainly in the elderly between 60 and 70 years of age. Involvement of the skin is more common than mucosal disease (Fig. 57.23). Intertriginous areas such as axillae and groin are frequently affected. In men, adhesions between glans and foreskin and phimosis may result. The vulva is rarely affected. Feared complications in women are ulceration and stenosis.

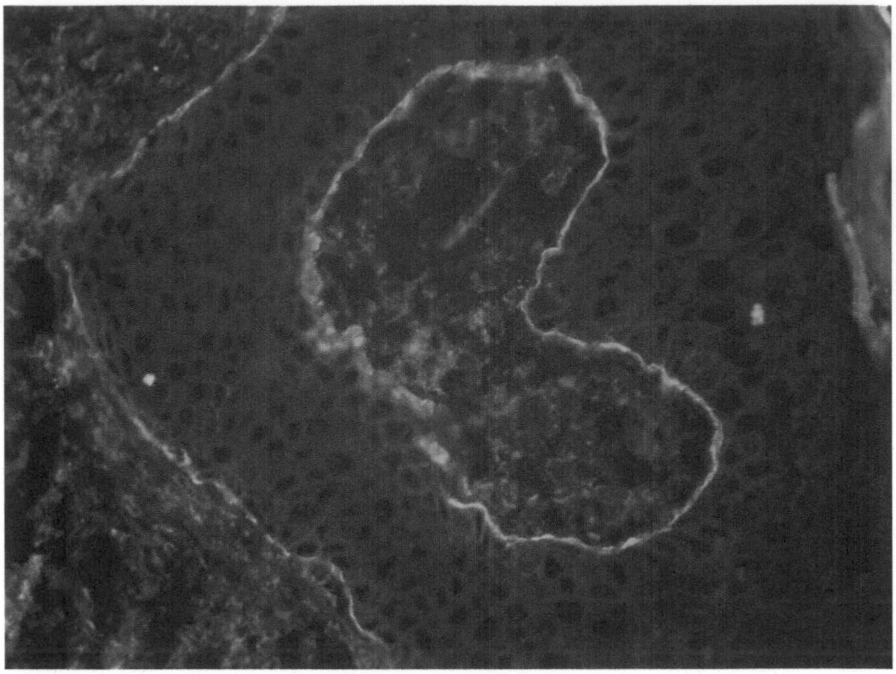

Fig. 57.22 Linear band of immunoglobulin G at the basement membrane: Direct immunofluoresence of bullous pemphigoid

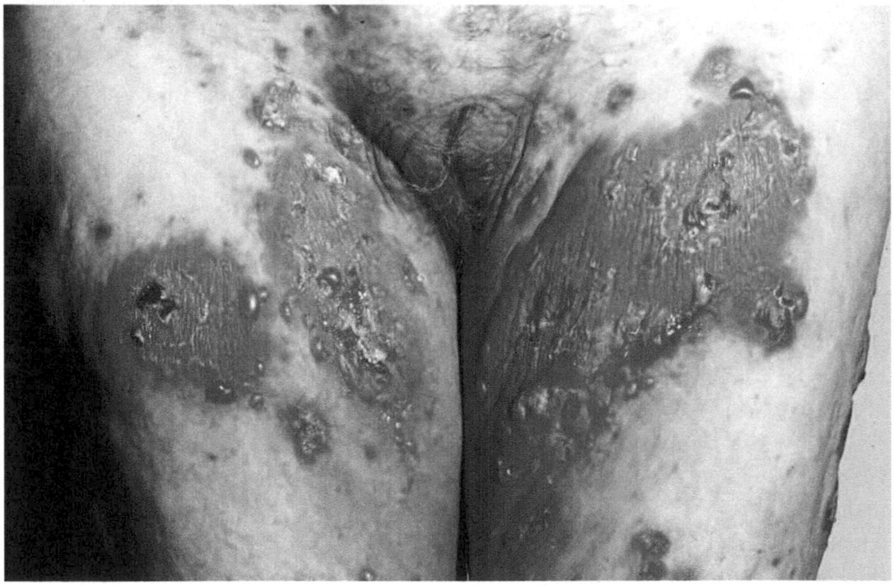

Fig. 57.23 Severe bullous pemphigoid on the upper legs

Diagnosis of bullous pemphigoid has become specific in the last years. Histology shows a subepidermal blister with varying amounts of eosinophils (Figs. 57.24 and 57.25). Direct immunofluorescence is necessary for confirmation of diagnosis (Fig. 57.22) Circulating IgG antibodies are directed toward the pemphigoid antigen in the lamina lucida of the basal membrane zone.

57.5.2 Cicatrical Pemphigoid

This autoimmune blistering disease occurs preferentially in 50- to 70-year-old women, targeting the mucous membranes of the mouth, the eyes, and frequently the genitalia. Chief complaints are vulvar pain and dyspareunia. The disease regularly leads to

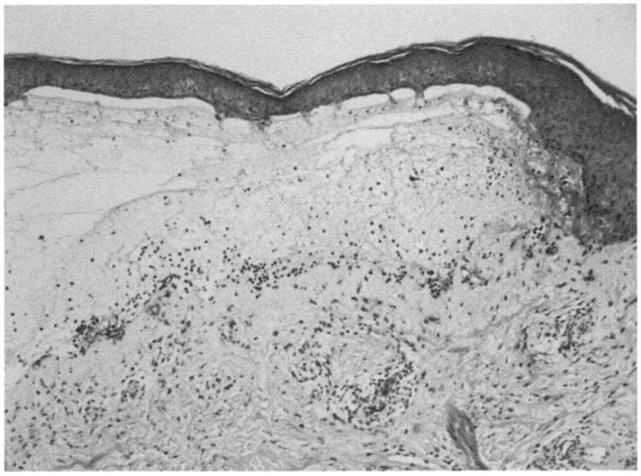

Fig. 57.24 Histology: subepidermal cleft and eosinophil-rich infiltrate in the upper dermis

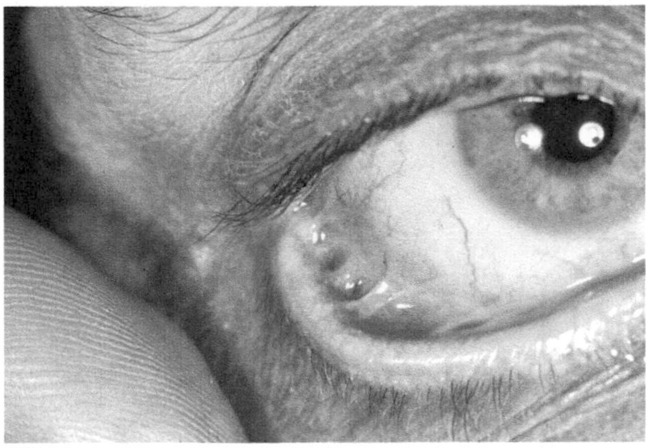

Fig. 57.26 Cicatrical pemphigoid with formation of symblepharon

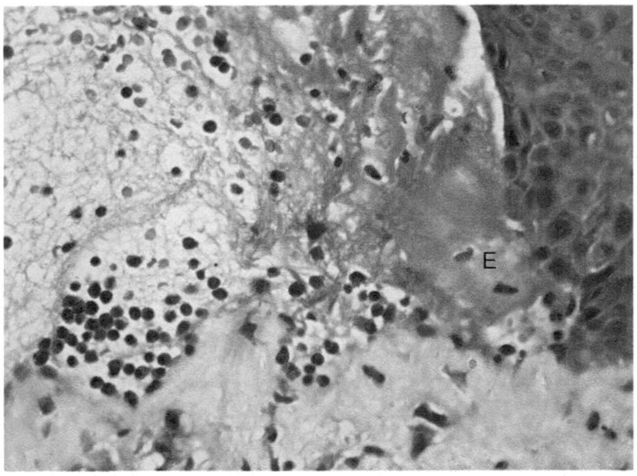

Fig. 57.25 Magnification from Fig. 57.24: Multiple eosinophils E=Epidermis

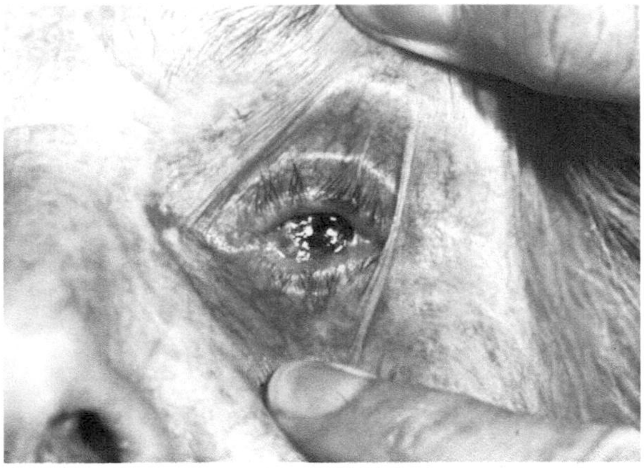

Fig. 57.27 Ocular involvement of cicatrical pemphigoid

scarring. A greatly feared dreaded ocular complication is symblepharon formation, keratitis, and blindness (Figs. 57.26 and 57.27). Therapy consists in topical corticosteroids and oral steroids.

57.5.3 Epidermolysis Bullosa Acquisita

This autoimmune blistering disease often presents with mucous membrane involvement [26]. Differentiation from bullous pemphigoid, which is histologically very similar, is made by demonstrating antibodies against type IV collagen in the patient's serum.

57.5.4 Pemphigus Vulgaris

Differential Diagnoses

- Bullous Pemphigoid

This rare severe chronic bullous eruption affects mucous membranes of mouth and genitalia as well as the skin. The blisters are located intraepidermally. Erosions are more common features than vesicles and bullae (Figs. 57.28–57.30).

Residual erosions cause pain and discomfort. In women, the vulva, the vagina, and the cervix may be affected. In men, especially the glans and the coronal sulcus are involved. Diagnosis is confirmed by biopsy and direct immunofluorescence (Fig. 57.31). In the blood, circulating autoantibodies are identified. Therapy consists in systemic corticosteroids and immunosuppressives.

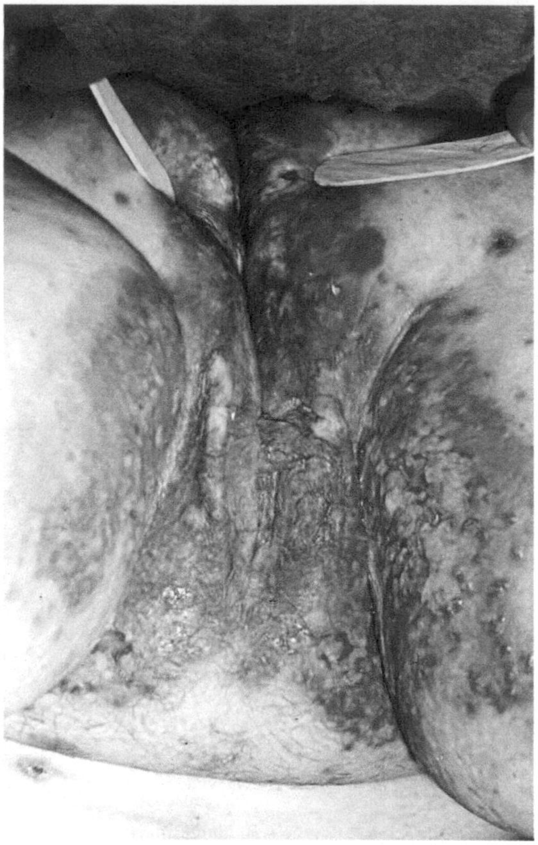

Fig. 57.28 Pemphigus vulgaris vegetans. Multiple confluent bullous lesions on the groins, the vulvar and perianal skin

57.6 Genetic Disorders

57.6.1 Benign Familial Chronic Pemphigus (Hailey-Hailey's Disease)

Differential Diagnoses

- Psoriasis inversa
- Eczema
- Darier's disease
- Condylomata acuminata

This dermatosis is rare and affects the genitoanal area of persons aged 20–40 years. However, other flexural areas, especially the axillae, may also be involved. Hailey-Hailey's disease consists in moist red papules with erosions and fissures. Pustules and vesicles may occur.

The lesions are sore and itching and may produce an impleasant smell. Exacerbations are seen in the context of heat, pregnancy, obesity, contact irritation, or allergy. Infection with bacteria, candida, or herpes simplex may also play a role.

Hailey-Hailey's disease is an important differential diagnosis of inverse psoriasis, irritated eczema, and Darier's disease. Rarely Hailey-Hailey disease is mistaken for genitoanal warts (Fig. 57.32). Histology is helpful to establish the correct diagnosis and examination of the extragenital skin sites will be helpful in many cases [12]. Characteristic histologic features are intraepithelial acanthosis and suprabasal cleft formation (Fig. 57.33). The disease is inherited autosomally and associated with a defect in keratinocyte adhesion.

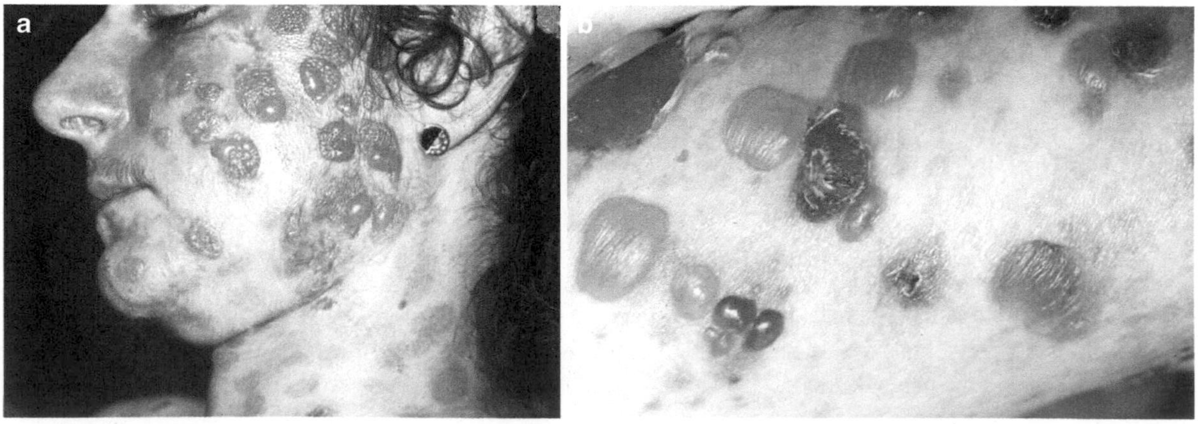

Fig. 57.29 (**a**) Pemphigus vulgaris. Multiple flaccid bullae on the face. (**b**) Hemorrhagic and eroded superficial bullous lesions

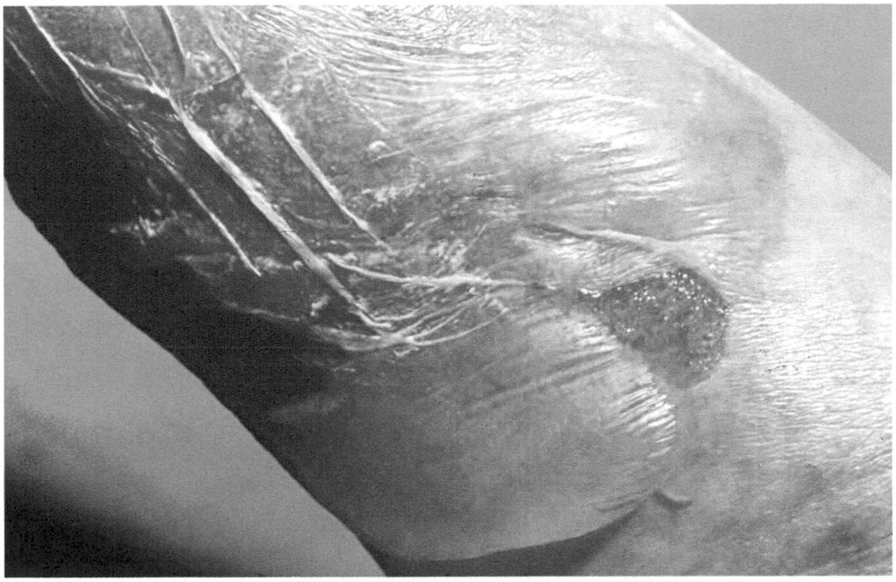

Fig. 57.30 Pemphigus vulgaris. Superficially located intraepithelial bulla and fresh erosion

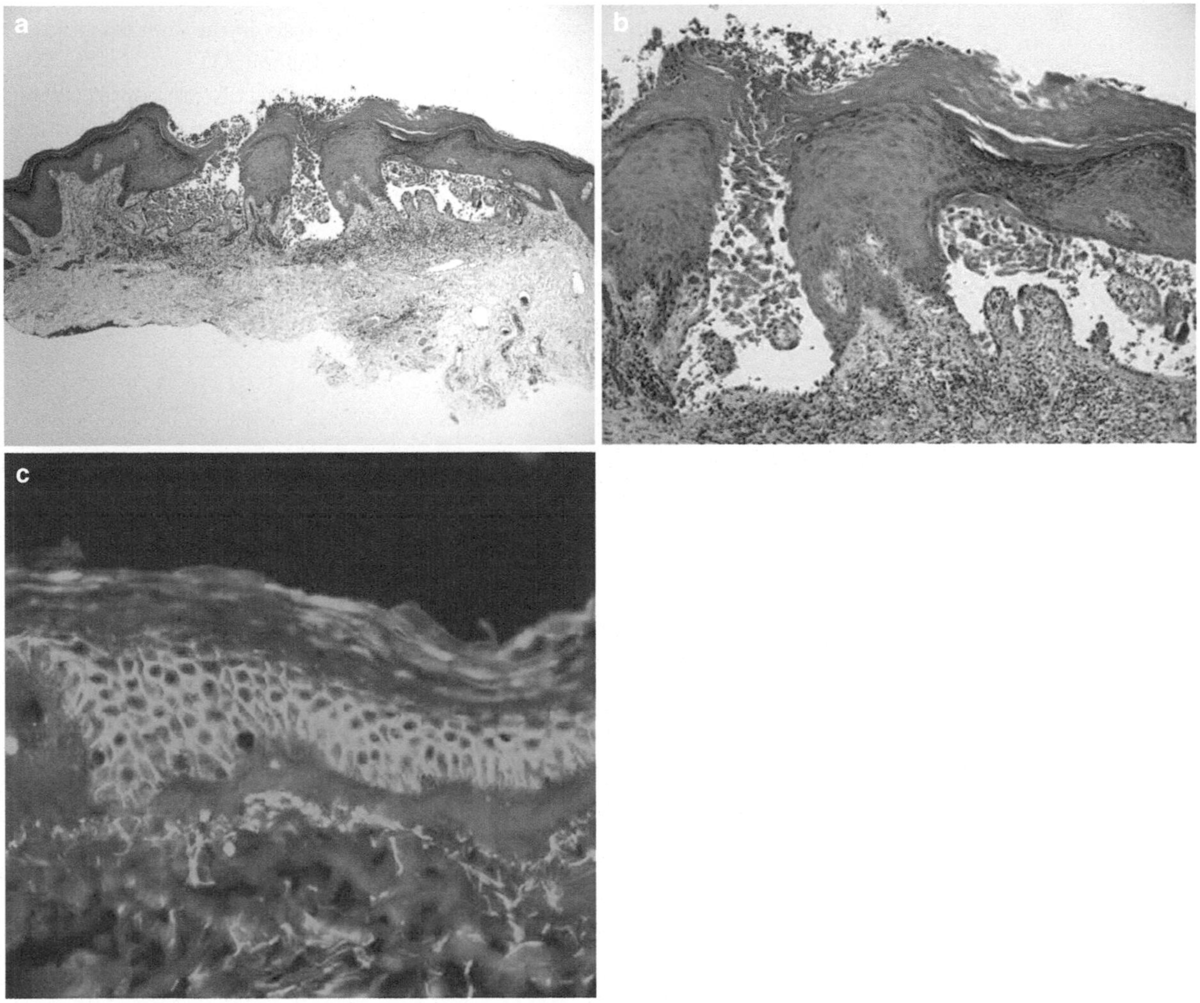

Fig. 57.31 (**a**) Histology of pemphigus vulgaris: Suprabasal acantholysis and formation of clefts. Papillomatous and acanthotic epidermis. (**b**) Magnification from (**a**). (**c**) Intraepidermal net-like direct immunofluoresence of IgG in the intercellular spaces

Treatment consists in topical steroids and antiseptics, long-term oral antibiotics and steroids. Some attempts have been made with oral cyclosporine [6], photodynamic therapy, and CO_2-laser [21], as well as with tacrolimus [39].

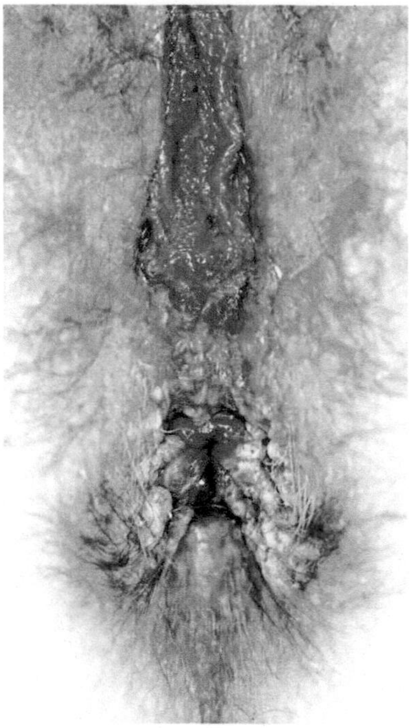

Fig. 57.32 Perivulvar and perianal aspect of benign familial chronic pemphigus (Hailey-Hailey)

57.6.2 Keratosis Follicularis (Darier's Disease)

Differential Diagnoses

- Hailey-Hailey's Disease
- Genital warts

Both Hailey-Hailey's disease and Darier's disease are chronic conditions. Darier's disease develops earlier, in childhood and adolescence. The initial lesions are horny papules involving the genitalia as well as other parts of the body. Lesions are seen particularly on the folds, the lower back, and other areas affected by seborrheic dermatitis such as the central face (Fig. 57.34). Important features are seen on the nails with longitudinal white and red lines, fragility, and splitting of the distal nail plate.

Histology is characterized by the presence of typical dyskeratotic keratinocytes, the so-called "corps ronds." There is acantholysis in the suprabasal layers and formation of clefts (Fig. 57.35).

Actual treatment of Darier's disease consists in oral acitretin. Its use is limited by severe side effects, particularly teratogenicity. For women of childbearing age, isotretinoin is an alternative with some better outcome. Other options are ablative therapies, such as laser, dermabrasion, photodynamic therapy, and topical 5-fluorouracil.

Other genetic dermatoses such as epidermolysis bullosa very rarely affect the genitoanal area and are not discussed here in detail.

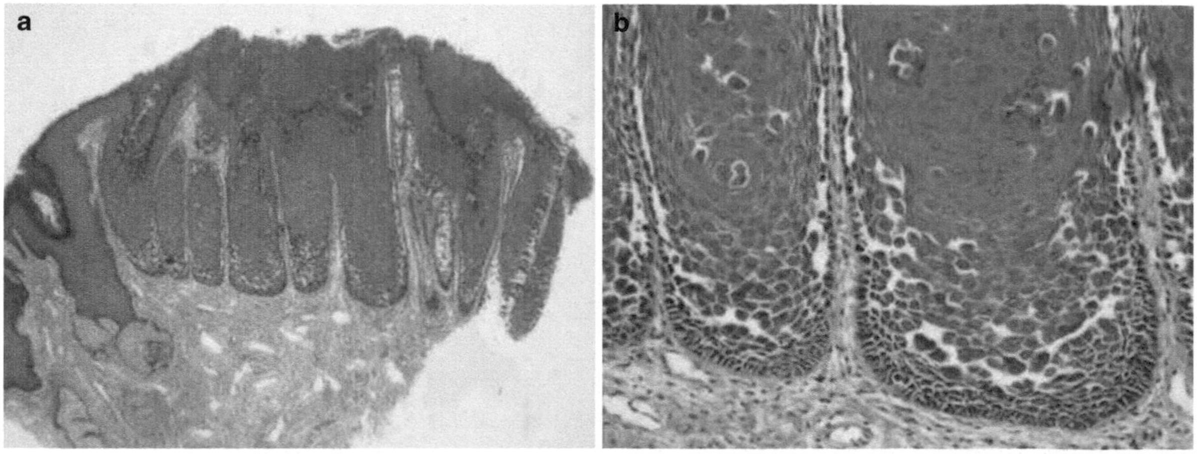

Fig. 57.33 Suprabasal acantholysis (magnification in Fig. 57.33b)

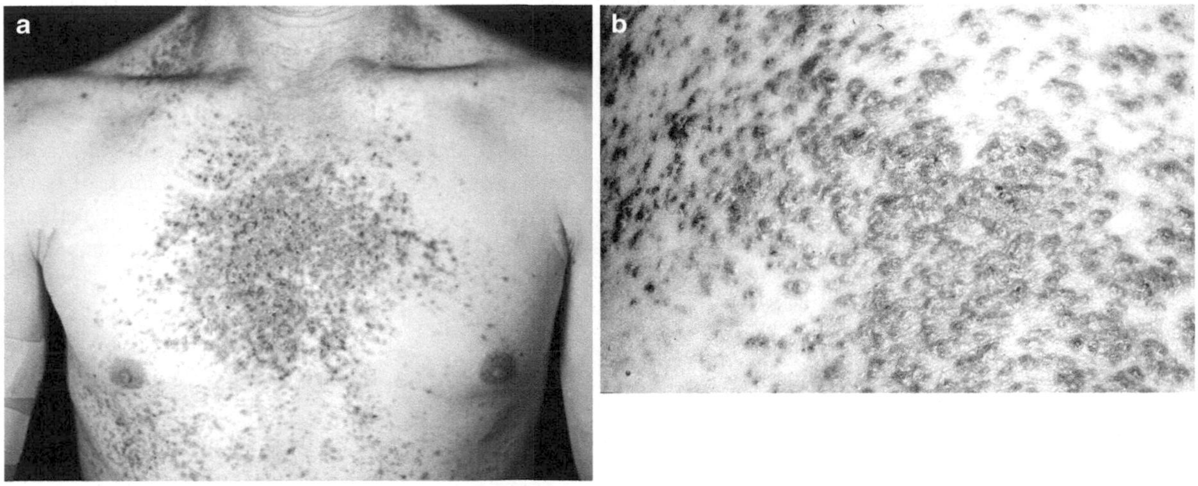

Fig. 57.34 (a) Keratosis follicularis (Darier's disease) on the breast. (b) Confluent horny papules

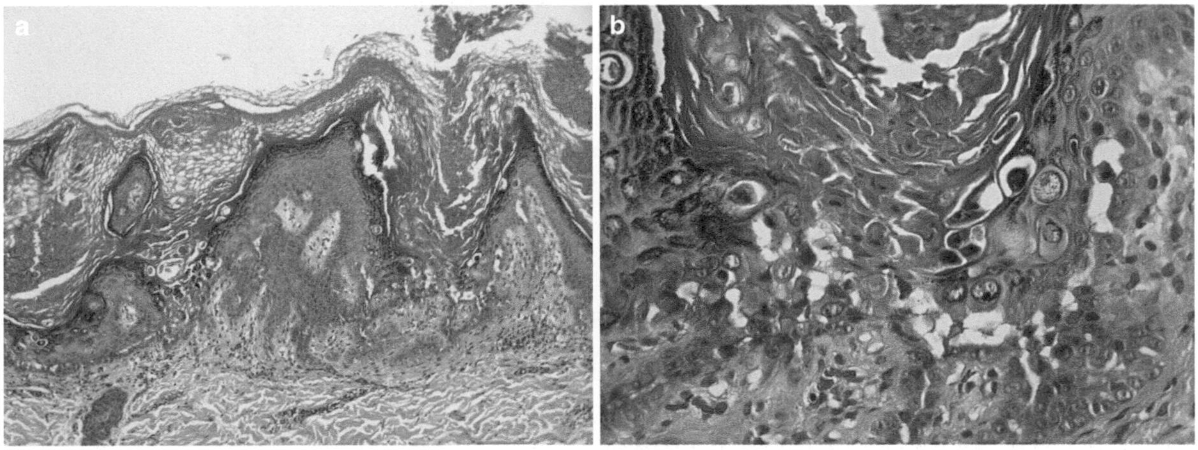

Fig. 57.35 (a) Histology: Dyskeratosis and circumscribed acantholysis. (b) "Corps ronds" within the basal epidermis (magnification from a)

57.7 Genitoanal Manifestations of Systemic Diseases

57.7.1 Necrolytic Migratory Erythema (Glucagonoma Syndrome)

Differential Diagnoses

- Pustular psoriasis
- Bullous dermatoses

Features of this disease are spreading painful periorificial erythematous and bullous lesions with healing in a serpiginous pattern. The eruption preferentially affects the lower abdomen and the genitoanal area of middle-aged persons with a female predominance. It has been associated with glucagonomas, which are rare alpha-cell tumors of the pancreas. The symptoms are weight loss, diabetes, anemia, stomatitis, and glossitis. The clinical picture can be mistaken with psoriasis and bullous dermatosis. Therapy consists in surgical removal of the tumor and symptomatic treatment.

57.7.2 Inflammatory Bowel Disease

57.7.2.1 Crohn's Disease

Differential Diagnoses

- Skin lesions in ulcerative Colitis
- Granulomatous disease
- Hidradenitis suppurativa
- Facticial disease
- Granuloma inguinale

In up to 30% of patients, intestinal Crohn's disease is accompanied by genitoanal erosions and ulceration, fistulae, and edema (Figs. 57.36–57.38). The so-called "knife-cut" fissures in the interlabial folds and the perianal skin are characteristic features of the disease.

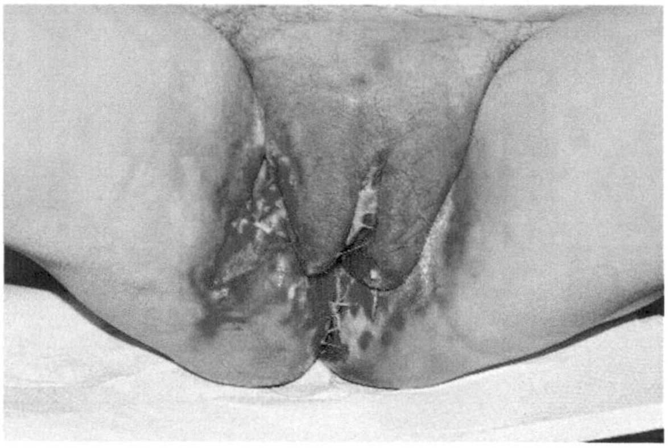

Fig. 57.36 Crohn's disease: Inguinal, perineal, and perianal ulcers and fistulation

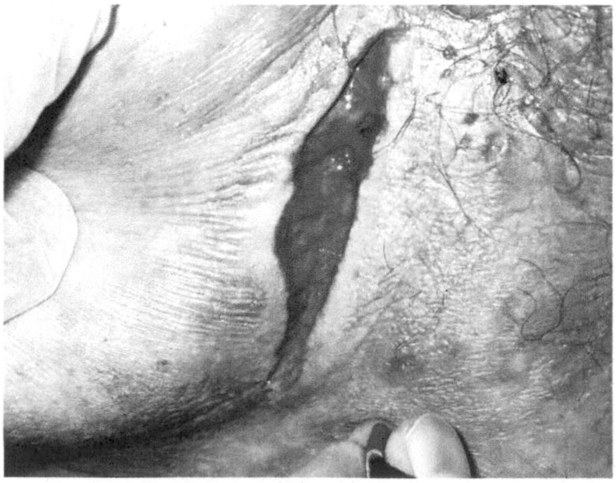

Fig. 57.37 Vulvar features of Crohn's disease: "Knife-cut" fissures

In the oral mucosa cheilitis and tag-like lesions are often present [18]. Healing of genitoanal lesions may result in scarring and chronic edema.

Histology consists in noncaseating granulomatous inflammation (Fig. 57.39). Cutaneous lesions of Crohn's disease may precede or follow the diagnosis of bowel disease. Early diagnosis of skin lesions at perianal, perineal sites, at the vulva and at the penis is as

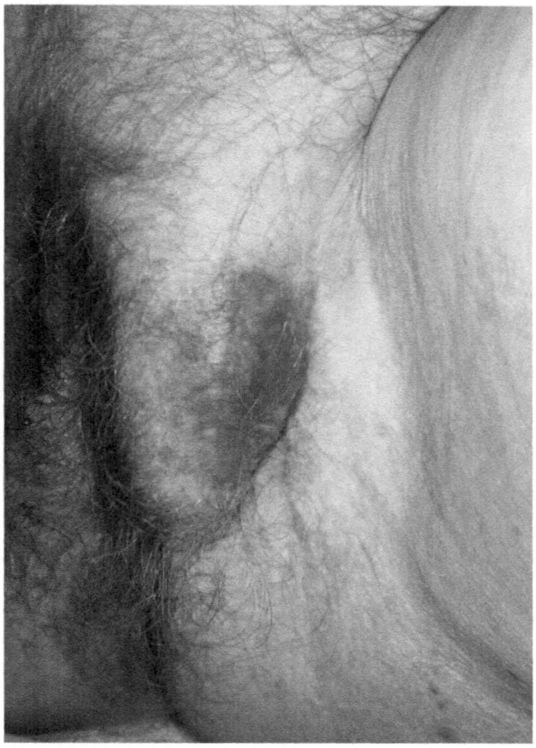

Fig. 57.38 Crohn's disease: edema of the left labium majus

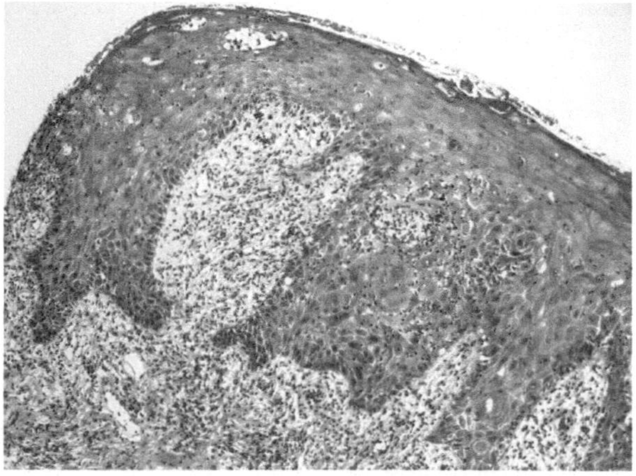

Fig. 57.39 Histology of Crohn's disease: Dense, granulomatous infiltrations with lymphocytes and giant histiocytes

mandatory as is the intestinal investigation. Therapy of genitoanal lesions linked to Crohn's disease depends on the activity of intestinal disease: Oral steroids, antibiotics such as metronidazole, sulfasalazine, and immunosuppressives. A further option seems to be infliximab as recently shown [4]. Topical therapies with steroids or tacrolimus are helpful only for superficial skin defects.

57.7.2.2 Ulcerative Colitis

Anogenital skin lesions are rarely seen in patients with ulcerative colitis. According to [19], genitoanal Behcet's disease and pyoderma gangrenosum may occur in patients suffering from inflammatory bowel disease.

57.8 Genitoanal Inflammatory Dermatoses

These conditions are the most frequently diagnosed genitoanal dermatoses (Table 57.1). Correct diagnosis often requires taking a biopsy for thorough histopathological investigation.

57.8.1 Intertrigo

Differential Diagnoses

- Tinea
- Candidiasis
- Eczema
- Erythrasma
- Psoriasis inversa

Table 57.1 Genitoanal Inflammatory dermatoses

• Intertrigo
• Lichen sclerosus
• Lichen planus
• Psoriasis
• Seborrheic dermatitis
• Plasma cell balanitis, plasma cell vulvitis
• Hidradenitis suppurativa
• Erythema multiforme
• Stevens–Johnson syndrome
• Fixed drug eruption
• Behcet's disease
• Eczema (atopic eczema, contact eczema)
• Lichen simplex

This is a nonspecific inflammation of the folds. Important differential diagnoses are tinea, candidiasis, psoriasis, and erythrasma. Intertrigo is caused by sweating and heat. Risk factors are diabetes, immobility, obesity, and incontinence. Superinfection with bacteria and candida is a regular finding.

The topical treatment is nonspecific with zinc ointment and mild corticosteroids combined with antibacterial or antifungal agents.

57.8.2 Lichen Sclerosus

Differential Diagnoses

- Intraepithelial neoplasia
- Lichen planus, erosive lichen planus
- Paget's disease
- Vitiligo
- Bullous pemphigoid

The etiology of lichen sclerosus is unknown. Historically Darier defined the disorder as a variant of lichen planus [10]. Today different hypotheses exist: infective origin, inheritance, and autoimmunity-related. Borrelia burgdorferi has been suspected. However, no spirochetes were found in vulvar lichen sclerosus tissue [13].

The disease affects all ages and all parts of the body. However, it is preferentially located in the anogenital area. The primary lesion is a white atrophic papule or macule (Fig. 57.40). The lesions may be disseminated

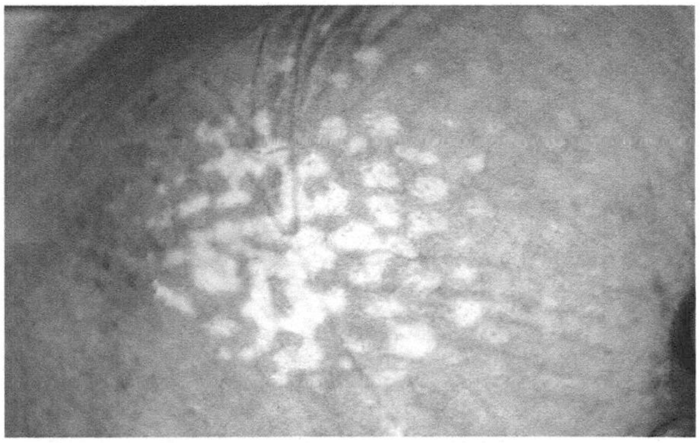

Fig. 57.40 Lichen sclerosus: Whitish maculopapular lesions

or confluent forming shiny white sclerotic plaques. Secondary bullae, atrophy, whitening of the skin as well as teleangiectasias, and purpura are frequently seen (Fig. 57.41). Lichen sclerosus is a condition where Köbner's phenomenon is common with new lesions at previous burns, surgical scars, and sites of pressure.

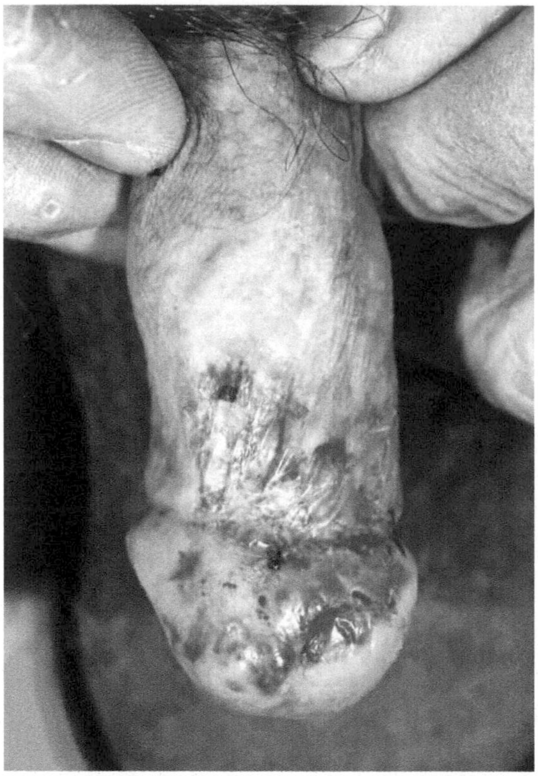

Fig. 57.41 Severe lichen sclerosus of the penis with hemorrhages and sclerotic lesions

There is a female preponderance. As many as 50% of affected patients have initial lesions before puberty. The more intense inflammation is the more intense pruritus. Gradual destruction of vulval tissue and perianal skin may lead to resorption of the labia minora and constriction of the introitus (Fig. 57.42). Severe vulval lichen sclerosus is known as kraurosis vulvae. In men, the glans and prepuce are involved with the consequence of meatal stenosis and phimosis (so-called balanitis xerotica obliterans) (Fig. 57.8).

The histology of lichen sclerosus is characterized by a flattened epidermis with hyperkeratosis and partially elongated rete ridges. The upper dermis is hyalinized. Liquefaction degeneration at the dermoepidermal junction with edema of the papillary layer may form clefts (Fig. 57.43). Dilated vessels and extravasated erythrocytes are further typical findings. A band-like aggregation of chronic inflammatory cells is seen in the middermis.

An important differential diagnosis is vitiligo. Both disorders, vitiligo and lichen sclerosus, may coexist. Scarring bullous disorders such as bullous pemphigoid may pose problems. The clinical picture of lichen sclerosus and lichen planus may be very similar. There is some overlap with regard to histology. Sometimes differentiation appears almost

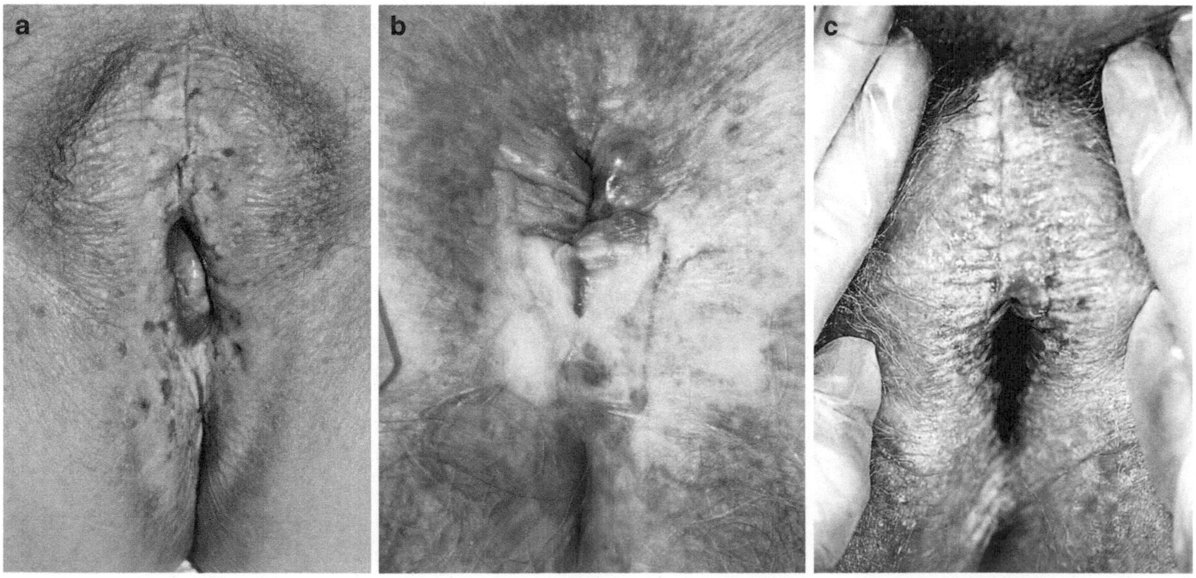

Fig. 57.42 (**a**) Vulvar lichen sclerosus with ecchymosis, scarring, and loss of the labia minora. (**b**) Sclerotic ivory-white skin with fissures. (**c**) Atrophic vulva: Defect of labia minora (Kraurosis vulvae)

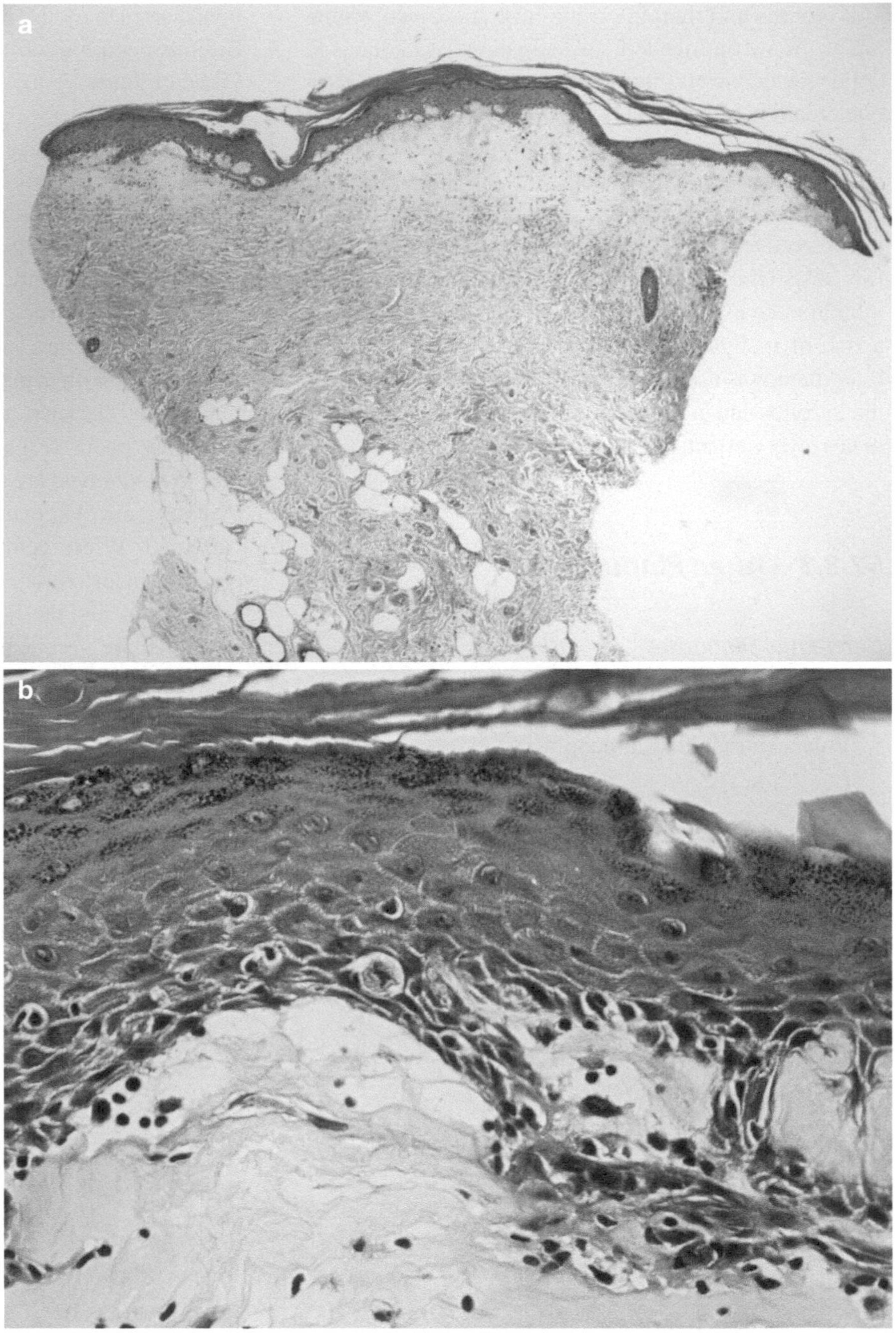

Fig. 57.43 (**a**) Histology of lichen sclerosus: Hyperkeratotic, flattened epidermal layer. Vacuolated degeneration of basal cells and subepidermal band-like aggregation of inflammatory cells in the mid-dermis. (**b**) Hyalinization and subepidermal cleft

impossible. Direct immunofluorescence may be of help (Fig. 57.52).

Chronic lichen sclerosus is a risk factor for squamous cell cancer of the vulva and of the penis. Apparently, vulvar and penile cancer have a dual etiology since high-risk HPV is detectable in about 40–50% of these malignancies. Regarding vulvar cancer, an association with oncogenic HPV types is seen in younger women. In older women, vulvar cancer lesions are preferentially associated with lichen sclerosus. The same seems to be true with regard to penile cancer [9, 15] (see Chaps. 35 and 37 page 457 and page 489).

The management of lichen sclerosus is primarily local with a potent corticosteroid ointment used nightly

1–2 months and then intermittently. A soap substitute has to be recommended. Investigations of Sideri and colleagues showed that neither estrogen nor testosterone cream is of help [41].

Another option seems to be topical retinoid, particularly in hyperkeratotic lichen sclerosus [43]. The calcineurin inhibitors tacrolimus and pimecrolimus should be reserved for acute disease where corticosteroids failed [36, 44]. Under no circumstances should calcineurin inhibitors be used as maintenance therapy since there is a risk of malignant transformation. Surgery including laser therapy is useful only in scarring and narrowing of the introitus and in preneoplastic and invasive lesions. In males a very effective therapy is circumcision.

57.8.3 Lichen Planus

Differential Diagnoses

- Lichen sclerosus
- Vulvar intraepithelial neoplasia
- Penile intraepithelial neoplasia
- Bullous pemphigoid
- Lichen nitidus
- Zoon's balanitis
- Zoon's vulvitis

Manifestation sites of this inflammatory, possibly autoimmune, dermatosis are the skin, the genital, and the oral mucous membranes. The lesions of lichen planus (Syn. lichen ruber planus) use to be very pruritus. The lesions are small, flat, polygonal, violaceous papules with white Whickham's striae on the top. Erosive, hypertrophic, atrophic, and annular lesions may occur (Figs. 57.44 and 57.45). Typical genital sites involved are the glans penis, prepuce, anal and vulvar areas. Vagina and vestibulum are generally not affected. While genital mucosal areas are rarely involved, skin lesions are frequently seen on the wrists, legs, forearms, and the sacral region (Fig. 57.46). The finger nails are frequently involved with nail dystrophy. In severe cases scarring may occur. Lichen planus is a self-limiting disease. Healing may lead to hyperpigmentation and atrophy (Fig. 57.47). In

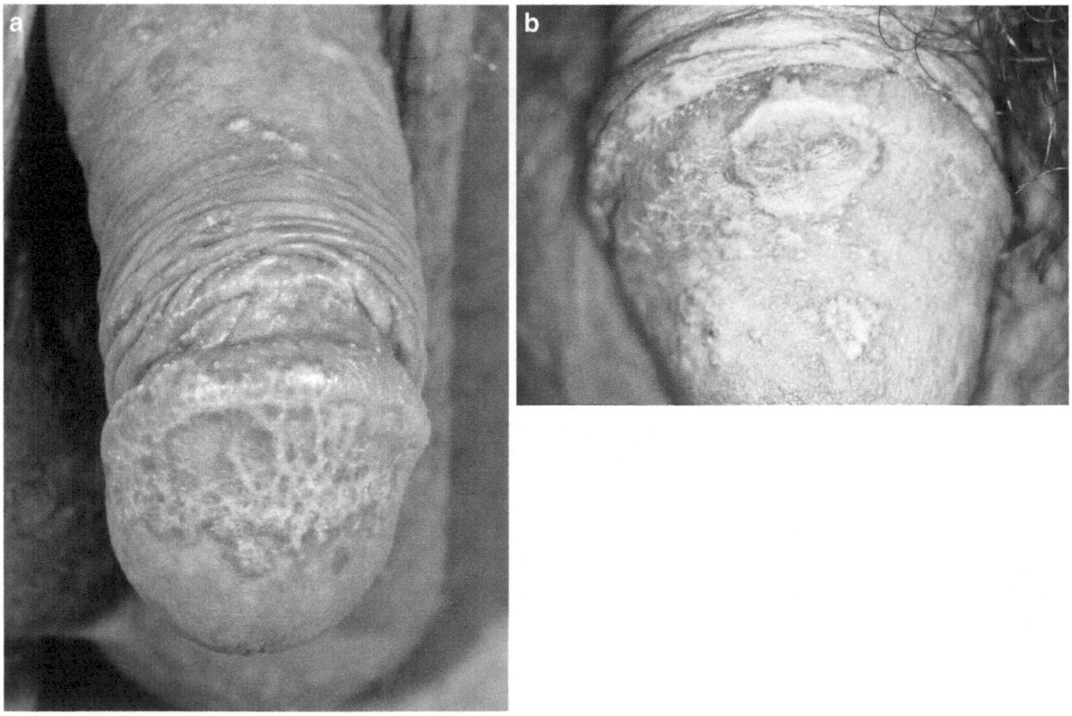

Fig. 57.44 (**a**) (Male). Lichen planus: reticular whitish lesions on the glans and coronal sulcus. (**b**) Anular lichen planus

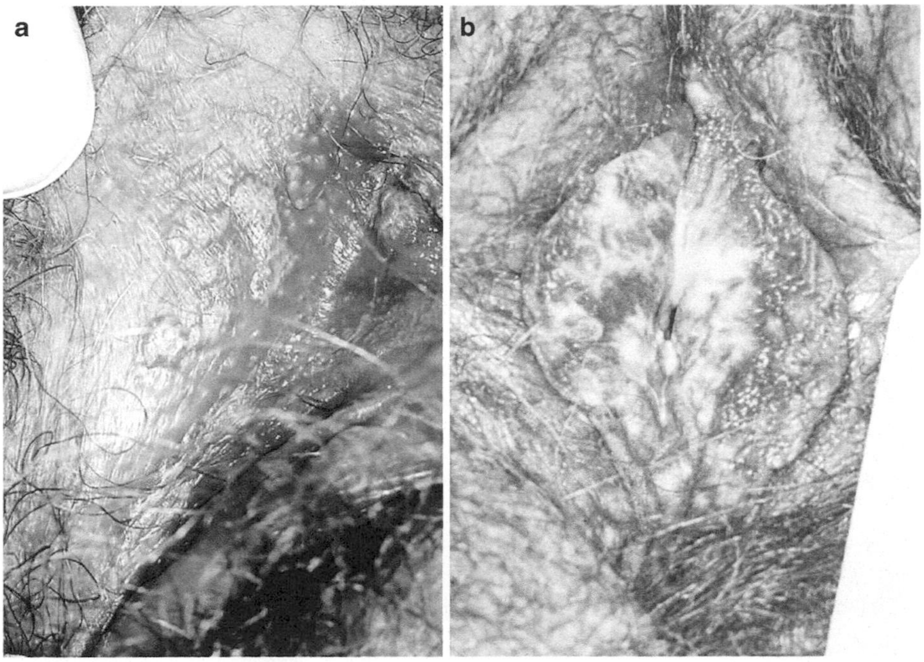

Fig. 57.45 (**a**) Vulval lichen planus with polygonal papules. (**b**) White reticulate papular lichen planus on the labia minora

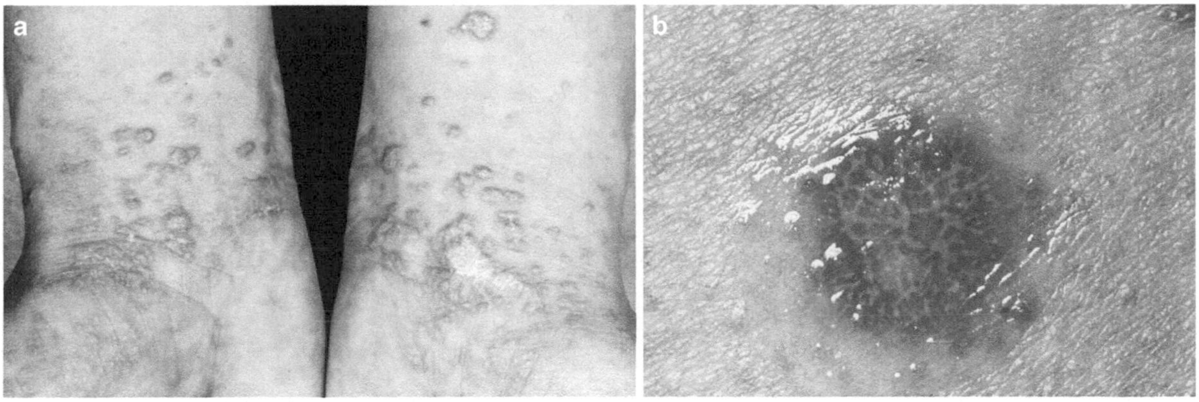

Fig. 57.46 (**a**) Papular lesions of lichen ruber on the wrist. (**b**) Wickham's striae under oil immersion

both genders the oral mucosa is a frequent target (Fig. 57.48).

Erosive lichen planus affects the inner aspects of the vulva and the vagina. It is the commonest form of lichen planus in the genital area of the female. Adhesions, fusions, and scarring of the labia minora and the clitoris may develop (Fig. 57.49) and mimic lichen sclerosus. Cutaneous lichen planus lesions, however, are infrequently seen. Coexisting oral lesions are common (Fig. 57.50).

The so-called vulvovaginal-gingival syndrome, which was described by Pelisse and coworkers [37], is characterized by burning and painful sensations as well as postcoital bleeding. Vaginitis and stenosis may occur. Less frequently, the perianal area and even the cervix can be affected [38]. Erosive oral lesions affect the buccal surfaces, the gingiva, and less frequently, the tongue (Fig. 57.50).

The course of lichen planus is generally good. However, erosive forms tend to become chronic. Both oral and genital lichen planus show an increased potential of malignancy. So far, a similar risk has been reported in the vulvovaginal-syndrome.

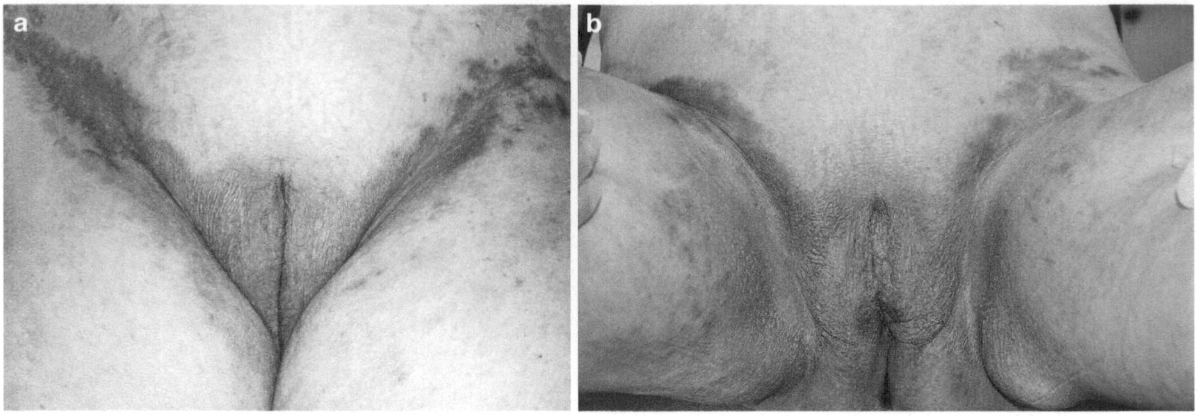

Fig. 57.47 Postinflammatory hyperpigmentation of lichen planus: (**a**) Dusky red to violaceous pigmented macular lesions on the groins. (**b**) Vulvar aspect

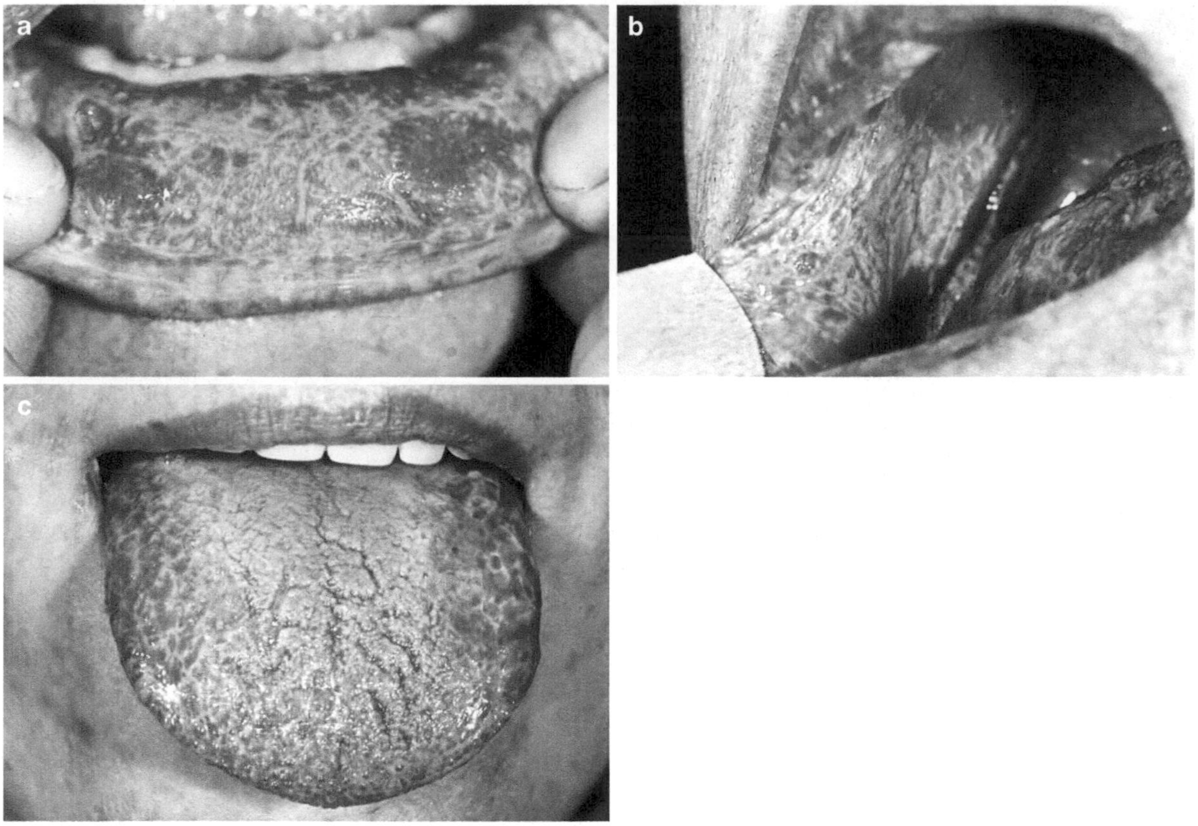

Fig. 57.48 (**a**) Lichen planus: involvement of the lips. (**b**) Reticular oral lichen planus on the buccal mucosa. (**c**) Lichen planus on the tongue

Histologically, lichen planus shows characteristic features of the epidermis with hyperkeratosis and a focal increase of the granular layer. Acanthosis is irregular with a sawtooth appearance of rete ridges (Fig. 57.51). In the superficial dermis, there is a band-like, mainly lymphocytic, infiltrate resulting in basal cell liquefaction. In erosive lichen planus, vacuolization of basal keratinocytes and

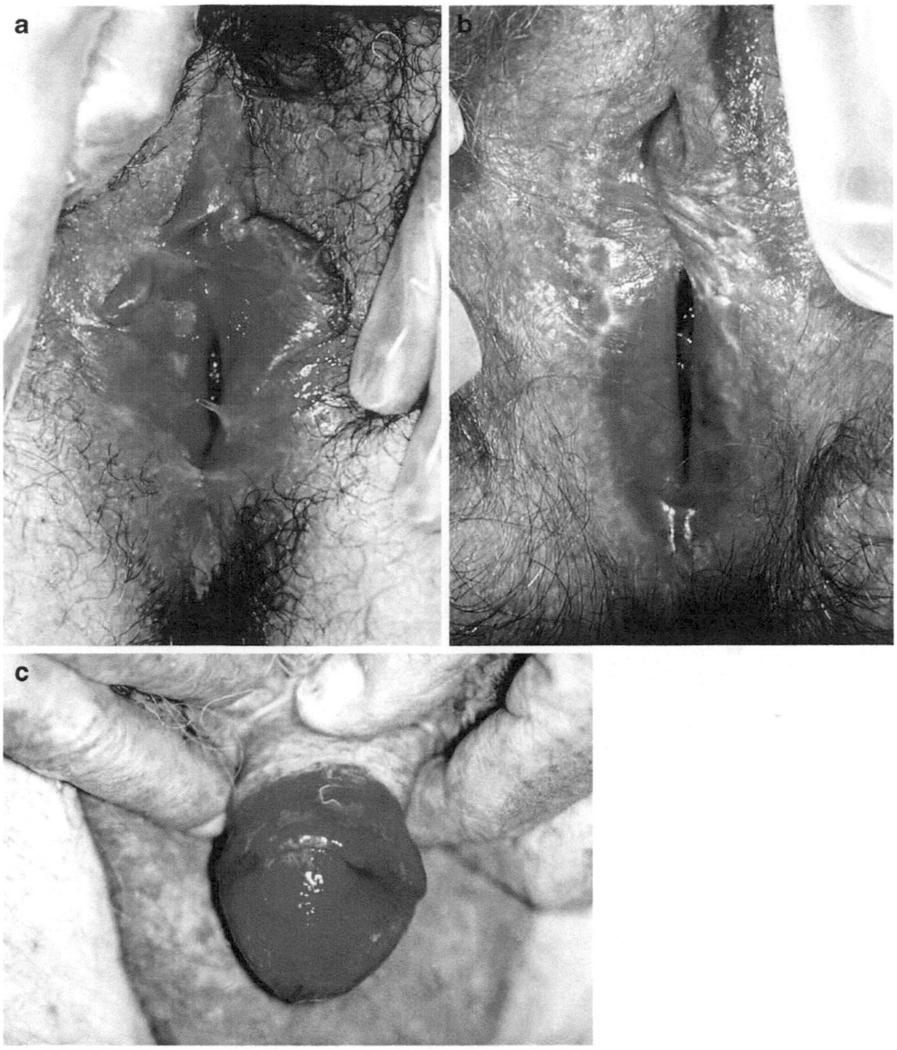

Fig. 57.49 (**a**) Mild erosive vulval lichen planus. (**b**) Initial scarring of erosive lichen planus. (**c**) Erosive lichen planus of the prepuce and glans

blister formation may be seen. A specific finding of lichen planus is the direct immunofluorescence staining for fibrinogen at the basement membrane zone (Fig. 57.52).

Clinically there are clear overlaps with lichen sclerosus. Differential diagnosis from intraepithelial neoplasia (VIN and PIN) as well as from lichen sclerosus and bullous pemphigoid is important and should always include taking a biopsy for histology and immunofluorescence.

Treatment is unsatisfactory. Drugs of choice are corticosteroids either locally or systemically. Erosive lichen planus is also primarily treated symptomatically by mild antiseptic and anti-inflammatory soaks and baths. The first-line treatment is a potent topical corticosteroid. For vulval and vaginal erosions suppositories and foam steroid preparations should be used. In patients with vulvovaginal-gingival-syndrome, attempts were made with topical cyclosporine and retinoic acid, however, without success. Again, only limited success was obtained with the calcineurin inhibitors tacrolimus and pimecrolimus [7, 24]. Treatment of nonresponsive cases is difficult. Oral steroids or cyclosporine appear to have some effect. Dapsone, azathioprine, chloroquine, and minocycline are of limited effect.

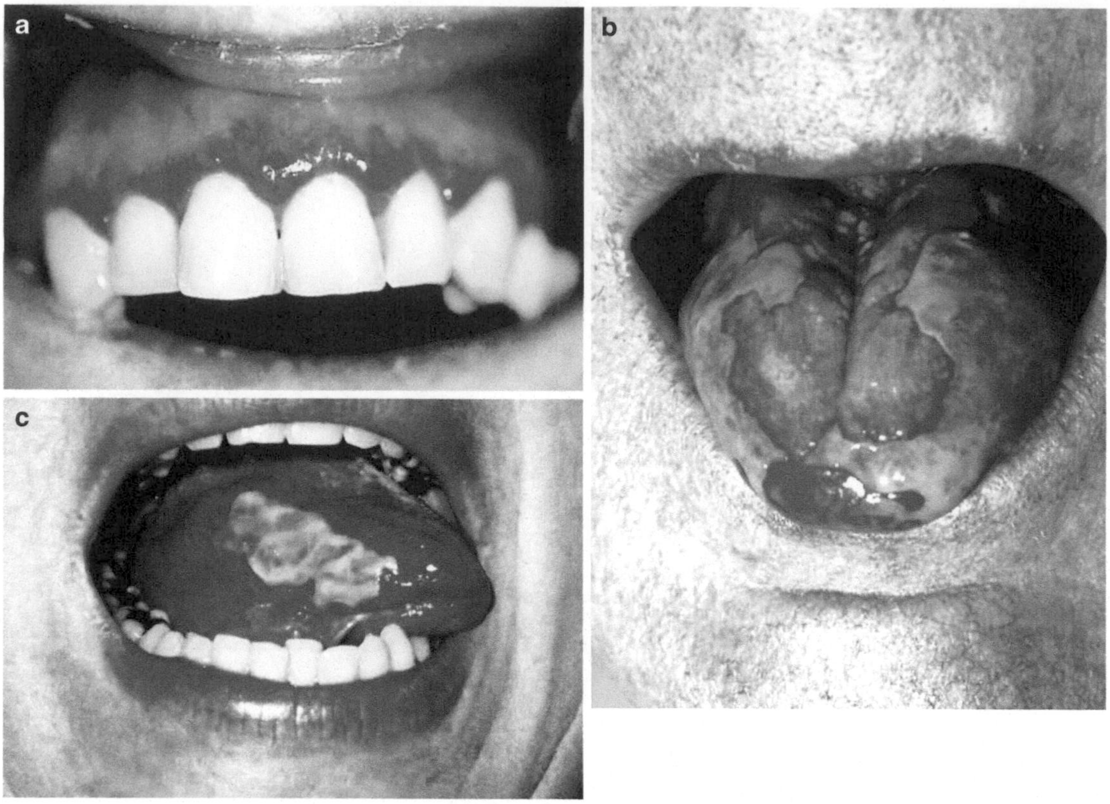

Fig. 57.50 (**a**) Erosive oral lichen planus: erosive gingivitis. (**b**) Desquamative lichen planus of the tongue. (**c**) Almost complete desquamation of epithelium of the tongue

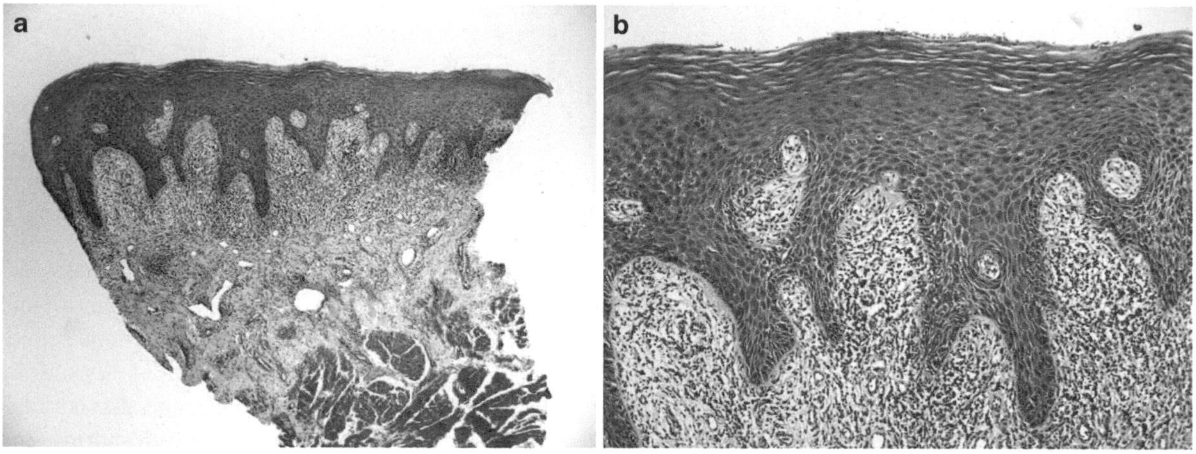

Fig. 57.51 (**a**) Histology of lichen planus: "Saw-tooth like" elongated rete ridges and subepidermal band-like lymphomatoid infiltration. (**b**) Magnification from (**a**)

57.8.4 Psoriasis

Differential Diagnoses

- Bowen's disease
- Erythroplasia of Queyrat
- Tinea
- Candidiasis
- Syphilis II
- Genital warts
- Reiter's disease
- Eczema

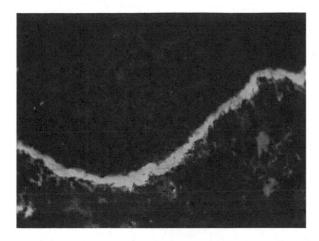

Fig. 57.52 Typical features of lichen planus. Direct immunofluoresence of the basement membrane zone for fibrinogen

The primary lesion of psoriasis is a itching, sharply outlined, erythematous papule, tending to growth and confluence. Lesions may be plaques with or without silvery scales on the penis, vulva, perineum, and the perianal skin (Fig. 57.53). The skin of the natal cleft often shows fissuring. Mucosal surfaces are not affected. Flexural psoriasis, also called psoriasis inversa, is very common. Psoriasis is an inherited disorder seen in about 3–5% of the population. Anogenital lesions may be the only manifestations. Psoriasis lesions at other parts of the body are helpful for diagnosis. Preferential sites involved are knees, elbows, sacrum, and scalp. At the nails, subungual hyperkeratosis, pitting and onychodystrophy are signs of psoriasis (Fig. 57.54). Individual trigger factors exist. Flexural lesions may be due to friction and occluding

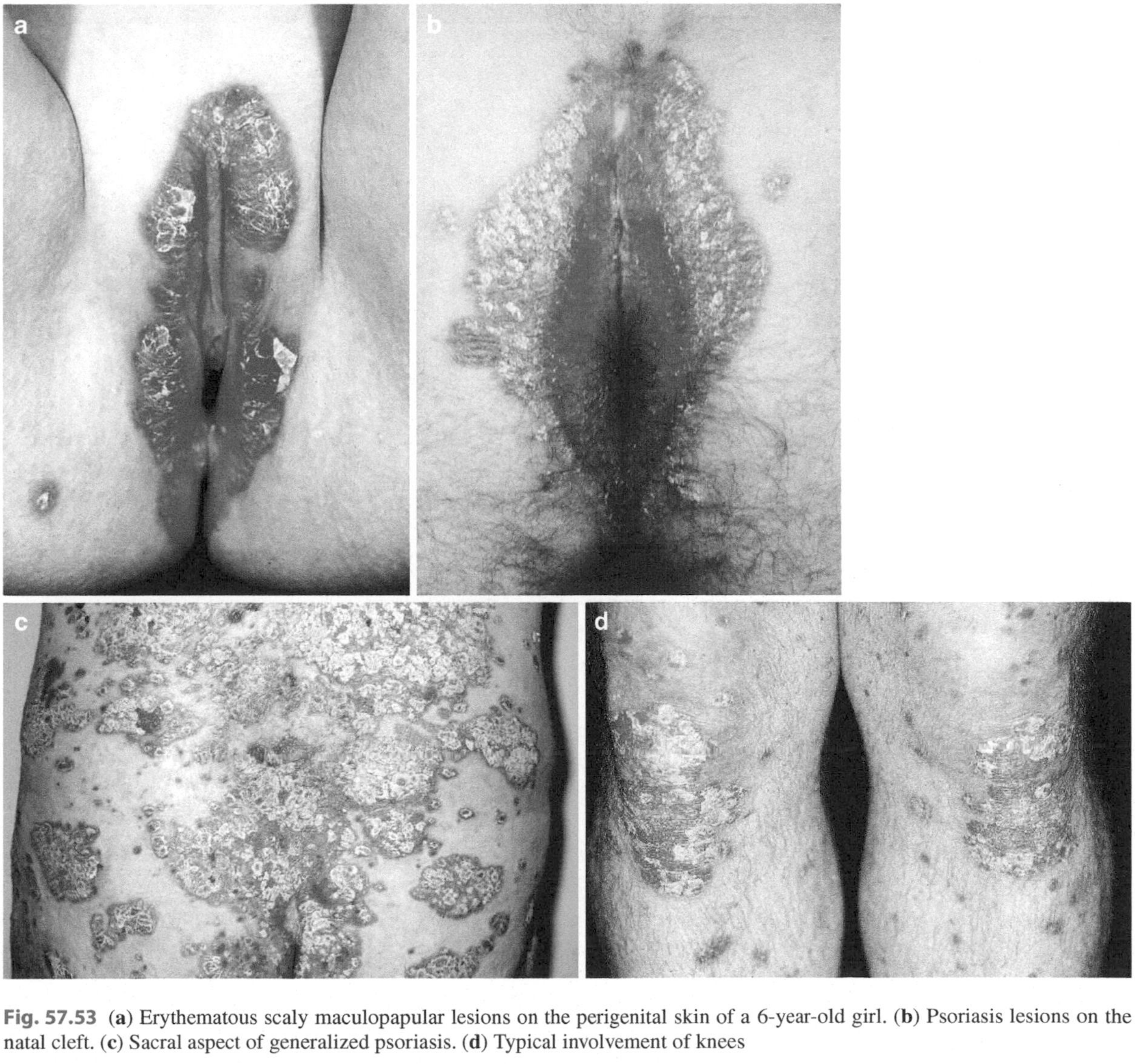

Fig. 57.53 (**a**) Erythematous scaly maculopapular lesions on the perigenital skin of a 6-year-old girl. (**b**) Psoriasis lesions on the natal cleft. (**c**) Sacral aspect of generalized psoriasis. (**d**) Typical involvement of knees

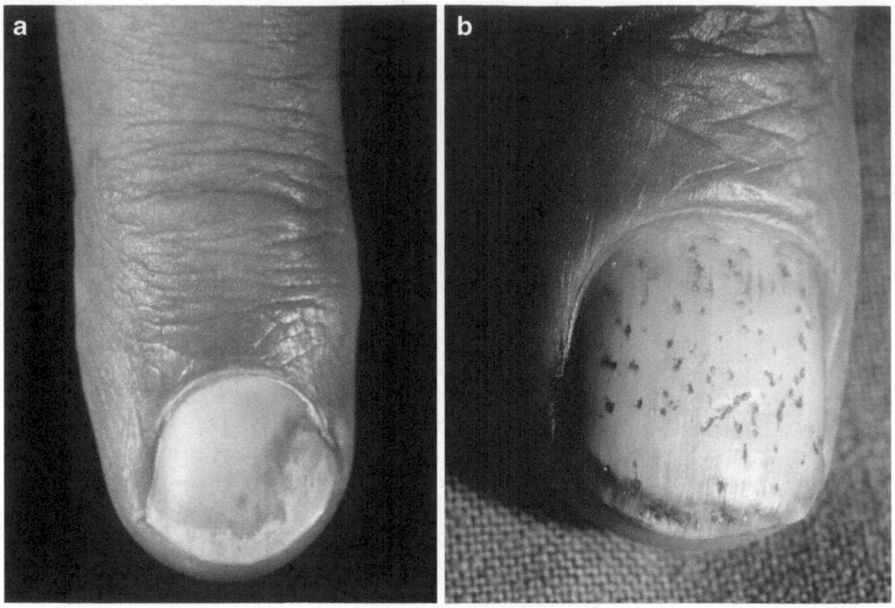

Fig. 57.54 Psoriatic nails. (**a**) subungual psoriasis. (**b**) Psoriasis pits of the nail plate

conditions at these sites. Lesions may appear at sites of trauma (so-called Koebner's phenomenon). Other trigger factors include streptococcal infections.

In Reiter's disease, nonsuppurative polyarthritis following an enteric and lower-genital tract infection psoriasiform skin lesions coexist with sexually transmitted infections (mainly Chlamydia), with urethritis or cervicitis and conjunctivitis together with so-called circinate balanitis (Fig. 57.55), rarely vulvitis and the so-called keratosis blennorrhagica. The latter consists in keratotic rupia-like lesions on the plantar aspect of the feet (see Chap 8 on Chlamydia trachomatis, page103). Histology is indistinguishable from pustular psoriasis. HIV-patients may exhibit more severe disease than individuals with normal immunity.

Histology of flexural psoriasis sometimes does not show the typical features of psoriasis which are parakeratosis, acanthosis with elongated rete ridges, thinned granular cell layer, and agglomerations of neutrophils in the corneal layer (Fig. 57.56).

Generally, systemic therapy of psoriasis with so-called "biologicals" has made immense progress in the last decade. Second-line systemic treatments are oral methotrexate, oral retinoids, or cyclosporine A.

In flexural psoriasis, however, such therapies have not yet proven as effective as at other cutaneous sites. Psoriasis at the genitoanal skin is effectively treated with a moderately potent topical corticosteroid. The

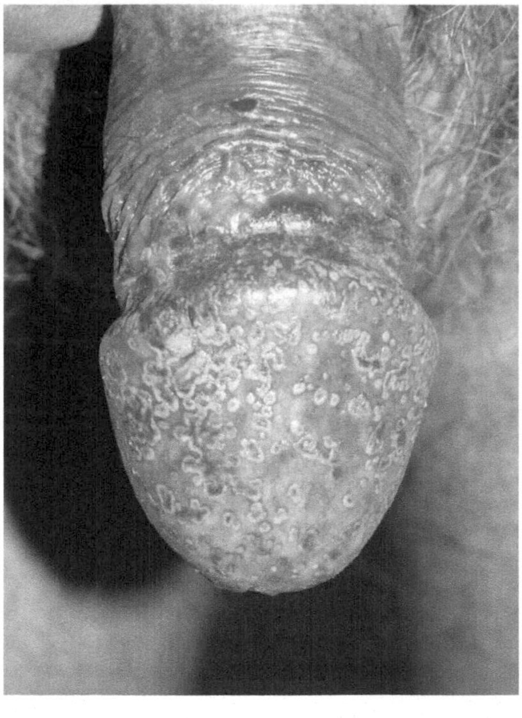

Fig. 57.55 Balanitis circinata associated with Reiter's disease

effective topical treatments of psoriasis at other areas of the skin such as dithranol, calcipotriol, and tar are irritant and not tolerated on the genitoanal skin. Tar and particularly ultraviolet radiation and psoralen UVA

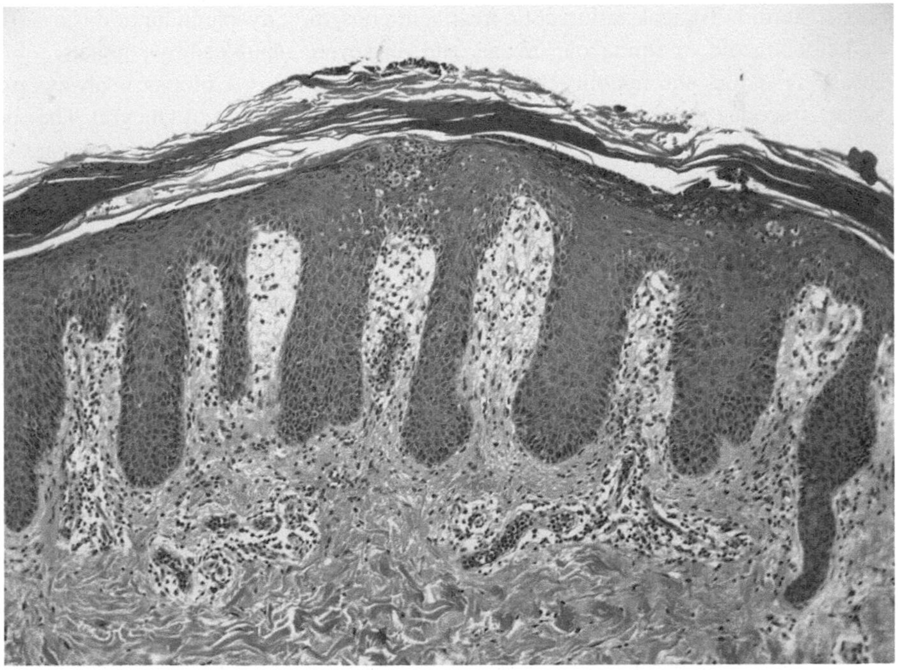

Fig. 57.56 Histology of psoriasis: acanthotic epidermis with parakeratosis and elongated rete ridges. Neutrophils in the corneal layer

psoralen plus UVA (PUVA) treatment of genitoanal skin sites is strictly contraindicated because of a possible risk of malignant conversion.

57.8.5 Seborrheic Dermatitis

Differential Diagnoses

- Psoriasis
- Intertrigo
- Candidiasis

Seborrheic dermatitis is a frequent finding in seborrheic areas, which are the scalp, the centrofacial skin and forehead, the ears, and the chest. The genitoanal and perianal folds are often involved by itchy pink-red erythematous lesions, covered with yellowish fatty scales (Fig. 57.57). It is assumed that seborrheic dermatitis is a genetically determined disease with *Pityrosporum ovale,* a commensal surface lipophilic yeast.

Histologically, eczematous and psoriasiform features are seen.

Differential diagnosis are psoriasis and intertrigo as well as candidiasis. Therapy is with a topical moderate

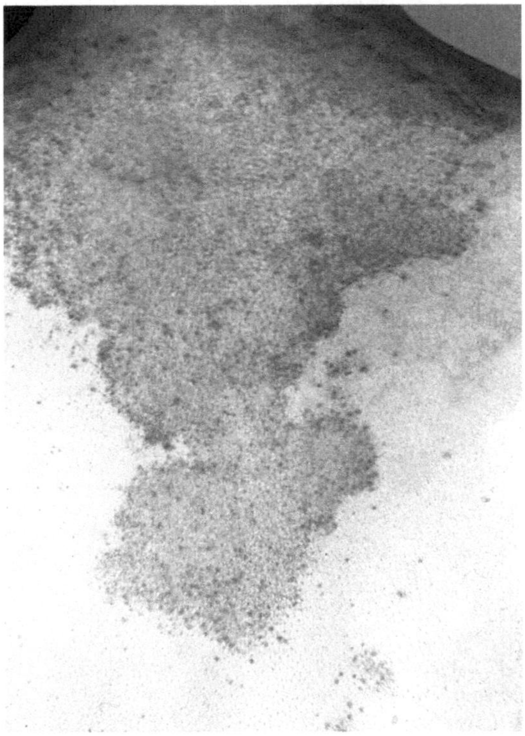

Fig. 57.57 Seborrheic dermatitis: orange-pink, discrete scaly lesions on the back

corticosteroid. Topical antimycotic treatment consists of ketoconazole or imidazole creams and, in severe cases, systemic antimycotic treatment with fluconazole, itraconazole, or ketoconazole.

57.8.6 Plasma Cell Balanitis and Plasma Cell Vulvitis

Differential Diagnoses

- Penile intraepithelial neoplasia
- Vulvar intraepithelial neoplasia
- Fixed drug eruption

Plasma cell balanitis (Zoon's balanitis) is diagnosed more frequently than plasma cell vulvitis [48]. Etiology has not been understood so far. There is some doubt whether plasma cell vulvitis is indeed a specific disease entity or some type of reaction pattern to another inflammatory process.

Clinical features in the male consist in red moist, shiny patches on the glans and the inner prepuce (Fig. 57.58). On the female genitalia, similarly, a circumscribed red patch is seen on the labia majora or minora. The lesions are burning. There may be dyspareunia or dysuria. In some cases bleeding occurs induced by contacts.

A biopsy is always mandatory to exclude erythroplasia of Queyrat. The epidermis appears flattened and basal keratinocytes are often elongated. A band-like plasma cellular infiltrate with exocytosis into the epidermis lies in the upper dermis. Capillaries are dilated with some hemosiderin deposits in the surrounding (Fig. 57.59).

Treatment consists in topical corticosteroid ointment. An alternative is topical clindamycin. The effect of imiquimod is not yet established in clinical studies.

57.8.7 Hidradenitis Suppurativa

Differential Diagnosis

- Folliculitis
- Deep bacterial and fungal infection
- Crohn's disease
- Lymphoma

The clinical features are those of acne of the flexures with bridged comedones, nodular lesions (Fig. 57.60), and bridged scars. It is a chronic inflammatory disease with the target of follicular epithelium rather than apocrine glands in the anogenital region, the axilla, breast,

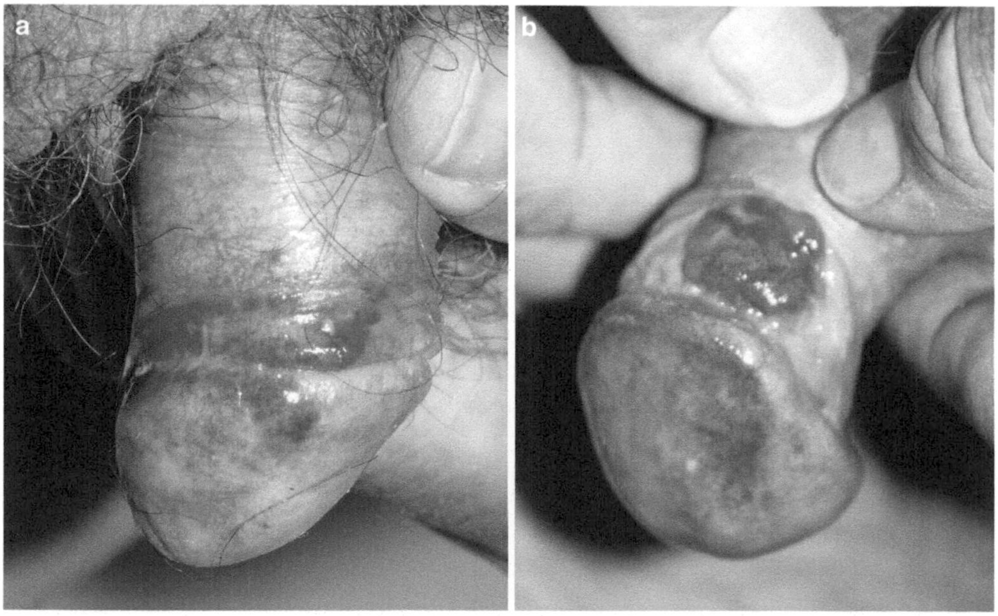

Fig. 57.58 (**a**) Zoon's balanitis with red macules. (**b**) Patches of balanitis plasmacellularis at the glans and foreskin

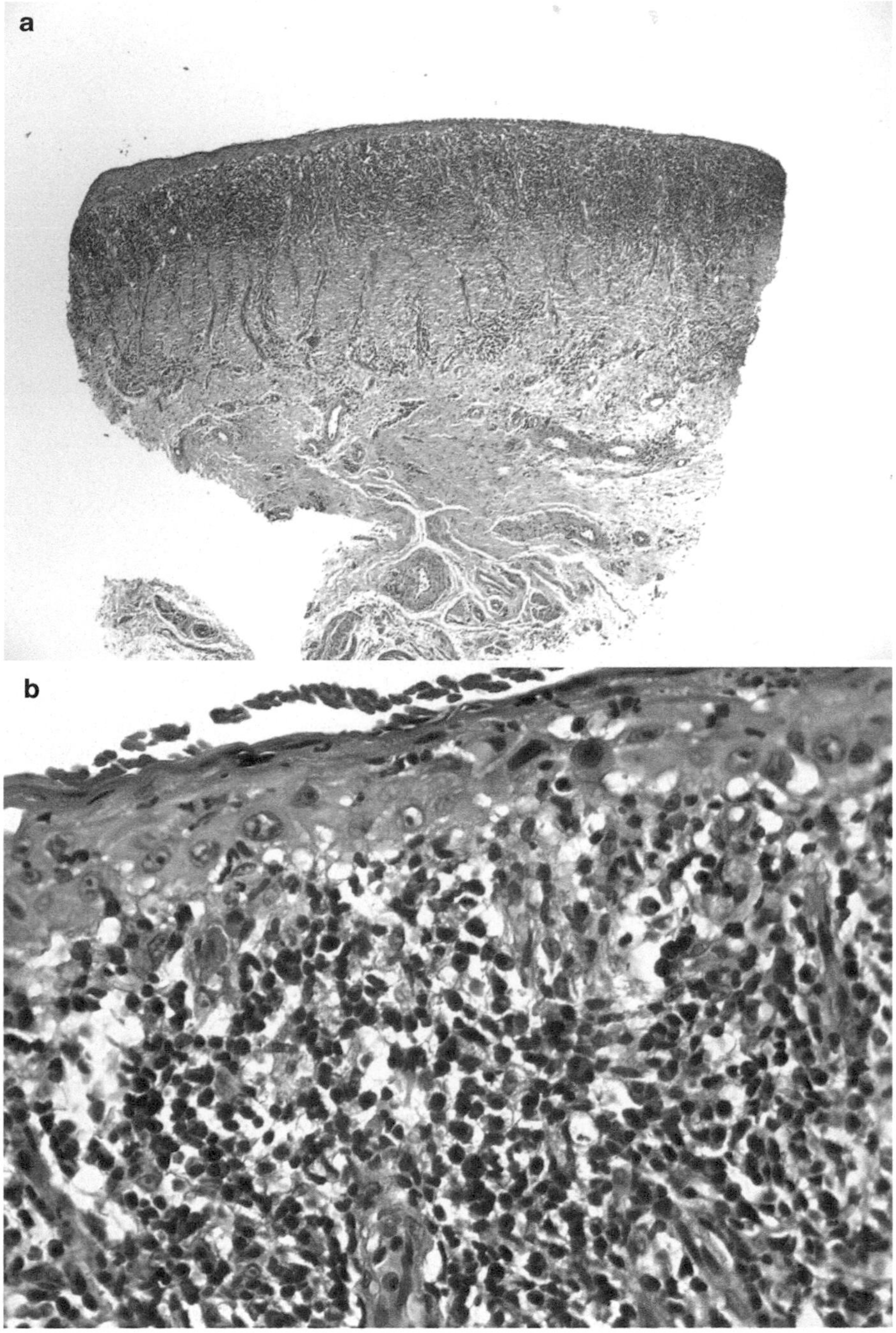

Fig. 57.59 Histology: Flattened epidermis with spongiosis and infiltrating plasma cells. Intense inflammatory subepidermal infiltrate

periumbilical skin, and neck. The triggering factor is not yet clearly defined. Bacterial infections are not regarded as causative. Hormonal factors such as elevated free testosterone seem to play a role. However, obesity also contributes. Most affected patients are strong smokers. Hidradenitis is not seen in prepubertal children and regression is frequent in postmenopausal women. The typical features are painful papules and

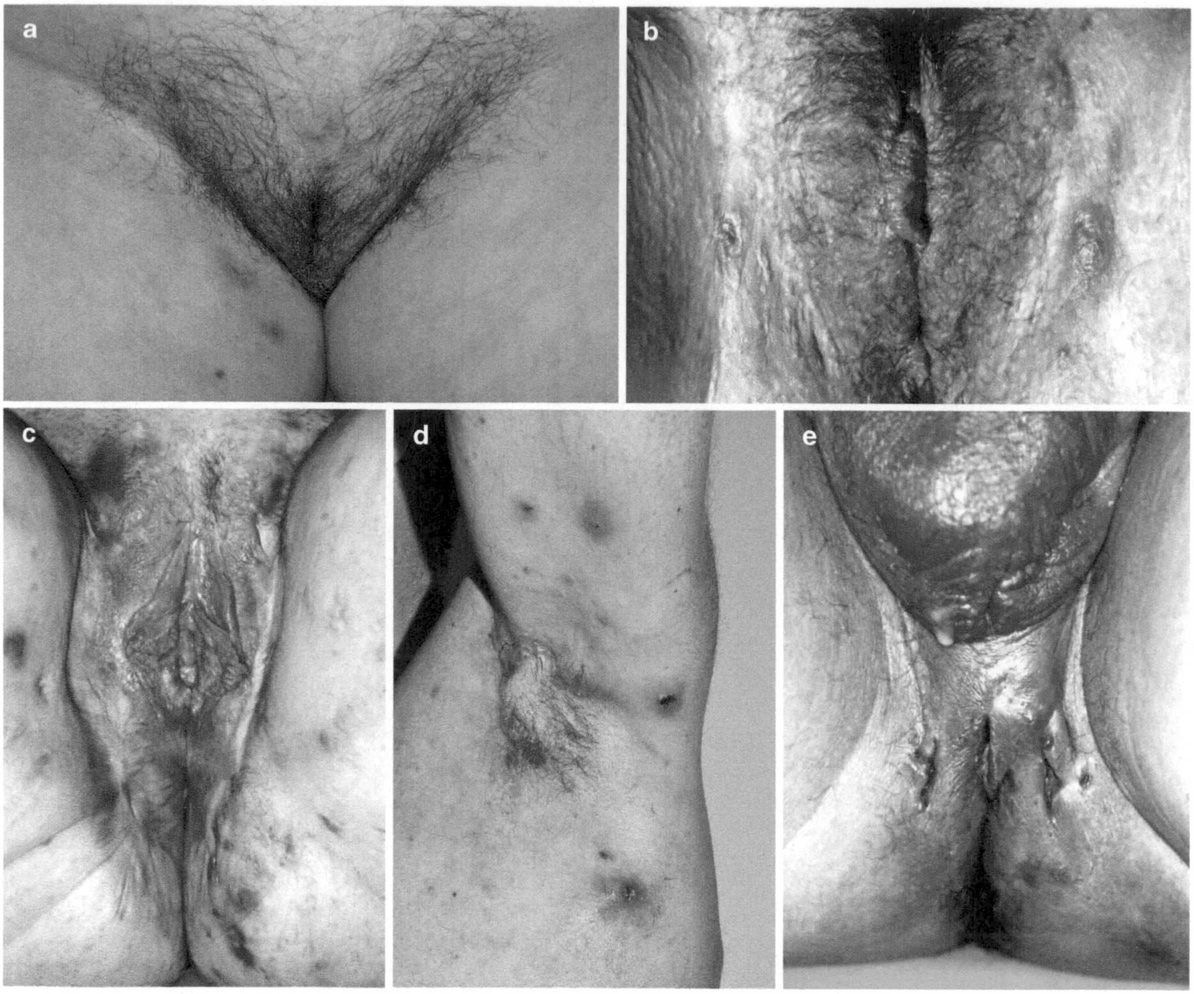

Fig. 57.60 Hidradentis suppurativa. (a) Comedones. (b) Nodular lesions. (c) Scarring at the vulva. (d) Axillar hidradenitis suppurativa. (e) Perianal and scrotal fistules and scars

nodules with abscess formation. Complications are fistulae, scarring, and edema. Severe disease may lead to amyloidosis [29], and there is a risk of squamous cell carcinoma.

Differential diagnoses comprise folliculitis, deep bacterial and fungal infections, and particularly Crohn's disease.

Primary treatment is weight-reduction and cessation of smoking. Antiseptic washing and topic or systemic antibiotics with tetracycline or clindamycin have been effective. Further systemic therapies are synthetic retinoids. Recently, new biologicals such as infliximab have been used with varying effects and sometimes severe side effects [30].

Alternatives are antiandrogen therapy and immunosuppression with such as cyclosporine. In recalcitrant disease therapy of choice is surgery. In large areas, secondary healing or closure by grafting is appreciated. A further option is intralesional corticosteroid.

57.8.8 Erythema Multiforme and Stevens–Johnson Syndrome

Differential Diagnoses

- Bullous pemphigoid
- Pemphigus
- Toxic epidermal necrolysis (Lyell's syndrome)

There is a minor form with target skin lesions and maculopapular or bullous lesions on the vulva and the buttocks as well as on the extremities (Fig. 57.61). Mucosal lesions are rarely seen. In Stevens–Johnson syndrome, which is the major form of erythema multiforme, however, mucous membranes of the mouth, eyes, and genitalia are particularly involved with painful erythematous urticarial and bullous lesions (Fig. 57.62). Other findings are fever and pulmonary and renal involvement. In severe cases scarring may occur. Frequently the disease is recurrent. In more than 60% of the cases the etiology remains unidentified.

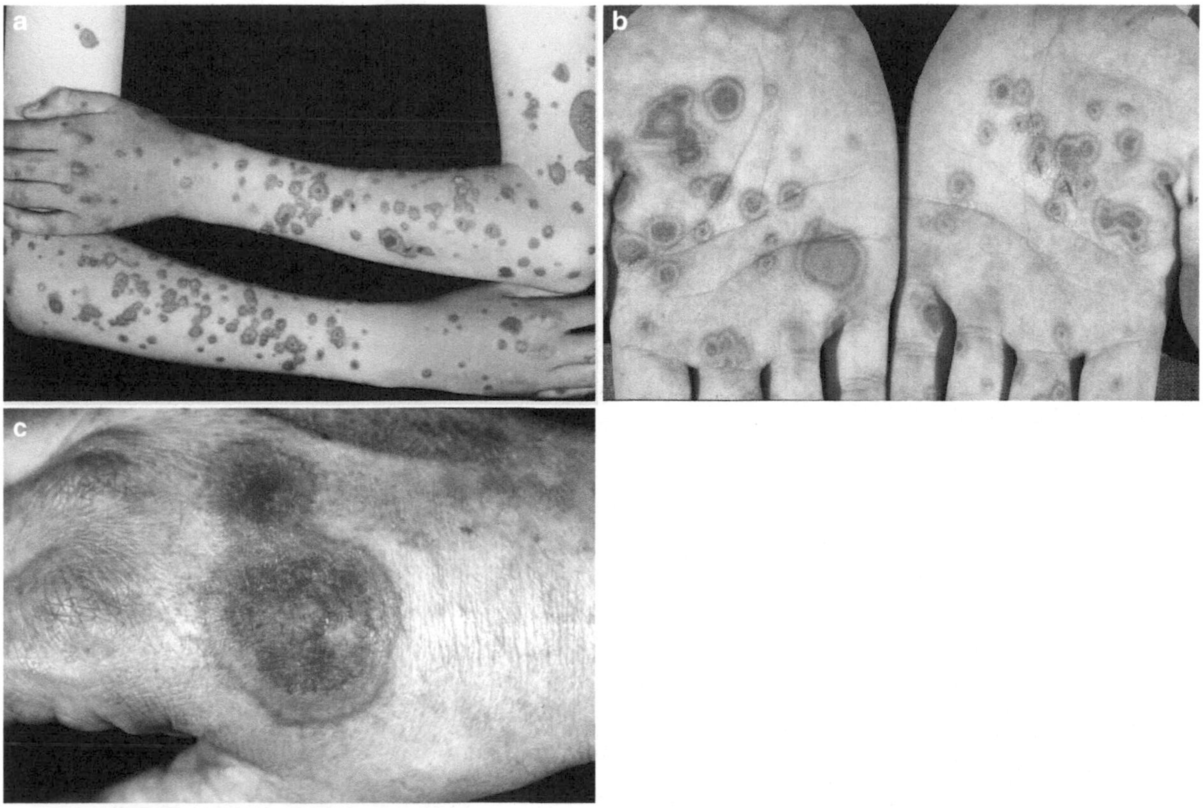

Fig. 57.61 (**a**) Erythema exsudativum multiforme (minor form) on the lower arms. (**b**) Target-like lesions on the palms. (**c**) Huge target-like lesions on the dorsal aspect of the hand

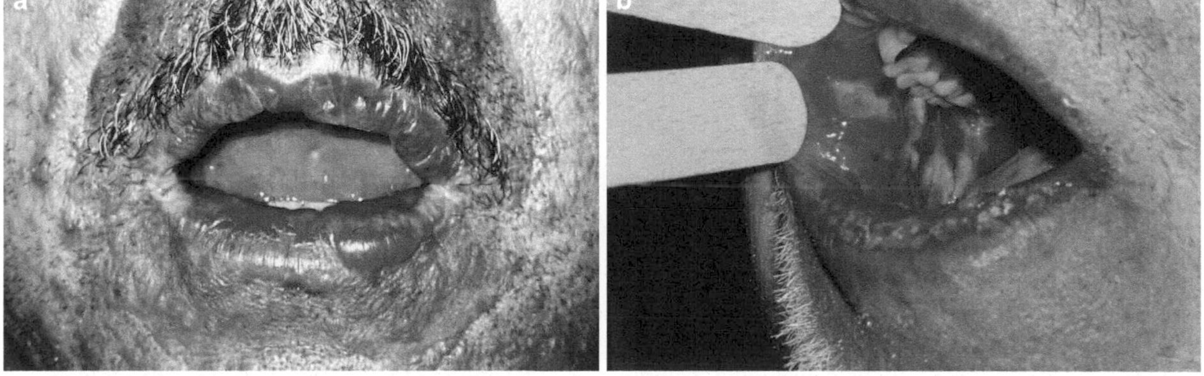

Fig. 57.62 (**a**) Bullous lesions of Stevens–Johnson syndrome on the lips. (**b**) Erosion on the oral mucosal. (**c**) Severe erosive lesions on the glans and inner foreskin. (**d**) Erosions and shallow ulcers of Stevens–Johnson syndrome on the vulvar and perianal skin

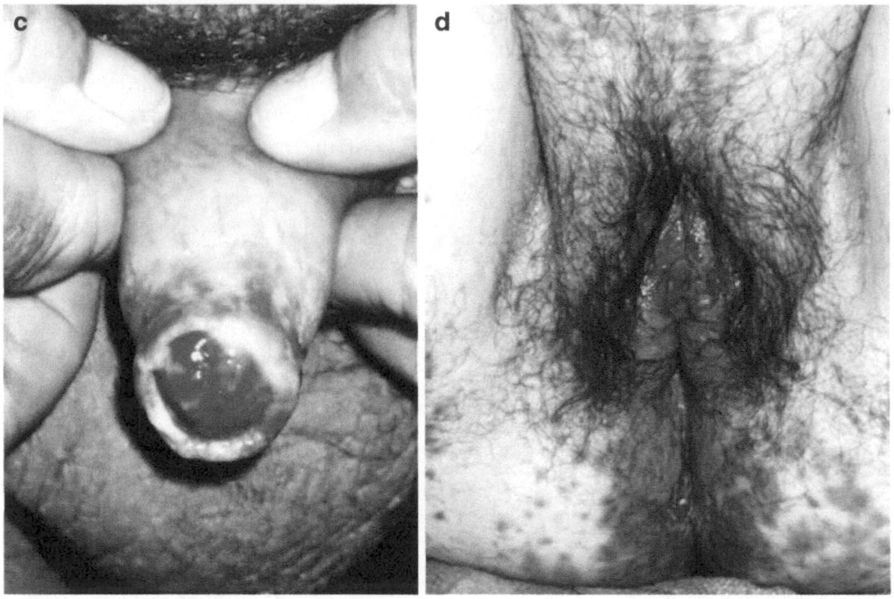

Fig. 57.62 (continued)

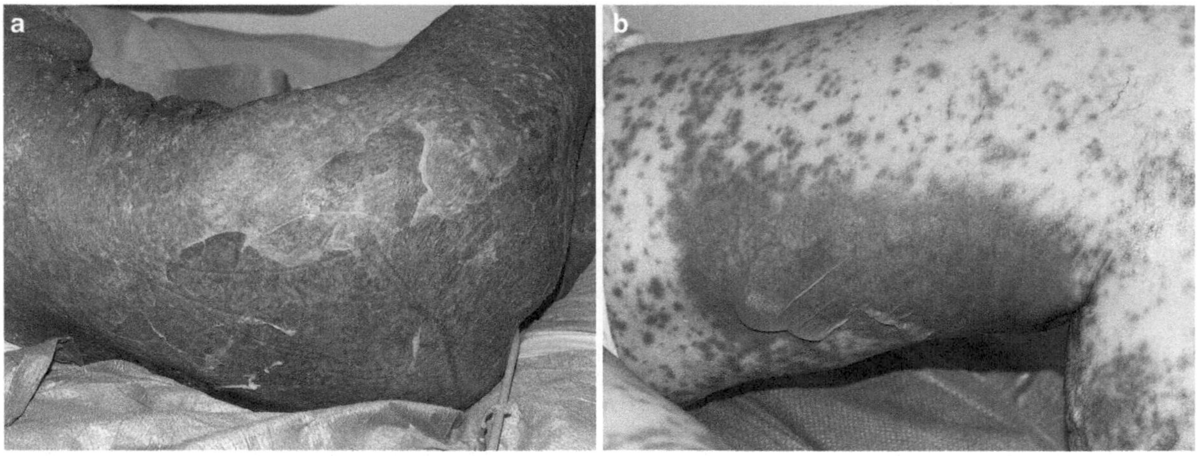

Fig. 57.63 Toxic epidermal necrolysis (Lyell's syndrome) (a) Extensive blistering and desquamation of the skin (b) solitary and confluent blister at the left high

It is well accepted that erythema multiforme is a hypersensitivity reaction. Suspected etiologic factors are viral infections, particulary HSV and mycoplasma infections as well as drugs such as sulphonamides, penicillins, and tetracyclines. Also neoplasias and autoimmune-diseases may be causative.

The list of differential diagnoses is long. Taking a biopsy and immunofluorescent staining is always required to differentiate bullous pemphigoid, pemphigus, and toxic epidermal necrosis (Lyell's syndrome), which is the most severe drug reaction of the skin (Fig. 57.63). Extensive blistering, erosions of Stevens–Johnson syndrome the skin and mucosal surfaces require intense care in a burns unit.

In the minor form of erythema multiforme, symptomatic treatment with antiseptic soaks is sufficient. Systemic prednisolone is necessary in together with oral antibiotics if prevention of additional infections is necessary.

Prevention of recurrence is done with avoidance of the causative drug or in case of recurrence of oral or genital herpes longtime continuous oral acyclovir.

57.8.9 Fixed Drug Eruption

Differential Diagnoses

- Herpes simplex
- Melanocytic lesion
- Vulvar intraepithelial neoplasia
- Penile and perianal intraepithelial neoplasia

In the genital area all types of drug reactions occur. Fixed drug eruption is more frequent on the male genitalia than on the vulva. It is characterized by an acute swelling with an erythematous patch, formation of blisters, and erosions (Fig. 57.64). Sometimes other typical lesions may coexist at extragenital sites. Recurrence of identical lesions after ingestion of the causative drug confirms the diagnosis. The lesion disappeard with desquamation and hyperpigmentation which may be long lasting. Implicated drugs are tetracyclines, cotrimoxazole, sulphonamides, barbiturates, nonsteroidal anti-inflammatory compounds, Cox 2-inhibitors, dapsone, salicylates, quinine, etc.

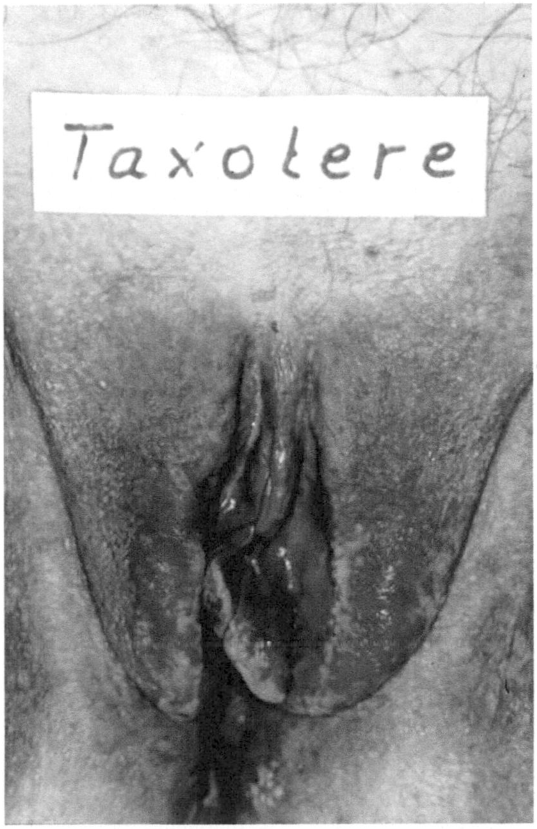

Fig. 57.64 Fixed drug eruption on the vulva: Focal dusky-red edema and erosions

Treatment consists in topical steroid application and strict avoidance of the triggering drug.

57.8.10 Behcet's Disease

Differential Diagnoses

- Herpes simplex
- Stevens–Johnson syndrome
- Recurrent aphthous disease

Diagnosis of Behcet's disease is established when a patient has painful oral ulcerations (Fig. 57.65) together with at least two of following features such as recurrent painful genital ulcerations (Fig. 57.66), eye lesions such as uveitis or retinal vasculitis, cutaneous lesions (folliculitis, papulopustular lesions, erythema nodosum), or a positive pathergy test. This is characterized by development of sterile pustules following a needle prick at an interval of 24–48 h. The etiology of Behcet's disease remains unidentified. Clinical features and histology are in favor of an autoimmune vascular response.

Behcet's disease is a chronic multiorgan disease with recurrent cutaneous, ocular, centralnervous, thrombotic aspects, bearing the risk of severe complications. The cutaneous and mucosal conditions have to be differentiated from herpes simplex, genital herpes,

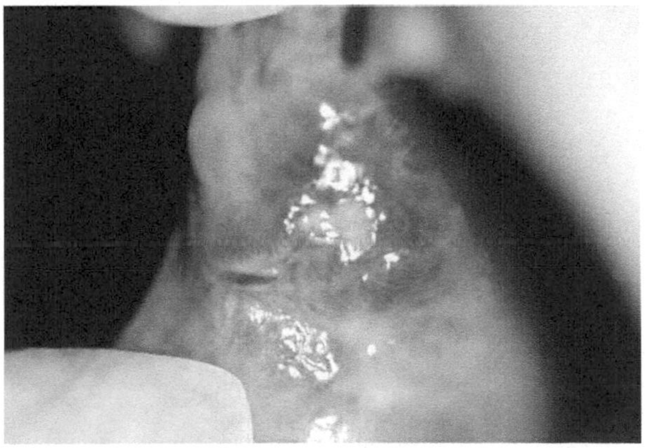

Fig. 57.65 Behcet's disease: large aphthous ulcer on the buccal mucosa

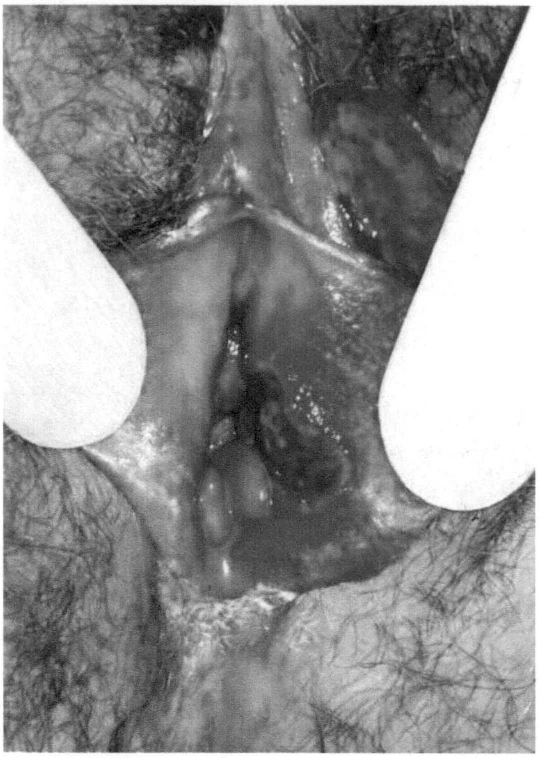

Fig. 57.66 Deep, giant aphthous ulcer on the labium majus

aphthosis, and rarely Stevens–Johnson syndrome. A broad interdisciplinary approach is mandatory.

Therapy is difficult. The list of treatments is long and consists of colchicine, steroids, dapsone, thalidomide, and immunosuppressive drugs. Local steroids are helpful only in superficial ulcers.

57.8.11 Eczema

Eczema (syn.: dermatitis) is likely to be underestimated in its frequency in the genitoanal skin.

Patients with genitoanal eczema suffer from intractable itching which regularly leads to scratching of the skin. Eczema has multiple causes. The lesions can be generalized or localized [14].

Acute eczema is characterized by erythema, papules, and vesicles (Fig. 57.67). The appearance of chronic eczema is variable according to the degree of scratching. It comprises mainly lichenification, which is thickening of the skin, excoriations, fissuring, and depigmentation (Figs. 57.69 and 57.70).

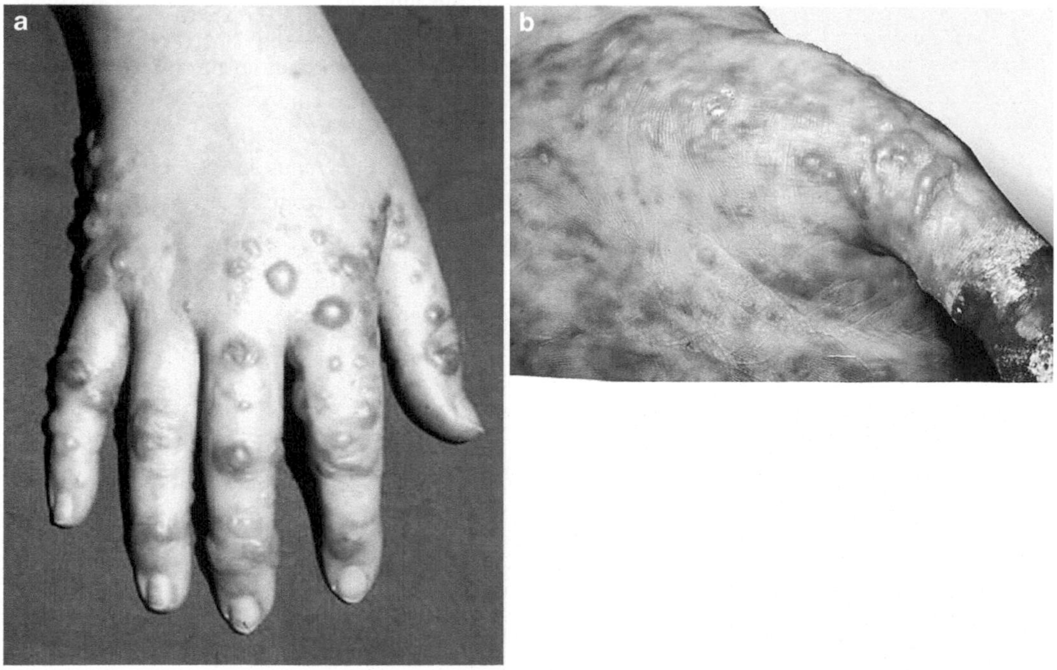

Fig. 57.67 (a) Acute eczema with multiple tense bullae and vesicles on the dorsal aspect of the hand. (b) Multiple partially confluent vesicles on the palm. (c) Subacute perianal eczema

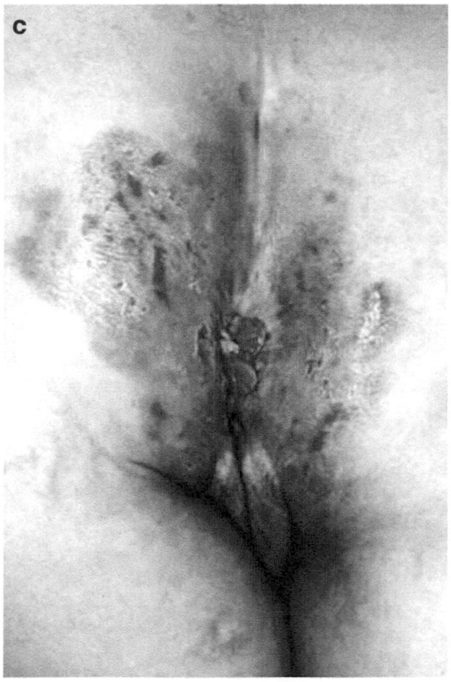

Fig. 57.67 (continued)

In women, the most common sites of involvement are the labia majora and the labia minora. In men, the scrotum and the proximal aspects of the penis are particular targets affected by eczematous lesions. Three major types of eczema can be differentiated: atopic eczema, allergic contact eczema, and irritant contact eczema.

57.8.12 Atopic Eczema

In contrast to widespread atopic eczema at other sites of the skin as the wrists, elbows, neck etc., the genitoanal area is the less severely affected. A simple erythema at the scrotum, at interlabial sites, at perianal skin, and in the natal cleft may be reminiscent of atopic eczema. Depending on the degree of inflammation, hyperpigmentation or hypopigmentation may occur (Fig. 57.70). A herpes simplex virus infection is rather frequent in atopic eczema and may lead to eczema herpeticum (so-called varicelliform eruption of Kaposi). This was a dangerous condition until antiviral treatment arrived (Fig. 57.71). Rarely this complication is found at the genitoanal skin.

Clinical features are helpful to diagnose atopic eczema. Patients often have asthma or hay fever. High levels of IgE antibodies to antigens such as staphylococcal and house mite proteins are frequently detectable. Atopic dermatitis patients show a white dermographism (Fig. 57.72), which reflects hyperreactivity of cutaneous vessels in these patients. Another frequent feature is palor of facial skin, periocular halo, and rarity of lateral eyebrows (Hertoghe-sign). Precipitating factors of atopic eczema are environmental substances such as, for instance, sweat and wool fibers and dust.

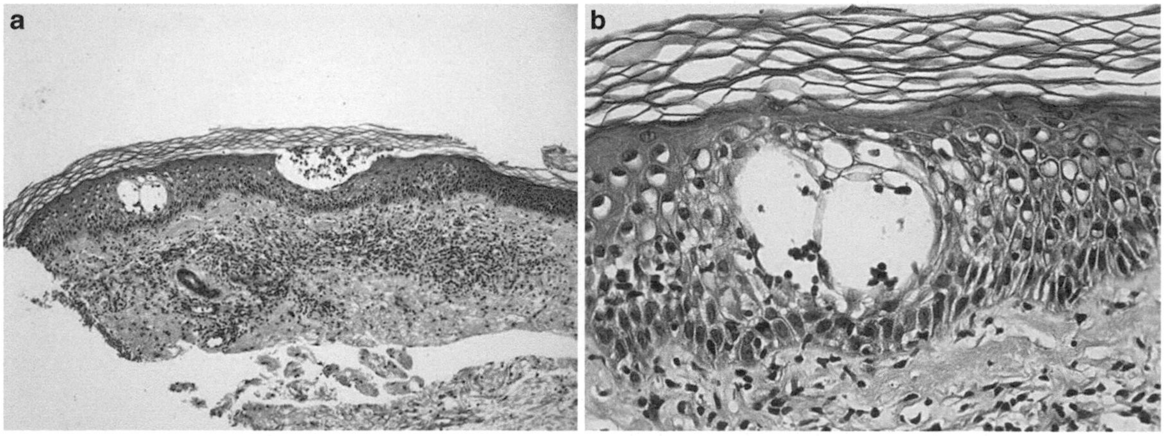

Fig. 57.68 (a) Histology: spongiotic epidermis with a spongiotic vesicle and inflammatory infiltrates in the upper dermis. (b) Magnification from (a)

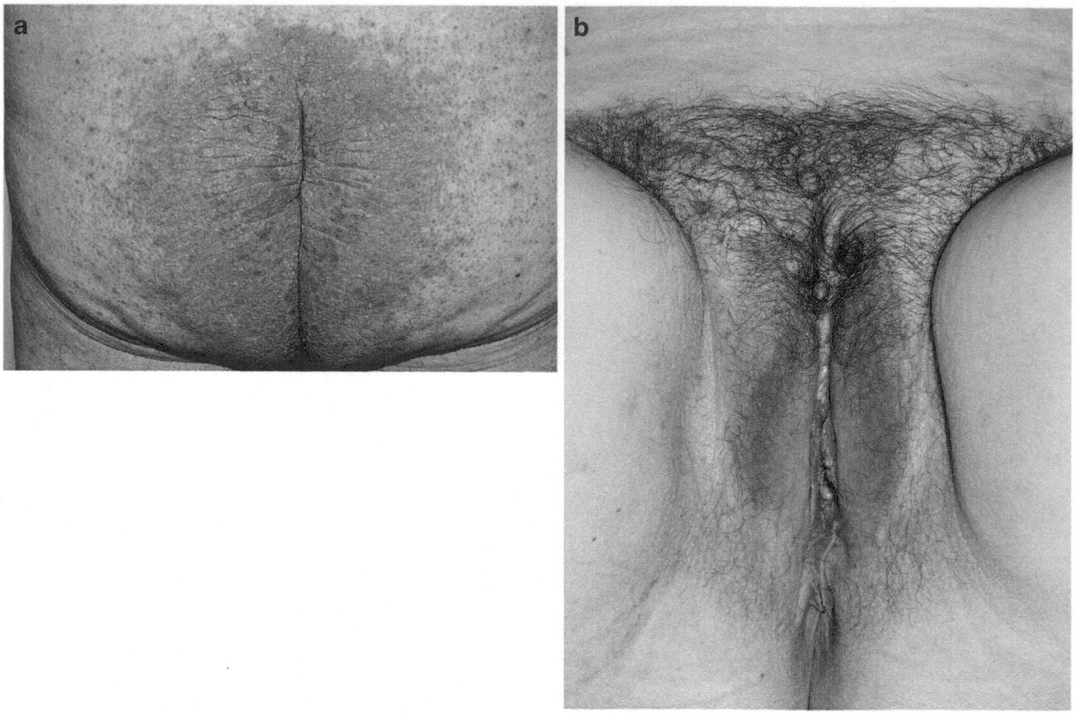

Fig. 57.69 Chronic eczema: (**a**) Excessive lichenification on the anal cleft. (**b**) Subacute vulvar eczema

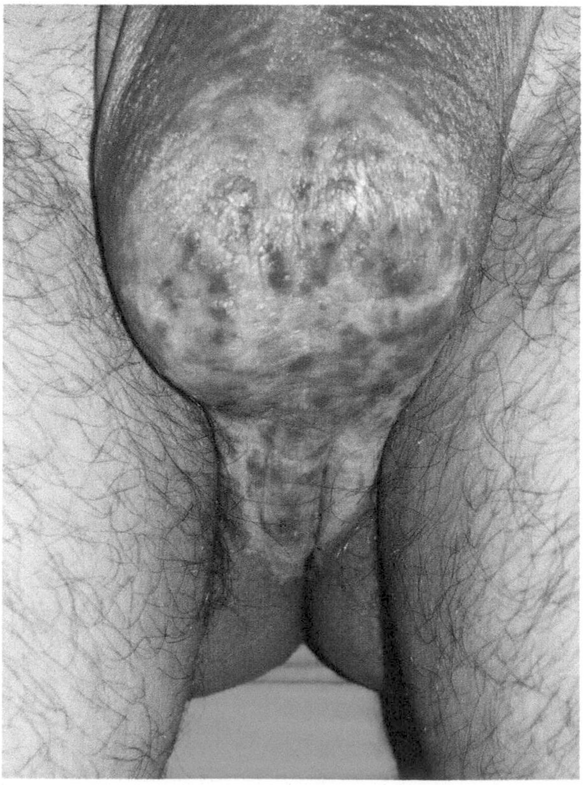

Fig. 57.70 Chronic eczema: Lichenification and hypopigmentation of scrotal skin

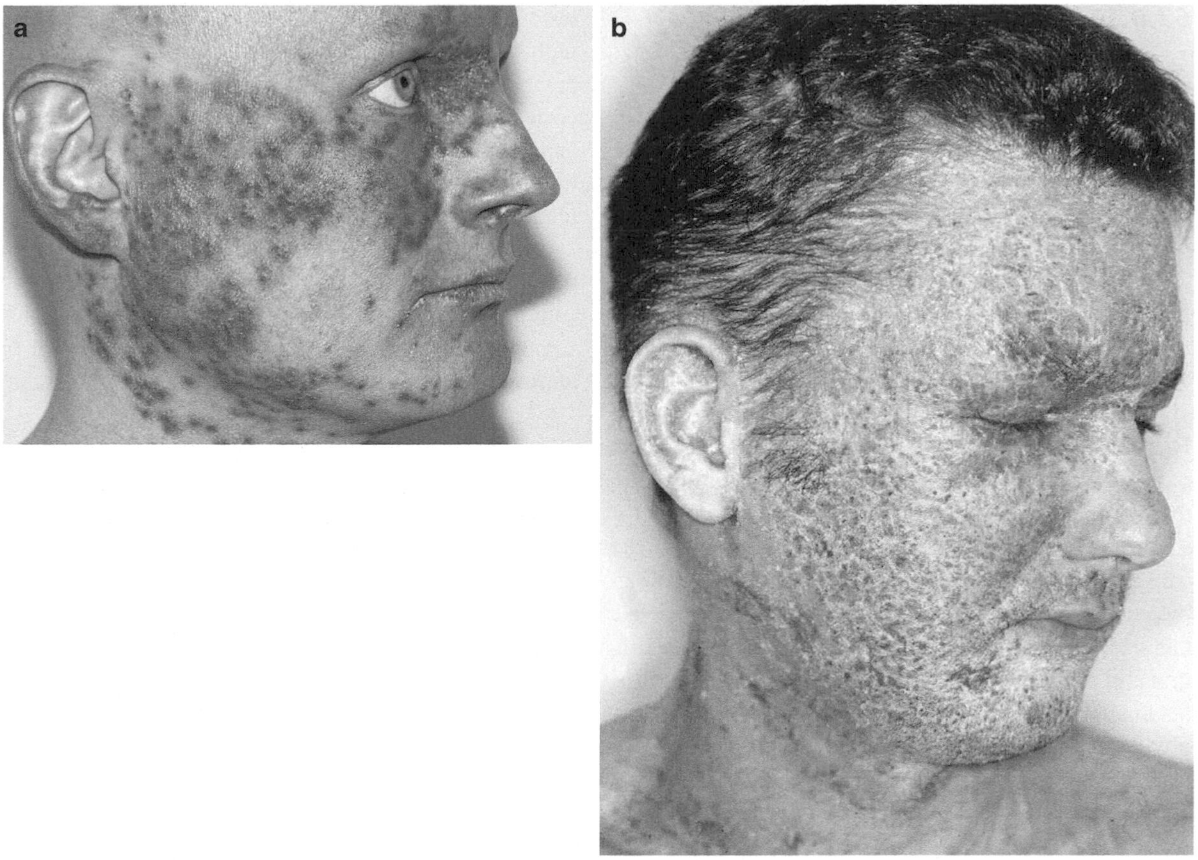

Fig. 57.71 Eczema herpeticum (so-called varicelliform eruption of Kaposi). (**a**) Acute dermatitis (**b**) Subacute eczema with crusted lesions on the face (after acyclovir therapy)

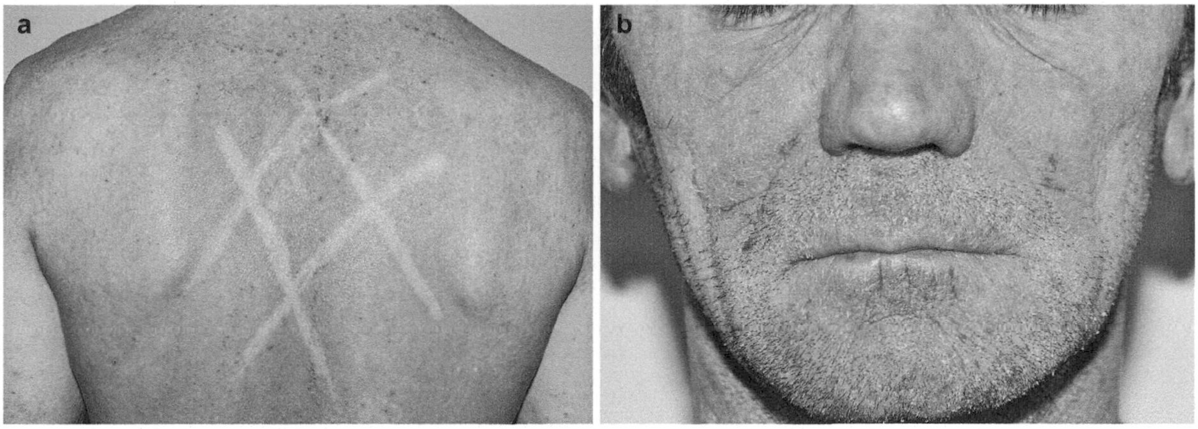

Fig. 57.72 (**a**) White dermographism (**b**) Palor of facial skin, periocular halo and dry skin

57.8.13 Contact Eczema

Differential Diagnoses

- Candida vulvovaginitis
- Candida balanitis
- Psoriasis
- Seborrhoeic dermatitis

Both irritant and allergic eczema may coexist [14]. The affected skin appears red, scaly, and often moist. The vulva and the male genitalia as well as the perianal skin may be involved without eczema at other sites. Histology is identical with acanthosis, spongiosis, and parakeratosis, as well as an inflammatory infiltrate in the upper corium. (see Fig. 57.68).

In case of *irritant contact eczema,* skin lesions are caused by contact with irritating chemicals or local treatments. There is no allergic mechanism involved. Clinically, there is diffuse erythema, sometimes maceration and erosion. A long list of topical treatments exists, leading to irritant eczema such as tar, podophyllin, podophyllotoxin, trichloracetic acid etc. Cosmetic preparations, cleaning with soap and hygiene products, deodorant spray and sanitary items etc. are all potentially irritant.

Allergic contact eczema, genitoanal itching and inflammation may be caused by a delayed (type IV) allergic reaction. This is a specific immunological reaction of the skin immune system to specific allergens. Particularly patients with perianal eczematous lesions have positive sensitivity reactions. The patients with genitoanal eczema very often react to medicaments such as local antibiotics, anesthetics, and corticosteroids; however, disinfectants, rubber products, and perfumes may be the origin of the allergic reaction. In all cases of eczema, a patch test is required to identify the causative allergen (Fig. 57.73).

Management is similar in all kinds of eczemas. In the acute stage, bathing or soaks with mild antiseptic solutions are very helpful. Topical corticosteroids sometimes as a combination with an antibacterial or antifungal agent are of value.

57.8.14 Lichen Simplex

Thickening of epithelium is caused by itching and subsequent scratching or rubbing. Characteristically, lichen simplex consists of asymmetrical localized solitary red or pale skin area which is slightly scaly. Sometimes erosions are seen (Fig. 57.74). Lichen simplex is regularly located in an area that can be reached by the dominant hand. Hyperacanthosis, hyperkeratosis and lengthened rete ridges of the epidermis, and a chronic inflammatory infiltrate are typical histological features.

Treatment is successful only with potent local steroids that have to be given together with oral antihistamines long enough until the symptoms have definitely disappeared.

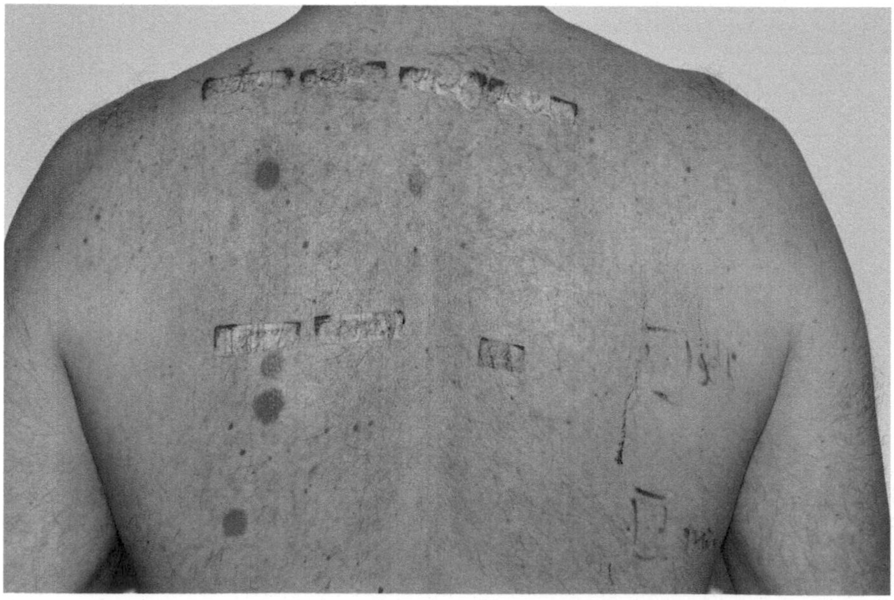

Fig. 57.73 Patch test. Positive test results after 72 h

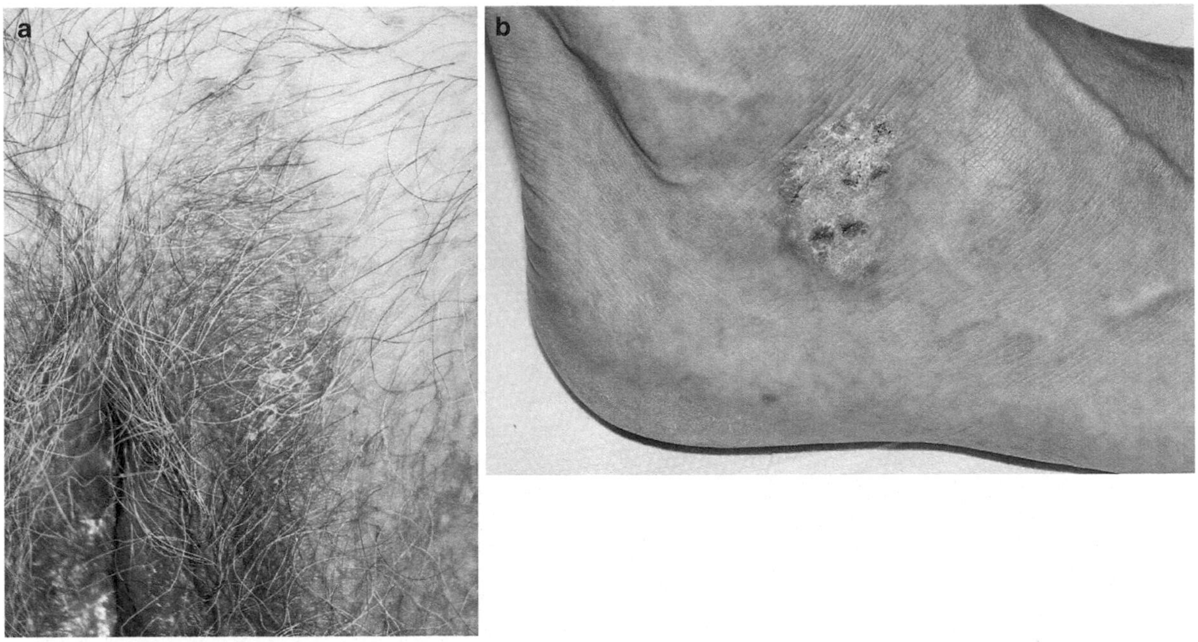

Fig. 57.74 (**a**) Vulvar lichen simplex involving the left labium majus. Thickening of the skin. (**b**) Circumscribed lichen simplex on the right ankle. Lichenification and slightly scaly skin with excoriations

57.9 Genitoanal Tumors

Patients frequently present with genitoanal-located papular lesions and tumors which may be the cause of fear of cancer or infertility. In general, any tumor can arise on the vulva, the penis, the scrotum, and the perianal skin. There is a large number of different tumor entities that may affect the genital area and the perianal and crural skin. The most common tumors, subdivided into benign tumors, premalignant lesions, and (invasive) malignant lesions, are listed in Table 57.2.

Table 57.2 Genitoanal tumors

Benign Tumors
Epidermal tumors • Seborrheic keratosis (seborrheic wart) • Fibroepithelial polyp (skin tag)
Epidermal appendages • Syringoma • Hidradenoma papilliferum • Fox–Fordyce disease
Cysts • Epidermal cysts • Bartholin's gland cysts
Melanocytic tumors (moles) • Junctional nevus • Compound nevus • Intradermal nevus • Other pigmented lesions • Benign juvenile melanomas • Lentigo simplex (melanosis genitalis) • Postinflammatory hyperpigmentation • Vitiligo
Mesodermal tumors • Fibroma, lipoma, fibrolipoma • Angiokeratoma • Capillary nevus • Hemangioma • Lymphangioma • Leiomyoma
Premalignant (intraepithelial) neoplasias • Multicentric (pigmented) Bowen's disease (bowenoid papulosis) • Bowen's disease • Erythroplasia of Queyrat • Paget's disease
Malignant (invasive) neoplasias • Squamous cell carcinoma • Basal cell carcinoma • Malignant melanoma • Other malignant neoplasias

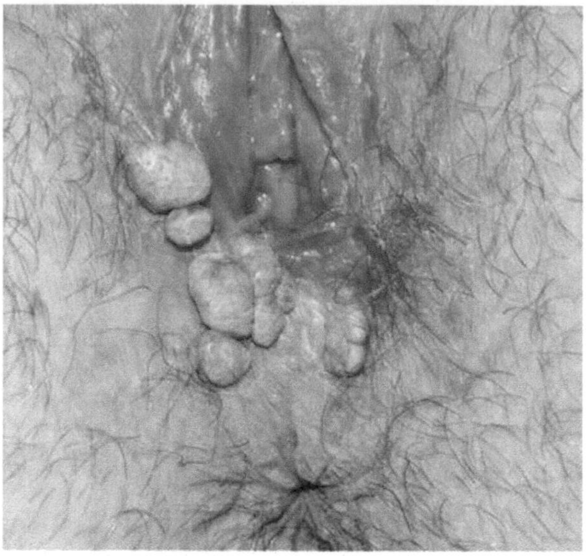

Fig. 57.75 Genital warts

A common diagnosis of benign tumors in young adults are condylomata acuminata which are also the most frequent sexually transmitted common disease of viral origin (Fig. 57.75) (see Chap. 37 page 489).

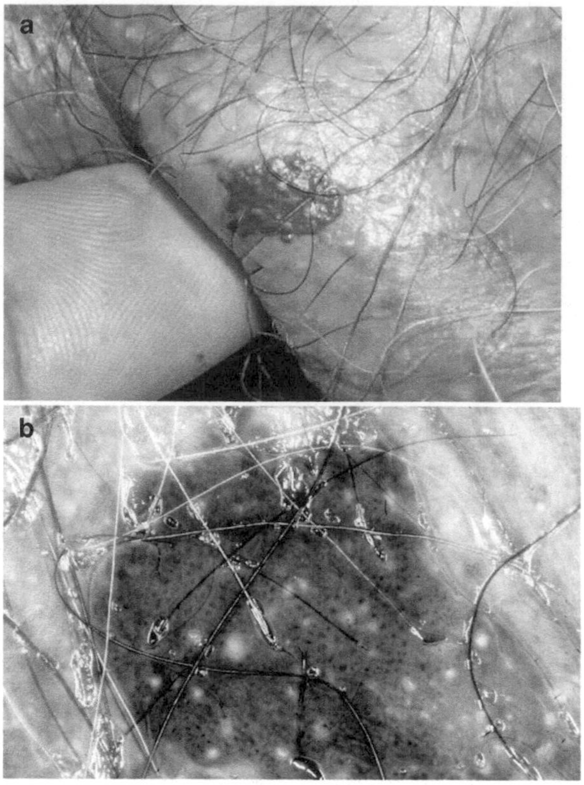

Fig. 57.76 (**a**) Seborrheic wart: waxy appearing flat papule. (**b**) Dermatoscopy: Detection of several cysts and pseudocysts

57.9.1 Benign Tumors

57.9.1.1 Seborrheic Keratosis (Syn. Seborrheic Warts)

Differential Diagnoses

- Melanocytic nevus
- Pigmented genital wart
- Pigmented Bowen's disease
- Pigmented basal cell carcinoma
- Malignant melanoma

Seborrheic keratoses are quite frequently found tumors in elderly patients located on the thoracic skin and the back. They are, however, less common on the genitoanal skin. They appear as a solitary pigmented papule with a waxy surface (Fig. 57.76). Histologically, basaloid cells form papillary formations together with pseudocysts. Variable amounts of melanin pigment are further typical features (Fig. 57.77).

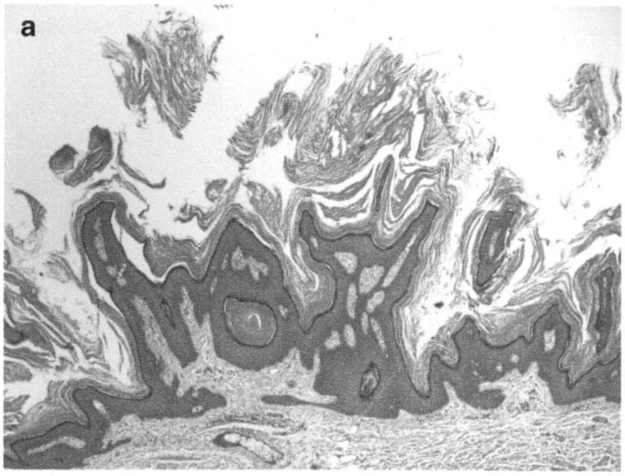

Fig. 57.77 (**a**) Histology of a seborrheic wart: pseudocysts within hyperpapillomatous and acanthotic epidermis. (**b**) Magnification from (**a**)

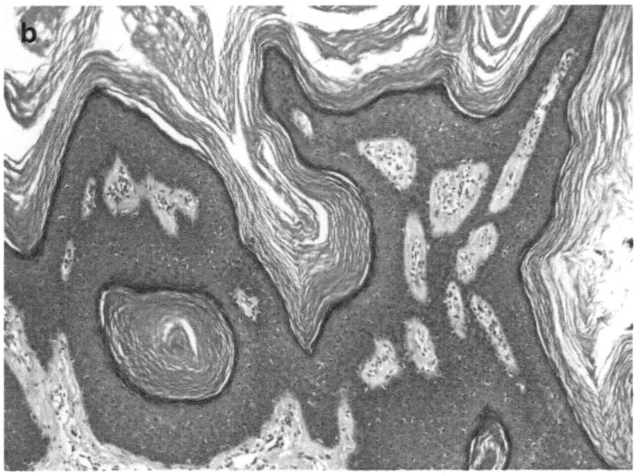

Fig. 57.77 (continued)

Therapy is done on a cosmetic base with ablative methods as scissor-snip excision or electrocautery. Suspect lesions have to be excised.

57.9.1.2 Skin Tags (Fibroepithelial Polyps)

Differential Diagnoses

- Neurofibroma
- Genital wart
- Dermal nevus

Macroscopically, these lesions present as sessile or pedunculated painless nodules on the penis, the scrotum, and prepuce and on the labia majora of the vulva. They are especially common in the genitocrural folds and the axillae. They are composed of a vascular connective tissue with an overlying squamous epithelium that may be acanthotic. A similar lesion is neurofibroma, which however is painful on pressure and has an association with café au lait spots at other skin sites. Simple scissor-snip excision or laser is the therapy of choice.

57.9.1.3 Tumors of the Epidermal Appendages

Apart from sebaceous retention cysts two sweat gland tumors have to be differentiated: Syringoma and hidradenoma papilliferum.

Syringoma

Differential Diagnoses

- Hidradenoma papilliferum
- Cyst
- Angioma

These are very small translucent papules which rarely involve the genital skin (vulva and penis), but the centrofacial aspect of the face. Women are affected by far more often than men.

Numerous cystic ducts ending in epithelial strands are typical histologic features. Treatment is not necessary. Allation with CO_2 laser may be helpful.

Hidradenoma papilliferum

Hidradenoma papilliferum is a rare benign tumor of apocrine sweat gland origin which is found on the interlabial fold of the vulva. It appears as skin-colored single nodule of a size of 1 cm or smaller. Mostly diagnosis is made by histology.

Fox–Fordyce Disease

Differential Diagnoses

- Acute contact eczema
- Atopic eczema

Fox–Fordyce disease is another condition of epidermal appendages. It is characterized by grouped conical pruritus papules around follicles in the axillae, around the nipples and the anogenital region. Women are affected about tenfold more often than men. The first lesions appear after puberty. Regression is often seen in postmenopausal women. Fox–Fordyce disease results from occlusion of apocrine sweat ducts with the consequence of apocrine anhidrosis. The intense pruritus leads to scratching and lichenification as well as alopecia. The major histological finding is a spongiotic vesicle within the follicular wall.

The treatments used are corticosteroid creams, estrogen cream, antihistamines, and oral contraceptives. If itching is unbearable, excision of involved areas is an option.

57.9.1.4 Cysts

In the genitoanal area of women, mainly two kinds of cysts have to be differentiated: Bartholin's cysts and epidermal cysts.

Epidermal Cysts

Differential Diagnosis

- Multiple epidermoid cysts in Gardner's syndrome
- Other cysts with and without metaplasia

In general, cysts are benign, common, and asymptomatic nonsolid tumors. The most common cysts are epidermal (epidermoid) cysts, which have an epidermal origin as do milia, comedones, and pilonidal cysts. Epidermal cysts affect the labia majora, penis, and scrotum (Fig. 57.78). The origins of epidermal cysts are obstructed hair follicles or a traumatic displacement of epidermis into the corium. Epidermal cysts may reach a size of 1–5 cm in diameter. Histology of the cystic wall shows squamous epithelium. The cysts are filled with keratinous material.

Therapy is not required unless inflammation or rupture occurs. Treatment is then surgical.

Bartholin's Gland Cysts

Differential Diagnoses

- Adenomas
- Malignancy

Bartholin's gland duct cysts occur in about 2% of women. The origin of these cysts is obstruction of the Bartholin's gland in the vestibular area. Inflammation and abscess formation may be caused by gonorrhea and trauma (see Chap. 6 page 77).

57.9.1.5 Benign Melanocytic Tumors

Differential Diagnoses

- Malignant melanoma
- Vascular nevi
- Pigmented seborrheic warts
- Pigmented basal cell carcinoma
- Histiocytoma
- Pigmented Bowen's disease
- Kaposi's sarcoma

Melanocytic nevi (moles) (Fig. 57.79) are benign melanocytic lesions as are lentigo simplex and postinflammatory hyperpigmentation (Table 57.2) that may occur

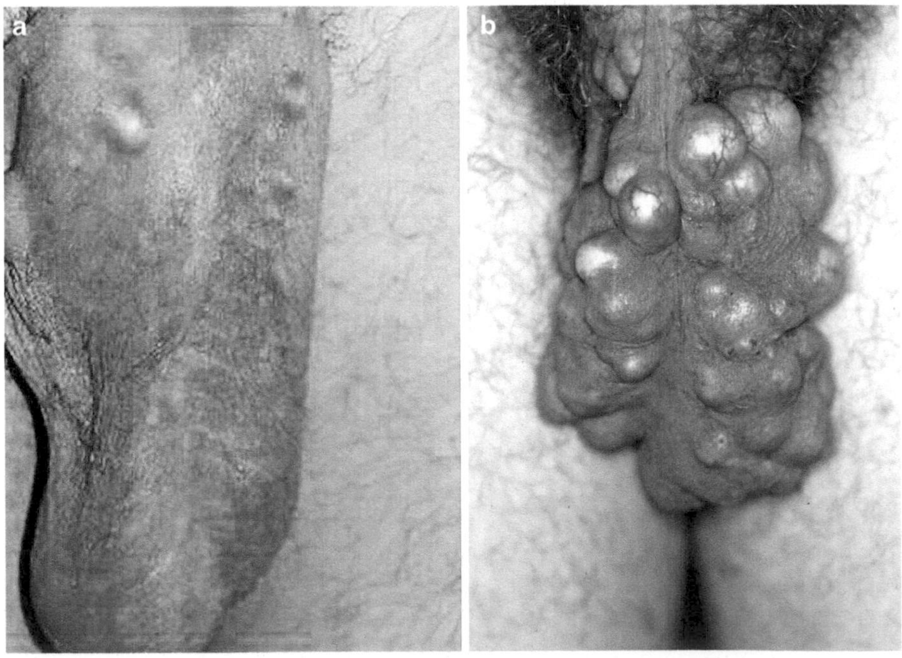

Fig. 57.78 (**a**) Scrotal cysts. (**b**) Multiple cysts involving the whole scrotal skin

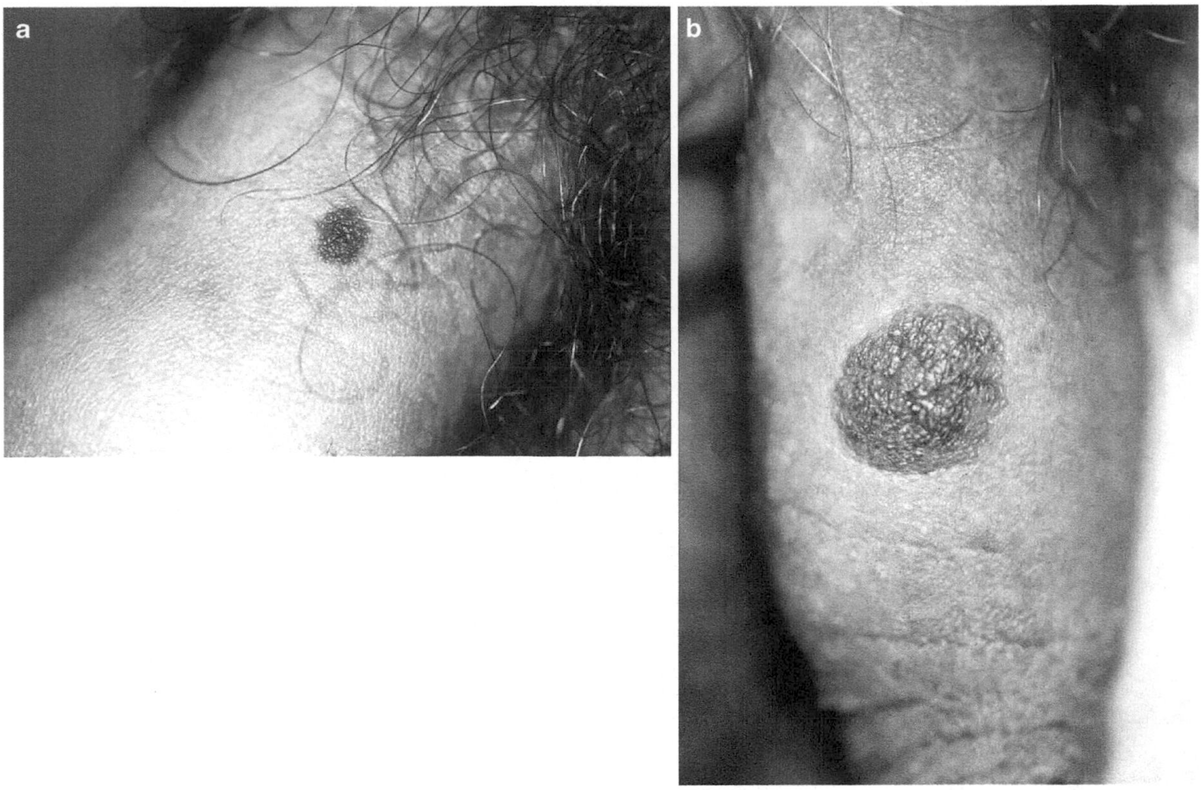

Fig. 57.79 (**a**) Junctional melanocytic naevi on the penile shaft. Symmetrical homogenously brownish macules. (**b**) Solitary large almost symmetrical maculopapular lesion

at any part of the vulva, the penis, the scrotum, and the perineo-perianal skin. Melanocytic nevi can be differentiated on histological grounds as junctional, compound, or intradermal (Fig. 57.80). On the genitalia, junctional and intradermal nevi are the most common types identified. Very rarely, the so-called juvenile benign melanoma, which is predominately seen on the face and extremities in children, arises in the genitalia. Clinically, it is a solitary dome-shaped small nodule, which has a reddish rather than a brown color due to sparsity of melanin.

Differentiation of moles and other circumscribed pigmented lesions from early malignant lesions is difficult especially on clinical grounds only. Patients with genitoanal pigmented lesions should always be referred to a dermatologist for further diagnosis. The best policy is to remove all such lesions completely and to investigate histologically.

The lesions may undergo malignant conversion. Multiple and grouped macular melanocytic lesions are characteristics of lentigines, which are then also called melanosis (Fig. 57.81). Rarely melanosis occurs at perianal sites and in the anal canal (Fig. 57.82). Clinical differentiation is almost impossible from pigmented intraepithelial neoplasia, postinflammatory inflammation, and idiopathic acquired pigmentation of Laugier as well as sometimes from malignant melanoma. Excision is mandatory. Histological interpretation can be difficult. A second opinion may be necessary. Postinflammatory hyperpigmentation is a common feature of destructive inflammation such as lichen sclerosus and lichen planus (Fig. 57.47). In some cases, multiple and grouped areas of pigmentation persist during months or years.

Postinflammatory hypopigmentation is a feature of lichen sclerosus. Rarely, herpes zoster may lead to circumscribed asymmetrical patches of hypopigmentation (Fig. 57.19) organized within a previously zoster-affected dermatome.

Vitiligo may affect the genitoanal skin in both genders with total and symmetrical depigmentation.

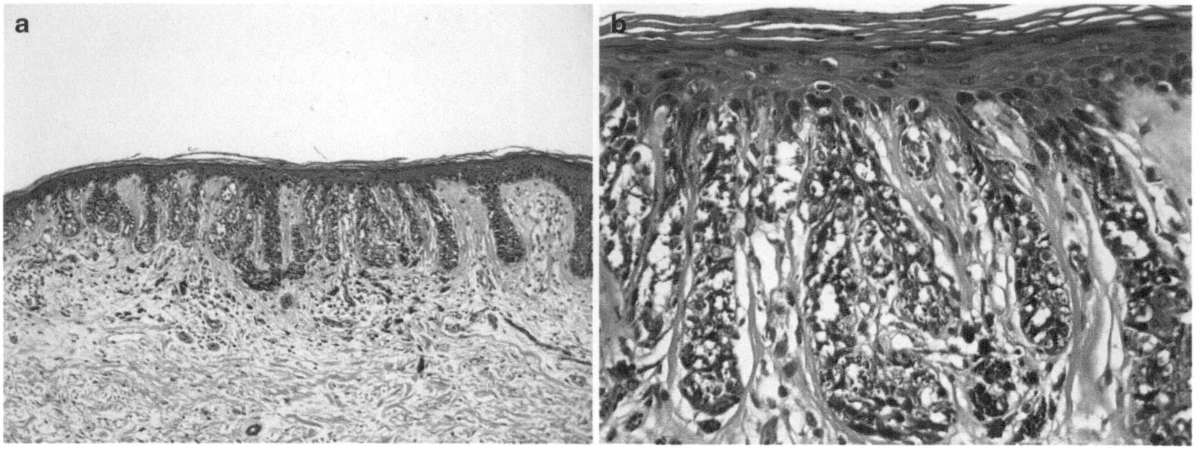

Fig. 57.80 (a) Histology: Flat epidermis with elongated rete ridges and numerous nests of melanocytes in the junctional area. (b) Magnification from (a)

57.9.1.6 Mesodermal Tumors

Differential Diagnoses

- Fibroma
- Lipoma
- Fibrolipoma
- Angiokeratoma
- Hemangioma
- Lymphangioma
- Other mesodermal tumors

Neoplasias of mesodermal origin are extremely uncommon on the external genital area. Accurate diagnosis on histological grounds sometimes requires immunohistochemistry. The most common benign mesodermal tumors are fibroma, lipoma, fibrolipoma, leiomyoma, and the neoplasmas of vascular tissue such as angiokeratoma, capillary nevus (port-wine nevus), hemangioma, angiomatous nevus, and lymphangioma. The other tumors of smooth muscle and striated muscle, fibroblastic tumors, and fibrohistiocytic tumors are very rare and are not discussed here.

Angiokeratoma

Differential Diagnoses

- Malignant melanoma (solitary)
- Anderson–Fabry disease (Angiokeratoma corporis diffusum universale) (disseminated)

Angiokeratomas are red or violaceous tiny papules consisting in dilated blood vessels covered by a hyperkeratotic epidermis. These tumors occur in particular on the scrotum, but the labia majora, the vulva, and the penis may be affected (Fig. 57.83). Normally they develop in adulthood until old age. If therapy is considered, diathermy or laser is an option.

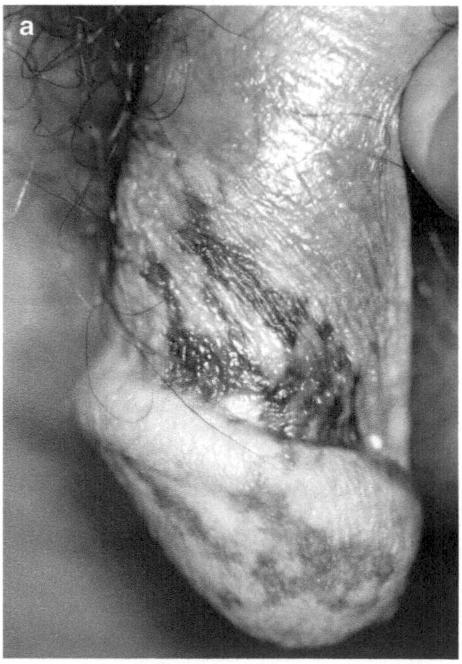

Fig. 57.81 (a) Reticular melanosis of the penis (coronal sulcus and inner part of the prepuce) (b, c) Histology: basal epidermis with increased number of melanocytes (c) Magnification from (b).

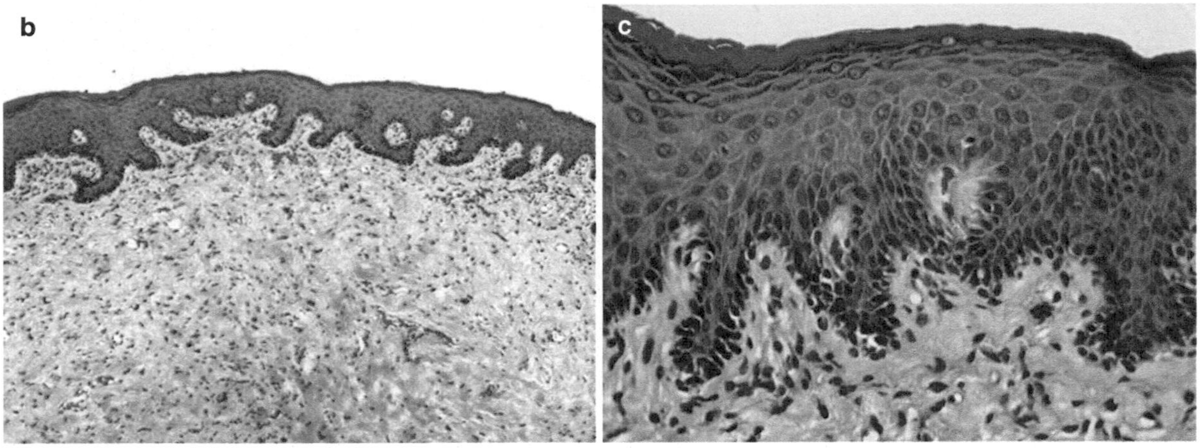

Fig. 57.81 (continued)

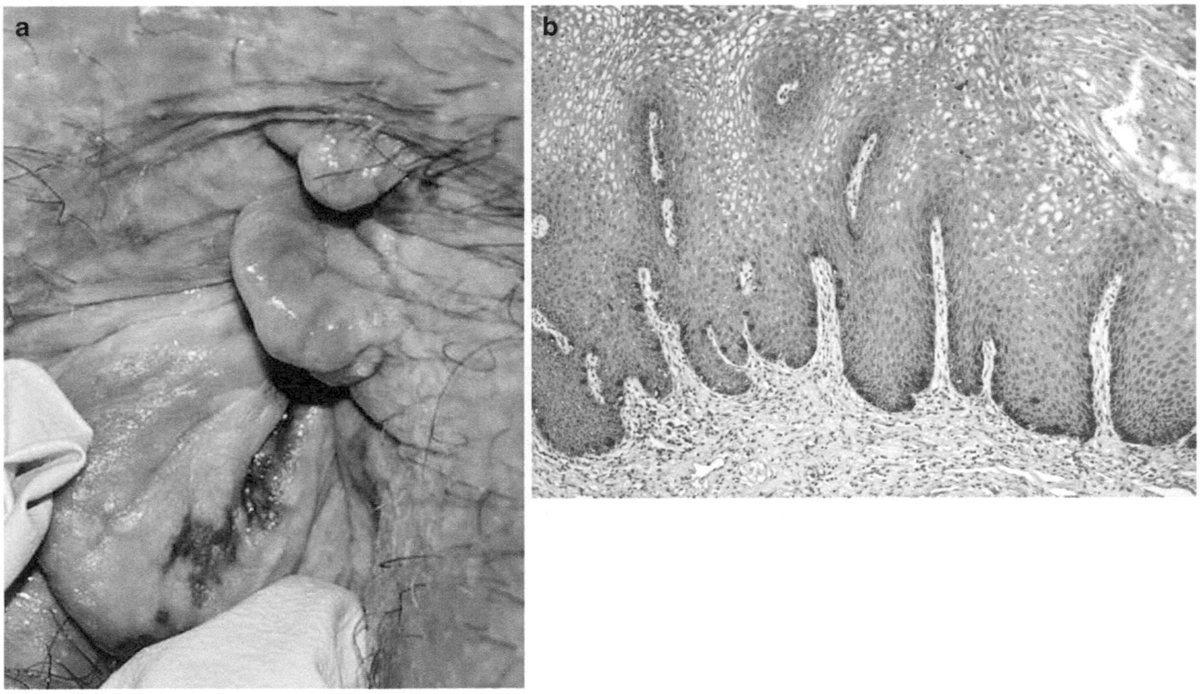

Fig. 57.82 (a) Linear pigmentation in a perianal tag extending into the anal canal. (b) Histology: Melanosis with hyperpigmented basal layer

Hemangioma

Differential Diagnosis

- Malignant melanoma

Hemangiomas develop shortly after birth. Clinically they are superficial subcutaneous bluish-red masses. Histologically, they consist of dilated capillaries with endothelial proliferations and cavernous spaces. Superficially located hemangiomas can be destroyed by laser coagulation. Proliferating capillary hemangioma (so-called pyogenic granuloma) (Fig. 57.84) is a rapidly enlarging small reddish papule that may bleed after minor trauma. As it can be mistaken for malignant melanoma, the lesion should be excised entirely and investigated histologically.

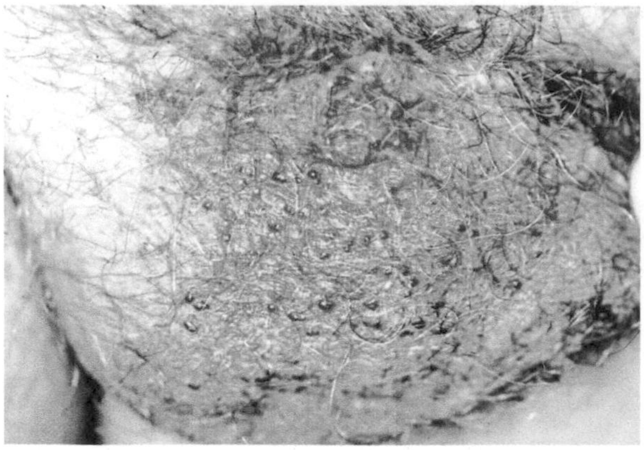

Fig. 57.83 Angiokeratoma on the scrotum

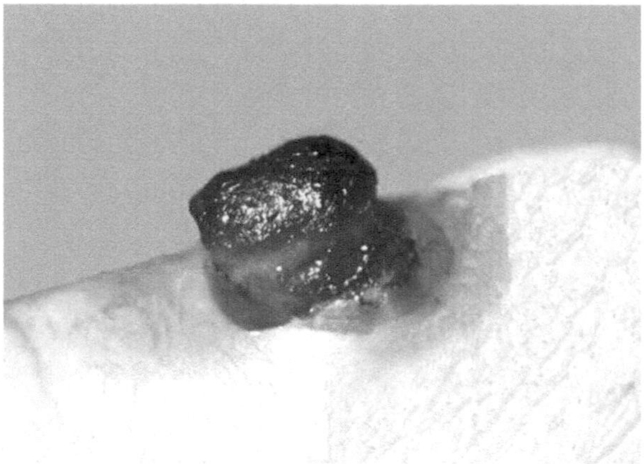

Fig. 57.84 Pyogenic granuloma: large hemorrhagic nodule

Lymphangioma

Differential Diagnoses

- Hemangioma
- Genital warts

Lymphangiomas are vascular neoplasias composed of lymphatic vessels. Lymphangioma circumscriptum is widely distributed with diffuse swelling of the vulva as a consequence of lymph stasis secondary to local occlusion, chronic infection (i.e. streptococcal infection in recurrent erysipelas), persistent lymphedema, or x-irradiation (Fig. 57.85). Treatment consists in wide excision or CO_2-laser [22]. Lymphedema may be complicated by cellulitis (see 57.4.1, on page 782). The so-called bicyclist's vulva [2] is a chronic lymphedema increasingly observed in women, which is caused by intense cycling.

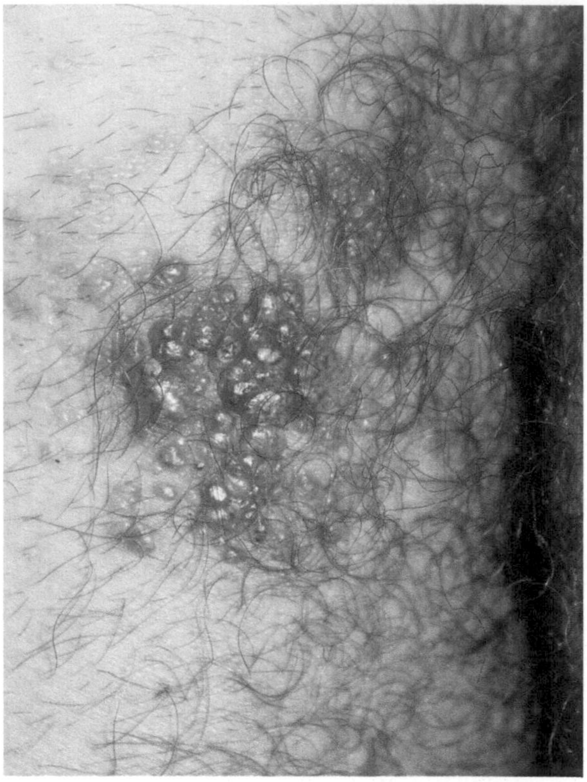

Fig. 57.85 Lymphangioma: focal aggregation of translucent confluent papules

57.9.2 Premalignant Intraepithelial Neoplasias

Intraepithelial neoplasias do not necessarily present as a tumor. Mostly macular or maculopapular lesions are observed. Histologically, squamous intraepithelial neoplasia of the vulva (VIN), the penis (PIN), and the perianal skin (PAIN) are defined by a loss of epithelial maturation and an associated atypia of the keratinocytes. According to the International Society of the Study of Vulvar disease (ISSVD) (Table 57.3) three grades of VIN (VIN I, VIN II, VIN III) have been differentiated [47]. Accordingly, PIN and PAIN have been subdivided into grade I, II, and III. VIN III, PIN III, and PAIN III have replaced to some degree the descriptive terms of bowenoid papulosis (multicentric (pigmented) Bowen's disease), Bowen's disease, and erythroplasia of Queyrat, respectively. Histologically all these conditions are indistinguishable. However, clinically and with respect to prognosis there are important differences. (For details refer to Chap 35 and 37 page 457 and 489).

Table 57.3 Classification of vulval disease

According to the International Society for the Study of Vulvar Disease (ISSVD) and the International Society of Gynaecological Pathologists (ISGP)
Benign • Lichen sclerosus • Squamous cell hyperplasia • Other dermatoses (psoriasis, lichen planus, eczema etc.)
Premalignant • Squamous
VIN I: Atypia lower one third of epidermis
VIN II: Atypia up to two thirds of epidermis
VIN III: Atypia > two thirds of epidermis or full thickness
• Nonsquamous Paget's disease Malignant melanoma in situ

57.9.2.1 Multicentric (Pigmented) Bowen's Disease (Bowenoid Papulosis)

Differential Diagnoses

- Genital warts
- Seborrheic keratoses
- Lichen nitidus
- Melanocytic tumors

Bowenoid papulosis is characterized clinically by multiple pigmented or erythematous papules of the penis, vulva, or perianal sites (Fig. 57.86) developing in young adults. There is a clear association with sexually transmitted high-risk HPV types mainly HPV 16 [17]. The risk of malignant conversion is generally low. Treatment is with local imiquimod, laser, electrocautery, and cryotherapy, rarely excision.

57.9.2.2 Bowen's Disease

Differential Diagnoses

- Invasive cancer
- Paget's disease
- Genital wart
- Psoriasis
- Eczema
- Malignant melanoma
- Seborrheic keratosis

Bowen's disease is seen in people over the age of 50. Clinically, this condition consists of a solitary plaque with centrifugal growth pattern in red, white, or brown (Fig. 57.87). Spontaneous regression does not occur. Progression to invasive cancer is regularly seen. Association with high-risk HPVs as HPV16 is comparable to bowenoid papulosis. Histologically, Bowen's disease is indistinguishable from bowenoid papulosis showing features of carcinoma in situ. Treatment with imiquimod is an option. In nonresponding cases excision is mandatory [42]. In rare instances, imiquimod, however, may lead to autoimmune disease such as pemphigus vulgaris [8].

57.9.2.3 Erythroplasia of Queyrat

Differential Diagnoses

- Balanitis plasma cellularis (Zoon's balanitis)
- Vulvitis plasma cellularis
- Lichen planus
- Psoriasis

Erythroplasia of Queyrat is histologically an intraepithelial neoplasia grade III of the foreskin, glans, penis, and the inner side of the vulva with features similar to Bowen's disease. Macroscopically, it consists of a maculopapular, solitary, eroded, or ulcerated plaque (Fig. 57.88). There is an association with high-risk HPV as in Bowen's disease.

Laser ablation or cautery as well as local therapy with imiquimod or 5-fluorouracil are optional therapies. Eroded or ulcerative lesions have to be excised entirely.

For further details on intraepithelial neoplasias refer to the chapter on page 35 and 37 on page 457 and 489.

57.9.2.4 Non-squamous Cell Intraepithelial Neoplasias

Differential Diagnoses

- Lichen simplex planus
- Candidiasis
- Eczema
- Bowen's disease

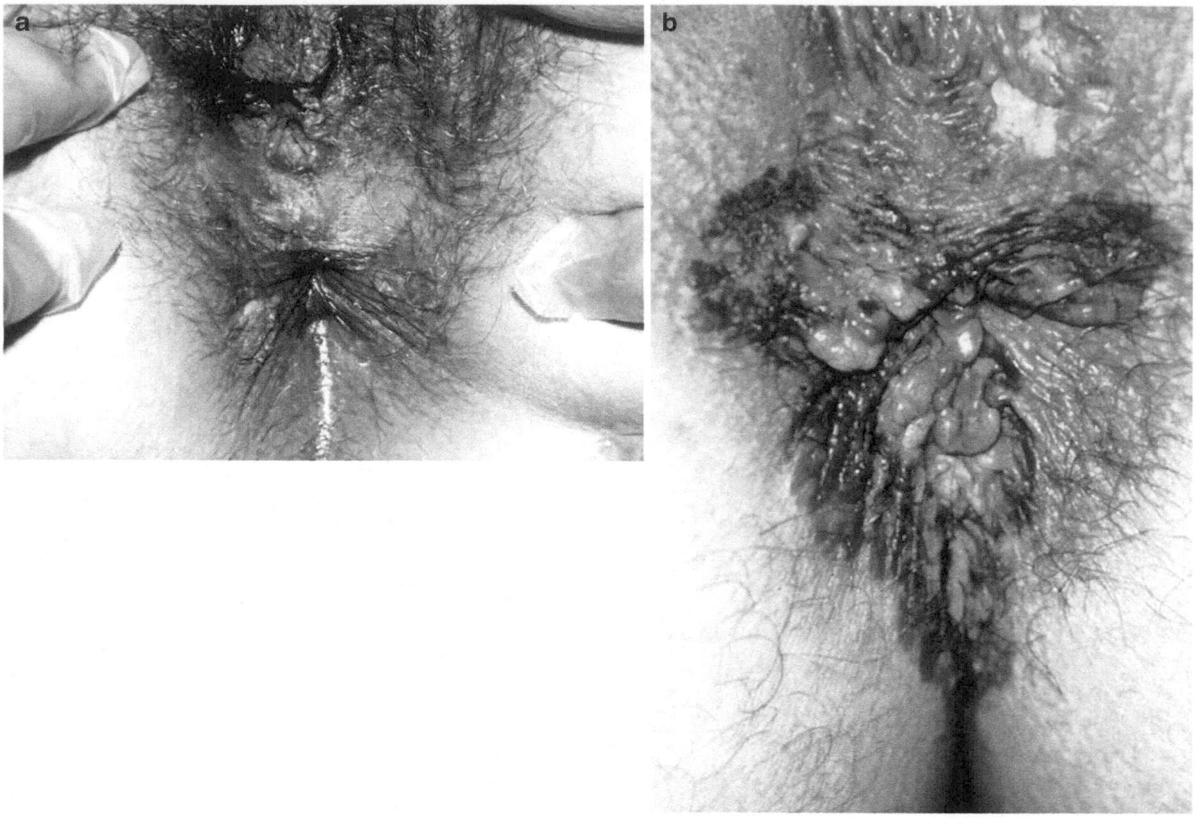

Fig. 57.86 Multicentric (pigmented) Bowen's disease (Bowenoid papulosis). (**a**) Perianal and perineal flat papular lesions. (**b**) Brownish, erythematous and depigmented maculo-papular lesions at the perianal skin and at the perineal skin (histology VIN III AND PAIN III)

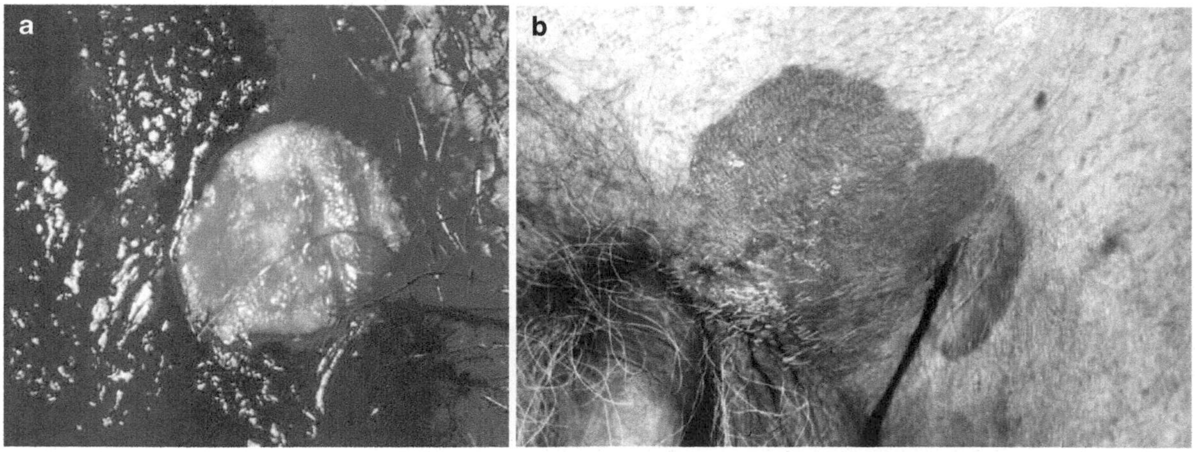

Fig. 57.87 Bowen's disease. (**a**) Solitary depigmented plaque. (**b**) Large reddish macular lesion on the pubic skin and in the groins

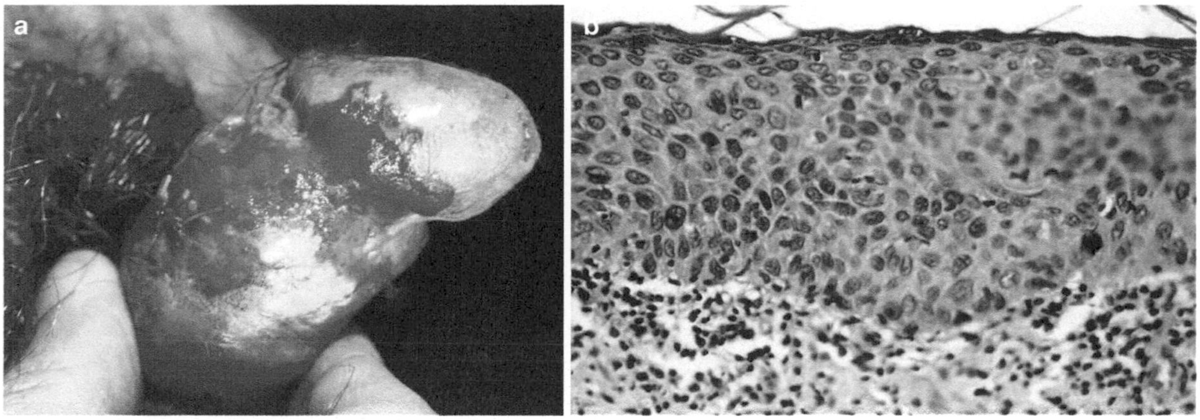

Fig. 57.88 Erythroplasia of Queyrat. (**a**) Solitary maculopapular partially eroded lesion on the penile shaft and the glans. (**b**) Histology: Penile intraepithelial neoplasia grade III

- Erythroplasia of Queyrat
- Malignant melanoma

These neoplasias comprise malignant melanoma in situ (see below) and extramammary Paget's disease (Table 57.2).

57.9.2.5 Paget's Disease

Extramammary paget's disease is a rare epithelial neoplasm of the apocrine gland-bearing areas such as the anus, the vulva, the penis, the pubic skin, the umbilicus, and the axillae seen in the elderly [16]. Men are affected less frequently than women (ratio of 1:3).

There are associations with distant carcinomas of the uterus, renal tract, breast, and gastrointestinal tract. The most common symptoms are itching and burning. The lesions are well-demarcated, moist, eczematoid pink to red plaques with ulcerations and hyperkeratosis. Such lesions spread extensively. Single or multiple plaques occur (Fig. 57.89). Diagnosis is made only by biopsy. The presence of vacuolated Paget's cells that are large clear cells staining with PAS, alcian blue, and CEA (Fig. 57.90) enables differentiation from malignant melanoma and squamous cell carcinoma. In all cases of extramammary Paget's disease, evaluation of the breasts, genitourinary tract, and anorectum has to be performed.

Therapy is primarily complete excision. In recurrent disease, imiquimod has shown to be effective according to case reports [45].

57.9.3 Malignant Neoplasias

57.9.3.1 Squamous Cell Carcinoma

Differential Diagnoses

- Keratoacanthoma
- Basal cell carcinoma
- Intraepithelial neoplasia

The majority of genitoanal malignant neoplasias are of the squamous type and develop close to or within a preexisting area of chronic lichen sclerosus. The role of HPV in vulval and penile squamous cell cancer is different from perianal and anal sites. Only 50%, in contrast to more than 80%, of the genital tumors have an evidence of an HPV infection. Age but also immunodeficiency are important risks of genitoanal cancer. There are a number of conditions of risk such as lichen sclerosus, being uncircumcised, erythroplasia of Queyrat, Bowen's disease, Paget's disease, exposure to PUVA, and genitoanal warts [15]. However, squamous cell cancer can arise from normal tissue. Macroscopically it is a solid tumor which may be ulcerated and pruritus (Fig. 57.91). Further symptoms may be bleeding and discharge as well as involved inguinal lymph nodes. Treatment is surgical. For further details refer to Chap. 37 and 38 on page 489 and page 511.

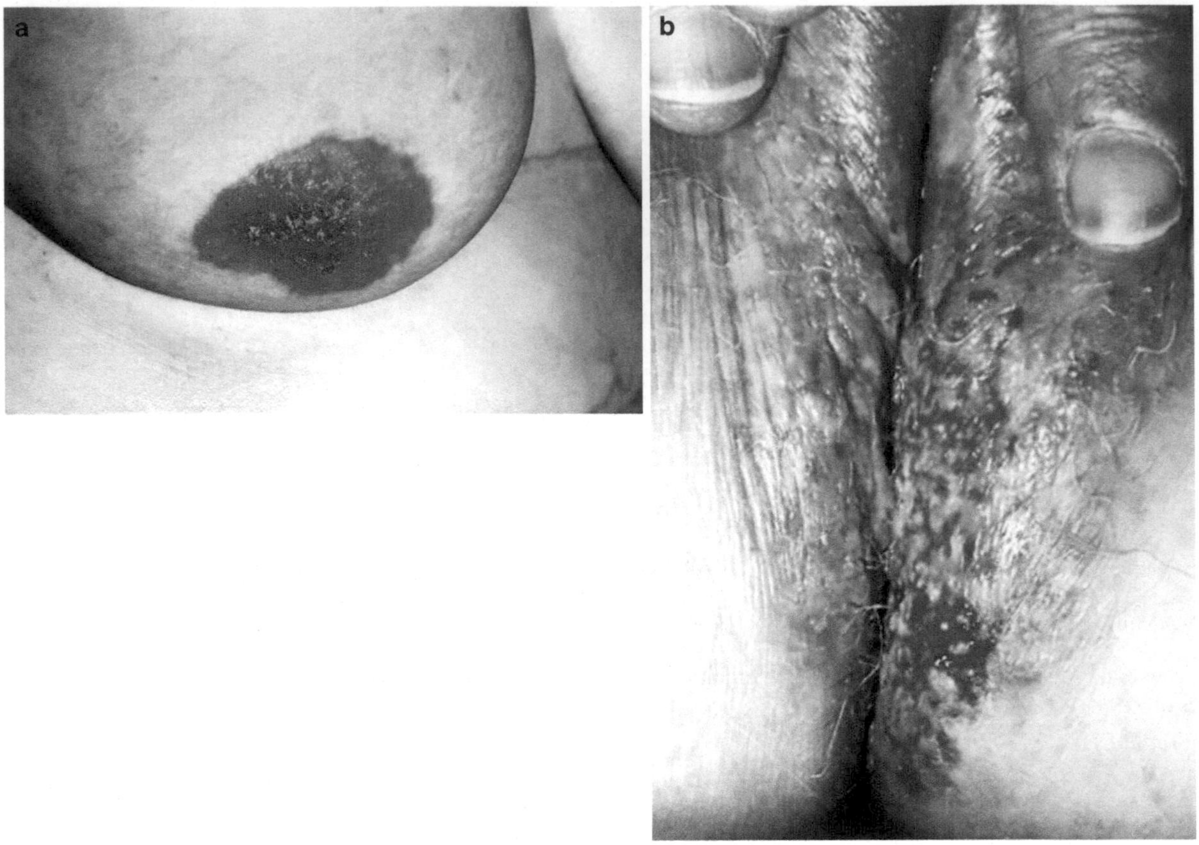

Fig. 57.89 (**a**) Mammary Paget's disease: crusting of the nipple and the areola. (**b**) Extramammary Paget's disease. Multicentric erythematous, erosive lesions on the vulva

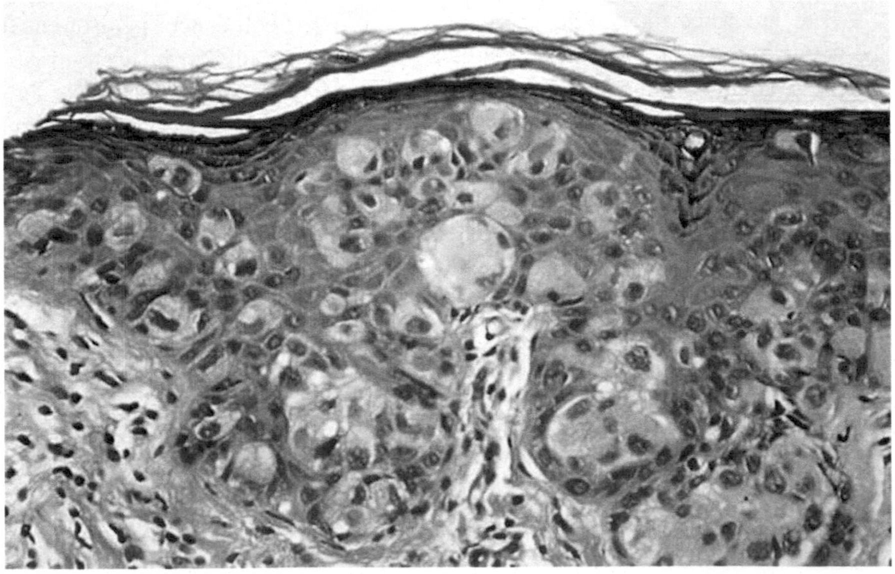

Fig. 57.90 Histology: Large pale-staining tumor cells infiltrating the epidermis. The tumor cells show large vesicular nuclei

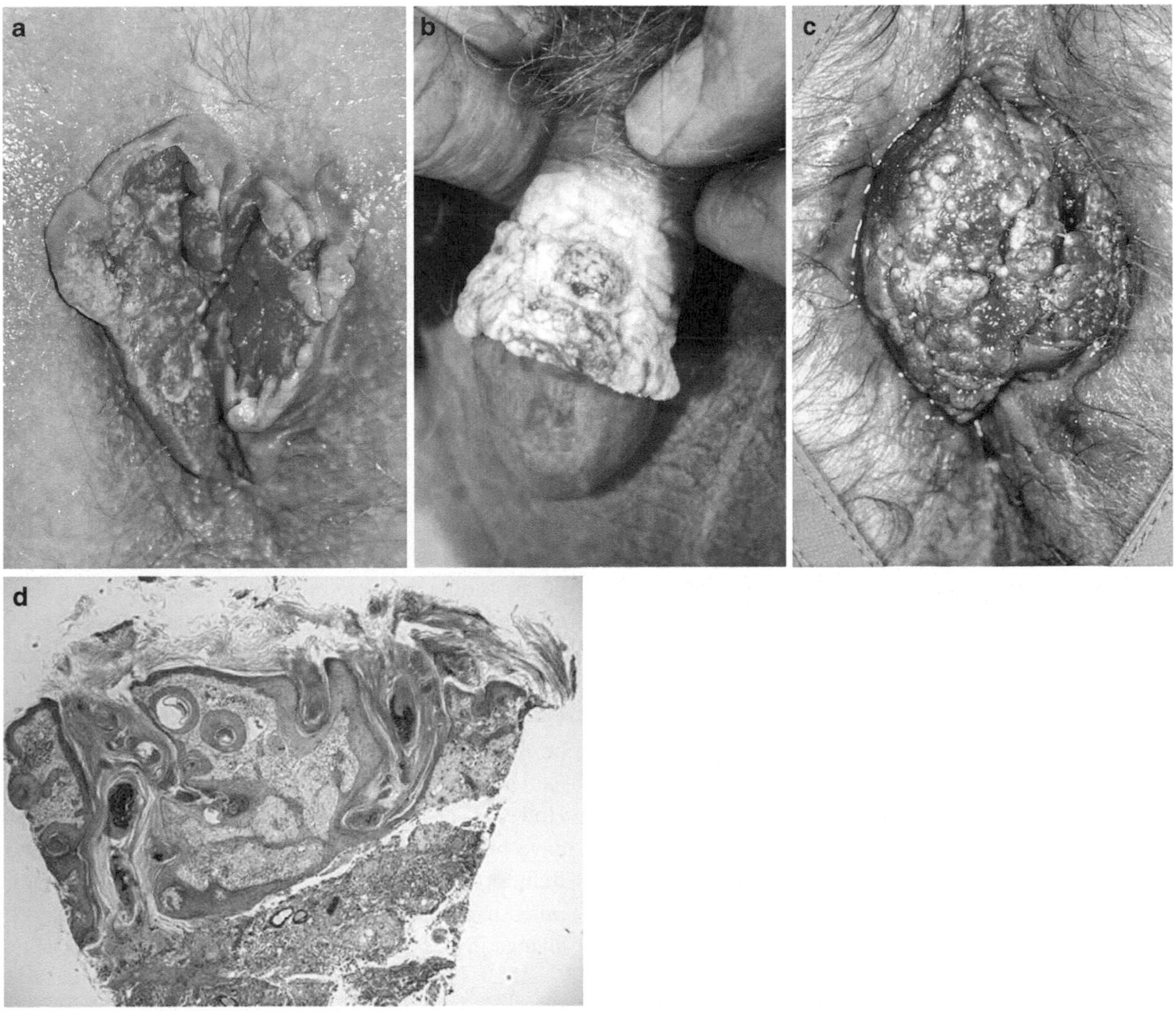

Fig. 57.91 Invasive squamous cell carcinoma. (**a**) Perianal giant fleshy, exulcerated tumor (HPV16 DNA positive). (**b**) Squamous cell carcinoma on lichen sclerosus of the prepuce. (**c**) Perianal verrucous carcinoma. (**d**) Histology: Well-differentiated squamous cell carcinoma (Histology from lesion in (**a**))

57.9.3.2 Basal Cell Carcinoma

Differential Diagnoses

- Cysts
- Benign tumors
- Malignant melanoma
- Seborrheic keratosis
- Melanocytic nevi

Basal cell carcinoma is an uncommon tumor on the genitoanal skin. As a rule, basal cell carcinomas are almost always solitary tumors. The male to female ratio of genitoanal basalioma is about 1:4. In women basal cell carcinomas occur on the hair-bearing skin of the labia majora. In men, tumors have been detected on the penis, the scrotum, and at the perianal skin. They appear nodular with a pearly edge and a centrally located depression or ulceration (Fig. 57.92). Most lesions are grayish with telangiectatic vessels on the surface. Pigmentation is a rare finding. As a rule basal cell carcinoma rarely metastasize. However, the tumors behave locally very destructive. Predisposing factors are UV-exposure, previous PUVA and radiation-therapy. A biopsy is required for diagnosis. Histology is identical to extragenital basal cell carcinomas and consists of basaloid proliferations with peripheral palisading (Fig. 57.93). Treatment is local excision with sufficient margins [33].

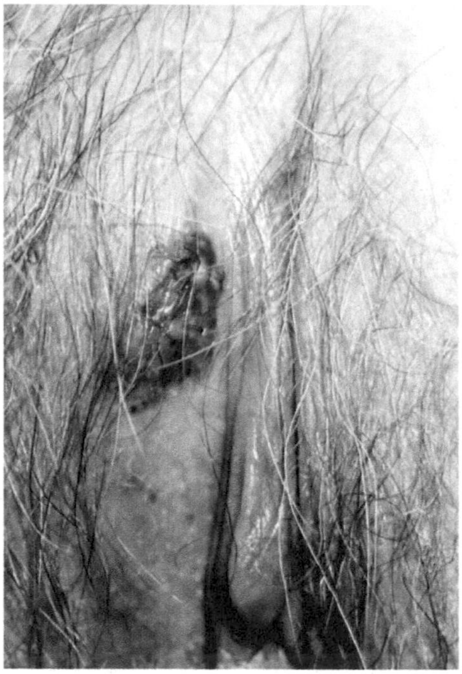

Fig. 57.92 Pigmented basal cell carcinoma on the right labium majus

57.9.3.3 Malignant Melanoma

Differential Diagnoses

- Pigmented nevus
- Pigmented basal cell carcinoma
- Pigmented seborrheic keratosis
- Melanosis
- Lichen sclerosus
- Kaposi's sarcoma

Malignant melanoma is uncommon on the male genitalia. However, vulvar malignant melanomas account for up to 10% of all vulvar malignant neoplasias [11, 49]. In both sexes genitoanal melanomas develop late in life (in the sixth to the seventh decade). The main site of involvement are the labia majora and in males glans and the coronal sulcus. Melanomas arise de novo directly from epidermal melanocytes. Others evolve from the junctional part of a melanocytic nevus. Malignant melanomas may occur on adjacent mucous membranes of the anus and even of the vagina, the cervix uteri, and the urethra. Genitoanal melanomas may be of the superficial spreading but also of the nodular variety. Most tumors are pigmented (Fig. 57.94). However, at genitoanal sites, amelanotic melanomas have been more frequently observed than elsewhere. Itching, ulceration, bleeding, and crusting should raise suspicion of malignant melanoma. Furthermore, change in size and pigmentation of a preexisting nevus

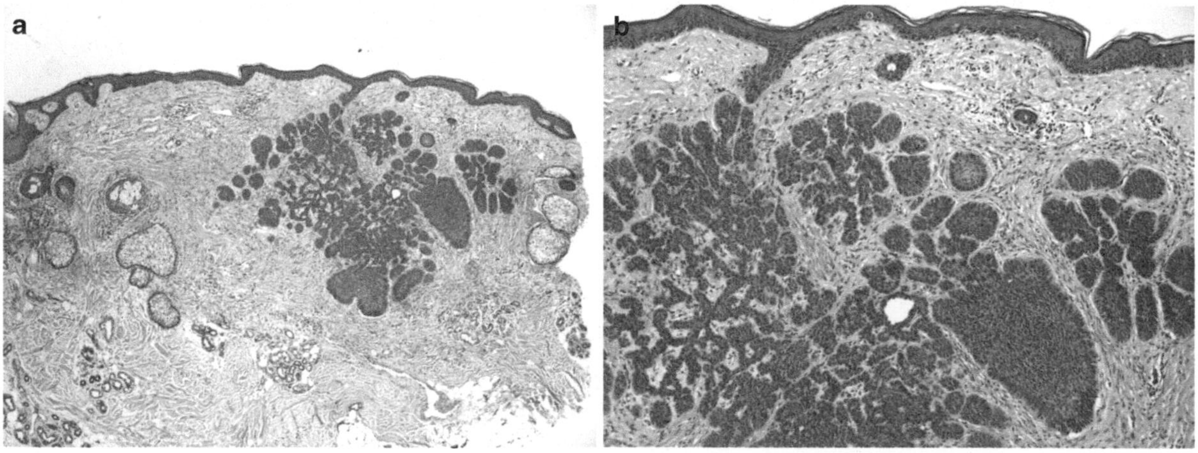

Fig. 57.93 (**a**) Histology: Basalioma. Basaloid tumor cell islands with peripheral palisading in the upper and middermis. (**b**) Magnification from (**a**)

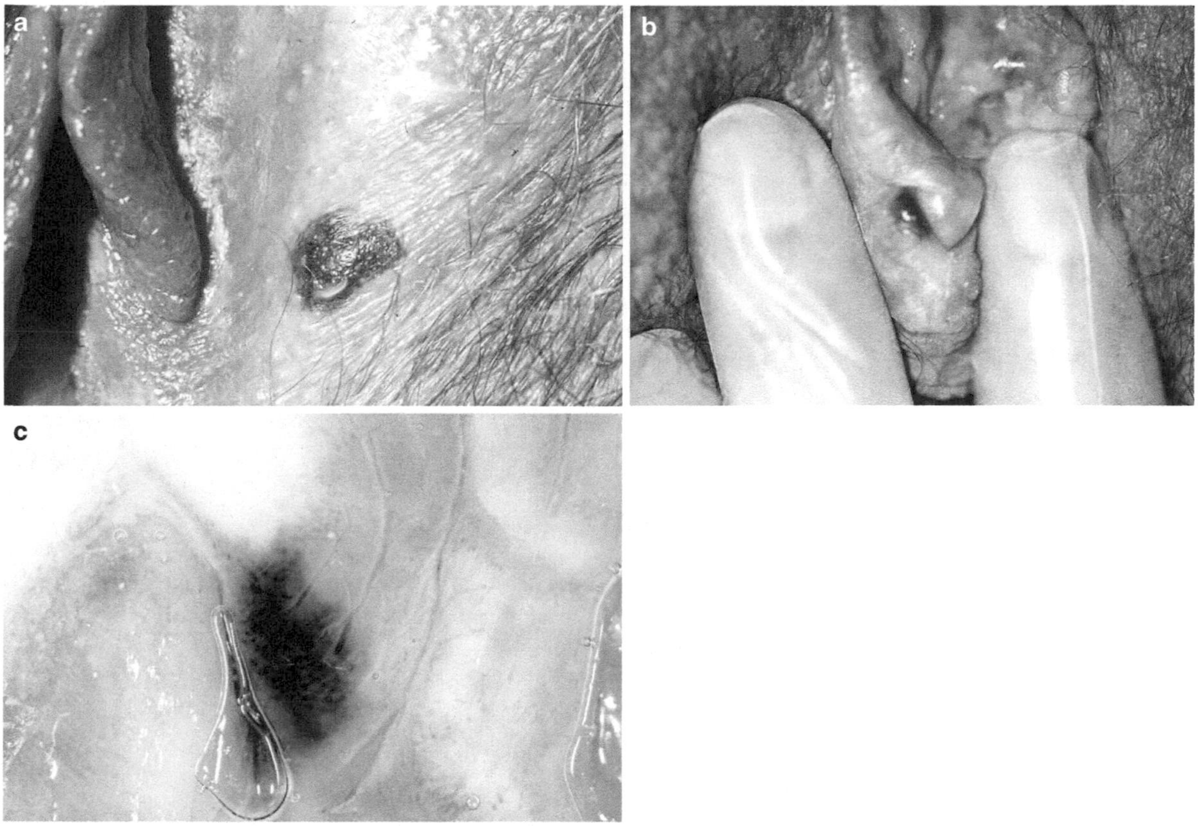

Fig. 57.94 (**a**) Malignant melanoma on the left labium majus. (**b**) Small brownish papule on the periclitoral skin. (**c**) Dermatoscopic aspect: grayish pigmentation abnormalities (magnification from **b**)

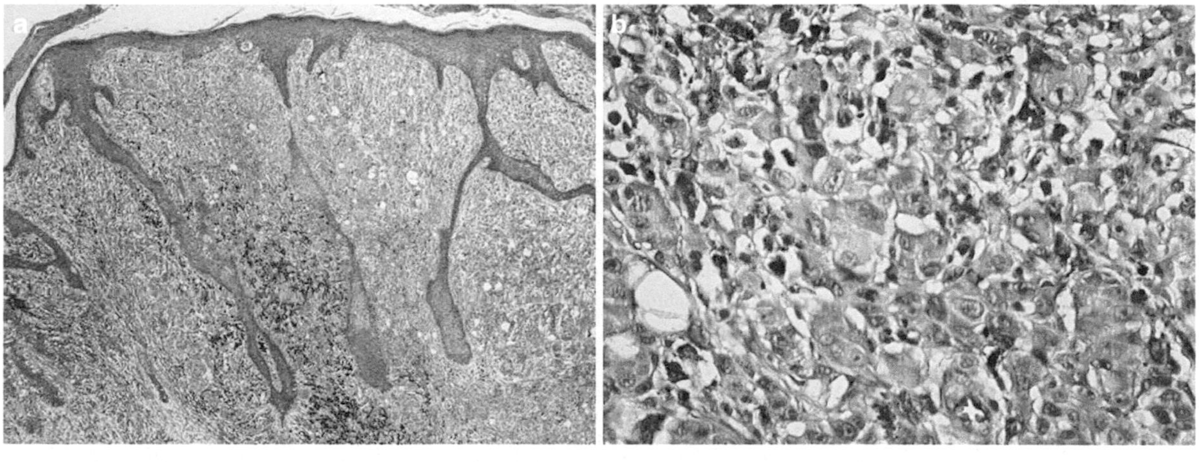

Fig. 57.95 Histology of nodular melanoma. (**a**) There is no melanocytic proliferation in the adjacent epidermis. (**b**) Atypical melanocytes with pleiotropic nuclei (Magnification from (**a**))

is suspicious. Prognosis of malignant melanoma is closely related to the depth of the lesion (Fig. 57.95). Untreated lesions metastasize rapidly to the regional lymph nodes. A good outcome can be obtained with wide local resection of a margin of 1–3 cm, according to the histologic depth of the tumor. Melanomas located at the clitoris have shown a poor prognosis [40]. Chemotherapy is of limited value.

57.9.3.4 Other Malignant Neoplasias

Differential Diagnoses

- Kaposi's sarcoma
- Malignant melanoma
- Hemangioma
- Melanocytic nevus

There are other malignant neoplasias that may generally affect the genitoanal area such as fibrosarcoma and leiomyosarcoma. Kaposi's sarcoma, which is proliferative and reactive rather than a malignant condition associated with human herpes virus type 8, may involve the genitoanal area as part of generalized skin disease. This is especially true for the rapidly disseminating disease in immunodeficient individuals (HIV-seropositive and transplant recipients). Macroscopically, the lesions are heterogeneous and consist in patches, plaques, or tumors of red violaceous colour. Local treatment consists in cryotherapy. Radiotherapy is an option for disseminated cutaneous lesions. Chemotherapy is indicated in systemic disease. Further details are discussed in Chap. 31 on page 405.

57.10 Genitoanal Pain

Infections of the skin and dermatological disorders may cause genitoanal pain. If pain is burning and stinging in nature, it can exist without abnormality. The assessment of affected patients includes a careful examination of the skin to rule out trauma, infection, inflammation, and tumor (Table 57.4). Only in patients with chronic pain, burning, and soreness without detectable cause, it is justified to diagnose vulvodynia (syn.: vulvar burning syndrome) or anodynia [25]. Apparently there are similarities between women and men. But the data collected on vulvodynia are by far more comprehensive than those on scrotodynia or penodynia.

Table 57.4 Disorders which frequently contribute to genitoanal pain

Dermatoses • Lichen planus, erosive lichen planus • Lichen sclerosus • Psoriasis • Autoimmune disease • Eczema
Infections • Yeast • HPV-infection • Herpesvirus infection • Postherpetic neuralgia • Vaginitis
Estrogen deficiency • Coinfections with bacteria and fungi

Secondary vulvar or perianal burning and pain may result from primary *Candida albicans* or other yeast infections, from bacterial infections, and secretions. Eczema is primarily itching but becomes painful due to scratching. Other dermatoses producing pain in a second step are lichen planus and erosive lichen planus as well as lichen sclerosus.

Herpes infections and postherpetic neuralgia may cause acute and chronic genitoanal pain. Less frequently, malignancies such as intraepithelial neoplasias and even genital warts may be the origin of a burning sensation. The most recent classification of vulvar pain established by The International Society for the Study of Vulvovaginal Disease is of 2003 [32]: Currently, three groups of vulvodynia have been recognized: *Vestibulitis, cyclic vulvitis, and dysaesthetic vulvodynia.*

Vulvar vestibulitis is a typically chronic severe pain. Clinically, there is erythema localized to the vestibulum, often at the site of openings of Bartholin's glands. The second symptom is tenderness on these sites. It can be tested with a cotton bud. The third symptom of the condition is dyspareunia.

In some women with vulvodynia, tiny papillae may be seen on the entire mucosal surface of the labia minora. Micropapillomatosis vulvae is frequently encountered in asymptomatic women (Fig. 57.3). Papillomatosis of the vulvar vestibulum is a nonspecific finding and is estimated as an anatomical variant in normal patients. Similar lesions in men are pearly penile papules (hirsuties) (Fig. 57.2) (see page 780) There has been no evidence for an association with HPV infection [5, 31]. Symptoms of vulvar vestibulitis are possibly linked to candidiasis, irritants, wart treatments, or other topical treatments.

Tricyclic antidepressants may lower the symptoms such as burning. Scrotal and penile pain requires similar clinical evaluation as vulvar pain. However, scrotodynia and penodynia are by far less frequently observed than vulvodynia. At first line, dermatological disorders and sexually transmitted diseases have to be ruled out carefully as have neurology problems related to herpes virus infection or other causes.

Intermittent tenderness related to the menstrual cycle, irritation, and pain following intercourse are symptoms of so-called *cyclic vulvitis*. In the acute phase a marked vulvar erythema may be present. Since a certain number of women respond favorably to an anticandidal treatment as nystatin *Candida albicans* is likely to be linked to this condition [28].

Another group of mostly older women suffer from constant burning of the entire vulva including the labia majora. On examination, no definite clinical sign is visible. Whether the origin of this condition called *dysaesthetic vulvodynia* is pudendal neuralgia or an abnormality of cutaneous perception has not yet been clarified. These patients often respond to tricyclic antidepressants such as oral amitriptyline.

In scrotodynia and penodynia, apparently psychological factors play an important role. Low-dose amitriptyline and other antidepressants have been used with some success.

Take-Home Pearls

- Correct diagnosis of genitoanal cutaneous and mucocutaneous conditions is the prerequisite for a successful therapy.
- Diagnosis of the majority of genitoanal cutaneous disorders requires dermatologic expertise.
- Primarily differential diagnosis is done by history taking and on a morphological basis. This includes clinical examination with a magnifying glass or colposcope and histology. Immunofluorescence staining is very helpful to diagnose autoimmune dermatoses.
- Genitoanal biopsy is one of the most efficient ways of making diagnoses.
- Genitoanal pain with and without clinically visible features always requires exclusion of an infection, an inflammatory condition, a tumor or a neurological cause.

References

1. Altmeyer, P., Chilf, G.N., Holzmann, H.: Hirsuties papillaris vulvae (Pseudokondylome der Vulva). Hautarzt **33**, 281–283 (1982)
2. Baeyens, L., Vermeersch, E., Bourgeois, P.: Bicyclist's vulva: observational study. BMJ **325**(7356), 138–139 (2002)
3. Bauer, A., Greif, C., Vollandt, R., Merker, A., Elsner, P.: Vulval diseases need an interdisciplinary approach. Dermatology **1999**(3), 223–226 (1999)
4. Bens, G., Laharie, D., Beylot-Barry, M., Vergier, B., Noblesse, I., Beylot, C., Amouretti, M.: Successful treatment with infliximab and methotrexate of pyostomatitis vegetans associated with Crohn's disease. Br. J. Dermatol. **149**(1), 181–184 (2003)
5. Bergeron, C., Ferenczy, A., Richart, R.M., Guralnick, M.: Micropapillomatosis labialis appears unrelated to human papillomavirus. Obstet. Gynecol. **76**(2), 281–286 (1990)
6. Berth-Jones, J., Smith, S.G., Graham-Brown, R.A.: Benign familial chronic pemphigus (Hailey-Hailey disease) responds to ciclosporine. Clin. Exp. Dermatol. **20**(1), 70–72 (1995)
7. Byrd, J.A., Davis, M.D., Rogers 3, R.S.: Recalcitrant symptomatic vulvar lichen planus: response to topical tacrolimus. Arch. Dermatol. **140**(6), 715–720 (2004)
8. Campagne, G., Roca, M., Martínez, A.: Successful treatment of a high-grade intraepithelial neoplasia with imiquimod, with vulvar pemphigus as a side effect. Eur. J. Obstet. Gynecol. Reprod. Biol. **109**(2), 224–227 (2003)
9. Crum, C.P., McLachlin, C.M., Tate, J.E., Mutter, G.L.: Pathobiology of vulvar squamous neoplasia. Curr. Opin. Obstet. Gynecol. **9**(1), 63–69 (1997)
10. Darier, J.: Lichen plan scléreux. Ann. Dermatol. Syph. **23**, 833–837 (1892)
11. Dunton, C.J., Kautzky, M., Hanau, C.: Malignant melanoma of the vulva: a review. Obstet. Gynecol. Surv. **50**(10), 739–746 (1995)
12. Ewald, K., Gross, G.: Perianal Hailey-Hailey disease: an unusual differential diagnosis of condylomata acuminata. Int. J. STD AIDS **19**(11), 791–792 (2008)
13. Farrell, A.M., Millard, P.R., Schomberg, K.H., et al.: An infective aetiology for lichen sclerosus: Myth or reality? Br. J. Dermatol. **50**, 25 (1997)
14. Goldsmith, P.C., Rycroft, R.G., White, I.R., Ridley, C.M., Neill, S.M., McFadden, J.P.: Contact sensitivity in women with anogenital dermatoses. Contact Dermat. **36**(3), 174–175 (1997)
15. Gross, G., Pfister, H.: Role of human papillomavirus in penile cancer, penile intraepithelial squamous cell neoplasias and in genital warts. Med. Microbiol. Immunol. **193**(1), 35–44 (2004)
16. Helwig, E.B., Graham, J.H.: Anogenital (extramammary) Paget's disease. A clinicopathological study. Cancer **16**, 387–403 (1963)
17. Ikenberg, H., Gissmann, L., Gross, G., Grussendorf-Conen, El., zur Haŭsen, H.: Human papillomavirus type-16-related DNA in genital Bowen's disease and in Bowenoid papulosis. Int. J. Cancer **32**(5), 563–565 (1983)
18. Kao, M.S., Paulson, J.D., Askin, F.B.: Crohn's disease of the vulva. Obstet. Gynecol. **46**(3), 329–333 (1975)

19. Kobashigawa, T., Okamoto, H., Kato, J., Shindo, H., Imamura, T., Iizuka, B.E., Tanaka, M., Uesato, M., Ohta, S.J., Terai, C., Hara, M., Kamatani, N.: Ulcerative colitis followed by the development of Behçet's disease. Intern. Med. **43**(3), 243–247 (2004)
20. Krol, A.L.: Perianal streptococcal dermatitis. Paediatr. Dermatol. **7**, 97–100 (1990)
21. Kruppa, A., Korge, B., Lasch, J., Scharffetter-Kochanek, K., Hunzelmann, N.: Successful treatment of Hailey-Hailey disease with a scanned carbon dioxide laser. Acta Derm. Venereol. **80**(1), 53–54 (2000)
22. Landthaler, M., Hohenleutner, U., Braun-Falco, O.: Acquired lymphangioma of the vulva: palliative treatment by means of laser vaporization carbon dioxide. Arch. Dermatol. **126**(7), 967–968 (1990)
23. Lin, H.C., Chien, C.W., Ho, J.D.: Herpes zoster and the risk of stroke. Neurology **74**, 792–797 (2010)
24. Lonsdale-Eccles, A.A., Velangi, S.: Topical pimecrolimus in the treatment of genital lichen planus: a prospective case series. Br. J. Dermatol. **153**(2), 390–394 (2005)
25. Lynch, P.: Vulvodynia: a syndrome of unexplained vulvar pain, psychologic disability and sexual dysfunction. J. Respond Med. **31**, 773–780 (1986)
26. Marren, P., Wojnarowska, F., Venning, V., Wilson, C., Nayar, M.: Vulvar involvement in autoimmune bullous diseases. J. Reprod. Med. **38**(2), 101–107 (1993)
27. Mattox, T.F., Ruttgers, J., Yoshimori, R.N., Bhatia, N.N.: Nonfluorescent erythrasma of the vulva. Obstet. Gynecol. **81**(5 (Pt 2)), 862–864 (1993)
28. Mc Kay, M.: Vulvodynia: diagnostic patterns. Dermatol. Clin. **10**, 423–426 (1992)
29. Montes-Romero, J.A., Callejas-Rubio, J.L., Sánchez-Cano, D., González-Martínez, F.J., Navas-Parejo, A., Ortego-Centeno, N.: Amyloidosis secondary to hidradenitis suppurativa. Exceptional response to infliximab. Eur. J. Intern. Med. **19**(6), e32–33 (2008)
30. Moschella, S.L.: Is there a role for infliximab in the current therapy of hidradenitis suppurativa? A report of three treated cases. Int. J. Dermatol. **46**(12), 1287–1291 (2007)
31. Moyal-Barraco, M., Leibowitch, M., Orth, G.: Vestibular papillae of the vulva. Lack of evidence for human papillomavirus etiology. Arch. Dermatol. **126**(12), 1594–1598 (1990)
32. Moyal-Barraco, M., Lynch, P.J.: 2003 ISSVD terminology and classification of vulvodynia: a historical perspective. J. Reprod. Med. **49**, 772–777 (2004)
33. Mulayim, N., Foster Silver, D., Tolgay, O.I., Babalola, E.: Vulvar basal cell carcinoma: two unusual presentations and review of the literature. Gynecol. Oncol. **85**(3), 532–537 (2002)
34. Murphy, R.: Training in the diagnosis and management of vulvovaginal diseases. J. Reprod. Med. **52**, 92–97 (2007)
35. Neri, L., Barduzzi, F., Nurzaduri, S., Patrizi, A.: Perianal streptococcal dermatitis in adults. Br. J. Dermatol. **135**, 796–798 (1996)
36. Nissi, R., Eriksen, H., Risteli, J., Niemimaa, M.: Pimecrolimus cream 1% in the treatment of lichen sclerosus. Gynecol. Obstet. Invest. **63**(3), 151–154 (2007)
37. Pelisse, M., Leibowitch, M., Sedel, D., Hewitt, J.: Un nouveau syndrome vulvo-vagino-gingival. Lichen plan erosive plurimuqueux. Ann. Dermatol. Vénéréol. **109**(9), 797–798 (1982)
38. Pelisse, M.: Erosive vulvar lichen planus and desquamative vaginitis. Semin. Dermatol. **15**, 47–50 (1996)
39. Sand, C., Thomsen, H.K.: Topical tacrolimus ointment is an effective therapy for Hailey-Hailey disease. Arch. Dermatol. **139**, 1401–1402 (2003)
40. Scheistrøen, M., Tropé, C., Koern, J., Pettersen, E.O., Abeler, V.M., Kristensen, G.B.: Malignant melanoma of the vulva. Evaluation of prognostic factors with emphasis on DNA ploidy in 75 patients. Cancer **75**(1), 72–80 (1995)
41. Sideri, M., Origoni, M., Spinaci, L., Ferrari, A.: Topical testosterone in the treatment of vulvar lichen sclerosus. Int. J. Gynaecol. Obstet. **46**(1), 53–56 (1994)
42. Van Seters, M., van Beurden, M., ten Kate, F.J., Beckmann, I., Ewing, P.C., Eijkemans, M.J., Kagie, M.J., Meijer, C.J., Aaronson, N.K., Kleinjan, A., Heijmans-Antonissen, C., Zijlstra, F.J., Burger, M.P., Helmerhorst, T.J.: Treatment of vulvar intraepithelial neoplasia with topical imiquimod. N Engl J. Med. **358**(14), 1465–1473 (2008)
43. Virgili, A., Corazza, M., Bianchi, A., Mollica, G., Califano, A.: Open study of topical 0.025% tretinoin in the treatment of vulvar lichen sclerosus. One year of therapy. J. Reprod. Med. **40**(9), 614–618 (1995)
44. Virgili, A., Lauriola, M.M., Mantovani, L., Corazza, M.: Vulvar lichen sclerosus: 11 women treated with tacrolimus 0.1% ointment. Acta Derm. Venereol. **87**(1), 69–72 (2007)
45. Wang, L.C., Blanchard, A., Judge, D.E., Lorincz, A.A., Medenica, M.M., Busbey, S.: Successful treatment of recurrent extramammary Paget's disease of the vulva with topical imiquimod 5% cream. J. Am. Acad. Dermatol. **49**(4), 769–772 (2003)
46. Waugh, M.: Herpes zoster of the anogenital area affecting urination and defaecation. Br. J. Dermatol. **90**(2), 235–238 (1974)
47. Wilkinson, E.J., Rico, M.J., Pierson, K.K.: Microinvasive carcinoma of the vulva. Int. J. Gynecol. Pathol. **1**(1), 29–39 (1982)
48. Zoon, J.J.: Balanitis and Vulvitis plasmacellularis. Dermatologica **111**, 157 (1955)
49. Chung, A.F., Woodruff, J.M., Lewis, J.L.: Malignant melanoma of the vulva: a report of 44 cases. Obstet Gynecol. **45**, 638–646 (1975)

STIs in Pediatrics, Perinatology and Reproduction

58

Amber R. Gill and Anita K. Shetty

Core Messages

- The incidence of many sexually transmitted infections (STIs) in women, including *Chlamydia trachomatis* and *Neisseria gonorrhoeae*, is greatest among those under the age of 25 years, a time when many women may become pregnant.
- STIs can have several effects on fertility and pregnancy, depending on the timing of the infection.
- Infection prior to pregnancy may contribute to infertility or ectopic pregnancy.
- Infection during pregnancy can cause spontaneous abortion, preterm labor, perinatal death, and fetal infection.
- The presence of STIs in children may be the result of transmission from the mother during childbirth, sexual abuse, or nonsexual contact.
- Screening and treating pregnant women for STIs continues to be an important step in reducing the transmission of many STIs to infants.
- In the future, new vaccines will decrease or eliminate the transmission of certain STIs to neonates and children prior to sexual contact.

A.R. Gill (✉)
School of Medicine, University of Texas Medical School at Houston, Houston, TX, USA
e-mail: amber.gill@uth.tmc.edu

A.K. Shetty
Center for Clinical Studies, Loyola University Medical Center, Division of Dermatology, Maywood, Illinois, USA
e-mail: anitaks@gmail.com

58.1 STIs in Pediatrics, Perinatology, and Reproduction

The incidence of many STIs in women, including *Chlamydia trachomatis* and *Neisseria gonorrhoeae*, is greatest among those under the age of 25 years (1). This is also an age at which many women will become pregnant. STIs can have several effects on fertility and pregnancy, depending on the timing of the infection. Infection prior to pregnancy may contribute to infertility or ectopic pregnancy, while infection during pregnancy can cause spontaneous abortion, preterm labor, perinatal death, and fetal infection.

58.2 Infertility

Many sexually transmitted infections of the genital tract can affect female fertility. Generally, infertility is defined as the inability to conceive after one year of regular intercourse without the use of contraceptives (2). Acute pelvic inflammatory disease (PID) has long been recognized as an important cause of tubal factor infertility, ectopic pregnancy, and chronic pelvic pain (3). A longitudinal cohort study in Lund Sweden, documented the reproductive outcomes of 1,844 women with laparoscopically diagnosed acute PID (4). In this study, 11% of those with PID subsequently developed tubal occlusions that left them infertile, compared to none of the controls without PID. The same study found that the number of acute PID episodes determined the risk of infertility. Having just one episode of acute PID was associated with an infertility rate of 8%, while two and three episodes raised the rate to 19.5% and 40%, respectively. In addition, the severity of the

G. Gross and S.K. Tyring (eds.), *Sexually Transmitted Infections and Sexually Transmitted Diseases*,
DOI: 10.1007/978-3-642-14663-3_58, © Springer-Verlag Berlin Heidelberg 2011

inflammation associated with the PID was correlated with rates of infertility. For the severe cases, the rate of infertility was 21% while the mild and moderate cases suffered from infertility rates of only 0.6% and 6.2%, respectively. In addition, early treatment of PID was found to improve the reproductive outcomes of these patients (5). Those who were treated within 2 days of onset of symptoms were less likely to become infertile compared to those who were treated later in the course of PID (8.3% compared to 19.2%).

Infections of the genital tract with *N. gonorrhoeae* and *C. trachomatis* have been associated with PID, and in areas where untreated gonococcal and chlamydial infections are common, tubal infertility is also more prevalent (6). Serological studies have identified antibodies against both *N. gonorrhoeae* and *C. trachomatis* in the sera of women with tubal damage. While the numbers vary, the presence of these antibodies is associated with a much greater incidence of tubal infertility (7, 8). In some areas, up to two-thirds of tubal infertility cases have been attributed to *C. trachomatis* infection (9).

Another complication associated with PID is ectopic pregnancy. A case control study of 112 women with ectopic pregnancies revealed that 50% of the women had tubal adhesions and 65% were seropositive for antichlamydial antibodies (10). In another study, 59% of patients with previous ectopic pregnancy had antibodies to *C. trachomatis* (11). A similar association has been reported with *N. gonorrhoeae*, albeit less extensively studied (12). Thus, *N. gonorrhoeae* and *C. trachomatis* are important causes of acute PID and contribute to infertility and ectopic pregnancy as supported by serologic data.

58.3 Perinatology

There are many changes that occur during pregnancy alter host defense mechanisms. It is thought that perhaps suppression of the maternal immune system is one reason a fetus is not generally rejected from womb (13). However, this immunosuppression may also leave the mother more vulnerable to infections, including STIs. The female reproductive tract also undergoes dramatic anatomical changes during pregnancy. First, the cervix hypertrophies and there is an increased area of cervical ectopy, exposing more columnar epithelium (14). This may make the cervix more susceptible to infection. The cervix also secretes thick mucus, which forms a plug and is believed to act as a barrier to microorganisms, possibly blocking ascending infections during pregnancy. There is also increased blood flow to the vagina and uterus during pregnancy, which would favor the growth of aerobic microbes. In addition, there is a much higher glycogen content in the vagina which leads to a more acidic environment and likely affects the normal vaginal flora (15). In fact, several studies suggest that during pregnancy the overall variety of bacterial species in the vagina decreases, especially the number of anaerobic bacteria, while the amount of lactobacilli increases (16).

Acute inflammation of the fetal membranes, or chorioamnionitis, has been found to be very strongly correlated with preterm birth (17–19). The prevalence of chorioamnionitis varies by gestational age. Chorioamnionitis was found in 95% of pregnancies at less than 25 weeks gestation, 35–40% of pregnancies for 25–32 weeks, 11% from 33 to 35 weeks and only 3–5% of full term pregnancies (20). Further, the mean birth weight for the group with chorioamnionitis was much lower than the control group (2,811 vs. 3,320 g, $p<0.001$), although the birth weights were appropriate for the gestational age and not attributable to intrauterine growth restriction (20). Several microorganisms have been isolated from the fetal membranes with histologic chorioamnionitis; the most frequently isolated are *U. urealyticum*, *Gardnerella vaginalis*, Group B Streptococcus (GBS), *Escherichia coli*, anaerobic gram positive cocci, *Bacteriodes* spp., *Prevotella bivia*, and *Fusobacterium nucleatum.* A similar correlation with gestational age is seen with infection of the amniotic fluid with intact membranes, although it is at a lower level (21–23). The microorganisms most frequently isolated from the amniotic fluid are similar to those isolated from fetal membranes. These data suggest that the fetal membranes are likely to be the site of primary infection with secondary infection of the amniotic fluid.

Animal models suggest that pro-inflammatory cytokines that are produced in response to infection of the amniotic fluid may be to blame for preterm delivery. In one study, increased levels of intraamniotic cytokines were detected between 9 and 18 h after inoculating pregnant rhesus monkeys with GBS. There was also an increase in prostaglandins, leading to uterine contractions 10–20 h after the increased cytokine levels were detected (24). In a similar study, intraamniotic infusion of the cytokine IL-1 without bacteria induced preterm labor in all treated animals, suggesting that cytokines, rather than bacteria, are to blame for the preterm labor (25). In addition, pro-inflammatory cytokines have also been associated with increased frequency of neonatal complications such as respiratory distress syndrome, intraventricular hemorrhage, and periventricular leukomalacia, even after adjusting for gestational age at delivery (26, 27).

Several lower genital tract infections, including *N. gonorrhoeae*, *C. trachomatis*, bacterial vaginosis, and *Trichomonas vaginalis* have been associated with increased risk of adverse pregnancy outcomes such as preterm premature rupture of membranes (PPROM), and premature birth (28, 29). Significantly, bacterial vaginosis has consistently been identified as a risk factor for both PPROM and preterm birth (30, 31). Systemic treatment for bacterial vaginosis has been shown to reduce the rate of preterm birth in cases where the risk for preterm birth was high (32, 33). *T. vaginalis* infection has also been associated with an increased risk of PPROM, preterm delivery, and low birth weight (34). Many bacterial species commonly found in the lower genital tract produce proteases, which have been shown to reduce the strength and elasticity of membranes in vitro (35, 36). In another study, adding *E. coli* or GBS to cultured fetal membranes reduced the pressure required for bursting (37). Similarly, in vitro studies have shown that *T. vaginalis* isolates decrease the elasticity and bursting tension of chorioamniotic membranes in an inoculum-dependent manner (38). These data suggest that genital tract infections and the resulting inflammatory response may directly damage the fetal membranes, resulting in PPROM.

58.4 Bacterial STIs

58.4.1 *Syphilis*

The clinical manifestations of syphilis in adults are not altered by pregnancy, but most women with syphilis are asymptomatic. While it is possible to transmit syphilis during delivery (39, 40), it is believed that most cases arise from transplacental infection (41–43). This is likely due to the invasive nature of *Treponema pallidum*, which has been shown to cross the placenta, most likely at intercellular junctions (44, 45). Congenital syphilis is entirely preventable with routine screenings in pregnant women, followed by appropriate treatment (46). The rate of transfer and the severity of complications during pregnancy depend on the stage of infection in the mother. Untreated primary or secondary syphilis affects virtually 100% of fetuses. In one study, 50% of the pregnancies ended in preterm delivery or perinatal death, while the other 50% developed congenital syphilis (47). With untreated early latent syphilis, 40% of the infants contracted congenital syphilis and there was a rate of 40% for prematurity or perinatal death, while the remaining 20% of infants were healthy. In cases of late latent syphilis, 70% of the infants were healthy, 11% died perinatally, 10% developed congenital syphilis, and 9% were born prematurely. Interestingly, there was no increase in the rate of prematurity in cases of late latent syphilis, compared to women without syphilis (47). Congenital syphilis can nearly be diagnosed by the distinct appearance of the placenta at birth. Characteristic findings in the placenta include hypercellular villi, proliferative vascular changes, and acute or chronic villitis (41, 43, 48–50). The placenta is an important clue in diagnosis of congenital syphilis as most infected infants are asymptomatic at birth (51–53).

Congenital syphilis is often divided into early and late disease, depending on the age at onset of symptoms. Early congenital syphilis comprises symptoms appearing in the first two years of life, while symptoms of late congenital syphilis typically appear around puberty. Symptoms of congenital syphilis are the consequence of infection with *T. pallidum* and the resultant inflammatory responses within the various tissues. Clinical manifestations can involve almost any fetal organ, with liver, kidneys, bone, pancreas, spleen, lungs, heart, and brain being the most frequently affected (54). Various mucocutaneous lesions are also common in congenital syphilis. The most common lesion is a large round pink macule that develops slowly over a period of weeks and resolves in 1–3 months without treatment, leaving residual pigmentation (51, 55). These lesions may be covered with a silvery scale and are typically distributed over the back, perineum, extremities, palms, and soles, sparing the anterior trunk. Another common cutaneous manifestation is a highly infectious vesiculobullous eruption, known as pemphigus syphiliticus (55). These lesions are most prominent on the palms and soles and are typically followed by desquamation upon rupture. Other characteristic findings of congenital syphilis include apical notching of the teeth, ocular lesions such as interstitial keratitis, neural deafness, nasal discharge, and ulceration and necrosis of the nasal septum leading to the characteristic "saddle-nose" deformity.

58.4.2 Gonorrhea

Gonorrhea infection during pregnancy has many implications for the outcome of the pregnancy, as well as the health of the neonate. Gonorrhea infection has been associated with several pregnancy complications, including PPROM, premature birth and low birth weight. In one case control study, *N. gonorrhoeae* was isolated from 13% of patients with PPROM but found in none of the term controls (56). Interestingly, all patients in this study had been screened, and if positive, treated for gonorrhea early in pregnancy. Other studies of women with untreated gonorrhea reported a three- to six-fold increased risk for preterm birth and low birth weight (57, 58). In general, untreated maternal gonococcal infections are associated with adverse pregnancy outcomes, including premature delivery, perinatal stress, and perinatal death (59–61).

Gonorrhea is generally transmitted to neonates at the time of birth when they come in contact with gonorrhea in the birth canal. Fetuses may also be exposed in utero to infected amniotic fluid. Unfortunately, the most common mode of acquiring gonorrhea in children after the newborn period, but before puberty, is sexual abuse (62, 63).

Gonococcal infections in pediatrics produce a wide range of manifestations that are age related. A well-recognized neonatal manifestation of exposure to maternal gonorrhea is gonococcal ophthalmia neonatorum, usually appearing 2–5 days after birth. In one study performed in Kenya, 42% of newborns not receiving prophylactic eye treatment acquired the ocular infection (64). However, prophylactic eye drops or ointment containing 1% silver nitrate, 0.5% erythromycin, or 1% tetracycline have been shown to reduce the incidence of gonococcal ophthalmia significantly (65, 66). Gonococcal ophthalmia may also be acquired in utero after premature rupture of membranes (PROM), and ocular prophylaxis administered at birth may not help in this situation (61, 67). If left untreated, gonococcal ophthalmia can lead to permanent corneal damage. Other localized gonococcal infections in the neonatal period include vaginitis, urethritis, rhinitis, anorectal infection, pharyngeal infection, and funisitis, all are attributable to exposure to infected amniotic fluid or contact in the birth canal (68–72). While dissemination is uncommon, septic arthritis is the most frequent manifestation of disseminated gonococcal infection in the neonatal period (73–75). However, *N. gonorrhoeae* has also been isolated from blood in the absence of arthritis (76).

The most common form of gonorrhea in children beyond the neonatal period is gonococcal vaginitis. The alkaline vaginal mucosa of prepubertal girls may make them susceptible to colonization with *N. gonorrhoeae*. Gonococcal vaginitis is generally a mild disease with few signs or symptoms other than a minor vaginal discharge. However, this infection may progress to a more serious condition involving the fallopian tubes or may disseminate to the pelvis, leading to perihepatitis and PID. Gonococcal urethritis is much less common than vaginitis in girls, but this condition can occur in prepubertal boys. Other manifestations of gonorrhea in children include pharyngeal infections and anorectal infections, generally resulting from sexual abuse (68, 77).

58.4.3 Chlamydia

Although results vary, chlamydial infections before and during pregnancy may be associated with adverse outcomes, including abortion, PPROM, low birth weight, stillbirth, and neonatal death (78–80). *Chlamydia trachomatis* infection is generally acquired by the neonate during passage through the birth canal (81, 82). Although rare, infection of the amniotic fluid with intact membranes and infection following a cesarean delivery have been reported (83). Infants who are exposed to *C. trachomatis* are often infected at more than one anatomical site, including the conjunctiva, nasopharynx, rectum and vagina. The most frequent site of infection is the nasopharynx. In one study, 78% of infants born to infected mothers had nasopharyngeal cultures positive for *C. trachomatis* (83). Most cases of nasopharyngeal infection are asymptomatic and may persist for up to 3 years (84). Only about one-third of infants with nasopharyngeal infection will subsequently develop chlamydial pneumonia, which is generally self-limiting (85). Nasopharyngeal infections may also lead to otitis media because the middle ear is contiguous with the nasopharynx (86).

While the nasopharynx is the most common site of infection, the most common clinical manifestation of neonatal chlamydial infection is conjunctivitis. It has been reported that between 15% and 37% of infants born to mothers with active, untreated chlamydial infections will develop conjunctivitis (81–83). About two-thirds of cases occur in both eyes and the infection usually presents within 5–14 days. Long-term sequelae of neonatal chlamydial conjunctivitis include corneal neovascularization and scarring, which may lead to blindness.

Like gonorrhea, chlamydial infections in older children are generally associated with sexual abuse (81, 82, 87). However, vaginal and rectal infections resulting from exposure to *C. trachomatis* during childbirth have been documented to persist for up to 3 years (84). This should be considered when investigating cases of suspected child abuse. Most chlamydial infections in children are asymptomatic.

58.5 Viral STIs

58.5.1 Cytomegalovirus

Cytomegalovirus (CMV) can be acquired before or during pregnancy by both sexual and nonsexual transmission. CMV is the most common cause of congenital viral infections and is likely transmitted to the fetus transplacentally. Primary CMV infections during pregnancy are more likely to be transmitted to the fetus than recurrent infections. Approximately 40% of pregnant women with primary CMV infection will transmit the virus to the fetus transplacentally and between 10% and 20% of these infants will show signs of infection at birth, including microcephaly, hepatosplenomegaly, and petechiae (88). In contrast, CMV is only transmitted in approximately 3.4% of women with recurrent infections during pregnancy (89). However, due to the high prevalence of CMV seropositivity throughout the world, it has been suggested that recurrent, rather than primary, infections during pregnancy may be the leading cause of intrauterine CMV infection (90). It has been reported that 90% of infants who are symptomatic for CMV at birth will subsequently die or suffer major morbidity, such as microcephaly, mental retardation, developmental delay, seizures, sensorineural hearing loss, and ocular abnormalities (88, 91). CMV may also be transmitted during vaginal childbirth or postpartum through breast milk (92). Intrapartum and postpartum transmission do not seem to have ill effects on full term infants. However, between 10% and 20% of premature infants who are infected through breast milk will subsequently develop sepsis-like symptoms or viral hepatitis (93–95).

58.5.2 Herpes Simplex Virus

Herpes simplex virus (HSV) infections of the genitals are caused by both HSV-2 and HSV-1, and both forms may be transmitted to neonates. It has been estimated that between 16.5% and 32% of pregnant women in the USA are HSV-2 seropositive, with the majority being unaware of their infection (96–98). Another study found that 21.4% of genital herpes cases among women were culture-positive for HSV-1 rather than HSV-2 (99). Approximately 85% of HSV infections in the neonate are transmitted in the birth canal, while only about 5% are transmitted transplacentally, and the other 10% are due to exposure from other sources, such as the lips of a caregiver (100). Primary HSV infection during pregnancy has been associated with an increased rate of transfer to the neonate when compared to recurrent infections. In five studies, 44% of infants born to mothers with primary HSV infections developed neonatal infections (98, 101–104). On the other hand, two studies found that only 0–3% of infants born to mothers with recurrent HSV infections developed neonatal HSV infections (104, 105). Primary HSV infection during pregnancy has also been associated with an increased rate of adverse effects such as spontaneous abortion, preterm labor, low birth weight, growth retardation, and neonatal HSV infection (101, 102). However, recurrent genital HSV does not seem to increase the risk for preterm birth or fetal growth retardation (106). Primary HSV infection may pose a greater risk to the neonate because the viral load in the birth canal is likely large, maternal antibodies are absent and not transferred to the fetus, and the neonate is likely to be immunologically immature at birth. On the other hand, neonates born to mothers with recurrent HSV infections are likely to acquire some protective immunity from maternal antibodies.

58.5.3 Human Papillomavirus

Human papillomavirus (HPV) is a relatively common STI and the highest rates of infection are found in 18–28 year olds (107). The majority of studies have found that HPV is upregulated during pregnancy, possibly due to suppression of the maternal immune system (108–111). The external manifestations of HPV are also more pronounced during pregnancy as genital warts tend to enlarge and become more vascular. Neonatal exposure to HPV most often occurs during passage through the birth canal and the most common manifestations of infection are laryngeal papillomas or genital warts in infancy or childhood (112). Laryngeal papillomatosis, a form of recurrent respiratory papillomatosis, is the most common tumor of the larynx in children. While laryngeal papillomas are rarely malignant, they are frequently recurrent and require multiple surgical procedures to protect the airway (113, 114). Studies have found that HPV types 6 and 11 account for most cases of laryngeal papillomas and genital warts (115).

Condylomata acuminata, or genital warts, are most often caused by HPV types 6 and 11 in adults, while warts on other areas of the body such as the hands (verruca vulgaris) are typically due to HPV type 2. In one study, 94% of genital warts in adults contained HPVs 6/11, while HPV 2 caused only 3% (116). The other 3% were caused by HPVs 42, 43, and 44. However, the same study found that 59% of warts on the genitals of children were caused by HPVs 6/11, while 41% were due to HPV 2 (116). Another study found HPV DNA of various types in 20 out of 110 girls who had no history of sexual activity or sexual abuse (117). These studies suggest that warts on the genitals of children may be true condyloma acuminata (HPV 6/11) acquired from passage through the birth canal of their infected mother or from sexual abuse, or verruca vulgaris (HPV 2), which is not sexually transmitted and likely caused by autoinoculation.

Vaccination against HPV types 6 and 11 could decrease the rates of these HPV types in women and decrease or eliminate the transmission of HPV to neonates in the future (118). The bivalent vaccine confers protection against HPV 16 and 18 only, while the quadrivalent vaccine, which is currently available in the USA, protects against HPV 6, 11, 16, and 18 (119, 120).

58.6 Conclusion

The incidence of many STIs is highest among women in their fertile years. STIs before pregnancy can affect fertility, while infection during pregnancy can cause spontaneous abortion, preterm labor, perinatal death, and fetal infection. The presence of STIs in children may be the result of transmission from the mother during childbirth, sexual abuse, or nonsexual contact. Symptoms associated with various STIs range from mild or asymptomatic to severe and debilitating. Screening and/or treating pregnant women continues to be an important step in reducing the transmission of many STIs to their infants. In the future, new vaccines will decrease or eliminate the transmission of certain STIs to neonates and children prior to sexual contact.

Take-Home Pearls

- The incidence of many STIs is highest among women in their fertile years.
- Becoming infected with STIs before pregnancy can adversely affect fertility.
- STI during pregnancy can cause spontaneous abortion, preterm labor, perinatal death, and fetal infection.
- STIs in children may be the result of transmission from the mother during childbirth, sexual abuse, or nonsexual contact.
- Screening and treating pregnant women for STIs is an important step toward reducing the transmission of many STIs to their infants.
- In the future, new vaccines will decrease or eliminate the transmission of certain STIs to neonates and children prior to sexual contact.

References

1. Centers for Disease Control and Prevention: Sexually Transmitted Disease Surveillance, 2004. Department of Health and Human Services, Atlanta, GA (2005)
2. Speroff, L., Fritz, M.A.: Clinical Gynecologic Endocrinology and Infertility, 7th edn, p. 1013. Lippincott Williams & Wilkins, Philadelphia (2005)
3. Westrom, L.: Effect of pelvic inflammatory disease on fertility. Venereology **8**, 219–222 (1995)
4. Westrom, L., Joesoef, R., Reynolds, G., Hagdu, A., Thompson, S.E.: Pelvic inflammatory disease and fertility. A cohort study of 1844 women with laparoscopically verified disease and 657 control women with normal laparoscopic results. Sex. Transm. Dis. **19**, 185–192 (1992)
5. Hillis, S.D., Joesoef, R., Marchbanks, P.A., Wasserheit, J.N., Cates, W., Westrom, L.: Delayed care of pelvic inflammatory disease as a risk factor for impaired fertility. Am. J. Obstet. Gynecol. **168**(5), 1503–1539 (1993)
6. World Health Organization Task Force on the Prevention and Management of Infertility: Tubal infertility: Serologic relationship to post chlamydial and gonococcal infection. Sex. Transm. Dis. **22**, 71–77 (1995)
7. Tijam, K.H., Zeilmaker, G.H., Alberda, A.T., et al.: Prevalence of antibodies to *Chlamydia trachomatis*, *Neisseria gonorrhoeae*, and *Mycoplasma hominis* in infertile women. Genitourin. Med. **61**, 175–178 (1985)
8. Miettinen, A., Heinonen, P.K., Teisala, K., Hakkarainen, K., Punnonen, R.: Serologic evidence for the role of *Chlamydia trachomatis*, *Neisseria gonorrhoeae*, and *Mycoplasma hominis* in the etiology of tubal factor infertility and ectopic pregnancy. Sex. Transm. Dis. **17**, 10–14 (1990)
9. Kosseim, M., Brunham, R.C.: Fallopian tube obstruction as a sequela to *Chlamydia trachomatis* infection. Eur. J. Clin. Microbiol. **5**, 584 (1986)
10. Svensson, L., Mardh, P.A., Ahlgren, M., Nordenskjold, M.: Ectopic pregnancy and antibodies to *Chlamydia trachomatis*. Fertil. Steril. **44**, 313 (1985)
11. Rowland, G.F., Moss, T.R.: In vitro fertilization, previous ectopic pregnancy, and *Chlamydia trachomatis* infection. Lancet **2**, 830 (1985)
12. Robertson, J.N., Hogston, P., Ward, M.E.: Gonococcal and chlamydial antibodies in ectopic and intrauterine pregnancy. Br. J. Obstet. Gynaecol. **95**, 711–716 (1988)
13. Suzuki, K., Tomasi, T.B.: Immune responses during pregnancy: Evidence of suppressor cells for splenic antibody response. J. Exp. Med. **150**, 898 (1979)
14. Ayra, O.P., et al.: Epidemiological and clinical correlates of chlamydial infection of the cervix. Br. J. Vener. Dis. **57**, 118 (1981)
15. Singer, A.: The uterine cervix from adolescence to the menopause. Br. J. Obstet. Gynaecol. **82**, 81 (1975)
16. Larsen, B., Galask, R.P.: Vaginal microbial flora: Practical and theoretic relevance. Obstet. Gynecol. **55**(Suppl 5), 1005 (1980)
17. Hillier, S.L., et al.: Case control study of chorioamnionic infection and chorioamnionitis in prematurity. N. Engl. J. Med. **319**, 972 (1988)
18. Cooperstock, M., et al.: Circadian incidence of labor onset hour in preterm birth and chorioamnionitis. Obstet. Gynecol. **70**, 852–855 (1987)
19. Guzick, D.S., Winn, K.: The association of chorioamnionitis with preterm delivery. Obstet. Gynecol. **65**, 11–15 (1985)
20. Russel, P.: Inflammatory lesions of the human placenta. 1: Clinical significance of acute chorioamnionitis. Am. J. Diagn. Gynecol. Obstet. **1**, 127 (1979)
21. Weibel, D.R., Randall Jr., H.W.: Evaluation of amniotic fluid in preterm labor with intact membranes. J. Reprod. Med. **30**, 777–780 (1985)
22. Skoll, M.A., et al.: The incidence of positive amniotic fluid cultures in patients in preterm labor with intact membranes. Am. J. Obstet. Gynecol. **161**, 813–816 (1989)
23. Romero, R., et al.: Infection and labor. V: Prevalence, microbiology, and clinical significance of intraamniotic infection in women with preterm labor and intact membranes. Am. J. Obstet. Gynecol. **161**, 317–324 (1989)
24. Gravett, M.G., et al.: An experimental model for intraamniotic infection and preterm labor in rhesus monkeys. Am. J. Obstet. Gynecol. **171**, 1660–1667 (1994)
25. Witkin, S.S., et al.: Induction of interleukin-1 receptor antagonist in rhesus monkeys after intraamniotic infection with group B streptococci or interleukin-1 infection. Am. J. Obstet. Gynecol. **171**, 1668–1672 (1994)
26. Hitti, J., et al.: Amniotic fluid infection, cytokines, and adverse outcome among infants at 34 weeks' gestation or less. Am. J. Obstet. Gynecol. **98**, 1080–1088 (2001)
27. Martinez, E., et al.: Elevated amniotic fluid interleukin-6 as a predictor of neonatal periventricular leukomalacia and intraventricular hemorrhage. J. Matern. Fetal Investig. **8**, 101–107 (1998)
28. Gravett, M.G., et al.: Independent associations of bacterial vaginosis and *Chlamydia trachomatis* infections with adverse pregnancy outcome. JAMA **256**, 1899 (1986)
29. Minkoff, H., et al.: Risk factors for prematurity and premature rupture of membranes: A prospective study of vaginal flora in pregnancy. Am. J. Obstet. Gynecol. **150**, 965–972 (1984)
30. Kurki, T., et al.: Bacterial vaginosis in early pregnancy and pregnancy outcome. Obstet. Gynecol. **80**, 173–177 (1992)
31. Hay, P.E., et al.: A longitudinal study of bacterial vaginosis during pregnancy. Br. J. Obstet. Gynecol. **101**, 1048–1053 (1994)
32. Hauth, J.C., et al.: Reduced incidence of preterm delivery with metronidazole and erythromycin in women with bacterial vaginosis. N. Engl. J. Med. **333**, 1732–1736 (1995)
33. McDonald, H.M., et al.: Impact of metronidazole therapy on preterm birth in women with bacterial vaginosis flora (*Gardnerella vaginalis*): A randomized, placebo controlled trial. Br. J. Obstet. Gynecol. **104**, 1391–1397 (1997)
34. Cotch, M.F., et al.: *Trichomonas vaginalis* associated with low birth weight and preterm delivery. Sex. Transm. Dis. **24**, 1–8 (1997)
35. McGregor, J.A., et al.: Bacterial protease-induced reduction of chorioamniotic membrane strength and elasticity. Obstet. Gynecol. **69**, 167–174 (1987)
36. Shoonmaker, J.N., et al.: Bacteria and inflammation cells reduce chorioamniotic membrane integrity and tensile strength. Obstet. Gynecol. **74**, 590–596 (1989)
37. Sbarra, A.J., et al.: Effect of bacterial growth on the bursting pressure of fetal membranes in vitro. Obstet. Gynecol. **70**, 107–110 (1987)

38. Draper, D., et al.: *Trichomonas vaginalis* weakens human amniochorion in an in vitro model of premature membrane rupture. Infect. Dis. Obstet. Gynecol. **2**, 267–274 (1995)
39. Dorfman, D.H., Glaser, J.H.: Congenital syphilis presenting in infants after the newborn period. N. Engl. J. Med. **323**(19), 1299–1302 (1990)
40. Sanchez, P.J., Wendel, G.D., Norgard, M.V.: Congenital syphilis associated with negative results of maternal serological tests at delivery. Am. J. Dis. Child. **145**(9), 967–969 (1991)
41. Benirschke, K.: Syphilis – the placenta and the fetus. Am. J. Dis. Child. **128**(2), 142–143 (1974)
42. Beck, A., Dailey, W.: Syphilis in pregnancy. Pub. Am. Assoc. Adv. Sci. **6**(101), 101–110 (1938)
43. Qureshi, F., Jacques, S.M., Reyes, M.P.: Placental histopathology in syphilis. Hum. Pathol. **24**(7), 779–784 (1993)
44. Peeling, R.W., Hook III, E.W.: The pathogenesis of syphilis: The Great Mimicker, revisited. J. Pathol. **208**(2), 224–232 (2006)
45. Thomas, D.D., Navab, M., Haake, D.A., Fogelman, A.M., Miller, J.N., Lovett, M.A.: *Treponema pallidum* invades intercellular junctions of endothelial cell monolayers. Proc. Natl. Acad. Sci. USA **85**(10), 3608–3612 (1988)
46. Mascuta, L., et al.: Congenital syphilis: Why is it still occurring? JAMA **252**, 1719 (1984)
47. Fiumara, N.J., Fleming, W.L., Downing, J.G., Good, F.L.: The incidence of prenatal syphilis at the Boston City Hospital. N. Engl. J. Med. **247**(2), 48–52 (1952)
48. Russel, P., Altshuler, G.: Placental abnormalities of congenital syphilis: A neglected aid to diagnosis. Am. J. Dis. Child. **128**(2), 160–163 (1974)
49. McCord, J.: Syphilis of the placenta: The histological examination of 1,085 placentas of mothers with strongly positive Wasserman reactions. Am. J. Obstet. Gynecol. **28**, 743 (1934)
50. Sheffield, J.S., Sanchez, P.J., Wendel Jr., G.D., et al.: Placental histopathology of congenital syphilis. Obstet. Gynecol. **100**(1), 126–133 (2002)
51. Nabarro, D.: Congenital Syphilis. E. Arnold, London (1954)
52. Brown, W.J., Moore Jr., M.B.: Congenital syphilis in the United States. Clin. Pediatr. (Phila) **2**, 220–222 (1963)
53. Ingraham, N.R.: The diagnosis of congenital syphilis during the period of doubt. Am. J. Syph. Neurol. **19**, 547 (1935)
54. Oppenheimer, E.H., Hardy, J.B.: Congenital syphilis in the newborn infant: Clinical and pathological observations in recent cases. Johns Hopkins Med. J. **129**(2), 63–82 (1971)
55. Stokes, J., et al.: Modern Clinical Syphilology. WB Saunders, Philadelphia (1934)
56. Alger, L.S., et al.: The association of *Chlamydia trachomatis*, *Neisseria gonorrhoeae*, and group B streptococci with preterm rupture of membranes and pregnancy outcome. Am. J. Obstet. Gynecol. **159**, 397–404 (1988)
57. Donders, G.G., et al.: The association of gonorrhea and syphilis with premature birth and low birth weight. Genitourin. Med. **69**, 98–101 (1993)
58. Elliott, B., et al.: Maternal gonococcal infection as a preventable risk factor for low birth weight. J. Infect. Dis. **161**, 531–536 (1990)
59. Israel, K.S., Rissing, K.B., Brooks, G.F.: Neonatal and childhood gonococcal infections. Clin. Obstet. Gynecol. **18**, 143 (1975)
60. Edwards, L., Barrada, M.I., Hamann, A.A., et al.: Gonorrhea in pregnancy. Am. J. Obstet. Gynecol. **132**, 637 (1978)
61. Rothbard, M.J., Gregory, T., Salerno, L.J.: Intrapartum gonococcal amnionitis. Am. J. Obstet. Gynecol. **121**, 565 (1975)
62. Neinstein, L.S., Golfenring, J., Carpenter, S.: Nonsexual transmission of sexually transmitted diseases: An infrequent occurrence. Pediatrics **74**, 67 (1984)
63. Kellogg, N., Committee on Child Abuse and Neglect: The evaluation of sexual abuse in children. Pediatrics **116**, 506 (2005)
64. Laga, M., et al.: Epidemiology of ophthalmia neonatorum in Kenya. Lancet **2**, 1145 (1986)
65. Laga, M., et al.: Prophylaxis of gonococcal and chlamydial ophthalmia neonatorum: A comparison of silver nitrate and tetracycline. N. Engl. J. Med. **318**, 653 (1988)
66. Hammerschlag, M.R., et al.: Efficacy of neonatal ocular prophylaxis for the prevention of chlamydial and gonococcal conjunctivitis. N. Engl. J. Med. **320**, 769–772 (1989)
67. Hompson, T.R., et al.: Gonococcal ophthalmia neonatorum: Relationship of time of infection to relevant control measures. JAMA **228**, 186 (1974)
68. Handsfield, H.H., Hodson, W.A., Holmes, K.K.: Neonatal gonococcal infection. 1. Orogastric contamination with *Neisseria gonorrhoeae*. JAMA **225**, 697 (1973)
69. Barton, L.L., Shuja, M.: Neonatal gonococcal vaginitis. J. Pediatr. **98**, 171 (1981)
70. Desenclos, J.C.A., Garrity, D., Scaggs, M., et al.: Gonococcal infection of the newborn in Florida, 1984–1989. Sex. Transm. Dis. **19**, 105 (1992)
71. Hunter, G.W., Fargo, N.D.: Specific urethritis (gonorrhea) in a male newborn. Am. J. Obstet. Gynecol. **38**, 520 (1939)
72. Kirkland, H., Storer, R.V.: Gonococcal rhinitis in an infant. Br. Med. J. **1**, 263 (1931)
73. Angevine, C.D., Hall, C.B., Jacox, R.F.: A case of gonococcal osteomyelitis. A complication of gonococcal arthritis. Am. J. Dis. Child. **130**, 1013 (1976)
74. Cooperman, M.B.: Gonococcus arthritis in infancy. Am. J. Dis. Child. **33**, 932 (1927)
75. Kohen, D.P.: Neonatal gonococcal arthritis: Three cases and review of the literature. Pediatrics **53**, 436 (1974)
76. Thadepalli, H., Rambhatla, K., Maidman, J.E., et al.: Gonococcal sepsis secondary to fetal monitoring. Am. J. Obstet. Gynecol. **126**, 510 (1976)
77. Ingram, G.L., Everett, N.O., Lyna, P.R., et al.: Epidemiology of adult sexually transmitted disease agents in children being evaluated for sexual abuse. Pediatr. Infect. Dis. J. **11**, 945 (1992)
78. Harrison, H.R., et al.: Cervical *Chlamydia trachomatis* and mycoplasmal infections: Epidemiology and outcomes. JAMA **250**, 1721–1727 (1983)
79. Martin, D.H., et al.: Prematurity and perinatal mortality in pregnancies complicated by maternal *Chlamydia trachomatis* infections. JAMA **247**, 1585 (1982)
80. Sweet, R.L., et al.: *Chlamydia trachomatis* infection and pregnancy outcome. Am. J. Obstet. Gynecol. **156**, 824 (1987)
81. Hammerschlag, M.R.: Infections due to *Chlamydia trachomatis* and *Chlamydia pneumoniae* in children and adolescents. Pediatr. Rev. **25**, 43 (2004)
82. Hammerschlag, M.R.: Chlamydia Infections. In: Feigen, R.D., Cherry, J.D., Demmler, G.J., et al. (eds.) Textbook of Pediatric Infectious Diseases, 5th edn. Saunders, Philadelphia (2004)

83. Bell, T.A., Stamm, W.E., Kuo, C.C., et al.: Risk of perinatal transmission of *Chlamydia trachomatis* by mode of delivery. J. Infect. **29**, 165 (1994)
84. Bell, T.A., Stamm, W.E., Wang, S.P., et al.: Chronic *Chlamydia trachomatis* infections in infants. JAMA **267**, 400 (1992)
85. Hammerschlag, M.R., Chandler, J.W., Alexander, E.R., et al.: Longitudinal studies of chlamydial infection in the first year of life. Pediatr. Infect. Dis. **1**, 395 (1982)
86. Tipple, M.A., Beem, M.O., Saxon, E.M.: Clinical characteristics of the afebrile pneumonia associated with *Chlamydia trachomatis* infection in infants less than 6 months of age. Pediatrics **63**, 192 (1979)
87. Beck-Sague, C.M., Solomon, F.: Sexually transmitted diseases in abused children and adolescent and adult victims of rape. Clin. Infect. Dis. **28**(suppl 1), S74 (1999)
88. Fowler, K.B., et al.: The outcome of congenital cytomegalovirus infection in relation to maternal antibody status. N. Engl. J. Med. **326**, 663–667 (1992)
89. Stagno, S., et al.: Congenital cytomegalovirus infection: Occurrence in an immune population. N. Engl. J. Med. **1254**, 296 (1977)
90. Stagno, S., et al.: Congenital cytomegalovirus infection: The relative importance of primary and recurrent maternal infection. N. Engl. J. Med. **945**, 306 (1982)
91. Pass, R.F., et al.: Outcome of symptomatic congenital cytomegalovirus infection: Results of long-term longitudinal follow-up. Pediatrics **758**, 66 (1980)
92. Stagno, S., et al.: Breast milk and risk of cytomegalovirus infection. N. Engl. J. Med. **1073**, 302 (1980)
93. Hamprecht, K., et al.: Epidemiology of transmission of cytomegalovirus from mother to preterm infant by breastfeeding. Lancet **513**, 357 (2001)
94. Meier, J., Lienicke, U., Tschirch, E., Kruger, D.H., Wauer, R.R., Prosch, S.: Human cytomegalovirus reactivation during lactation and mother-to-child transmission in preterm infants. J. Clin. Microbiol. **43**, 1318 (2005)
95. Doctor, S., et al.: Cytomegalovirus transmission to extremely low birthweight infants through breast milk. Acta Paediatr. **53**, 94 (2005)
96. Boucher, F.D., et al.: A prospective evaluation of primary genital herpes simplex virus type 2 infections acquired during pregnancy. Pediatr. Infect. Dis. J. **499**, 9 (1990)
97. Frenkel, L.M., et al.: Clinical reactivation of herpes simplex virus type 2 infection in seropositive pregnant women with no history of genital herpes. Ann. Intern. Med. **414**, 118 (1993)
98. Brown, Z.A., et al.: The acquisition of herpes simplex virus during pregnancy. N. Engl. J. Med. **509**, 337 (1997)
99. Lafferty, W.E., et al.: Herpes simplex virus type 1 as a cause of genital herpes: Impact on surveillance and prevention. J. Infect. Dis. **1454**, 181 (2000)
100. Whitley, R., et al.: A controlled trial comparing vidarabine with acyclovir in neonatal herpes simplex virus infection. N. Engl. J. Med. **324**, 444–449 (1991)
101. Nahmias, A.J., et al.: Perinatal risk associated with maternal genital herpes simplex virus infection. Am. J. Obstet. Gynecol. **825**, 100 (1971)
102. Brown, Z.A., et al.: Effects on infants of a first episode of genital herpes during pregnancy. N. Engl. J. Med. **1246**, 317 (1987)
103. Arvin, A., et al.: Failure of antepartum maternal cultures to predict the infant's risk of exposure to herpes simplex virus at delivery. N. Engl. J. Med. **796**, 315 (1986)
104. Brown, Z.A., et al.: Neonatal herpes simplex virus infection in relation to asymptomatic maternal infection at the time of labor. N. Engl. J. Med. **1247**, 324 (1991)
105. Prober, C.G., et al.: Low risk of herpes simplex virus infection in neonates exposed to the virus at the time of vaginal delivery to mothers with recurrent genital herpes simplex virus infection. N. Engl. J. Med. **240**, 316 (1987)
106. Brown, Z.A., et al.: Asymptomatic maternal shedding of herpes simplex virus at the onset of labor: Relationship to preterm labor. Obstet. Gynecol. **483**, 87 (1996)
107. Koutsky, L.A.: Epidemiology of genital human papillomavirus infection. Am. J. Med. **3**, 102 (1997)
108. Fife, K.H., et al.: Cervical human papillomavirus deoxyribonucleic acid persists throughout pregnancy and decreases in the postpartum period. Am. J. Obstet. Gynecol. **1110**, 180 (1999)
109. Nobbenhuis, M.A.E., et al.: High-risk human papillomavirus clearance in pregnant women: Trends for lower clearance during pregnancy with a catch-up postpartum. Br. J. Cancer **75**, 87 (2002)
110. Ziegler, A., Kastner, C., Chang-Claude, J.: Analysis of pregnancy and other factors on detection of human papillomavirus (HPV) infection using weighted estimating equations for follow-up data. Stat. Med. **2217**, 22 (2003)
111. Hernandez-Giron, C., et al.: High-risk human papillomavirus detection and related risk factors among pregnant and nonpregnant women in Mexico. Sex. Transm. Dis. **613**, 32 (2005)
112. Sinal, S.H., Woods, C.R.: Human papillomavirus infections of the genital and respiratory tracts in young children. Semin. Pediatr. Infect. Dis. **306**, 16 (2005)
113. Reeves, W.C., et al.: National registry for juvenile respiratory papillomatosis. Arch. Otolaryngol. Head Neck Surg. **976**, 129 (2003)
114. Syrjanen, S., Puranen, M.: Human papillomavirus infections in children: The potential role of maternal transmission. Crit. Rev. Oral Biol. Med. **259**, 11 (2000)
115. Gissmann, L., et al.: Human papillomavirus types 6 and 11 DNA sequences in genital and laryngeal papillomas and in some cervical cancers. Proc. Natl. Acad. Sci. USA **560**, 80 (1983)
116. Aguilera-Barrantes, I., Magro, C., Nuovo, G.J.: Verruca vulgaris of the vulva in children and adults: A nonvenereal type of vulvar wart. Am. J. Surg. Pathol. **31**(4), 529–535 (2007)
117. Doerfler, D., Bernhaus, A., Kottmel, A., Sam, C., Koelle, D., Joura, E.A.: Human papilloma virus infection prior to coitarche. Am. J. Obstet. Gynecol. **200**(5), 487.e1–487.e5 (2009)
118. Govan, V.A.: A novel vaccine for cervical cancer: Quadrivalent human papillomavirus (types 6, 11, 16 and 18) recombinant vaccine (Gardasil). Ther. Clin. Risk Manag. **4**(1), 65–70 (2008)
119. Prescribing Insert, Gardasil®,Whitehouse Station, NJ, USA: Merck & Co. 2008.
120. Prescribing Insert, Cervarix®, Rixensart, Belgium: GlaxoSmithKline Biologicals. 2007.

59 Female Genital Mutilation and Risk for Transmission of STIs

Aldo Morrone, Roberta Calcaterra, and Gennaro Franco

Core Messages

- Female genital mutilation (FGM) is a traditional cultural practice, but also a form of violence against girls, which affects their lives as adult women. FGM comprises a wide range of procedures: the excision of the prepuce; the partial or total excision of the clitoris (clitoridectomy) and labia; or the stitching and narrowing of the vaginal orifice (infibulation). The number of girls and women who have been subjected to FGM is estimated at around 137 million worldwide and 3 million girls per year are considered at risk. Most of the females who have undergone mutilation live in 28 African countries.
- International migration has led to an increased presence of circumcised women in Europe and developed countries. Healthcare specialists need to be made aware of and trained in the physical, psychosexual, and cultural aspects and effects of FGM and in the response to the needs of genitally mutilated women.

59.1 Introduction

The migration of millions of people from southern areas of the world to affluent countries in search of a better future for themselves and their children has produced cultural and social changes, in addition to remarkable effects from a medical viewpoint.

Diseases such as tuberculosis, malaria, leprosy, and tropical dermatoses, considered to have been eradicated in industrialized countries, are reappearing.

Migrations to northern industrialized countries have exposed the populations to different cultures and habits. In recent years, the phenomenon of Female Genital Mutilation (FGM) has been encountered in the European Union, the US, Canada and Australia.

The presence of an increasing number of refugees and immigrants from countries in which this procedure is practiced has aroused much interest in the issue. As a result, several countries have passed laws against FGM. In some countries, programs have been started to increase awareness of the issue, and alert health and social services to protect girls at risk of FGM [1–7].

59.2 Historical Data

The ritual cutting and alteration of the genitalia of female infants, girls, and adolescents have been traditional practices since antiquity. The origin of the practice is unknown, and there is no certain evidence to indicate how and when it began and propagated.

Apparently, in all communities in which female circumcision is carried out, male circumcision is also present. Male circumcision is portrayed in some reliefs of the Egyptian tomb of Ankh-Ma-Hor (sixth dynasty, 2340–2180 BC) and other representations concerning

A. Morrone (✉), R. Calcaterra, and G. Franco
National Institute for the promotion of migrants' health and the control of poverty-related diseases – San Gallicano, Via di San Gallicano 25/a, 00153, Rome, Italy
e-mail: morrone@inmp.it; r.calcaterra@yahoo.it; gefranco@libero.it

G. Gross and S.K. Tyring (eds.), *Sexually Transmitted Infections and Sexually Transmitted Diseases*,
DOI: 10.1007/978-3-642-14663-3_59, © Springer-Verlag Berlin Heidelberg 2011

different dynasties. It is not known whether excision and infibulations shared a parallel development. With regard to the first millennium, however, the practice is documented as existing in Egypt. The most ancient authority reporting circumcision was Herodotus (484–424 BC). He asserted that the Phoenicians, Hittites and Ethiopians, as well as the Egyptians, practiced excision. At about 25 BC, the Greek geographer and historian Strabone related that the Egyptians circumcised boys and practiced excision on girls.

Other testimonies are brought in the ancient medical literature. Sorano, a working Greek physician between the I sec and the II sec BC to Alexandria of Egypt and to Rome, describes in details the intervention and the used techniques, reporting moreover that it was practiced for decreasing the female sexual desire. Later, Ezio (527–565 BC) and Paul of Egina (625–690 BC) brought an analogous description: they approved the same operation, maintaining that the clitoris had to necessarily be ablated because it could have an erection like the masculine sex, and would allow the lesbian venery.

The term "infibulation" comes from the ancient Latin language. In the ancient Rome, the term "fibula" was for a pin used to hold the peplum. When the fibula was tight, it was not possible to take the pelum off and therefore, no sexual intercourse was possible.

In modern Europe, we find again many references to the custom of the exercise of rigid control of the female sexuality. Remember the use in medieval times of the belt of chastity, imported by the Crusaders during the twelfth century, with which the fidelity of the young brides during their husbands' long periods of absence was checked. After all, the European physicians of the middle ages and '600 had founded their own education and their own philosophical thought upon the platonic and Aristotelian theories related to the role and the function of the female body. The great explorers of the eighteenth century tell us of the same things when they had been exposed to people who practiced FGM. Carsten Niebuhr (1733–1815) the only survivor of the first scientific consignment in Arabia and in Egypt, brings us the news of an excision on the female genital, which happened in 1767. Sir Richard Burton (1821–1890), a known British explorer who lived in the nineteenth century, devoted a good part of his writings to the study of the sexuality of the populations that he considered primitive. He noticed that while the intent of the practice was to inhibit female sexual desire, its effects were revealed to be the opposite. According to Burton, the excision gave a greater sexual desire to the women, but at the same time a smaller possibility to satisfy it.

During the 18th century and the early 19th century, many physicians – aiming at personal profits - spread out the idea that the clitoridectomia, could have originated by the biblical story of Onan. So, the idea of the so called "therapeutic mutilations" – the masturbation, especially female causes several diseases of the brain from the epilepsy to the folly, and clitoridectomia as the only way to the possibility of recovery - diffused across France, Germany and England.

59.3 Religious, Health Beliefs And Cultural Aspects

It is not known when or where the tradition of FGM originated, and a variety of reasons (sociocultural, psychosexual, hygienic, aesthetic, and religious) have been given for its maintenance. FGM is practiced by followers of a number of different religions, including Muslims and Christians (Catholics, Protestants, and Copts), by animists and Jews (Falashas in Ethiopia), and by nonbelievers in the countries concerned. The practice is deeply embedded in local traditional belief systems. In some countries, the practice seems to be more common among Muslim groups, and many people falsely believe that Islam requires FGM. In the Ivory Coast, 80% of Muslim versus 16% of Christian women have been genitally cut; in Burkina Faso, Muslim women have undergone FGM due to the belief that God does not listen to the prayers of uncut women. Debate has been ongoing among Islamic scholars as to whether or not Islamic teaching mandates FGM. It is now generally conceded by many Islamic authorities that there are no authenticated Islamic texts requiring the practice.

FGM represents one of the many "harmful traditional practices" (HTP); in fact, there are a number of HTPs specifically directed at women, such as early marriage, marriage by abduction, shaking a woman after delivery, food discrimination, bleeding after expulsion of the placenta. Furthermore, there are other practices that are degrading to women such as those related to "woman and blood." A woman who is bleeding either as a result of her menstrual period or after child birth is considered unclean or polluted and is not allowed to join in religious or social services such as entering the church (Orthodox Church) or carrying out the "Solat" for Muslim women.

It is important to stress, however, that even though communities are aware that it is not a religious requirement, the practice continues because it serves as a way of controlling women's sexuality. It is therefore necessary to work with women first, before approaching religious leaders, so that they become convinced of the need to stop FGM due to health consequences.

FGM is done for various reasons in various communities. It is interrelated with other cultural elements such as marriage; interclan relationships, and several other sociocultural elements. With respect to marriage, for example, FGM is a prerequisite for marriage, in most societies in Africa. It is believed to ensure fertility and preserve virginity until marriage. In this way, it is essential to study how FGM is interrelated with other parts of a culture, what role it plays in maintaining the social organization of a community and how it contributes to enhancing social integration. Attempts to abolish FGM will impact marriage and a number of other social systems. The community believes that FGM ensures fertility, preserves virginity, and creates the norms of interaction in the community and trust between the couple. How, with the change, is the community going to develop trust between the boy and his fiancée? How can the community confirm that girls will not be easily raped in communities such as Affar and Somali, where girls have to stay outside the home watching animals in the bush? Affar and Somali people believe, in fact, that it is not easy to rape infibulated girls in the bush. Rape leads to unwanted pregnancies and illegal children; pregnancy and delivery before marriage is taboo among several ethnic groups, for example, in Ethiopia and may lead to interfamily or even interclan feuds. Thus, it could mean that by eliminating a harmful tradition, the community may be reinforcing another one. This is not to advocate the retention of a harmful tradition but to illustrate the complexity of the task.

The challenge in bringing about a deliberate change in an element of a given culture, therefore, is to understand the function and role of that specific cultural element in the integrity of a "whole."

59.4 Definition

Today confusion still persists regarding the classification of this practice.

The terminology used for FGM procedures varies considerably, depending on the regional and ethnic group. In the international arena, the term "female genital mutilation" is widely used. At the local level, the term "female circumcision" is commonly used, or a woman is referred to as being "open" or "closed." In analogy with male circumcision, the term "female circumcision" could be used to describe excision of the prepuce. A number of researchers have expressed disagreement with this definition, however, because the term "circumcision" is used to describe a specific male procedure, which is less invasive. Analogous operations for men would involve the partial or complete removal of the penis rather just removal of the foreskin [4]. Also used is the expression "ritual female genital surgery," which refers to the nontherapeutic nature of the procedures and has a less emotional connotation than "female genital mutilation" [2, 11].

It is because of the severity and irreversibility of the damage inflicted on a girl's body that the procedure has been termed "female genital mutilation." This is the term currently used in all official documents of the United Nations.

59.5 Classification

The traditional practice of FGM has attracted increasing international attention over the past 15 years. The joint statement on FGM issued in April 1997 by the World Health Organization (WHO), United Nations International Children's Emergency Fund (UNICEF) and United Nation Population Fund (UNFPA) referred to FGM as "all procedures involving partial or total removal of the external female genitalia or other injury to the female genital organs whether for cultural, religious or other nontherapeutic reasons" [27].

There are different types of female genital mutilation known to be practiced today. They include:

- Type I – excision of the prepuce, with or without excision of part or the entire clitoris (Fig. 59.1)
- Type II – excision of the clitoris with partial or total excision of the labia minora (Fig. 59.2)
- Type III – excision of part or all of the external genitalia and stitching/narrowing of the vaginal opening (infibulation) (Fig. 59.3)
- Type IV – unclassified; this includes a variety of procedures, most of which are self-explanatory (Fig. 59.4)

There is considerable evidence in the literature that the classification of these procedures can only be done theoretically. Categorizing the different types of FGM in an anatomically precise and simplified system is only an attempt to help clinicians and researchers standardize their descriptions of a multitude of operations (Figs. 59.5 and 59.6).

The most common type of FGM is excision of the clitoris and the labia minora, accounting for up to 80% of all cases; the most extreme form is infibulation, which constitutes about 15% of all procedures (Figs. 59.7 and 59.8).

Traditional practitioners – generally, elderly women specially designated for this task, or traditional birth attendants, usually perform FGM. The operation lasts about 15–20 min, is carried out with special knives, scissors, scalpels, pieces of glass, or razor blades. The instruments may be reused without cleaning. Anesthetics and antiseptics are not generally used, and pastes containing herbs, local porridge, or ashes are frequently rubbed on the wounds to stop bleeding. Unintended additional damage is often caused because of the crude tools, poor light, poor eyesight of the practitioner, and septic conditions, or because of the struggling of the girls or women during the procedure.

In some countries, health professionals – trained midwives and physicians – are increasingly being used to perform FGM. In Egypt, for example, preliminary results from the 1995 Demographic and Health Survey indicated that the proportion of women who reported having been "circumcised" by a doctor was 13%.

In our series, enrolled at the Department of Preventive Medicine for Migration, Tourism and Tropical Dermatology of San Gallicano Institute in Rome, from January 2005 to December 2007, we observed more than 16,000 patients, of which women represent more than 50% and among them, 8,457 came from countries where FGM is widely performed. Out of these, 6,678 gave the informed consent to a clinical examination. It revealed that 4,477 women (70.9% range 18–46 years) presented FGM, with the 81% coming from Somalia, Ethiopia and Eritrea.

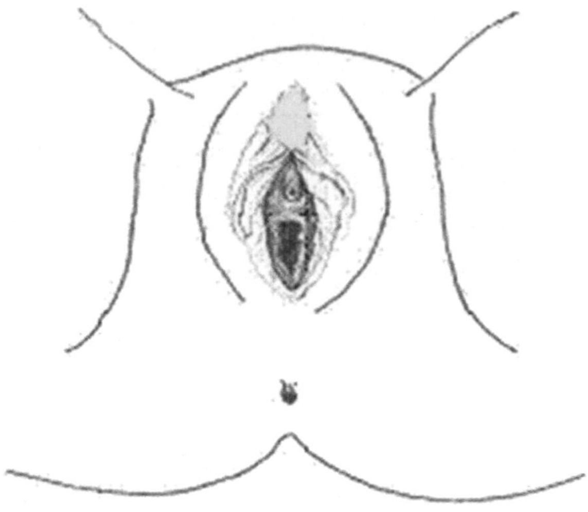

Fig. 59.1 Type I female genital mutilation

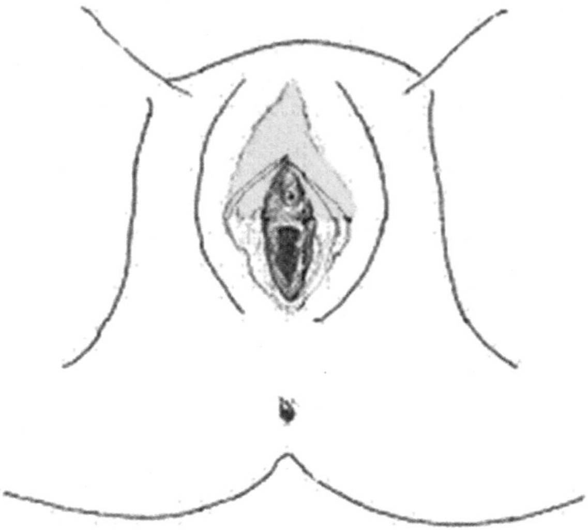

Fig. 59.2 Type II female genital mutilation

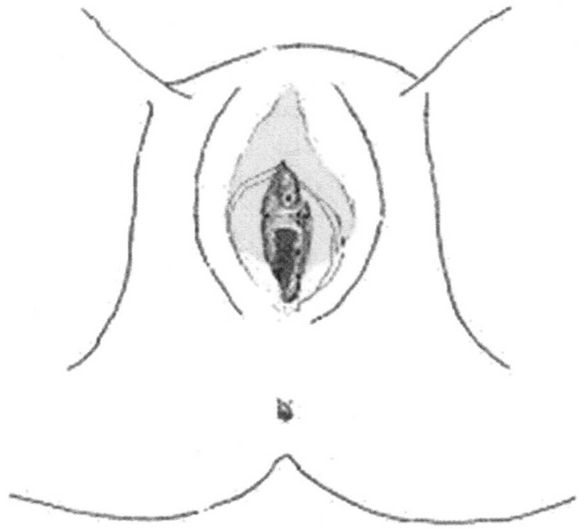

Fig. 59.3 Type III female genital mutilation

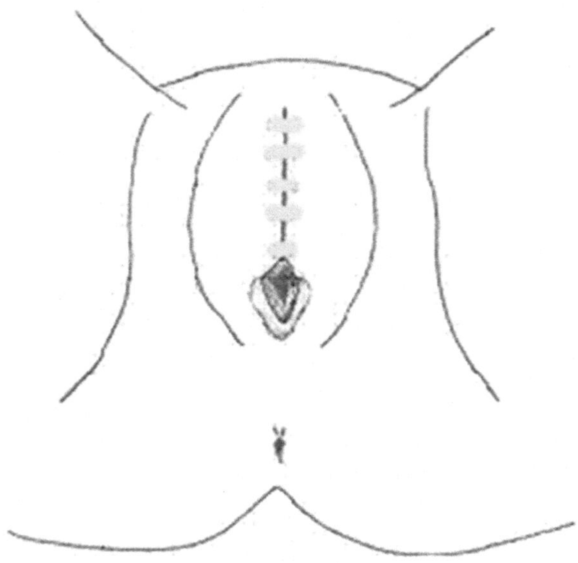

Fig. 59.4 Type VI female genital mutilation

The prevalence of the types of FGM was 66.6% for type I, 28.2% for type II and 5.2% for type III.

59.6 Prevalence

WHO estimates that between 100 million and 140 million girls and women worldwide have been subjected to one of the first three types of female genital mutilation.

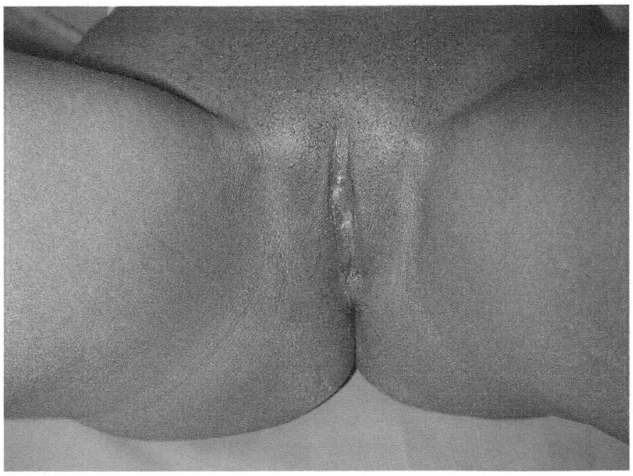

Fig. 59.5 Type II female genital mutilation

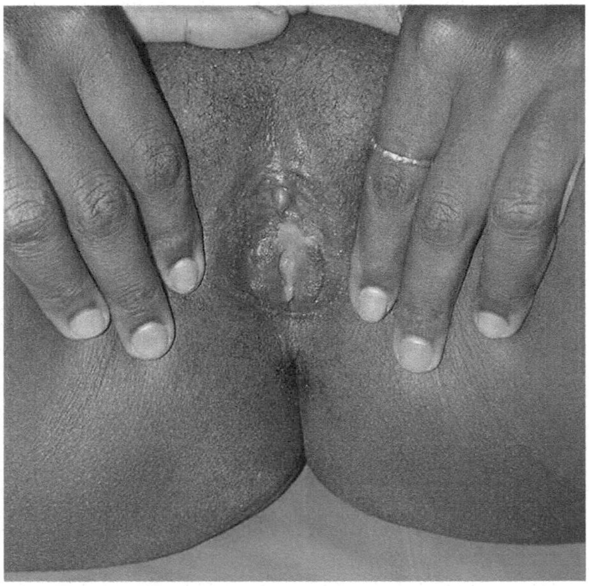

Fig. 59.6 Type II female genital mutilation

Estimates based on the most recent prevalence data indicate that 91.5 million girls and women above 9-years old in Africa are currently living with the consequences of female genital mutilation. There are an estimated three million girls in Africa at risk of undergoing female genital mutilation every year.

Type I, II and III female genital mutilation have been documented in 28 countries in Africa, and in a few countries in Asia and the Middle East. Growing migration has increased the number of girls and women living outside their country of origin who have

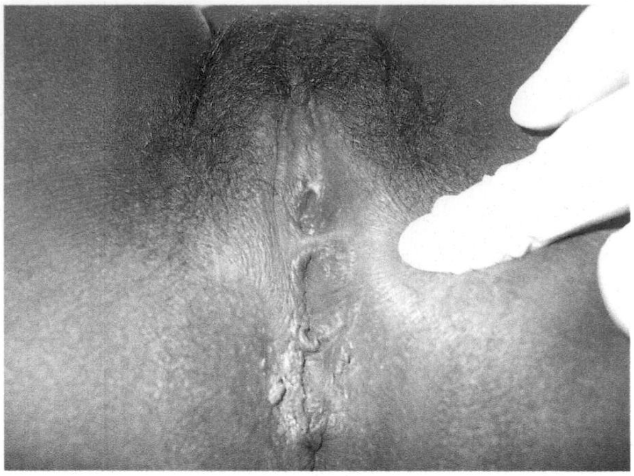

Fig. 59.7 Type II female genital mutilation and genital warts

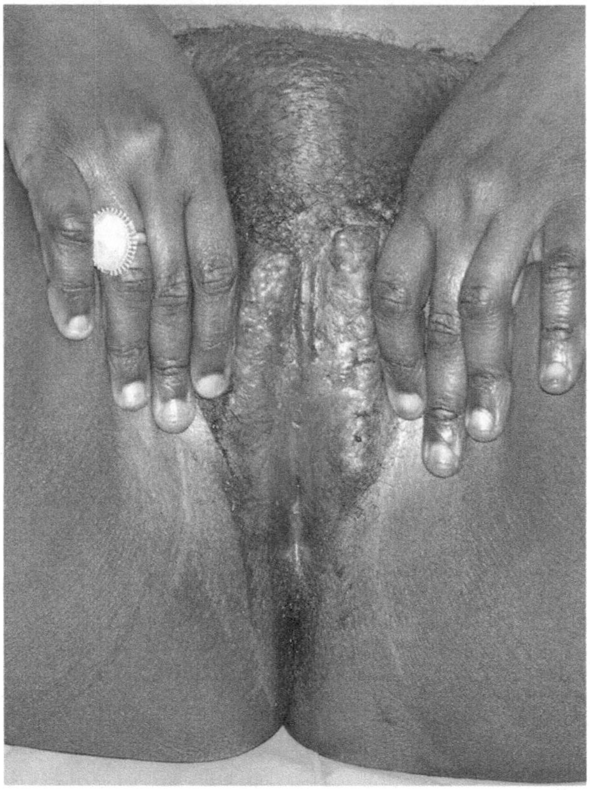

Fig. 59.8 Type III female genital mutilation

undergone female genital mutilation or who may be at risk of being subjected to the practice [24].

Estimates on prevalence of female genital mutilation come from large-scale, national surveys, which have so far been conducted in 18 African countries, asking women aged 15–49 years if they have themselves undergone the practice. The prevalence varies considerably, both between and within regions and countries, with ethnicity as the most decisive factor. In seven countries, the national prevalence is almost universal (more than 85%); four countries have high prevalence (60–85%); medium prevalence (30–40%) is found in seven countries; and low prevalence (0.6–28.2%) is found in nine countries. There is often marked variation in prevalence in different parts of any given country (Fig. 59.9).

Some communities on the Red Sea coast of the Yemen are also known to practice FGM and reportedly, though to a limited extent, FGM is practiced in Jordan, Oman, the Palestinian Territories (Gaza) and in certain Kurdish communities in Iraq. The practice has also been reported among population groups in India, Indonesia and Malaysia [9, 23].

FGM is also practiced among immigrant communities throughout the world. Families from Benin, Chad, Guinea, Mali, Niger and Senegal tend to migrate to France, where they continue the practice, whereas those from Kenya, Nigeria and Uganda generally settle in the United Kingdom. In the 1970s, refugees fleeing war and civil unrest in Eritrea, Ethiopia and Somalia brought FGM to several countries of Western Europe, including Norway, Sweden and Switzerland. Canada and the USA in North America, and Australia and New Zealand in Australasia also host women and children who have been subjected to FGM [25, 26].

59.7 Health Consequences

Female genital mutilation is associated with a series of health risks and consequences [6]. Almost all who have undergone it experience pain and bleeding. The intervention itself is traumatic as usually girls are physically held down during the procedure. Those who are infibulated often have their legs bound together for several days or weeks thereafter. Other physical and psychological health problems occur with varying frequency. Generally, the risks and complications associated with Types I, II and III are similar, but they tend to be significantly more severe and prevalent the more extensive the procedure. Immediate consequences that have been documented include severe pain, shock, excessive bleeding, and difficulty in passing urine,

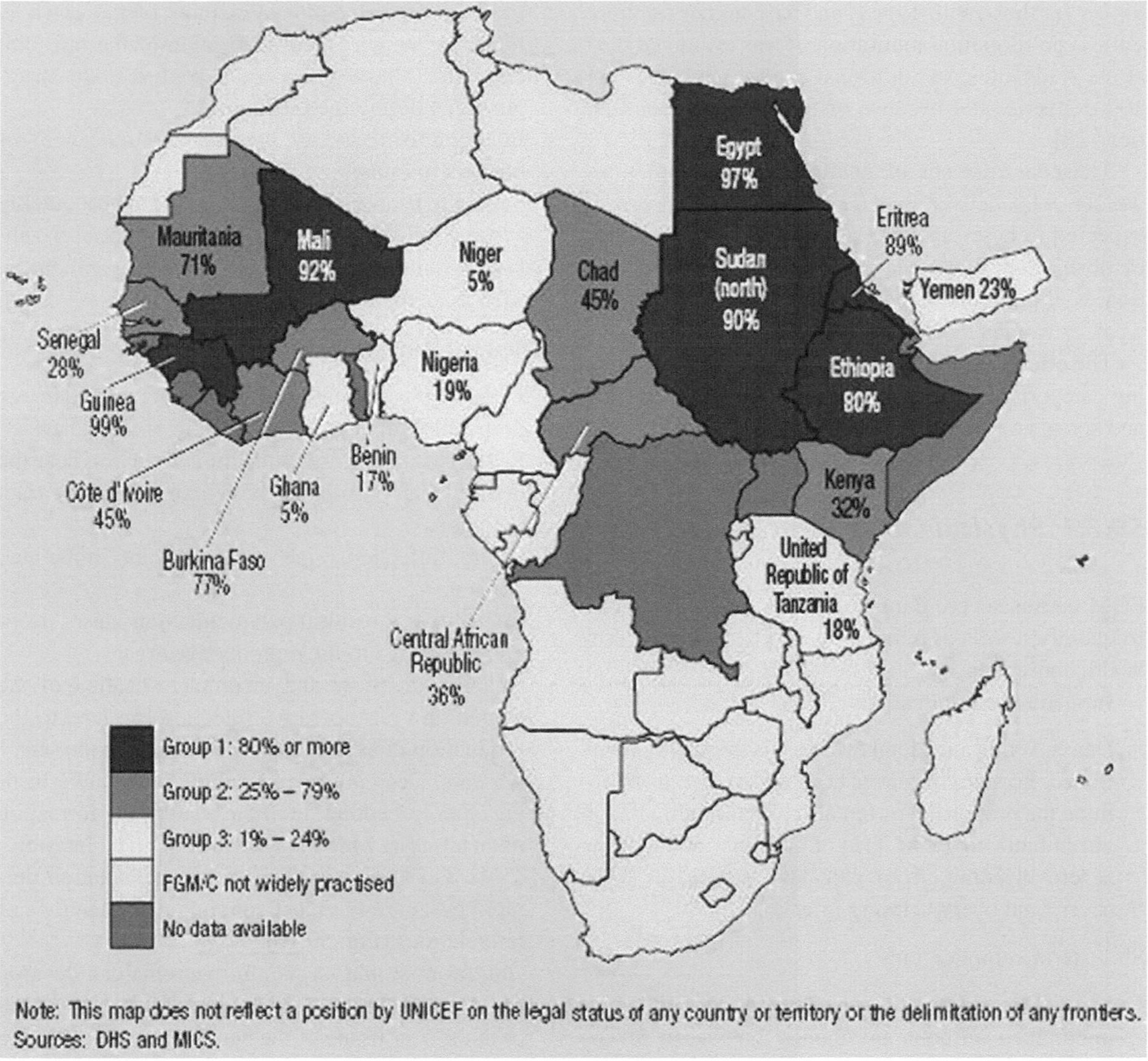

Fig. 59.9 Female genital mutilation prevalence among women aged 15–49 (Source: FGM a statistical exploration. New York, NY, UNICEF; 2005)

infections, death and psychological consequences. Since such complications usually only are documented if the girl or woman seeks hospital treatment, the true extent of immediate complications is unknown. Long-term consequences that have been documented include chronic pain, infections, cysts and abscesses, decreased sexual enjoyment, infertility, posttraumatic stress disorder and dangers in childbirth [25].

Findings from a WHO multi-country study in which more than 28,000 women participated, confirm that women who had undergone genital mutilation had significantly increased risks for adverse events during childbirth. Higher incidences of caesarean section and postpartum hemorrhage were found in the women with Type I, II and III genital mutilation compared to those who had not undergone genital mutilation, and the risk increased with the severity of the procedure.

A striking new finding from the study is that genital mutilation of mothers has negative effects on their newborn babies. Most seriously, death rates among babies during and immediately after birth were higher for those born to mothers who had undergone genital mutilation compared to those who had not: 15% higher for those whose mothers had Type I, 32%

higher for those with Type II and 55% higher for those with Type III genital mutilation. It was estimated that, at the study sites, an additional one to two babies per 100 deliveries die because of female genital mutilation [28].

The consequences of genital mutilation for most women who deliver outside the hospital setting are expected to be even more severe. The high incidence of postpartum hemorrhage, a life threatening condition, is of particular concern where health services are weak or women cannot easily access them.

The effects of FGM may be divided into the following categories: physical consequences, sexual, mental and social consequences.

59.7.1 Physical Consequences

FGM causes severe damage to girls and women and frequently results in immediate, short-, and long-term health consequences.

Immediate complications

- Death. While anecdotal evidence is frequently mentioned, no study has ever been undertaken to determine the proportion of female child mortality that is attributable to FGM [13]. Death can result from severe bleeding, from pain and trauma, or from severe and overwhelming infection.

Short-term complications

- Pain. The majority of mutilation procedures is undertaken without anesthetics and cause severe pain.
- Injury to adjacent tissue of the urethra, vagina, perineum, and rectum sometimes occurs.
- Hemorrhage. Excision of the clitoris involves cutting the clitoral artery, which has a strong flow and high pressure.
- Shock. Immediately after the procedures, the girl may develop shock, because of the sudden blood loss (hemorrhagic shock) and severe pain and trauma (neurogenic shock), which can be fatal.
- Tetanus can occur due to the use of unsterilized equipment and the lack of tetanus toxoid injection.
- Acute urine retention can result from swelling and inflammation around the wound, the girl's fear of the pain of passing urine on the raw wound, or injury to the urethra.
- Fracture or dislocation. Fractures of the clavicle, femur, or humerus, or dislocation of the hip joint can occur if heavy pressure is applied to the struggling girl during the operation.
- Infection is the most common consequence for obvious reasons.
- Failure to heal. The wounds may fail to heal quickly because of infection, irritation from urine or rubbing when walking, or an underlying condition, such as anemia and malnutrition.

Long-term complications

- Difficulty in passing urine can occur due to damage to the urethral opening or scarring of the meatus.
- Recurrent urinary tract infection. Infection near the urethra can result in ascending urinary tract infections.
- Pelvic infections are common in infibulated women.
- Infertility can result if pelvic infection causes irreparable damage to the reproductive organs.
- Keloid scar. Slow and incomplete healing of the wound and postoperative infection can lead to the production of excess connective tissue in the scar.
- Abscess. Deep infection resulting from faulty healing or an embedded stitch can result in the formation of an abscess, which may require surgical incision.
- Cysts and abscess of the vulva. Implantation dermoid cysts are the most common complications of infibulations (Fig. 59.10).
- Clitoral neuroma. A painful neuroma can develop because of trapping of the clitoral nerve in a stitch or in the scar tissue of the healed wound, leading to hypersensitivity and dyspareunia.

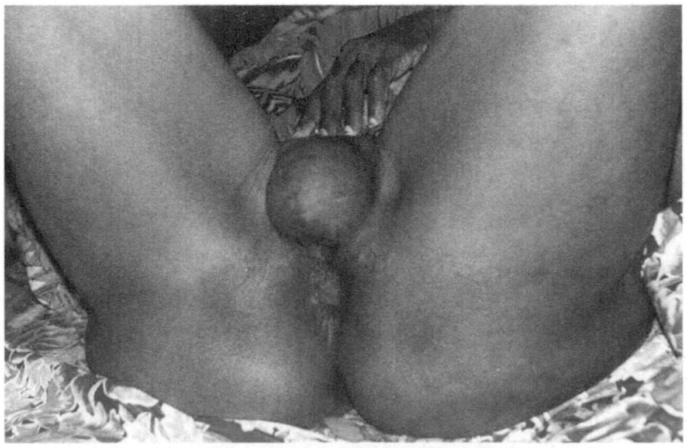

Fig. 59.10 Dermoid cyst in female genital mutilation

- Difficulties in menstruation can occur because of partial or total occlusion of the vaginal opening. Calculus formation in the vagina can occur because of the accumulation of menstrual debris and urinary deposits in the vagina or in the space behind the bridge of scar tissue formed after infibulations.
- Fistulae (holes or tunnels) between the bladder and the vagina (vesicovaginal) and between the rectum and vagina (rectovaginal) can form because of injury during mutilation, deinfibulation, or reinfibulation, sexual intercourse, or obstructed labor.
- Development of a "false vagina" is possible in infibulated women if, during repeated sexual intercourse, the scar tissue fails to dilate sufficiently to allow normal penetration.
- Dyspareunia is a consequence of many forms of FGM because of scarring, reduced vaginal opening, and complications such as infection.
- Sexual dysfunction can result in both partners because of painful intercourse, difficulty in vaginal penetration, and reduced sexual sensitivity following clitoridectomy.
- Difficulties in providing gynecologic care. The scarring resulting from type III mutilation may reduce the vaginal opening to such an extent that an adequate gynecologic examination cannot be performed without cutting.
- Problems in pregnancy and childbirth are common, particularly following type III mutilation, because the tough scar tissue that forms causes partial or total occlusion of the vaginal opening and prevents dilation of the birth canal.

59.7.2 Psychosexual, Mental, and Social Consequences

Little research on the psychologic, sexual, and social consequences of FGM has been conducted. The personal accounts of women who have suffered ritual genital procedures, however, recount anxiety before the event, terror at being seized and forcibly held during the event, great difficulty during childbirth, and lack of sexual pleasure during intercourse [17].

Catania et al., demonstrated, that in infibulated women, some erectile structures fundamental for orgasm have not been excised. Cultural influence can change the perception of pleasure, as well as social acceptance. Every woman has the right to have sexual health and to feel sexual pleasure for full psychophysical well-being of the person. In accordance with other research, the present study reports that FGM/C women can also have the possibility of reaching an orgasm. Therefore, FGM/C women with sexual dysfunctions can and must be cured; they have the right to have an appropriate sexual therapy [5].

59.8 Fgm And Sexually Transmitted Infections

FGM has been said to lead to increased risk of acquiring Sexually Transmitted Infections (STIs) and their complications, such as pelvic inflammatory diseases (PID), but still little is known about the relation of this practice and STIs [22].

As we know, STIs are an important public health problem worldwide. The global incidence of STIs is estimated by the WHO to be in excess of 125 million per year, mainly affecting developing countries [1, 15]. The most common bacterial cause of STIs is *Clamydia trachomatis* [20]. Studies in Africa have shown seroprevalence of chlamydial antibodies ranging from 8% to 91% [8, 15]. *Neisseria gonorrhoeae* is highly prevalent in much of sub-Saharan Africa. As many as 59% of women attending antenatal clinics and family planning clinics in Ethiopia were seropositive for gonococcal antibodies, but still little is known about the situation in Sudan [7]. Studies on syphilis in Africa have shown different figures. In Tanzania, a 2.5% prevalence was found among women attending antenatal clinics [10]. Various studies in Mozambique, where FGM is generally not practiced, have shown prevalence ranging from 4% to 18% [15].

PID is considered one of the complications of FGM [19]. A study in Sudan has shown that the incidence of PID in patients with type III FGM was more than three times higher than in patients with type I FGM [21]. Another study among women attending family planning and antenatal care clinics at three hospitals in Nigeria has shown that the women with FGM were significantly more likely to have experienced repeated symptoms of reproductive tract infections [22].

In spite of the known complications and the potential for HIV transmission through FGM, there are very limited studies reviewing this practice currently and presenting perspective on the probability of FGM leading to HIV transmission [18]. Biologically, any sexually related viral or bacterial pathogen has increased propensity for transmission, given trauma or preexisting laceration to the vaginal epithelium. FGM increases the risk of vaginal epithelial damage and consequently increases the probability of HIV transmission. HIV transmission from this FGM practice is enhanced through shared instruments and blood products during the practice of genital cutting as well as damage to the vaginal epithelium associated with the trauma, inflammation and complications. Other modes of HIV transmission, as well as other HIV risk factors may occur in association with this practice, making it difficult to ascertain whether FGM is the sole predisposing risk factor, as well as a contributing variable to the cumulative incidence of HIV in sub-Saharan Africa. Similarly, if approximately 6,000 young girls undergo FGM daily and about two million young girls are at risk of being genitally mutilated in a year, the odds of FGM as a risk factor to HIV transmission needs to be assessed [12, 16–18].

A recent article revealed the transmission of HIV to girls who have a non-perforated hymen (virgins) and that 97% of the time, the same instrument could be used on 15 to 20 girls [17]. This data suggest the possibility of FGM procedure as a risk variable in HIV transmission. Female genital mutilation may predispose women to HIV in many other ways. For example, the increased need for blood transfusions due to hemorrhage either when the procedure is performed, at childbirth, or a result of vaginal tearing during defibulation and intercourse. These tears would tend to make the squamous vaginal epithelium similar in permeability to the columnar mucosa of the rectum, thus facilitating the possibility of HIV transmission [12]. In addition, many women with type III (pharaonic) mutilation experience dyspareunia, as well as repeated tissue damage and bleeding. Difficult and painful vaginal intercourse in some of these women eventually lead to anal intercourse with heterosexual partners, further increasing the HIV risk in these women. Thus, it is plausible that HIV transmission may be enhanced by the widespread practice of FGM [3, 12–14]. In spite of this biologic casual plausibility, there are no epidemiologic data associating HIV transmission with FGM.

59.9 Trends

Although prevalence data obtained over the last decade have shown little change in the frequency of FGM, they do reveal several trends. Possibly as a result of an emphasis on the negative health implications of FGM, there has been a dramatic increase in the proportion of FGM operations carried out by trained healthcare personnel. Today, 94% of women in Egypt arrange for their daughters to undergo this "medicalized" form of FGM, 76% in Yemen, 65% in Mauritania, 48% in Côte d'Ivoire, and 46% in Kenya. This approach may reduce some of the immediate consequences of the procedure (such as pain and bleeding) but as WHO and UNICEF point out, it also tends to obscure its human rights aspect and could hinder the development of long-term solutions for ending the practice.

There has also been a lowering in some countries of the average age at which a girl is subjected to the procedure [29]. This could be to some extent the result of anti-FGM legislation: the younger the girl, the easier it is to elude legal scrutiny. Another possible adverse effect of legislation is, as often occurs with abortion, its tendency to drive FGM underground or encourage a cross-border movement of women from a country where the practice is illegal to a neighboring country where it is allowed.

One encouraging trend seen consistently in countries for which data from at least two surveys are available is that women aged 15–19 years are less likely to have been submitted to FGM than are women in older age groups. In almost all of these countries, support for the discontinuation of the practice is particularly high among younger women.

59.10 Conclusions

FGM is a problem unfamiliar to most Western physicians and dermatovenereologists. In addition to a lack of clinical knowledge of FGM procedures and complications, information about the underlying sociocultural beliefs and traditions is incomplete. For example, in many communities in which FGM is a traditional practice, women are reluctant to discuss sexual matters with health personnel and are shy to complain about painful intercourse or inability to consummate marriage.

In northern Sudan, women have a defibulation procedure performed immediately after marriage. This procedure is carried out by a local midwife or birth attendant and facilitates the consummation of marriage. The physiologic, psychosexual, and cultural aspects of FGM should be incorporated into the training of healthcare personnel working with immigrant communities who practice FGM.

European politicians need to create an environment that does not contribute to the further marginalization of refugees and immigrants. This means that they must evaluate current social policies and statements about immigrants in this context.

For example, immigration and asylum laws should be assessed as to how they affect identity and for which the potential links of the immigrants are infavar of FGM. Women should be able to request political asylum on their own and not only as dependants of men. Girls should be made aware of the possibility of seeking help and refuge, for example, through telephone help lines, social services, and battered women's shelters.

It is the responsibility of politicians to meet with communities; these consultations can be employed to identify important issues, which can then be used as a basis for developing a policy framework to tackle the medical, economic, social, and legislative aspects of FGM. Immigrant and refugee workers need to be supplied with systematic information on groups that still perform FGM and on groups that provide services to deal with FGM. Policy makers should stress that a holistic approach is needed towards immigrants and that immigrant women have rights too. Funds should be raised in order to tackle more than one aspect of immigrant women's lives. Dermatovenereologists, anthropologists, educators, social assistants, and health operators should be able to reach villages and districts and inform practitioners about the dangers of FGM. In order to successfully eliminate this practice, it will be necessary to act with great delicacy, as cultural beliefs are very strongly held.

We consider FGM to be more than a health problem; it is also a social means of controlling women's sexuality. We therefore do not strive for the eradication of FGM as such.

Instead, we wish to label it as a social behavior, using gender as a basis. This means that our message is not just "do not practice FGM;" rather, we aim to facilitate social and economic change. We consider that FGM is a form of gender-based violence, while recognizing that it is not an intentional and deliberate effort to produce injury.

Take-Home Pearls

› The presence of FGM and eventually STIs should be considered in the approach to women with genital diseases, who come from areas where FGM is practiced.

References

1. Adler, M.W.: Sexually transmitted diseases control in developing countries. Genitourin. Med. **72**, 83–88 (1996)
2. Asali, A., Khamaysi, N., Aburabia, Y., et al.: Ritual female genital surgey among Bedouin in Israel. Arch. Sex. Behav. **24**, 573–577 (1995)
3. Brady, M.: Female genital mutilation: complications and risk of HIV transmission. AIDS Patient Care STD **13**(12), 709–716 (1999)
4. Carr, D.: Female Genital Cutting. Findings from the Demographic and Health Surveys Programme, pp. 7–9. Macto International, Calverton (1997)
5. Catania, L., Adbulcadir, O., Puppo, V., et al.: Pleasure and orgasm in women with female genital mutilation/cutting (FGM/C). J. Sex. Med. **4**(6), 1666–1678 (2007)
6. Dirie, M.A., Lindmark, G.: The risk of medical complications after female circumcision. East Afr. Med. J. **69**, 479–482 (1992)
7. Duncan, M.E., Reimann, K., Tibaux, G., et al.: Seroepidemological study of gonorrhea in Ethiopian women. 1. Prevalence and clinical significance. Genitourin. Med. **67**, 485–492 (1991)
8. Duncan, M.E., Jamil, Y., Tibaux, G., et al.: Chlamydial infection in a population of Ethiopian women attending obstetric, gynaecological and mother and child health clinics. Cent. Afr. J. Med. **42**, 1–14 (1996)
9. El Dareer, A.A.: Epidemiology of female circumcision in the Sudan. Trop. Doct. **13**, 41–45 (1983)
10. Elmusharaf, S., Elkhidir, I., Hoffmann, S., et al.: A case-control study on the association between female genital mutilation and sexually transmitted infections in Sudan. BJOG **113**, 349–374 (2006)
11. Grisaru, N., Lazer, S., Belmaker, R.H.: Ritual female genital surgery among Ethiopian Jews. Arch. Sex. Behav. **26**, 211–215 (1997)
12. Hrdy, D.B.: Cultural practices contributing to the transmission of HIV in Africa. Rev. Infect. Dis. **9**(6), 1109–1117 (1987)
13. Kun, K.E.: Female genital mutilation: the potential for increased risk of HIV infection. Int. J. Gynecol. Obstet. **15**, 153–155 (1997)

14. Linke, U.: AIDS in Africa. Science **231**, 203 (1986)
15. Machungo, F., Zanconato, G., Persson, K., et al.: Syphilis, gonorrhea and chlamydial infection among women undergoing legal or illegal abortion in Maputo. Int. J. STD AIDS **13**, 326–330 (2002)
16. Monjok, E., Essien, E.J., Holmes, L.: Female genital mutilation: potential for HIV transmission in sub – Saharan Africa and prospect for epidemiologic investigation and intervention. Afr. J. Reprod. Health **11**(1), 33–42 (2007)
17. Morrone, A., Hergocova, J., Lotti, T.: Stop female genital mutilation: appeal to the international dermatologic community. Int. J. Dermatol. **41**, 253–263 (2002)
18. Mutenbei, I. B., Mwesiga, M.K.: The impact of obsolete traditions on HIV/AIDS rapid transmission in Africa: the case of compulsory circumcision on young girls in Tanzania. Int Conf on AIDS. **12**, 436(abstract 23473) (1998)
19. Okonofu, F.E., Larsen, U., Oronsaye, F., et al.: The association between female genital cutting and correlates of sexual and gynecological morbidity in Edo State, Nigeria. BJOG **109**, 1089–1096 (2002)
20. Paavonen, J., Eggert-Kruse, W.: Chlamydia trachomatis: impact on human reproduction. Hum. Reprod. Update **5**, 433–447 (1999)
21. Rushwan, H.: Etiologic factors in pelvic inflammatory disease in Sudanese women. Am. J. Obstet. Gynecol. **138**, 877–879 (1980)
22. Shandall, A.: Circumcision and infibulations of females. Sudan Med. J. **5**, 178–212 (1967)
23. Toubia, N.: Female Genital Mutilation: A Call for Global Action, 2nd edn, pp. 35–44. Rainbo, New York (1995)
24. UNICEF: Female Genital Mutilation/Cutting: A Statistical Exploration. UNICEF, New York (2005)
25. WHO study group on female genital mutilation and obstetric outcome, Banks, E., Meirik, O., Farley, T., et al.: Female genital mutilation and obstetric outcome: WHO collaborative prospective study in six African countries. Lancet. **367**(9525), 1835–1841 (2006)
26. World Health Organization. Female genital mutilation. Report of a WHO Technical Working Group, 17–19 July 1995, pp. 3–4. World Health Organization, Geneva (1996)
27. World Health Organization. Female genital mutilation: a joint WHO/UNICEF/UNFPA statement, pp.1–6. World Health Organization, Geneva (1997)
28. World Health Organization: Female genital mutilation – new knowledge spurs optimism. Progress in sexual and reproductive health research. WHO **72**, 2–8 (2006)
29. Yoder, P.S., Abderrahim, N., Zhuzhuni, A.: Female Genital Cutting in the Demographic Health Surveys: A Critical and Comparative Analysis. ORC Marco, Calvelton (2004)

Other Sexually Transmitted Infections

60

Miguel Sanchez

Core Messages

- Some infections can be transmitted through sexual practices.
- Patients who practice oral-genital-anal sex are at-risk for infection with enteric pathogens.
- Sexual contact may be an importance source of transmission of pathogens, such as MRSA.

60.1 Introduction

There are a number of infections for which sexual activity may not be the primary form of transmission but, is an important method of spread. The source of infection by parasites, bacteria and viruses causing enteritis is usually contaminated food or water. However, sexual transmission of these diseases is significant in homosexual men, particularly those who engage in ano-genital or oro-anal practices. Considering the increasing popularity of these sexual acts in the heterosexual population, it is expected that sexually acquired enteric infections will also become more prevalent in this group of persons. If these infections are, indeed, not more common, it is probably because sexual activity may be delayed during the time when a person is actively ill with symptoms such as loose stool. Practitioners of group sex are particularly vulnerable to these infections as they may engage in genito-oro-anal sex with different partners, one or more of whom may be infected, although these pathogens may also be shed in the feces during asymptomatic periods. In a study, one or more species of protozoan was detected in (57%) of men attending a Scotland STD clinic. Giardia intestinalis was identified in 5 (3%) and Blastocystis hominis in 46 (26%). Infection with the latter was not associated with diarrhea [1]. A problem in these studies is the reluctance of gay men to divulge details of their sexual practices to researchers. The use of condoms during oral-genital or anal-genital contact, dental dams during oral-anal contact, and gloves during digital-anal contact can reduce sexual transmission of these enteric pathogens. Persons who engage in sexual contact that exposes them or their sex partners to fecal material should wash their hands and anal-genital regions with soap and water before and after sexual activity.

Other infections are presumably acquired through the close skin-to-skin contact and tissue friction experienced during sexual activity.

60.2 Shigellosis

Infection with the gram-negative, aerobic, nonmotile, facultative intracellular bacteria of the genus, *Shigella* (*S. dysenteriae, S. flexneri, S. sonnei, S. boydii*) is a salient cause of enteritis worldwide. Since the organism can pass intact through the stomach, a low inoculum of only 10 to 200 bacteria can cause symptomatic disease [2]. For this reason, person-to-person contact is a particularly effective means of transmission, though ingestion of contaminated food and water is the most common source of infection. The incubation period averages 3 days (range: 1–7 days) after which time patients develop abdominal pain, mucoid, watery

M. Sanchez
Department of Dermatology, New York University School of Medicine, NY, USA
e-mail: miguelrsmd@aol.com

G. Gross and S.K. Tyring (eds.), *Sexually Transmitted Infections and Sexually Transmitted Diseases*,
DOI: 10.1007/978-3-642-14663-3_60, © Springer-Verlag Berlin Heidelberg 2011

and bloody diarrhea; and in 30–40% fever and vomiting. Complications are rare but include proctitis, rectal prolapse, toxic megacolon, colonic perforation, intestinal obstruction, bacteremia, dehydration and metabolic disturbances [3]. Reactive arthritis and hemolytic-uremic syndrome have been reported [4].

Although sexually acquired shigellosis has long been recognized in gay men [5], the disease has "reemerged" as a sexually transmitted infection [6]. Outbreaks of shigellosis have been reported in men who have sex with men, many of whom admitted to oral-genital or oral-anal contact during the week before diagnosis with Shigella infection [7, 8]. Identical plasmid profiles demonstrated that the same strain infected all the cases [9, 10]. In one such outbreak in Chicago, the organism was found to be *Shigella flexneri* serotype 3 [11]. However, an earlier but similar outbreak in San Francisco was caused by *S. sonnei* [12].

Definitive diagnosis is made through culture, preferably from a stool sample rather than a swab, immediately plated or transported in buffered glycerol saline, since the bacteria is particularly fastidious [13]. Polymerase chain reaction tests have been developed.

Patients who appear ill and present with diarrhea should be treated, especially if they are immunocompromised, HIV-infected, or elderly. Food handlers as well as health care or pediatric day care center workers should also receive treatment.

Resistance to ampicillin precludes continued use of this antibiotic so a fluoroquinolone such as ciprofloxacin, 500 mg twice a day, usually for 3 days, but for at least 5 days in HIV-infected individuals, is recommended although resistance in South Asia is significant. An alternative therapy is a tablet of trimethoprim (160 mg)-sulfamethoxazole (800 mg) twice daily for 5 days. Although data is scare, rifaximin, a semisynthetic, rifamycin-based nonabsorbed oral-antibiotic, at a dose of 200 mg three times a day for 3 days, seems to be an effective alternative [14]. Antidiarrheal drugs (paregoric, diphenoxylate) are prescribed to control intestinal motility.

60.3 Campylobacteriosis

This infection is caused by highly infectious species of the gram-negative bacteria genus, *Campylobacter*, most commonly *C. jejuni* and *C. coli*. A leading cause of enteric illness in many countries including the United Sates, the organism infects the small and usually also the large intestine. Depending on the size of the inoculum and various other factors, the incubation period ranges from 1 to 7 days (average 3 days). Since stomach acidity destroys the bacteria, infection is facilitated by antacid medications.

The symptoms include profuse diarrhea, which is often bloody, abdominal cramps and nausea but less than one in five patients vomit. The symptoms are self-limiting and resolve in about 1 week in 80–90% of cases but the bacteria continues to be present in feces for a mean of 5 weeks, up to 10 weeks [15]. Acute complications such as peritonitis, cholecystitis, pancreatitis and urticaria are rare and even rarer still are late sequelae, such as arthritis and the Guillain-Barré syndrome. Most cases are acquired through ingestion of undercooked meat (especially chicken) or food contaminated by raw meat during the preparation process, by drinking well or surface water, or from contact with infected animals.

The risk of infection in HIV-infected persons, especially men who have sex with men, is 39-times higher than in HIV-negative people. Oral-anal sex has long been considered a route of *Campylobacter* transmission [16]; however, others have found that at least in HIV-infected individuals, food contamination, and not sexual activity, is the usual means of transmission [17]. Immunodeficient patients with HIV infection or hypogammaglobulinemia develop more severe and persistent symptoms [18, 19].

Diagnosis is made by culture in selective media incubated in a gas mixture of 5–10% oxygen and 1–10% carbon dioxide at 42°C, or much less effectively by direct microscopic examination of stained specimens of watery stool.

Patients treated within the first 3 days respond better to treatment but altogether antibiotics reduce symptoms by only 1.3 days [20]. So only immunocompromised, seriously ill, elderly, and pregnant cases are treated with antibiotics. The treatment of choice is oral erythromycin ethylsuccinate 400 mg twice a day, or a 1 g single dose of azithromycin or, erythromycin stearate 500 mg twice daily for 5 days.

Fluoroquinolones and tetracyclines are usually effective but the rate of resistance to these drugs is escalating [21].

60.4 Cryptosporidiosis

Symptomatic disease with the highly infectious Apicomplexa protozoans of the genus *Cryptosporidium* results in diarrhea, which is self-limited (1–2 weeks, rarely up to 10 weeks) in immunocompetent people but can be profuse and persistent in immunocompromised persons with diseases such as AIDS, especially those with CD_4 counts lower than 150 cells/uL.

Cryptosporidium hominis, infests only humans while *Cryptosporidium parvum*, also infects cattle. The protozoan's hardy oocysts are excreted in the stool and can endure environmental rigors (including chlorination, disinfectants, and water filtering). Infection usually occurs through ingestion of contaminated water and food. In addition to common venues like swimming pools, transmission via fecal-oral sexual activities have been demonstrated. Those at greatest risk are immunocompromised adults and children, especially those with AIDS, children in day care, travelers to endemic regions, dairy or cattle farm workers or their families or contacts, household contacts of cases or carriers, and possibly owners of infected dogs or cats or their neighbors.

Risk factors for symptomatic cryptosporidial infection in gay and bisexual men reportedly include sexual intercourse with multiple partners, insertive anal sex and attending a sex venue one or more times [22]. Attending a spa or sauna has been related to serological response to cryptosporidial antigens [23].

Watery stools, often accompanied by intestinal cramps and occasionally low-grade fever, begin 2–10 days after infection. Other complications that can afflict immunosuppressed persons include sclerosing cholangitis, and acalculous cholecystitis. Uncommonly, pancreatitis can develop even in otherwise healthy patients because of biliary disease. Respiratory tract infections have been reported in HIV-infected patients.

Many persons are asymptomatic carriers. Approximately 30% of US adults are seropositive for cryptosporidial antibodies and the organism is found in about 4% of stools sent for parasitologic examination (versus 13% of fecal specimens in developing countries) [24].

Diagnosis is made by acid-fast stained microscopic examination of stool specimens, which show the red-stained oocysts. Immunofluorescent, immunochromatography, enzyme-linked immunosorbent, and polymerase chain reaction assays are all even more sensitive. Patients should be clinically and chemically evaluated for dehydration and systemic involvement. Biliary infection is likely when the alkaline phosphatase and glutamyl transpeptidase, but not the total bilirubin, are elevated. Further evaluation can be performed with abdominal ultrasonography or endoscopic retrograde cholangiopancreatography.

The most promising treatment is the oral synthetic nitrothiazolyl-salicylamide derivative, nitazoxanide. In a randomized, double-blind, multicenter, placebo-controlled study of 56 Egyptian outpatients 12 years of age and older from the Nile Delta region of Egypt, 96% of the cases treated with 500 mg of oral nitazoxanide in tablet or liquid twice daily for three consecutive days responded clinically versus 41% of the control group. Stool samples showed eradication of oocytes in 93% of the treated but in only 37% of the untreated groups [25]. Comparable results were obtained in a similar prospective, placebo-controlled study of adults and children [26]. The dose may be doubled to 1 g twice daily in patients with AIDS for 3 or more days until symptoms resolve.

Cryptosporidiosis is hard to eradicate in patients with AIDS, but combination antiretroviral therapy that includes an HIV protease inhibitor produces dramatic improvement in many cases. Because nucleoside antiretrovirals are not well absorbed in chronic cryptosporidiosis, pretreatment with nitazoxanide or paromomycin combined with azithromycin is warranted. Protease inhibitors have a direct inhibitory effect on Cryptosporidium infection. Avoidance of dietary lactose and symptomatic relief with antimotility agents are also recommended [27]. Because the oral nonabsorbed aminoglycoside, paromycin, is only partially active in cryptosporidiosis, it is often paired with another agent. The dose is 25–35 mg/kg/day orally given in 2–4 daily doses for 28 days, and then reduced to 500 mg twice daily for maintenance.

Azithromycin at a dose of 600 mg daily orally for 5 days is effective in many cases. In AIDS patients, this dose produced symptomatic improvement in all, but persistent stool shedding continued in 60% of cases even after treatment was prolonged to 14 days [28]. In severely immunosuppressed and symptomatic HIV-infected patients, a regimen consisting of the oral nonabsorbed aminoglycoside, paromomycin (1.0 g twice a day) plus azithromycin (600 mg once a day) for 4 weeks, followed by paromomycin alone for 8 weeks has been reported to be curative or to significantly reduce diarrhea [29].

60.5 Giardiasis

The most frequently diagnosed protozoan intestinal infection is caused by ingestion of *Giardia* cysts, which are so resilient that they remain intact in cold water for 2–3 months. About 15% of infected patients evacuate cysts only and have no symptoms. However, around half of infected patients develop symptoms, such as acute watery diarrhea, which occurs in 90% of symptomatic cases. Approximately three out of four patients who develop symptoms complain of abdominal cramping, flatulence and bloating. Chronic diarrhea can lead to malabsorption, weight loss, and deficiencies of protein and vitamins. Up to 40% of cases develop lactose deficiency following infection.

Most persons become infected through ingestion of *G. lamblia* cysts in contaminated water or food and through routine person-to-person contact. Infection is particularly common in travelers to developing countries. Sexual transmission has been recorded and may be common in persons who practice genito-anal or oro-anal sex or partner coprophagia [30]. Infection is inevitable after ingestion of 25 cysts but can develop after consumption of as few as 10 cysts.

Microscopic examination of stool specimens (usually three) examined fresh, or preserved in polyvinyl alcohol or in formalin, remains the diagnostic gold standard and confirms the diagnosis in 80–85% of cases. Stool enzyme-linked immunosorbent assays are also reliable with specificities between 87 and 100% and sensitivities ranging from 88% to 98%. Aspiration of duodenal contents for trophozoites, though more invasive, has a lower diagnostic yield.

Cases of giardiasis are particularly common in gay men, most of whom are HIV-negative [30]. Notably, in one study of HIV-infected persons, recovery of Giardia was strongly associated with anal-penile intercourse but no other sexual practice [31].

Symptomatic patients should be treated with metronidazole, 250 mg three times a day for 5 days, which is 85–95% effective or a single oral 2 g dose of tinidazole, which is equally efficacious. Other therapies include albendazole, 400 mg daily for 5 days or furazolidone, 100 mg four times a day for 7–10 days. Longer courses and higher doses, such as metronidazole 750 mg three times daily for 10 days are administered to patients who relapse. Tinidazole has the advantage of efficacy at a single oral dose of 2 g given with food. Nitazoxanide at an oral dose of 500 mg BID for 3 days inhibits growth of trophozoites. Paromomycin 30 mg/kg/day in 3 divided doses for 7 days is preferred for symptomatic infection in pregnant women [32].

60.6 Amebiasis

Worldwide, the protozoan Entamoeba histolytica infects about 50 million people. In 90% of the cases, the infection is asymptomatic, but the rest develop diarrhea, dysentery or less often peritoneal disease or extra intestinal (hepatic, pulmonary, cardiac, brain) which results in 40,000 deaths annually [33]. Peritonitis is a serious complication that occurs in only 0.5% of cases but is fatal in 40% of them [34]. The course of the infection is determined by host factors such as genetic susceptibility, age and immune status [35].

Infection usually follows ingestion of food and water that is contaminated by amebic cysts, but fecal-oral sexual transmission has been well-documented [33].The prevalence of amebiasis is high in indigent areas of India, Africa, Mexico and Central or South America, but in industrialized nations, this infection is mainly seen in immigrants and travelers from endemic regions, men who have sex with men, and institutionalized patients [33, 36]. In a retrospective study, 48% of 27 Japanese symptomatic men with amebiasis affirmed homosexual or bisexual practices and over a third of the rest had never married [37]. HIV infection is not considered a risk factor for amebiasis [38], but invasive disease has been reported as a complication among HIV-immunocompromised men from Taiwan and Japan [39].

Symptoms such as diarrhea that can be mild or profuse and bloody (dysentery), abdominal pain, fever and weight loss begin after an incubation period of 1–3 weeks. In some patients, a nondysentery form of the disease produces chronic abdominal cramps and intermittent symptoms which can last for years.

Detection of amebic trophozoites and cysts in stool specimens of asymptomatic gay men does not mandate treatment since in the United States and Europe most of these cases reflect colonization with *E. dispar* and occasionally *E. moshkovskii*, neither of which is pathogenic. *E. histolytica* is more often found in gay men from Asian countries such as Japan and Taiwan. Antigen detection tests (ELISA, radioimmunoassay, immunofluorescence) distinguish between *E. histolytica* and nonpathogenic species and have higher sensitivities than microscopy, which misses two-thirds of cases of *E. histolytica* infection [40]. PCR tests have been developed and are highly specific[40]. Serum antibodies to *E. histolytica* are reactive within a week of acute infection but remain detectable for years. So serology is most valuable to exclude disease.

With a cure rate of about 90%, the gold standard for amebic enteritis remains metronidazole at a dose of 500–750 mg orally three times daily for 7–10 days. For those who cannot tolerate metronidazole, tinidazole, 2 g daily for 3 days or nitazoxanide can be administered. A second agent (paromomycin – 25–50 mg/kg/day in three divided doses for 7 days, or diiodohydroxyquin, for 600 mg three times daily for 20 days, or diloxanide for 500 mg three times a day for 10 days) is recommended to eliminate cysts [32].

60.7 Human T-Lymphotropic Virus Type I (HTLV-I)

Between 10 and 20 million people throughout the world are infected with the retrovirus HTLV-1. Most of these persons will never have symptoms but 2–5% eventually develop adult-T-cell leukemia/lymphoma (ATL) and less than 2% will be affected by HTLV-1-associated myelopathy (tropical spastic paraparesis) [41, 42]. Other clinical manifestations associated with HTLV-I infection include neuropathy, chronic inflammatory arthropathy, Sjogren's syndrome, polymyositis, lymphocytic alveolitis, idiopathic thrombocytopenic purpura, and uveitis [43]. An infective dermatitis consisting of weeping, eczematous plaques mainly distributed on the scalp, face, axillae and groin has been described predominantly in young children from the Caribbean, South America, and Japan. Watery nasal exudate and nare crusting are common. The skin lesions are often infected with Staphylococcus aureus or Beta hemolytic streptococci. Asymptomatic patients have been found to have dermatophytosis, seborrheic dermatitis and acquired ichthyosis more frequently [44].

HTLV-1 is endemic in southern Japan where it is most often detected in the elderly and also in Papua-New Guinea, Central and South Africa, the Middle East, the Melanesian islands, and South America. In some regions, such as the Caribbean and Peru, the retrovirus affects younger people, some of whom are present with skin disease.

The routes of virus transmission/acquisitions include mother-to-child transmission, sexual contact, blood transfusion, and intravenous drug use [45]. After age 30, women are infected twice as often as men, presumably because of the higher risk of viral transmission through sexual activity in women, especially those with cervicitis and genital ulcerations [46, 47]. A number of reports have implicated unprotected sex as a risk factor for HTLV-I infection. In various studies of nondrug using female sex workers, prevalence between 3.2 and 21.8% was found in endemic areas [48]. However, in some countries such as the US, sexual transmission in women is associated with a male partner who has histories of intravenous drug use and sexually transmitted infections [46].

The diagnosis of HTLV-I infection is made with an ELISA and confirmed by Western blot testing. Polymerase chain reaction-based tests have been developed and are used to differentiate HTLV-I from HTLV-II infection.

Treatment is not recommended for asymptomatic patients. Combinations of antiretroviral agents containing a nucleoside analogue reverse transcriptase inhibitor such as lamivudine, zidovudine and other antiretrovirals reduce proviral logs but do not significantly improve neurologic or hematologic disease [49]. Patients should be advised against needle shedding and breast-feeding.

60.8 Human T-Lymphotropic Virus Type II (HTLV-II)

Initial reports associating HTLV II infection with hairy cell and large granular lymphocytic leukemia were subsequently disproven [50]. Although further publications have continued to implicate this retrovirus with the development of neurologic disease, especially myelopathy, lymphoma, pneumonia, bronchitis, tuberculosis, arthritis, asthma, and dermatitis, a true association with any pathologic process remains to be determined [51–53]. However, HTLV-II infected persons may be at risk of earlier death [54]. More rapid deterioration of immunosuppression, as well as enhanced progression of HTLV-II–associated lymphoma in patients with HIV has been reported in HTLV-II and HIV coinfected persons [55, 56].

Transmission is similar to that of HTLV-I. Venereal risk factors consist of sex with multiple partners or with a current or former intravenous drug user. High prevalence has been found in Europe, Africa, and South and Central America. In North America, HTLV-II is predominantly found in American Indians and intravenous drug users, particularly those who are African American [57, 58].

60.9 MRSA

Infection with community-acquired methicillin-resistant Staphylococcus aureus (CA-MRSA) was reported initially among drug users in the 1980s. Since then, numerous reports have documented a precipitous rise in CA-MRSA infections in the general population, especially among prison inmates, team sport players, postpartum women and their newborn infants, military personnel, healthcare facilities staff and patients, and men who have sex with men (MSM). HIV patients with more advanced immunodeficiency have higher rates of MRSA colonization. In a retrospective study, 7% of HIV-seropositive patients developed a CA-MRSA infection during a 1-year period. CA-MRSA accounted for 37% of all wound cultures and 65% of all staphylococcal isolates. Although CA-MRSA infection has been correlated with worsening immunodeficiency and a history of syphilis [59], Lee found only associations with high-risk sex, use of illicit drugs, and environmental exposures but not with immune status [60]. Presumably, sexual transmission of MRSA among heterosexuals has also been described in couples in whom one partner had folliculitis or abscesses in the pubic area, groin or buttocks [61].

The usual findings are abscesses, furuncles, or cellulitis in the buttocks, genitals, or perineum. Unlike traditional MRSA strains, CA-MRSA strains often produce Panton-Valentine leukocidin, a pore-forming cytotoxin associated with increased tissue destruction [62].

USA300A is a widely disseminated, multidrug-resistant clone of CA-MRSA that can cause unusually severe disease, including necrotizing fasciitis, sepsis, endocarditis, and pneumonia even among healthy individuals who lack traditional risk factors for MRSA [63]. In a study from San Francisco, this strain was most prevalent in areas highly populated by male same-sex couples residents, suggesting that in this population, sexual transmission is a major risk factor independent of HIV status [64]. Other risk factors associated with the spread of USA300 CA-MRSA among MSM include skin abrading sex, promiscuity (multiple partners, group sex parties), sexual partnering through the Internet, use of recreational drugs such as methamphetamine, and previous sexually transmitted diseases [60].

In one longitudinal study, bullous impetigo was present in 9% of recently HIV-seroconverted men as well as 9% of HIV-seronegative men who had engaged in unprotected anal intercourse with an HIV-infected man [65].

If a localized abscess is fluctuant, it should be surgically drained. Needle aspiration or ultrasonography can help to locate a collection of pus that is not clinically apparent. Additional administration of antibiotics has not been demonstrated to improve outcomes in patients with uncomplicated abscesses and do not need to be routinely prescribed in healthy cases without co-morbidities, preexisting medical conditions, or signs of systemic infection [66]. If the abscess cannot be drained adequately, if there is surrounding cellulitis, or if the patient has medical conditions that may interfere with clearing of infection, antibiotics should be started. Recent reports suggest that antibiotics may be beneficial in abscesses due to CA-MRSA. A large retrospective cohort study found that 95% of abscesses caused by CA-MRSA healed with treatment that included surgical drainage and active antibiotics in contrast to 87% of cases in whom antibiotics were withdrawn [67]. Antibiotics with incision and drainage also seem to be the treatment of choice for abscesses larger than 5 cm in diameter [68]. Unlike hospital-associated MRSA strains, which are resistant to multiple antibiotic classes, CA-MRSA strains are typically resistant to only β-lactams and one or two other drug classes, and are often sensitive to clindamycin, a tetracycline antimicrobial, or trimethoprim–sulfamethoxazole. Therefore, these antibiotics may be initially administered for uncomplicated skin and soft tissue infections, pending results of the antibiotic sensitivities of cultured organisms [69].

However, culture of lesions is imperative as clusters of infection caused by multidrug resistant bacteria have been reported [70].

Examination of sexual partners of persons with MRSA infection for transmission of CA-MRSA should be considered and treatment provided if there is laboratory or clinical evidence of infection.

60.10 Conclusion

Sexual activity is becoming recognized as an important means of transmission for several pathogens, thus expanding the roster of sexually acquired diseases beyond genital infections. Physicians who treat sexually transmitted infections, especially those who provide health care for men-who-have-sex-with men, need to be aware of the symptoms associated with these infections, know effective treatments, and counsel at-risk patients on preventive measures.

Take-Home Pearls

- › Acute or recurrent gastrointestinal symptoms may be caused by pathogenic bacteria or protozoa transmitted through oral-anal-genital sexual practices.
- › Men who engage in high-risk sex with multiple male partners over time or at group sex parties are especially prone to enteric infections.
- › Although most commonly associated with men who have sex with men, heterosexual persons may also engage in oral-anal-genital sexual practices.
- › As is the case with HIV (previously called HTLV-III) infection, sexual intercourse appears to be a less effective but significant means of transmission of HTLV-I and HTLV-II viruses.
- › Sexual contact can result in *S. aureus* pyoderma of the anogenital area and may be the means of MRSA transmission in sex partners of persons from high risk groups for MRSA.

References

1. Pakianathan, M.R., McMillan, A.: Intestinal protozoa in homosexual men in Edinburgh. Int. J. STD AIDS **10**(12), 780–784 (1999)
2. DuPont, H.L., Levine, M.M., Hornick, R.B., Formal, S.B.: Inoculum size in shigellosis and implications for expected mode of transmission. J. Infect. Dis. **159**, 1126–1128 (1989)
3. Bennish, M.L.: Potentially lethal complications of shigellosis. Rev. Infect. Dis. **12**(Suppl 4), 319–324 (1991)
4. Barret-Connor, E., Connor, J.D.: Extraintestinal manifestations of shigellosis. Am. J. Gastroenterol. **53**, 234–245 (1970)
5. Quinn, T.C., Goodell, S.E., Fennell, C., et al.: Infections with *Campylobacter jejuni* and *Campylobacter*-like organisms in homosexual men. Ann. Intern. Med. **101**, 187–192 (1984)
6. Outbreak of *Shigella flexneri* and *Shigella sonnei* enterocolitis in men who have sex with men, Quebec, 1999–2001. Can. Commun. Dis. Rep. **/31**, 85–90 (2005)
7. Tauxe, R.V., McDonald, R.C., Hargrett-Bean, N., et al.: The persistence of *Shigella flexneri* in the United States: increasing role of adult males. Am. J. Public Health **78**, 1432–1435 (1988)
8. Bader, M., Pedersen, A.H., Williams, R., et al.: Venereal transmission of shigellosis in Seattle-King County. Sex. Transm. Dis. **4**, 89–91 (1977)
9. Marcus, U., Zucs, P., Bremer, V., et al.: Shigellosis-a re-emerging sexually transmitted infection: outbreak in men having sex with men in Berlin. Int. J. STD AIDS **15**, 533–537 (2004)
10. O'Sullivan, B., Delpech, V., Pontivivo, G., et al.: Shigellosis linked to sex venues, Australia. Emerg. Infect. Dis. **8**, 862–864 (2002)
11. Shigella flexneri serotype 3 infections among men who have sex with men – Chicago, Illinois, 2003–2004. MMWR, Centers for Disease Control and Prevention. **54**(33), 820–822 (26 Aug 2005)
12. CDC. Shigella sonnei outbreak among men who have sex with men – San Francisco, California, 2000–2001. MMWR. **50**, 922–926 (2001)
13. Edwards, B.H.: Salmonella and Shigella species. Clin. Lab. Med. **19**(3), 469–487 (1999)
14. Taylor, D.N., McKenzie, R., Durbin, A., et al.: Rifaximin, a nonabsorbed oral antibiotic, prevents shigellosis after experimental challenge. Clin. Infect. Dis. **42**(9), 1283–1288 (2006)
15. Kapperud, G., Lassen, J., Ostroff, S., et al.: Clinical features of sporadic Campylobacter infections in Norway. Scand. J. Infect. Dis. **190**, 1150–1157 (2004)
16. Paulet, P., Stoffels, G.: Sexually-transmissible anorectal diseases. Rev. Méd. Brux. **10**(8), 327–331 (1980)
17. Kent, C., Reingold, A., Anderson, G., et al.: Risk factors for Campylobacter infections in men with AIDS/ARC. Int. Conf. AIDS. **6**, 255 (1990) (abstract no. Th.B.533)
18. Melamed, I., Bujanover, Y., Igra, Y.S., et al.: Campylobacter enteritis in normal and immunodeficient children. Am. J. Dis. Child. **137**, 752 (1983)
19. Tee, W., Mijch, A.: Campylobacter jejuni bacteria in Human Immunodeficiency Virus (HIV) infected and non-infected patients; comparison of clinical features and review. Clin. Infect. Dis. **26**, 91–96 (1998)

20. Ternhag, A., Asikainen, T., Giesecke, J., et al.: A meta-analysis on the effects of antibiotic treatment on the duration of symptoms caused by infection with Campylobacter species. Clin. Infect. Dis. **44**, 696–700 (2007)
21. Moore, J.E., Barton, M.D., Blair, I.S., et al.: The epidemiology of antibiotic resistance in Campylobacter. Microbes Infect. **8**(7), 1955–1966 (2006)
22. Hellard, M., Hocking, J., Willis, J., et al.: Risk factors leading to Cryptosporidium infection in men who have sex with men. Sex. Transm. Infect. **79**(5), 412–414 (2003)
23. Caputo, C., Forbes, A., Frost, F., et al.: Determinants of antibodies to Cryptosporidium infection among gay and bisexual men with HIV infection. Epidemiol. Infect. **122**(2), 291–297 (1999)
24. Amin, O.M.: Seasonal prevalence of intestinal parasites in the United States during 2000. Am. J. Trop. Med. Hyg. **66**(6), 799–803 (2002)
25. Rossignol, J.F., Kabil, S.M., el-Gohary, Y., et al.: Effect of nitazoxanide in diarrhea and enteritis caused by Cryptosporidium species. Clin. Gastroenterol. Hepatol. **4**(3), 320–324 (2006)
26. Rossignol, J.F., Ayoub, A., Ayers, M.S.: Treatment of diarrhea caused by Cryptosporidium parvum: a prospective randomized, double-blind, placebo-controlled study of Nitazoxanide. J. Infect. Dis. **184**(1), 103–106 (2001)
27. Rossignol, J.F.: Nitazoxanide in the treatment of acquired immune deficiency syndrome-related cryptosporidiosis: results of the United States compassionate use program in 365 patients. Aliment. Pharmacol. Ther. **24**(5), 887–894 (2006)
28. Allam, A.F., Shehab, A.Y.: Efficacy of azithromycin, praziquantel and mirazid in treatment of cryptosporidiosis in school children. J. Egypt Soc. Parasitol **32**, 969–978 (2002)
29. Cron, S.N.H., Valdez LM, S., et al.: Combination drug therapy for cryptosporidiosis in AIDS. J. Infect. Dis. **178**(3), 900–903 (1998)
30. Kean, B.H., William, D.C., Luminais, S.K.: Epidemic of amoebiasis and giardiasis in a biased population. Br. J. Vener. Dis. **55**, 375–378 (1979)
31. Esfandiari, A., Jordan, W.C., Brown, C.P.: Prevalence of enteric parasitic infection among HIV-infected attendees of an inner city AIDS clinic. Cell. Mol. Biol. **41**(Suppl 1), 19–23 (1995)
32. The Medical Letter On Drugs and Therapeutics: Drugs For Parasitic Infections Handbook, 2nd edition, Abramowicz M (ed),The Medical Letter Inc, New Rochelle, New York, pages 3–22 (2010)
33. Huston, H.R., CD, H.M., et al.: Amebiasis. N Engl. J. Med. **348**, 1565–1573 (2002)
34. Van Hal, S.J., Stark, D.J., Fotedar, R., et al.: Amebiasis: current status in Australia. Med. J. Aust. **186**(8), 412–416 (2007)
35. Stanley, S.L.: Protective immunity to amebiasis, New insights and new challenges. J. Infect. Dis. **184**, 504–506 (2001)
36. Weinke, T., Friedrich-Janicke, B., Hopp, P., Janitschke, K.: Prevalence and clinical importance of Entamoeba histolytica in two high-risk groups: Travelers returning from the tropics and male homosexuals. J. Infect. Dis. **161**, 1029–1031 (1990)
37. Ohnishi, K., Murata, M.: Present characteristics of symptomatic amebiasis due to Entamoeba histolytica in the east-southeast area of Tokyo. Epidemiol. Infect. **119**(3), 363–367 (1997)
38. Moran, P., Ramos, F., Ramiro, M., et al.: Infection by the human immunodeficiency virus-1 is not a risk factor for amebiasis. Am. J. Trop. Med. Hyg. **73**, 296–300 (2005)
39. Hung, C.C., Deng, H.Y., Hsiao, W.H., et al.: Invasive amebiasis as an emerging parasitic disease in patients with human immunodeficiency virus type 1 infection in Taiwan. Arch. Intern. Med. **165**, 409–415 (2005)
40. Haque, R., Ali, I.K., Akther, S.: Comparison of PCR, isoenzyme analysis, and antigen detection for diagnosis of Entamoeba histolytica infection. J. Clin. Microbiol. **36**(2), 449–452 (1998)
41. Matsuoka, M.: Human T-cell leukemia virus type I (HTLV-I) infection and the onset of adult T-cell leukemia (ATL). Retrovirology **2**, 27 (2005)
42. Gessain, A., Barin, F., Vernant, J.C., et al.: Antibodies to human T-lymphotropic virus type I in patients with tropical spastic paraparesis. Lancet **2**, 407–410 (1985)
43. Silva, M.T., Harab, R.C., Leite, A.C., et al.: J. Clin. Infect. Dis. **44**(5), 689–692 (2007)
44. LaGrenade, L., Hanchard, B., Fletcher, V., et al.: Infective dermatitis of Jamaican children: a marker for HTLV-I infection. Lancet **336**(8727), 1345–1347 (1990)
45. Hisada, M., Maloney, E.M., Sawada, T., et al.: Virus markers associated with vertical transmission of human T lymphotropic virus type 1 in Jamaica. Clin. Infect. Dis. **34**(12), 1551–1557 (2002)
46. Manns, A., Hisada, M., La Grenade, L., et al.: Human T-lymphotropic virus type I infection. Lancet **353**, 1951–1958 (1999)
47. Zunt, J., Dezzuti, C.S., Montano, S.A., et al.: Cervical shedding of human T cell lymphotropic virus type 1 is associated with cervicitis. J. Infect. Dis. **186**, 1669–1672 (2002)
48. Gotuzzo, E., Sánchez, J., Escamilla, J., et al.: Human T cell lymphotropic virus type I infection among female sex workers in Peru. J. Infect. Dis. **169**, 754–759 (1994)
49. Balestrieri, E., Forte, G., Matteucci, C., et al.: Effect of lamivudine on transmission of human T-cell lymphotropic virus type 1 to adult peripheral blood mononuclear cells in vitro. Antimicrob. Agents Chemother. **46**, 3080 (2003)
50. Pawson, R., Schulz, T.F., Matutes, E., et al.: The human T-cell lymphotropic viruses types I/II are not involved in T prolymphocytic leukemia and large granular lymphocytic leukemia. Leukemia **11**(8), 1305–1311 (1997)
51. Safaeian, M., Wilson, L.E., Taylor, E., et al.: HTLV-II and bacterial infections among injection drug users. J. Acquir. Immune Defic. Syndr. **24**(5), 483–487 (2000)
52. Roucoux, D.F., Murphy, E.L.: The epidemiology and disease outcomes of human T-lymphotropic virus type II. AIDS Rev. **6**(3), 144–154 (2004)
53. Murphy, E.L., Wang, B., Sacher, R.A., et al.: Respiratory and urinary tract infections, arthritis, and asthma associated with HTLV-I and HTLV-II infection. Emerg. Infect. Dis. **10**(1), 109–116 (2004)
54. Orland, J.R., Wang, B., Wright, D.J., et al.: Increased mortality associated with HTLV-II infection in blood donors: a prospective cohort study. Retrovirology **24**, 1–4 (2004)
55. Poiesz, B., Dube, D., Dube, S., et al.: HTLV-II-associated cutaneous T-cell lymphoma in a patient with HIV-1 infection. N Engl J. Med. **342**(13), 930–936 (2000)

56. Hershow, R.C., Galai, N., Fukuda, K., et al.: An international collaborative study of the effects of coinfection with human T-lymphotropic virus type II on human immunodeficiency virus type 1 disease progression in injection drug users. J. Infect. Dis. **174**(2), 309–317 (1996)
57. Lee, H.H., Weiss, S.H., Brown, L.S., et al.: Patterns of HIV-1 and HTLV-I/II in intravenous drug abusers from the middle atlantic and central regions of the USA. J. Infect. Dis. **162**(2), 347–352 (1990)
58. Hjelle, B., Zhu, S.W., Takahashi, H., et al.: Endemic human T cell leukemia virus type II infection in southwestern US Indians involves two prototype variants of virus. J. Infect. Dis. **168**, 737–740 (1993)
59. Crum-Cianflone, N.F., Burgi, A.A., Hale, B.R.: Increasing rates of community-acquired methicillin-resistant Staphylococcus aureus infections among HIV-infected persons. Int. J. STD AIDS **18**, 521–526 (2007)
60. Lee, N.E., Taylor, M.M., Bancroft, E., et al.: Risk factors for community-associated methicillin-resistant *Staphylococcus aureus* skin infections among HIV-positive men who have sex with men. Clin. Infect. Dis. **40**, 1529–1534 (2005)
61. Cook, H.A., Furuya, E.Y., Larson, E., et al.: Heterosexual transmission of community-associated methicillin-resistant *Staphylococcus aureus*. Clin. Infect. Dis. **44**, 410–413 (2007)
62. Moellering, R.C.: The growing menace of community-acquired methicillin-resistant Staphylococcus aureus. Ann. Intern. Med. **144**, 368–370 (2006)
63. Miller, L.G., Perdreau-Remington, F., Rieg, G., et al.: Necrotizing fasciitis caused by community-associated methicillin-resistant *Staphylococcus aureus* in Los Angeles. N Engl J. Med. **352**, 1445–1453 (2005)
64. Diep, B.A., Chambers, H.F., Graber, C.J., et al.: Emergence of multidrug-resistant, community-associated, methicillin-resistant Staphylococcus aureus clone USA300 in men who have sex with men. Ann. Intern. Med. **148**(4), 249–257 (2008)
65. Donovan, B., Rohrsheim, R., Bassett, I., et al.: Bullous impetigo in homosexual men–a risk marker for HIV-1 infection? Genitourin. Med. **68**(3), 159–161 (1992)
66. Moellering, R.C., Kamitsuka, P.: Management of skin and soft-tissue infection. N Engl. J. Med. **59**, 1063–1067 (2008)
67. Ruhe, J.J., Smith, N., Bradsher, R.W., et al.: Community-onset methicillin-resistant Staphylococcus aureus skin and soft-tissue infections: impact of antimicrobial therapy on outcome. Clin. Infect. Dis. **44**, 777–784 (2007)
68. Lee, M.C., Rios, A.M., Aten, M.F., et al.: Management and outcome of children with skin and soft tissue abscesses caused by community-acquired methicillin-resistant Staphylococcus aureus. Pediatr. Infect. Dis. J. **23**, 123–127 (2004)
69. Szumowski, J.D., Cohen, D.E., Kanaya, F., et al.: Treatment and outcomes of infections by methicillin-resistant *Staphylococcus aureus* at an ambulatory clinic. Antimicrob. Agents Chemother. **51**, 423–428 (2007)
70. Han, L.L., McDougal, L.K., Gorwitz, R.J., et al.: High frequencies of clindamycin and tetracycline resistance in methicillin-resistant *Staphylococcus aureus* pulsed-field type USA300 isolates collected at a Boston ambulatory health center. J. Clin. Microbiol. **45**, 1350–1352 (2007)

Sexual Abuse

61

Wolfgang Harth

Core Messages

- Sexual abuse denotes sexual acts that violate the sexual self-determination of a person who has not reached a certain age, is in a particular relationship to the abuser, or is not able to defend himself or herself physically or emotionally.
- It is certain, however, that based on the consistently high prevalence of sexual abuse, every doctor is consciously or unconsciously confronted with this problem area and thus with the particular demands of sexually transmitted diseases as well as the diagnostics and management of psychosomatic disorders.
- Directly after sexual abuse there are injuries in the genital area, even more often to the body and psychosomatic disturbances.
- Long-term consequences arising from sexual abuse including worse mental and physical health may occur years later, initially not associated with the trauma.
- The localization of a dermatosis in the genital area, as well as an atypical morphology, false-positive laboratory tests or false history in the framework of neurotic-psychotic illnesses may lead to the incorrectly presumed suspicion of sexual abuse.
- When investigating a potential case of sexual abuse, it is necessary to avoid traumatizing diagnostic procedures.
- The approach in cases of sexual abuse must be extremely sensitive. The protection of the patient must be foremost.
- A multidisciplinary approach is recommended to adequately evaluate and treat child abuse victims.
- The doctor must be careful on the one hand and carry out the necessary exclusion diagnostics cautiously, but on the other hand refer the patient immediately to a special care center if necessary.

Definition

Sexual abuse denotes sexual acts that violate the sexual self-determination of a person who has not reached a certain age, is in a particular relationship to the abuser, or is not able to defend himself or herself physically or emotionally [6, 9].

61.1 Incidence/Prevalence

Retrospective studies shows that a high percentage of the population have been subject to some sort of sexual abuse.

In Germany (82.5 million inhabitants), 56,784 criminal acts violating sexual self-determination were

W. Harth
Clinic for Dermatology and Phlebology, Vivantes Clinc, Spandau Berlin, Germany and
Klinik für Dermatologie und Allergologie, Vivantes Klinikum Spandau, Neue Bergstraße 6, 13585, Berlin, Germany
e-mail: wolfgang.harth@vivantes.de

G. Gross and S.K. Tyring (eds.), *Sexually Transmitted Infections and Sexually Transmitted Diseases*,
DOI: 10.1007/978-3-642-14663-3_61, © Springer-Verlag Berlin Heidelberg 2011

recorded in 2008, of which the absolute numbers were 7,292 cases of rape and 12,052 cases of sexual abuse of children [19].

Results of a national telephone survey conducted in 2001–2003 indicate that 1 in 59 US adults (2.7 million women and 978,000 men) experienced unwanted sexual activity in the 12 months preceding the survey and that 1 in 15 US adults (11.7 million women and 2.1 million men) have been forced to have sex during their lifetime [3]. Findings suggest that victimization rates have remained consistent since the 1990s.

Sociological studies assume, however, that the number of unreported cases is vastly greater. The prevalence figures of sexual abuse show a broad scattering with estimates of 9–38% for women and from 9% to 16% for men [15, 23, 27]. Comparison is only possible to a limited extent due to the varying observation periods of the individual studies and the nonuniform definition of sexual abuse.

It is certain, however, that based on the consistently high prevalence of sexual abuse, every doctor is consciously or unconsciously confronted with this problem area and thus with the particular demands of venereological diseases as well as the diagnostics and management of psychosomatic disorders.

61.2 Classification

In practice, three principal areas can be differentiated in the context of sexual abuse (Table 61.1).In addition to the acute effects, the latent long-term consequences and the consequences of unnecessary examinations in unconfirmed suspected diagnoses require careful attention.

Table 61.1 Classification of medical consequences after sexual abuse [9]

1. Acute direct consequences of sexual abuse Injuries Sexually transmitted diseases Pregnancy Emotional symptoms
2. Long-term consequences of sexual abuse Physical function impairments Psychosomatic/psychiatric diseases
3. Imitations and misdiagnoses Specific skin diseases mimicking sexual abuse Iatrogenically induced, reactive emotional symptoms

61.3 Acute Consequences of Sexual Abuse

Directly after sexual abuse there are injuries in the genital area, even more often to the body and psychosomatic disturbances. Some cases of assault show no evidence of trauma. The most common manifestations of child abuse are cutaneous [13]. Injuries are found at buttocks, back, genitals, inside of the upper thigh, and show conspicuous patterns of the clinical picture.

In women, injury is most likely to be observed in cases of violent assault, or in virgins (hymenal tears, laceration, fissures).

Genital injury in boys may also be the result of abuse, which may be physical or sexual in nature [10]. Anal penetrative assault can show acute signs of forced entry, such as tears, fissures and laceration, swelling, erythema, and venous congestion. Chronic changes are lichenification, reduction of anal sphincter tone.

After corresponding incubation, the entire spectrum of sexually transmitted diseases (STDs) can be found: syphilis, gonorrhea, chancroid, herpes genitalis, condylomata acuminata, chlamydia urethritis, trichomonas vaginalis, pediculosis pubis, scabies, and HIV are reported in the literature [7, 15]. Attention must be paid to the different sexual and nonsexual transmission possibilities (during birth, hetero-, autoinoculation) especially in cases of human papillomavirus (HPV) infections.

Sexual abuse must also be considered in the case of pregnancy in very young girls.

Acute psychosomatic consequences of sexual abuse differ widely and depend mainly on the age of the person affected, the intensity and dangerousness of the abuse, relationship to the abuser and, especially in children, from the frequency and length of time of the trauma.

The direct consequence is often depression and reduction of self-esteem, acute stress disorder, anxiety, shame, or feelings of guilt [1]. Frequently reported changes in emotional behavior among children include disrupted development, difficulties in learning, excessive sexualization including masturbation, touching the genitals of other children, running away, truancy and enuresis, self-injury, insomnia, eating disorders, or suicidal tendencies [6]. A strong association between abuse and urinary frequency, urgency, and nocturia was shown [14]. Many abused children show characteristic traits in interaction, such as the so-called frozen smile, or frozen alertness. In addition, fears are evident in situations that are reminiscent of the abuse context, such as bathing and showering, or fear of physical examinations.

61.4 Long-Term Consequences of Sexual Abuse

Long-term consequences arising from sexual abuse including worse mental and physical health may occur years later, initially not associated with the trauma [28].

Scars or functional impairment occur only in the most rare cases as long-term consequences of sexual abuse.

Consideration should be given to psychosomatic long-term sequelae of sexual abuse in the history of patients, self-injuries to the lower arms, borderline disorders, or anorexia nervosa [8, 18]. Especially self-inflicted dermatoses may be based on an emotional disturbance in former years, reflecting a reactivation of injuries experienced in childhood and may contain an appeal function.

In some cases, a possible comorbidity can be proven with urticaria [4], dys- and hyperhidrosis, alopecia areata, perioral dermatitis, vulvar eczema, vulvodynia, pruritus, and body dysmorphic disorders [5].

Sexual abuse, particularly childhood sexual abuse, has been linked to chronic pelvic pain and to sexual dysfunction [22]. Especially men who reported having experienced sexual, physical, or emotional abuse had increased prevalence for symptoms of chronic prostatitis/chronic pelvic pain syndrome [11].

Significantly higher levels of global mental health problems, hostility, paranoid ideation, and psychosis were found [29]. Often psychosomatic long-term consequences of sexual abuse are only nonspecific depressive symptom (83%) or additionally sleep disorders, headache, dyspareunia, chronic gastritis, somatoform pain disorders, phobia, eating disorders, addictions, suicidal thoughts, self-injury, frequent consultation of doctors, increased divorce rates, sexual disorder including greater sexual risk behavior, promiscuity or prostitution, more sexual partners, unprotected sex and alcohol use for men, and drug use for women [1, 16, 24].

Women reported higher levels of dissociation, confusion regarding self-identity, and relationship problems [2]. As coping or defense mechanisms against the traumatizing situation, the patients develop splitting phenomena and long-term dissociative disorders up to and including borderline personality disorders or posttraumatic stress disorders, and psychoses may occur.

The therapy for long-term consequences of the medical symptoms or disease is usually only successful when the emotional disorder resulting from the trauma is taken into account.

61.5 Misdiagnosis

Due to the variability of clinical findings and the broad spectrum of normal variants, the diagnostic of sexual abuse of children is difficult. The localization of a dermatosis in the genital area, as well as an atypical morphology, false-positive laboratory tests or false history in the framework of neurotic-psychotic illnesses may lead to the incorrectly presumed suspicion of sexual abuse (Table 61.2).

Table 61.2 Imitations: differential diagnoses of sexual abuse [9]

Dermatoses in the genital area	Allergic-toxic contact dermatitis (phytodermatitis) Atopic vulvar dermatitis Hemorrhagias, vasculitis Blistering diseases/Behcet disease Lichen sclerosus atrophicans (hemorrhagic after minimal trauma with toilette paper) Lichen planus Psoriasis
Infections	Bacterial Fungal Viral (varicellae, herpes, condylomata acuminata) Parasitic
Neoplasm	Papilloma Carcinoma/Sarcoma
Congenital deformities	Vascular deformity (hemangiomas) Syndrome (Klippel Trenaunay) Epispadia, Infantile perineal protrusion
Trauma	Irritations Fall, accident Cultural (circumcision)
Systemic diseases	Morbus Crohn Megacolon Fistulae

Misdiagnosis may arise in cases with easily confused morphology that may mimic sexual abuse, especially vulvar and/or perianal diseases such as lichen sclerosus et atrophicus, Behcet's syndrome, bullous diseases, contact dermatitis, or neoplastic lesions [20].

Infantile perineal protrusion is a relatively newly recognized condition. Based on the typical anatomic location and prevalence in prepubertal children, the morphologic features may be mistaken for sexual abuse [12].

The group of sexually transmitted diseases (STDs) pose particular difficulties.

Studies of larger numbers of patients conclude that sexual abuse cannot be directly proven in the majority of children with condylomata acuminata and that other causes are possible. HPV has become one of the most common sexually transmitted diseases in adults, but anogenital warts in children may be also acquired perinatally. Vertical transmission from mother to infant during birth is well recognized. Postnatal acquisition by nonsexual transmission can occur [25]. The transmission of genital papilloma virus infections or herpes infections can occur by smear infection. On the other side, routine screening for HSV-2 in sexually abused children does not have a high yield [21]. There is an unacceptably high rate of false-positive results.

When investigating a potential case of sexual abuse, it is necessary to avoid traumatizing diagnostic procedures. Differential diagnosis must be undertaken with special and extraordinary tact in this situation. One must warn against prematurely pronouncing a suspected diagnosis without strong evidence, and the resulting negative effect upon the family situation. There is no specific test or behavior which would rule out or confirm sexual abuse at the physical or emotional level. Moreover, negative statements about the child's abuser should be avoided since the children have an ambivalent relationship to this person, especially when it is a person of the family. Accusations of guilt, aggressive confrontations, or reproaching the parents are contraindicated. A suspected diagnosis and the corresponding diagnostic measures to rule out sexual abuse may lead to distrust and annoyance on the part of the patient involved, the partner, or the family, as well producing reactive emotional disturbances.

Involving the police is a decision with serious consequences which should be a team decision whenever possible.

61.6 Management

Proof of sexual abuse is very difficult and only possible by means of time-consuming history-taking, physical examination, medical tests, and thorough psychological examination. The approach in cases of sexual abuse must be extremely sensitive. The protection of the patient must be foremost [2].

The forensic examination following rape has two primary purposes: to provide health care and to collect evidence and also has a forensic significance in that injuries are linked to the outcome of legal proceedings [26]. Occasionally, abuse is simulated, and this must be ruled out.

This is normally performed in special regional centers, usually in cooperation with the investigative authorities and specialized clinics or gynecological centers.

Recording gynecological findings is quickly required in suspected sexual abuse when there is a possibility of obtaining sperm traces shortly after the fact, or if acute injury must be treated. Sexually transmitted infections and characteristic injuries in the genital and anal areas are important guiding symptoms in the confirmation of sexual abuse.

Venereal disease is generally found rarely in children. If one of the classical venereal diseases is diagnosed in a child or there are specific gynecological findings, these are attributable with high probability to sexual abuse. Sexually transmitted diseases must be treated according to the guidelines.

Physical injuries need treatment so that they heal without adverse consequences. Sexual-medical queries, especially in connection with possible sexual abuse, require in all cases psychosomatic primary care or more intensive psychotherapeutic measures. If an acute stress disorder is present, anxiolytics and sedatives may be necessary. In the case of long-term sequelae, therapy with antidepressive drugs or neuroleptics is indicated, depending on the dominant comorbidities. Long-term consequences, especially in the presence of factitious disorders, posttraumatic stress disorders, dissociative disorders, or borderline personality disorders, can often not initially be interpreted as late sequelae of sexual abuse and patients often show great resistance to revealing this information, and need psychological diagnostics or a long-term psychotherapy.

In this case, the doctor should be particularly aware of unconscious reactivation of previous trauma during diagnostic clarification with physical examination, gynecological examinations of children, including smears and introduction of the speculum.

In conclusion, a multidisciplinary approach is recommended to adequately evaluate and treat child abuse victims; however, the responsibility often lies with the family physician to recognize and treat these cases at first presentation to prevent significant morbidity and mortality.

The doctor must be careful on the one hand and carry out the necessary exclusion diagnostics cautiously, but on the other hand refer the patient immediately to a special care center if necessary to prevent child maltreatment although home visitation programs have been effective [17].

Take-Home Pearls

- Sexual abuse denotes sexual acts which violate the sexual self-determination of a person
- Every doctor is consciously or unconsciously confronted with this problem area
- In practice, three principal areas can be differentiated in the context of sexual abuse:
  1. Acute direct consequences of sexual abuse include
     - Injuries
     - Sexually transmitted diseases
     - Pregnancy
     - Emotional symptoms
  2. Long-term consequences of sexual abuse include
     - Physical function impairments
     - Psychosomatic/psychiatric diseases
  3. Imitations and misdiagnoses include
     - Specific skin diseases mimicking sexual abuse
     - Iatrogenically-induced, reactive emotional symptoms
- The approach in cases of sexual abuse must be extremely sensitive
- A multidisciplinary approach is recommended
- The doctor must be careful on the one hand and carry out the necessary exclusion diagnostics cautiously, but on the other hand refer the patient immediately to a special care center if necessary

References

1. Bachmann, G.A., Moeller, T.P., Benett, J.: Childhood sexual abuse and the consequences in adult woman. Obstet. Gynecol. **71**, 631–642 (1988)
2. Bailey, H.N., Moran, G., Pederson, D.R.: Childhood maltreatment, complex trauma symptoms, and unresolved attachment in an at-risk sample of adolescent mothers. Attach. Hum. Dev. **9**, 139–161 (2007)
3. Basile, K.C., Chen, J., Black, M.C., Saltzman, L.E.: Prevalence and characteristics of sexual violence victimization among U.S. adults, 2001–2003. Violence Vict. **22**, 437–448 (2007)
4. Brosig, B., Niemeier, V., Kupfer, J., Gieler, U.: Urticaria and the recall of a sexual trauma. Dermatol. Psychosom. **1**, 53–55 (2000)
5. Didie, E.R., Tortolani, C.C., Pope, C.G., Menard, W., Fay, C., Phillips, K.A.: Childhood abuse and neglect in body dysmorphic disorder. Child Abuse Negl. **30**, 1105–1115 (2006)
6. Egle, T., Hoffmann, S.V., Joraschky, P.: Sexualer Mißbrauch, Misshandlung, Vernachlässigung. Schattauer, Stuttgart/New York (1997)
7. Folland, D.S., Burke, R.E., Hinman, A.R., Schaffner, W.: Gonorrhea in preadolescent children: an inquiry into source of infection and mode of transmission. Pediatrics **60**, 153–156 (1977)
8. Gupta, M.A., Gupta, A.K.: Dermatitis artefacta and sexual abuse. Int. J. Dermatol. **32**, 825–826 (1993)
9. Harth, W., Linse, R.: Dermatological symptoms and sexual abuse: a review and case reports. J. Eur. Acad. Dermatol. Venereol. **14**, 489–494 (2000)
10. Hobbs, C.J., Osman, J.: Genital injuries in boys and abuse. Arch. Dis. Child. **92**, 328–331 (2007)
11. Hu, J.C., Link, C.L., McNaughton-Collins, M., Barry, M.J., McKinlay, J.B.: The association of abuse and symptoms suggestive of chronic prostatitis/chronic pelvic pain syndrome: results from the Boston Area Community Health survey. J. Gen. Intern. Med. **22**(11), 1532–1537 (2007)
12. Khachemoune, A., Guldbakke, K.K., Ehrsam, E.: Infantile perineal protrusion. J. Am. Acad. Dermatol. **54**, 1046–1049 (2006)
13. Kos, L., Shwayder, T.: Cutaneous manifestations of child abuse. Pediatr. Dermatol. **23**, 311–320 (2006)
14. Link, C.L., Lutfey, K.E., Steers, W.D., McKinlay, J.B.: Is abuse causally related to urologic symptoms? Results from the Boston Area Community Health (BACH) survey. Eur. Urol. **52**, 397–406 (2007)
15. Lowy, G.: Sexually transmitted diseases in children. Pediatr. Dermatol. **9**, 329–334 (1992)
16. McDonagh-Coyle, A., McHugo, G.J., Friedman, M.J., Schnurr, P.P., Zayfert, C., Descamps, M.: Psychophysiological reactivity in female sexual abuse survivors. J. Trauma. Stress **14**, 667–683 (2001)
17. McDonald, K.C.: Child abuse: approach and management. Am. Fam. Physician **75**, 221–228 (2007)
18. van Moffaert, M.: Localization of self-inflicted dermatological lesions: what do they tell the dermatologist? Acta Derm. Venereol. Suppl. (Stockh) **156**, 23–27 (1991)
19. Bundeskriminalamt: Polizeiliche Kriminalstatistik 2008 Bundeskriminalamt, Wiesbaden (2009)

20. Porzionato, A., Alaggio, R., Aprile, A.: Perianal and vulvar Crohn's disease presenting as suspected abuse. Forensic Sci. Int. **155**, 24–27 (2005)
21. Ramos, S., Lukefahr, J.L., Morrow, R.A., Stanberry, L.R., Rosenthal, S.L.: Prevalence of herpes simplex virus types 1 and 2 among children and adolescents attending a sexual abuse clinic. Pediatr. Infect. Dis. J. **25**, 902–905 (2006)
22. Randolph, M.E., Reddy, D.M.: Sexual abuse and sexual functioning in a chronic pelvic pain sample. J. Child Sex. Abus. **15**, 61–78 (2006)
23. Satin, A.J., Paicurich, J., Millman, S., Wendel, G.D.: The prevalence of sexual aussault: a survey of 2404 puerperal woman. Am. J. Obstet. Gynecol. **167**, 973–975 (1992)
24. Senn, T.E., Carey, M.P., Vanable, P.A., Coury-Doniger, P., Urban, M.A.: Childhood sexual abuse and sexual risk behavior among men and women attending a sexually transmitted disease clinic. J. Consult. Clin. Psychol. **74**, 720–731 (2006)
25. Sinal, S.H., Woods, C.R.: Human papillomavirus infections of the genital and respiratory tracts in young children. Semin. Pediatr. Infect. Dis. **16**, 306–316 (2005)
26. Sommers, M.S.: Defining patterns of genital injury from sexual assault: a review. Trauma Violence Abuse **8**, 270–280 (2007)
27. Spencer, M.J., Dunklee, P.: Sexual abuse of boys. Pediatrics **78**, 133–138 (1986)
28. Springer, K.W., Sheridan, J., Kuo, D., Carnes, M.: Long-term physical and mental health consequences of childhood physical abuse: results from a large population-based sample of men and women. Child Abuse Negl. **31**, 517–530 (2007)
29. Young, M.S., Harford, K.L., Kinder, B., Savell, J.K.: The relationship between childhood sexual abuse and adult mental health among undergraduates: victim gender doesn't matter. J. Interpers. Violence **22**, 1315–1331 (2007)

Part XII

Psychosocial Issues

Psychosocial Issues

62

Kurt Seikowski

Core Messages

The 4 levels of prevention models:

Level 1 – Health prophylaxis

› To maintain emotional and physical health
› Including health education and health consultation (which appeal primarily to the emotional side of the person, because emotionally processed knowledge usually leads to changes in attitudes and behavior)

Level 2 – Primary prevention

› Education in clubs, schools and clinics has been found to be particularly effective at reducing the occurrence of venereal disease; also successful in drug therapies
› Involving the uninfected partner in the treatment process

Level 3 – Secondary prevention

› 4 step concept:
  1. Phase of acceptance with the intention of *emotional calming*
  2. Provide information and knowledge
  3. Detailed consultation about various possible treatments
  4. Therapeutic measures (e.g., involving a psychologist and psychotherapist)
› Therapeutic measures: interventions to reduce depressions and other emotional fluctuations (people with depression, emotional dysfunction in the sense of fluctuating moods and unstable lifestyle suffer more recurrences)

Level 4 – Tertiary prevention

› Medicinal interventions and psychological therapies reduces danger of recurrence

62.1 Prevention Model as a Frame of Reference

In the framework of disease prevention, differentiation is made between four levels of prevention models: *Level 1 – In health prophylaxis*, the objective is to keep diseases from occurring at all. The means of providing information about prevention play a very particular role, especially in sexually transmitted diseases. It is repeatedly assumed that sexual abstinence is utopian. Thus, the point is to protect oneself and to have the knowledge of how one can protect oneself against sexually transmitted diseases. *Level 2 – In primary prevention*, elimination of disease-promoting risk factors is in the foreground. With respect to sexually transmitted diseases, the attempt is repeatedly made to identify such risk factors in order to develop appropriate prevention programs. *Level 3 – Secondary prevention* attempts to prevent the outbreak of disease. This is particularly relevant in HIV infection since the HIV infection itself does not initially cause symptoms/complaints and there are clear indications that safer-sex and antiviral therapies can stop AIDS. In *Level 4 (tertiary prevention)*, coping with the disease is in the foreground. This applies not only to AIDS, but also to permanently recurring diseases such as genital herpes. At the center is the realization of having to live with the disease.

K. Seikowski
Department of Dermatology, Venerology and Allergology, University of Leipzig, Philipp-Rosenthal-Str. 23-25, 04103 Leipzig, Germany
e-mail: kurt.seikowski@medizin.uni-leipzig.de

G. Gross and S.K. Tyring (eds.), *Sexually Transmitted Infections and Sexually Transmitted Diseases*, DOI: 10.1007/978-3-642-14663-3_62, © Springer-Verlag Berlin Heidelberg 2011

62.2 Health Prophylaxis

Health prophylaxis is taken to mean activities directly influencing individual persons or groups to maintain emotional and physical health [19]. It includes health education and health consultation. With respect to sexually transmitted diseases, the objective is to alter sexual convictions, attitudes, and norms. This should begin in late childhood and adolescence. Recent studies in the USA show how important this is. The studies demonstrated that 40% of all persons with new HIV infections were younger than 25 years of age [2]. There is an enormous need for research on the sexual behavior of adolescents and young adults [5, 8]. There are no current studies on this topic, although they are necessary if education and consultation are to be kept up to date. For example, there are practically no reliable studies on whether the Internet alters the sexual behavior of this age group. There are, for example, chat rooms in which dates can be made for anonymous sex. On the other hand, the question can be posed whether there is, in fact, less real sexual contact because of masturbation in front of the computer thanks to Internet sex pages?

Among adolescents, simply having the knowledge that sexual abstinence and condoms provide protection does not help much since the knowledge is often not applied [12] or because the learning effects are not stable [25]. Here, the goal is to seek possibilities for consultation and education that appeal primarily to the emotional side of the person. Emotionally processed knowledge typically leads to changes in attitudes and behavior.

A health-awareness lifestyle consists of:

1. Health and prevention behavior by means of informal education and educative training programs. The latter can also be easily integrated into everyday life at school.
2. Imparting health-relevant guidance orientations. Among these are sense of coherence and subjective theories of health and disease. If, for example, someone is of the opinion that his HIV infection is his fate and he deserves to be sick, he will protect himself less and accept reinfections as inevitable.
3. Personal competencies. These consist of the ability to adequately process and apply information – having problem-solving abilities even in the case of long-lasting disease (coping) and making use of social resources through social contacts (social support).

62.3 Primary Prevention

There are many studies on the risk factors for sexually transmitted diseases, all of which have similar results. In a meta-analysis by Darbes [6], unprotected sexual intercourse takes first place in the onset of sexually transmitted diseases. Couples should be advised to consciously make use of contraception as protection [13]. Drug consumption, especially of methamphetamines, is another risk factor [21]. However, political, structural, and institutional factors also influence the occurrence of these diseases. Poverty is among these factors [1].

As representative of many other studies, the following risk factors were identified in a very complex study of 14,322 persons between 18 and 27 years of age who were tested for venereal diseases [4]:

- Housing insecurity
- Exposure to crime
- Having been arrested
- More lifetime partners
- Earlier sexual debut
- Childhood sexual abuse
- Gang participation
- Frequent alcohol use
- Depression
- Sexual risk behavior

Education concerning sexually transmitted diseases in clubs, schools, and clinics with special centers for venereal diseases has been found to be particularly effective in reducing infection rates [16]. In addition, when sex education was coupled with drug therapy, the occurrence of venereal disease was reduced [22]. The same applies to involving the uninfected partner in the treatment process [9].

62.4 Secondary Prevention

At this prevention level, those involved are already infected. Initially, communication of the diagnosis is especially important. In a different context, Bosse [3] developed a four-step concept of dermatological procedures for patients with atopic dermatitis. The concept can also be applied to patients with other chronic diseases. Bosse first defined a *phase of acceptance* by the patient, during which the physician's intention is emotional calming when the diagnosis is made known. For many patients, it is alarming to have a venereal disease. They become agitated and this leads to processes of selective perception. These are filters that typically only allow negative information in cases of agitation. Conducting an educative and informational interview in this phase would mean a loss of information to the patient as he can only adequately take in important information when he is emotionally calm.

The second phase involves *providing information and knowledge* with the goal of giving the patient an orientation for his treatment. The venereal disease is precisely explained to the patient. He can also ask about anything that is unclear. This phase is followed by a *detailed consultation about various possible treatments,* the results of which lead to the initiation of *therapeutic measures* (for example, involving a psychologist and psychotherapist). Rather than a purely medical therapy, the psychologist/psychotherapist practices supportive medicine: supporting – acting (speaking), waiting (listening), and observing (oriented to the therapeutic value rather than to a quick cure).

Among the therapeutic measures are also interventions to reduce depressions and other emotional fluctuations. Psychological studies of genital herpes are interesting in this respect. It was found that highly depressive people suffer more recurrences [11, 15, 28]. Emotional dysfunctions in the sense of fluctuating moods and an instable lifestyle also influence the frequency of recurrence [23].

Secondary prevention programs have been especially valuable to HIV patients [7, 27]. Compliance with functions presented in these programs is lower among depressive or drug-dependent persons, who require additional specific therapies [10]. Recently, anonymous audio-computer-assisted self-interviews have been found effective for HIV-positive patients [17].

The possibility for consultation concerning a wish for children among HIV-infected persons must also be mentioned [26].

62.5 Tertiary Prevention

Medicinal interventions are not the only therapeutic measures. Psychological therapies can also reduce the danger of recurrence.

Psychological group interventions, for example, in genital herpes were most effective among depressive and mood-instable persons; however, a lower number of recurrences could only be achieved in *structured* group therapies, as compared to thematic group therapy [20]. This was not the case in pure "*social support groups*" [14, 15].

In AIDS, the topic "death" is in the foreground. The care of these persons focuses on the following aspects [18]:

1. Orientation to the physical symptoms in the sense of symptomatic relief
2. Promotion of education and decisional autonomy (Status of prognosis, providing realistic information)
3. Reflection of dignity and identity
4. Integration in a social network
5. Integration offer for family members/significant others

62.6 The Value of Psychotherapy

First of all, in many countries, there is the availability of individual consultation and therapy in all phases of prevention at help centers specializing in sexually transmitted diseases [24].

Psychotherapy is always useful when anxieties and fears are involved [29]. This applies for persons who have developed venerophobias. As a result of venerophobias, some do not dare to have sexual contact and they are even afraid to touch objects that others have touched because those other people could be infected. Others have pathologically dealt with sexual contacts based on an anxious personality and observation of their own bodies. They fear the onset of symptoms, often perceive such symptoms, and then go from one doctor to another. Behavior-therapeutic measures for the treatment of phobias are particularly successful in such cases.

In people who are already infected, psychotherapy helps cope with anxiety in relationships. For example, when someone was infected by a stranger and must now tell his/her partner. Anxiety about the future is foremost in HIV infections, where depression may result. Here, too, it is helpful to develop coping strategies that make it easier to maintain a positive attitude toward life despite the diagnosis.

Palliative care is foremost in people with AIDS who do not have long to live.

Take-Home Pearls

- Value of Psychotherapy
- Psychotherapy is always useful when anxieties and fears are involved – for uninfected or infected people

References

1. Aiello, A.E., Simanek, A.M., Galea, S.: Population levels of psychological stress, herpesvirus reactivation and HIV. AIDS Behav.: PM:18264753 (2008)
2. Benton, T.D., Ifeagwu, J.A.: HIV in adolescents: what we know and what we need to know. Curr. Psychiatry Rep. **10**, 109–115 (2008)
3. Bosse, K.: Psychosomatische Gesichtspunkte bei der Betreuung atopischer Ekzematiker. Z. Hautkr. **65**, 422–427 (1990)
4. Buffardi, A.L., Thomas, K.K., Holmes, K.K., Manhart, L.E.: Moving upstream: ecosocial and psychosocial correlates of sexually transmitted infections among young adults in the United States. Am. J. Public Health **98**, 1128–1136 (2008)
5. Celentano, D.D., Sirirojn, B., Sutcliffe, C.G., Quan, V.M., Thomson, N., Keawvichit, R., Wongworapat, K., Latkin, C., Taechareonkul, S., Sherman, S.G., Aramrattana, A.: Sexually transmitted infections and sexual and substance use correlates among young adults in Chiang Mai, Thailand. Sex. Transm. Dis. **35**, 400–405 (2008)
6. Darbes, L., Crepaz, N., Lyles, C., Kennedy, G., Rutherford, G.: The efficacy of behavioral interventions in reducing HIV risk behaviors and incident of sexually transmitted diseases in heterosexual African Americans. AIDS **22**, 1177–1194 (2008)
7. Deribe, K., Woldemichael, K., Wondafrash, M., Haile, A., Amberbir, A.: Disclosure experience and associated factors among HIV positive men and women clinical service users in Southwest Ethiopia. BMC Public Health **8**, 81 (2008)
8. DiClemente, R.J., Crittende, C.P., Rose, E., Sales, J.M., Wingood, G.M., Crosby, R.A., Salazar, L.F.: Psychosocial predictors of HIV-associated sexual behaviors and the efficacy of prevention interventions in adolescents at-risk for HIV infection: what works and what doesn't work? Psychosom. Med. **70**, 598–605 (2008)
9. Goldsworthy, R.C., Fortenberry, D.J.: Patterns and determinants of patient-delivered therapy uptake among healthcare consumers. Sex. Transm. Dis.: PM:18779762 (2008)
10. Kalichman, S.C.: Co-occurrence of treatment nonadherence and continued HIV transmission risk behaviors: implications for positive prevention interventions. Psychosom. Med. **70**, 593–597 (2008)
11. Kemeny, M.E., Cohen, F., Zegans, L.S., Conant, M.A.: Psychological and immunological predictors of genital herpes recurrence. Psychosom. Med. **51**, 195–208 (1989)
12. Kourtis, A.P., Kraft, J.M., Gavin, L., Kissin, D., McMichen-Wright, P., Jamieson, D.J.: Prevention of sexually transmitted human immunodeficiency virus (HIV) infection in adolescents. Curr. HIV Res. **4**, 209–219 (2006)
13. Kraft, J.M., Harvey, S.M., Thorburn, S., Henderson, J.T., Posner, S.F., Galavotti, C.: Intervening with couples: assessing contraceptive outcomes in a randomized pregnancy and HIV/STD risk reduction intervention trial. Womens Health Issues **17**, 52–60 (2007)
14. Longo, D.J., Clum, G.A., Yaeger, N.J.: Psychological treatment for recurrent genital herpes. J. Consult. Clin. Psychol. **56**, 61–66 (1988)
15. McLarnon, L.D., Kaloupek, D.G.: Psychological investigation of genital herpes recurrence: prospective assessment and cognitive-behavioral intervention for a chronic physical disorder. Health Psychol. **7**, 231–249 (1988)
16. Sales, J.M., Milhausen, R.R., DiClemente, R.J.: A decade in review: building on the experiences of past adolescent STI/HIV interventions to optimise future prevention efforts. Sex. Transm. Infect. **82**, 431–436 (2006)
17. Schackman, B.R., Dastur, Z., Ni, Q., Callahan, M.A., Berger, J., Rubin, D.S.: Sexually active HIV-positive patients frequently report never using condoms in audio computer-assisted self-interviews conducted at routine clinical visits. AIDS Patient Care STDs **22**, 123–129 (2008)
18. Schroeder, C.: Psychosoziale Arbeit im Rahmen der palliativ-medizinischen Versorgung. In: Braehler, E., Strauss, H. (eds.) Handlungsfelder in der Psychosozialen Medizin, pp. 407–424. Hogrefe, Göttingen/Bern/Toronto/Seattle (2002)
19. Schroeder, H.: Gesundheitserziehung und Gesundheitsfoerderung. In: Berth, H., Balck, F., Braehler, E. (eds.) Medizinische Psychologie und Medizinische Soziologie von A bis Z, pp. 181–184. Hogrefe, Goettingen/Bern/Wien/Paris/Oxford/Prag/Toronto/Cambridge/Amsterdam/Kopenhagen (2008)
20. Seikowski, K.: Medizinisch-Psychologische Problemfelder in der Dermatologie. Westdeutscher Verlag, Opladen/Wiesbaden (1999)
21. Semple, S.J., Zians, J., Strathdee, S.A., Patterson, T.L.: Methamphetamine-using felons: psychosocial and behavioral characteristics. Am. J. Addict. **17**, 28–35 (2008)
22. Shoptaw, S., Klausner, J.D., Reback, C.J., Tierney, S., Stansell, J., Hare, C.B., Gibson, S., Siever, M., King, W.D., Kao, U., Dang, J.: A public health response to the methamphetamine epidemic: the implementation of contingency management to treat methamphetamine dependence. BMC Public Health **6**, 214 (2006)
23. Silver, P.S., Auerbach, S.M., Vishniavsky, N., Kaplowitz, L.G.: Psychological factors in recurrent genital herpes infection: stress, coping style, social support, emotional dysfunction, and symptom recurrence. J. Psychosom Res. **30**, 163–171 (1986)
24. Forschung, S.P.I.: Sexuell übertragbare Krankheiten. Asanger, Heidelberg und Kröning (2004)
25. Stanton, B., Harris, C., Cottrell, L., Li, X., Gibson, C., Guo, J., Pack, R., Galbraith, J., Pendleton, S., Wu, Y., Burns, J., Cole, M., Marshall, S.: Trial of an urban adolescent sexual

risk-reduction intervention for rural youth: a promising but imperfect fit. J. Adolesc. Health **38**, 55 (2006)
26. Tandler-Schneider, A., Sonnenberg-Schwan, U., Gingelmaier, A., Meurer, A., Kremer, H., Weigel, M., Vernazza, P., Schmied, B., Klumb, S., Schafberger, A., Kupka, M., Friese, K., Brockmeyer, N.H.: Diagnostik und Behandlung HIV-betroffener Paare mit Kinderwunsch. J. Reproduktionsmed Endokrinol **5**, 186–192 (2008)
27. Temoshok, L.R., Wald, R.L.: Integrating multidimensional HIV prevention programs into healthcare settings. Psychosom. Med. **70**, 612–619 (2008)
28. VanderPlate, C., Aral, S.O., Magder, L.: The relationship among genital herpes simplex virus, stress, and social support. Health Psychol. **7**, 159–168 (1988)
29. Wicks, L.A.: Psychotherapy and AIDS: The Human Dimension. Taylor & Francis, Washington (1997)

Part XIII

Economical and Political Issues

Economic and Political Issues Associated with Sexually Transmitted Diseases

63

Viviane Brunne

Core Messages

- Although not easily measured, STIs, including HIV/AIDS, do have macroeconomic consequences, which may add up over time.
- Companies may face direct, indirect and systemic costs as a consequence of heightened STI infection rates (including HIV/AIDS); while employers tend to be reactive, an increasing number of business coalitions offer assistance at the international, regional and national level.
- The international policy framework for sexual reproductive health, including STIs, was agreed upon at the International Conference on Population and Development (ICPD) 1994 in Cairo.
- The Cairo Programme of Action emphasized contextual factors of STIs, such as poverty, and advocated a rights-based approach aiming at empowering men and women to make informed decisions about their sexual reproductive health.
- Issues discussed at the ICPD and other important international conferences at the time were later merged into a set of eight Millennium Development Goals, of which goal 6 specifically addresses HIV/AIDS.
- Implementation of internationally agreed policy frameworks related to STIs may be hindered by political considerations, including sensitivities of certain interest groups.
- Given the interdependence of political and economic factors impacting the STI policy regime, measures have to be pursued that merge the resources of public and private actors, for example, in the form of public–private partnerships.

63.1 Introduction

Sexually transmitted infections (STIs) and reproductive tract infections are responsible for considerable ill health throughout the world. Each year, there are an estimated 340 million new cases of curable STIs, as well as some five million new HIV infections. STIs are infections that are spread primarily through person-to-person sexual contact. There are more than 30 different sexually transmissible bacteria, viruses and parasites.[1] To different degrees, medicine is able to offer treatment to either cure or alleviate the effects of the disease. However, STIs are not merely medical phenomena. They occur in social, cultural, political and economic contexts that play a major role in how much certain groups of society or certain regions of the world may be affected. These contexts determine

V. Brunne
Genève, Switzerland
e-mail: viviane.brunne@rub.de

[1] http://www.who.int/reproductive-health/stis/index.htm; http://www.who.int/topics/sexually_transmitted_infections/en/.

Disclaimer: All statements made in this article are made in the author's private capacity and are in no way related to her work at UNAIDS.

G. Gross and S.K. Tyring (eds.), *Sexually Transmitted Infections and Sexually Transmitted Diseases*,
DOI: 10.1007/978-3-642-14663-3_63,

which coping strategies are chosen and to what extent they may be successful. This article shall explore economic and political factors that are of relevance in connection with STIs. It shall help to see the bigger picture and understand the context of different prevalences of STIs among certain populations and in some regions rather than in others. The analysis shall also help to show how economic and political factors influence the ability to define appropriate strategies and how the interdependence of economic and political factors strongly suggests collaborative approaches, prominently involving both public and private partners.

Before looking at the economic and political factors themselves, a brief reflection shall be helpful on what is actually meant by "political" and "economic" factors. Literature suggests that the "political" is generally concerned with government, the state and public affairs, with conflict and its resolution and with the sources and the exercise of power. Complementary to that, economics is focused on systems of production and exchange, on rational behavior directed towards the maximization of utility through optimal allocation of scarce resources and the accumulation and distribution of wealth ([1], pp. 389–390). The political usually pertains to the public sphere; the economic is associated with the private sphere, guided by the rules of the market. Public actors are defined as fulfilling a public task, as producing public goods and protecting individual rights as well as a more general public interest. The public sphere is responsible for preventing discrimination or exploitation of structurally disadvantaged groups and for preserving continuity of the availability of certain public services and enhancing social cohesion. All other actors belong to the private sphere that is concerned with efficiency concerns and generating and maximizing profits ([2], p. 37; [3], p. 32; [4], p. 218).

In reality, the political and the economic are closely intertwined and influence one another: "states dispose of substantial material resources while production and exchange can hardly take place without some framework of security" ([1], p. 389). As a field of scientific analysis, Political Economy studies these interdependencies between the economy and politics. Different scientific schools of thought within the political economy approach have been in favor of different balances between the political and the economic in order to achieve the most favorable governance results ([5], p. 723). Taking into account that more and more problems observed at the national level have international causes and/or consequences, a new field of International Political Economy has emerged. It studies the "relationship between political and economic changes and their impact on global and domestic political, market, and production activities. It covers a wide range of issues among countries, as well as public and private institutions in both domestic and global arenas" ([6], p. 5). This perspective offered by International Political Economy as a discipline is useful when looking at STIs and their differentiated impact on regions. Understanding the underlying dynamics is a crucial prerequisite for devising effective response strategies.

In order to better understand how these considerations apply to STIs, their economic and political implications will now be focused on in turn. First, the economic dimension will be outlined and second, the political framework of STI-related policymaking will be described to show how both have to be seen as interdependent when devising strategies.

63.2 Economic Issues Associated with STIs

Precise data about the economic impact of STIs are not easily obtained. The biggest body of evidence can be derived from the economic analysis of HIV/AIDS, bearing in mind that HIV unlike some other STIs cannot be cured. Although therapy today allows people living with HIV/AIDS to lead productive lives for decades after infection, in many of the most affected areas of the world, appropriate therapies are not readily available to all who need them. People living with HIV die earlier and the economic consequences may be more significant than in the more developed world. Therefore, experiences from HIV/AIDS, which is in fact currently causing the biggest economic burden of all STIs, will especially be focused on. At the same time, HIV/AIDS is closely related with other STIs, as with preexisting STIs – often unrecognized or untreated out of shame or lack of access to treatment – the likeliness of HIV infection increases significantly.

STIs, and AIDS in particular, can have economic implications on different levels, in particular on the macroeconomy and on companies and their workforce. On the macroeconomic level, the impact of an HIV/AIDS epidemic is difficult to measure. Most models show a moderate decline of the gross domestic product (GDP). However, even a GDP decline of only 1–2% per year results in a situation where after 25 years the GDP is about 30% lower than without an epidemic. The impact of the epidemic becomes more visible when looking at the health sector specifically. In some countries, the funds required to sustain complex programs in response to HIV/AIDS may be higher than the amount previously available for the entire public health budget. In South Africa, for example, when the government first planned to bring 80% of all patients in need into therapy, the estimated cost of 45 billion South African Rand (4.7 billion euros) exceeded the total previous health budget by 20% ([7], p. A2933). Later, while implementing the programs, shortages in funding threatened to interrupt the availability of antiretroviral drugs for patients already on treatment in some provinces [8]. The global financial crisis has made the shortages in funds for HIV/AIDS and STIs more dramatic as donor countries downscale funding or refrain from scaling up as needed to achieve universal access to treatment [9].

HIV/AIDS epidemics may also affect the attractiveness of a country for foreign direct investment. Higher public expenditure for health and redirected public budgets – away from infrastructure or other business-friendly policies – as well as reduced demands for certain goods (as household income decreases due to disease or income is reallocated to health related goods and services) may make certain locations look less attractive. International rating agencies may classify countries strongly affected by HIV/AIDS less favorably. South African companies, for example, have been burdened with a higher risk premium. This however, has not led to any visible decrease in economic investment. A South African study showed that 90% of companies had not been influenced in their investment decisions by the HIV situation ([10], p. 49). Nevertheless, it remains difficult to measure business opportunities lost as companies refrain from new investments *because* a country is burdened with an AIDS epidemic, since other factors such as high crime rates or lack of skilled staff may also come into the equation. At the same time, business confidence into a location may be increased by a proactive government response.[2] An issue of concern, however, is that new epidemics are currently developing in countries occupying key positions in the international economy such as China or India ([7], p. A2934).

The impact of the STI situation and an AIDS epidemic can also be felt on the individual company level. Direct, indirect and systemic costs can be distinguished. Among the direct costs are increasing expenses for health programs, for social and health insurance, for recruitment and education of replacement staff. Indirect costs may incur through absenteeism or less productivity due to sickness. Systemic costs are the combined negative effects of disease on workplace coherence or strained atmosphere and less motivation in the work environment. Systemic costs may also be incurred by a general decrease in levels of education and experience as well as the availability of internal tacit knowledge.

In general, companies seem to react in a more intuitive than calculated manner to these challenges. A survey of the World Economic Forum (WEF) among more than 10,000 business leaders in 117 countries revealed that only about 9% of companies had carried out a quantitative risk analysis on the impact of HIV/AIDS on their companies. However, the survey also revealed growing concern. Close to every second participant (46%) in the survey expected an impact of the epidemic on their operations over the coming 5 years, 17% of which expected a strong impact. The WEF report showed that only when national prevalence of HIV is higher than 20%, that is, when the epidemic becomes more visible, do more companies start to take action. They may draft policy papers on HIV in the workplace and may introduce programs on prevention, counseling, testing and therapy targeting their workforce. At the same time, companies in Western European countries with low HIV prevalence have hardly been concerned with STIs or HIV/AIDS. Outside the hardest hit countries, only 6% of the companies surveyed had written AIDS policies [11]. Thanks to Highly Active Antiretroviral Therapy (HAART), people living with HIV/AIDS in those

[2]Prof. Dr. Michael Grimm: "Die ökonomischen Konsequenzen der AIDS Epidemie. Mögliche Wirkungskanäle und empirische Evidenz," Satellitenkonferenz "AIDS & Economy," 27.6.2007, http://www.doeak2007.de/pdf/aids_economy/02_Michael_Grimm.pdf.

countries are well integrated into working life. A Swiss study showed that 70% of people living with HIV were in paid employment, 68% of which were in full-time ([12], p. 327). For Germany, data from the Competence Network for HIV/AIDS provide the most comprehensive evidence. Within this cohort, 48.7% of men and 23.4% of women are working full time, that is, at least 35 h a week. Another 5.2% of men and 14.3% of women worked part-time (15–34 h/week) and 2.9% of men and 4.9% of women worked less than 15 h/week, while 34.7% of men and 48.4% of women were not working at all (the status of 6.5% of men and 7.3% of women was not known) (Competence Network HIV/AIDS, 2009, personal communication). As the Swiss study highlights, people living with HIV tend to keep their infection secret from their employer. Employers in turn do not see that HIV is an issue in their workforce, although integration of HIV-patients can be a real win-win situation: Productive participation in the work environment can have positive effects on disease progression. Patients report that they are more satisfied and integrated into society. This may eventually even decrease health spending and companies may profit from a highly motivated workforce ([7], p. A2933).

Increasingly, international forums offer assistance to companies to better handle their AIDS risk and situation. In addition to the Global Business Coalition against HIV/AIDS, TB and Malaria there are several regional and more than 40 national business coalitions supporting the private sector to address HIV-related issues. According to the needs in an individual country or a region, they offer services such as coordinating the national private sector treatment program (Malawi Business Coalition Against HIV/AIDS), assisting small, medium and micro enterprises in developing HIV workplace programs (the South African Business Coalition on HIV and AIDS), initiating staff capacity-building and community outreach to customers or monitoring and evaluating workplace programs (Coalition des Entreprises de Côte d'Ivoire contre le sida). The UNAIDS Corporate and Private Sector Team, among others, works with business coalitions around workplace issues ([13], p. 17).

In summary, it can be seen that STIs may have an impact on the macroeconomy and the individual company level, the exact extend of which may be difficult to measure. Given its economic consequences – how does the political level react, which policy frameworks have been put in place to address these issues?

63.3 Political Issues Associated with STIs

The issue of STIs is embedded in the policy framework of sexual reproductive health as part of population policies. The concept of sexual reproductive health includes five core components: the improvement of antenatal, perinatal, postpartum and newborn care; the provision of high-quality services for family planning, including infertility services; the elimination of unsafe abortions; the prevention and treatment of sexually transmitted infections, including HIV/AIDS, reproductive tract infections, cervical cancer and other gynecological morbidities and the promotion of a healthy sexuality ([14], pp. 1595–1607). The policy level can be divided into international and national policymaking. As national policies generally have to be interpreted in relation to the international strategy discussion, the latter shall be set out first.

63.3.1 The International Policy Framework

The International Conference on Population and Development (ICPD) 1994 in Cairo was an important milestone for the development of the international population regime. The ICPD Programme of Action, sometimes referred to as the Cairo Consensus, emphasized the interrelationship of population, development and individual well-being. It broadened the approach to sexual and reproductive health and took a more contextual attitude, including poverty and sustainable economic development, the education of girls and equal gender rights, the protection of the family, the decrease of maternal mortality as well as mortality of babies and children below 5 years, access to reproductive health services, family planning and sexual health. The needs of the individual were placed above reproductive targets. Following a new rights-based approach, women and men should be enabled to make informed decisions about their lives. At the same time, the Cairo programme emphasized health sector reforms with the aim of achieving better service delivery, multisectorality and community involvement. The Cairo approach explicitly called for decentralization and partnerships with NGOs and the private sector ([15], pp. 74–75, 82;

[16], pp. 195–205).[3] The 1995 Fourth World Conference on Women in Beijing confirmed many of the issues discussed in Cairo, in particular, the importance of women's rights and empowerment. Sexual self-determination was advocated as a human right. The empowerment of women was interpreted as an expansion of choices in all areas, including education, employment and health ([17], pp. 215–225).

In 2000, different threads of activity of social development were merged into a common set of goals that should henceforth provide overarching guidance for the whole UN system – the Millennium Development Goals (MDGs). These eight interlinked goals each with several associated targets were derived from the Millennium Declaration, adopted by the General Assembly in 2000 [18]. They consisted of time-bound goals with the overarching aim of reducing poverty by half until the year 2015. The goals merged commitments made at a series of international conferences in the 1990s, in particular those on children, population and development, human rights, women, social development, HIV/AIDS and financing for development.[4] Several of the goals are related to sexual reproductive health: Goal number 3 is concerned with the promotion of gender equality and the empowerment of women, number 4 with the reduction of child mortality and number 5 with the improvement of maternal health. Most directly linked to STIs is goal number 6, which demands to "combat HIV/AIDS, malaria and other diseases." Associated targets are to have halted and begun to reverse the spread of HIV/AIDS by 2015, to achieve universal access to HIV treatment by 2010 and to have halted and begun to reverse the incidence of malaria and other major diseases by 2015.[5] Although STIs other than HIV have not directly been mentioned they are closely related to this goal.

However, critics have remarked that the MDGs have been adversarial to the comprehensive reproductive health approach that aims to enable women to achieve autonomy over their reproductive lives ([19], pp. 1550–1551). They criticize that these issues have declined on the international agenda as they have not explicitly been included into the MDG framework and that funding for sexual reproductive health has decreased in favor of increased attention for HIV/AIDS ([14], pp. 1595–1607). In this context, the World Health Assembly has helped to reemphasize the importance of STIs in their own right by endorsing its Global Strategy for the Prevention and Control of STIs ([19], pp. 1550–1551; [20]). At the same time, the UN General Assembly included the ICPD goal of "Universal access to reproductive health by 2015" as a new associated target to goal 5 "Improve maternal health" in the MDG framework that aims to reduce poverty ([21], pp. 1565–1566). This addition reasserts the concept of Cairo that poverty and development are closely linked to sexual reproductive health ([14], pp. 1595–1607). In recent years, the general trend in international policymaking has moved more towards reintegrating efforts related to HIV/AIDS, STIs and reproductive health in prevention, care and support, the setting of quality standards and the development of protocols as well as staff training [22].

With this policy framework agreed upon, the implementation on the country level is supported by agencies of the UN, such as UNFPA, WHO or the UNAIDS Secretariat. Their main aim is to help governments work towards internationally adopted targets and to enhance their capacities to meet them. Looking at the realities of implementing these internationally agreed policy frameworks, Glasier and Gülmezoglu ([19], pp. 1550–1551) remarked: "Most governments do have appropriate population and family planning policies, but without international encouragement do not have the motivation to implement them alongside HIV/AIDS prevention and promotion of safe motherhood." Even though there has been a recent move to reinsert them into the policy debate, STIs other than HIV/AIDS have been somewhat eclipsed – despite the amount of disease, death and misery they are causing. The social repercussions of infertility, for example, are often underestimated. In Asian and African societies, women often blame themselves and are blamed by their partners or his family for not producing a child or not producing a son. This may result in threatening divorce, their relocation to the parents' home, the remarrying of the partner, physical and verbal abuse by the husband or the in-laws ([14], pp. 1595–1607). Infertility can be a result of untreated or unrecognized STIs. Although it may be proven cost-effective to deal with STIs, the widespread distaste for them is a high barrier to be overcome. When it comes to issues such as abortion, sexual health services for adolescents or sexual activity

[3]Vgl. auch http://www.unfpa.org/icpd/index.htm.

[4]http://www.unfpa.org/icpd/index.htm.

[5]http://www.unfpa.org/icpd/about.htm.

outside marriage, sexual reproductive health becomes indeed political. Some of the success achieved since 1994 also lead to reduced funding for family planning services, although worldwide many still do not have access to such services. This has been accompanied by a general trend to emphasize abstinence and faithfulness ([19], pp. 1550–1551). Glasier et al., have stated that the "[t]he increasing influence of conservative political, religious, and cultural forces around the world threatens to undermine progress made since 1994, and arguably provides the best example of the detrimental intrusion of politics into public health" ([14], pp. 1595–1607).

Clearly, when looking at the implementation of the international policy framework, political factors come into play. "They can determine which sexual and reproductive health issues are included in national policy agendas, which evidence is examined (or excluded), which policy alternatives are considered (and ultimately adopted), and the degree to which they are implemented," as Buse et al., ([23], p. 2101) confirm. The politics of an issue are particularly at stake when "a subject is culturally taboo [...]; if an intervention could adversely affect some interest groups [...]; if the intervention is perceived to be difficult to administer (e.g., the complexity of sexual and reproductive health care services being used as an argument against integration of such services); or if the benefits would accrue mainly to those with little political influence, such as poor people, women, and girls" (ibid.). In this context, the authors make out four levels that are central to policy making: "opportunities and constraints within the policy context of a specific sexual and reproductive health issue; the formal and informal processes by which decisions are made; the stakeholders who might be affected by a proposed reform; and the influence, interests, positions, and degree of commitment of various stakeholder groups in relation to a specific policy for sexual and reproductive health" ([23], p. 2102). They therefore conclude: "Evidence of the technical feasibility of affordable, cost-effective interventions to address a health problem might not be sufficient to ensure that relevant policies are formulated or adopted. Indeed, in some cases policies have been adopted in the absence of sufficient evidence, in contradiction to the evidence, or even when the data suggest that the proposed intervention might not work – because political factors have outweighed the available scientific evidence" ([23], p. 2101). In order to better understand such issues and obstacles, it shall be helpful to look at an example of how internationally agreed policies can become issues of contention at the national level.

63.3.2 The National Policy Level

The extent of implementation of the outlined global public policy frameworks vary. In many cases, dealing with STIs on a national policy level is anything but straight forward. How an STI can be political is best illustrated with the example of the public discourse around HIV/AIDS that long dominated the public debate in South Africa. Time and again conflicts between the South African government and other forces in society made it into the news headlines of Western European media. What was behind the controversy and how has HIV/AIDS – now well treatable in the West – become so politicized in the first place?

The politicization of AIDS in South Africa revolved around the controversies between advocates of the orthodox view about HIV/AIDS – a view on which Western European practice of AIDS treatment and prevention is based – and defenders of the so-called dissident view. The dissidents were a group of scientists and other individuals of which some believed that HIV was not the cause of AIDS and others that HIV did not exist. Therefore, they questioned the efficiency of antiretroviral drugs; some claimed that this therapy only caused AIDS because of the toxicity of the drugs. Others maintained that the promotion of antiretroviral therapy was merely furthering the interests of pharmaceutical industry. These assumptions cast doubt on the scientific evidence of the existence of HIV, which could be shown to cause immune suppression resulting in AIDS ([24], p. 226).

Sympathies with the dissident views on the highest ranks of government resulted in political resistances against the introduction of antiretroviral medicine as a solution to the HIV/AIDS epidemic in South Africa. Instead, emphasis was put on prevention. At the International AIDS Congress in Durban in 2000, President Thabo Mbeki announced that a single virus could not be responsible for the large numbers of AIDS casualties. He believed that AIDS was a syndrome of several known diseases caused by poverty and bad nutrition. In response, several thousand scientists signed a petition against these views. A public debate incurred in which Mbeki argued that claims about the extent of the epidemic and its causes were based on racist stereotypes of a violent sexuality of black men ([24], pp. 226–227). Contrary to the Western biomedical discourse that emphasized behavior and risk, Mbeki focused on the social conditions of disease. Youde explains: "While it is true that certain behaviors will place individuals at a higher risk of contracting HIV, it is also true that certain economic and social conditions may place a person in a situation where they are forced to make that choice. [...] They [people] make choices, though they may increase exposure to HIV, because they lack the funds or social status to choose otherwise" ([25], pp. 430–431).

Against this bias towards emphasizing social contexts and prevention alone, a strong civil movement formed demanding access to therapy and thus advocating the orthodox medical perspective. The Treatment Action Campaign (TAC) most prominently represented this movement. Strong lobbying finally lead to the introduction of a government plan to make antiretroviral treatment available for all. However, the implementation of this plan was once more characterized by resistances. The controversy left many people unsure about what to believe, how to protect themselves and how to treat those infected. Energies were diverted from finding solutions and effective strategies to debating about the existence of the problem ([24], pp. 231–237).

This politicization of HIV/AIDS had several underlying dimensions. *Firstly*, the argument was one of denial. The amount of death was conflicting with the paradigm of an African Renaissance that wanted to transport a picture of an aspiring dynamic continent. Media reports of an African catastrophe were considered damaging and therefore denied. Having only just achieved the liberation of Apartheid, the country was not ready to accept that it was hit by yet another problem before it has even started to benefit from new freedom ([26], pp. 28, 35–36).

Secondly, the denial was also an expression of the dogmas of the Apartheid state and its colonial fears of an "untamed black sexuality" ([26], p. 12). Sexuality and marriage across racial divides was previously strongly regularized, driven by the motivation of the white minority to protect themselves against the more numerous "black masses." The liberation from Apartheid therefore also meant a sexual liberation, which found its expression in a rapid increase of the presence of sexual images; sexual policies were publicly discussed in a manner previously unheard of. This was illustrated by the new constitution, which was the most advanced in the world when it came to legalizing pornography for adults, rights of sexual orientation, rights of gender equality and the right of freedom from violence in marriage ([26], pp. 12–14). The liberation from the multifaceted restrictions of the past became equal to the liberation from the restraints of the Apartheid state and the moral values of the parent generation at the same time ([26], p. 16). This new symbol of sex as freedom collided with the message of sex as a threat because of AIDS and was therefore denied ([26], p. 25).

Thirdly, public health issues in South Africa were automatically interpreted in the context of the former Apartheid system, which used them to establish and sustain its order, as Youde explains: "Starting in the 1870s, fear of disease like cholera, plague, and smallpox rationalized calls among whites to segregate blacks and Indians" ([25], p. 424). The Public Health Action of 1883 gave local authorities the power to establish quarantines and sanitary corridors. Later, in connection with the worldwide plague epidemic of 1894 to 1901, public health measures were again used to establish segregationist policies, when African populations were moved into "native locations" ([25], pp. 424–425). Those crowded settlements that lacked adequate sanitary infrastructure soon became breeding grounds for disease themselves. This in turn reinforced the argument in favor of segregating the African population ([25], p. 425). Given that AIDS seemed to affect black South Africans more strongly than the white population, the issue became immediately contested. Black South Africans resisted being told by white South Africans how to change their behavior. Any paradigm that suggested that "the black man" was connected with something threatening and infectious was automatically denied. Rumors circulated that the disease was deliberately spread in order to reduce the African population ([25], p. 425). Such suppositions were enhanced when police officers admitted during the hearings before the South African Truth and Reconciliation Commission that they deliberately deployed HIV-positive men in mining camps to spread the disease so as to keep the "black enemy" under control ([25], p. 427).

Fourthly, the politicization of AIDS in South Africa was connected to negative experiences with Western public health campaigns and with the wish "to find African solutions to African problems" ([25], p. 422). Mbeki made it his point to emphasize the uniquely African character of the epidemic. In a letter written in 2000 to a number of world leaders, he emphasized the differences between the African and the Western AIDS epidemics: In Africa, several million deaths had incurred as opposed to limited numbers in the West. In Africa, numbers were increasing, while in the West they decreased. Therefore, taking over solutions coming from the West was seen as "absurd and illogical" ([25], pp. 429–430) and "African solutions" were to be preferred. The crises should be used to foster a distinct African identity ([25], p. 427; [27], p. 151; [28], p. 86). In the meantime the new South Africa president Jacob Zuma and the new Minister of Health Aaron Motsoaledi have both made tackling HIV and AIDS according to international standards a public health priority [29,30]. However, catching up on implementation will not happen from one day to another.

63.4 Conclusion: STIs – Interdependence of Economic and Political Factors

When looking at both economic and political factors associated with STIs, it becomes clear that they are in fact closely interrelated. For example, the way young women are able to protect themselves from STIs is an expression of both their economic status and the political framework. At the same time, the extent to which a government can build trust in its ability to control STIs also affects the work environment and productivity of their companies and their attractiveness to foreign investment. Making funds available for prevention and treatment of STIs is eventually a political question as is the decision to address economic and social determinants of disease proliferation. However, if policies are not implemented, companies affected by a public health issue may start to become proactive by offering services to their employees themselves, thus setting examples and putting pressure on government to start addressing the issue. The private sector can help depoliticize sensitive issues around STIs by pursuing hands-on approaches. Where on the political level there was much debate in South Africa, companies were starting health programs even contrary to the official government position to protect their businesses. The private sector may not be genuinely responsible for providing health programs. In several countries however, it has a share in offering services that are otherwise unavailable.

Both public and private sectors have valuable resources to contribute to effective STI management. Government can set policy frameworks, coordinate the response of different actors and set tax or other incentives for implementers on the ground. They may facilitate complementary contacts with the health sector or build capacity. Private sector can make financial resources available and contribute management skills or communication chains to target groups that may otherwise be difficult to reach. Therefore, international policymakers have increasingly advocated public-private partnerships (PPP) to better address the political and economic aspects of public health problems. In fact, this approach goes back to the Cairo Programme of action, which advocated closer collaboration with private sector and civil society organizations already at the time. A prominent example of a PPP is the Global Fund to Fight AIDS, Malaria and Tuberculosis, the so-called poverty-related neglected diseases. Again, STIs are not explicitly included, but AIDS programs may involve components beneficial for STI prevention. The Global Fund is designed as a PPP in that government, private sector and civil society are represented on the board and in that it addresses all three parties in its fundraising endeavors. At the same time, applicants have to form Country Coordinating Mechanisms (CCMs), which have to include all three parties to jointly develop proposals. Also on other levels private sector is integrated into achieving public health policy gains. The Campaign "Product Red" has drawn some attention. Several companies selling brand names have developed red prototypes and profits generated from their sales are partly handed over to the Global Fund. Among the participating companies are GAP und Armani; Apple has developed a red iPod, Motorola contributed a red cell phone and American Express offers a credit card where clients can opt to donate 1% of their transaction volume to the Fund ([7], p. A2934).

The Global Fund also announced a Corporate Champions initiative that commits corporations to donate around US$ 30 million to top-up grants approved by the fund. Companies thereby co-finance projects where they can profit from the infrastructure put in place by the Global Fund ([31], p. 986). Furthermore, UNAIDS has also become active as a broker of public–private arrangements and helps to identify opportunities for co-investment, which it defines as a harmonized and coordinated joint investment of public and private resources with the common objective to improve equitable access to and provision of HIV/AIDS services." Often this approach is used in connection with workplace programs of companies who want to make additional services available to the communities in the vicinity of their locations [32]. UNAIDS also assists in making technical expertise available and in creating monitoring und evaluation systems. Many of the cosponsors of UNAIDS have also become active in public–private partnerships. For example, the UN Office on Drugs and Crime (UNODC) has started partnering with the Egyptian Business Coalition on HIV/AIDS. Together with other stakeholders, they have taken a joint initiative to produce an Egyptian Partnership Menu, a tool to link private sector companies with innovative AIDS partnership opportunities. The menu provides potential donors with a list of AIDS projects they can sponsor. Projects include HIV prevention and care among injecting drug users and initiatives on harm reduction. Furthermore, workshops have been organized in order to provide the private sector with technical expertise on how to develop workplace policies and to organize HIV training sessions for their employees. UNODC and its task force partners participated in a series of regional consultations coordinated by the UNDP HIV/AIDS Regional Programme for the Arab States, which led to the development of the AIDS Business Coalition in the Arab Region (ABCAR) ([33], pp. 16–17).

Public–private partnership approaches also exist on the South African national level. For example, mining companies have started making periodic presumptive treatment for STIs available to commercial sex workers in the area of the mines. With the help of government, they have set up mobile clinics where sex workers can be counseled, tested and treated. Often, mining towns attract young men from remote rural villages who migrate for work. They live in hostels, far away from their families. Their disposable income attracts women as commercial sex workers or to try and form secondary families with the miners. While miners may be receiving good treatment in the hospitals of their employers, commercial sex workers are usually less well treated, so that miners frequently become reinfected. This was the rationale for mining companies to start cooperating with the public sector on women's health issues near their operations. However, given the effects of the global economic crises on the mining sector, it remains to be seen whether previous activity levels can be sustained.

As can be seen, political and economic aspects are very relevant in defining the phenomenon and strategies against STIs, more prominently so around HIV/AIDS but also more generally for STIs. Political and economic actors are closely interdependent and therefore both have to be integrated in strategy making. Partnerships between the public and private sector are certainly no panacea, but require intensive work. Misunderstandings between such heterogeneous actors may be frequent and both sides have to develop a better understanding of each other's attitudes and organizational cultures. Some encouraging examples both on the international as on the national level have instilled hopes that such integrated approaches may help to address these issues more effectively (cf. [34]). In any case, support is there to set the framework on the highest level to encourage public and private actors to walk together: In the words of former UN Secretary-General Kofi Annan: "Now we know that peace and prosperity cannot be achieved without partnerships involving governments, international organizations, the private sector and civil society. In today's world we depend on each other" ([13], p. 14). Also his successor, current UN Secretary-General Ban Ki-moon has confirmed the necessity to form partnerships: "Whether in the workplace or in the wider community, through advocacy and branding, prevention, care and treatment programs for employees, or financial, scientific and technical commitment, the role of the private sector is indispensable" ([13], p. 12). Given the massiveness of the challenges involved in reproductive health including HIV/AIDS, these statements will likely set the tone for the years to come in addressing not only HIV/AIDS but in trying to develop a more balanced agenda that looks at sexual reproductive health in a more comprehensive manner.

Take-Home Pearls

- The political and the economic spheres are interdependent and they both have an influence on the significance of STIs on the public health agenda as well as the ability to develop effective response strategies.
- Although the economic impact of STIs, including HIV/AIDS, may be difficult to measure, there is some indication that companies and macroeconomists tend to underestimate the true dimensions and that activities at company level remain reactive and start relatively late.
- Comprehensive policy frameworks have been developed in the framework of the international conferences of the 1990s, which were later merged into the Millennium Development Goals; however, implementation remains difficult when faced with certain sensitivities or strong adversarial political interest groups.
- The knowledge about a strong interdependence of economic and political factors will have to be taken into consideration more actively when devising strategies. Public-private partnerships should be used more consciously and factors contributing to their effectiveness should be studied more in-depth.

Abbreviations

ABCAR	AIDS Business Coalition in the Arab Region
AIDS	Acquired Immunodeficiency Syndrome
CCM	Country Coordinating Mechanism
GDP	Gross Domestic Product
GHI	Global Health Initiative
HAART	Highly Active Antiretroviral Therapy
HIV	Human Immunodeficiency Virus
ICPD	International Conference on Population and Development
MDGs	Millennium Development Goals
PPPs	Public-private partnerships
STIs	Sexually Transmitted Infections
TAC	Treatment Action Campaign
UNODC	United Nations Office on Drugs and Crime
WEF	World Economic Forum
WHO	World Health Organization

References

1. McLean, I.: Concise Dictionary of Politics. Oxford University Press, Oxford (1996)
2. Carroll, P., Steane, P.: Public-private partnerships. Sectoral perspectives. In: Osborne, S.P. (ed.) Public-Private Partnerships. Theory and Practice in International Perspective, pp. 36–56. Routledge, London/New York (2000)
3. Roggencamp, S.: Public Private Partnership. Entstehung und Funktionsweise kooperativer Arrangements zwischen öffentlichem Sektor und Privatwirtschaft, Europäische Hochschulschriften, Reihe V, Volks- und Betriebswirtschaft, Bd. 2410, Frankfurt am Main u. a.. (1999)
4. Rosenau, P.V.: The strengths and weaknesses of public-private policy partnerships. In: Rosenau, P.V. (ed.) Public-Private Policy Partnerships, pp. 217–241. MIT Press, Cambridge/London (2000)
5. Nohlen, D., Schultze, R.O.: Lexikon der Politikwissenschaft. München C.H. Beck (2004)
6. Pearson, F., Payaslian, S.: International Political Economy. Houghton, Boston (1999)
7. Brunne, V.: Wie Aids die Weltwirtschaft schwächt. Ärzteblatt **104**(43), A2932–A2934 (2007)
8. Magamdela, P.: Lack of funds threatens ARV programmes, health-e, 26 Sept 2009, http://www.health-e.org.za/news/article.php?uid=20032518 (2009)
9. Bodibe, K.: Consequences of less funding for AIDS, health-e, 19 Nov 2009, http://www.health-e.org.za/news/article.php?uid=20032576 (2009)
10. BER/SABCOHA: The impact of HIV/AIDS on selected business sectors in South Africa. http://www.sabcoha.org/research/what-is-the-impact-of-hiv-aids-on-the-south-african-economy-4.html (2005)
11. WEF: Business & HIV/AIDS: a healthier partnership? A global review of the business response to HIV/AIDS 2005–2006. http://www.weforum.org/en/initiatives/globalhealth/index.htm (2006)
12. Pärli, K., et al.: AIDS. Recht und Geld, Zürich/Chur (2003)
13. UNAIDS: AIDS is everybody's business. UNAIDS & Business: working together. http://data.unaids.org/pub/Agenda/2007/unaids_private_sector_en.pdf (2007b)
14. Glasier, A., et al.: Sexual and reproductive health: a matter of life and death. Lancet **368**(9547), 1595–1607 (2006)
15. Mayhew, S.H.: The impact of decentralisation on sexual and reproductive health services in Ghana. Reprod Health Matters **11**(21), 74–87 (2003)
16. Woiwod, C.: Die internationale Konferenz über Bevölkerung und Entwicklung in Kairo 1994: Vom Nil zu neuen bevölkerungspolitischen Ufern?. In: Messner, D., Nuscheler, F. (eds.) Weltkonferenzen und Weltberichte, pp. 195–205. Bonn J.H.W. Dietz Nachfolger (1996)
17. Klingebiel, R.: Weltfrauenkonferenz in Beijing 1995: Aktion für Gleichberechtigung, Entwicklung und Frieden? In: Messner, D., Nuscheler, F. (eds.) Weltkonferenzen und Weltberichte, pp. 215–225. J.H.W. Dietz Nachfolger Bonn (1996)
18. United Nations: 55/2. United Nations Millennium Declaration, A/RES/55/2 (2000)
19. Glasier, A., Gülmezoglu, A.M.: Putting sexual and reproductive health on the agenda. Lancet **368**(9547), 1550–1551 (4 Nov 2006)

20. WHO: Global strategy for the prevention of sexually transmitted infections 2006–2015, Geneva. http://www.who.int/reproductive-health/publications/stisstrategy/stis_strategy.pdf (2006)
21. Greer, G.: Defending and debating sexual and reproductive rights. Lancet **368**(9547), 1565–1566 (4 Nov 2006)
22. UNFPA: ICPD/15 Desk review. Of progress, challenges and lessons learned in implementing the ICPD programme of action in Eastern Europe and Central Asia, New York (2009)
23. Buse, K., et al.: Management of the politics of evidence-based sexual and reproductive health policy. Lancet **368**(9552), 2101–2103 (2006)
24. Brunne, V.: HIV und AIDS in Südafrika. Die Public-Private Partnership-Strategie. Nomos, Baden-Baden (2008)
25. Youde, J.: The development of counter-epistemic community: AIDS, South Africa, and International Regimes. Int Relations **19**(4), 421–439 (2005)
26. Posel, D.: Die Kontroverse um HIV/AIDS in Südafrika. Zur Politisierung von Sexualität nach der Apartheid. Peripherie **24**(93/94), 8–41 (2004)
27. Schneider, H.: On the fault-line: the politics of AIDS policy in contemporary South Africa. Afr Stud **61**(1), 145–167 (2002)
28. Van der Vliet, V.: South Africa divided against AIDS: a crisis of leadership. In: Kauffman, K.D., Lindauer, D. (eds.) AIDS and South Africa. The Social Expression of a Pandemic, pp. 48–96. Palgrave Macmillan, Houndmills/Basingstoke (Hampshire)/New York (2004)
29. Health-e: Health Minister promises responsible action on AIDS, 13 Nov 2009. http://www.health-e.org.za/news/article.php?uid=20032569 (2009a)
30. Health-e: Zuma delivers historic AIDS speech, 31 Oct 2009. http://www.health-e.org.za/news/article.php?uid=20032543 (2009b)
31. Buse, K., et al.: Corporate champions: doing good more effectively. Lancet **371**(9617), 986 (22 Mar 2008)
32. GTZ/GBC: Making co-investment a reality, Eschborn (2005)
33. UNAIDS: AIDS is everybody's business. Partnerships with the private sector: a collection of case studies from UNAIDS. http://data.unaids.org/pub/Report/2007/unaids_private_sector_case_studies_en.pdf (2007a)
34. Buse, K., Harmer, A.M.: Seven habits of highly effective global public-private health partnerships: practice and potential. Soc Sci Med **64**(2), 259–271 (2007)

Index

G. Gross and S.K. Tyring (eds.), *Sexually Transmitted Infections and Sexually Transmitted Diseases*,
DOI: 10.1007/978-3-642-14663-3, © Springer-Verlag Berlin Heidelberg 2011

D

O

T

Printed by Printforce, the Netherlands